T0290233

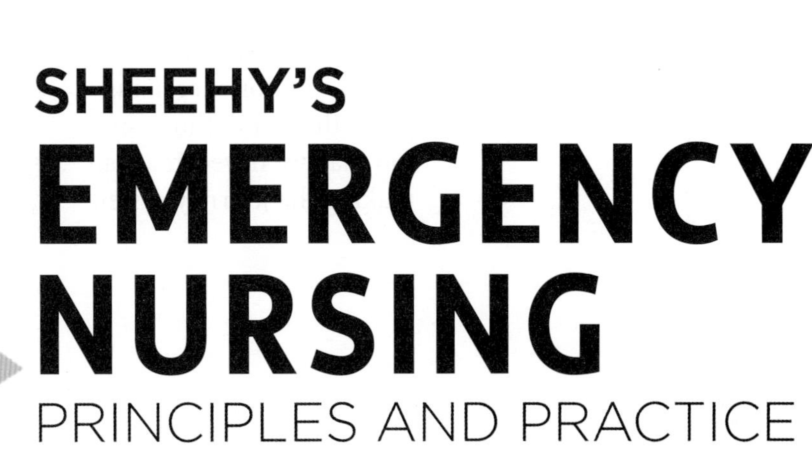

SHEEHY'S

EMERGENCY NURSING

PRINCIPLES AND PRACTICE

For the amazing emergency nurses who taught us,
thank you and may we have learned well.

For those making a difference beside us,
may we support each other through
the good times and the tough times.

For the next generation,
thank you for energizing
us with your enthusiasm
and may we have left a trail
making the journey easier.

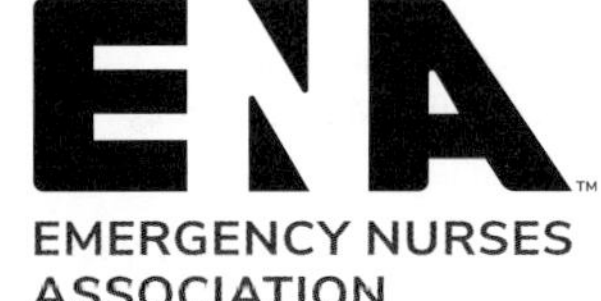

SHEEHY'S

EMERGENCY NURSING

PRINCIPLES AND PRACTICE

SEVENTH EDITION

Edited by

Vicki Sweet, MSN, RN, CEN, FAEN
ALS/CQI Coordinator, Emergency Medical Services, County of Orange,
Health Care Agency
Santa Ana, CA
Associate Faculty, Health Sciences & Human Services
Saddleback College, Mission Viejo, CA

Andi Foley, DNP, RN, ACCNS-AG, CEN, TCRN
Emergency Services Clinical Nurse Specialist
CHI Franciscan: St Francis Hospital.

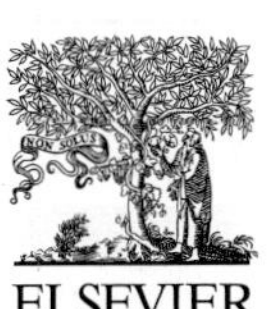

Elsevier
3251 Riverport Lane
St. Louis, Missouri 63043

SHEEHY'S EMERGENCY NURSING: PRINCIPLES AND PRACTICE,
SEVENTH EDITION
ISBN 978-0-323-48546-3

Library of Congress Control Number: 2019940505

Content Development Manager: Laurie Gower
Content Development Specialist: Elizabeth Kilgore & Elizabeth McCormac
Content Strategist: Sandra Clark
Publishing Services Manager: Deepthi Unni
Project Manager: Bharat Narang
Cover Design: Patrick Ferguson

Printed in India

Last digit in the printer: 9 8 7 6 5 4 3

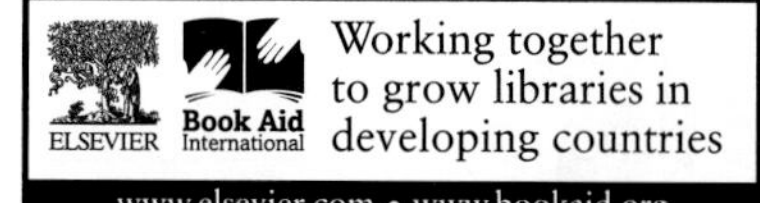

CONTRIBUTORS

Sherri Lynne Almeida, Dr.PH, MSN, M.Ed,RN, CEN, FAEN
Nurse Executive, Clinical Practice Office
Michael E. DeBakey, VA Medical Center
Houston, Texas

Vicki Bacidore, DNP, APRN, ACNP-BC, CEN
Assistant Professor, Niehoff School of Nursing
Loyola University Chicago
Emergency Nurse Practitioner, Emergency Medical Services
Loyola University Medical Center
Maywood, Illinois

Jessica Balcom, MSN, FNP
Family Nurse Practitioner, Emergency Department
Banner Payson Medical Center
Payson, Arizona
Adjunct Nursing Instructor
Grand Canyon University
Phoenix, Arizona

Cynthia S. Baxter, DNP
Chief Nurse Ambulatory Care, Nursing Services
VA Medical Center
Clinical Instructor
College of Nursing
University of Kentucky
Lexington, Kentucky

Sarah Berry, DNP, RN, AGCNS-BC, CEN
Clinical Nurse Specialist, Nursing Education and Research
Beaumont Hospital
Troy, Michigan

Cynthia Blank-Reid, MSN, RN, CEN, TCRN
Trauma Clinical Nurse Specialist, Department of Trauma and Surgical Critical Care
Surgical Clinical Reviewer - National Surgical Quality Improvement Program
Performance Improvement Department
Temple University Hospital
Philadelphia, Pennsylvania

Nancy Bonalumi, DNP, MS, BSN
President
NMB Global Leadership LLC
Lancaster, Pennsylvania

Beth Broering, MSN, RN, CEN, CCRN, TCRN, CCNS, CAISS, FAEN
Trauma/Burn Program Director, Trauma Center
VCU Medical Center
Richmond, Virginia

Gina Carbino, BSN, RN, CEN, CPEN, TCRN, CCRN, PCCN, SANE-A
Clinical Education Manager - Emergency Care Center
Patient Care Operations
The University of Vermont Health Network - Champlain Valley Physicians Hospital
Plattsburgh, New York

Mary Jo Cerepani, DNP, FNP-BC, ENP-C, FAANP, FAEN
Adjunct Faculty, School of Nursing
University of Pittsburgh
Nurse Practitioner
MyHealth@Work/Emergency Medicine
The University of Pittsburgh Medical Center
Pittsburgh, Pennsylvania

Garrett K. Chan, PhD, APRN, FAEN, FPCN, FCNS, FNAP, FAAN
President & CEO
HealthImpact
Oakland, California
Associate Clinical Professor, School of Nursing
University of California, San Francisco
San Francisco, California
Clinical Associate Professor, School of Medicine
Stanford University
Stanford, California

Sharon Saunderson Coffey, DNP, FNP-C, ACNS-BC, FAEN
Clinical Assistant Professor, College of Nursing
University of Alabama in Huntsville
Huntsville, Alabama
Nurse Practitioner
Athens-Limestone Hospital
Athens, Alabama

Kierstin Jeana Cohen, BSN, RN
Staff Nurse, Pediatric ICU
Children's National Medical Center
Washington DC

Michael De Laby, MSN, CCRN, CFRN, TCRN, EMT-P
Assistant Director, Emergency Medical Services
County of Orange, Health Care Agency
Santa Ana, California

Nancy J. Denke, DNP, RN, ACNP-BC, FNP-BC, CEN, CCRN, FAEN
Toxicology Consultants of Arizona
Scottsdale, Arizona
Associate Faculty
Arizona State University
Phoenix, Arizona

Angela Dillahunty, BSN, RN, CA-CP SANE, SANE-A, SANE-P
Forensic Nurse Examiner, Program Coordinator
CHRISTUS Health St. Elizabeth
Beaumont, Texas

Andi Foley, DNP, RN, ACCNS-AG, CEN, TCRN
Emergency Services Clinical Nurse Specialist
CHI Franciscan: St Francis Hospital

Chris M. Gisness, RN, MSN, BC FNP-C, ENP-C, CEN, TCRN, FAEN
Emory University, Department of Emergency Medicine
Emory University
Atlanta, Georgia

Randy Hamm, DNP, RN, CEN, CCRN
Assistant Professor, School of Nursing
Barton College
Wilson, North Carolina

Amy Herrington, DNP
Assistant Faculty, Nursing
University of Saint Augustine for Health Sciences
Saint Augustine, Florida

Renee Semonin Holleran, FNP-BC, PhD, CEN, CCRN (emeritus), CFRN and CTRN (retired), FAEN
Nurse Practitioner, Pain Management
Veterans Health Administration
Salt Lake City, Utah
Former Chief Flight Nurse
University Air Care, University Hospital
Cincinnati, Ohio
Former Manager of Adult Transport
Intermountain Life Flight, Intermountain Health Care
Salt Lake City, Utah
Family Nurse Practitioner
Hope Free Clinic
Midvale, Utah

Patricia Kunz Howard, PhD, RN, CEN, CPEN, TCRN, NE-BC, FAEN, FAAN
Enterprise Director, Emergency Services
University of Kentucky HealthCare
Lexington, Kentucky

Kathleen Sanders Jordan, DNP, MS, RN, FNP-BC, ENP-C, SANE-P, FAEN
Clinical Associate Professor, School of Nursing
University of North Carolina at Charlotte
Nurse Practitioner, Emergency Medicine
Mid-Atlantic Emergency Medical Associates
Charlotte, North Carolina

Betty Kuiper, DNP, APRN, ACNS-BC, CEN
Research Manager
Baptist Health Paducah
Paducah, Kentucky

Lorie Ledford, MSN, BSN
Staff Nurse, Emergency Department
Mayo Clinic Arizona
Chairperson
Board of Directors
Board of Certification for Emergency Nursing
Oak Brook, Illinois
Flight Nurse
Alia MedFlight
Phoenix, Arizona

Katherine Logee, RN, MSN, FNP-BC, CPNP, CNE
Registered Nurse
Emergency Department
Adventist Plus/Rideout
Marysville, California

Heather Martin, DNP, RN, PNP-BC
Senior Pediatric Emergency Medicine Nurse Practitioner
University of Rochester Medical Center
Rochester, New York

Lisa Matamoros, DNP, RN-BC, CEN, CHSE, CPEN
Senior Simulation Education Specialist
Johns Hopkins All Children's Hospital
St. Petersburg, Florida

Tamara C. McConnell, MSN, RN, LNC, PHN
Director, Emergency Medical Services
County of Orange, Health Care Agency
Santa Ana, California

Nancy McGowan, PhD
Associate Professor, School of Nursing
The University of Texas Health Science Center at San Antonio
San Antonio, Texas

Terri McGowan Repasky, APRN, CNS, MSN, BSN, EMT-P, CEN
Clinical Nurse Specialist Emergency/Trauma
Heart & Vascular Nurse Manager Accreditation
Tallahassee Memorial Hospital
Tallahassee, Florida

Joanne Ingalls McKay, RN, MSN, CEN
Healthcare Consultant
McKay Healthcare Consulting
Dearborn, Michigan

Laurie Nolan-Kelley, DNP, MSN, BA
Clinical Nurse Leader, Trauma and Orthopedics
Dartmouth-Hitchcock Medical Center
Lebanon, New Hampshire
Associate Professor, School of Nursing and Health Professions
Colby-Sawyer College
New London, New Hampshire

Colleen Mary Pedrotty, BSCH, MSHA, MSN
Clinical Education Specialist
St Mary Medical Center
Langhorne, Pennsylvania
SANE
NOVA
Warwick, Pennsylvania

Wanda S. Pritts, BSN, MSN
Clinical Nurse Specialist, CEN, CCRN
Clinical Education
Placentia-Linda Hospital
Placentia, California

Catherine T. Recznik, BSN, MSN, PhD, RN, CEN, CPEN
Assistant Professor
Nursing
Franciscan University
Steubenville, Ohio
Senior Professional Staff Nurse, Casual
Emergency Department
UPMC St. Margaret
Pittsburgh, Pennsylvania

Paul C. Reid, MSN, RN, CEN
LVRS Nurse Coordinator
Lung Center
Temple University Hospital
Philadelphia, Pennsylvania

Ruthie Robinson, PhD, RN, CNS, FAEN, CEN, NEA-BC
Director, Graduate Nursing Studies
JoAnne Gay Dishman School of Nursing
Lamar University
Beaumont, Texas

Bill Schueler, MSN, RN, CEN, CPPS, WVTS
Patient Safety Specialist
Quality Management & Medical Staff Services
Providence Health & Services
Portland, Oregon
Owner
WJS Services, LLC
Beaverton, Oregon

Vicki Sweet, MSN, RN, CEN, FAEN
ALS/CQI Coordinator, Emergency Medical Services, County of Orange
Health Care Agency
Santa Ana, CA
Associate Faculty, Health Sciences & Human Services
Saddleback College, Mission Viejo, CA

Colleen Vega, MSN, CNS, ACHPN
Clinical Nurse Specialist
Palliative Care
Stanford Healthcare
Stanford, California
Clinical Nurse Specialist
Palliative Care/Emergency Room
El Camino Hospital
Mountain View, California
Lecturer
Nursing
San Francisco State University
San Francisco, California

Amy Waunch, RN, MSN, FNP
Trauma Program Manager
Children's Hospital of Orange County
Orange, California

Patricia Weismann, MSN, RN, CEN, TCRN, CPPS
Director of Patient Safety
Methodist Texsan Hospital
Associate Director of Emergency Services
Adult Emergency Department
Methodist Hospital
San Antonio, Texas

Joni Lee Winter, DNP, MSN, FNP-BC, AGACNP-BC, ENP, CEN
Lead Nurse Practitioner
Hospital Medicine
EAMC-Lanier
Valley, Alabama
Nurse Practitioner
Emergency Department
Wellstar West Ga (Apollo MD)
LaGrange, Georgia
Nurse Practitioner
Inpatient Surgical Unit
CTCA-SERMC
Newnan, Georgia

Gordon H. Worley, MSN, RN, FNP-C, ENP-C, CEN, CFRN, EMT-P, FAWM
Assistant Clinical Professor
Betty Irene Moore School of Nursing
University of California Davis
Sacramento, California
Nurse Practitioner
Emergency Department
Sutter Amador Hospital
Jackson, California
Nurse Practitioner
Urgent Care
Western Sierra Medical Clinic
Grass Valley, California

Cheryl Wraa, MSN, RN, TCRN, FAEN
Director
TCAR Programs
VisionEm
Sacramento, California

Kimberly Zaky, MSN, RN, FNP-C
Base Hospital Coordinator
Emergency Trauma Department
Children's Hospital of Orange County
Orange, California

REVIEWERS

Michon Colette Dohlman, MSN, RN
Registered Nurse
Mayo Clinic
Rochester, Minnesota

Jenna Hannity, MSN, RN, CEN, TCRN
Trauma Program Coordinator
Emergency/Trauma Services
St. Francis Hospital
Federal Way, Washington

Janet D. Magnani, RN, MSN
Director of Patient Relations, Retired
St. Jude Medical Center
Fullerton, California

Karen L. Sharp, MSN, RN
Director, Patient Relations. Retired
Emergency Services & Advanced Wound Healing/Hyperbaric Medicine Center
MemorialCare Saddleback Medical Center
Emergency Department
Laguna Hills, California

PREFACE

The seventh edition of Sheehy's Emergency Nursing: Principles and Practice continues the tradition of defining emergency nursing practice. We synthesized current practice, evidence and clinical guidelines to provide you with a resource reflecting best practices in emergency care. Authors shared their knowledge to enhance the clinical outcomes of the patients in your care. The expertise of the professional nurses writing or revising chapters represents geographic diversity and spans all emergency nursing practice areas.

New to this edition are chapters on Ethical Considerations, Workplace Violence, Geriatric Emergencies and Geriatric Trauma. The seventh edition chapters of Emergency Nursing Practice, Communicable Diseases, Fluids and Electrolytes, Obstetrical Trauma, and Abuse and Neglect are the result of combining similar content from chapters in the previous edition. In response to the dynamic and evolving nature of emergency nursing practice, significant enhancements have been made to all chapters. Many chapters have been streamlined to focus on the unique challenges and practices of emergency nursing and valuable illustrations, including a section of images in color have been added.

It is our hope that the seventh edition will enhance your ability to provide safe practice and safe care.

Vicki Sweet and Andi Foley

ACKNOWLEDGMENTS

We were honored to be asked to co-edit the seventh edition of this renowned emergency nursing resource. To that end, we acknowledge the original work of Sue Sheehy and her generosity in giving this text to the Emergency Nurses Association.

No project gets done in isolation and this edition is no exception. Without the efforts of individual chapter authors, reviewers, Emergency Nurses Association staff, and Elsevier staff, this edition could not have been written.

Authors and contributors, we applaud your perseverance through unique and challenging personal trials and tribulations. We repeatedly asked you to meet challenging deadlines and you rose to the challenge with grace and excellence. Your willingness to write, edit, and rewrite will be remembered for years to come as a gift to your emergency nursing colleagues, both present and future.

We would also like to acknowledge our co-workers who have tolerated distracted multitasking in our attempt to do it all. Your support means a lot to each of us and we thank you for tolerating and working with us the past 2 years.

Most importantly, we recognize the time we have taken away from those closest to us—our friends and family. We are humbled by your constant willingness to let us do things to benefit others.

We hope this edition gives each of you what you need in your practice to continue your commitment to caring for our patients and for each other.

Vicki & Andi

CONTENTS

UNIT IV Medical and Surgical Emergencies

UNIT V Trauma Emergencies

UNIT I

Foundations of Emergency Nursing

1

Emergency Nursing Practice

Sarah Berry

A BRIEF HISTORY OF EMERGENCY NURSING

After World War II, the practice of medicine and the focus of hospitals were changing. At the time, most care was delivered in the community, and prehospital care was ill-defined. Private hospital emergency departments (EDs) were underutilized and staffed on an "as-needed" basis. Only public hospitals, serving predominately indigent patients, devoted staff resources to their EDs. Interns and resident physicians in training provided most of the medical care. In the 15 to 30 years after World War II, an increase in use of EDs was due to the changing dynamics of health care. The prewar medical practice of the "family doctor" primary care provider model changed into one of directing patients to EDs for after-hours care. Hospitals were becoming a community resource for help and information instead of institutions only for the seriously ill and injured.[1] As more patients arrived in EDs, hospitals were forced to assign increasing numbers of nursing staff to provide care. Even though the role of ED nursing was not well defined, only the most experienced nurses were selected for ED "duty" because of the unexpected, episodic nature and acuity of patient care.

At the same time EDs were becoming more recognized as prominent care delivery areas in hospitals, transport of patients to hospitals for care was also gaining attention. Community leaders and the medical community realized that the lessons learned from World War II and the Korean conflict about triage, field care, and rapid transport could be translated into civilian practice. The military had developed training programs for field medics to initiate care and had refined transport strategies. In addition to use of ground ambulances, helicopter transport of injured soldiers was initiated in Korea. Legislation was created in the 1960s to establish community and educational programs leading to modern emergency medical services. Development of space-age technology, such as telemetry and portable defibrillators, also contributed to the growth of emergency care. As a result of these historical dynamics, emergency medicine and emergency nursing became recognized specialties.

A NEW NURSING SPECIALTY: DEFINING THE SCOPE OF PRACTICE

By definition, emergency nursing is the care of individuals of all ages with perceived or actual physical, emotional, or psychological alterations of health that may be undiagnosed or require further interventions.[2] Emergency nursing care is episodic, primary, and usually acute and occurs in a variety of settings.[3]

Alliance or affiliation with a specific body system, disease process, care setting, age group, or population defines most specialty nursing groups. In contrast, emergency nursing is defined by diversity of knowledge, patients, and disease processes. Emergency nurses care for all ages and populations across a broad spectrum of diseases and injury prevention and lifesaving and limb-saving measures while addressing crisis intervention, forensic, palliative, and end-of-life issues.[2] Emergency nursing practice requires a unique blend of generalized *and* specialized assessment, intervention, and management skills. The multiple dimensions of emergency nursing specify roles, behaviors, and processes inherent in the practice and delineate characteristics unique to the specialty. Practice area, patient population, and the variety of those who provide care are as diverse in emergency nursing as in the nursing profession as a whole. Emergency nursing practice is systematic and includes nursing process, nursing diagnosis, decision making, and analytic and scientific thinking and inquiry. Professional behaviors inherent in emergency nursing practice require acquisition and application of a specialized body of knowledge and skills, accountability and responsibility, communication, autonomy, and collaborative relationships with others.

The scope of emergency nursing practice encompasses assessment, diagnosis, treatment, and evaluation. Resolution of problems may require minimal care or advanced life support measures, patient and/or family education, appropriate referral, and knowledge of legal implications. Care delivery occurs whenever and wherever a person requires rapid assessment and stabilization of illness and injury that could be related to multiple aspects of the person's self.[2] Box 1.1 identifies multiple practice areas for emergency nursing.

Nursing roles include patient care, research, management, education, consultation, and advocacy. Emergency nursing practice is defined through specific role functions, as delineated in the Emergency Nurses Association's (ENA's) *Emergency Nursing Scope and Standards of Practice*.[2]

BOX 1.1 Emergency Nursing Practice Settings.

Hospital-based emergency department (ED)
Freestanding ED
Prehospital services
Air and ground transport services
Military-based centers
Urgent care center
Retail health clinic
Health maintenance organization
Ambulatory services
Schools and universities
Business/industry
Correctional institution
Occupational health clinics
Clinical decision units
State and federal disaster management response teams
Mobile-integrated health care
Telemedicine
Poison centers

BOX 1.2 History of the Emergency Nurses Association.

In 1968, Anita M. Dorr, RN, and Judith C. Kelleher, RN, working at opposite sides of the United States, perceived a need for nurses involved in emergency health care to pool their resources to set standards and develop improved methods of effective emergency nursing practice. In addition, they wished to provide continuing education programs for emergency nurses as well as a united voice for nurses involved in emergency care. By 1970, Ms. Dorr had formed the Emergency Room Nurses Organization on the East Coast and Ms. Kelleher had formed the Emergency Department Nurses Association on the West Coast. The two groups joined forces, and the Association was initially incorporated as the Emergency Department Nurses Association (EDNA) in Rochester, NY, on December 1, 1970. The first National Association meeting was held in New York in 1971.

THE EMERGENCY NURSES ASSOCIATION

The development of emergency nursing as a specialty is intertwined with the rich history of the Emergency Department Nurses Association (EDNA; later called the Emergency Nurses Association), which was chartered in 1970 (Box 1.2 and Fig. 1.1). Rapid growth of association membership, interest in defining emergency nursing, and recognition from community, medical, and legislative groups led to many initiatives. Within 5 years of its inception, EDNA developed a core curriculum for emergency nurse education, taught emergency nurse courses, and participated in every major program dealing with emergency care throughout the country.[4] In the mid-1970s, the status of the specialty of emergency nursing continued to grow within the nursing community. EDNA published seminal works, the first *Core Curriculum, Standards of Emergency Nursing Practice* (with the American Nurses Association), and the *Journal of Emergency Nursing.* By 1978, EDNA had determined that independent management for the organization was essential and established its own office with dedicated staff in Chicago, Illinois. At the end of this busy decade, EDNA continued to validate the specialty of emergency nursing by funding a certification committee to begin the development process for a national certification credential.[5] ED nurses were beginning to further define their roles in flight nursing, mobile intensive care nursing, and advanced practice. Master of science in nursing programs with an emergency nursing major were established for specializing in advanced practice, administration, and education and in providing much-needed research.

In 1985, the association name was changed to the Emergency Nurses Association (ENA), recognizing the practice of emergency nursing as role-specific rather than site-specific. The *Standards of Emergency Nursing Practice* were updated, and the certification committee evolved into the Board of Certification for Emergency Nursing.[6] Another important educational program, the Trauma Nursing Core Course (TNCC), was developed, which standardized the core level of knowledge needed in implementing the trauma nursing process. TNCC became one of the ENA's most successful programs, creating a model for measuring competency. As other countries adopted TNCC, the ENA established liaisons with other emergency nursing organizations internationally. In the latter part of the decade, the ENA created Emergency Nurses Day and began to explore the formation of an Emergency Nursing Foundation for the purpose of education and research.

As emergency nursing entered the 21st century, practice problems of ED crowding, holding patients, rising costs, safety in the workplace, and a nursing shortage continued. In addition to EDs, new practice areas included urgent care centers, clinical decision units, and occupational care centers. Protecting and providing resources to emergency nurses was a major focus of the ENA. Internet technology expedited communication and resource acquisition. Important new education programs, such as the Geriatric Emergency Nursing Education (GENE), were introduced. After the events of 9/11, bioterrorism and weapons of mass destruction became new professional and educational initiatives for emergency nurses and the emergency care community. In addition, the topics of five-level triage and staffing and productivity in EDs were among the many issues addressed by position statements.[7] In the past decade, growing national issues affecting health care have been addressed by the ENA, such as the assessment and identification of human trafficking victims, the use of mobile devices and social media, the opioid crisis, and behavioral health care. To meet future challenges, the ENA once again examined itself and reorganized around the core competencies of administration, advocacy, membership, professional development, research, and practice. Originally aimed at teaching and networking, the organization has evolved into an authority, advocate, lobbyist, and voice for emergency nursing. The ENA continues to grow, with members representing more than 32 countries around the world.

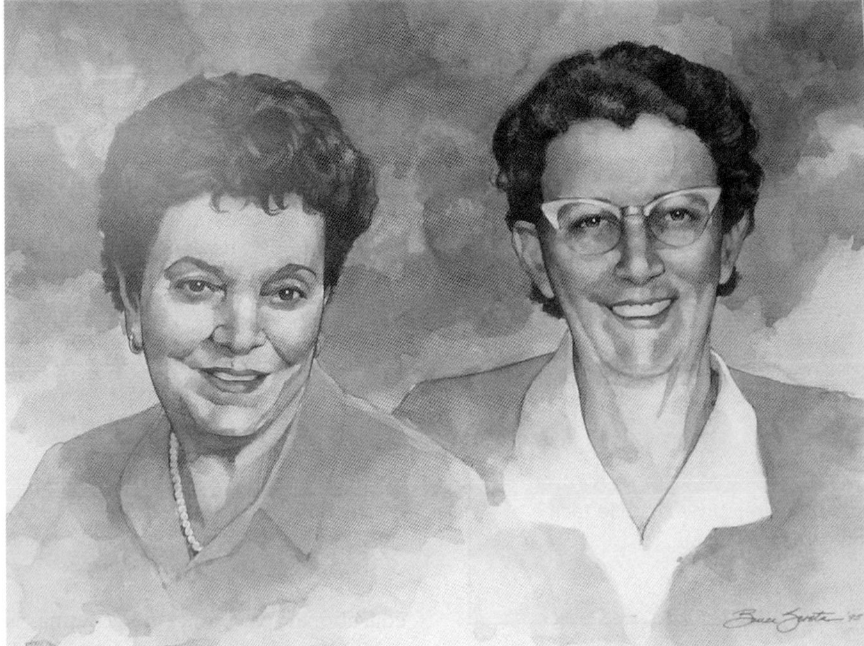

Fig. 1.1 Emergency Nurses Association Cofounders Judy Kelleher *(left)* and Anita Dorr *(right)*. (*ENA Archives;* artwork by Bruce Sereta [brucesereta.com].)

NURSING PRACTICE MISSION AND VALUES

The specialty practice of emergency nursing is guided by the association's vision and mission statement to "advocate for patient safety and excellence in emergency nursing practice." The ENA's vision is to be the global emergency nursing resource and advocate for "Safe Practice and Safe Care." The vision and mission are accomplished by standards of emergency nursing practice, which include standards of practice and professional performance.

STANDARDS OF EMERGENCY NURSING PRACTICE

The following standards of emergency nursing practice are authoritative statements developed by the ENA that (1) reflect the values, priorities, and duties for emergency nurses; (2) provide direction for professional emergency nursing practice; and (3) provide a framework for evaluation of the practice.[8] The standards of emergency nursing are categorized in two areas: Practice and Professional Performance. Practice standards include assessment, diagnosis, outcomes identification, planning, implementation, and evaluation. Professional performance standards include ethics, culturally congruent practice, communication, collaboration, leadership, education, evidence-based practice and research, quality of practice, professional practice evaluation, resource utilization, and environmental health. Each standard has accompanying competencies in which proficiency is expected, and the competencies are evidence of compliance with the standard. Competencies for the standards are defined by the role of registered nurses (RNs), graduate-level prepared RNs, and advanced practice registered nurses (APRNs).

COLLABORATIVE PRACTICE

The achievement of a healthy work environment is multifactorial and requires the support of the health care workers through an environment of positive commitment and coworker satisfaction. Collaborative practice brings together health care professionals with distinct and complementary knowledge and skills (e.g., prehospital providers, ED physicians and nurses, trauma surgeons, respiratory therapists, radiologists, and pharmacists) to enhance the delivery of emergency care.[9] This practice can address complex patient needs within a framework of quality, cost, and access. The primary commitment is to the patient, family, groups, and the community.[10]

Coalitions are fundamental for creating successful changes within patients, families, groups, and communities. Commonly, a joint purpose or activity or clinical dilemma may result in the formation of a permanent or temporary team that is likely to embrace collaborative practice. Coalitions may be built around any issue and on any scale, from neighborhood to national impact. The ENA has successfully drafted several position statements and department guidelines after the formation of a coalition of professional organizations. Successful coalition building is more likely to occur when the following are present[10]:

- Goals are similar and compatible.
- Working together enhances the ability of all to reach their goals.
- Benefits of coalescing are greater than costs.

POSITION STATEMENTS AND CLINICAL PRACTICE GUIDELINES

The ENA provides national and international leadership in emergency nursing care by identifying the standards of

BOX 1.3 ENA Position Statements and Clinical Practice Guidelines.

Position Statements

Access to Quality Health Care (July 2016)
Advanced Practice in Emergency Nursing (February 2012)
Care of patients with chronic/persistent pain in the emergency setting (January 2014)
Crowding, Boarding, and Patient Throughput (December 2017)
Cultural Diversity in the Emergency Setting (May 2012)
Healthy Work Environment (March 2013)
Human Trafficking Patient Awareness in the Emergency Center (February 2015)
Intimate Partner Violence (August 2015)
Mobile Electronic Device Use in the Emergency Setting (September 2013)
Mitigating Violence in the Workplace (January 2015)
Palliative and End-of-Life Care in the Emergency Setting (September 2013)
Patient Transfers and Handoffs (March 2018)

ENA Clinical Practice Guidelines

Family Presence During Invasive Procedures and Resuscitation (2012)
Intranasal Medication Administration (2016)
Geriatric Emergency Department Guidelines (2013)

Emergency Nurses Association. *ENA position statements.* https://www.ena.org/practice-resources/resource-library/position-statements. Accessed July 26, 2018.

quality care. This leadership is set forth in the form of position statements and clinical practice guidelines, which are used to support the improvement of patient care at all levels. The position statements listed in Box 1.3 represent the organization's official stand on a variety of issues; the full listing may be accessed at http://ena.org.

COMMUNITY EDUCATION

Emergency RNs are active in prevention education and harm reduction in the clinical setting and within the community. Emergency nurses are actively involved in community education programs because they serve to reduce the risk and consequences of disease, illness, and injury. The ultimate outcome is achieved through primary, secondary, and tertiary prevention[11]:

- Primary prevention attempts to avert disease or injury by reducing risk factor levels (e.g., child safety seat distribution and education).
- Secondary prevention aims to detect disease early to control or limit its effects (e.g., human immunodeficiency virus [HIV] and sexually transmitted infection [STI] testing for those with risky behaviors).
- Tertiary prevention focuses on treating disease and injury in an effort to reduce disability and preserve function (e.g., referral to treatment programs for substance use).

PATIENT SAFETY CONCEPTS[12]

The Joint Commission's Board of Commissioners annually publishes and updates a list of National Patient Safety Goals (NPSGs). The NPSGs are developed after a systematic review of the literature and available databases by patient safety experts and clinicians in a variety of health care settings. Emergency nurses integrate these safety goals into the care delivered to their ED patients. Table 1.1 provides an abbreviated list of the approved 2018 NPSGs for hospitals.

Quality, Safety, and Injury Prevention[13]

The ENA's Institute for Quality, Safety and Prevention (IQSIP) focuses on issues related to practice, quality, safety, injury prevention, and wellness. Charged with developing resources, programs, and leading projects, the IQSIP collaborates with local, regional, and national organizations. The IQSIP Advisory Council consists of member experts who participate on committees, including ED operations, a Position Statement, and the Lantern Award and Annual Achievement Awards. The scope of practice for the IQSIP includes developing evidence-based practice resources; raising awareness on issues of quality, patient/staff safety, and injury prevention; and advocating for ED nurses in discussions with external stakeholders and organizations.[12]

EMERGENCY NURSING VALIDATION OF KNOWLEDGE

Nursing is both a scientific discipline and a profession. Nursing science is a domain of knowledge concerned with the adaptation of individuals to actual or potential health problems, the environments that influence health, and the therapeutic interventions that promote health and affect the consequences of illness.[14] Emergency nursing is clearly one area of specialization in which there are specific clusters of phenomena of concern. The knowledge required for nursing can be seen as a synthesis of what is known about the person, environment, health, and nursing. Therefore, the discipline has a unique perspective, a distinct way of viewing all phenomena, which ultimately defines the limits and nature of its inquiry and knowledge.

Two established venues to validate specialty nursing knowledge are through certification and further education. Professional nursing certifications are increasingly viewed as a standard assurance that the nurse has acquired the specific body of knowledge to practice in the specialty. Furthering education may include a bachelor's degree or graduate program, such as a master's degree or APRN certification from established institutions, such as universities.

VALIDATION OF KNOWLEDGE THROUGH CERTIFICATION

One means of validating emergency nursing knowledge is through certification. The opportunity for certification in a nursing specialty dates back to 1945, when the American

TABLE 1.1 2019 National Patient Safety Goals.

Goal 1	**Identify patients correctly.**
NPSG.01.01.01	Use at least two ways to identify patients. For example, use the patient's name and date of birth. This is done to make sure that each patient gets the correct medicine and treatment.
NPSG.01.03.01	Make sure that the correct patient gets the correct blood when he or she gets a blood transfusion.
Goal 2	**Improve staff communication.**
NPSG.02.03.01	Get important test results to the right staff person on time.
Goal 3	**Improve the safety of using medications.**
NPSG.03.04.01	Before a procedure, label medicines that are not labeled. For example, medicines in syringes, cups, and basins. Do this in the area where medicines and supplies are set up.
NPSG.03.05.01	Take extra care with patients who take medicines to thin their blood.
NPSG 03.06.01	Record and pass along correct information about a patient's medicines. Find out what medicines the patient is taking. Compare those medicines with new medicines given to the patient. Make sure the patient knows which medicines to take when he or she is at home. Tell the patient it is important to bring his or her up-to-date list of medicines every time he or she visits a doctor.
Goal 6	**Use alarms safely.**
NPSG 06.01.01	Make improvements to ensure that alarms on medical equipment are heard and responded to on time.
Goal 7	**Reduce the risk of health care-associated infections.**
NPSG.07.01.01	Use the hand cleaning guidelines from the Centers for Disease Control and Prevention or the World Health Organization. Set goals for improving hand cleaning. Use the goals to improve hand cleaning.
NPSG.07.03.01	Use proven guidelines to prevent infections that are difficult to treat.
NPSG.07.04.01	Use proven guidelines to prevent infection of the blood from central lines.
NPSG.07.05.01	Use proven guidelines to prevent infection after surgery.
NPSG 07.06.01	Use proven guidelines to prevent infections of the urinary tract that are caused by catheters.
Goal 15	**Identify patient safety risks.**
NPSG.15.01.01	Find out which patients are at risk for suicide.
Universal Protocol	**Prevent mistakes in surgery.**
UP.01.01.01	Make sure that the correct surgery is done on the correct patient and at the correct place on the patient's body.
UP.01.02.01	Mark the correct place on the patient's body where the surgery is to be done.
UP.01.03.01	Pause before the surgery to make sure that a mistake is not being made.

Modified from The Joint Commission. Patient safety. The Joint Commission website. http://www.jointcommission.org/patientsafety/nationalpatientsafetygoals. Accessed April 24, 2019.

Association of Nurse Anesthetists first initiated certification. Most certifications in nursing, however, were established within the past three decades. An increase in the number of nursing specialty organizations has been a major factor in the proliferation of nursing certifications.

The Board of Certification for Emergency Nursing (BCEN) identifies an additional purpose, which is to validate, based on predetermined standards, an individual's qualifications and knowledge for practice in a defined functional or clinical area of nursing.[15]

Consequently, the certification process benefits both the individual nurse and the employer while serving society's interest. Achieving certification may lead to greater respect from employers and colleagues, salary increases, and perhaps greater self-esteem and a sense of professional pride. Employers and potential employers also benefit from nursing certification. Certification provides an objective measure of an employee's knowledge base and valuable information about prospective employees.

The nursing profession, as a whole, benefits from certification. Because of the certification process, bodies of specialty nursing knowledge are defined and examined. Certification demonstrates to other health care disciplines that nurses are able to articulate a defined body of knowledge and establish levels of specialty competence based on that knowledge. An individual's preparation for the certification examination also benefits nursing. Successful certification requires thorough study of the body of knowledge of the specialty. Certification renewal encourages the practicing nurse to remain current in all aspects of specialty nursing practice.

There are three ways to obtain certification. One method is certification by a state or government agency. State certification represents legal endorsement of a nurse's ability to function in certain expanded nursing roles. Certification by a state usually refers to a specific aspect of nursing practice beyond the level addressed in a state board examination for registration. State certification is often based on prior certification by a nurse certification body, completion of an educational program, or both. In some instances, a certifying examination is administered by a state agency. Requirements for state certification vary, so certification by one state may not be recognized by another. Examples of state certifications include emergency communications registered nurse (ECRN), mobile intensive care nurse (MICN), and trauma nurse specialist (TNS).

Certification may also occur through an institution. The institution may be a health care facility or an educational system. This type of certification is usually based on successful completion of an educational offering, often varying in length and characteristics. Most often, the state or profession does not control content or requisites for such certification. Because of program variability and lack of oversight by a national body, this type of certification may have limited appeal or applicability outside of the particular certifying institution.

The most common way to obtain certification in a nursing specialty is through a professional organization. Many types of certifications are offered by the American Nurses Credentialing Center (ANCC). Most nursing specialty organizations have also developed, or are in the process of developing, a certification process in their specialty. These efforts are testimony to the belief that knowledge beyond the level of safe basic nursing practice is required for specialty nursing practice.

EMERGENCY NURSING CERTIFICATION

The first emergency nursing certification examination was administered on July 19, 1980. Approximately 1400 nurses took the first examination, with 900 successfully passing and obtaining the certification. The examination was composed of 250 questions, all of which were calculated into the score. The correct number necessary for a passing score and certification was consistent at 175. Over time, the certification examination has evolved into a more sophisticated measure of emergency nursing knowledge. All question-and-answer sets are now pretested on actual examinations for accuracy, clarity, and reliability before inclusion in the test bank. This process tests the validity and reliability of the proposed certification examination questions. Items being pretested are not included in scoring of the examination. Currently, each examination contains 25 pretest items and 150 scored items. The Accreditation Board for Specialty Nursing Certification (ABSNC) has 18 standards that must be met for a certification to be accredited. These standards address board structure, testing security, test development, autonomy, the appeals process, and proof of specialty practice. In February 2002, ABSNC approved the CEN certification for accreditation and was most recently reaccredited in 2017.

Certification and Renewal

To ensure that the certification examination reflects current emergency nursing practice, role delineation studies (RDSs) are completed by the BCEN. The RDSs are research studies, also known as a practice analysis or job analysis, that are conducted by examination committees of subject matter experts. The most recent RDS results[15] were published in 2015. The blueprint for the examination is based on clinical categories. Within each of those categories, questions may focus on aspects of assessment, analysis/diagnosis, intervention, or evaluation.

The BCEN is responsible for receiving and approving all applications for the CEN examination. Successful examination candidates will receive a card and a certificate that are valid for 4 years. These individuals may use the certification mark "CEN." Unsuccessful candidates are eligible to reapply for the examination 3 months after the initial date of testing. CEN certification renewal may be achieved by completing one of two options: (1) examination—successfully passing the computer-based test offered through the network of testing centers, or (2) continuing education—submitting a log listing 100 continuing education hours, with a minimum of 75 hours of clinical content. More information on CEN certification, as well as the certified flight registered nurse (CFRN) certification, the certified transport registered nurse (CTRN) certification, the certified pediatric emergency nurse (CPEN) certification, and the newly developed Trauma Certified Registered Nurse (TCRN) certification, is available at https://bcen.org/.

Advanced Practice Certification

General skills and competencies for two APRN roles, clinical nurse specialist (CNS) and nurse practitioner (NP), often utilized in emergency settings have been established by professional organizations, such as the ENA.[16] Education, accreditation, and certification are necessary components of an overall approach to preparing the APRN for practice. However, the licensing of APRNs is governed by state regulations and statutes. Each state independently determines the APRN legal scope of practice, the roles that are recognized, the criteria for entry into advanced practice, and the certification examinations accepted for entry-level competence assessment.[17] APRN practice requires specialized knowledge and skills gained through graduate-level education. Certification of APRNs is gained through successful completion of a rigorous examination, granting the credential of "board certified" in the practice specialty. For the emergency setting, APRNs can practice effectively in an emergency environment and use their abilities, knowledge, and specialized skills to meet the needs of patients and their families at the point of crisis or need, and they should be involved with extending their responsibilities to community outreach, including prevention of injury and illness.[18]

SUMMARY

Emergency nursing practice has evolved and become recognized as a specific specialty practice area for medicine and nursing. Nursing has formally defined the scope of practice and specialization in the ANA social policy statement. Emergency nursing has further defined the specialization through research and has outlined the standards of practice in the ENA's *Scope and Standards of Practice.* The practice of emergency nursing results in an empowerment of our discipline to significantly affect the health needs of society.

Emergency nursing continues to become more complex and demanding. An increasing demand for emergency care, for both critically ill and noncritical patients, requires innovations in care methodology and technology. As emergency nurses care for more critically ill patients for longer periods, the need for sophisticated monitoring equipment increases. Technology previously reserved for the critical care unit is now commonplace in the ED. As care becomes more complex, the emergency nurse's knowledge must continue to expand to make increasingly complex decisions about patient care.

The development of the ENA as a cohesive professional organization has truly played a tremendous role in advancing emergency nursing as a specialty and providing guidance on best practice. The resources that the ENA offers include practice guidelines, educational courses, and community and policy advocacy opportunities to further enhance emergency nursing practice. Validation of knowledge for emergency nursing can be done through professional certification in several categories and advanced graduate-level education with board certification.

The nursing profession and how it is perceived will continue to evolve. As nursing becomes more active in the decision-making process and speaks with a single voice, these changes in health care become shining opportunities. Emergency nurses must continue to join together with new energy, speak with inspired voices, and maintain their prominence as partners in the emergency health care arena.

REFERENCES

1. Weinerman ER, Edwards HR. "Triage" system shows promise in the management of emergency department load. *Hospitals.* 1964;38(22):55.
2. Emergency Nurses Association. *Emergency Nursing Scope and Standards of Practice.* 2nd ed. Des Plaines, IL: Emergency Nurses Association; 2017.
3. Emergency Nurses Association. *Emergency Nursing Scope and Standards of Practice.* Des Plaines, IL: Emergency Nurses Association; 2011.
4. Kelleher J. In the beginning we were "roadrunners." *ENA Connect.* 2005;29(3):1.
5. Fadale J. The growing years. *ENA Connect.* 2005;29(4):1.
6. Board of Certification for Emergency Nursing. About exams. Board of Certification for Emergency Nursing website. https://www.bcencertifications.org/Get-Certified/CEN/About-Exams. Accessed July 16, 2018.
7. Emergency Nurses Association. The new millennium. *ENA Connect.* 2005;29(9):1.
8. McPhail E. Overview of emergency nursing. In: Newberry L, ed. *Sheehy's Emergency Nursing.* 5th ed. St Louis, MO: Mosby; 2003.
9. Emergency Nurses Association. Position statement: healthy work environment. https://www.ena.org/docs/default-source/resource-library/practice-resources/position-statements/healthyworkenvironment.pdf?sfvrsn=a4170683_12. Accessed July 16, 2018. Published 2013.
10. Spangler B. Coalition building beyond intractability. Beyond Intractability website. http://www.beyondintractability.org/essay/coalition_building. Accessed August 14, 2008. Published June, 2003.
11. Fazio J. Emergency nursing practice. In: Kunz-Howard P, Steinmann RA, eds. *Sheehy's Emergency Nursing.* 6th ed. St Louis, MO: Elsevier; 2010.
12. The Joint Commission. National hospital inpatient reporting measures. https://www.jointcommission.org/assets/1/6/HIQR_Release_Notes_5_4.pdf. Accessed June 24, 2018. Published November 27, 2017.
13. Emergency Nurses Association. Institute for Quality, Safety, and Injury Prevention (IQSIP) summary description. www.ena.org.
14. Donaldson SK, Crowley DM. The discipline of nursing. *Nurs Outlook.* 1978;26:113.
15. Board of Certification for Emergency Nursing. A national role delineation study of the emergency nurse executive summary. https://www.bcencertifications.org/BCENMain/media/CEN/2015-BCEN-Emergency-Nurse-Executive-Summary.pdf. Accessed July 16, 2018.
16. Wolf L, Delao A, Perhats C, et al. The experience of advanced practice nurses in US emergency care settings. *J Emerg Nurs.* 2017;43(5):426–434.
17. APRN Consensus Work Group, the National Council of State Boards of Nursing APRN Advisory Committee. Consensus model for APRN regulation: licensure, accreditation, certification & education. https://www.ncsbn.org/Consensus_Model_for_APRN_Regulation_July_2008.pdf. Accessed July 16, 2018. Published July 7, 2008.
18. Emergency Nurses Association. Position statement: advanced practice in emergency nursing. https://www.ena.org/docs/default-source/resource-library/practice-resources/position-statements/advpracticeernursing.pdf?sfvrsn=e4186f66_18. Accessed July 16, 2018. Published 2012.

2

Legal and Regulatory Constructs

Tamara C. McConnell

The health care industry is one of the most highly regulated sectors in the United States, as evidenced by the vast array of laws and regulations related to health care access, quality, licensing, eligibility, safety, and cost. Health care regulations are developed and enforced by all levels of government—federal, state, and local—and also by private organizations. Each state has its own regulatory structure reflective of various public-private partnerships comprising working professionals with technical expertise and governmental oversight agencies. Several layers of law have blended to form statutes, rules, regulations, case law, codes, and opinions that vary between states and other jurisdictions. It is incumbent upon emergency nurses to understand the general principles of law related to the industry, recognize professional standards of care, and have the ability to access appropriate state or federal laws applicable to their practice setting.

SOURCES OF LAW

Legal issues relevant to emergency nursing are predicated on a variety of sources of law. The sources of law having an effect on nursing include constitutional law (federal and state), common (case) law, statutory law (federal and state), ordinances, and administrative (regulatory) law (Table 2.1). To maintain a balance of power and prevent abuse, the US Constitution divides the federal government into three branches: the legislative branch (to write laws), the executive branch (to execute laws), and the judicial branch (to interpret laws). The legislative branch[1] is Congress, divided into the House of Representatives and the Senate. The executive branch[2] consists of the president and the administration. The judicial branch[3] is composed of the court systems. Each branch plays a constitutionally determined role in determining the law and is prevented from becoming too powerful by the checks and balances provided by the other two branches. Each state system mirrors that of the federal system with its governor, legislature, and court system.

At the federal level, Congress proposes laws that, once enacted, become statutes that are controlling throughout the nation. The statutes may be accompanied by federal funding, such as the Homeland Security Act or Medicare and Medicaid, or they may be "unfunded mandates," such as the Emergency Medical Treatment and Active Labor Act (EMTALA) and the Health Insurance Portability and Accountability Act of 1996 (HIPAA). State legislatures propose and enact state laws in the same manner.

The president and governors are responsible for enforcing the laws, and such enforcement is performed in large part through administrative agencies.[4] Agencies such as the Drug Enforcement Agency (DEA), the Federal Bureau of Investigation (FBI), the Environmental Protection Agency (EPA), and the National Transportation Safety Board (NTSB) have considerable political influence and are able to promulgate, interpret, and enforce agency rules. In contrast to federal agencies, the states also have administrative agencies for state-specific issues, such as education, public health, transportation, labor law, and so on. These agencies are mirror images of the respective federal agencies but are not entitled to create rules and regulations that go against those created by their federal counterparts.

Federal agencies such as the Centers for Medicare and Medicaid Services (CMS), the Occupational Safety and Health Administration (OSHA), the National Labor Relations Board (NLRB), and the Food and Drug Administration (FDA) are responsible for oversight of issues that affect emergency departments (EDs). At the state level, state licensing boards, state health departments, offices of the attorney general, and child protective services are examples of state agencies regulating many issues that affect emergency nursing.

The judicial system is divided into federal and state courts. The federal courts resolve disputes regarding federal law or the US Constitution and are divided into district courts sitting in each state. Each district court's decisions may be appealed to one of 10 respective circuit courts. The US Supreme Court is the final authority for circuit court conflicts. Again, the state systems mirror the federal system, with trial, appellate, and final appeals courts. State courts hear disputes regarding state laws, including civil cases such as medical malpractice.

EMERGENCY MEDICAL TREATMENT AND ACTIVE LABOR ACT

As an amendment to the larger Consolidated Omnibus Budget Reconciliation Act (COBRA), Congress enacted EMTALA[5] in 1986. The statute was intended to prohibit the practice of "patient dumping," which involved hospitals' refusal to undertake emergency screening and stabilization for patients who sought emergency care, typically because of

TABLE 2.1 **Sources of Law and Regulation.**

Type of Law	Source	Focus	Examples
Supreme	US Constitution	Supreme law of the land Individual rights Checks and balances of authority	Right to free speech HIPAA
Statute	Congress or state legislature	Describes protections available to citizens	State privacy laws EMTALA
Common (Case)	Judicial branch	Formed by judicial decision in various courts Judgments evolve as society and decisions may become precedents to support or oppose points of law	Individual lawsuits
Regulations	Executive branch federal and state Administrative agencies	Enact and enforce federal and state laws	Nurse Practice Act

EMTALA, Emergency Medical Treatment and Active Labor Act; *HIPAA*, Health Insurance Portability and Accountability Act.

insurance status, inability to pay, or other grounds unrelated to the patient's need for services or the hospital's ability to provide them. CMS, a division of the Department of Health and Human Services (DHHS), administers the Medicare program and enforces EMTALA regulations. CMS defines an emergency department (ED) as a "specially equipped and staffed area of the hospital used a significant portion of the time for initial evaluation and treatment of outpatients for emergency medical conditions." Private medical offices and outpatient clinics may refer patients to the nearby ED to satisfy EMTALA. However, EMTALA does apply to hospital-owned treatment areas that accept unscheduled visits for over one-third of their visits, or where the name implies emergency services, or when hospital advertising or signage holds the location out to the public as a place to come for emergency services. EMTALA imposes on all Medicare-participating hospitals a legally enforceable duty of care, entitling all individuals who seek care at a hospital ED to a medical screening examination (MSE) and to either stabilizing treatment or a medically appropriate transfer if an emergency medical condition is identified. There are no restrictions on transferring patients without emergency medical conditions.[9]

An MSE is an ongoing process beginning at triage and continued until a patient is stabilized, admitted, or transferred. At a minimum, an MSE should include vital signs, history, documented physical examination of the involved area or system (if needed), ancillary tests and specialists available through the hospital (e.g., laboratory test, diagnostic tests and procedures, computed tomography scans or other imaging services), and continued monitoring. Hospitals generally specify who may conduct the MSE, such as a physician, nurse practitioner, or physician assistant. In most cases, triage is not considered an MSE. The hospital also must maintain an on-call list of medical staff available to provide the screening examination and stabilizing treatment. It is expected that hospitals strive to provide adequate specialty on-call coverage consistent with the services provided at the hospital, and there is flexibility in establishing on-call coverage.[9]

Under regulation 42 CFR 489.24(b), a patient who is stable for transfer means that no material deterioration of condition is likely, within a reasonable medical probability, to result from transfer or, for a pregnant woman, no delivery of child and placenta is likely to result from transfer. Under interpretive guidelines,[7] a patient who is stable for transfer means that an emergency medical condition has resolved, even though an underlying medical condition may persist. For psychiatric conditions, the patient is protected and prevented from harming themselves or others.

If the patient is not stabilized, the hospital may not transfer or discharge the patient unless either one of the following occurs: the patient or guardian requests transfer or the physician certifies that the medical benefit outweighs the medical risks of transfer. The transfer of an unstable patient must be "appropriate" and the following criteria must be met: the transferring hospital has stabilized the patient to the extent possible within its capacity; the patient requires the services of the receiving facility; the medical benefits outweigh the medical risks of transfer; the risk/benefit analysis is documented in a medical certificate by a physician; the receiving hospital has accepted the transfer and has the facilities and personnel to provide the necessary treatment; the transferring hospital sends the relevant records available at the time and additional records as soon as practicable; and the transfer is effected through qualified personnel with proper equipment, including life support measures.

Physicians signing the medical certificate for transfer are subject to EMTALA's penalties if they knew or should have known that the benefits of transfer were in fact outweighed by the risks of transfer and in so knowing misrepresented the patient's condition or the ED's obligations under the law. On-call physicians who refuse to appear when called by the ED may also be liable under EMTALA and may subject the hospital to a penalty in the process.

Under 42 CFR 489.24(d)(4), a hospital cannot delay examination or treatment to inquire about payment and cannot seek preauthorization from an insurer until after the examination is conducted and stabilizing treatment initiated. It should not be suggested to patients that they should leave or obtain services elsewhere at less cost, or that insurance may not cover the treatment.

Hospitals with "specialized services" must accept transfers if they have the capacity, such as specialized equipment or personnel (mental health, neonatal intensive care, burn, trauma, etc.). The recipient hospital may refuse transfers if the transferring hospital has similar capabilities, the transferring hospital admitted the patient as an inpatient, or the transfer is from outside the United States. Receiving hospitals must also report EMTALA violations when receiving patients transferred in an unstable condition.

Initially under EMTALA, hospital-owned ambulances were required to transport patients to that particular hospital, regardless of another hospital's proximity. In 2003, the regulations were amended to allow hospital-owned ambulances to transport patients to a different facility as long as they are integrated within local emergency medical services (EMS). EMTALA allows hospitals to deny access to patients in non–hospital-owned ambulances while the ED is on diversion for staffing or facility inadequacies. Even if there has been radio or telephone contact with the ED, EMTALA does not consider the patient in a non–hospital-owned ambulance to have "come to the emergency department" before its arrival.

EMTALA violations are found in about one-quarter of investigations. Financial penalties against hospitals have reached $150,000 for multiple violations, and hospitals are required to compensate the patient (or family) for damages. EMTALA violations are also reported to the Department of Justice to consider Hill-Burton Act violations (loss of federal funding to improve the hospital); to the Office of Civil Rights to consider discrimination implications; to the Internal Revenue Service for evaluation of tax-exempt status; and to third-party accrediting organizations. Hospitals and/or physicians with multiple or flagrant violations may also be terminated from Medicare participation.

Unlike HIPAA, EMTALA does allow for a civil right of action, meaning that patients may directly sue hospitals for EMTALA violations. The statute establishes two types of "dumping" claims: "(1) failure to conduct an appropriate medical screening examination to determine the existence of an emergency medical condition, and (2) failure to stabilize the emergency condition or to provide an appropriate transfer." There are no limits on such claims unless liability caps are established by state law."[8] The statute of limitations for an EMTALA claim is 2 years. Courts have held that EMTALA's private right of action allows patients to sue hospitals, but not individual physicians, for EMTALA violations.[9,10]

Patients with psychiatric conditions or problems related to chemical dependency are entitled to the same EMTALA protections as those with medical conditions. EDs must carefully screen for medical emergencies associated with intoxication and psychiatric illness.[11] Intoxication may mask head injuries, which must be ruled out. A psychiatric patient is considered stable for purposes of discharge under EMTALA when he or she is no longer considered to be a threat to himself or herself or others. Table 2.2 lists definitions of key EMTALA provisions as they are stated in the statute and have evolved through case law interpretation.

HEALTH INSURANCE PORTABILITY AND ACCOUNTABILITY ACT

On August 21, 1996, Congress enacted the Health Insurance Portability and Accountability Act (HIPAA) of 1996 amid concerns about health care fraud and abuse, the portability of health insurance, and the potential for compromising patient privacy regarding personal medical information through the use of electronic media for collecting claims data and payments. HIPAA required DHHS to adopt national standards for electronic patient health information, code sets, unique health identifiers, and security to protect the confidentiality and integrity of individually identifiable health information.

Pursuant to HIPAA's mandate, DHHS was to promulgate rules to be effective in February 1998, with compliance required by 2000, later modified in August 2002. A final Privacy Rule in December 2000 set national standards for the protection of individually identifiable health information by three types of covered entities: health care providers, health plans, and health care clearinghouses. In February 2003, a final Security Rule 2003 set national standards for protecting the confidentiality, integrity, and availability of electronic health information. The rules underwent many revisions, however, and the final version of the privacy regulations was not issued until December 2000. They went into effect[6] on April 14, 2001, with compliance not required until April 14, 2003.

HIPAA's privacy regulations require that covered entities protect personal health information (PHI) from disclosure and that access to PHI be limited to authorized entities, with access restricted to the information necessary. Covered entities are health care providers conducting certain transactions in electronic form, health care clearinghouses, and health plans.

HIPAA provides patients with the right to access and make changes in their medical records while restricting access by others. Patients also have the right to information regarding how their records have been accessed. Formal notices of an institution's privacy practices are required. In addition, covered entities are required to assign a privacy officer who is responsible for administering the institutional privacy program and ensuring compliance. Covered entities are also required to educate all workers on privacy policies and procedures and to discipline infractions of those policies and procedures.

Hospitals are required to update their systems so that PHI is protected. When instituting an electronic medical record, it is necessary to design computerized systems in a manner that limits medical record access to authorized persons through password protection or data encryption. Policies and procedures must be developed to protect the systems and their

TABLE 2.2 **Key EMTALA Provisions.**

Provision	Description/Definition
Hospital campus	CMS requires hospital staff to respond to emergencies anywhere on the campus. The medical center campus includes the main building and other structures located within 250 yards of the main buildings.
Participating hospitals	Hospitals with emergency departments and Medicare provider agreements.
MSE	Performed by a "qualified medical provider," as determined by hospital bylaws, policies, and procedures, to determine if an emergency medical condition exists. **Note: Triage does not constitute a medical screening examination. Triage determines in what order a patient is seen by a physician, not if he or she is seen by one.**
EMC	• CMS defines an EMC as a condition manifested by acute, severe symptoms (including severe pain) such that the absence of immediate medical attention could reasonably be expected to result in placing the individual's health (or that of an unborn child) in serious jeopardy, or when serious impairment to bodily functions, or serious dysfunction of bodily organs, could occur. • An EMC exists with a pregnant woman having contractions when there is inadequate time to effect a safe transfer to another hospital before delivery, or when the transfer may pose a threat to the health or safety of the woman or unborn child.
Stabilization	Treatment of the EMC to reasonably ensure that the condition will not further deteriorate upon transfer or discharge. If a patient's condition is not clearly stabilized, the patient can still be transferred if the medical benefits exceed the risk, or upon the patient's request.
On-call requirements	Hospitals are required to maintain an on-call roster (conspicuously posted in the emergency department) such that usual patient needs are met. Specialists are not required to be on call at all times, although the hospital must have reasonable policies that dictate what happens when a physician cannot respond.
Transfer	CMS defines "transfer" as whenever a patient leaves the hospital campus, including discharge, unless the patient makes an informed decision to leave against medical advice.
"Appropriate" transfer	An "appropriate" transfer relates less to what the MSE constitutes and more to the requirement that there must be a uniform evaluation of patients (regardless of insurance status). All of the following are required: • Patient has been treated at the transferring hospital and stabilized as far as possible within the limits of its capabilities. • Patient needs treatment at the receiving facility, and the medical risks of transferring him or her are outweighed by the medical benefits of the transfer; the weighing process as described above is certified in writing by a physician. • Receiving hospital has been contacted and agrees to accept the transfer and has the facilities to provide the necessary treatment to the patient. • Patient is accompanied by copies of his or her medical records from the transferring hospital. • Transfer is effected with the use of qualified personnel and transportation equipment, as required by the circumstances, including the use of necessary and medically appropriate life support measures during the transfer. • Receiving facility has available space and qualified personnel and agrees to accept the patient in transfer.
Patient refusal	• A hospital has met the requirement of a medical screening if the patient is offered further medical examination and treatment and if the patient or another on his or her behalf is informed of the risks and benefits of the offered examination and treatment. • Upon patient refusal to consent to the examination and treatment, the medical record contains a description of the examination and/or treatment that was refused. The hospital must take reasonable steps to secure the refusal in writing and obtain a document signed by the patient stating that the patient or person acting on his or her behalf has been informed of the risks and benefits of refusing examination or treatment.
Physician certification	A physician is required to certify that medical benefits outweigh the risks of the transfer. Certification must contain a summary of risks and benefits upon which the certification is based.
Transfer records	• All available medical records pertaining to the individual's emergency condition, including copies of the H&P, observation notes, preliminary diagnosis, results of diagnostic studies, treatment and response to treatment, informed written consent of the individual or his or her designated representative, written physician certification, and name and address of any on-call practitioner who refused or failed to appear within a reasonable time to provide necessary stabilizing treatment after being requested to do so by the emergency physician or by the treating physician. • Any records not available at the time of transfer are sent as soon as possible. • Vital signs are recorded on the transfer form immediately before transfer.

Continued

TABLE 2.2 **Key EMTALA Provisions.—cont'd**

Provision	Description/Definition
Nondiscrimination	A participating hospital with specialized capabilities or facilities shall not refuse to accept an appropriate transfer of an individual who requires such specialized capabilities or facilities if the hospital has the capacity to treat the individual.
EMTALA statute of limitations	A claim must be brought within 2 years of the alleged violation.
Financial inquiries	• A participating hospital may not delay appropriate medical screening examinations to inquire about the individual's method of payment or insurance status or to seek MCO preauthorization. • Stabilization must begin before financial inquiries.

CMS, Centers for Medicare and Medicaid Services; *EMC,* emergency medical condition; *EMTALA,* Emergency Medical Treatment and Active Labor Act; *H&P,* history and physical; *MCO,* managed care organization; *MSE,* medical screening examination.

information. Confidentiality statements should be included in all e-mail or fax transmissions. Security measures must be instituted to verify users.

HIPAA does not create a private right of action, meaning that patients cannot directly sue providers for HIPAA violations.[6] The law does create both criminal and civil sanctions, however, for improper use or disclosure of PHI. Patients may make formal complaints to the Office of Civil Rights (OCR). The OCR reviews evidence about the complaint and may determine that there was no Privacy Rule violation. If the evidence indicates that there was a violation, the OCR attempts to resolve the complaint by obtaining voluntary compliance, a corrective action plan, or a resolution agreement.

The OCR may refer complaints to the Department of Justice for criminal investigation in cases involving the knowing disclosure or obtaining of PHI. Noncompliant organizations can be fined up to $100 per violation and up to $25,000 in a calendar year. "Knowingly" obtaining or disclosing PHI can lead to fines of up to $50,000, as well as 1 year in prison. Using false pretenses to commit offenses can allow for penalties of up to $100,000 in fines and up to 5 years in prison. Committing offenses with the intent to sell, transfer, or use PHI for commercial advantage, personal gain, or malicious harm can allow for fines of $250,000 and up to 10 years in prison.[13]

Between April 14, 2003, when the law went into effect, and May 31, 2018, the OCR received more than 183,458 HIPAA complaints, 96% of which were resolved. The five compliance issues investigated the most were as follows:

- impermissible uses and disclosures of protected health information,
- lack of safeguards of protected health information,
- lack of patient access to their protected health information,
- lack of administrative safeguards of electronic protected health information, and
- use or disclosure of more than the minimum necessary protected health information.

Confusion and misinterpretation of the Privacy Rule have resulted in the inappropriate withholding of information.[8] HIPAA does not prohibit the disclosure of PHI in all circumstances and explicitly allows disclosure when required by law and for health oversight, law enforcement, crime reporting, military and veterans' activities, national security and intelligence activities, organ and tissue donation, abuse and neglect reporting, judicial and administrative proceedings, public health surveillance, public health and safety, public benefits programs, treatment, payment, health care fraud reporting, health plan audits, health care operations, and certain research purposes.[14]

The US Constitution specifically dictates that when there is conflict between federal and state law, federal law prevails when preemption is the clear and manifest purpose of Congress. As federal law, HIPAA supersedes state privacy statutes. However, HIPAA only establishes minimum privacy protections and outlines basic principles for protecting PHI while recognizing that state law may impose more stringent requirements. State privacy laws are not preempted by HIPAA when the state law offers greater privacy protection or when the state law requires reporting.[13]

Reportable Situations

Individual states have legally defined certain situations that require health care professionals to breach patient confidentiality and report the situation to a specified agency or individual. Because of variances by state, each ED needs to obtain copies of its particular state laws related to mandatory reporting requirements. Examples of mandatory reporting include homicide or suicide attempts, child maltreatment, elder abuse, rape, communicable diseases, and deaths within 48 hours of hospital admission.

If the situation requires either a physician or a nurse to report the incident, nurses should not assume that the physician will be the person responsible; the nurse shares equally in this legal responsibility. If the nurse believes in good faith that the incident meets the statutory reporting requirements but the physician disagrees, it remains the nurse's responsibility to report to the designated authority or to document that social services have assumed responsibility for the case.[15]

MEDICAL RECORDS

A medical record must be initiated and maintained on every individual who seeks emergency care, and it serves as a communication system for health care professionals providing care to document and chronicle the patient's treatment, progress, and disposition. Records of patient care are kept to meet legal, regulatory, managed care, and billing requirements. In the event of a malpractice lawsuit, the medical record is also used as evidence of the care provided. State law may dictate the minimum requirements of what is included in medical records.

ED records must be legible and clearly demonstrate the chronology of treatment. Every entry must be dated, timed, and signed. Dates, times, and signatures must be complete; signatures must be complete and include licensure—RN, LPN; and so forth. Triage notes must indicate level of distress and duration of complaint to justify classification. All appropriate forms and consents must be included in the medical record.

Providers must be identified by last name. Entries such as "MD aware," "supervisor notified," and "report to floor" do not adequately indicate that information has been transmitted. Policy and procedure manuals must reflect current practice and provide guidance on documentation methods. Chart audits should be performed on a regular basis to ensure compliance with regulatory standards and best documentation practices. Abbreviations are error-prone and should be restricted to those on the institution's approved list.

All communication or attempted communication with physicians, supervisors, or administrators regarding the patient's status should be documented; failure to follow the chain of command to benefit the patient is the focus of many lawsuits. Documentation must reflect compliance with state laws (e.g., evidence of organ request in the case of death and documentation of the patient's decision regarding life support for the patient admitted from the ED).

Critically ill or injured patients should have documented evidence that intensive nursing care, through the frequent recording of vital signs or interventions, was being performed.

Unusual occurrences or events that are not part of routine care or operations and result in, or have the potential to result in, harm to the patient should be documented in objective, factual terminology in the medical record. If pertinent, provide a description of the environment (e.g., "side rails up and locked" or "water on floor.") Do not document in the medical record that an unusual occurrence form was completed. If a problem is found (e.g., esophageal intubation), resolution should also be documented (e.g., endotracheal tube replaced into trachea with equal breath sounds present).

Every discharged patient should receive written and verbal discharge instructions. Documentation that discharge instructions were discussed with the patient and that the patient indicated understanding must be included in the record as well as a copy of the discharge instruction. The language of the discharge instructions should not be more complex than a sixth-grade reading level and should be available in the predominant language of the patient. Claims of inadequate discharge instructions are frequent issues in ED lawsuits.

Electronic Medical Records

Electronic medical record (EMR) systems are defined as:

> *an electronic record of health-related information on an individual that can be created, gathered, managed and consulted by authorized clinicians and staff within one health care organization. These systems can facilitate workflow, improve the quality of patient care and patient safety and allows organizations to meet regulatory standards and patient needs more effectively than traditional paper systems. Interoperable systems streamline information flow, reduce medical errors, eliminate illegibility, allow EDs to be compliant with regulatory and accreditation standards, facilitate data collection for quality improvement, interconnect clinical data, provide bio-surveillance capability, and save provider time. They may also reduce health care costs, enhance liability protection, and inform clinical practice.*[16]

Implementation of an EMR requires careful planning and involvement of the institution's HIPAA compliance officer to address privacy concerns, as discussed in the next sections. Frontline personnel are crucial in the planning stages because the expertise of the end users is necessary in design. It may be necessary to phase in the system with flexible implementation timelines. Significant time may be required for education because productivity can be affected by long learning curves. Staff readiness should be carefully assessed before going live with the EMR system. Postimplementation assessment is necessary to detect problems, revise the system, and support staff. Whether using traditional paper systems or EMR, the ED records are hospital property, but patients have the right to review and make copies of their own charts and to make corrections in the records.[5] Each hospital must have a policy and a procedure for responding to patient requests for their records.

CONSENT

The law recognizes that mentally competent adults have the right to control decisions relating to their own health care, including decisions to have life-sustaining treatment withheld or withdrawn and to be free from unauthorized touching. Standards for consent rose as part of the 2009 CMS and Joint Commission mandate that required hospitals to provide "culturally competent patient-centered care" and to "honor the patient's right to give or withhold informed consent" by considering "patient needs and preferences" as well as legal requirements.[8] That said, major therapeutic and diagnostic procedures require informed consent.

The informed consent process is intended to ensure the protection of the rights of patients and is a fundamental principle of American ethics and the right of patient autonomy in medical decision making. In 1914, the New York State Supreme Court held that adults of sound mind have the right to make medical decisions. The process of "informed consent" requires three elements: determination of decisional capacity, delivery of information, and voluntary consent from the patient. Informed consent means the patient understands the risks, benefits, and alternatives to the proposed treatment. The patient has been given the opportunity to ask questions, and those questions have been answered to the patient's satisfaction. Generally, the emergency physician is responsible for explaining risks, benefits, and alternatives, although nurses may be called upon to witness the patient's signature. In the absence of consent, treatment may be considered assault or battery, even if clinically appropriate.

There are three basic types of informed consent: express, implied, and consent implied in law (emergency). Express consent is when a patient specifically agrees to an intervention. Implied consent is consent that is implied by the patient's conduct, for example, when a patient willingly holds an arm out to have blood drawn. Consent implied in law[17] is emergency treatment to save life or preserve health for patients who are unable to give consent in life-threatening situations. It removes liability for the treatment of life-, limb-, or organ-threatening conditions. In an emergency situation, an incapacitated person or minor may be treated under the assumption that a reasonable person would consent to care. Second opinions regarding the need for immediate intervention may provide further protection. Court orders for treatment may be obtained when time permits.

Adults lacking capacity are unable to consent to treatment. Capacity can be lacking from altered consciousness, unconsciousness, mental illness, or chemical influences. In the absence of an emergency, consent must be obtained from the next of kin, legal guardian, health care proxy, or person with durable power of attorney for health care decisions. Court orders can also be obtained for treatment. Psychiatric consultation can be helpful in determining capacity.

For incompetent individuals, involuntary consent is often used by physicians, psychiatrists, and law enforcement to ensure that mentally incompetent individuals receive treatment. If an incompetent individual refuses to consent to necessary medical treatment and the care required exceeds 48 hours, most states require a hearing before a judge with a psychiatric evaluation to assess mental capacity.

Minors (persons under the age of legal consent as defined by state law) often require care in the ED. Under most circumstances, parental consent is required for the medical evaluation and treatment of minor children. As long as the parent or legal guardian possesses medical decision-making capacity, he or she has the right to refuse medical care for the child but is required to act in the best interest of the child. Other responsible adults, such as school officials acting with parental permission or child welfare authorities, may have legal authority to authorize treatment for minors. Parents may not refuse life-, limb-, or organ-saving treatment on behalf of their children for religious reasons. In 1944, the US Supreme Court held, "[P]arents may be free to become martyrs themselves. But it does not follow they are free, in identical circumstances, to make martyrs of their children before they have reached the age of full and legal discretion when they can make that choice for themselves."[18]

If the legal guardian refuses to consent to care that is necessary and likely to prevent death, disability, or serious harm, law enforcement may intervene under local and state child abuse and neglect laws.

Many states allow minors to consent to treatment in specific areas (e.g., mental health services, pregnancy-related care, contraception, testing for and treatment of sexually transmitted diseases, and treatment for drug and alcohol addiction).

The courts and states recognize a "mature minor doctrine" that allows a minor to consent or refuse to consent to medical treatment if it is established that the minor is sufficiently mature to understand, discern, and appreciate the benefits and risks of the proposed medical treatment.[19] States vary in terms of whether a physician makes this determination or whether a judicial determination is required.

An emancipated minor is considered an adult for consent purposes and may authorize treatment without parental consent or notification. Each state identifies criteria for emancipation, but most states recognize minors to be emancipated if they are married, economically self-supporting and living apart from parents, or on active-duty status in the military.

If a patient refuses medically indicated treatment, it is essential that a determination be made regarding the patient's mental competency to make such a decision. If the patient is deemed competent, the emergency physician must provide a comprehensive explanation of the risks involved in refusing treatment; the details of the patient conference, as well as the patient's understanding, must be thoroughly documented in the medical record. Patients should be requested to sign a "release of responsibility" form; if a patient refuses to sign the form, document the refusal in the medical record.[15]

If a patient's refusal of treatment puts the patient at risk and there is a question of the patient's competency, contact the hospital administrator or designee to consider court-ordered treatment and obtain a psychiatric consultation to evaluate mental capacity. Hospitals should have policies related to patient consent, refusal of care, and elopements.

In general, consent for treatment of patients in the custody of law enforcement remains with the individual, not law enforcement personnel. Conflict may occur if a patient is in custody for suspected alcohol or drug intoxication or ingestion. State law governs whether the individual in custody can refuse consent for withdrawal of blood and other body fluid specimens for police or forensic purposes. A court order may be obtained in the absence of patient consent. Invasive surgical procedures to remove suspected ingested balloons or bags of illegal drugs generally require a court order if the patient refuses removal. The court may not order the removal because of the risk associated with the surgery; the court weighs the interests of the state and the individual in custody. An exception to this is if the physician believes within a reasonable degree of medical certainty that the patient is in imminent danger, thus creating a medical emergency. Legal counsel should be consulted for specific direction for policy development.

EDs must have policies and procedures regarding consent for law enforcement evidence collections and photographs as well as refusal of treatment and leaving against medical advice (AMA). Documentation for AMAs must include a discussion and the patient's understanding of the risks of leaving before formal discharge. Patients who elope or leave the ED without informing providers that they are leaving may need to be recalled, and the ED must have a policy for determining when this is necessary and how it is performed. EMTALA, discussed earlier, also mandates ED responsibilities with AMAs.[20]

AFFORDABLE CARE ACT

The Patient Protection and Affordable Care Act (PPACA), also known as the Affordable Care Act (ACA),[6] was signed into law to reform the health care industry by President Barack Obama on March 23, 2010, and upheld by the Supreme Court on June 28, 2012. The ACA expands the affordability, quality, and availability of private and public health insurance through consumer protections, regulations, subsidies, taxes, insurance exchanges, and other reforms and went into effect on January 1, 2014. Its enactment and implementation have not been without controversy, as each of America's 50 states decided to either create a state-run health insurance exchange or follow a federally operated exchange.

HOSPITAL ACCREDITATION ORGANIZATIONS

Hospitals seek accreditation services for three primary reasons: (1) each of the private accreditation organizations develops sets of standards to help hospitals demonstrate they have voluntarily gone beyond minimum federal standards related to quality, health, and safety; (2) for teaching hospitals, accreditation is mandatory for practicing interns; (3) accreditation helps hospitals to meet the necessary reimbursement criteria under the CMS Conditions of Participation (CoPs).[21]

For more than 40 years, there were two federally approved programs. However, after the enactment of the Medicare Improvements for Patients and Providers Act (MIPPA) of 2008, oversight shifted. The accrediting organizations maintain oversight for participating hospitals, and CMS maintains oversight for them.

Currently, there are four hospital programs with deeming authority to determine compliance with corresponding CMS regulations: The Joint Commission; the Health Care Facilities Accreditation Program (HFAP); Det Norske Veritas (DNV GL) National Integrated Accreditation for Healthcare Organizations; and the Center for Improvement in Healthcare Quality (CIHQ).

NEGLIGENCE AND MALPRACTICE

Negligence is the failure to act in a manner in which a reasonably prudent person would act in the same or similar circumstances. Medical malpractice claims are sought when a patient or their agent alleges improper, illegal, or negligent professional activity or treatment. A registered nurse is negligent when he or she fails to use the level of skill, knowledge, and care in diagnosis and treatment that other reasonably careful registered nurses would use in the same or similar circumstances.[22] This level of skill, knowledge, and care is referred to as "the standard of care." In the context of a nurse-patient relationship, a medical malpractice claim must prove four elements of negligence[23]: duty, breach of duty, proximate cause, and damages (Table 2.3).

A duty must be owed to the patient and usually occurs when the nurse accepts responsibility for the care and treatment of that patient. In *Lunsford v. the Board of Nurse Examiners*, 648 SW 2d 391 (Tex.App.3 Dist., 1983), the court held that nurses have a duty to patients just as physicians owe a duty, and that duty stems from the privilege granted by the state in nurse licensure.[24]

A breach of duty (standard) occurs when the care rendered was below the acceptable standard of care (the nurse departed from the standard of care), thereby causing injury. A direct causal relationship must exist between the breach of duty and

TABLE 2.3 Elements of Nursing Malpractice.

Element	Description	Example
Duty	Duty occurs when the nurse accepts responsibility for the care and treatment of a patient.	*Lunsford v. the Board of Nurse Examiners,* 648 SW 2d 391 (Tex. App. 3 Dist., 1983): Court held that nurses have a duty to patients just as physicians owe a duty, and that duty stems from the privilege granted by the state in nurse licensure.
Breach of duty	Departure from the standard of care that a reasonable, prudent nurse would exercise in the same or similar circumstances.	An intravenous infusion set requires a special filter to be used to prevent an air embolism, but if the nurse fails to set up the system properly by omitting the filter, a breach has occurred.
Proximate cause	A causal connection between the breach of duty and the harm or damages that occurred.	But for the departure from the standard of practice, the injury would have not occurred.
Damages	Monetary damages or injuries suffered by the patient due to the breach.	Pain and suffering; past, present and future medical expenses; disfigurement; premature death; loss of life.

the injury and is referred to as proximate cause. But for the departure from the standard of care (lack of using appropriate intravenous tubing), the injury (air embolism) would not have occurred.

Finally, the patient must demonstrate that a physical, psychological, or financial injury (damages) occurred because of the negligence of the nurse. Damages may include compensation for pain and suffering, medical expenses, and lost wages. If allowed, a patient's estate may seek punitive damages, meant to punish or deter wrongful conduct.

Expert witnesses are generally not required in simple negligence lawsuits because reasonably intelligent laypeople are able to anticipate the consequences of negligent behavior. However, malpractice is a form of negligence that requires expert witness testimony because it pertains to professional standards. Standard of care testimony is presented in court through the use of expert witnesses and documents such as the Nurse Practice Act, institutional policies and procedures, professional standards of practice, professional position statements, and learned treatises.[25] It is imperative that ED policy and procedure manuals are regularly updated to reflect current practice, and they are routinely demanded and evaluated as part of the discovery process.

Although most malpractice lawsuits are against physicians, surgeons, and institutions and not nurses, claims against nurses do occur. Common causes of lawsuits against emergency nurses include medication errors; inadequate patient monitoring and failure to report; failure to observe and report; substandard documentation; inadequate references to patient condition and changes in condition; insufficient notations of treatment rendered and responses to treatment; lack of noting transfer of care to another health care professional; inconsistent timing of entries and chronology of events; and patient falls.

Under a theory of liability called *respondeat superior,* employers have vicarious liability for negligent actions of their employees acting within the scope of their employment. The hospital employer is legally liable for acts of its staff members while they are performing duties. An employer may be required to pay a settlement for an employee found liable for professional negligence. If so, the employer may require the employee to repay the employer for money lost (indemnification).

Typically, hospitals provide malpractice insurance for nurses to cover costs associated with litigation of professional negligence cases and expenses of a settlement or verdict. These policies cover the nurse for malpractice within the scope of the nurse's employment. Malpractice insurance is available and recommended for nurses as a means to manage risk and actions contrary to employer policies and procedures, licensure actions, and out-of-hospital events.

Another concept in negligence is called *res ipsa loquitor* and is derived from the Latin phrase meaning, "The thing speaks for itself." These claims occur when (1) the injury does not normally occur without negligence; (2) the plaintiff is ruled out as the cause of the injury; and (3) the type of negligence clearly falls within the scope of the defendant's duty to the patient.

SUMMARY

The legal aspects of health care have an effect on the manner in which emergency nursing care is delivered. Because nursing care poses a risk of harm to the public if practiced by professionals who are negligent or incompetent, the government, through its enforcement powers, is required to protect its citizens from harm. Federal and state laws and other regulatory requirements define the scope of practice and identify the oversight authority for each jurisdiction. It is essential for emergency nurses to stay up to date on legislative changes that may affect their practice and to be aware of all of the standards of practice through their respective professional organizations.

REFERENCES

1. U.S. Constitution—Article 1 Section 1. U.S. Constitution Website. https://www.usconstitution.net/xconst_A1Sec1.html. Accessed June 1, 2018.
2. U.S. Constitution—Article 2 Section 1. U.S. Constitution Website. https://www.usconstitution.net/xconst_A2Sec1.html. Accessed June 1, 2018.
3. U.S. Constitution—Article 3 Section 1. U.S. Constitution Website. https://usconstitution.net/xconst_A3Sec1.html. Accessed June 1, 2018.
4. USLegal. Administrative agencies. USLegal website. https://system.uslegal.com/administrative-agencies/. Accessed June 26, 2018.
5. 1395dd. https://www.cms.gov/Regulations-and-Guidance/Legislation/EMTALA/index.html. Accessed June 26, 2018.
6. US Department of Health and Human Services. Summary of the HIPAA Privacy Rule. https://www.hhs.gov/hipaa/for-professionals/privacy/laws-regulations/index.html. Accessed June 26, 2018.
7. US Department of Health & Human Services, Centers for Medicare & Medicaid Services. Transmittal #60: Revisions to Appendix V—Interpretive Guidelines—Responsibilities of Medicare participating hospitals in emergency care. https://www.cms.gov/Regulations-and-Guidance/Guidance/Transmittals/2017Downloads/R176SOMA.pdf. Accessed April 07, 2019. Published July 16, 2010.
8. The Joint Commission. The Joint Commission 2009 requirements related to the provision of culturally competent patient-centered care hospital accreditation program (HAP). https://www.jointcommission.org/assets/1/6/2009_CLASRelated-StandardsHAP.pdf. Accessed June 28, 2018.
9. Emergency Medical Treatment and Active Labor Act (EMTALA). (suppl. 1995). Title 42, U.S.C.A. section. (1995). https://www.cms.gov/Regulations-and-Guidance/Guidance/Transmittals/2017Downloads/R176SOMA.pdf.

10. *King of Ahrens*, 16 F3d 265 (8th Cir 1994).
11. *Fed Regist*. 2000;65(250):82566. http://www.hhs.gov/ocr/part3.pdf. Accessed June 27, 2018.
12. Federal law, EMTALA, and state law enforcement: Conflict in the ED? https://www.ahcmedia.com/articles/120641-federal-law-emtala-and-state-law-enforcement-conflict-in-the-ed. Accessed June 27, 2018.
13. Pre-emption of state law. 45 CFR Part 160, subpart B.
14. Uses and disclosures for which an authorization or opportunity to agree or object is not required. 45 CFR 164.512.
15. Emergency Nurses Association. *Emergency Nursing Core Curriculum*. 7th ed. St Louis, MO: Elsevier; 2018;675–684.
16. US Department of Health and Human Services. Electronic medical record systems, Agency for Healthcare Research and Quality website. https://healthit.ahrq.gov/key-topics/electronic-medical-record-systems. Accessed June 26, 2018.
17. Rozovsky FA. *Consent to Treatment: A Practical Guide: Supplement*. 2nd ed. Boston, MA: Little, Brown; 1995.
18. US. *Prince v Massachusetts*. 1944;321:158.
19. Will JF. My God my choice: the mature minor doctrine and adolescent refusal of life-saving or sustaining medical treatment based upon religious beliefs. *J Contemp Health L Policy*. 2006;22:233. http://scholarship.law.edu/jchlp/vol22/iss2/2. Accessed June 26, 2018.
20. 42 CFR 489.24(d)(3), (5). Special Responsibilities for Medicare Hospitals.
21. Field RI. Why is health care regulation so complex? *Pharm Ther*. 2008;33(10):607–608. http://www.ncbi.nlm.nih.gov/pmc/articles/PMC2730786/. Accessed June, 2018
22. California Judicial Branch. Judicial Council of California civil jury instructions. https://www.courts.ca.gov/partners/317.htm. Accessed April 06, 2019.
23. Brent NJ. *Nurses and the Law: A Guide to Principles and Applications*. 2nd ed. Chicago, IL: W.B. Saunders; 2000.
24. Lunsford v. *Board of Nurse Examiners. 648 SW 2d 391, Tex. App. 3 Dist*; 1983.
25. McConnell T, Vaughn S. Standards for nurse expert witnesses: a recommendation. *J Legal Nurse Consult*. 2010;21(3):5–9.

Approaching Diversity

Heather Martin

As human beings, we are all diverse—each one of us is different from the other. As health care professionals, we care for patients who have recently arrived in this country and others whose families have been here for generations. We may or may not share attributes with our patients and fellow staff members. We may identify with a group that is not the dominant society. Many health care professionals have taken cultural sensitivity courses and learned basic information about different cultural or ethnic groups. Most likely, some of the learned information did not fit for all members of those groups. It is impossible to know everything about all the groups (patient populations) we serve. There is often as much diversity within groups as there is between them. Some individuals will identify closely with their country of origin or religion, whereas others will not. Health care professionals have an obligation to address and respect issues of diversity. There is always an opportunity to learn from patients and colleagues. As a way to begin, it is important for all health care professionals to examine their own beliefs and attitudes regarding diversity.

Understanding cultural diversity is an essential tool that health care providers should possess when caring for patients. The way of life for a group of people with regard to their beliefs, behavior practices, attitudes, rituals, and customs is what defines an individual's identified culture.[1] Diversity has been defined as the fact or quality of being diverse, differing one from another, made up of differences, or composed of distinct characteristics, qualities, and elements.[2] These differences include visible and invisible value and belief patterns, as well as characteristics such as age, class, culture, ethnicity, gender, nationality, race, religion, sexual orientation, and marginalization. It is important that health care professionals recognize and accept the differences in themselves and in us all.

AREAS OF DIVERSITY

When asking questions related to a patient's diversity, it is imperative to "ask the questions that need to be asked." These are questions that seek information needed to further assess the patient's condition and the patient's ability to complete the needed treatment. Questions that show a bias or that are derogatory can only hamper the patient-staff relationship. "Why" questions such as "Why are you homeless?" will not assist in determining whether a patient can follow a plan of care or other needed treatment. Asking questions that are not pertinent to the patient's evaluation and are asked out of curiosity are inappropriate and may cause patient distrust. For example, asking a transgender person about their reassignment surgery when they present for a toothache is not necessary and will not add any value to their medical evaluation. Outlining the plan in a nonjudgmental, objective manner and enlisting the patient's help in ascertaining if the care plan is feasible based on his or her individual circumstances would be more beneficial.

A thorough patient assessment includes a diversity assessment. The diversity assessment seeks to identify the patient's language preference, information about who may assist the patient in decision making, and what the patient believes are his or her most pressing medical needs. During this assessment the health care professional should be keenly aware of the effect of nonverbal communication. Eye contact, personal space issues, and tone of voice may directly affect the ability of the patient to trust the health care professional. All the areas of diversity have unique characteristics that may or may not identify an individual patient as a member of that particular group.

Age

Age is defined as the length of existence from the beginning to any given time or one's stages of life.[3] There are obvious anatomic, physiologic, and behavioral changes at every stage of life. The health care plan should be based on the effect of these stages and how these will affect the patient's response. The Joint Commission[4] requires hospitals and health care organizations to provide ongoing education, training, and competency validation to ensure safe and effective age-specific and culturally sensitive patient care.

Staff attitudes can affect the quality of care available to the older adult. The Age Discrimination Act of 1975 is a national law that prohibits discrimination on the basis of age in any program that receives federal financial assistance.[5]

Generational differences can explain a patient's need for care and reaction to that care. Advancing age is commonly associated with comorbidities; infants are completely dependent on caregivers for meeting their self-care needs. The older adult may have greater expectations of common courtesy, such as expecting staff members to knock before entering and to introduce themselves. Younger adults are more likely to be involved in traumatic events. When caring for pediatric patients, there can be increased anxiety within the family and staff.

Class

Class identifies a group of people whose members share the same attributes, such as social rank or socioeconomic status, and adhere to traditional roles and principles.[6] Socioeconomic status may have more to do with how individuals are judged by others than any other area of diversity. Socioeconomic status is a strong predictor of health. Race and culture may often be blamed when socioeconomic status or poverty is actually the causative factor. Differences commonly seen with patients living in poverty directly affect access to care, transportation, and the ability to provide self-care when needed. Poverty is a fact of life for every racial/ethnic group.[7] Many people have come to the United States to escape war or long-time military rule. Poverty was the way of life in their home countries. They may arrive here with minimal resources or education.

Culture

Culture includes patterns of behavior and thinking that persons living in social groups learn and share.[1] Culture is closely related to the identified ethnic background. Culture may affect the way a patient responds to health concerns, such as in response to crisis or grief. Negative attributes may be associated with being part of one's culture, when actually the effects of a lower socioeconomic status cause violence and/or criminal activities.

Culture is handed down from generation to generation. You may see one age-group that follows their parents' culture more closely than another, younger group might. Culture can also be self-identified. A patient may identify more with a culture because of an affinity for the group's traits. Asking open-ended questions about culture, without judgment, can aid in understanding.

Ethnicity

A person's ethnicity can be seen as a conscious choice of his or her identity based on beliefs, values, practices, and loyalty to a certain group or groups.[8] Ethnicity is generally related to heritage or country of origin of one's ancestors. An individual's ethnic identity may be an area of invisible diversity to someone not of that group. Statements such as "You don't look like someone from that ethnic group" are perceived as ignorant and unkind. Not all people from each group look alike. All ethnic groups have variations in skin color, hair color, and the color of their eyes. Some groups have pronounced features that may or may not be easily identified. There are, of course, many people whose mother and father come from different ethnicities. Such an individual may or may not identify with either or both groups. A patient's last name may not be one normally identified as part of a particular ethnic group. If information about ethnicity is pertinent, the health care professional should ask open-ended questions without making initial assumptions. If the health care professional finds it necessary to identify a person according to his or her ethnicity, it is most appropriate to ask the patient what he or she prefers. Table 3.1 lists terms used by certain groups that may or may not be used as identifiers by all members of those groups.

Gender

Gender is one's self concept of being a male or female. This seems to be an easy question to answer, but it may not always be apparent. We usually do not use biologic markers (e.g., DNA) to identify if a person is male or female, but make assumptions regarding their gender based on their gender markers, such as what clothing they wear or their hairstyle or voice.[9] The use of a form that asks basic demographic information with a gender checkbox is helpful. Transgender patients identify with a gender other than the one that was applied to them at birth. Transgender patients may or may not have had reassignment surgery, but this does not change the fact that the patients identify their own gender. The name and gender the patient describes should be used as identifiers. Ask what pronouns they would like to referred to by (he, she, they, etc.) and note these in their medical record for future reference.

There continue to be stereotypic presentations pertaining to gender. A health care professional is less likely to expect a male sexual assault victim than one who is female. Heart disease can be misdiagnosed in women who do not present with

TABLE 3.1 Terms Used to Describe Groups (Always Ask What the Person Would Prefer).[17]

African American	Black, African American, Afro American, colored (older people)
Arab	Arab, Middle Eastern, by country of origin *When asked about country of origin, some may respond with the city where they were born.*
Chinese	Chinese or Chinese American
Puerto Rican	Puerto Rican, Puertorriqueño(a), Boricua
Japanese	Japanese American
Mexican	Mexican, Mexican American, Latino(a), Chicano(a) *Acculturated Mexican Americans may prefer American.*
American Indians	Tribal names are often used: Chippewa, Hopi, Seneed, Colulle, Native Americans, American Indians *Tribal affiliation names such as Navaho are not the real names.*
Vietnamese	Vietnamese (English speakers), ngõi, Viet Nam *It is derogatory to use the term refugee.*

the classic signs and symptoms. The health care professional must consider gender issues and how they affect the care of a patient.

Sexual Identity

Sexual orientation, identity, and preference all refer to our attraction to others and what characteristics of individuals we find sexually attractive.[9] Some individuals may also identify as being asexual—not being attracted to either sex. Health care professionals may unintentionally offend a gay or lesbian patient by assuming that he or she is heterosexual. A routine question when information about sexual activity is needed would be, "Are you sexually active with males, females, both, or neither?" All questions should be asked in an open, nonjudgmental manner with an emphasis on maintaining privacy for the patient when asking such questions. The term "homosexual" should be avoided in conversation because it is seen as being offensive because of the past negativity in the medical establishment.[9] Multiple individuals in the LGBTQ community have expressed their avoidance of emergency departments due to fear of discrimination, negative past experiences, lack of privacy, and repetitiveness of questions regarding their gender and sexual identity that led to feelings of embarrassment, frustration, and disempowerment.[9] As stated in the Emergency Nurses Association Cultural Diversity Position Statement, all nurses (and health care providers) should treat each patient with compassion and respect for human dignity and the uniqueness of the individual.[10]

Race

Race is defined as a group of people united or classified together on the basis of common history, nationality, or geographic distribution.[11] Other definitions of race include characteristics that are visible and identifiable to that group. These definitions include skin color and facial feature similarities. There is much debate about what constitutes a race. Often race and ethnicity are used interchangeably.

Anthropologists in the 17th and 18th centuries proposed racial classifications based on observable characteristics such as skin color, hair type, body proportions, and skull measurements. The traditional terms for these populations are *Caucasoid, Mongoloid,* and *Negroid.* In certain circumstances the use of these terms is seen as offensive. Current-day anthropologists now consider race to be more a social construct than an objective biologic fact.

Religion

Religion is an organized or unorganized system of religious attitudes, beliefs, and practices that an individual possesses.[12] Patients may identify with a religion even if they do not actively participate in that religion. Staff should not impose their own religious beliefs but should take their cues from what the patient or family wishes. It is not uncommon for staff and patients to have religious beliefs in conflict. This is particularly true when the patient's religious belief prohibits a planned health intervention. Staff must remember that the patient has the right to consent or decline care even if his or her decision is not what the staff believes to be prudent. Issues where conflict may occur include use of contraception, organ donation, blood administration, and decisions regarding death. Staff members should discuss concerns they have with their management if there are religious issues that may affect their ability to care for certain patient groups. Managers should make provisions for staff to switch assignments or have another staff member care for that particular patient.

Marginalization

Individuals seen as possessing relatively little social power or deemed unimportant are of a marginalized status, or experience marginalization.[13] These are people whose diversity is assumed to be "wrong" or "unworthy" by some members of the dominant society. Individuals who perform criminal acts or are incarcerated are often viewed as dispensable. Overweight individuals pose a challenge for health care professionals because the additional needs of the overweight patient can elicit ill feelings in staff members. A homeless person may be viewed as someone who chooses his or her lifestyle and thus is not deserving of services. Health care professionals may feel that a homeless patient misuses emergency services for non–health care-related issues, such as food or shelter. A patient with a history of mental illness may have difficulty articulating his or her medical concerns and therefore is categorized as just a "psych" patient. Frequently these patients are discharged or referred to psychiatric services only to return to the emergency department with a medical condition that was overlooked. A developmentally delayed individual may be seen as a difficult patient because of communication barriers and self-care issues. The patient's caregiver can be instrumental in assessing baseline status and the patient's ability to assist with the health care plan.

The effect of a marginalized status must be recognized. There should be an objective review of how the marginalized status affects the plan of care. The health care professional should examine any bias he or she may have and ensure that it does not negatively affect patient care.

THE DIVERSITY PRACTICE MODEL

There must be a realization that the delivery of quality health care includes an appreciation and respect for patient and staff diversity. Caring for diverse populations in a sensitive manner implies that there is recognition of differences and individual differences are not seen as wrong or unworthy of respect.[14] Health care professionals should ask those questions that need to be asked and are pertinent to the medical plan of care. These questions would further understanding and assist in formulating the patient care plan. Questions out of curiosity should be avoided.

The Diversity Practice Model (Table 3.2) was developed by the Emergency Nurses Association Diversity Task Force to provide a framework to use when discussing diversity issues.[15] The model uses an ABCDE mnemonic to guide relevant ideas and questions.

TABLE 3.2 Diversity Practice Model.[15]

A	Assumptions	The act of taking for granted or supposing that a thought or idea about a group is true.
B	Beliefs	Beliefs are shared ideas about how a group operates.
C	Communication	The two-way sharing of information that results in an understanding between the receiver and the sender.
D	Diversity	The ways in which people differ and the effect that these differences have on health perception and health care.
E	Education	The act of attaining knowledge about diversity.

TABLE 3.3 Pertinent Questions When Discussing Diversity.[15]

Assumptions	What do we assume or take for granted about this individual or community that they come from?
Beliefs/Behavior	How does my belief system affect the care I provide for the patient? Are my beliefs mirrored in the way I act toward a patient?
Communication	How does the patient communicate? If they do not speak English, is there a translator available? Can the patient see and hear?
Diversity	Which aspects of diversity are present? Some characteristics of diversity are visible; some are invisible. Reminder: age, class, culture, ethnicity, gender, race, religion, sexual identity, and marginalization
Education/Ethics	What educational recommendations do you have?

The Diversity Practice Model can be used to discuss sensitive issues or when presenting patient-based case reviews. Table 3.3 contains the fundamental questions to ask when using the model. The model begins with staff examining their assumptions about the patient. Assumptions are ideas or thoughts that may or may not be true and are usually based on little factual information. This is a time in the discussion to recognize that everyone makes assumptions. It is what we do with those assumptions and how they can negatively affect patient care that should be examined.

The model then moves to an examination of beliefs. Beliefs are long-held ideals and may be based on assumptions. In the professional health care arena, facilities have belief statements or mission statements that outline the organizational philosophy. These documents can be helpful to show how those initial assumptions may be incongruent with the beliefs of the organization. Generally, there is a statement of the fundamental rights of patients and how they should be treated equally regardless of their diversity. In one example, we can look to the forefathers of the United States and relate the beliefs of the preamble of the Declaration of Independence: "We hold these truths to be self-evident, that all men are created equal, that they are endowed by their Creator with certain unalienable Rights, that among these are Life, Liberty and the pursuit of Happiness."[16]

If one believes that all men and women are created equal, then the standard of health care has to be the same for everyone. This belief, whether it be from a governmental document, a facility mission statement, or a group consensus, should override any implied negative assumptions.

The third step of the model involves a discussion of communication, which is the transfer of information from a sender to a receiver. It is imperative that we know if our communication has been received and understood. When obtaining informed consent, diversity issues must be considered. Table 3.4 gives some general information on how different groups may approach consent.

A patient must have an avenue to ask questions, and in turn the patient must be able to understand the answers. The goal when discussing communication is to ensure that the patient understands the plan of care. In hospitals, certified translators should be used whenever a patient requests or a staff member determines that a translator is needed to facilitate communication. Translators should be trained and their fluency in the identified language(s) evaluated. When using a translator, the health care professional should always be present. The health care professional should direct his or her questions to the patient. Even if the words are not understood, a caring tone and professional manner of speech assist the patient in trusting the health care professional.

The model continues with a focus on the patient's areas of diversity. The health care professional can ask questions such as "What do you believe caused your illness?" This may encourage the patient to discuss his or her views on health. The patient's view may be rooted in his or her cultural/ethnic background. Another question may be "What have you done to treat yourself?" The patient may then disclose the use of folk medicine practices. This may include the use of herbs or rituals. When the patient is asked, "What is most important in your ability to recover from this illness?" the response may reveal a strong religious or spiritual belief or give the health care professional more information about the patient's family structure. Family structure is extremely important when communicating about serious illness.

Table 3.5 identifies how families and patients may respond to discussions about serious illness. It is interesting that most of the described groups respond in a similar manner. Most families would prefer not to tell a patient about a serious illness or diagnosis. This would not be congruent with the health

TABLE 3.4 Considerations When Obtaining Consent.[17]

African American	Avoid using medical jargon. Elicit feedback to check understanding. Involve the family in the consent process.
Arabic	Written consent may be problematic. Verbal consent based on trust is more acceptable. There is a dislike of listening to all possible complications before the procedure. Explain the need for written consent while emphasizing positive consequences.
Chinese	Involve the oldest male family member during consent explanations, especially if the patient is a young girl or a woman.
Puerto Rican	Prefer verbal consent to signed consent if feasible. Nodding affirmatively may not necessarily mean agreement or understanding. Provide an option for language preference for either verbal or written information. Allow time for the reading of material or the sharing of information with other family members.
Japanese	Explain the procedure clearly. Stop to elicit feedback and understanding. Patients may be uncomfortable asking questions. Nisei may be more likely to consent than Sansei and Yonsei because of the recommendation of the health care professional.
Mexican	Undocumented immigrants tend to be suspicious of any type of consent, especially written consent. A Latino health care provider may be helpful in obtaining consent. Language preference and reading level must be considered. Important decisions may require consultation among the entire family.
American Indians	Discuss consent with the patient while explaining the roles of all involved, including the family. Ask if the patient needs to consult anyone before consenting. Some individuals may be unwilling to sign written consents based on political and personal history of documents being misused.
Vietnamese	The patient may nod affirmatively although not understanding or approving of what is said. The patient may not ask questions publicly; allow for private time with the patient. Assess understanding by asking the patient to verbalize what was discussed. Allow the patient to discuss forms with a spouse or trusted friend.

TABLE 3.5 Patient/Family Response to Serious Illness.[17]

African American	Have a family conference or talk with a family elder or family-identified minister. The patient may have an older relative reveal a poor prognosis.
Arabic	Family members buffer the sick person from knowing the whole truth about his or her health situation. Discuss with the family spokesperson about the best way to provide information to the patient. Accommodate family needs for the gradual and prolonged disclosure of information.
Chinese	Some families may prefer to be present when discussing serious illness. The head of household should be involved.
Puerto Rican	Terminal illness is often kept secret from the patient. The family does this as a protective mechanism to provide the best quality of life for the patient. On admission, ask the patient if someone else has the responsibility for health care decisions.
Japanese	The family may filter information for the non–English-speaking patient. Families may be reluctant to divulge a terminal diagnosis. Consult with family members.
Mexican	The clinician should inform the patient and family together and as soon as possible. Ask the patient who should be included in the discussion.
American Indians	The health care team may suggest a family meeting to discuss the condition and course of treatment.
Vietnamese	The family may not want the patient informed without consulting the head of the family. It is believed that the patient will experience more stress and worry.

care practice of informing a patient. This is an area where the health care professional should work with the family/patient to discover a common ground that allows all parties to fully participate in the health care plan.

Identifying the pertinent areas of diversity and how those areas affect care is vital. Is there conflict with the staff because of a misunderstood gesture? Does that conflict have to do with the staff's not understanding how the area of diversity (age, class, culture, ethnicity, gender, race, religion, sexual identity, and marginalization) directly affects care?

Health care professionals should be prepared to address the differences between them and their patients. The goal is harmony and better understanding for all.

The model ends with a plan for education. Staff members may decide that formal presentations are needed and will then invite representatives from a particular group to speak. A needs assessment can be performed to assess staff response to diversity issues. It may highlight areas that require further staff education, such as religious groups and their wishes to refuse blood transfusion. Questions can be geared to reveal bias, such as toward individuals who are not able to pay their medical bills. Staff can then receive additional information (e.g., about poverty and government or hospital programs that can assist patients with payment) to help overcome those biases.

There are many ways that staff can share information with each other. One might document a case study in a newsletter or e-mail format to let other staff members benefit from the discussion session on a diversity issue. Even a potluck meal with foods from different regions can serve to celebrate diversity.

SUMMARY

The delivery of competent care is enhanced by an appreciation and understanding of those qualities that define us as individuals, as well as those qualities we share. Regardless of personal views, each patient should be treated with dignity and respect. Ethnocentrism, prejudice, bias, stereotypes, and ignorance of cultural differences negatively affect relationships with both our patients and our colleagues. Approaching diversity in a positive, nonjudgmental, and sensitive manner will only aid in our ability to deliver quality patient care.

REFERENCES

1. Mitchell AM, Fioravanti M, Founds S, Hoffman RL, Libman R. Using stimulation to bridge communication and cultural barriers in health care encounters: report of an international workshop. *Clin Simul Nurs.* 2010;6(5):193–198.
2. Diversity. *Merriam-Webster's Online Dictionary.* Merriam-Webster.com website. https://www.merriam-webster.com. Accessed June 26, 2018.
3. Age. *Merriam-Webster's Online Dictionary.* Merriam-Webster.com website. https://www.merriam-webster.com. Accessed June 26, 2018.
4. The Joint Commission. *A crosswalk of the National Standards for Culturally and Linguistically Appropriate Services (CLAS) in Health and Health Care to The Joint Commission Ambulatory Health Care Accreditation Standards.* https://www.jointcommission.org/assets/1/6/Crosswalk_CLAS_AHC_20141110.pdf. Published 2014. Accessed June 25, 2018.
5. US Department of Health and Human Services. *OCR Fact Sheet: Know About the Federal Law that Protects Against Age Discrimination.* https://www.hhs.gov/sites/default/files/ocr/civilrights/resources/factsheets/age.pdf. Accessed June 25, 2018.
6. Class. *Merriam-Webster's Online Dictionary.* Merriam-Webster.com website. https://www.merriam-webster.com. Accessed June 26, 2018.
7. US Census Bureau. *Race and Hispanic Origin of the Foreign-Born Population in the United States.* https://census.gov/library/publications.html. Published 2007. Accessed April 07, 2019.
8. Ethnicity. *Merriam-Webster's Online Dictionary.* Merriam-Webster.com website. https://www.merriam-webster.com. Accessed June 26, 2018.
9. Eliason MJ, Chinn PL. *LGBYQ Cultures: What Health Care Professionals Should Know About Sexual and Gender Diversity.* 3rd ed. New York, NY: Wolters Kluwer; 2018.
10. Emergency Nurses Association. *Emergency Nurses Association Position Statement: Cultural Diversity in the Emergency Setting.* https://www.ena.org/docs/default-source/resource-library/practice-resources/position-statements/culturaldiversity.pdf?sfvrsn=e85dc130_14. Published 2012. Accessed June 25, 2018.
11. Race. *Merriam-Webster's Online Dictionary.* Merriam-Webster.com website. https://www.merriam-webster.com. Published 2012. Accessed June 26, 2018.
12. Religion. *Merriam-Webster's Online Dictionary.* Merriam-Webster.com website. https://www.merriam-webster.com. Accessed June 26, 2018.
13. Marginalization. *Merriam-Webster's Online Dictionary.* Merriam-Webster.com website. https://www.merriam-webster.com. Accessed June 26, 2018.
14. Newberry L, Criddle L. *Sheehy's Manual of Emergency Care.* 6th ed. St Louis, MO: Mosby; 2005:27–32.
15. Emergency Nurses Association Diversity Task Force. Approaching diversity: an interactive journey. Unpublished work, 1996–1998.
16. US Declaration of Independence: annotated text of the declaration. https://en.wikipedia.org/wiki/United_States_Declaration_of_Independence#Annotated_text_of_the_engrossed_declaration. Accessed September 4, 2007.
17. Lipson JS, Dibble SL, Minarik PA. *Culture and Nursing Care: A Pocket Guide.* San Francisco, CA: UCSF Nursing Press; 1996.

UNIT II

Professional Practice

4

Evidence-Based Practice

Sharon Saunderson Coffey, Kierstin Jeana Cohen

Beginning with Florence Nightingale (1820–1910), and continuing today, nursing has been on the battlefields, at the bedside, and in the research laboratories, collecting the facts, analyzing the facts, and translating those facts, so the care and treatment we give to our patients are not based on opinions of how to do something but rather facts based on the scientific data. Florence Nightingale was a systematic thinker and passionate about facts, and statistics. During her time, she not only used statistics but also developed tools that were vetted by other professionals and experts to help her validate answers to questions or observations and to push for social reform.[1–2] She was also a pioneer in translating statistics into layman's terms through color pie charts and graphs, enabling politicians, many without medical or nursing knowledge, to better understand the data and thus direct social health reform by using the data Nightingale presented.[3]

Nightingale had the spirit of inquiry. It was her drive to inquire and search for evidence to validate observations, which ultimately changed what nurses did at the bedside. In essence, Florence Nightingale was the first nurse to use evidence to validate and change clinical practice. Today, this spirit of inquiry is referred to as evidence-based practice (EBP) and is described as a problem-solving approach that integrates the best evidence from high-quality research studies and patient care data and combines that into a patient-centered clinical care approach.[1]

More than 100 years of nursing practice has passed since Nightingale first used evidence to change clinical nursing practice, and nurses are still seeking answers to questions regarding what they do at the bedside. Nurses want to know that what they do at the bedside does make a difference in patient outcomes. But what is evidence? What is *quality* evidence? What evidence is necessary before a practice can be changed? These questions continue to constitute much of the work of bedside nurses, nurse leaders, nurse researchers, and nurse scholars. Nurses, along with physicians and other health care providers, are clearly in the infancy of developing a practice based on evidence.[4]

Some examples of evidence-based changes in nursing practice are using saline flushes instead of heparin flushes for peripheral intravenous lines;[5] discontinuing the common practice of placing patients in Trendelenburg's position for hypotension,[6] highlighting that volume replacement and the supine position with the head of the bed flat are the most beneficial interventions for patients with hypovolemia; and discontinuing the common practice of aspirating during an intramuscular injection. All these changes are due to lack of evidence to support the old practice.[7,8]

WHAT IS EVIDENCE-BASED PRACTICE?

One of the most prolific authors and leaders in the use of EBP in health care is David Sackett from the University of Oxford in England. He describes EBP as "the conscious, explicit and judicious use of current best evidence in making decisions about the care of individual patients."[4] The implementation of evidence into health care practice was initiated by Dr. Archie Cochrane, a British epidemiologist. He believed that people should not pay for health care if the care was not supported by evidence. As a result of his actions, the Cochrane Collaboration was founded with the purpose of assisting individuals to make educated health care decisions based on the evidence from updated systematic reviews of health care interventions.[9,10]

Nursing and health care leaders are asking for research-based evidence to guide clinical practice. EBP does direct care and treatment, lead to higher quality of care, improve patient outcomes, reduce health care costs, and improve satisfaction of both the health care provider and the patient.[11] The Institute of Medicine's Roundtable on Evidence-Based Medicine has a 2020 goal of having 90% of clinical decisions be supported by accurate, timely, and up-to-date clinical information and reflect the best available evidence.[12] This is a lofty goal, as many values in health care organizations still do not consistently support the implementation of EBP into clinical settings. Each hospital or organization will have their own unique reasons for using or not using EBP. Determining the barriers and the strengths of EBP utilization will aid in beginning and sustaining an EBP culture supporting nurses in all aspects of clinical care. EBP will further support the delivery of professional nursing care integrated with clinical experience, patient values and preferences, and the best scientific evidence available.

The *Case Scenario for EBP: Handoff Communication* (Box 4.1) will provide a context for understanding and applying EBP into the emergency department (ED) clinical setting. It will be used throughout this chapter as we explore the steps of EBP and implementation of our findings in the ED setting.

BOX 4.1 Case Scenario for EBP: Handoff Communication Tool.

You are a staff nurse in a busy emergency department (ED). In a recent multidisciplinary quality meeting, ED hospital data were presented showing that over a 3-month period, 11 patients who were admitted after having been seen and treated in the ED had a reportable adverse event within 1 hour of admission. Of those 11 patients, 6 had medication errors and 3 had falls. All were attributed to floor or intensive care unit staff not having enough information about their newly admitted patient. In a recent peer-reviewed nursing journal, you found an article that discusses the evidence showing a reduction in adverse patient events with a standardized handoff reporting communication tool. You are excited about this information and decide to inquire further on the idea of a standardized communication tool that the ED nurses could use to improve communication and reduce adverse patient events.

Through this case scenario, you will see the steps to EBP and how-to implementation of EBP in the clinical ED setting.

Evidence consists of both knowledge gained from clinical experience and knowledge gained from scientific studies or research. The blending of clinical experience and science provides a solid foundation from which care decisions can be made.[13] External evidence comes from several sources such as from rigorously designed studies such as randomized control trials (RCTs), meta-analyses, or metasynthesis data. Internal evidence is typically generated from knowledge found in the clinical experience, quality review data, or quality improvement projects.

EVIDENCE-BASED PRACTICE MODELS

Several EBP nursing models have been developed to help guide the design and implementation of EBP. Forty-seven prominent EBP models can be identified in the literature, and they can be placed into four categories: (1) EBP and knowledge transformation processes, (2) strategic change to promote adoption of new knowledge, (3) knowledge exchange and synthesis for application and inquiry, and (4) designing and interpreting dissemination research.[14]

One such EBP nursing model is the Academic Center for Evidence-Based Practice (ACE) Star Model of Knowledge Transformation (Fig. 4.1).[15] The ACE Star Model is an interdisciplinary strategy for transferring knowledge into nursing and health care practice to meet the goal of quality improvement. This model addresses both translation and implementation aspects of the EBP process.[15]

Likewise, the function of clinical practice guidelines is to guide practice.[16] Important new knowledge resources have been developed and advanced owing to the EBP movement. Although resources were available for Point 1 on the ACE Star Model, only recently have resources been developed for the knowledge forms on Points 2, 3, 4, and 5 of the Model.[16] These resources are outlined in Table 4.1.

Although the Star Model is well developed and many articles can be found on EBP implementation projects using this model, a summary of other popular models can be found in Table 4.2. There are various formally recognized models of EBP summarized in this chapter. Each has a varying number of steps outlined.

The Advancing Research and Clinical Practice Through Close Collaboration (ARCC) model has been used in hospital and community practice settings and has been researched as a strategy for improving practice outcomes. The emphasis on identifying organizational strengths and barriers to EBP and identifying mentors to work with direct care staff contributes to an organizational culture supporting EBP. The ARCC Model focuses on building resources and training mentors who play a central role in facilitating and sustaining EBP at the point of care and throughout the organization. The ARCC model uses seven steps, beginning with motivating nurses to begin to ask or inquire.[17,18] The seven sequential steps are:

1. Cultivate a spirit of inquiry.
2. Develop the clinical question in a PICOT format (discussed later in this chapter) to assist in determining how to search and find the most relevant and best evidence.
3. Search for the most current, most applicable evidence using the most rigorous research methods to lead toward the best answers for the clinical question.
4. Critically appraise and synthesize the evidence found in the search. Determine how "good" the evidence is by appraising the evidence for points such as validity, reliability, and applicability. Synthesis includes combining the appraised evidence to determine whether an EBP recommendation exists.
5. Integrate synthesized recommendations into clinical practice through a well-developed implementation plan, considering the risks and benefits and feasibility of implementation.
6. Evaluate outcomes after implementation to ensure the implementation plan is meeting the set goals.
7. Dissemination is the final step and can be done formally or informally. Venues to share your outcomes include nursing rounds; hospital research days; and local, national, or international conferences.

ASKING THE CLINICAL QUESTION: SPIRIT OF INQUIRY—PICOT QUESTION

In thinking about the handoff scenario, spirit of inquiry is in place as the ED staff have already started to ask questions about communication between the ED and the units/floors when patients are admitted[1]. Developing a well-built clinical question is key to finding the answer to the questions that you or staff in the ED may be asking. One method to do this is to use the PICOT format when developing the research question. PICOT is an acronym for the five elements used to develop a sound clinical question: (P) *p*opulation to be looked at; (I) *I*ntervention, *i*nnovation, or *i*ssue of interest; (C) comparison or *c*urrent intervention or issue of interest; (O) *o*utcome(s) related to clinical idea; and (T) *t*ime it takes for the intervention to achieve an outcome or time desired to evaluate the effectiveness of an intervention (Box 4.2).[19] Using the PICOT format will guide the team in a consistent and step-wise manner to

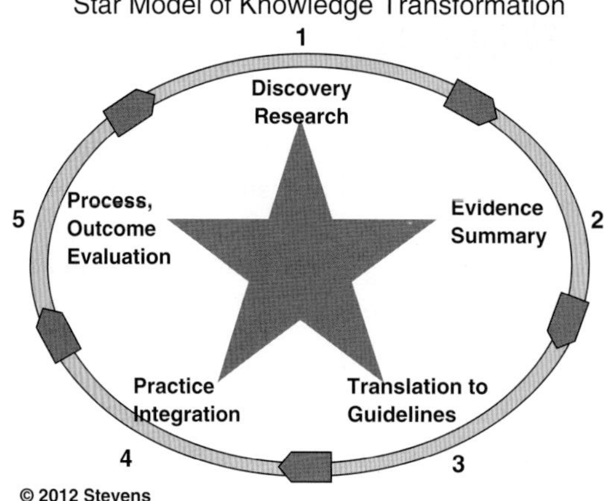

Fig. 4.1 Stevens Star Model of Knowledge Transformation © 2015. http://nursing.uthscsa.edu/onrs/starmodel/star-model.asp

TABLE 4.1 Resources for Forms of Knowledge in the Star Model.

Form of Knowledge	Description of Resources
Point 1. Discovery	Bibliographic databases such as CINAHL provide single research reports and, in most cases, multiple reports.
Point 2. Evidence Summary	Cochrane Collaboration Database of Systematic Reviews provides reports of rigorous systematic reviews on clinical topics. See www.cochrane.org/
Point 3. Translation into Guidelines	National Guidelines Clearinghouse, sponsored by the Agency for Healthcare Research and Quality, provides online access to evidence-based clinical practice guidelines. See www.guideline.gov
Point 4. Integration into Practice	Agency for Healthcare Research and Quality Health Care Innovations Exchange-sponsored, by the Agency for Healthcare Research and Quality, provides profiles of innovations and tools for improving care processes, including adoption the guidelines and information to contact the innovator. See http://innovations.ahrq.gov/
Point 5. Evaluation of Process and Outcome	National Quality Measures Clearinghouse, sponsored by the Agency for Healthcare Research and Quality, provides detailed information on quality measures and measure sets. See http://qualitymeasures.ahrq.gov/

TABLE 4.2 Common EBP Models.

Models of Evidence-Based Practice	
Iowa Model:	The Iowa Model guides a clinician through the process of asking a question, forming a team to investigate the question, and assessing whether there is sufficient evidence to move forward with an evidence-based decision, followed by implementation on small and large scales. Originally published in 2001 and implemented at the University of Iowa.
ARCC Model (Advancing Research and Clinical Practice Through Close Collaboration)	A model integrating control and cognitive behavioral theories works to build a cadre of EBP mentors to advance EBP in a system. Detailed in the popular EBP text by the model's authors, *Evidence Based Practice in Nursing & Healthcare.*[14]
PARIHS (Promoting Action on Research Implementation in Health Services) Framework	This developing model incorporates elements and subelements, including research, clinical experience, patient experience, local information, culture, and leadership.
Johns Hopkins Nursing Evidence-Based Practice Model	This model incorporates several directive steps and an evidence rating scale that incorporates a multitude of article types.
Clinical Scholar Model	The work of Alyce Schultz, this is another mentorship-based model.

BOX 4.2 Template for Writing PICOT Questions.

INTERVENTION
In _______________ (P), how does _______________
(I) compared
To _______________ (C) affect _______________
(O) within _______________ (T)?

THERAPY
In _______________ (P), what is the effect of
_______________ (I) compared with _______________ (C)
on _______________ (O) within _______________ (T)?

PROGNOSIS/PREDICTION
In _______________ (P) how does _______________ (I)
compared with _______________ (C)
Influence _______________ (O) over _______________ (T)?

DIAGNOSIS OR DIAGNOSTIC TEST
In _______________ (P) are/is _______________ (I)
compared with _______________ (C) more accurate
in diagnosing _______________ (O)?

ETIOLOGY
Are _______________ (P), who have
_______________ (I) compared with
those without _______________ (C) at _______________
risk for/of _______________ (O) over _______________
(T)?

MEANING
How do _______________ (P) with
_______________ (I) perceive
_______________ (O) during _______________ (T)?

Adapted from Ellen Fineout-Overholt. PICOT Questions Template; 2006. This form may be used for education.

fully identify the elements related to the clinical topic of interest. How the question is written, specifically, the words chosen for the PICOT elements, will guide the literature search.

In our case scenario questioning the idea of a standardized handoff communication tool ED nurses could use to improve communication and reduce adverse patient events, consider using the PICOT method to formulate a clinical question on this topic. A PICOT question on this topic might look like this: *In ED patients being transferred to an inpatient unit, (P), how does the use of a standardized handoff communication tool (I) compared with not using a standardized communication handoff tool (C) reduce adverse patient events (O) within the first 24 hours after transfer (T)?* This type of PICOT question is an intervention question because it compares two interventions: the use of a standardized handoff communication tool versus not using a standardized tool.

FINDING THE EVIDENCE

Conducting a literature review takes time, a great deal of research knowledge, and mastery of the art of reviews. Many health care organizations employ research librarians who can be an invaluable resource to nurses conducting a search for evidence. The review must be conducted in an organized and systematic manner. The first step of the literature review is writing the PICOT question to provide clear direction for the literature search. Many databases can be searched to find evidence for the topic of interest; for example, our scenario with standardized handoff communication. Nursing literature is commonly found in the Cumulative Index to Nursing and Allied Health Literature (CINAHL), whereas medical journals are indexed commonly in PubMed. Your search might take you into PsychInfo for mental health literature or ERIC for education literature. After determining which databases to search, keywords to be used when searching the databases need to be selected. Because different databases index different publications, searching many databases will reduce the possibility of missing relevant evidence or articles.[20]

Once databases have been chosen, the PICOT question provides search terms. From our PICOT question, "In ED patients being transferred to an inpatient unit, how does the use of a standardized handoff communication tool compared with not using a standardized communication handoff tool reduce adverse patient events within the first 24 hours after transfer?", each keyword can be searched individually or by combining words or phrases with the Boolean connector "AND," which will often result in articles relevant to our PICOT question.[20] An example might be to search CINAHL by using the keywords handoff communication tool AND adverse events. An additional strategy is to eliminate articles written in non-English languages or articles published more than 5 years ago.

Levels of Evidence

A commonly used hierarchy for evaluating evidence[21] is found in Fig. 4.2. The level and quality of the evidence inherently are important to clinicians because trustworthy evidence provides the confidence needed to use the evidence to make clinical decision.[22] There are eight different levels of research designs included in the hierarchy in Fig. 4.2, with level 1 being the highest level of evidence at the top of the pyramid and level 8 being the lowest level of the pyramid and having the least validity and reliability. The type of research considered to be at the top of the hierarchy is systematic reviews and meta-analysis of RCTs. The type of research considered to be at the bottom rung of the hierarchy, although still important, includes expert opinion, background information, and reports from expert committees.[21]

Once evidence is collected on a specific topic, it is then evaluated for scientific rigor, and each study is appraised for applicability to the current topic. Determining the level of evidence is an important step in evaluating the evidence. There are several other factors to consider when evaluating the current science of a particular topic, which will not be covered in detail in this chapter. Understanding statistical reporting is a very important skill that nurses must acquire to evaluate research and to determine whether the research study is good evidence or flawed evidence.

General Appraisal Considerations

After briefly reading the articles of interest, the next step is to critically appraise the evidence contained in each individual

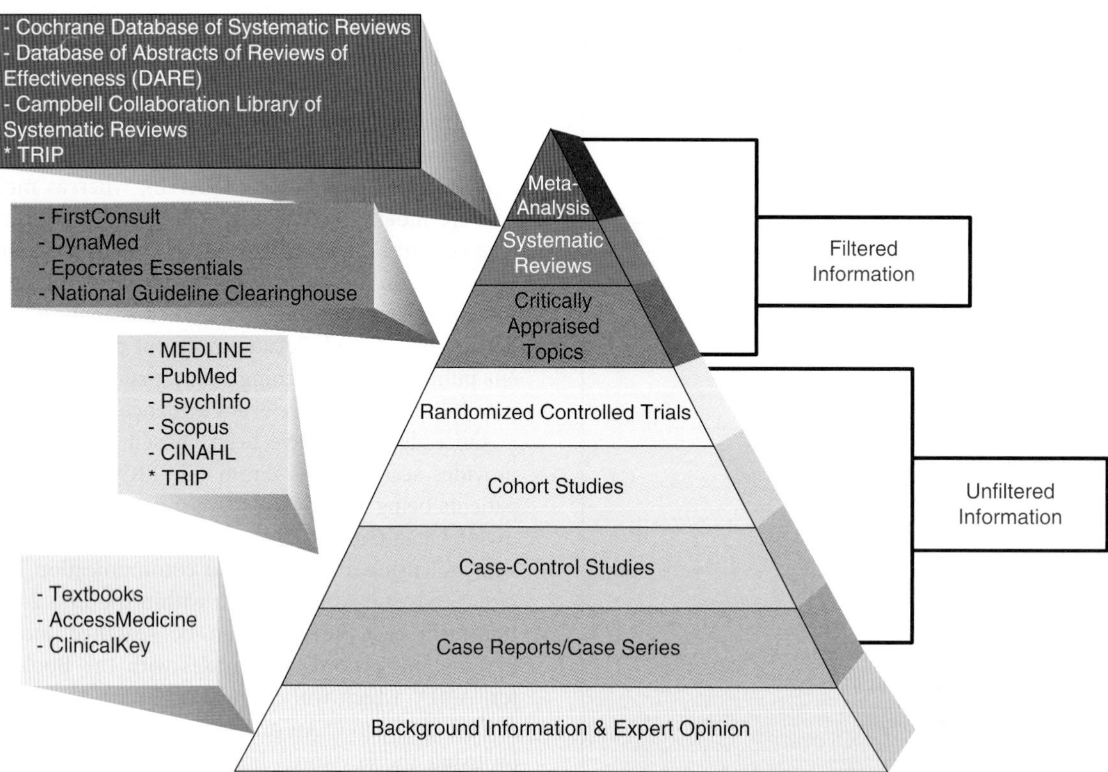

Fig. 4.2 Levels of Evidence. (Data from Sackett DL, Straus SE, Richardson WS, et al. Evidence-based medicine: how to practice and teach EBM. 2d ed. Edinburgh: Churchill Livingstone, 2000.)

article. Determine how "valuable" the evidence is by appraising the evidence for the following:

- Validity (Do the results seem real/true?). Research validity is all about the rigors of the study's methodology. For example, did the researchers use instruments that measured or performed what they were supposed to? Did they randomly select those to be included into the intervention group versus those who will be in the control group?
- Reliability (Could we get the same results time after time?)
- Applicability (Could the outcomes apply to my question?)
- Feasibility (Could we do the project in my department or hospital?)

Evidence Appraisal: Statistical Analysis

A basic understanding of common statistical references is important in appraising the evidence. The first number the nurse should pay attention to is the number of subjects involved in the study. The number of subjects will vary depending on the design. For descriptive, qualitative studies, the number of subjects in the study is generally small; however, for RCTs the numbers are usually large enough to allow for randomization, a control group, and for the variables and variances found in the study.[23] If there are too few subjects in the study, there may not be enough subjects to show any difference between those who received the intervention and those who did not. Many studies are published with 100 or fewer subjects; however, at least 400 subjects is generally considered the minimum for an RCT study.[24] Statistical significance is driven by numbers of participants. Clinical significance is driven by outcomes of the study and its effect on the subjects. An example would be a study on patient falls. A study may not show statistical significance due to low numbers of patient falls, but if the hospital implemented a fall reduction program resulting in no patient falls for 2 years, the clinical significance is high.

Although statistical data can be intimidating to most nurses, there are only a few statistics critical to evaluation. This section will give a brief overview of some that are integral in evaluating research: the alpha statistic (*p*-value), number needed to treat (NNT), and confidence intervals (CI). See also Research in Chapter 5 for common statistical tests.

p-Value

The *p*-value, represented by the Greek letter alpha (α) and indicating significance, informs the researcher of the probability the results found in the study are due only to chance and have nothing to do with the intervention. A *p*-value reported as $<.05$ means there is less than a 5% chance the reported results are due to something other than the study variable. Of course, most clinicians want a *p*-value of $< .00001$, meaning the probability is less than 1 out of 100,000 that the finding is due purely to chance. In reality, most scientists accept a *p*-value of $< .05$ as being a statistically significant finding.[23] Of course, if an intervention has life-threatening implications, a much lower *p*-value will be required before the findings are used to change practice. For example, if a drug is being examined that has a life threat, the clinician will want to have a *p*-value much lower than .05, meaning that fewer than 5 out of

100 people may be at risk for death from the drug. Therefore the acceptable p-value is directly tied to the life-threatening implications of the study. Because many studies are not dealing with life-and-death matters, a p-value of <0.05 is generally accepted as representing a statistically significant finding. A p-value $>.05$ means that, although the information may be interesting, there is no statistically significant difference found between the experimental group and the control group. Again, the results may still have clinical significance.

Number Needed to Treat

Number needed to treat (NNT) is a very clinically useful statistic. NNT is the number of patients who must be treated to prevent one patient from having an adverse outcome over a given period of time.[24,25] Another way to look at this is to indicate how many patients would need to be treated with the experimental therapy to achieve benefit over the standard care. Using an example of a drug trial comparing Drug A with Drug B (standard therapy), if 25% of the people benefited from therapy from drug A, NNT is 1/25%, or 1/0.25, or 4. This indicates four patients would need to be treated with Drug A to have one positive outcome. The most enviable, sought-after NNT for an experimental study is 1, meaning for every time you treated a patient with Drug A, there was a positive outcome. An NNT of 10 or less is usually considered acceptable.[13]

Confidence Intervals

The confidence interval (CI) informs the reader about the degree of precision involved in the findings and the degree within which the true difference in treatment would occur.[26] In other words, CI is the degree to which the research author is sure of making a correct assumption.[26] For example, with a CI of 95%, the reader would know the probability that the experiment reported correct findings is 95%. This means that there would be a 5% chance that the findings are wrong. Most clinicians require a CI of 95% to 99% for them to consider using the intervention espoused by the study.[23] The second piece to reporting the CI is to report the range in which the reported findings reach 95% accuracy. When CIs are reported, two numbers are generally reported with the CI, and these numbers represent the lowest and highest range the 95% CI represents. For example, consider a study that reports findings of incidence of lead poisoning among 200 inner-city children. The report states lead poisoning was found among 33 inner city children (95% CI, 20, 50). This means that the number of children with lead poisoning that fell within the 95% CI ranged between 20 and 50.[26]

CRITICAL APPRAISAL OF THE EVIDENCE

Once the evidence has been gathered and interpreted, the nurse will have to decide the overall meaning of the evidence. There are many facets to interpreting scientific reports. McAlister and colleagues examined the quality of evidence cited to support cardiovascular risk management recommendations and found the results of internally valid RCTs were not always applicable to the populations, interventions, or outcomes specified in a guideline recommendation.[27] This study highlights the importance of evaluating the evidence for overall quality and applicability to one's setting. Now that we know a bit more about statistics, additional questions we can ask when appraising the overall value of the evidence may include the following:

- Is the study design appropriate to the research questions?
- What is the number of subjects in the study?
- Are the numbers sufficient?
- Are the studies published in a peer-reviewed journal?
- What are the qualifications of the researchers?
- Is the study population similar to the population in which the results will be implemented?
- Is the treatment feasible in one's practice setting?
- Are the study findings realistic, are they too costly, or is the regimen too difficult for patients to adhere to?
- Where was the study conducted, and is the geographic difference a problem?
- Would the outcome matter to one's patient population?

Finally, synthesize what was found to determine whether your findings are applicable to clinical practice and, most important, will help answer the clinical question. Creating a study evaluation table may assist with the appraisal of the literature found in the search (see Box 4.1). Once the critical appraisal of the research is complete, the nurse or the team of health care workers translates the findings into practice recommendations.

EBP Implementation

Once the critical appraisal of the literature is completed and the information has been synthesized, it is hoped that the PICOT question can be answered. From the literature on standardized handoffs from our scenario, it was determined the use of a standardized handoff communication tool did reduce adverse patient events within the first 24 hours after patient transfer from the ED to any inpatient unit.

With these findings known, the next step is the development of an implementation plan for the use of a standardized handoff tool in the ED. The initial planning for implementation starts with determining how to collect baseline data on the outcome of patient adverse events within 24 hours of a patient transfer from the ED to an inpatient unit. Evaluation of before and after implementation data will help illustrate the true effect of standardized handoff tool implementation. Performing a SWOT (strengths, weakness, opportunities, and threats) assessment may help determine where challenges may lie ahead that also may need some planning to overcome.[28] Success of the implementation project is not only dependent on good evidence but also a well-thought-out implementation plan.[29] Originating a plan for a systematic way to implement change is integral to the success of the project. To assist with this planning, consider reviewing the ARCC model of EBP. Some of the steps of the ARCC model have already been completed, but several others require action.

For an implementation plan to be successful, think of all the weaknesses or threats in the SWOT analysis and incorporate solutions in the implementation plan. Part of the implementation plan for this project is to create an educational program and possibly a competency so all staff are trained on the use of the selected standardized handoff. Other questions to think about are whether the standardized handoff tool is to be incorporated into the medical record. If the handoff tool is to be contained within the electronic health record, then the computer/information technology department might have to work on incorporating it into the electronic health record. In some institutions, the tool might have to gain approval through a hospital or organizational committee. Again, the more details are thought through, the better the chance for implementation success. This chapter has been an overview of EBP process change with an intent to demonstrate the many and varied steps involved in a thorough EBP implementation plan.

EVALUATION

Last, but still very important, is to determine whether the use of the standardized handoff tool did reduce patient adverse incidences. Was the change effective, and were the results in alignment with the intended outcome of reducing patient adverse events within 24 hours after a patient was transferred from the ED to an inpatient unit? Are patients and staff satisfied with the change? Evaluation is just as important as the appraisal and implementation phase of EBP.

Evaluation must elicit reviews from the stakeholders and be instrumental in the decision to adapt, adopt, or reject the change based on feedback. The change should be evaluated for feasibility, usability, satisfaction, and risk/benefit analyses.

DISSEMINATION

Along with the plan for evaluation, there must be a plan for disseminating the results of the evaluation and a plan for ongoing assessment and change. Dissemination can take one or more of the "3Ps": poster, presentation, or publication. Posters can be formal or informal and shared in local, regional, national, or international venues. Presentations have similar local through international venues. Publications can be as varied as a department newsletter through a professional organization's peer-reviewed journal. Regardless of the method of dissemination, celebrating successes also recognizes work done to accomplish EBP changes.

SUMMARY

As health care change agents and leaders, nurses are instrumental in translating the evidence found in the research to its application into clinical practice. This translation is the key to improvement in outcomes for all our patients. Since the time of Florence Nightingale, nurses have been on the front lines asking questions, analyzing practice, and promoting better patient outcomes. No longer are nurses complacent with their clinical practice. Every day nurses are challenging the ways to provide excellent clinical care, and with the understanding and use of EBP and EBP implementation models, nurses are practicing to the full extent of their education and scope of practice to be full partners with all health care professionals in advancing health care and outcome improvement.

REFERENCES

1. Nightingale F. *Notes on Nursing: What It Is, and What It Is Not.* New York, NY: Appleton-Century; 1946.
2. McDonald L. Florence Nightingale and the early origins of evidence-based nursing. *EBN.* 2001;4(July):68–69.
3. Nightingale F. *Notes on Matters Affecting the Health.* St. Martin's Lane, WC: Harrison and Sons, Efficiency and Hospital Administration of the British Army; 1946.
4. Sackett DL, Rosenberg WM, Gray JA, Haynes RB, Richardson WS. Evidence based medicine: what it is and what it isn't. *Br Med J.* 1996;312(7023):71–72.
5. Goossens GA. Flushing and locking of venous catheters: available evidence and evidence deficit. *Nurs Res Pract.* 2015;2015:985686. https://doi.org/10.1155/2015/985686.
6. Castiglione SA, Landry T. What evidence exists that describes whether the Trendelenburg and/or modified Trendelenburg positions are effective for the management of hospitalized patients with hypertension? *Rapid Review Evidence Summary.* Montreal, QC: McGill University Health Centre; 2015.
7. Mekis NZ, Kamenik M. The influence of Trendelenburg position on haemodynamics: comparison of anaesthetized patients with ischaemic heart disease and healthy volunteers. *J Int Med Res.* 2011;39(3):1084–1089.
8. Sisson H. Aspirating during the intramuscular injection procedure: a systematic literature review. *J Clin Nurs.* 2015;24(17-18):2368–2375.
9. Jadad AR, Haynes RB. The Cochrane Collaboration—Advances and challenges in improving evidence-based decision making. *Med Decis Making.* 1998;18(1):2.
10. Jadad AR, Cook DJ, Jones A. Methodology and reports of systematic reviews and meta-analyses: a comparison of Cochrane reviews with articles published in paper-based journals. *JAMA.* 1998;280(3):278.
11. Titler MG. The evidence for evidence-based practice implementation. In: Hughes RG, ed. *Patient Safety and Quality: An Evidence-Based Handbook for Nurses.* Rockville, MD: Agency for Healthcare Research and Quality; 2008. Chapter 7. https://www.ncbi.nlm.nih.gov/books/NBK2659/. Accessed April 12, 2019.
12. Institute of Medicine Roundtable on Evidence-Based Medicine. *Leadership Commitments to Improve Value in Healthcare: Finding Common Ground: Workshop Summary.* Washington, DC: National Academies Press; 2009. https://www.ncbi.nlm.nih.gov/books/NBK52847/. Accessed April 12, 2019.
13. Sackett DL, Rosenberg WM, Gray JA. Evidence based medicine: what it is and what it isn't. 1996. *Clin Ortho Relat Res.* 2007;455:3–5.
14. Mitchell SA, Fisher CA, Hastings CE, Silverman LB, Wallen GR. A thematic analysis of theoretical models for translational science in nursing: mapping the field. *Nurs Outlook.* 2010;58(6):287–300. https://doi.org/10.1016/j.outlook.2010.07.001.

15. Stevens KR. Ace star model of EBP: knowledge transformation. Academic Center for Evidence-Based Practice. The University of Texas Health Science Center at San Antonio. www.acestar.uthscsa.edu. Accessed April 12, 2019.
16. Institute of Medicine (US). Committee on standards for developing trustworthy clinical practice guidelines. In: Graham R, Mancher M, eds. *Clinical Practice Guidelines We can Trust.* Washington, DC: National Academies Press; 2011.
17. Melnyk B, Fineout-Overholt E, Stillwell SB, Williamson KM. The seven steps of evidence-based practice. *AJN.* 2010;110(1):51–53.
18. Melnyk BM, Fineout-Overholt E. ARCC (Advancing Research and Clinical practice through close Collaboration): a model for system-wide implementation and sustainability of evidence-based practice. In: Rycroft-Malone J, Bucknall T, eds. *Models and Frameworks for Implementing Evidence-Based Practice: Linking Evidence to Action.* John Wiley & Sons; 2011:169–184.
19. Riva JJ, Malik KMP, Burnie SJ, Endicott AR, Busse JW. What is your research question? An introduction to the PICOT format for clinicians. *J Canadian Chiropractic Assoc.* 2012;56(3):167–171.
20. Stillwell SB, Fineout-Overholt E, Melnyk BM, Williamson KM. Evidenced-based practice, step by step: searching for the evidence. *Am J Nurs.* 2010;110(5):41–47.
21. Puro A. *Levels of Evidence Pyramid from Complementary and Alternative Medicine (CAM): Evaluating Evidence;* 2014. https://guides.himmelfarb.gwu.edu/c.php?g=27780&p=170382 . Accessed April 13, 2019.
22. Burns PB, Rohrich RJ, Chung KC. The levels of evidence and their role in evidence-based medicine. *Plast Reconstr Surg.* 2011;128(1):305–310. https://doi.org/10.1097/PRS.0b013e318219c171.
23. Polit DF, Beck CT. *Nursing Research: Generating and Assessing Evidence for Nursing Practice.* New York, NY: Lippincott Williams & Wilkins; 2008.
24. Flaherty RJ. A simple method for evaluating the clinical literature. *Fam Pract.* 2004;11(5):47.
25. Barratt A, Wyer PC, Hatala R. Tips for learners of evidence-based medicine: relative risk, absolute risk reduction and number needed to treat. I. *CMAJ.* 2004;171(4):353.
26. Montori M, Kleinbart H, Newman TB. Tips for learners of evidence-based medicine, II. Measures of precision (confidence intervals). *CMAJ.* 2004;171(6):611.
27. McAlister FA, van Diepen S, Padwal RS. How evidence-based are the recommendations in evidence-based guidelines? *PLoS Med.* 2007;4:e250.
28. Blayney DW. Strengths, weaknesses, opportunities, and threats. *J Oncol Pract.* 2008;4(2):53. https://doi.org/10.1200/JOP.0820501.
29. Gallagher-Ford L, Fineout-Overholt E, Melnyk BM, Stillwell SB. Evidenced-based practice, step by step: implementing an evidence-based practice change. *Am J Nurs.* 2011;111(3):54–60.

5

Research

Ruthie Robinson

The number of published research studies related to health care each year is staggering. And yet, nurses are expected to be able to read, critique, and implement changes in practice based on this research. The ability to successfully understand research is critical to continued improvements in patient care, patient outcomes, and the work environment. The focus of this chapter is to provide the emergency nurse with an overview of the research process as a basis to become a better consumer of research and to understand how to incorporate research findings into practice.

USING RESEARCH IN CLINICAL PRACTICE: COMPARING RESEARCH, EVIDENCE-BASED PRACTICE, AND QUALITY IMPROVEMENT

Nurses are often confused by the terms research, evidence-based practice (EBP), and quality improvement. This is not surprising considering the considerable overlap in terms. Chapter 4 looked at EBP in detail. This chapter will discuss research in greater depth in later sections. Very simply stated, nursing research is a systematic process of inquiry using guidelines intended to answer questions about nursing practice.[1] EBP is often defined in a variety of ways. However, most definitions include the following three components: (1) research information, (2) clinical expertise, and (3) patient preferences. So, EBP is based on current, high-quality research studies, the expertise of the practitioner, and preferences of the patient. EBP is the application of research and other evidence designed to improve practice.[2] Stated another way, EBP is the translation of research evidence and other evidence and applying it to clinical decisions.[3] According to the National Quality Forum,[4] clinical quality improvement is intended to raise standards for preventing, diagnosing, and treating poor health and is a systematic approach to improving outcomes. See Table 5.1.

COMPONENTS OF THE RESEARCH PROCESS

What is research? According to Polit and Beck,[5] research is a systematic method used to answer questions or solve problems. The goal of research is to develop and expand knowledge. However, conducting research and achieving meaningful discoveries will not help nurses or patients if these findings are not translated into practice. This chapter will also review how to use research in clinical practice.

Steps of the Research Process

Because research is a systematic method of inquiry, a systematic process is needed. See Table 5.2. The steps of the research process are generally as follows:

1. Problem identification
2. Literature review
3. Theoretical or conceptual framework
4. Purpose or research questions or hypotheses
5. Methodology (including design, sampling, data collection, data measurement, and data analysis)
6. Results
7. Discussion (including conclusions, limitations, and recommendations)

Research Step 1: Problem Identification

The initial step of the research process is defining the research question or research problem. The research question or problem reflects an identified problem related to patient care, nursing education, nursing administration, or any issue of nursing interest. Patient care or nursing practice problems generally address practice differences and what is ideal or desirable. Researchable questions often reflect clinical experiences, such as (1) How effective are sepsis guidelines in improving mortality rates in sepsis patients? (2) What type of pain management can be used for pediatric patients undergoing procedures in the emergency department (ED)?, or (3) How can education on human trafficking help in the identification of victims in the ED? Research studies often make recommendations for future studies when summarizing implications of the current study, and those can be another source for research ideas. Researchable questions or clinical problems yet to be addressed are often identified when nurses review research articles on the current state of the science. In addition, several nursing and federal organizations have published recommendations for potential research studies. The Emergency Nurses Association, American Association of Critical Care Nurses, American Nurses Association, Sigma, and the National Institute of Nursing Research are examples of organizations that have identified and published research priorities. The research question defines what the researcher is trying to discover and will drive the research design.

TABLE 5.1 **Evidence-Based Practice, Quality Improvement, and Research.**

Evidence-Based Practice (EBP)	Quality Improvement (QI)	Research
The translation of research evidence and other evidence and applying it to clinical decisions	A systematic approach to improving outcomes	A systematic process of inquiry using guidelines intended to answer questions about nursing practice
Examples of EBP models: • Iowa Model • Stetler Model • Johns Hopkins Nursing Model • ACE Star Model of Knowledge Transformation	Examples of QI models: • Plan, Do, Study, Act • Lean/Six Sigma • Total quality management	Examples of study designs: • Meta-analysis • Randomized control trials • Cohort study • Cross-sectional study • Qualitative designs
Examples of EBP projects: • Implementing best practices to reduce falls in the emergency department • Implementing a sepsis protocol to decrease hospital mortality rates	Examples of QI projects: • The implementation of advanced practice nurses in triage to reduce length of stay in the emergency department • Using code simulation to improve nursing performance during cardiac arrests	Examples of research: • Patient knowledge of discharge instructions • Comparison of temperature assessment methods

TABLE 5.2 **Components of the Research Study.**

Components of a Research Study	Overview of the Components
Problem identification	Identifies the "problem" that will be answered by the research study.
Literature review	Synthesizes current literature to summarize how current study can contribute to current body of literature on the topic.
Theoretical or conceptual framework	In theoretically driven studies, sets the context for the propositions or relationships related to the variables in the study.
Purpose or research questions or hypotheses	What the study intends to accomplish.
Methodology • Design • Sampling • Data collection • Data measurement • Data analysis	The methods section communicates what approaches will be used by the researcher to answer the research questions or hypotheses.
Results	Reports the results obtained in the analyses of data.
Discussion of the findings • Conclusions • Limitations • Recommendations	Discussion of the findings includes the drawing of conclusions based on what the results mean, explaining why results were obtained, and how results can be used in practice.

Research Step 2: Literature Review

The purpose of the literature review is to explore work conducted in a particular area of interest to further formulate or clarify the research problem. After critiquing previous research in a particular area, the researcher summarizes what has been previously studied and delineates how a proposed study will contribute to the state of the science. A good literature review critiques and summarizes other studies to see how they fit into the scope of the study being conducted. A thorough review reinforces the need for the study in light of what has already been done and adds credence to the importance of the proposed research topic.[1]

Information sources for literature reviews may include both primary and secondary resources. A primary source of information is the description of an investigation written by the person who conducted it. A secondary source is a description of a study prepared by someone other than the original researcher. Literature reviews are very useful for examining the body of evidence for best clinical practices, as well as for identifying the existing gaps in a given area of content.

Research Step 3: Theoretical and Conceptual Frameworks

Theories and conceptual frameworks provide a structure or blueprint to guide the study of clinical problems. A theoretical framework defines the concepts and proposes relationships between those concepts to provide a systematic view of a phenomenon. It further enables the researcher to link the findings to a body of knowledge. This framework consists of the definition of concepts and propositions about the relationships of those concepts, a way to organize rules or beliefs about what is observed, and a systematic method to organize information about a particular aspect of interest in a research study.[5]

Conceptual frameworks represent a less formal, less well-developed system for organizing phenomena. They contain concepts representing a common theme but lack the deductive system of propositions to identify the relationship among concepts. Conceptual frameworks are more or less a map for the proposed study.[5] The groundwork for more formal theories often evolves from conceptual frameworks.

Research Step 4: Research Questions or Hypotheses

Before a problem is researched, it must be narrowed, refined, and made feasible for study. The research interest can be stated as a research question or a hypothesis. The research question in a study should identify key independent and dependent variables. An independent variable is what is assumed to cause or thought to be associated with the dependent variable. Changes in the dependent variable are presumed to depend on the effects of the independent variable. The dependent variable is what a researcher wants to explain or understand. Research questions should be specific and not attempt to measure too much, because data analysis may be complex and be confusing to interpret.[1] For example, a research question might be, Will the use of a validated violence prediction checklist help decrease violence in mental health patients in the ED? The dependent variable is episodes of violence, and the independent variable is the use of a validated violence prediction checklist. The dependent variable is explained through its relationship with the independent variable. Many factors affect violence in mental health patients, but only one independent variable (the use of a validated violence prediction checklist) is intended to be measured in the proposed research question.

A hypothesis expands upon a research question, because it is a prediction of the relationship or differences between two or more variables and should stem directly from the research question. This prediction of expected outcomes is the basis of the research process. Hypotheses, which often stem from theories, are possible solutions or answers to research problems. The hypothesis is a prediction of the nature of the relationship between several variables intended to be identified before the initiation of the research study. For example, consider the research question: What is the effect on a patient liaison in the ED on patient satisfaction scores? The research hypothesis would be: A patient liaison in the ED will result in higher patient satisfaction scores, whereas the null hypothesis would be: A patient liaison in the ED will not have any effect on patient satisfaction scores.

Research Step 5: Methodology

The methods section of a research study reflects how the researcher plans to implement or did implement the research study to answer the research questions or hypotheses. The components of the methodology section include research design, subjects, measures used to collect data, and study procedures. There are two major categories of *research designs:* quantitative (numbers) and qualitative (trends in words). (See Tables 5.3 and 5.4.) In the context of this chapter, the focus will be on quantitative studies.

Institutional Review Board approval. Institutional Review Board (IRB) approval of research studies is a necessity. The purpose of IRB approval is to safeguard the rights and welfare of subjects, ensure appropriate procedures for informed consent, and allow subjects to make independent decisions about risks and benefits.[6] Box 5.1 delineates the components to be included in a consent form. There are circumstances when emergency consent is needed, without having the prior approval of the IRB. The determinants of the waiver to informed consent for emergency research are listed in Box 5.2.

Sampling. Subjects sampled for a research study will depend on the population to be studied and the estimated number of subjects needed to demonstrate a significant difference between experimental and control groups. The definition of a population is not restricted to human subjects. A population can consist of records, blood samples, actions, words, organizations, numbers, or animals. Regardless of the unit to be studied or sampled, a population is always made up of specific elements of interest. Often it is not feasible to include large populations because of expense and time involved for data collection. Generally, a study limits the population sampled to a representative sample. Samples should typify a portion of the entire population to be studied to ensure the sample is representative of a specific population. The sample should mirror the population to be studied to avoid sampling bias. Sampling error can result from sampling bias, which is the tendency to select a sample with particular characteristics, rather than the sample being representative of the population to be studied. For example, if one were studying the effect of a new triage education technique on ED nurses, selecting only experienced triage nurses may lead to a bias in results. On the other hand, selecting only new graduate nurses in the ED would also introduce bias into the study results.

Researchers use probability and nonprobability sampling techniques when designing studies. Probability sampling is the use of some form of random selection to choose the subjects or units to be sampled. Random sampling is not the same thing as random assignment. Random assignment involves randomly assigning a group of participants into different groups within the study. There are four basic types of probability sampling: simple random, stratified random, cluster, and systemic random.[7]

Nonprobability sampling does not include random selection, and samples may be less representative of a population when using this strategy. Common types of nonprobability sampling include convenience sampling, quota sampling, purposive sampling, snowball sampling, and theoretic sampling. Convenience sampling is choosing a population because they are available and is the most common sampling strategy used in nursing research.[7]

Data collection and data measurement. Data collection simply refers to a description of the processes used to implement the study and gather data. The key to successful data collection is using appropriate measures to accurately describe the variables in the study. Measurement tools have some common characteristics: (1) they are objective, (2) they are standardized measures (uniform items, response, and scoring), (3) items of measurement should be clearly defined, (4) types of items on any one test should have a limited number of variations, (5) items should not provide irrelevant cues, (6) measures requiring complex operations are avoided, (7) the measurement tool should encompass the defined variable, and (8) the measure must demonstrate a relationship between performance on the tool and a subject's behavior.[5,8]

Some of the more common types of data collection measures include (1) physiologic and biophysical measurements, (2) observational measurements, (3) interviews and questionnaires, (4) scales, and (5) records or available data. Physiologic measurements are those used to measure characteristics of subjects being studied, such as temperature, weight, height, cardiac output, muscle strength, and biochemical levels (e.g., hemoglobin, blood glucose, and potassium). Advantages of physiologic measurements are objectivity, preciseness, and sensitivity because the data are not influenced by the person performing the study.

TABLE 5.3 Overview of Common Types of Quantitative Research Designs.

Research Design	Characteristics of Research Design
EXPERIMENTAL AND QUASI-EXPERIMENTAL	
Experimental Examples of experimental research designs: • Nonequivalent control • After-only nonequivalent group • One-group (pretest-posttest)	• Manipulation of independent variable • Randomization of subjects (subjects randomly assigned to control and experimental groups) • Control or comparison group (one of the groups in the study does not receive "experimental" treatment but receives normal or routine care)
Quasi-Experimental Examples of quasi-experimental research designs: • Nonequivalent control • After-only nonequivalent group • One-group (pretest-posttest) • Time-series	• Manipulation of independent variable • Lacks control group or randomization
NONEXPERIMENTAL	
Survey Examples of survey nonexperimental research designs: • Descriptive • Exploratory • Comparative	• Collect and describe existing data • Helps describe the characteristics of subjects or a group • No intervention is performed • May identify trends and possibly help identify future needs
Relationship/Differences Examples of relationship/differences nonexperimental research designs: • Correlational • Developmental • Cross-sectional • Longitudinal and prospective • Retrospective and ex post facto	• Overall goal is to determine whether there is a relationship or difference between variables *Correlational* • Examining the relationship between two or more variables • Cannot imply causal relationships • Able to determine the "strength" of a relationship between variables *Cross-sectional* • Examines data at one point in time *Longitudinal and prospective* • Collects data from the same group at different time points *Retrospective and ex post facto* • Variations of independent variable in the natural course of events • This type of design also referred to as explanatory, causal-comparative, or comparative
Other Types of Quantitative Research Designs	
Methodological	• A controlled investigation related to ways of obtaining or organizing data • Addresses development, validation, and evaluation of research tools or techniques
Meta-analysis	• Analyzes the results from many studies on a specific topic • Combines data from many studies, usually randomized control clinical trials • Synthesizes findings and statistically summarizes data to obtain a precise estimate of the treatment effectiveness (effect size) and statistical significance

When researchers observe the research aspect of interest, direct observation measurements are used. For example, a researcher wants to observe the response of parents to casting or suturing procedures performed on their children. The observation method is most useful for entities difficult to measure, such as interactions, nursing process, changes in behavior, or group processes.

A third type of data collection is the use of interviews and questionnaires, which allows subjects to report data for or about themselves. The purpose of questioning participants is to seek direct data, such as age, religion, or marital status, or indirect data, such as level of intelligence, anxiety, and pain.

Measurement scales can be used to make distinctions among subjects concerning the degree to which they possess a certain trait, attitude, or emotion. Scales also permit comparisons in dimensions of interest. For example, a researcher interested in knowing whether a nerve block or a local injection of anesthetic is more effective for relieving pain during fracture reduction would use a pain scale to measure pain. Finally, use of records or available data refers to the researcher collecting data from existing databases, such as the electronic patient record.

TABLE 5.4 Overview of Common Types of Qualitative Research Designs.

Research Design	Characteristics of Research Design
Phenomenological	• Learning occurs through dialogue with persons representative of the population of interest to be studied • Construct meaning from the "lived" experience
Grounded theory	• Goal is to derive a theory about social processes • Uses inductive reasoning approaches, with theory arising from the data to reflect the social processes being studied
Ethnography	• Goal is to understand, scientifically describe, and interpret cultural or social groups and systems
Case study	• Overall goal is to study the uniqueness and commonalities of a specific case • Natural conditions are studied and variables related to history, current characteristics, interactions, or problems • Usually focuses on why the subject feels, thinks, and behaves in a particular manner
Historical	• An approach used to understand the past through a critical appraisal of facts

Data measurement validity and reliability. When instruments or tools are used for measuring subjects, the validity and reliability of tools should be addressed by the researcher to help establish trustworthiness. Validity is the degree to which an instrument measures what it is intended to measure. Reliability of a measure or an instrument refers to its ability to consistently and accurately measure a criterion. In other words, an instrument is reliable if it yields the same results with different populations and in different settings.[7,9]

Research Steps 6 and 7: Results/Discussion

Data analysis. After completing data collection, the researcher summarizes the data through statistical procedures. The purpose of analysis is to answer the study questions or hypotheses. Researchers who use quantitative methods for data collection should also have a data analysis plan in place before beginning data collection. Statistical tests give meaning to quantitative data because they reduce, summarize, organize, evaluate, interpret, and communicate numeric data. One does not need to know how to conduct all of the statistical tests to understand the common principle of data analysis. Specifically, it is more important to be able to determine whether the findings are statistically significant. This means the findings are probably valid and replicable with a new sample of subjects. The level of statistical significance is an index of the probability of reliability of the findings. For example, if a study indicates findings are significant at the .05 level, this means 5 out of 100 times there is a risk the result would be different from the reported finding, or possibly due to chance; in other words, 95 out of 100 times the findings would be the same.

Statistical tests are referred to as either descriptive or inferential. Descriptive statistics describe and summarize data. Examples are mode, median, mean, average, percentage, and frequency. Inferential statistics are used to draw conclusions

BOX 5.1 Key Components of an Informed Consent Form for Research.

- Statement involving research, explanation of purposes of the research, delineation of expected duration of subject's participation, description of procedures to be expected, and identification of any procedures that are experimental
- Description of any reasonably foreseeable risks or discomforts to the subject
- Description of any benefits to the subject or to others that may reasonably be expected from the research
- Disclosure of appropriate alternative procedures or courses of treatment, if any, that may be advantageous to the subject
- A statement describing to what extent, if any, confidentiality of records identifying the subject will be maintained
- For research involving more than minimal risk, an explanation as to whether any medical treatments are available if injury occurs and if so, what they consist of or where further information may be obtained
- An explanation of whom to contact for answers to pertinent questions about the research and the subject's rights and whom to contact in the event of a research-related injury to the subject
- A statement that participation is voluntary, refusal to participate will not involve any penalty or loss of benefits to which the subject is otherwise entitled, and the subject may discontinue participation at any time without any penalty or loss of otherwise entitled benefits

BOX 5.2 Key Components of Informed Consent Waiver.

- The patient has a life-threatening condition.
- Available treatments are unsatisfactory or unproven.
- The patient is not capable of giving informed consent (due to his or her medical condition), or the patient's legal representative is not available.
- Participation in the research may have direct benefit to the patient.
- The research could not feasibly be carried out without the waiver of informed consent.
- The investigator defines the length of therapeutic window and how the investigator will attempt to contact the legal representative.
- This includes summarizing the efforts to contact the patient's legal representative.
- Other provisions:
  - The Institutional Review Board had reviewed and approved the informed consent.
  - There has been community consultation regarding the proposed research study.
  - Public disclosure has occurred.
  - There is an independent data monitoring committee.

TABLE 5.5 Commonly Used Statistical Tests.

Parametric Test	Example of an Equivalent Nonparametric Test	Purpose of the Statistical Test
Two-sample (unpaired) *t*-test	Mann-Whitney *U*-test	Compares two independent samples drawn from the same population
One-sample (paired) *t*-test	Wilcoxon matched pairs test	Compares two sets of observations on a single sample
One-way analysis of variance (*F*-test) using total sum of squares	Kruskal-Wallis analysis of variance by ranks	Effectively, a generalization of the paired *t*-test or Wilcoxon matched pairs test where three or more sets of observations are made on a single sample
Two-way analysis of variance	Two-way analysis of variance by ranks	Effectively, a generalization of the paired *t*-test or Wilcoxon matched pairs test where three or more sets of observations are made on a single sample; tests the influence and interaction of two different covariates
Chi-square (χ^2)	Fisher's exact test	Tests the null hypothesis that the distribution of the discontinuous variable is the same in two (or more) independent samples
Pearson's *r* (product moment correlation coefficient)	Spearman's rank correlation coefficient	Assesses the strength of the straight-line association between two continuous variables
Regression by least squares method	Nonparametric regression	Describes the numerical relation between two quantitative variables allowing one value to be predicted from the other
Multiple regression by least squares method	Nonparametric regression	Describes the numerical relation between a dependent variable and several predictor variables (covariates)

about a large population based on a sample from a study, to make judgments, and to generalize information. Inferential statistics are then used to test the hypotheses to determine whether they are correct.

Two categories of inferential statistics are nonparametric and parametric. Most statistical tests are parametric tests, which focus on population parameters, require measurements on at least one interval or ratio scale, and make assumptions about distribution of the variables. Nonparametric tests are used when measured variables are nominal or ordinal. These tests do not make assumptions about distribution of variables.[5] Table 5.5 provides an overview of commonly performed statistical tests, both nonparametric and parametric, based on the level of measurement and variables in the study. Nurses often collaborate with biostatisticians to determine the appropriate statistical analyses to be used and obtain assistance with the data analyses for the research studies they undertake.

Results, conclusions, discussion, and recommendations. Results of the study are often organized by the research aims or hypotheses of the study and are often reported in the form of tables and graphs. Data summarized in graphs and tables can be more easily interpreted and compared with research questions or hypotheses and the theoretical framework. On the basis of the findings of the study, the researcher draws conclusions. Study conclusions provide the foundation for the discussion section of the research report or manuscript. The researcher should attempt to give meaning to "why" the findings occurred by interweaving previous studies done related to the study topic. Recommendations stem from changes the researcher plans in sample, design, or analysis if the study is repeated. Other explanations for results should be discussed so progress can be made in future studies of the research problem. Implications of research, such as how findings can be used to improve nursing or how to advance knowledge through additional research, should be provided.

USING RESEARCH FINDINGS IN PRACTICE

Factors Promoting Research in the Clinical Setting

Many barriers to and facilitators of the use of research in the clinical setting have been identified. Often-mentioned barriers include a lack of time, a lack of resources, a lack of knowledge, perceptions of lack of authority to change practice, and an unsupportive organizational culture. Frequently cited facilitators include a supportive organizational culture, staff "buy in" of research and EBP, education and mentorship, organizational resource support, individual staff incentives, and the presence of shared governance.[7,10–11]

Other facilitators for research utilization in clinical practice revolve around staff education and skill development, as well as the actual efforts going into the implementation of relevant research and EBP. A key strategy is the implementation of an educational plan to update the nurses' skill sets related to research using a variety of formats (e.g., continuing education, self-paced modules, and web-based tutorials). It is recommended the education include both a dissemination component (e.g., discussing benefits of research for practice) and implementation strategies to update the nurses' skill set

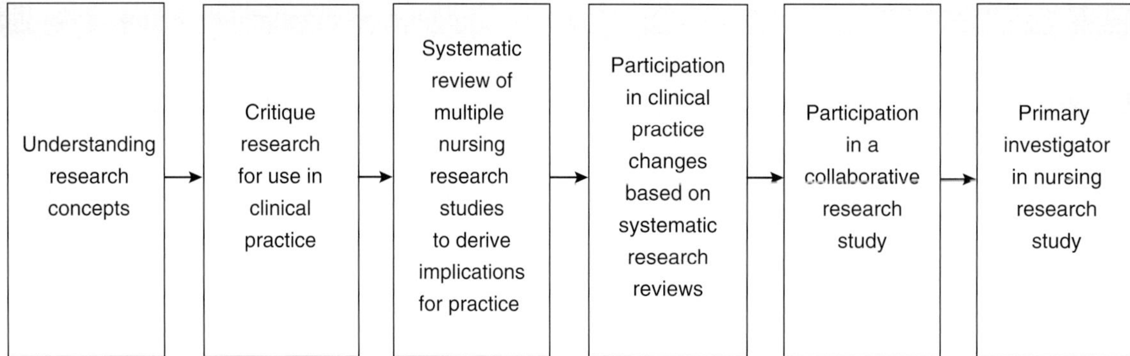

Fig. 5.1 Continuum of nursing research.

related to use of research (e.g., reading the research literature, understanding and appraising the research findings, and conducting systematic reviews).[12] In addition to the education component to promote research utilization, additional strategies include using collaborative teams who use cooperative learning approaches, providing opportunities for nurse-to-nurse collaboration, and having role models and mentors to support research utilization efforts by staff nurses (e.g., clinical nurse specialists). Specifically finding ways to incorporate the process of research into day-to-day practices is another key strategy. Approaches can include patient rounds to discuss supporting research and evidence for treatment interventions and decisions, using "teachable" moments on the nursing unit for problem solving, establishing protocols, using consistent methods to systematically review and appraise research, collecting information and data in daily work, and having staff lead practice reviews.[1]

The other major research utilization issue to be addressed is designing a consistent method for implementing practice changes. Once staff begin generating practice changes based on research utilization, it is vital that changes be made in a consistent manner to promote adoption and sustain the practice change. Useful strategies include planning the implementation, pilot testing in the clinical setting, reevaluating the effectiveness of the implementation plan, modifying the processes to implement the recommended clinical practice changes throughout all clinical settings in the organization, and using an accepted EBP model.[1]

SUMMARY

This chapter has provided an overview of nursing research processes and the importance of integrating research findings into clinical practice. Nurses' participation in the research process can vary along a continuum. At one end, participation can be reflected by a nurse's understanding of research concepts, whereas at the other end of the spectrum, participation is exemplified by the nurse being a primary investigator in a research study. The overview of the continuum of nursing research participation is depicted in Fig. 5.1. Regardless of the level of participation, all nurses have the opportunity to participate in research. The key role for all nurses is to strive for more integration of research into clinical practice.

REFERENCES

1. Houser J. *Nursing Research: Reading, Using, and Creating Evidence*. 4th ed. Burlington, MA: Jones & Bartlett Learning; 2018.
2. Schmidt NA, Brown JM. *Evidence-Based Practice for Nurses: Appraisal and Application of Research*. 4th ed. Burlington, MA: Jones & Bartlett Learning; 2017.
3. Seger BM. Evidence-based practice, research and quality improvement: using three initiatives to foster high-quality care. *The Voice of Nursing Leadership*. 2018:4–6.
4. National Quality Forum. *Phrase Book: A Plain Language Guide to NQF Jargon*. National Quality Forum. http://public.qualityforum.org/NQFDocuments/Phrasebook.pdf. Published 2018. Accessed May 2, 2018.
5. Polit DF, Beck CT. *Nursing Research: Generating and Assessing Evidence for Nursing Practice*. 10th ed. Philadelphia, PA: Lippincott Williams & Wilkins; 2017.
6. US Department of Health and Human Services. *Revised Common Rule*. HHS.gov website. https://www.hhs.gov/ohrp/regulations-and-policy/regulations/finalized-revisions-common-rule/index.html. Published 2018. Accessed May 18, 2018.
7. Boswell C, Cannon S. *Introduction to Nursing Research: Incorporating Evidence-Based Practice*. 4th ed. Burlington, MA: Jones & Bartlett Learning; 2017.
8. Creswell JW. *Research Design: Qualitative, Quantitative, and Mixed Methods Approaches*. 5th ed. Thousand Oaks, CA: Sage Publications; 2018.
9. Pajo B. *Introduction to Research Methods: A Hands-On Approach*. Thousand Oaks, CA: Sage Publications; 2018.
10. Cline GJ, Burger KJ, Amankway EK, Goldenberg NA, Ghazarian SR. Promoting the utilization of science in healthcare (PUSH) project: a description of the perceived barriers and facilitators to research utilization among pediatric nurses. *J Nurses Prof Dev*. 2017;33(3):113–119.
11. Sanjari M, Baradaran HR, Aalaa M, Mehrdad N. Barriers and facilitators of nursing research utilization in Iran: a systematic review. *Iran J Nurs Midwifery Res*. 2015;20(5):529–539.
12. Melnyk BM, Fineout-Overholt E. *Evidence-Based Practice in Nursing & Healthcare: A Guide to Best Practice*. 3rd ed. Philadelphia, PA: Wolters Kluwer; 2015.

6

Ethical Considerations

Lisa Matamoros

Ethics is a branch of philosophy in which a systematic approach exists to determine how to behave ideally. It is about defining what is right and wrong, good and bad, admirable and deplorable. It is derived from the Greek word "ethos," which means character. Different views exist on what is considered ethical, and ethics is based on how we were brought up and what was considered to be normal or acceptable behavior within our family, community, and society. One would view this as morals or values. Ethics is about what is right or wrong based on reason, whereas morals is about what is right or wrong based on social norms.[1–3]

Ethical theories and principles provide a foundation to analyze and guide decision making. When there are competing interests, these theories and principles can help justify decisions and actions. Four main ethical principles in health care guide behavior: autonomy, beneficence, nonmaleficence, and justice.

Autonomy is recognition of people's right to make their own decisions. It addresses personal freedom and self-determination. Patients have the right to choose their destiny by making informed decisions about their care and treatment, whether caregivers agree with the decision or not, as long as the decision does not affect the rights of another person. To be able to make a decision, the patient needs to be given the necessary information to make an educated decision. Information cannot be withheld because of a concern that it might cause the patient to make a decision we do not agree with.[1–3]

Beneficence is doing what is good for others, what will benefit them, prevent harm, or improve a situation. The benefits must be balanced against the risks. The patient's preferences, beliefs, values, and culture should be considered; otherwise, what one person may see as good may in fact be harmful.[1–3]

Nonmaleficence is to avoid causing harm. It is not concerned with doing good but instead concerns avoiding the infliction of harm, such as through pain, suffering, or injury. This is the core of ethical behavior.[1–3]

Justice is about treating people fairly and equally. It is making decisions based on fair and equal distribution and free from bias or prejudice. Everyone is entitled to the same goods and services, regardless of their contribution and who they are.[1–3]

NURSING ETHICS

Ethics has been a part of nursing since the 1800s. Nursing ethics is unique in that a wide variety of issues exist in relationships with nurses and patients, families, physicians, coworkers, and other professionals who are part of the health care team.[4] Early in nursing history, there was no formal code of ethics, and nurses used the Nightingale Pledge to guide practice. The American Nurses Association (ANA), along with other professional nursing associations, has developed guidelines for nurses to follow that address these relationships and how to practice with integrity.

The nursing code of ethics provides standards, or norms, for nursing practice. These standards are formal statements accepted as the professional code of conduct by the ANA's members and serve to provide guidance for actions. The code of ethics also serves to inform others of the minimum acceptable standard of behavior, which can be used to judge one's actions as right or wrong, good or bad, admirable or deplorable.

In 1926, the ANA published a "suggested" code of behavior. The purpose of the code was to guide nurses in their practice, conduct, and relationships. It outlined the relation of the nurse to the patient, to the medical profession, to the allied health profession, to other nurses, and to the nursing profession. Between 1926 and 2015, multiple reviews and revisions of the ANA Code of Ethics occurred, resulting in today's document.

The ANA Code of Ethics for Nurses With Interpretive Statements is considered to be a living document, changing and updating with changes to society, technology, health care delivery, and the world. The most current edition of the ANA Code of Ethics was released in 2015. It has nine provisions, which discuss the ethical responsibilities of nurses along with interpretive statements to provide guidance in everyday practice.

On the international front, the International Council of Nurses (2012), a group of more than 100 nursing associations, also adopted a code of ethics in 1953. Like the ANA's code of ethics, this document has been updated periodically to reflect changes to the world, with the most recent update[5] occurring in 2012.

EMERGENCY NURSING CODE OF ETHICS

Emergency nurses make ethical decisions every day. Emergency nurses make decisions about life and death, pain and suffering, and allocation of resources. All of these decisions require emergency nurses to examine their own values and beliefs. Emergency nurses not only act as individuals, examining their own values and beliefs, but also act as members of a profession and the organization they work for. Therefore emergency nurses must consider organizational missions and polices along with professional codes and standards of practice.

Emergency nursing has been officially recognized as a nursing specialty by the ANA. One of the requirements to be recognized as specialty is to have a scope and standards of practice. The Emergency Nurses Association (ENA) developed a scope and standards for emergency nursing and has adopted the ANA's nine provisions of the Nursing Code of Ethics. Those provisions are as follows:[6–11]

1. The nurse practices with compassion and respect for the inherent dignity, worth, and unique attributes of every person.
2. The Right to Self-Determination. Patients have the right to make their own decisions. The nurse's primary commitment is to the patient, whether an individual, family, group, community, or population.
3. The nurse promotes, advocates for, and protects the rights, health, and safety of the patient.
4. The nurse has authority, accountability, and responsibility for nursing practice; makes decisions; and takes action consistent with the obligation to promote health and to provide optimal care.
5. The nurse owes the same duties to self as to others, including the responsibility to promote health and safety, preserve wholeness of character and integrity, maintain competence, and continue personal and professional growth.
6. The nurse, through individual and collective effort, establishes, maintains, and improves the ethical environment of the work setting and conditions of employment that are conducive to safe, quality health care.
7. The nurse, in all roles and settings, advances the profession through research and scholarly inquiry, professional standards development, and the generation of both nursing and health policy.
8. The nurse collaborates with other health professionals and the public to protect human rights, promote health diplomacy, and reduce health disparities.
9. The profession of nursing—collectively, through its professional organizations—must articulate nursing values, maintain the integrity of the profession, and integrate principles of social justice into nursing and health policy.

EMERGENCY NURSING STANDARDS OF PRACTICE

The ENA's Scope and Standards of Practice provides guiding principles and standards for actions and decisions involved in the care of patients. These standards are essential to providing safe, quality care for patients. Six standards address practice and 11 standards address professional performance. Standard seven addresses ethics and describes the competencies necessary for emergency nurses to practice ethically. Ethical standards emergency nurses are held to include integrating the Code of Ethics to guide nursing practice; practicing with compassion and respect; advocating for all patients' rights; seeking guidance in any potential ethical conflict, understanding patient priority regardless of setting or situation; maintaining therapeutic relationships and professional boundaries; taking appropriate action to manage and mitigate unprofessional behavior; safeguarding privacy and confidentiality of patients and their protected health information; practicing with professional accountability; maintaining professional competence; demonstrating commitment to holistic wellness (of the nurse); contributing to a safe, quality ethical health care environment; collaborating with the entire health care team and the public to protect human rights and reduce health disparities; maintaining personal and professional integrity; integrating principles of social justice into nursing; guiding others in improving clinical or ethical decision-making processes; and advocating for universal patient access to health care resources within systems and throughout the community.[8]

MORAL DISTRESS

Emergency nurses work in stressful, fast-paced, high-acuity, high-demand, technology-driven, and resource-intensive environments. Emergency nursing involves situations potentially leading to moral distress. Ethical theories, principles, and codes help guide nurses to make ethically sound decisions in the best interest of the patient. At times, conflicts arise that lead to moral distress. Moral distress is when a discrepancy exists between what the nurse knows is the right thing to do and being able to do it. The nurse may be limited by organizational policy, unavailability of resources, inability or refusal of others, subordination or legal considerations, or by the nurses' personal beliefs.[2,3,12–14]

Nursing publications first identified the problem of moral distress[2,12–15] in 1984. Researchers have gone on to describe moral distress as the physiologic, emotional, and psychosocial disturbances that nurses experience when their actions are not consistent with what they believe.[2,12–15] Studies have revealed that emergency nurses develop distress over an inability to provide the quality of patient care they believe patients deserve.[12,13,16] The effects may be felt in symptoms such as palpitations, disturbances in sleep, increased or decreased food intake, panic attacks, headaches, gastrointestinal distress, fatigue, high blood pressure, anger, frustration, sadness, guilt, denial, shame, grief, depression, helplessness, self-blame, and loss of self-worth.[14–16] These symptoms can create job dissatisfaction and lead a nurse to become disengaged, uncaring, or cynical to patients or to leave the profession altogether, increasing turnover.[13,15]

Many situations encountered by emergency nurses create ethical dilemmas that may result in moral distress. These situations involve the concepts of autonomy, justice, beneficence, and nonmaleficence. Many have been discussed in the literature and recognized by the ENA along with other national organizations such as the American College of Emergency Physicians. These situations include access and crowding (justice), public health emergencies and disasters (justice, beneficence, and nonmaleficence), pain management (beneficence and nonmaleficence), resuscitation decisions and end-of-life care (autonomy), and decisional capacity (autonomy).

ETHICAL CONCERNS IN EMERGENCY NURSING

Crowding

Federal laws such as the Emergency Medical Treatment and Active Labor Act (EMTALA) prohibit emergency departments (EDs) from turning patients away because of acuity, volume, insurance, or ability to pay for care. The law imposes requirements for hospitals to provide a medical screening examination for anyone presenting to the ED with an emergency medical condition, to administer stabilizing treatment if an emergency medical condition exists, and if unable to provide the necessary services the patient may require, to provide for a safe transfer.[17] EMTALA is based on the principle of justice, fair and equitable care for all. (See Chapter 2, Legal and Regulatory Constructs.)

Data from the National Hospital Ambulatory Medical Care Survey have shown a dramatic increase in ED visits nationally in the past 10 years.[18] With increased volume comes throughput issues. These issues are directly related to the volume of patients who present to the ED and the number of available resources, such as ED staff, ancillary services, specialty services, and inpatient hospital beds. An imbalance occurs between the need for emergency care and the available resources. Increased volume causes increased utilization of these resources, which can cause scarcity of the resources or delays (or both). Wait times also increase as volume goes up. Examples include delays in seeing an ED provider, therefore delaying diagnosis and treatment, boarding of admitted patients because of lack of inpatient beds, delayed treatment and/or discharge from the ED because of delays in diagnostic studies, and patients with behavioral health problems either being boarded in the ED or having delayed treatment because of limited community psychiatric resources.[19]

Emergency nurses have identified environmental challenges as a source of moral distress.[16] Crowding contributes to delayed patient care, increased census, and increased acuity resulting in higher nurse–patient ratios, which contributes to work overload for emergency nurses and risks patient safety and quality.[13,16] Studies have demonstrated that crowding and boarding in the ED increases delays in treatment interventions, increases medical errors or adverse events, and increases mortality rates.[20–23] Situations such as delays in triage, stroke imaging, administration of antibiotics for sepsis, and pain management; increased mortality; and higher rates of patients leaving without being seen often create ethical dilemmas or moral distress. There is increased pressure nationally from regulatory agencies and employers to meet benchmarking criteria related to wait times and throughput times, which puts added pressure and stress on nurses. Emergency nurses are aware of the need to provide timely, quality, safe care, but are often constrained from doing so under existing conditions, leading to moral distress.

Emergency nurses play a vital role in creating healthier work environments and developing measures to minimize the distress associated with crowding. Emergency nurses assist ED and hospital administrators to collect data regarding wait times, throughput times, staffing, patient volume, and acuity. Nurses can then participate on interdisciplinary ED and hospitalwide teams using data to identify problems and to develop strategies to improve throughput, increase resources, and improve patient care.[13,18]

Public Health Emergencies and Disasters

Emergency management and disaster management are based on the theory of utilitarianism, doing the greatest good for the greatest number of people. They are also based on the principles of justice, beneficence, and nonmaleficence. The expectation in a disaster is that emergency nurses will provide the best care for patients, will prevent harm (beneficence), will avoid causing harm (nonmaleficence), and will improve a situation (beneficence). Additionally, emergency nurses are expected to deliver care fairly and equitably (justice).

Mass casualty, disaster-type situations are one such extreme where lives are at risk. These events can be caused by humans or by natural events. They include bioterrorism, acts of war, chemical exposures, radiation incidences, hurricanes, tsunamis, wildfires, earthquakes, volcanic eruptions, epidemics, and pandemics. The focus in these types of events will shift from saving individuals' lives to saving the largest number of lives. (See Chapter 17, Health Emergency Management.)

Several ethical issues exist related to disaster response and have been discussed in the literature.[24] Two ethical challenges arising from such events for nurses are duty to care and duty to self.[25–27] Disaster situations will quickly deplete resources (supplies, equipment, and personnel) and will require nurses to ration or reallocate resources to provide the greatest good for the greatest number of people, creating moral distress for the nurse.[28] According to the ANA Code of Ethics, nurses also have an obligation to care for themselves as they would. Emergency nurses may be required to work long hours in adverse conditions, such as those with scarce food, water, sanitation and shelter resources, and to leave their families and loved ones (who may also be in danger). In addition, a nurse may feel threatened in a particular situation either for personal health and/or physical well-being. Distress arises for nurses as to whether they should put themselves in harm's way for others.[25,29]

The Institute of Medicine (IOM) published a 2009 report offering guidance for local and state public health officials in establishing crisis standards of care for use in disaster situations. The IOM's recommendations are based on the understanding that a disaster scenario would stress the limits of health care systems and, as a result, the usual standards of care would need to change to meet the demand for critical resources. The IOM defined crisis standards of care as:

> *a substantial change in usual health care operations and the level of care it is possible to deliver, which is made necessary by a pervasive (e.g., pandemic influenza) or catastrophic (e.g., earthquake or hurricane) disaster. The change in the level of care delivered is justified by specific circumstances and is formally declared by a state government, in recognition that crisis operations will be in effect for a sustained period. The formal decision that crisis standards of care are in operation enables special legal/regulatory powers and protections for health care providers in necessary tasks of allocating and using scare medical resources and implementing alternate care facility operations.*[30]

IOM guidelines may assist health care professionals to provide fair and equitable care and possibly minimize distress associated with decision making when resources are scarce.

Emergency nurses personally and professionally prepare for disasters by participating in planning. Planning can potentially help alleviate or minimize moral distress associated with disasters. Personally, nurses should make plans for themselves and their families in an attempt to minimize risk to their physical and emotional well-being. Developing a communication plan, a shelter plan in the event of evacuation, and anticipating specific food, water, medication, child/dependent care, and pet needs is important, along with knowing employers' emergency response plans and role expectations. In the professional environment, emergency nurses should advocate for systems, protocols, and guidelines addressing fair and equitable care during times of limited resources.[25,29]

Pain Management

A common role for the emergency nurse is the treatment of pain. Pain is the cause of four of the top 10 reasons for US ED visits, and analgesics are the primary medication type dispensed in the ED.[18] Emergency nurses have an ethical obligation to treat a patient's pain based on the principles of beneficence and nonmaleficence. Managing the patient's pain will benefit them, improve the situation (beneficence), and avoid inflicting harm by alleviating suffering (nonmaleficence). The principle of nonmaleficence may also lead the nurse to moral distress. The nurse may avoid treating pain with medications such as opioids for fear of causing harm through addiction or dependency.

National attention has been drawn to the growing opioid crisis. This crisis, along with national standards regarding time to treatment in the ED and patient experience regarding the treatment of their pain, creates an ongoing dilemma for nurses. Nurses experience moral distress when faced with a delay in providing care to patients in pain or an inability to effectively treat pain, or when they perceive the treatment may cause harm, as with the case of addiction or dependency.[14,16]

There are steps nurses can take to limit the amount of distress experienced when treating pain in the ED. A joint statement created by the ENA, in collaboration with other emergency medicine colleagues, recommends using a multimodal approach to the treatment of pain in the ED that includes both pharmacologic (opioid and other) and nonpharmacologic approaches. In addition, steps discussed earlier for overcrowding can play a role in improving treatment times for patients. Emergency nurses should also educate themselves on current, evidence-based guidelines for pain management so they can collaborate with the health care team to provide effective pain management to patients. (See Chapter 10, Pain.)

Resuscitation Decisions and End-of-Life Care

Patients have the right to make decisions about their care (autonomy). This includes the right to refuse lifesaving treatment such as resuscitation. Emergency nurses are frequently faced with assisting patients, families, or both with making decisions about resuscitation care. Moral distress exists for emergency nurses either because a decision is made not to provide resuscitation and the nurse believes it is in the best interest of the patient to provide resuscitation, or the patient or family request that resuscitation be initiated and the nurse believes it will prolong pain/suffering.[3,13]

In either of these situations, the emergency nurse must work with the health care team to educate the patient/family about the risks and benefits to providing resuscitation. Emergency nurses should use other resources within the organization to assist, such as social workers, pastoral care, the ethics department, palliative care, risk management, or all of these. Emergency nurses should respect and support the patient's autonomy and the family's role and support and carry out the plan based on the patient's/family's wishes. If the patient and the family are in disagreement, the nurse should access appropriate hospital resources to assist in resolution.

Decisional Capacity

Patients leaving the ED against medical advice account for 1% to 3% of patients.[18] Patients who leave against medical advice have been shown to have a higher rate of repeated visits and adverse outcomes.[31,32] Emergency nurses are able to affect these statistics by taking the time to discuss decisions with the patient and advocate for them.

Autonomy is not a simple matter of making a decision about one treatment over another; it is also about the capacity of the person to make the decision, and the assurance they have received the necessary information to make the decision. To make an autonomous decision, the patient must have the ability to fully understand the choices and be educated on the pros and cons of the decision.[1–3] Capacity is demonstrated by four essential components: understanding the information, appreciation of how the decision will affect the person, reasoning through the information, and expression of choice.[31,32]

Several situations present themselves in the ED regarding capacity. Patients presenting to the ED may have impaired capacity as the result of conditions such as unconsciousness; impaired consciousness from alcohol, drugs, or head trauma; or cognitive disorders or mental health conditions, such as psychosis or anxiety.[31,32]

Emergency nurses, although not directly responsible for obtaining informed consent, are frequently involved in the process. They can play a key role in determining the capacity for decision making and communicate this with the health care team. Nurses can identify patient behaviors requiring a more thorough investigation to determine capacity. Moral distress is encountered when the nurse believes the patient does not have capacity and the patient refuses care; the nurse believes the refusal will lead to harm. Medicolegal considerations come into play when a patient refuses care and decision-making capacity is impaired. Detaining the patient comes with risks, and allowing the patient to leave comes with equally concerning risks.

Organizations can take steps to minimize the risks associated with impaired decision-making capacity by developing guidelines on how to deal with these types of situations. Nurses should be familiar with organizational policies along with state laws regarding decision-making capacity, and intervene accordingly. Emergency nurses should also use other resources within the organization when faced with this dilemma. Social services, pastoral care, risk management, and psychiatric services can also be of assistance.

Moral Resilience

Moral resilience is a concept recently defined in the literature. Lachman defines it as "the ability and willingness to speak and take right and good action in the face of an adversity that is moral/ethical in nature."[33] Several authors have described moral resilience and how to create a path to recover from moral distress.[33,34] They suggest that through practice, education, research, and policy, nurses can recover from moral distress. In practice, nurses should participate in shared governance initiatives and collaborate with other health care professionals to assist in identifying situations that can lead to moral distress, to develop ethical values, and to develop guidelines and policies to address ethical conflicts. Organizations can assist by developing ethics committees and adopting decision-making frameworks to help nurses resolve ethical dilemmas.[2,3] Nurses should advocate for and seek out opportunities to educate themselves on situations leading to moral distress, and strategies to cope with the distress. Nurses should also encourage and participate in research initiatives related to ethics, moral distress, and the development of resilience.

SUMMARY

Ethical dilemmas present themselves to emergency nurses every day. When there is a discrepancy between what is believed to be the right thing to do and being able to do it, nurses experience moral distress. Moral distress has physical, psychological, and emotional consequences for nurses. Strategies to deal with moral distress have been discussed. Nurses can play an active role in their recovery by implementing these actions.

REFERENCES

1. Chiduku A. Ethics in nursing. *Nurs Update.* 2016;41(6):58–59.
2. Guido GW. *Legal and Ethical Issues in Nursing.* 6th ed. Boston, MA: Pearson; 2014.
3. Ferrell KG. *Nurse's Legal Handbook.* 6th ed. New York, NY: Wolters Kluwer; 2016.
4. Epstein B, Turner M. The nursing code of ethics: its value, its history. *Online J Iss Nurs.* 2015;20(2):Manuscript 4. http://www.nursingworld.org/MainMenuCategories/ANAMarketplace/ANAPeriodicals/OJIN//TableofContents/Vol-20-2015/No2-May-2015/The-Nursing-Code-of-Ethics-Its-Value-Its-History.html?css=print. Accessed April 8, 2019.
5. International Council of Nurses. The ICN code of ethics for nurses. 2012. http://ethics.iit.edu/ecodes/sites/default/files/International%20Council%20of%20Nurses%20Code%20of%20Ethics%20for%20Nurses.pdf. Accessed April 8, 2019.
6. American Nurses Association. *Code of Ethics for Nurses with Interpretive Statements.* 2nd ed. Silver Spring, MD: American Nurses Association; 2015.
7. Gurney D, Gillespie GL, McMahon M. Nursing code of ethics: provisions and interpretive statements for emergency nurses. *J Emerg Nurs.* 2017;43(6):497–503.
8. Emergency Nurses Association. *Emergency Nursing Scope and Standards of Practice.* Des Plaines, IL: Emergency Nurses Association; 2017.
9. Emergency Nurses Association 2017 Code of Ethics Work Team. Nursing code of ethics: provisions and interpretive statements for emergency nurses. *J Emerg Nurs.* 2017;43(6):497–503.
10. Winland-Brown J, Lachman VD, O'Connor Swanson E. The new 'code of ethics for nurses with interpretive statements' (2015): practical clinical application, part I. *Medsurg Nurs.* 2015;24(4):268–271.
11. Lachman VD, O'Connor Swanson E, Winland-Brown J. The new 'code of ethics for nurses with interpretative statements' (2015): practical clinical application, part II. *Medsurg Nurs.* 2015;24(5):363–368.
12. Robinson R, Stinson CK. Moral distress: a qualitative study of emergency nurses. *Dimens Crit Care Nurs.* 2016;35(4):235–240.
13. Fernandez-Parsons R, Rodriguez L, Goyal D. Moral distress in emergency nurses. *J Emerg Nurs.* 2013;36(6):547–552.
14. McCarthy J, Gastmans C. Moral distress: a review of the argument-based nursing ethics literature. *Nurs Ethics.* 2015;22(1):131–152.
15. Rathert C, May DR, Chung HS. Nurse moral distress: a survey identifying predictors and potential interventions. *Int J Nurs Stud.* 2016;53:39–49.

16. Wolf LA, Perhats C, Delao AM, Moon MD, Clark PR, Zavotsky KE. "It's a burden you carry": describing moral distress in emergency nursing. *J Emerg Nurs.* 2016;42(1):37–46.
17. Centers for Medicare and Medicaid Services. Emergency Medical Treatment and Active Labor Act. CMS.gov website. https://www.cms.gov/Regulations-and-Guidance/Legislation/EMTALA/index.html. Accessed April 8, 2019.
18. US Department of Health and Human Services, Centers for Disease Control and Prevention. National Hospital Ambulatory Medical Care Survey: 2006-2015 emergency department summary tables. 2006-2015. https://www.cdc.gov/nchs/ahcd/web_tables.htm. Accessed April 8, 2019.
19. Emergency Nurses Association. Position statement: crowding, boarding, and patient throughput. 2017. https://www.ena.org/docs/default-source/resource-library/practice-resources/position-statements/crowdingboardingandpatientthroughput.pdf?sfvrsn=5fb4e79f_4 Accessed April 8, 2019.
20. Carter EJ, Pouch SM, Larson EL. The relationship between emergency department crowding and patient outcomes: a systematic review. *J Nurs Scholarship.* 2014;46(2):106–115.
21. George F, Evridiki K. The effect of emergency department crowding on patient outcomes. *Health Sci J.* 2015;9(1):1–6.
22. Reznek MA, Murray E, Youngren MN, Durham NT, Michael SS. Door-to-imaging time for acute stroke patients is adversely affected by emergency department crowding. *Stroke.* 2017;48(1):49–54.
23. Van der Linden MC, Meester B, Van der Linden N. Emergency department crowding affects triage processes. *Int Emerg Nurs.* 2016 Nov;29:27–31.
24. Leider J, DeBruin D, Reynolds N, Koch A, Seaberg J. Ethical guidance for disaster response, specifically around crisis standards of care: a systematic review. *Am J Public Health.* 2017;107(9):e1–e9.
25. American Nurses Association. Who will be there? Ethics, the law and a nurse's ethical duty to respond in a disaster. Issue brief. https://www.nursingworld.org/~4af058/globalassets/docs/ana/ethics/who-will-be-there_disaster-preparedness_2017.pdf. Published 2017. Accessed April 8, 2019.
26. Wagner JM, Dahnke MD. Nursing ethics and disaster triage: applying utilitarian ethical theory. *J Emerg Nurs.* 2015;41(4):300–306.
27. Doubler A. Exploring the laws and ethics with disaster nursing. *Ohio Nurs Rev.* 2014;89(2):6–7.
28. Perry F. The ethics of resource allocation in disasters: anticipate ethical issues before a crisis occurs. *Healthcare Execut.* 2015;30(3):54–55.
29. Casey D. Ethical considerations during disaster. *Medsurg Nurs.* 2017;26(6):411–413.
30. Institute of Medicine. Guidance for establishing crisis standards of care for use in disaster situations: A Letter Report. Report brief. https://www.phe.gov/coi/Documents/Guidance%20for%20Est%20CSC%20for%20Use%20in%20Disaster%20Situations%20A%20Letter%20Rpt.pdf. Published September 2009. Accessed April 8, 2019.
31. Marco CA, Brenner JM, Kraus CK, McGrath A, Derse AR, ACEP Ethics Committee. Refusal of emergency medical treatment: case studies and ethical foundations. *Ann Emerg Med.* 2017;70(5):696–703.
32. Mitchell MA. Assessing patient decision-making capacity: it's about the thought process. *J Emerg Nurs.* 2015;41(4):307–312.
33. Lachman VD. Moral resilience: managing and preventing moral distress and moral residue. *Medsurg Nurs.* 2016;25(2):121–124.
34. Rushton CH, Schoonover-Shoffner K, Kennedy MS. A collaborative state of the science initiative: transforming moral distress into moral resilience in nursing. *Am J Nurs.* 2017;117(2 Suppl 1):S2–S6.

7

Workplace Violence

Bill Schueler

The very nature of the emergency nursing profession places emergency department (ED) nurses in harm's way. EDs frequently experience the highest rates of violence in a hospital.[1] This problem has increasingly gained national attention, and it is likely that ED nurses will be exposed to workplace violence (WPV) at some point in their career. Some nurses say the problem has been around for decades and is finally being addressed as a top priority. Whether WPV is a new or long-standing issue, evidence suggests that emergency nurses are at a higher risk for violence, and the risk will not be going away anytime soon. Interacting with the ill and injured, the anxious and agitated, and the acutely psychotic will continue to expose ED nurses to episodes of violence.

Many current WPV prevention strategies have their limitations and have not been shown to significantly decrease risk. Because of the current model of emergency care, nurses have limited time and knowledge about their patients, which may result in misinterpreting glaring clues of escalating behavior, causing nurses to get caught off guard when violence occurs.[2–4] Busy ED environments cannot provide adequate care for personality traits and disorders requiring constant attention, as personnel and resources are limited.[5] The current practice of placing patients in department hallways provides high stimulation, a lack of privacy, and feelings of neglect that may escalate agitated patients. No matter how hard we try, the high quality and safe care ED nurses provide does not always meet patients' expectations.

To address WPV, we should universally acknowledge the complex problem of violence in health care. By bringing the problem to light, we realize we have an urgent issue to be addressed. There is much work to be done, and greater efforts can be made to abate health care WPV. It is not as simple as adding more security staff or another policy. The emergency nurse, the caregiver on the front line of patient care, can have a significant effect on creating a safer workplace, lowering the risk of preventable violence. Zero occurrences of violence in the ED might not be achievable, as we are interacting with a variety of people and illnesses. However, we can implement the philosophy and actions supporting a position recognizing preventable violence is not part of the job and is not acceptable in the hospital. Through influence and action, emergency nurses are uniquely positioned to be at the forefront of efforts to reduce WPV and mitigate its effects. This chapter highlights WPV issues from the scientific literature and expert opinion, as well as practical strategies for the emergency nurse, as shown in Box 7.1.

Health care and social services have a rate of violence quadruple that of any other business in the private sector. According to the Bureau of Labor Statistics 2016 data, the incidence of injuries from violence requiring days away from work for all businesses in the private sector was 3.8 per 10,000 full-time employees.[6] In the health care and social services sector, the same incidence rate was 14.3. More specifically, RNs had an incidence rate of 12.7 injuries per 100 full-time workers.[6] Keep in mind these data are from mandatory injury reporting requiring days away from work as reported to federal and state agencies and not from every health care WPV report filed at every hospital. The Emergency Nurses Association's *Emergency Department Violence Surveillance Study* revealed that 54.5% of emergency nurses experienced physical violence and verbal aggression in the past 7 days.[7] More recent studies have indicated that 88% to 100% of emergency nurses have experienced verbal aggression and 43% to 96% have experienced physical violence.[1,8-10] Eighty percent of violence against health care workers is perpetrated by patients, with the remaining 20% coming from visitors, family members, coworkers, and others.[11] Risk factors for violence in health care are highlighted in Table 7.1.

The cost of WPV is significant. The estimated violence response strategies cost US hospitals and health systems $2.7 billion[12] in 2016. Total costs include the following:

- $280 million for preparedness and prevention
- $852 million for unreimbursed medical care for victims of violence
- $1.1 billion for security and training
- $429 million for medical care, staffing, indemnity, and other costs

When broken down, it is estimated that an average hospital paid $481,596 for violence-related costs in 2016. The annual costs to a hospital can range from approximately $94,000 to $270,000 for injured health care staff.[12,13] Violence can also contribute to significant costs related to increased turnover, overtime, temporary staffing, and deterioration of productivity and morale.

Violence is not a problem solely reserved for the United States. About a third of nurses worldwide are physically assaulted, bullied, or injured, and a quarter of nurses are sexually harassed.[14] Different regions of the world also seem to present unique WPV issues. The highest rates of physical

BOX 7.1 Practical Advice for the Emergency Department Nurse.

1. Make your personal safety a priority. Do not rely on other people or systems to keep you safe.
2. Participate fully in workplace violence prevention training. Commit to refreshing your skills annually at a minimum.
3. Delay care of violent patients until the risk of harm to the emergency department nurse or the patient has decreased or ceased. (Except for life-threatening situations.)
4. Never wear the stethoscope around your neck. Place it in a pocket or use a holster specifically designed for stethoscopes.
5. When entering the room of a violent or potentially violent patient, remove all potential weapon items from your person (pens, trauma shears, watches, earrings, necklaces, and name badge).
6. Know your emotional and physical limitations, and do not take insults personally.
7. Assess the patient's room with the mindset of potentially weaponizing anything easily available. Remove possible risks from the room, including oxygen stored on the gurney and, if possible, remove the gurney as well.
8. Never perform patient care alone with a violent or potentially violent patient.
9. Support nurse colleagues who are survivors of violence. Do not assign blame. For many nurses, this is a life-altering event.
10. Know your hospital's violence prevention policies and procedures. Advocate for improving these policies and procedures if there are deficiencies.
11. Establish a relationship with your local enforcement agency.
12. Know your hospital security officers. Train with them. If your hospital does not have security officers, get to know the people who are in charge of safety.
13. Know your violence reporting process. If your hospital does not have a reporting system or process, advocate for its creation and implementation.
14. Commit yourself to report every incident of verbal aggression and physical violence to your hospital's violence reporting system, even if there was no injury. Hold your colleagues accountable to do the same. Ask your leader for follow-up information after you report.
15. Know violence data and trending in your hospital. If the data are not readily available, ask for them.
16. Advocate for state and national legislation to promote safer emergency nursing care.
17. If you want to know how to safely handle weapons discovered on a patient, learn to do so from a trusted professional.
18. If you have a burning question about workplace violence in emergency departments, design a study. You can reach out to your local research institute or the Emergency Nurses Association Institute of Emergency Nursing Research for assistance.
19. Become your emergency department's (better yet, your hospital's) expert on violence prevention.
20. Support a culture of safety in the emergency department by doing all the previously mentioned activities.

TABLE 7.1 Risk Factors for Violence.[5,9,11,15,20,37]

People	Physical Environment	Systems and Processes
Staff's inability to recognize warning signs of violent behavior	Unrestricted access to hospital	Long wait times
Lack of deescalation application or training for staff	Placement in a hallway	Inefficient emergency department throughput
Preceding events before arrival to the emergency department/hospital	Crowding	Understaffing
Being a male caregiver	Presence of firearms or weapons	Inadequate security presence and/or training
Loss of dignity, privacy or control over personal rights	Poor lighting	Poor communication
Medical diagnosis	Lack of duress/panic alarms	Use of hospitals in lieu of jail
Altered mental status	Lack of easy egress/escape	Patients under custody of law enforcement
Intoxication and/or substance abuse or withdrawal	Hospitals considered "soft targets" for terrorism	Working in isolation
Reacting to bad news		Lack of or inconsistent procedure/policy
Gang activity		Lack of mental health personnel and community mental health care
Domestic disputes		
Loss of coping mechanisms		

and sexual harassment occur in Anglo regions (Australia, Canada, England, Ireland, New Zealand, Scotland, and the United States). Worldwide, the ED represents the highest risk for violence to nurses.

Compared with hospitals in Israel, US hospitals could be considered easy targets for violence, including terrorism.[15] A study of Washington State EDs revealed nearly 63% of EDs have 24-hour security officer coverage and 45% of ED staff reported their current security staffing as inadequate. Only 26% of ED staff felt their current security staffing was adequate to respond to a surge or mass-casualty event.[16] In security and law enforcement language, easy targets are called "soft targets." On the other hand, "hard targets" in health care would be those hospitals with a strong and visible security presence, surveillance, and swift response. Many US hospitals do not have the training or capability to quickly improve patient flow, lock down the hospital, or coordinate with local law enforcement. Combine facility challenges with the open environment of hospitals and with EDs operating at capacity, and the resulting risk for violence is high. The current culture in US health care is to have an open and welcoming hospital. A very strong security presence, almost to a militarized level, is not the current trend as it would not appear to support the open hospital environment. In other words, US hospitals are not well prepared to handle extreme forms of violence.

Although WPV in health care is gaining national attention, mitigation strategies are on the horizon. As of 2018, there is no national regulation requiring violence prevention programs and education in health care facilities. For workplace safety, the Occupational Safety and Health Administration (OSHA) enforces the "General Duty Clause," which states an employer must provide a work environment safe from known risks and hazards.[17] Although not widely enforced, there has been increased attention to the safe practice standard in the health care setting. A 2017 OSHA directive has provided clarification and guidance for the investigation of WPV in health care, which is considered high risk.[18] In late 2016, OSHA publicized a request for information for the consideration of a national standard for violence prevention education in the health care and social services sector.[19] A public hearing was conducted in early 2017 with emergency nurses presenting their testimony and support of the OSHA proposed standard.

The Joint Commission, an accrediting agency for many US hospitals, has a sentinel event category specifically related to violence in hospitals. A sentinel event is a serious safety event requiring an immediate investigation, root cause analysis, and corrective actions. The violence sentinel event category is defined as a "rape, assault (leading to death, permanent harm, or severe temporary harm), or homicide of a staff member, licensed independent practitioner, visitor or vendor while on site at the hospital."[20] The Joint Commission's sentinel event data revealed 68 incidents fitting into this sentinel event category, or an average 8.5 events per year, for an 8-year period.

In early 2018, the first legislative bill addressing health care WPV prevention was introduced in the US House of Representatives. The Health Care Workplace Violence Prevention Act, also known as H.R. 5223, was introduced by California Representative Ro Khanna.[21] The act, if passed, will require OSHA to develop and regulate mandatory violence prevention education to every US hospital receiving Medicare and Medicaid funding. Other unique aspects of the act included the requirement of nurses' participation in the development of the WPV prevention program, nonretaliation for health care workers reporting incidents of WPV, and nonretaliation for nurses requesting help from local emergency responders (i.e., calling 9-1-1 for a work-related violence event). Emergency nurses and other nursing organizations started to lobby for congressional support of this bill in early 2018.

Even with this greater recognition and national attention to WPV, barriers to violence prevention in health care abound,[22] as shown in Table 7.2. A common belief of violence in health care as part of the job persists. This theme is perpetuated by some judicial systems, prosecuting attorneys, and health care leaders, as well as caregivers themselves. The definition of WPV violence varies, leading to increased confusion. Is WPV solely intentional violence? Or does it include both intentional and unintentional violence? Is it limited to verbal aggression and threats? Does it include bullying or lateral violence between colleagues? There does not seem to be a consensus nationally on WPV, and its definition is largely left to each hospital or health care entity to decide.

Evidence suggests ED nurses have some ownership in WPV. ED nurses can be desensitized to verbal aggression and may not set behavioral boundaries, which might allow the behavior to continue, according to a conversation with I. Giske, MSN, Behavioral Health Unit Nurse Manager, on June 6, 2018. There might be complacency to defer personal safety practices to security officers, physical barriers, and system strategies.[4] Elements of WPV prevention might make ED nurses feel safe but might not reduce the risk of a violent assault. ED nurses' perceptions of safety might differ greatly from the reality of violence risk. Nursing perception of generalized safety and confidence in personal abilities may increase risk of injury from violence.[4] ED nurses may even consider

TABLE 7.2 Barriers to Violence Prevention.[4,22,25]

Emergency department RNs might not know their patients	Inconsistent definitions of workplace violence
Tolerance of abusive behaviors	Inadequate workplace violence prevention program
Emergency department is open 24/7	Lack of leadership accountability
Highly stressful and emotional environment	Focus on customer service
Lack of reporting of violent or assaultive behavior	Poorly funded mental health and social services
Lack of administrative support and resources	Normalization of violence

elements of community risk factors for violence, such as high crime, that are not necessarily associated with high violence in the ED.[23] What nurses think makes them safe, such as adequate security resources, timely security response to violence, and a low volume of verbal abuse, are not shown to be predictive of assault rates.[4]

Nurses consider reporting violent incidents to be a waste of time and vastly underreport them.[2,22,24] Reasons include a lack of leadership support, perceptions of no changes occurring after filing a report, lack of perceived significant injury, fear of retaliation, fear of being perceived as weak or incompetent, and the "the customer is always right" expectations or culture. Sixty-four percent of ED nurses agree verbal and physical violence is an expected part of the job and demonstrate a higher tolerance to violence.[25] ED nurses may normalize the violent behavior of a person in crisis with contributing factors ranging from having a bad day to true psychosis. Leadership may not support or allow the nurse paid time to complete violence reports, or there may not be a violent event reporting system. Nurses may consider a verbal report to their manager as a formal report. A lack of clear procedures for reporting WPV also contributes to underreporting. Even so, available data indicate reporting all physically violent and verbally assaultive events can be as low as 3%.[25] Concerningly, no evidence supports the idea of reduced violence from incident reporting.[26] However, reporting is essential for data gathering to assist in identifying trends. Reporting is an essential component of evaluating a WPV prevention program and can also assist in procuring essential resources, such as equipment and additional staffing.

PREVENTION OF WORKPLACE VIOLENCE

Surprisingly, there are deficiencies in the scientific literature for violence prevention strategies currently recommended and in use throughout the nation. It is unknown how widely throughout the health care sector current recommendations are implemented. As of this writing, only nine states have mandatory violence prevention education for health care workers.[27,28] Abatement strategies are largely recommended by governmental and regulatory agencies. This presents a significant opportunity to study the various violence prevention methods in practice. Currently, the standard is to have a WPV prevention program. A comprehensive program can be complex, with many elements recommended by regulatory agencies, as shown in Box 7.2.

BOX 7.2 Elements of a Workplace Violence Prevention Program.[11,20,29]

- Definition of workplace violence
- Reporting systems for workplace violence incidents
- Capture, trending, and tracking all reports of workplace violence
- Executive and leadership commitment
- Caregiver participation
- Worksite hazard and risk assessment and analysis
- Identified hazard and risk prevention and control
- Root cause analysis of violent incidents
- Safety training program for risk identification, behavior escalation and interventions, policies/procedures, current data and trends, reporting procedures, postincident debriefings, and survivor support for health caregivers
- Ongoing evaluation of hazards, training

OSHA highlights four types of WPV that appear in the following list.[18] An unofficial fifth type of WPV has recently been considered because of increases in active shooter events and terrorism.[29,30]

1. ***Criminal intent:*** There is no legitimate relationship with the perpetrator to the business or employee. Acts of robbery, shoplifting, trespassing, active shooters, and terrorism would fit into this type.
2. ***Patient/customer:*** The violent person is a patient, visitor, or family member. This is the largest category in which health care violence incidents apply.
3. ***Worker-on-worker:*** This type of violence is committed by current or past employees.
4. ***Personal relationship:*** This includes domestic violence. The perpetrator does not have a relationship with the business, but with an employee.
5. ***Ideological:*** This type is targeted toward people or an organization for religious, ideological, or political reasons. The perpetrators feel justified by their beliefs.

The physical hospital environment can influence the safety of emergency nurses. Simple, often overlooked, design elements such as desk height and depth, physical barriers between staff and patients, locked doors, adequate lighting, curved mirrors for corners, heavy chairs, aligning chairs in open rows, egress (escape) routes, and clear sight lines have been shown to influence safety.[31] Options enhancing ED physical environment safety can include design elements such as bullet-proof glass, metal detectors, and systems to lock down the ED with a simple push of a button. Silent panic/duress alarms to quickly alert security or local law enforcement to an emergent situation are widely in use, although their efficacy in violence prevention has not been proved.[26,32] Duress alarms may improve ED nurses' confidence and decrease fears, but each ED setting might require a different alarm system. Environmental strategies tailored to the EDs assessed or anticipated risk can help mitigate long-term issues.

Studies on metal detectors have not demonstrated their effectiveness in decreasing violent events in hospitals. Although risk of violence perpetrated with weapons may decrease, most violence in health care has been shown to occur without a weapon. Hitting, kicking, or biting are examples of nonweapon violence. In the studies, metal detectors were not used to screen for weapons on every patient and visitor entering the hospital and ED.[33,34] A study on hospital active shooter events postulated that only 30% to 36% of hospital active shooter events could have been prevented by metal detectors.[35]

Nurses are often not comfortable asking patients about weapons.[10,26] If such questions are to be part of the nurse's assessment, consideration must include actions to take when a weapon is discovered. Is there an established procedure to place the weapon in storage? Is there training on weapon handling, whether it be a gun or knife? Even if weapons are identified and removed from persons entering the ED, nurses must know how to respond to violent encounters. Metal detectors are not a substitute for deescalation and physical skills training and therefore have limited effectiveness for decreasing violence in health care. This highlights the importance of a well-thought-out violence prevention education plan.

The idea hospitals in high-crime areas would have a higher problem of violence is not necessarily true. Blando et al. found small hospitals in high-crime neighborhoods had more assaults within the hospital (2 to 5 times higher) than larger hospitals in high-crime areas.[23] The study highlighted that the local community crime rate does not influence assaults in hospitals; instead, resources and training of hospital security officers have the most influence. Gang activity and violence have opportunity to enter the ED. Hospitals are not considered neutral territory by gangs.[35] The emergency nurse should address known gang members with honesty and respect, as they would any other patient. Gang awareness training for hospitals in known gang territories should be part of a comprehensive WPV prevention program.

A strong security program reduces the risk of injury to health care employees. A recent study of Washington State EDs revealed only 63% of EDs have 24-hour security officer coverage, and 45% of ED staff reported current security staffing as inadequate.[16] Hospital security officers who have adequate training and resources and are strategically placed can influence the safety of ED nurses. Security officers stationed near the ED entrance can allow for quick, active intervention and give a psychological benefit of physical presence.[31,37] Security officers might be limited in their response to violent events, either by policy, physical abilities, or interventional tools and strategies, such as being limited only to verbal deescalation or a "hands-off" approach.[37] Limitations can decrease an appropriate physical response when deescalation has failed or is not appropriate. Without properly trained security officers, patients, visitors, and health care workers are at increased risk for injury.[38] Security officers may act as ambassadors for the hospital, enforcing policies and behavioral expectations of patients and visitors.[38] Security officers can also enhance relations with local law enforcement.[29] As with any volatile situation, adding additional personnel or the presence of an audience, including security officers, may actually escalate a potentially violent situation. Interdisciplinary training with both ED nurses and security officers is of the utmost importance to adequately and safely respond to violent events in the ED.[37]

Although patient characteristics, physical environment deterrents, and individual nurse responses influence ED violence, systems factors have been shown to affect WPV. ED crowding is a known contributor to ED violence. The efficiency of ED patient throughput is inversely related to physical violence in the ED.[19] The more inefficient the work processes and patient throughput in the ED and the hospital, the higher the ED risk for physical violence. Because ED crowding is a hospitalwide problem, any efforts to increase the efficiency and throughput in the hospital could theoretically decrease WPV.

Safe staffing in EDs is a concern to nurses. According to The Joint Commission, understaffing is a risk factor for violence in hospitals.[20] A study by Hyland et al. reported that 66% of ED nurses felt a lack of support in managing patients with challenging behaviors.[9] ED nurses are a limited resource, and understaffing negatively influences the care of agitated and potentially violent patients.[5]

VIOLENCE PREVENTION

Currently, even though most elements are largely based on expert consensus, the best strategy recommended to address and prevent WPV is a comprehensive violence prevention program.[5,20,40] Box 7.2 presents the essential violence prevention program elements. In one study, an ED experienced a 50% decline in violence as a result of their WPV program. The keys to this success were attributed to enthusiastic support from leadership and implementation of program elements that included environmental changes, supportive policies and procedures, and a high rate of employee participation.[41] The study also highlighted the importance of evaluating and updating the WPV prevention program on an ongoing basis and having a work culture supporting employee safety as a top priority. There is insufficient scientific evidence to show what type of training is effective in preventing WPV, yet training is an essential element to violence prevention,[42] as shown in Box 7.2.

Consistent use of agitation/aggression assessment tools predicts risk for violence.[26] Many aggression risk assessment tools are available, with varying degrees of validity and reliability.[43] Currently the Brøset Violence Checklist (www.riskassessment.no) is the most prevalent in the literature and shows the best validity.[42] Assessment tools offer an opportunity for identification of patient needs and early intervention to reduce escalation of aggressive behavior. Hospitals and organizations are encouraged to select an assessment tool appropriate for the patient population and unit dynamics.

A comprehensive violence prevention plan should consider a team response to violence and not rely on ED nurses to handle violent situations alone. A team response offers a show of support to both the agitated person and the staff and decreases the rate of placing patients in restraint or seclusion.[28,44] ED nurses should never have to face violent patients alone. In Oregon, state law supports a nurse refusing to care for a patient who has been violent if the employer cannot provide another staff member for safety.[44] A team response to violence may be difficult because of the ad hoc nature of ED teams, with their changing membership and interpersonal dynamics.[5] An interdisciplinary ED team approach to violence can help break silos and encourage collaboration.

The educational portion of a comprehensive WPV prevention program, at a minimum, should contain elements of deescalation, self-defense, and responses to emergency codes.[20] Other considerations could include early recognition of escalating behaviors, hospital-specific data and trends, and policies. Educational programs are viewed favorably by caregivers even though no evidence shows which type of commercial program is best. Programs studied did not contain all of the recommended elements,[46] which are listed in Box 7.2. WPV prevention programs could counteract some of the deleterious effects of WPV, such as stress and burnout.[46] Educational programs should include training on the identification of and response to escalating behaviors and violence, including active shooter situations and crisis intervention.[28]

There is always a cause for aggressive behavior, whether from personality, emotional distress, or physical illness. Other potential causes include personal freedom restrictions, the physical environment, and the attitudes and behaviors shown by staff or bystanders.[47] The ED nurse can assume aggression indicates that a person in crisis is trying to communicate unmet needs or that their coping abilities have been exceeded. Remember, a crisis is unique to each individual, and there is an increased risk for aggression and violence for those in crisis, according to a conversation with I. Giske on June 6, 2018.

Nurses can successfully deescalate agitated persons, but there is a process and many considerations.[26] Taking a few extra minutes to speak with the patient or visitor, as highlighted in Box 7.3, can save valuable time.[48] Deescalation skills vary from nurse to nurse. Sometimes deescalation is successful, and other times medications to treat agitation might be the best option, according to a conversation with I. Giske on June 6, 2018. Deescalation cannot be the sole focus, as not all persons can be deescalated and it might not be appropriate based on the situation. If a person is trying to attack a nurse, the appropriate response in the moment is to exit or use breakaway techniques to safely escape from the encounter and call for help. Like many nursing procedures, deescalation is a skill; ongoing practice and experience are required.

There is always a chance deescalation might not be successful, even when practical.[39] Effective physical skills training is necessary to successfully control, restrain, and respond to violent situations. Concerns with physical skills include the risk of being too aggressive (combined with inadequate training), resorting to whatever skill the caregiver has or has not learned in the past, and the perception of a preference by the employer to pay worker's compensation rather than train employees in applicable physical control, restraint, and/or break-away (self-defense) skills. Assessing the differences between physical intervention training and "nontouch" interventions would most likely support physical intervention in violent situations.[49]

Common physical skills training includes techniques for controlling, for restraining, and break-away techniques for hand grabs, clothing grabs, chokes, hair pulls, strangle holds, kicks, strikes, and bear hugs.[46] Depending on the training, prone restraint is sometimes an option, which can create significant risk to the restrained person's breathing. Patient control and restraint in the prone position should be temporary.[3] Studies do suggest an increase in confidence and safety when physical skills are taught to caregivers.[45,49,50]

BOX 7.3 Deescalation Considerations for Agitated Persons.

Respect their personal space and your own.
Be polite and introduce yourself.
Do not be provocative.
Only have one person talking to the patient.
Be concise and keep it simple.
Repeat your message.
Identify their needs, wants, and feelings.
Use active listening.
Agree or agree to disagree.
Establish rules and set clear limits.
Coach the person on controlling his or her behavior.
Offer choices and hope/optimism.
Debrief the situation with the patient and involved staff.

Adapted from Richmond J, Berlin J, Fishkind A, Holloman G, Zeller S, Wilson M, et al. (2012). Verbal de-escalation of the agitated patient: consensus statement of the American Association for Emergency Psychiatry Project BETA De-escalation Workgroup. *West J Emerg Med.* 13(1):17–25.

Conversely, multiple studies have demonstrated the issue of physical skill attrition.[50,51] A consideration raised by nurses is one of maintaining physical skill, as well as ongoing competency. Training, including the specific physical skill(s), might not be recalled during a violent encounter, the breakaway technique might not be successful, or the skill might not be used as taught.[51] These gaps highlight the importance of the continual physical skill practice to enhance retention, recall, and effectiveness of these individual skills. One study suggests up to 66% of nurses felt physical skills had helped them avoid or escape an assault.

Part of a strong WPV prevention program can be the clear procedures outlining the plan, prevention strategies, and postincident response and support. All policies should include strategies to address and respond to domestic violence, staff-on-staff violence, WPV, rape or sexual assault, and active shooter situations. A well-rounded policy will also contain procedures for the support and care of survivors of violence.[28]

Zero tolerance for violence is a common component in WPV prevention policies. Because of the Emergency Medical Treatment and Active Labor Act (EMTALA), EDs cannot turn away potential patients because of violent behavior. Zero tolerance enforcement might be more appropriate for family members, visitors, and employees, including physicians, as consequences can be more easily applied.[25] Policies are not preventive, as the consequences outlined in the policy are placed into effect after a violent event has occurred. Current zero tolerance policy strategies are not demonstrating effectiveness in decreasing violence. Violence prevention should focus on risk assessment, response, and resource allocation instead of zero tolerance. The unique circumstance of providing care yet facing violence presents an ethical conundrum to caregivers known as the "patient care paradox." The same actions increasing patient safety can simultaneously increase personal danger for the emergency nurse. This paradox is known to influence stress, dissatisfaction, and burnout.[5] A better strategy could include communicating behavioral expectations and consequences to those with the capacity to understand the policy and also hold them accountable for their behavior.

There are multiple modes of violence risk notification, depending on the audience. For the public, including patients and visitors, the display of signage explaining behavioral expectations while in the ED and in the hospital could help reinforce the WPV plan. Because hospital procedures are not readily available to patients and the public, signage can bridge the gap. Staff, supervisors, management, leadership, and other members of the public could easily point out these signs when a person's behavior is escalating and becoming abusive or disruptive. Depending on hospital procedure and state laws, signage could highlight the consequences for assaultive behavior, including ejection from the facility and punishment to the fullest extent of the law.

The best predictor of violent behavior is a history of violence. Use of the electronic health record could help communicate this risk to all members of the health care team. Although many violent patients/visitors are discharged from the ED, many others are admitted into the hospital, where their violent behavior will likely continue. Appropriate use of alerts or displayable banners in the electronic health record can serve as a continual reminder of the increased risk of violence throughout the patient's continuum of care. Alerts placed on doors or doorways could also provide an additional visual alert to caregivers, ancillary staff, and visitors.

Physical control, restraint, and breakaway techniques are learned through motor skills training and repetition, all of which should be included in a WPV prevention program. Although there is no guarantee, successful performance requires specific knowledge and practice to decrease the risk of physical harm to both the patient/visitor and the health care team. Physical techniques have not been studied to show which are more effective than others. Depending on the WPV program and theoretical model, differing physical skills will be selected and taught to caregivers. Professional opinion has heavy sway on which physical control, restraint, and self-defense skills are appropriate for the health care setting. The emergency nurse must practice the physical skills included as part of their WPV prevention program to avoid the high risk of skill attrition.[50]

STRATEGIES DURING VIOLENT ENCOUNTERS

When a patient is violent, it is appropriate to delay their care while improving safety, not only for the emergency nurses' safety but also for safety of the patient. Whenever a physical altercation is taking place, whether one is responding to violent behavior or applying restraints, the risk of injury is high, both to the caregivers and the patient. This is the time where the retention of education and physical skills training provides the chance of a successful outcome and lack of injury. Although there is no guarantee of outcome, the use of verbal deescalation and physical skills is essential to the safety of the emergency nurse.

BOX 7.4 Effects of Workplace Violence.[1,2,53]

Acute and permanent injuries
Lingering trauma
Posttraumatic stress
Becoming fearful of work in the emergency department
Lost work time
Change in relationship with colleagues—from a desire to withdraw to feelings of betrayal
Change in relationship with patient—from mild hypervigilance to apathy
Intention to leave position
Feelings of abandonment
Intention to change career
Withdrawing from work
Lessening self-fulfillment from work

AFTER VIOLENCE

Hospitals with a culture of workplace safety are more likely to offer support to health care workers after a violent incident.[52] According to studies, 42% of health care workers receive post-incident support. The negative effects of WPV are serious and far-reaching, as presented in Box 7.4. Nurses have reported feeling a lack of support and even betrayal by their own colleagues, their leadership, and the judicial system.[2,53]

The current recommendation is for all WPV prevention programs to include strategies to support caregivers after violent events. Immediate medical attention must be provided for any physical injury to the caregiver. Caregivers may choose to use their employer's worker's compensation program, and many organizations offer an employee assistance program. To deal with the more immediate psychological side effects of WPV, a well-designed peer-to-peer support program, stress debriefing, psychological counseling, or trauma-informed care should be offered.[20] In following the recommendations from the Centers for Medicare and Medicaid Services, debriefing should also be offered to the patient and family after a violent event, including for incidents resulting in restraints or seclusion, according to a conversation with J. Flynn, Nurses Service Organization Health Risk Manager, and L. Pierce, RN, CNA, Healthcare Risk Control Director, on May 31, 2018.

Incidents of violence should be reviewed closely to determine the root cause and facilitate knowledge.[20] Learnings should then be shared, and violence prevention efforts may be adjusted as necessary to prevent recurrence. If nursing performance is to be considered as part of the event, the hospital should endorse a just and fair culture that promotes professional accountability yet realizes systems and processes can be responsible for unfortunate events. Every verbal assault and violent event should be reported to the hospital for tracking and trending. As stated previously, violent incident reports help gather data and can provide justification for additional training and resources.

The emergency nurse must also remember that one person intentionally assaulting another person is a crime, whether it be in the hospital setting or not, and crime should be reported to law enforcement. The emergency nurse should report the incident to law enforcement. A manager, leader, or security officer cannot do it for them. There are mitigating circumstances in which violence might not be considered a crime, such as the organic causes of violence, which can include traumatic brain injury, hypoxemia, sepsis, shock, and psychosis. In these circumstances, violence could be considered a manifestation of the illness.

Although reporting assaults is important, nurses might be discouraged by their employer from reporting violence to law enforcement and may experience fear of retaliation and blame. Violent acts reported to law enforcement might not be addressed by hospital administration or prosecuted in court, reducing any possible legal accountability on the part of the offender. Nurses employed by small, rural hospitals may also be reluctant to report to law enforcement for fear of retaliation by people within the community. Small-town politics might also limit the effectiveness of reporting to law enforcement.[54] It is beneficial to build relationships with local law enforcement to enhance mutual understanding of WPV incidents and reporting processes.

The court of law can be helpful in determining whether the violent act was purposeful or unintentional. The process starts with a report to local law enforcement. The task then falls to the local district prosecuting attorney to press criminal charges against the offender. The survivor may be asked for more details and may also be asked or ordered to attend court hearings and sentencing. The legal process can be daunting as the emergency nurse shifts roles from caregiver to victim. Legal proceedings might require days off work and may not include legal support from the hospital. Although 60% of states currently provide enhanced penalties for assaults against health care workers,[2] no scientific data show these laws prevent violence in health care, and data suggest enhanced penalties are not applied consistently to violent offenders, according to a conversation with S. Alexander, RN, MBA, Clinical Risk Manager, on May 25, 2018. Professional relationships with local law enforcement and prosecuting attorneys can help the nurse advocate for the fair application of laws pertaining to WPV.

A hospital has a liability risk if it lacks some standard of WPV prevention. Hospital risk management trends include reports of increasing support of nurses after assault. Nurses are provided assistance for law enforcement reporting and provision of legal assistance if the nurse is required to appear in court. The next trend may include RNs hiring private attorneys if they have not felt supported by their health care employer or if they feel their rights have been violated, according to a conversation with M. Seidl, Civil Litigation Attorney, on May 29, 2018. Emergency nurses can decrease their liability risk by following hospital policies and procedures for WPV and reporting each assault through the facility's reporting program. Injuries from WPV are typically covered under worker's compensation programs. A nurse's supplemental insurance policy might also help compensate for injuries and counseling.[54]

A disturbing trend is disciplinary action, not excluding termination, for a nurse involved in a violent patient interaction (M. Seidl, personal communication). Some hospitals expect nurses to function as security officers and have blamed nurses for violent incidents even though the nurse was performing within the scope of training. In some instances, the hospital has not provided adequate training and is not following state law for violence prevention. Hospitals are grappling with institutional fatigue because of a lack of behavioral health resources and financial decision-making practices, leaving safety and security as a low priority. The current laws in place for violence prevention are only as effective as the hospitals complying with them and the agencies enforcing them.

Caring for nurses after an assault should be a top priority. Yet some hospitals have used the debriefing process not as an avenue to support nurses but instead as a way to investigate the event and start the disciplinary process. This only increases liability for the hospital, especially if the nurse feels he or she was wrongly terminated from employment. These unfair practices only serve to increase disengagement, burnout, and turnover.

Compassionate care for the nurse after a significant violent event can decrease the potential negative effects of violence. And yet nurses are sometimes their own worst enemy in not seeking help. Self-care, for some, is not a high priority. Nurses can find themselves in a lonely mental or emotional state if they are not supported by their colleagues or their employer. Hospitals and nurses have a duty not only to care for their patients but also to care for nurses who are survivors of violence.

SUMMARY

Violence in health care is a complex problem. The emergency nurse has a unique opportunity to contribute to the science and study of the various violence prevention methods currently in practice. A more active role in helping your ED achieve a robust safety culture and a positive violence prevention climate can make a difference to patients, visitors, and staff. Addressing the personal risk factors and prioritizing bigger systems problems, such as crowding and throughput, will help foster a positive violence prevention climate.[40] Collaboration with local law enforcement and active engagement with hospital administration and legal platforms are essential in changing the culture of safety in EDs across the nation. If ED nurses do not feel safe, they cannot ensure the patients' safety. Every emergency nurse has the right to work in a facility free from violence.

REFERENCES

1. Rosenthal LJ, Byerly A, Taylor AD, Martinovich Z. Impact and prevalence of physical and verbal violence toward healthcare workers. *Psychosomatics*. 2018;59(6):584–590. http://doi.org/10.1016/j.psym.2018.04.007.
2. Wolf LA, Delao AM, Perhats C. Nothing changes, nobody cares: understanding the experience of emergency nurses physically or verbally assaulted while providing care. *J Emerg Nurs*. 2014;40(4):305–310. http://doi.org/10.1016/j.jen.2013.11.006.
3. Wright S, Sayer J, Parr A, Gray R, Southern D, Gournay K. Breakaway and physical restraint techniques in acute psychiatric nursing: results from a national survey of training and practice. *J Forensic Psychiatr Psychol*. 2005;16(2):380–398. http://doi.org/10.1080/14789940412331270735.
4. Blando JD, O'Hagan E, Casteel C, Nocera M, Peek-Asa C. Impact of hospital security programmes and workplace aggression on nurse perceptions of safety. *J Nurs Manage*. 2013;21(3):491–498. http://doi.org/10.1111/j.1365-2834.2012.01416.x.
5. Wong AH, Ruppel H, Crispino LJ, Rosenberg A, Iennaco JD, Vaca FE. Deriving a framework for a systems approach to agitated patient care in the emergency department. *Jt Comm J Qual Patient Saf*. 2018;44(5):279–292. http://doi.org/10.1016/j.jcjq.2017.11.011.
6. Bureau of Labor Statistics. *Workplace Injuries and Illnesses Database in Illnesses, Injuries and Fatalities*. https://www.bls.gov/iif/#data. Published 2017. Accessed April 14, 2019.
7. Emergency Nurses Association. *Emergency Department Violence Surveillance Study*. Des Plaines, IL: Emergency Nurses Association; 2011. https://ena.org/docs/default-source/default-document-library/practice-resources/work-place-violence/enaedvsreportnovember2011.pdf?sfvrsn=ff262d3d_2. Published November 2011.
8. Partridge B, Affleck J. Verbal abuse and physical assault in the emergency department: rates of violence, perceptions of safety, and attitudes towards security. *Australas Emerg Nurs J*. 2017;20(3):139–145.
9. Hyland S, Watts J, Fry M. Rates of workplace aggression in the emergency department and nurses' perceptions of this challenging behaviour: a multimethod study. *Australas Emerg Nurs J*. 2016;19(3):143–148. http://doi.org/10.1016/j.aenj.2016.05.002.
10. Renker P, Scribner SA, Huff P. Staff perspectives of violence in the emergency department: appeals for consequences, collaboration, and consistency. *Work*. 2015;51(1):5. http://doi.org/10.3233AVOR-141893.
11. Occupational Safety and Health Administration. *Workplace Violence in Healthcare: Understanding the Challenge*. OSHA 3826. https://www.osha.gov/Publications/OSHA3826.pdf. Published 2015. Accessed April 14, 2019.
12. Van Den Bos J, Creten N, Davenport S, Roberts M. *Cost of Community Violence to Hospitals and Health Systems: Report for the American Hospital Association*. Milliman Research Report. https://www.aha.org/system/files/2018-01/community-violence-report.pdf. Published July 26, 2017. Accessed April 14, 2019.
13. Speroni KG, Fitch T, Dawson E, Dugan L, Atherton M. Incidence and cost of nurse workplace violence perpetrated by hospital patients or patient visitors. *J Emerg Nurs*. 2014;40(3):218–228. http://doi.org/10.1016/j.jen.2013.05.014.
14. Spector P, Zhou Z, Che X. Nurse exposure to physical and nonphysical violence, bullying and sexual harassment: a quantitative review. *Int J Nurs Studies*. 2014;51(1):72–84.
15. Golabek-Goldman M. Adequacy of US hospital security preparedness for mass casualty incidents: critical lessons from the Israeli experience. *J Public Health Manag Pract*. 2016;22(1):68–80. https://doi.org/10.1097/PHH.0000000000000298.
16. Weyand JS, Junck E, Kang CS, Heiner JD. Security, violent events, and anticipated surge capabilities of emergency departments in washington state. *West J Emerg Med*. 2017;18(3):466–473.
17. Occupational Safety and Health Administration. *OSH Act of 1970*. https://www.osha.gov/laws-regs/oshact/toc. Accessed April 14, 2019.
18. Occupational Safety and Health Administration. *Directive Number: CPL 02-01-058. Enforcement Procedures and Scheduling for Occupational Exposure to Workplace Violence*; 2017. https://www.osha.gov/OshDoc/Directive_pdf/CPL_02-01-058.pdf. Published 2017. Accessed April 14, 2019.
19. Occupational Safety and Health Administration. *Prevention of Workplace Violence in Healthcare and Social Assistance: A Proposed Rule by the Occupational Safety and Health Administration on 12/7/2016*. https://www.federalregister.gov/documents/2016/12/07/2016-29197/prevention-of-workplace-violence-in-healthcare-and-social-assistance. Published 2016. Accessed April 14, 2019.
20. The Joint Commission. Physical and verbal violence against health care workers. *Sentinel Event Alert*. 2018;17(59):1–9. https://www.jointcommission.org/assets/1/18/SEA_59_Workplace_violence_4_13_18_FINAL.pdf. Accessed April 14, 2019.
21. *Health Care Workplace Violence Prevention Act*. 2018. H.R. 5223, 115th Cong. https://www.congress.gov/bill/115th-congress/house-bill/5223. Accessed April 14, 2019.
22. Blando J, Ridenour M, Hartley D, Casteel C. Barriers to effective implementation of programs for the prevention of workplace violence in hospitals. *Online J Issues Nurs*. 2015;20(1):1.
23. Blando JD, McGreevy K, O'Hagan E, Worthington K, Valiante D. Emergency department security programs, community crime, and employee assaults. *J Emerg Med*. 2012;42(3):329–338. http://doi.org/10.1016/j.jemermed.2008.06.026.
24. Gacki-Smith J, Juarez AM, Boyett L, Homeyer C, Robinson L, MacLean SL. Violence against nurses working in US emergency departments. *J Nurs Adm*. 2009;39(7–8):340–349. http://doi.org/10.1097/NNA.0b013e3181ae97db.
25. Copeland D, Henry M. Workplace violence and perceptions of safety among emergency department staff members: experiences, expectations, tolerance, reporting, and recommendations. *J Trauma Nurs*. 2017;24(2):65–77. http://doi.org/10.1097/JTN.0000000000000269.
26. Morphet J, Griffiths D, Beattie J, Velasquez Reyes D, Innes K. Prevention and management of occupational violence and aggression in healthcare: a scoping review. *Collegian (Australian Journal of Nursing Practice)*. 2018;25(6):621–632. https://doi.org/10.1016/j.colegn.2018.04.003.
27. Occupational Safety and Health Administration. *Workplace Violence Prevention and Related Goals: the Big Picture*; 2015. OSHA 3828. https://www.osha.gov/Publications/OSHA3828.pdf. Published December 2015. Accessed April 14, 2019.
28. SIA Health Care Security Interest Group, International Association for Healthcare Security & Safety Foundation. *Mitigating the Risk of Workplace Violence in Health Care Settings*. https://www.securityindustry.org/wp-content/uploads/2017/11/Workplace-Violence-In-Health-Care-Settings-IAHSS.pdf. Published August 2017. Accessed April 14, 2019.
29. Pennfield W. The Five Types of Workplace Violence. [blog]. https://www.everbridge.com/five-types-workplace-violence/. Published January 24, 2017. Accessed April 14, 2019.

30. Lenaghan PA, Cirrincione NM, Henrich S. Preventing emergency department violence through design. *J Emerg Nurs.* 2018;44(1):7–12. https://doi.org/10.1016/j.jen.2017.06.012.
31. Perkins C, Beecher D, Aberg D, Edwards P, Tilley N. Personal security alarms for the prevention of assaults against healthcare staff. *Crime Science.* 2017;6(11). http://doi.org/10.1186/s40163-017-0073-1.
32. Rankins R, Hendey G. Effect of a security system on violent incidents and hidden weapons in the emergency department. *Annals Emerg Med.* 1999;33(6):676–679.
33. Malka S, Chisholm R, Doehring M, Chisholm C. Weapons retrieved after the implementation of emergency department metal detection. *J Emerg Med.* 2015;49(3):355–358.
34. Kellen G, Catlett C, Kubit J, Hsieh Y. Hospital-based shootings in the United States: 2000–2011. *Annals Emerg Med.* 2012;60(6):790–798. http://doi.org/10.1016/j.annemergmed.2012.08.012.
35. Moore CS. Gangs and healthcare security: preparation and education are the keys. *J Healthc Protect Manage.* 2012;28(2):65–71.
36. Menendez CC, Gillespie GL, Gates DM, Miller M, Howard PK. Emergency department workers' perceptions of security officers' effectiveness during violent events. *Work.* 2012;42(1):21–27.
37. Brubaker TW. Use of force in the healthcare setting. *J Healthc Protect Manage.* 2015;31(1):73–80.
38. Maas J. Hospital security: "protecting the business." *J Healthcare Protect Manage.* 2013;29(1):65–73.
39. Arnetz J, Hamblin L, Sudan S, Arnetz B. Organizational determinants of workplace violence against hospital workers. *J Occup Environ Med.* 2018;60(8):693–699.
40. Gillespie GL, Gates DM, Kowalenko T, Bresler S, Succop P. Implementation of a comprehensive intervention to reduce physical assaults and threats in the emergency department. *J Emerg Nurs.* 2014;40(6):586–591. http://doi.org/10.1016/j.jen.2014.01.003.
41. Martindell D. Violence prevention training for ED staff. *Am J Nurs.* 2012;112(9):65–68.
42. Calow N, Lewis A, Showen S, Hall N. Literature synthesis: patient aggression risk assessment tools in the emergency department. *J Emerg Nurs.* 2016;42(1):19–24. http://doi.org/10.1016/j.jen.2015.01.023.
43. Kelley EC. Reducing violence in the emergency department: a rapid response team approach. *J Emerg Nurs.* 2014;40(1):60–64. http://doi.org/10.1016/j.jen.2012.08.008.
44. Safety of Health Care Employees. *Ore Rev Stat. §654.* 2017;423:418–654. https://www.oregonlegislature.gov-/bills_laws/ors/ors654.html. Accessed April 14, 2019.
45. Lamont S, Brunero S. The effect of a workplace violence training program for generalist nurses in the acute hospital setting: a quasi-experimental study. *Nurse Educ Today.* 2018;68:45–52. http://doi.org/10.1016/j.nedt.2018.05.008.
46. Harwood R. How to deal with violent and aggressive patients in acute medical settings. *J R Coll Physicians Edinb.* 2017;47(2):176–182.
47. Richmond J, Berlin J, Fishkind A, Holloman G, Zeller S, Wilson M, et al. Verbal de-escalation of the agitated patient: consensus statement of the American Association for Emergency Psychiatry Project BETA De-Escalation workgroup. *West J Emerg Med.* 2012;13(1):17–25.
48. Southcott J, Howard A. Effectiveness and safety of restraint and breakaway techniques in a psychiatric intensive care unit. *Nurs Stand.* 2007;21(36):35–41.
49. Lamont S, Brunero S, Woods K. Breakaway technique training as a means of increasing confidence in managing aggression in neuroscience nursing. *Australian Health Rev.* 2012;36(3):313–319. http://doi.org/10.1071/AH11001.
50. Dickens G, Rooney C, Doyle D. Breakaways in specialist secure psychiatry. *J Psychiatr Mental Health Nurs.* 2012;19(3):281–284. http://doi.org/10.1111/j.1365-2850.2011.01825.x.
51. Shea T, Cooper B, De Cieri H, Sheehan C, Donohue R, Lindsay S. Postincident support for healthcare workers experiencing occupational violence and aggression. *J Nurs Scholarsh.* 2018;50(4):344–352. http://doi.org/10.1111/jnu.12391.
52. Lamothe J, Guay S. Workplace violence and the meaning of work in healthcare workers: a phenomenological study. *Work.* 2017;56(2):185–197. http://doi.org/10.3233/WOR-172486.
53. US Department of Health and Human Services. *Centers for Medicare and Medicaid State Operations Manual.* 42 CFR §482.13 Conditions of participation: patient's rights; 2017. https://www.gpo.gov/fdsys/pkg/CFR-2017-title42-vol5/pdf/CFR-2017-title42-vol5-sec482-13.pdf. Published 2017. Accessed April 14, 2019.
54. Emergency Nurses Association. *Gearing Up for Advocacy: A Toolkit For ENA State Council Government Affairs Chairpersons.* Des Plaines, IL: Emergency Nurses Association; 2018:1–22.

UNIT III

Clinical Foundations of Emergency Nursing

8

Triage

Andi Foley

Emergency triage is the complex complaint-based process of sorting patients to ensure the right patient sees the right provider at the right time in the right place for the right reason. The element of basing an assessment on complaint compared with assessment based on diagnosis creates a recognized emergency nursing specialty.[1] The triage nurse must quickly differentiate patients who need to be seen immediately from patients who are safe to wait for care. Statistics from 2015 report almost 140 million emergency department (ED) visits.[2] Each visit resulted in at least one triage decision. This important decision must be based on a brief patient assessment leading the triage nurse to assign an acuity rating. In many EDs, the triage nurse may also decide ultimate placement of the patient within the department.

Additionally, hospital crowding has increased internationally which, in turn, has increased focus on triage and ED intake processes.[3–5] Novel throughput strategies in many facilities have led to the work of the triage nurse and the triage team as it is today.

The triage concept dates back to the French military, who designated a "clearing hospital" for wounded soldiers. After World War II, triage came to mean the process quickly identifying those most likely to return to battle after medical intervention. This sorting process directed medical resources toward soldiers who could fight again. During subsequent military conflicts, triage was refined to accomplish the "greatest good for the greatest number of wounded or injured men."[6]

The concept of ED triage was introduced in the 1950s when the volume of patients seeking emergency care started increasing. More and more patients were presenting with nonurgent complaints, and the process of seeing patients according to time of arrival was no longer feasible. Because EDs manage an increased number of patients seeking emergency care, a system for rapid, accurate triage upon presentation is critical to patient safety.

In 2017, with the publication of the second edition of *Emergency Nursing: Scope and Standards of Practice*[1] and for the first time in the history of nursing, the American Nurses Association approved a variation to typical nursing standard formatting by allowing the inclusion of triage as a formal standard, unique to emergency nursing practice. Competencies in the triage standard include understanding triage legalities, prioritizing patients using a valid and reliable system, communicating and collaborating with the ED team to enhance patient care, educating patients, and improving triage processes both in the moment as needed and long-term when appropriate.[1] The rest of this chapter addresses considerations specific to triage standards and competencies as found in *Emergency Nursing: Scope and Standards of Practice*.[1]

LEGAL CONSIDERATIONS

Emergency Medical Treatment and Active Labor Act

In 1986 the US Congress passed the Emergency Medical Treatment and Labor Act (EMTALA)[7] to ensure access to emergency care regardless of an individual's ability to pay. EMTALA was enacted in response to reports of hospitals "dumping" or transferring patients to other facilities because of the inability to pay for care. EMTALA obligates hospitals receiving Medicare funding to provide a medical screening examination (MSE) to every patient presenting for care to determine whether an emergency medical condition exists. The Centers for Medicare and Medicaid Services define medical screening examination as being separate from the triage process.[8] Facility bylaws must clearly identify individuals approved to complete the MSE. Allowing ED RNs to perform MSE depends on state nursing scope of practice, hospital medical bylaws, and training. If an emergency condition is identified, the patient must be stabilized within the facility's capabilities before transfer. If the patient cannot be stabilized and requires care beyond the hospital's capabilities or the patient requests a transfer, an appropriate transfer can be arranged.

Health Insurance Portability and Accountability Act

In 1996 the Health Insurance Portability and Accountability Act (HIPAA)[9] was enacted to protect certain aspects of health information, including the privacy and security of patient's personal health record. Privacy protection extends to information shared verbally and via technology such as fax transmissions and electronic health records. Triage nurses need to be aware of HIPAA protections when working in public spaces, such as the hallway care or reassessments in the waiting room. Calling a patient's name aloud in a crowded waiting room is NOT a HIPAA violation. Once the patient responds, asking about the complaint while walking to a treatment space might be a violation. The triage nurse must be aware of HIPAA laws and make every attempt to maintain patient privacy, including protected information.

ABILITY TO PRIORITIZE

The ability to prioritize patient care begins with qualifications of the triage nurse. Triage is not just an ED nursing staff assignment. It is a specialized role performed best by an experienced nurse who has also had a formal orientation with didactic and clinical components.

The triage nurse is a vital member of the ED health care team who is the first clinician greeting more than 80% of ED patients.[10] On the basis of a brief triage assessment, the triage nurse determines who goes directly to care and who waits to be seen. This decision has patient safety implications; undertriage can delay needed patient care, and overtriage may use a treatment space needed more urgently by someone else. Therefore the triage nurse must have the knowledge, experience, and temperament necessary to function in a high-stress role.

The triage nurse must remain professional at all times and manage multiple tasks simultaneously while communicating with patients, visitors, staff, and the ED charge nurse. The triage nurse has the opportunity to provide reassurance, begin to address the patient and family's/caregiver's concerns, and set expectations about time to treatment. To function effectively, the triage nurse must possess expert assessment skills, demonstrate competent interview and organizational skills, maintain an extensive knowledge base of diseases and injuries, and use past experiences to identify subtle clues to patient acuity. Patients with an obvious critical condition do not present the greatest challenge to the triage nurse. The true test of a competent triage nurse is his or her ability to think critically and to recognize the subtle signs and symptoms of a low-volume but high-risk presentation.

The complexity of the triage role led to the recommendation from the Emergency Nurses Association (ENA) for a nurse to have at least 1 year of emergency nursing experience before being oriented to the triage role.[11] The emergency nurse functioning in the triage role should have successfully completed continuing education in trauma, cardiac, and pediatric care, as well as verification in subspecialty courses, which may include advanced life support, geriatric, obstetric, neurologic, burn, and/or mental health care. In addition, obtaining emergency nursing certification is preferred.[11]

The ENA's position statement on triage qualification and competency suggests formal evidence-based triage orientation to improve the triage nurse's effectiveness and comfort in the role.[11] Written protocols assist in decision making, and a clinical orientation with an experienced triage preceptor gives the novice triage nurse an opportunity to ask questions, review cases, and become comfortable with the role. Ongoing competency evaluation includes observation, chart review, continuing education, and remediation, as needed.

In addition to emergency nursing experience and formal training recommendations, a triage nurse may be more successful if he or she is aware of anchoring, stigma, and bias.[12] Because the triage nurse is often the first ED staff member to ask questions and clarify patient concerns, decisions made during triage can affect the trajectory of the entire ED visit. If a triage nurse anchors to a part of a patient complaint, the entire team could be subject to following the initial triage direction. Whether unconscious, intentional, or perceived, unfair beliefs causing stigma or bias can similarly lead to over- or undertriage and jeopardize quality patient care.[12]

Triage Process

The triage process is the rapid collection of relevant subjective and objective data so that the triage nurse can assign an accurate acuity rating. It should be brief and occur soon after the patient arrives at the ED. The triage process begins with an across-the-room assessment. The triage nurse uses all senses to gather vital information: sight, hearing, and smell. See Table 8.1. Occasionally the patient's need for immediate care is determined from the across-the-room assessment. At that point, the triage process is over and the patient is taken directly to the treatment area. This generally occurs for only a small number of patients. Most other patients receive a triage interview to collect further information about the patient's concern and condition.

In a two-tiered triage system, the first nurse is performing an across-the-room assessment as well as determining the patient's chief complaint. On the basis of this information, the first triage nurse decides whether the patient needs to be taken directly to a care area or is stable enough to participate in a triage interview, step two of a two-tiered triage process.

Triage Interview

The patient is brought to a dedicated room or area where the triage interview helps gather additional information about the patient's illness or injury. The triage interview should begin with the nurse confirming the patient's identity, introducing himself or herself to the patient, and explaining the purpose of the triage process.

The patient's chief complaint should be documented in his or her own words using quotation marks. Some patients need to be asked directly, "What made you come to the emergency department today?" or "What made you call the ambulance?" Once the chief complaint has been determined, the triage nurse can proceed with a brief interview to elicit information about the chief complaint, including relevant signs and symptoms.

Gathering appropriate subjective information is vital to making the correct triage acuity rating decision. If the triage nurse does not clearly understand the patient, follow-up questions and clarification are needed. Obtaining information can be a challenge when the patient provides vague or global reasons for the visit: "I've been so sick," or "My doctor told me to come here." The triage nurse must focus the investigation on the history of the complaint and the related symptoms and signs. The PQRST mnemonic is one example of a systematic approach to patient assessment. See Table 8.2.

TABLE 8.1 **Across-the-Room Assessment.**

Sense	Category	Examples or Specifics
Sight	Sick or not sick	
	Obvious deformities/amputations	Child with a craniofacial abnormality Severe kyphosis
	Method of arrival	Walked in, carried, wheelchair
	Body habitus	Tall, short, cachectic, thin, obese
	Dress	Appropriate Clean, disheveled
	Chronic illness	Bald due to chemotherapy, pursed-lip breathing from chronic obstructive pulmonary disease
	Activity level	Walking with no difficulty, walking bent over, holding abdomen Using an assistive device (e.g., cane)
	Obvious blood on clothing, skin	
	Breathing	Obvious respiratory distress, working hard Using home oxygen
	Skin color	Severe jaundice
	Level of consciousness	Crying, moaning, laughing, talking, lethargic
Hearing	Breathing	Wheezing, stridor, grunting
	Speech	Tone, cadence, volume, language spoken, slurred
Smell	Stool, urine, vomit	Incontinence, illness related
	Ketones	Diabetic
	Alcohol, cigarettes	
	Poor hygiene	Living situation may need assessment
	Pus	Infection
	Chemicals	Exposure—skin, clothing

The triage nurse should use a variety of open (eliciting feelings and perceptions) and closed (factual, "yes/no") questions to obtain information. Closed-ended questions such as, "Do you have any allergies?" are helpful for obtaining basic information. To elicit details, open-ended questions are more effective. See examples in Tables 8.2 and 8.3. Restating, verbalizing observations, sharing information, actively listening, and summarizing are important communication strategies. The nurse's style will vary with each patient and situation.

A medical interpreter should be used when the patient does not speak English or is more comfortable speaking in his or her native language. All hospitals must provide medical interpreters, either in person or using technology such as telephone or video services for non–English-speaking patients.[13] Using family members can be problematic because the family member may not understand medical terminology and the patient is sharing personal, potentially private information. The triage nurse should document when a professional medical interpreter or family member was used to gather the history.

The triage process lasts only minutes. Organized and efficient assessment is critical. The triage nurse must be able to multitask or delegate specific tasks to ancillary personnel.

When sufficient information has been obtained about the chief complaint and related symptoms, the triage nurse may need to obtain other information to determine a triage acuity, such as current medications, past medical history, allergies, last menstrual period, or immunizations. Medication usage needed to determine a triage acuity could include prescribed or over-the-counter medications, herbal preparations, or home remedies.

TABLE 8.2 **PQRST Mnemonic.**

Component	Sample Questions
P (provokes)	What provokes the symptom? What makes it better? What makes it worse?
Q (quality)	What does it feel like?
R (radiation)	Where is it? Where does it go? Is it in one or more spots?
S (severity)	If we gave it a number from 0 to 10, with 0 being none and 10 being the worst you can imagine, what is your rating?
T (time)	How long have you had the symptom? When did it start? When did it end? How long did it last? Does it come and go?

At this point, the triage nurse will perform a brief, focused physical assessment based on the patient's current injury or

TABLE 8.3 Examples of Patient Interview Questions.

Event	Triage Questioning
Minor burn	• Cause or mechanism of the burn • Location and depth of the burn • Extent of the burn • Treatment before arrival
Motor vehicle collision, not life-threatening	• When did the event occur? • Ambulatory at the scene? • Speed of the vehicle • Driver, passenger front or back • Seat belt use, airbag deployed • Vehicle damage • Current complaints
Fall	• When did this occur? • Current complaints • Fall—from what onto what? • Why do you think you fell? (e.g., dizzy before fall)
Sports-related injury	• Describe what happened • Were you wearing a helmet or other protective equipment? • Loss of consciousness? • Ambulatory at the scene? • Current complaints

TABLE 8.4 Examples of Focused Physical Assessment.

Chief Complaint	Focused Assessment
Short of breath	Respiratory rate, depth, effort Accessory muscle use Skin color Oxygen saturation Peak flow Level of consciousness Position Ability to talk in full sentences Abnormal sounds
Injured arm	Deformity, angulation Color, capillary refill, pulse Sensation Movement—ROM
Finger laceration	Wound length, depth, location Shape, swelling CSM, tendon involvement Evidence of foreign material Bleeding, bruising
Itchy eyes	Signs of inflammation, drainage Tearing, photophobia Visual acuity
Arm weakness	Level of consciousness Glasgow Coma Scale Facial symmetry Pronator drift Speech clarity and articulation Hand grasp strength Pupils—size and reaction

CSM, Circulation, sensation, and motor; *ROM,* range of motion.

illness. See Table 8.4. The purpose of the assessment is to gather additional information supporting the triage nurse's decision. The triage assessment is brief and should not require the patient to undress. The primary ED nurse will do a more in-depth assessment when the patient is taken to a treatment area.

Vital Signs and Triage

EDs have traditionally required a full set of vital signs on all patients as part of the triage process. Even so, care should never be delayed because vital signs have not been obtained, and patients with emergent needs must be taken immediately to a treatment area. Alternately, some EDs have chosen to document a full set of vital signs on all lower acuity patients. Documentation of stable vital signs provides additional data to support the triage acuity rating. In the most recent study of its kind, vital signs changed the level of triage acuity in only 8% of cases.[14] The triage nurse must be aware of normal parameters for age, the effect of medications, and certain disease processes.

VALID RELIABLE TRIAGE SYSTEMS

There is no single type of triage system used by all EDs. On the basis of an "across-the-room assessment," brief patient interview, and focused examination, the triage nurse assigns an acuity rating. As triage has evolved, recognition of high interrater reliability as a necessary characteristic of an effective triage acuity rating system has increased. With the publication of research questioning the reliability of a three-level acuity rating system and concerns about ED crowding, the American College of Emergency Physicians (ACEP) and the ENA convened a five-level triage task force to review the evidence on five-level triage scales. As a result of this effort, both ACEP and ENA recommend the use of a validated five-level triage acuity tool.[1,11,15] Although many are available and even more are being developed worldwide, there four commonly used triage tools: Australasian Triage Scale (ATS), Canadian Triage Acuity Scale (CTAS), Emergency Severity Index (ESI), and Manchester Triage Scale (MTS).

Australasian Triage Scale

ATS has been in use in all Australian EDs since 1994. Triage acuity levels in ATS are based upon patient's presenting complaints and related assessment. The five levels are associated with maximum waiting times spanning from immediate needs to waiting 120 minutes at the fifth and least urgent level.[16] With strong studies supporting reliability and validity,[17] ATS also includes special considerations for reevaluation, as well as pediatric, obstetric, ophthalmic, and mental health patients. Training materials are available from the Australian Department of Health.

Canadian Triage Acuity Scale

The CTAS, which is based on the Australasian Triage Scale, was developed by a group of Canadian emergency physicians working with the National Emergency Nurses Association (Canada).[18] All Canadian EDs use this valid, reliable five-level acuity rating system.[19] The system mandates that every patient presenting for care should be at least visually assessed within 10 minutes of presentation. For each triage level, there is a list of presenting complaints or conditions. The ED RN assigns acuity based on the chief complaint and a focused subjective and objective assessment. CTAS identifies time to physician for each triage level but recognizes that meeting this time objective 100% of the time is not realistic.[18] Reassessment times are identified for each of the five triage acuity levels. Training materials are available from the Canadian Association of Emergency Physicians (http://ctas-phctas.ca).

Emergency Severity Index

The ESI is a five-level triage scale categorizing patients initially by acuity for emergent and high-risk patients and then by expected resource consumption required for providers to make a disposition decision for the lower acuity levels.[20] Research has demonstrated ESI as a valid and reliable system.[21] ESI, unlike other five-level triage systems, does not recommend times associated with each acuity level and does not specifically associate each level with a standard color.[20] Training materials, including the algorithm and implementation handbook with pediatric-specific considerations, are available free of charge from the ESI Triage group, (https://www.esitriage.com/educational-materials/).

Manchester Triage Scale

The MTS, developed in England, is widely used throughout Europe. MTS includes 52 complaint-specific charts assisting the triage nurse by guiding questioning from most critical to least urgent for each complaint.[22] Despite the marked difference associated with using complaint-based charts, MTS has been shown to be a reliable and valid triage acuity rating scale.[23] As with ATS and CTAS, MTS assigns time goals for provider evaluation after arrival and assigns standardized colors to each acuity level. Training materials are available from the Manchester Triage Group (https://www.triagenet.net/classroom/).

IMMEDIATE BEDDING

Whether because of an across-the-room assessment of a critically ill patient or because there is space and a provider available, the next step is getting the patient to the right place. Immediate bedding requires communication with the department's patient placement person. In some cases, this may be a specialized role, or it may be done by the charge nurse. Some departments use the triage nurse to place patients.

Once a location has been determined, it is also the responsibility of the triage nurse to facilitate the patient reaching the treatment area. This may involve physically escorting the patient and family to the treatment space or delegating the task to another member of the team.

"Pull-Until-Full" Immediate Bedding

When physical ED treatment spaces are available, a throughput measure to decrease the time between ED arrival and ED provider evaluation is direct bedding, also referred to as a pull-until-full system. The ENA's *Topic Brief* on ED throughput[24] suggests that a pull-until-full method also increases the triage team's availability to provide direct patient care.

TRIAGE DOCUMENTATION

How much information should the triage nurse gather and document about each patient? This is a question many EDs struggle with because of requests for increased screening of patients who present to the ED for care. Requested screenings include fall risk, smoking, drug and alcohol use, suicidality, human trafficking, and domestic violence. Every ED should have a documentation policy or guideline detailing departmental required screening elements. At a minimum, the triage nurse should document enough information to support the triage acuity rating assigned to the patient. The elements of triage documentation generally include

- time and date of triage interview
- two patient identifiers (guided by hospital policy)
- chief complaint
- brief subjective and objective assessment based on complaint
- vital signs, usually including pain scores (for lower-acuity patients)
- triage acuity rating
- interventions initiated, including medications, laboratory testing, or imaging
- RN signature, if using a paper-based system

For stable patients who do not need to go directly to a treatment area, the triage nurse may gather more detailed information, such as

- allergies
- weight
- last menstrual period
- medications—including prescriptions, over-the-counter, and herbals
- past medical history
- immunization status
- mode of arrival

Triage documentation is often standardized through the use of an electronic medical record. This method may eliminate duplication of information because the data flow throughout the continuum of care. Electronic documentation may force entry of certain data elements to advance to the next screen. If a paper record is being used for triage, the form should be as user-friendly as possible to expedite patient care by saving time in the documentation process. Check boxes in documentation may serve as reminders to triage nurses about certain information to gather. Regardless of the system, triage documentation provides a "snapshot" of the patient's chief complaint, appearance, and acuity upon arrival.

SPECIAL CONSIDERATIONS

Changing Triage Acuity Score

A concept often causing confusion is that of changing the initial triage acuity score assignment. Remember, the purpose of triage is to provide a snapshot of the patient's condition upon arrival. The need for a triage acuity score is over when the provider evaluates the patient. If the patient's condition improves before provider evaluation, the presentation did not change and therefore the initial triage acuity should not be changed. Regardless of the triage system being used, triage acuity scores should not get changed UNLESS the patient's condition deteriorates while waiting. If diagnostic interventions return concerning results BUT the patient's condition has not changed, the triage acuity does not get changed.[25] Triage acuity scores are not intended to be used as department census tracking. Again, triage acuity scores provide a glimpse of the patient's condition upon ED arrival.

Infection Prevention

One role of the triage nurse is to identify the patient with a potential infectious disease, institute the appropriate infection control measures, document the situation, and then work with the charge nurse to get the patient to an appropriate treatment area.

The Joint Commission National Patient Safety Goals focus on reduction of the risk for health care–associated infections.[26] Infection prevention begins during triage with strict adherence to hand hygiene guidelines. Hand hygiene with soap and water or an alcohol-based hand rub is essential before and after every patient contact.

To prevent the spread of any respiratory infection, the Centers for Disease Control recommends all patients presenting to the ED with a cough should be asked to wear a surgical or procedure mask to prevent the spread of droplets to others.[27] In addition to hand hygiene, respiratory hygiene and cough etiquette must be emphasized. Having waiting rooms with tissues available for patients and visitors, as well as a place to dispose of any waste, are ways of working toward effective infection prevention. Waiting rooms with toys must have an established system for cleaning to prevent the spread of infection.

Infectious disease screening is a routine part of any triage assessment. Does this person potentially have an infection easily transmitted to other patients, staff, or visitors? Does the patient have symptoms of tuberculosis? Does the patient have a cough, fever, and diarrhea or a possibly communicable rash? Has the patient been traveling out of the country recently or exposed to anyone else who has a communicable disease?

Some ED patients are immunosuppressed from chemotherapy, radiation, or a disease process, making them more susceptible to infection. Every effort should be made to protect and isolate them from patients in the general waiting room. They should be separated from potentially ill patients and taken as quickly as possible to a treatment room with appropriately instituted isolation precautions.

Ambulance Triage

In 2015 about 15% of patients seen in US EDs were transported by ambulance.[2] Most EDs have a separate ambulance triage area. The triage process for ambulance patients should be exactly the same as it is for "walk-in" patients: an across-the-room assessment, followed by a brief subjective and objective assessment, and assignment of an acuity rating. The triage nurse should assess the ambulance patient who does not need to be seen immediately and decide if it would be appropriate for the patient to wait in the waiting room. Method of transportation to an ED should not determine how quickly the patient is seen.

The Pediatric Patient

The triage nurse must be able to rapidly and accurately identify children who need immediate care. Infants and children are small and portable, so when they are seriously ill or injured, they may be brought to the ED by car rather than by ambulance. For a variety of reasons, emergency nurses often feel uncomfortable triaging children, which can lead to either overtriage or undertriage.[28] To safely triage the pediatric population, the triage nurse must understand normal growth and development to quickly identify deviations.[29] Knowledge of developmental milestones assists the triage nurse with both subjective and objective assessments. A school-age child can tell the nurse if he or she is having pain. An adolescent can give the triage nurse a detailed history. The triage nurse must be familiar with illnesses or injuries prevalent in the pediatric age group.

The ENA Emergency Nursing Pediatric Course outlines the components of comprehensive pediatric triage. This includes the pediatric assessment triangle, the history, and physical examination.[29]

The pediatric assessment triangle is the first step of the assessment process and is a more clearly defined across-the-room assessment. The triage nurse uses his or her senses, forms a general impression, and then assesses work of breathing and circulation to the skin, usually without the child being aware of being observed.[29] See Table 8.5. This quick assessment is used to decide whether the child goes directly to a treatment area or is stable enough to continue the triage process.

If no life-threatening emergencies are identified using the pediatric assessment triangle, the triage nurse will begin the subjective and objective assessment. The Emergency Nursing Pediatric Course identifies the components for the history, primary assessment, and secondary assessment. This concept is no longer taught in ENPC. Please remove sentence. The 5th edition was released after submitting the final file.[29] The triage nurse also needs to be familiar with common pediatric red flags indicating a serious problem when found during the triage assessment. See Box 8.1. The history is obtained from the parent or caregiver who knows the infant or child best and can share with the triage nurse his or her concerns and impressions. For the child with disabilities, it is the caregiver who is most likely to notice subtle signs or changes suggesting a problem. The verbal child can answer specific questions

TABLE 8.5 The Pediatric Assessment Triangle.

General impression	Does the child look ill? Is the child playful? Is the child aware of surroundings? Is the child alert? Crying? Sleepy or unresponsive? What is the child's interaction with the environment and caregiver?
Work of breathing	What is the position of comfort to facilitate air entry? Are there audible airway sounds? Is the child coughing? Drooling? How is the child breathing? Is the respiratory rate slow, normal, or rapid for age? Are there signs of accessory muscle use?
Circulation to skin	Is the child's skin color pale, dusky, cyanotic, mottled, or flushed? Is here any obvious bleeding? Is the child diaphoretic?

Emergency Nurses Association. *Emergency Nursing Pediatric Course: Provider Manual.* 5th ed. Des Plaines, IL: Emergency Nurses Association; 2020.

posed by the triage nurse such as, "What happened?" or "Does it hurt?"

Finally, before assigning a triage acuity, the triage nurse must evaluate vital signs and question whether they are within the normal range for this infant or child. If they are abnormal, can the variation be readily explained? For example, a heart rate of 160 beats per minute is normal in a neonate, but this same rate in a toddler, even an ill or injured toddler, is a major concern.

The Geriatric Patient

People aged 65 and older in 2015 made up under 10% of the US population but accounted for over 30% of all ED visits.[2] The average life expectancy for both males and females is continuing to increase, and many are living with chronic medical problems requiring complex polypharmaceutical therapy. The triage interview may be more difficult as the older adult patient may have multiple complaints or vague complaints, or may not be able to tell the triage nurse why the ambulance was called.[30] Additional information should be obtained from emergency medical services, the sending facility, or the family.

- Older adults will often present with atypical signs and symptoms of common medical problems. For example, a change in level of consciousness may be the first sign of an infection.
- The effect of medications on vital signs must be considered.
- Interactions during triage are also an opportunity to screen for elder abuse and neglect.

BOX 8.1 Pediatric Red Flags.

In addition to abnormal vital signs, the triage nurse should be aware of the following pediatric red flags:

- Abnormal airway sounds such as stridor
- Grunting
- Increased work of breathing (using accessory muscles or retracting)
- Capillary refill greater than 2 seconds
- Sunken or bulging fontanel
- Change in level of consciousness
- Severe pain or distress
- Petechiae

Emergency Nurses Association. *Emergency Nursing Pediatric Course: Provider Manual.* 5th ed. Des Plaines, IL: Emergency Nurses Association; 2020.

Patients With Behavioral Health Concerns

Patients with a behavioral health history or new onset of symptoms usually present to the ED when coping mechanisms fail. They may self-present or may be brought in by family, friends, or police. Occasionally, the patient arrives in handcuffs or is restrained to an ambulance stretcher. This patient typically goes directly to a secure treatment area.

Triage of the behavioral health patient begins with the across-the-room assessment, which can provide the triage nurse important information. Bizarre dress, loud or rapid speech, odor of alcohol, demeanor, and activity level can be determined. On the basis of the across-the-room assessment, the triage nurse decides if the patient goes directly to a treatment area or if the patient can go through a more comprehensive triage assessment. The priority concern with impulsive patients is staff and patient safety: Is this patient a danger to himself or herself, others, or the environment? The experienced triage nurse will have security on standby in the ED, will quickly establish rapport with the patient, and will assess for both patient and staff safety. Questions may include the following[31]:

- Have you thought about hurting yourself or others?
  - If the answer is yes, determine whether the patient has a plan and whether the patient has the means to carry out the plan.
  - Use of a valid, reliable suicide risk assessment tool is highly recommended.[32]
- Do you have anything with you that can hurt you or me?
- Have you ever been hospitalized for any medical or emotional problems?
- What medications do you take, and are you taking them?
- When asking about substances: How much? How often? Last used or last drink?
  - Occasionally patients presenting to the ED decided to stop drinking or using drugs and may already be tachycardic and showing signs of withdrawal.
- When auditory, tactile, or visual hallucinations are suspected, confirm with the patient.
- Is the patient making any paranoid statements?

- Describe the patient's appearance, behavior, motor activity, and speech.
  - For example, is the patient making eye contact and answering questions appropriately?

The Obstetric Patient

Triage of the patient with obstetric concerns can be standardized or as varied as the nurse providing care. Some EDs have collaborated with obstetric partners to standardize triage care and decision making. This may include protocols for brief ED screening leading to intrafacility transfer to the obstetric unit OR may include protocols for fetal heart tones done in the ED for patients early in pregnancy.

The American College of Obstetricians and Gynecologists recommends use of a standardized, valid, reliable tool, such as the Maternal–Fetal Triage Index (MFTI) developed by Association of Women's Health, Obstetric and Neonatal Nurses.[33] MFTI is a five-level triage tool incorporating vital signs, life-threatening presentations, imminent delivery, or a need for a higher level of care.[33] Regardless of the triage tool used, the triage nurse's awareness of obstetric complications during all stages of pregnancy enhances the safety of both the patient and the unborn patient.

IMPLEMENTING DIAGNOSTICS AND INTERVENTIONS

Triage Care

The extent of care provided by the triage team varies from one ED to another and often depends on the availability of an appropriate treatment area. The triage nurse will not only often provide initial interventions for patients (such as ice, elevation, and immobilization of an injured extremity) but also may be expected to obtain patient information about the ED care to expect during the visit. When patients present with a bloody cloth wrapped around an injury or wound, the triage nurse should remove the makeshift dressing, assess the extent of the wound, and apply an appropriate dressing. Implementing specific complaint-based interventions for waiting ED patients is recommended by ENA[1,11,34] when allowed by local and state rules.

Many EDs have nurse-initiated triage protocols or standing orders authorizing nurses to initiate care before a provider evaluation. Protocols may include diagnostic testing (laboratory, radiographs, and electrocardiograms [ECGs]) or can be for the administration of medications for fever or pain if the patient meets predetermined criteria. Triage protocols are developed by the department and approved by the medical staff. Once the triage assessment is complete, the triage nurse may choose to implement an appropriate protocol. The goal of protocols is to decrease the patient's length of stay, increase patient and staff satisfaction, and decrease the number of patients who choose to leave without being seen.[34]

REASSESSMENT OF PATIENTS WAITING

In this era of crowding and longer wait times, EDs must have a recheck or reassessment protocol ensuring that patients waiting have not experienced a deterioration of condition. When the waiting room is full, the department is busy; a triage reassessment policy stating all patients will be reassessed within a specific time frame may be unrealistic. Each ED should have a process for reassessing and documenting patients waiting to be seen.

MODIFYING THE TRIAGE PROCESS

At times, ED circumstances require a modification from standard procedure. Once the triage acuity is determined, the triage nurse advocates for the patient's needs and works to create space for those needs. This fluid just-in-time process improvement is called "finding the momentary fit."[35] The triage nurse finds momentary fit because of capacity issues, when confronting colleagues disagreeing with a triage decision, or when reassessment causes an up-triage.

Telephone Triage

Telephone calls eliciting medical advice are problematic for EDs because evaluation of patients by telephone is difficult. Most EDs have a strict policy directing staff to inform the caller to hang up and dial 9-1-1 for a life-threatening condition. For other questions, the caller can be politely informed the ED does not provide medical advice over the telephone and the patient is welcome to come to the ED to be seen. The ENA position statement on telephone triage states that nurses do not give advice over the phone unless formal training and protocols are in place.[36]

Disaster Triage

In the event of a catastrophic occurrence, when the number of incoming patients exceeds the capabilities of a department, a system of disaster triage is activated. Disaster triage begins at the scene of the disaster and patients are retriaged upon arrival to the hospital. Standard ED triage systems are not the same as disaster triage systems, such as START triage.[37] Disaster triage is similar to military triage with a goal of providing the greatest good for the greatest number of ill or injured. In a disaster, the triage process is very rapid and includes a brief assessment of airway, breathing, perfusion, and mental status. Through an algorithm that overrides clinical judgment, patients are assigned to one of four categories.[37,38] The disaster triage team must be aware of limited resources, understanding that some patients are not salvageable. See Chapter 17.

TRIAGE PROCESS IMPROVEMENT

EDs should closely examine their intake or "front-end" process to ensure that it provides for patient and staff safety while maximizing efficiency. Delays at triage can lead to a longer patient length of stay. ED leadership must measure and evaluate throughput issues and multiple time metrics such as triage acuity accuracy, left without being seen (LWBS) rates, door to provider, and door to diagnostics, including ECGs. Every ED should continually look at each step of its entry process for ways to increase efficiency and facilitate flow of patients into the department.

SUMMARY

EDs continue to be the safety net of the US health care system. The role of the triage nurse will continue to be vital to safety and efficiency. The triage nurse remains the initial contact for the patient and family in their ED experience and, more importantly, can directly affect patient outcome. Although approaches vary, the common ingredient of successful triage requires an experienced, competent ED RN.

REFERENCES

1. Emergency Nurses Association. *Emergency Nursing: Scope and Standards of Practice*. 2nd ed. Des Plaines, IL: Emergency Nurses Association; 2017.
2. Centers for Disease Control and Prevention. *National Hospital Ambulatory Medical Care Survey: 2015 Emergency Department Summary Tables*. Centers for Disease Control and Prevention website. https://www.cdc.gov/nchs/fastats/emergency-department.htm. Accessed April 8, 2019.
3. Yarmohammadian MH, Rezaei F, Haghshenas A, Tavakoli N. 2017. Overcrowding in emergency departments: a review of strategies to decrease future challenges. *J Res Med Sci*. 2017;22:23.
4. Barish RA, Mcgauly PL, Arnold TC. Emergency room crowding: a marker of hospital health. *Trans Am Clin Climatol Assoc*. 2012;123:304.
5. Staines M. New figures reveal record hospital overcrowding in 2017. https://www.newstalk.com/Irish-hospitals-continue-to-face-record-overcrowding. Published Aug 9, 2017. Accessed April 8, 2019.
6. US Department of Defense. *Emergency war surgery*. Washington, DC: U.S. Government Printing Office; 1975.
7. Centers for Medicare and Medicaid Services. Emergency Medical Treatment and Active Labor Act (EMTALA). Centers for Medicare and Medicaid Services website. https://www.cms.gov/Regulations-and-Guidance/Legislation/EMTALA/. Published March 26, 2012. Accessed April 8, 2019.
8. Centers for Medicare and Medicaid Services. *State Operations Manual, Appendix V—Interpretive Guidelines—Responsibilities of Medicare Participating Hospitals in Emergency Cases*. https://www.cms.gov/Regulations-and-Guidance/Guidance/Manuals/Downloads/som107ap_v_emerg.pdf. Published July 16, 2010.
9. US Department of Health and Human Services. *Summary of the HIPAA Security Rule*. US Department of Health and Human Services website. https://www.hhs.gov/hipaa/for-professionals/security/laws-regulations/index.html. Published July 26, 2013.
10. Augustine JJ. *Emergency Medical Services Arrivals, Admission Rates to the Emergency Department Analyzed*. ACEP Now. ACEP Now website. https://www.acepnow.com/article/emergency-medical-services-arrivals-admission-rates-emergency-department-analyzed/. Published December 17, 2014.
11. Emergency Nurses Association. *Triage Qualifications and Competency*. https://www.ena.org/docs/default-source/resource-library/practice-resources/position-statements/triagequalificationscompetency.pdf?sfvrsn=a0bbc268_8. Published 2017.
12. Foley AL, James-Salwey J. Stigma, anchoring, and triage decisions. *J Emerg Med*. 2016;42(1):87–88. https://doi.org/10.1016/j.jen.2015.09.014.
13. US Department of Justice. *ADA Requirements: Effective Communication*. https://www.ada.gov/effective-comm.htm. Published January 2014. Accessed April 8, 2019.
14. Cooper R, Flaherty H, Lin E, et al. Effect of vital signs on triage decisions. *Ann Emerg Med*. 2002;39(3):223.
15. American College of Emergency Physicians and the Emergency Nurses Association. *Triage Scale Standardization*. https://www.ena.org/docs/default-source/resource-library/practice-resources/position-statements/supported-statements/triage-scale-standardization.pdf?sfvrsn=a940caa_4. Published September 2017. Updated January 2017. Accessed April 8, 2019.
16. Australian Government Department of Health. ATS categories. http://www.health.gov.au/internet/publications/publishing.nsf/Content/triageqrg~triageqrg-ATS. Updated January 21, 2013.
17. Ebrahimi M, Heydari A, Mazlom R, Mirhaghi A. The reliability of the Australasian triage scale: a meta-analysis. *World J Emerg Med*. 2015;6(2):94.
18. Canadian Association of Emergency Physicians. *The Canadian Triage and Acuity Scale Combined Adult/Paediatric Educational Program: Participant's Manual*. 2012. http://ctas-phctas.ca/wp-content/uploads/2018/05/participant_manual_v2.5b_november_2013_0.pdf.
19. Mirhaghi A, Heydari A, Mazlom R, Ebrahimi M. The reliability of the Canadian Triage and Acuity Scale: meta-analysis. *N Am J Med Sci*. 2015;7(7):299. http://ctas-phctas.ca/wp-content/uploads/2018/05participant_manualv2.5b_november_2013_0.pdf%20https://www.ncbi.nlm.nih.gov/pmc/articles.PMC4525387/.
20. Gilboy N, Tanabe P, Travers DA, et al. *Emergency Severity Index, Version 4: Implementation Handbook* AHRQ publication No. 05-0046-2. Rockville, MD: Agency for Healthcare Research and Quality; 2012.
21. Mirhaghi A, Heydari A, Mazlom R, Hasanzadeh F. 2015. Reliability of the emergency severity index: meta-analysis. *Sultan Qaboos Univ Med J*. 2015;15(1):e71.
22. *Manchester Triage System*. https://www.triagenet.net/classroom/. Published August 9, 2018. Accessed April 8, 2019.
23. Mirhaghi A, Mazlom R, Heydari A, Ebrahimi M. The reliability of the Manchester Triage System (MTS): a meta-analysis. *J Evid Based Med*. 2017;10(2):129–135.
24. Emergency Nurses Association. Topic brief: Emergency department throughput. https://www.ena.org/docs/default-source/resource-library/practice-resources/topic-briefs/ed-throughput.pdf. Published May 2017. Accessed April 8, 2019.
25. Foley A. Triage process and department practice are different. *J Emerg Nurs*. 2017;43(2):185–186.
26. The Joint Commission. *Hospital National Patient Safety Goals*; 2018. https://www.jointcommission.org/assets/1/6/2018_HAP_NPSG_goals._final.pdf. Accessed April 8, 2019.
27. Centers for Disease Control and Prevention. Respiratory hygiene/cough etiquette in healthcare settings. Centers for Disease Control and Prevention website. https://www.cdc.gov/flu/professionals/infectioncontrol/resphygiene.htm. Published February 27, 2012. Accessed April 8, 2019.

28. Hewes HA, Christensen M, Taillac PP, Mann NC, Jacobsen KK, Fenton SJ. Consequences of pediatric undertriage and overtriage in a statewide trauma system. *J Trauma Acute Care Surg*. 2017;83(4):662–667.
29. Emergency Nurses Association. *Emergency Nursing Pediatric Course: Provider Manual*. 4th ed. Des Plaines, IL: Emergency Nurses Association; 2012.
30. Buchanan GS, Kahn DS, Burke H, et al. Trauma team activation for geriatric trauma at a level II trauma center: are the elderly under-triaged? *Marshall J Med*. 2017;3(3):51.
31. Emergency Nurses Association. *Emergency Nursing Core Curriculum*. 7th ed. Des Plaines, IL: Emergency Nurses Association; 2017.
32. The Joint Commission. Quality and Safety. *Perspectives Preview: Special Report: Suicide Prevention in Health Care Settings: Recommendations Regarding Environmental Hazards for Providers and Surveyors*. 2017. https://www.jointcommission.org/issues/article.aspx?Article=GtNpk0ErgGF%2B7J9WOTTkXANZSEPXa1%2BKH0/4kGHCiio%3D. Published October 25, 2017. Accessed April 8, 2019.
33. American College of Obstetricians and Gynecologists. Committee opinion: Hospital-based triage of obstetric patients. https://www.acog.org/Clinical-Guidance-and-Publications/Committee-Opinions/Committee-on-Obstetric-Practice/Hospital-Based-Triage-of-Obstetric-Patients. Updated 2018. Accessed April 8, 2019.
34. Emergency Nurses Association. Position statement: use of protocols in the emergency setting. https://www.ena.org/docs/default-source/resource-library/practice-resources/position-statements/useofprotocolsined.pdf?sfvrsn=43f282ab_6. Published 2015. Accessed April 8, 2019.
35. Reay G, Rankin JA, Then KL. Momentary fitting in a fluid environment: a grounded theory if triage nurse decision making. *Int Emerg Nurs*. 2015. https://doi.org/10.1016/j.ienj.2015.09.006.
36. Emergency Nurses Association. *Telephone Triage*. 2015. Archived by ENA in 2018.
37. US Department of Health and Human Services. *START Adult Triage Algorithm*. 2017. https://chemm.nlm.nih.gov/startadult.htm. Published September 29, 2017.
38. Hong R, Sexton R, Sweet B, Carroll G, Tambussi C, Baumann BM. Comparison of START triage categories to emergency department triage levels to determine need for urgent care and to predict hospitalization. *Am J Disas Med*. 2017;10(1):13–21.

9

Patient Assessment

Vicki Sweet

Emergency nurses, no matter their practice environment, are faced with every possible medical, surgical, traumatic, social, and behavioral health condition. Not only must emergency nurses be competent in managing a broad spectrum of human conditions, but they must also be comfortable in caring for patients who span the age spectrum, from prenatal and neonates to centenarians. Assessment is the first step in the nursing process and is crucial to identifying the nature of each patient's presenting illness or injury, the severity of the problem, and the patient's perception of the issue and their need for and response to intervention. The ability to perform a rapid assessment of both the physical and the behavioral condition of the patient as a whole person is a skill necessary for all emergency nurses. Cultural diversity and sensitivity are also important pieces of patient assessment.

Assessment usually begins when the nurse first visualizes the patient, but it may also begin before the patient's arrival, based on either a report from incoming providers or by simply listening as a patient makes their way to the emergency department (ED). A systematic, standardized approach to the initial evaluation of each patient is essential for immediate recognition of life-threatening conditions, identification of signs or symptoms of specific illness and/or injury, and determination of priorities of care. Box 9.1 describes such a standardized approach to initial assessment using the A-to-I mnemonic as taught in the Emergency Nurses Association's *Trauma Nursing Core Course* (TNCC) and *Emergency Nursing Pediatric Course* (ENPC).

Information collected during the assessment process is both subjective and objective. Subjective data is the information provided by the patient themselves or by the patient's family or significant other. This information may provide a person's perception of the problem. Nurses should be aware that the information the patient or family member has chosen to share may not always be factual; people may omit critical information that assists in the identification and management of the presenting problem. (For example, a patient presenting with tachycardia may or may not volunteer that the pain was precipitated by illicit drug use.) Objective data are considered factual. These are observed or measured findings. Objective assessment data are obtained through the physical assessment process—inspection, auscultation, palpation, percussion, smell—as well as from physiologic measurements, laboratory tests, and other diagnostic studies. Many objective signs are manifestations of specific illnesses and disorders and may indicate the need for a more specific or focused assessment. Objective data may provide an opportunity to clinically validate the patient's subjective information; however, absence of objective data does not necessarily mean that illness or injury does not exist. A thorough emergency nursing assessment will include interpersonal skills, knowledge of anatomy and physiology, and physical assessment skills as well as the ability to apply critical thinking to each patient's unique situation.

This chapter will review general guidelines to be applied to every patient encounter. Detailed assessment and management considerations for specific patient illnesses, injuries, or disorders will be found in the corresponding chapters of this text.

INITIAL ASSESSMENT

Initial assessment is divided into two phases: the primary and secondary assessments (see Box 9.1). The primary assessment is done quickly to ensure that any potentially life-threatening conditions are immediately identified and managed through sequential evaluation of airway, breathing, circulation, disability, and exposure of the patient (the ABCDE portion of the A-I mnemonic). The goal of the secondary assessment, then, is to identify any clinical indicators of illness or injury (the FGHI portion of the mnemonic). Both the primary and secondary assessments can be completed within minutes unless resuscitative measures are required.

Primary Assessment

A general impression of the patient is often formed in the first seconds of the initial contact based on observations of the patient's general appearance (manner of dress, hygiene, color of skin, facial expression), posture and motor activity, quality of speech (normal, slurred, silent, unable to speak), affect and mood, and apparent degree of distress. The nurse makes a quick determination of "sick or not sick." Any unusual odors should be reported as certain conditions are associated with specific odors. Experienced ED nurses are often able to identify gastrointestinal bleeding, diabetic ketoacidosis, or certain infections based on smell alone. Components of the primary assessment are summarized in Table 9.1.

Airway

Evaluation of airway patency includes assessment for vocalization or sounds appropriate for age. If the patient is able to respond to verbal commands, ask the patient to open the mouth for inspection. Otherwise, perform a jaw thrust or a chin lift to observe for tongue obstruction, presence of foreign material, or other visible debris. Evaluate for edema of the lips, mouth, oropharynx, or neck; drooling; and dysphagia and abnormal airway sounds (i.e., stridor). If the airway is obstructed, either partially or totally, immediate intervention is required to restore airway patency. The airway may be maintained using adjuncts such as nasogastric or orogastric tubes or supraglottic airways or by endotracheal intubation. Any compromise in airway patency must be addressed before proceeding to assessment of breathing. Spinal protection is required if cervical spine injury is suspected. In such cases, all airway maneuvers must be accomplished while maintaining the cervical spine in neutral alignment.

BOX 9.1 Components of the Initial Assessment.

Primary Assessment

A Airway with simultaneous cervical spine protection for trauma patients
B Breathing effectiveness
C Circulation effectiveness
D Disability (brief neurologic assessment)
E Exposure/environmental control

Secondary Assessment

F Full set of vitals, focused adjuncts (cardiac monitor, continuous pulse oximetry), facilitate family presence
G Give comfort measures/Get resuscitation adjuncts: LMNOP
- L—Laboratory studies
- M—Monitor cardiac rate and rhythm
- N—Consider placement of nasogastric or orogastric tube
- O—Oxygen and ventilation
- P—Assess pain

H History and head-to-toe assessment
I Inspect posterior surfaces

Breathing

Assessment of breathing includes noting the presence of spontaneous respirations. Evaluate the rate and pattern of breathing as well as the presence of symmetric chest rise and fall. Increased work of breathing is indicated by nasal flaring, retractions, or use of accessory muscles. Note chest wall integrity and skin color, which is an indicator of perfusion. If breathing is absent or ineffective, assisted ventilation is required. Supplemental oxygen should be provided, and the patient should be positioned to maximize ventilation. Address any open chest wounds and ensure interventions to relieve tension pneumothoraces in cases of trauma. Any life-threatening compromise to respiratory status and ventilation must be addressed before proceeding to assessment of circulation.

Circulation

Initial evaluation of circulatory status includes assessment of skin color, temperature, and moisture. Palpate both central and peripheral pulses for rate and quality, especially if circulation appears compromised. If circulation is ineffective, consider the need for chest compressions depending on the clinical condition. Cardiac monitoring and vascular access should be established. In cases of trauma, control external hemorrhage.

Disability

In the primary survey, a brief neurologic assessment should be done to determine the patient's level of consciousness. The AVPU mnemonic is a simple, rapid screening tool:

A Alert: Patient is awake, alert, and responsive to voice and is oriented.
V Verbal: Patient responds to voice but is not fully oriented.
P Pain: Patient does not respond to voice but responds to a painful stimulus.
U Unresponsive: Patient does not respond to voice or painful stimulus.

The pupils should be assessed for size, symmetry, and reactivity to light. If an altered level of consciousness is noted, the nurse should consider possible causes, including medications,

TABLE 9.1 Assessment of the ABCDs.

Component	Description	Action
Airway	Appraise airway patency.	Identify and remove any partial or complete airway obstruction; position airway to maintain patency; insert oropharyngeal or nasopharyngeal airway; protect cervical spine.
Breathing	Determine presence and effectiveness of respiratory efforts. Identify other abnormalities in breathing (e.g., abnormal pattern, abnormal sounds, break in chest wall integrity).	Assist breathing with oxygen therapy, mouth-to-mask ventilation, or bag-mask ventilation; intubate when necessary.
Circulation	Evaluate pulse presence and quality, character, and equality; assess capillary refill, skin color and temperature, and the presence of diaphoresis.	Initiate chest compressions, defibrillation, synchronized cardioversion and medications as indicated; treat dysrhythmias, control bleeding, establish intravenous access, replace lost volume with isotonic crystalloids or blood products.
Disability	Determine level of consciousness.	Identify potential cause of altered level of consciousness, and treat as indicated; assess pupil size and reactivity.

illness, trauma, or behavioral conditions. Specific assessment findings will be covered in later chapters. Any alteration in consciousness requires further investigation during the secondary assessment.

Exposure and Environmental Control

The patient's clothing should be removed during the primary survey so that the nurse can thoroughly examine and identify any signs of illness or injury. It is crucial to provide environmental control, such as warm blankets or increased ambient temperature, to prevent heat loss. Covering the patient maintains dignity and privacy as well as reducing loss of body heat.

Secondary Assessment

Following the pattern of the A-I mnemonic, once emergent needs are addressed, the nurse can complete a secondary assessment. This phase includes measuring vital signs, conducting a pain assessment, taking a history, and performing a head-to-toe assessment, including the posterior surfaces. See Box 9.1.

Full Set of Vital Signs

Vital signs are objective indicators of the patient's current physiologic status. Vital signs are an important part of the continuum and should be measured on an ongoing basis to identify trends. A full set of vital signs may vary according to facility policy, but it usually includes temperature, pulse, and respiratory rates as well as blood pressure (BP), oxygen saturation, and weight. Vital signs may be obtained before the secondary assessment, especially when a team of providers is simultaneously involved in a resuscitation scenario. The astute emergency nurse will recognize and report both subtle and significant alterations in vital signs. When interventions are initiated, appropriate vital signs should be reevaluated to assess the efficacy of treatment. If vital signs are abnormal, the assessment of them should be repeated, especially before a decision is made about the disposition of the patient from the ED.

Temperature. Body temperature is affected by many factors, including physical activity, disease conditions, environmental factors, inflammation, infection, and injury. Temperature measurement should be mandatory for all patients in the ED because deviation from normal temperature may be the only indication of a significant medical problem. Institutional preference for temperature measurement (oral, tympanic, rectal, etc.) as well as the patient's age and condition should be considered when choosing an appropriate measurement site. Some situations may necessitate core temperature measurement via urinary catheter thermistors or esophageal probes. An abnormally high or low temperature reading should always be confirmed by an alternate route, thermometer, or observer.

Pulse. Assessment of the pulse is a physical measurement and involves determination of the heart rate and rhythm (regular or irregular). Note the quality (bounding, normal, weak and thready, or absent) and the equality of the central and peripheral pulses. Reliance on the cardiac monitor gives no indication of the quality or other characteristics of pulses. Cardiac monitors are important because rhythm disturbances may not be identified unless seen on the cardiac monitor. In combination with other objective physical findings, the pulse is an important indicator of cardiovascular function. A slight change in pulse rate is often the first sign that compensatory mechanisms are occurring to maintain homeostasis. In early volume depletion, a healthy person with an intact autonomic nervous system can maintain normal systolic pressures with only one subtle change—a slight increase in pulse rate. Any deviation from the normal range for the patient's age not related to psychological or environmental factors should be considered an indication of an abnormal physiologic condition until proved otherwise.

Respirations. Assess the rate, rhythm, and depth of respirations and the work of breathing. Signs of increased respiratory effort include nasal flaring; suprasternal, intercostal, or substernal retractions; accessory muscle use (neck and abdominal muscles); an inability to speak in complete sentences; and the presence of adventitious sounds. With inspiration, the chest should expand symmetrically on both sides. When pulmonary or chest wall conditions exist, the chest may rise asymmetrically during ventilation. This asymmetry can be seen only with the chest exposed. Other changes in chest contour include funnel chest, pigeon chest, kyphosis, and kyphoscoliosis. Anatomic changes in contour may interfere with normal lung inflation and may exacerbate respiratory conditions.

Oxygen saturation. Oxygen saturation measurement using pulse oximetry is essential for patients with any respiratory or hemodynamic compromise, an altered level of consciousness, or serious illness/injury. Establish a baseline value and continue with ongoing monitoring to detect subtle changes. To ensure accuracy, the pulse oximetry reading should be compared with the radial or apical pulse rate. The readings should always be correlated with the patient's clinical presentation. Inaccurate pulse oximetry readings may occur with hypotension, anemia, extreme peripheral vasoconstriction, hypothermia, carbon monoxide poisoning, and methemoglobinemia. Readings may also be affected by artificial nails and nail polish, particularly with blue, red, or bright polish.

Blood pressure. BP is a parameter reflecting cardiac contractility, heart rate, circulating volume, and peripheral vascular resistance. Systolic blood pressure (SBP) reflects cardiac output; diastolic blood pressure (DBP) is a measure of peripheral vascular resistance. The pulse pressure is the difference between SBP and DBP and represents approximate stroke volume. It is easily calculated and should be considered in certain situations, such as shock or head injury. A narrowing pulse pressure indicates a drop in cardiac output and a compensatory rise in peripheral vascular resistance. Pulse pressure is much more sensitive to hypovolemic changes in early shock than SBP is. A widening pulse pressure may indicate increased intracranial pressure.

BP can be obtained in a variety of ways, including auscultation, palpation, noninvasive BP monitors, or through Doppler ultrasound. Selecting the proper cuff size is essential to obtaining an accurate measurement. If the cuff is too small, falsely elevated readings will occur. A cuff that is too large results in erroneously low readings. A single BP recording yields little or no information. Serial blood pressures should be taken and documented. Normal pressures measured in the ED are not necessarily an indication that all is well, just as abnormal blood pressures may not indicate a problem. A healthy person may not demonstrate a drop in SBP despite significant volume loss until all compensatory mechanisms (i.e., the ability to increase heart rate and vasoconstrict) have been exhausted. If the patient is undergoing antihypertensive therapy, the values obtained during the ED visit may represent a significant deviation relative to the patient's "normally abnormal" pressure. Situations such as pain, fear, or anxiety may cause elevated blood pressures.

Orthostatic vital signs. Orthostatic vital signs may be indicated for patients presenting with syncopal episodes or suspected volume depletion. They are sometimes referred to as postural vital signs. When evaluating patients for orthostatic changes, the nurse records BP and pulse rate after the patient has been supine for 2 to 3 minutes. BP, pulse, and symptoms are then recorded after the patient has been sitting for 1 minute; the patient is assisted to a standing position, and after 1 minute the BP, pulse, and symptoms are again reassessed. The test may be considered positive if the pulse rate increases 30 beats/min or more in an adult and symptoms suggesting cerebral hypoperfusion with position change (i.e., dizziness or syncope) occur. A supine-to-standing measurement may be more accurate than a supine-to-sitting measurement. Follow your facility's protocol for obtaining orthostatic or postural vital signs.

Weight. Pediatric patients should be weighed at each ED visit to obtain an accurate measurement. In pediatrics, because fluid resuscitation and medications are dosed by kilogram of body weight, weight should always be recorded in kilograms. In many cases, adult weights should also be obtained, especially in cases where medications are weight-based or dosage is based on ideal body weight. Reported weights are subject to error; however, unless the patient requires weight-based medications (e.g., vasopressors or fibrinolytic infusions), this subjective measure may be adequate.

Give Comfort Measures

Pain is commonly referred to as "the fifth vital sign." Although pain is a subjective experience, all patients presenting to the ED should be queried about the presence of pain during the initial assessment, noting any self-reports or behavioral cues suggesting discomfort. Chapter 10 will cover pain assessment and pain management.

History

Obtaining a relevant history is an important component of the patient assessment. The patient interview is often done while the head-to-toe assessment is being conducted. Historical data include the patient's chief complaint, history of the present illness or injury, past medical history, current medications (prescription, over-the-counter, herbal supplements, and recreational substances), and allergies. It is important to listen to the patient's description of the problem. Documentation of the patient's complaint, in his or her own words, should be done. Sometimes patients cannot describe their symptoms or reason for coming to the ED (e.g., if a patient is unresponsive or a preverbal child). Attempts should be made to gather information from a witness to either the event or the onset of illness.

The AMPLE mnemonic is helpful for organizing and obtaining an adequate history. Table 9.2 summarizes pertinent historical data to be obtained using the AMPLE mnemonic. The questions, although open ended, should be directed by the chief complaint and build on information offered by the patient. If possible and pertinent, a family and social history may be elicited. Special communication needs related to vision, hearing, or language should be identified and addressed. If the patient can respond to questions, any history obtained from others should be validated by the patient. Previous medical records may be helpful, if available; with electronic health records and health information exchanges, these records are often immediately accessible. However, treatment should never be delayed until a history is available.

In addition to the data described, many facilities use a variety of screening tools as part of the assessment process for stable patients. Patients may be asked a series of questions regarding immunization status and signs and symptoms of tuberculosis or exposure to other communicable diseases (e.g., chickenpox). Screening for interpersonal violence, suicidal risk, or alcohol and tobacco use may be performed. With emerging infectious diseases, many facilities also ask about foreign travel.

General Head-to-Toe Assessment

A complete head-to-toe assessment is necessary for all critically ill or injured patients, especially those who are unresponsive. Patients presenting with minor illness or injury or symptoms isolated to one body system, may only require a rapid general evaluation and then a focused assessment on the specific problem. More information on assessment of specific conditions or injuries will be found in later chapters.

Head and face. The head and face should be inspected and palpated for any signs of surface trauma, rashes, ecchymosis, or edema. Any discharge from the nose, ears, or eyes should be noted. In cases of trauma, the bones of the head and face should be palpated, noting any bony deformity or crepitus, asymmetry, and tenderness. The oral mucosa may be assessed for color, hydration status, inflammation, swelling, and bleeding. Patients presenting with ocular complaints should have visual acuity measured. They should be questioned about any recent visual changes.

For patients presenting with neurologic complaints or deficits (e.g., headache, dizziness, seizure, altered mental status, loss of consciousness, or syncope), a focused neurologic

TABLE 9.2 Pertinent Historical Data Using the AMPLE Mnemonic.

	Description	Interview Questions
A	Allergies	Is the patient allergic to any medications? (Record type and severity of reaction.)
		Any adverse reactions to medications?
		Food allergies?
		Environmental allergies?
M	Medications	Current medications (prescribed or unprescribed, over-the-counter, herbals, and recreational)
		When was medication last taken?
P	Past health history	Pertinent medical history
		Has this problem ever occurred before?
		If so, was a medical diagnosis made? What was it?
		Has the patient ever had surgery? For what reason? What was the result?
		Is there any family medical history that may influence the patient's present complaint?
		Are there psychosocial factors that may be influencing the patient's condition?
		Does the patient have a private physician? (Obtain full name and where the physician practices if possible.)
		When was the last tetanus immunization? (if open wounds/eye injuries involved)
		When was the last normal menstrual period? (for females) Any possibility of pregnancy?
L	Last meal eaten	History of dietary intake?
		Last ingestion of fluids? Solids?
		Last void? Last bowel movement?
E	Events leading to the illness/injury	History of present illness or injury
		How and when injury or illness first occurred
		Influencing factors
		Travel within days or weeks of symptom onset
		Illness of household contacts
		Symptom chronology and duration
		Related symptoms
		Location of pain or discomfort
		What, if anything, the patient has done about the symptoms

assessment should be performed. The most important indicator of cerebral function is the patient's level of consciousness. Box 9.2 offers a mnemonic for investigating potential causes of an altered level of consciousness. The patient's orientation to time, place, person, and situation is evaluated. The Glasgow Coma Scale and the National Institutes of Health stroke scale are standardized tools used to measure and communicate neurologic status and provide trending over time. Some facilities also may use the FOUR Score Coma Scale. Pupil size, shape, and reactivity should be evaluated. More detailed neurologic assessment includes evaluation of muscle strength and tone, sensation, and cranial nerve function. These will be covered in later chapters.

Neck. The neck should be observed for any signs of soft-tissue injury, bony deformity or crepitus, edema, rashes, lesions, and masses. Depending on the presenting condition, the appearance of jugular veins may be evaluated. In cases of injury, the cervical spine should be palpated for the presence of point tenderness, bony crepitus, or step-offs. Complaints of dysphagia (difficulty swallowing) and hoarseness should be noted, depending on the chief complaint.

BOX 9.2 Causes of Altered Level of Consciousness: AEIOU-TIPPS.

A Alcohol
E Epilepsy/electrolytes
I Insulin (hypoglycemia or hyperglycemia)
O Opiates
U Uremia
T Trauma
I Infection
P Poison
P Psychosis
S Syncope

Chest. Assessment of the chest involves clinical evaluation of both pulmonary and cardiac function. Chest assessment will depend on the presenting complaint or condition.

Respiratory rate and depth, degree of effort, symmetry of chest wall expansion, use of accessory or abdominal muscles, and any paradoxical chest wall movement should be recorded. The chest should be inspected for injuries or abnormalities. The presence of central venous access devices, pacemakers, implantable cardioverter-defibrillators, and medication patches should be noted. Breath sounds should be auscultated for bilateral equality (normal, decreased, or absent), noting any adventitious sounds such as wheezes, crackles, and rhonchi. Further assessment is required for patients with dyspnea and abnormal breath sounds. Heart sounds can provide information about the integrity of heart valves, atrial and ventricular muscles, and the conduction system. Patients presenting with suspected ischemic chest pain require further assessment, including continuous cardiac monitoring and an immediate 12-lead ECG.

Abdomen. The contour of the abdomen should be inspected for abnormalities. The presence or absence and character of bowel sounds should be assessed. All four quadrants of the abdomen are gently palpated for rigidity, tenderness, and guarding. Palpation of the abdomen should always be done as the final step and is initiated away from the site of any reported pain or tenderness. Emesis or stool should be tested for blood and other laboratory diagnostics performed as ordered by the physician. Patient complaints of constipation, diarrhea, nausea, vomiting, indigestion, abdominal pain, and gastrointestinal bleeding require further evaluation.

Pelvis/perineum. If indicated, the pelvis and perineal area should be observed for lacerations, abrasions, rashes, lesions, edema, or bleeding from the meatus. Drainage or discharge from the vagina or penis should be described in patients presenting with genital concerns. If vaginal bleeding is noted, the character and amount of blood loss or saturated pads used should be reported. Priapism, if present, is indicative of pathologic conditions such as sickle cell crisis or spinal cord injury. Patients presenting with urinary complaints should be queried about pain or burning with urination, frequency, hematuria, decreased urination, dribbling, and flank tenderness. A urine sample should be obtained for analysis. For female patients of reproductive age, the possibility of an unknown pregnancy should be considered and a careful menstrual history obtained; a urine pregnancy test may be performed. If the patient is pregnant, fetal heart tones are assessed for presence, location, and rate.

Extremities. All four extremities should be assessed for redness, edema, rashes, lesions, or scars; pulse quality, movement, and sensation should be noted. In cases of injury, neurovascular status distal to the site of injury requires evaluation of pulse quality and skin temperature (with the injured extremity compared with the uninjured site), capillary refill, sensation, and movement.

Posterior surfaces. The patient's back and posterior aspects of the arms and legs should be evaluated for the presence of bleeding, abrasions, wounds, hematomas, ecchymosis, rashes, lesions, and edema. Focused assessment is done as indicated by the presenting condition.

ONGOING ASSESSMENT

Ongoing assessment is essential to identify the patient's response to interventions as well as to determine improvement or deterioration in patient status. Reassessment intervals should be based on the patient's clinical status. Facility protocols may offer guidelines for specific situations, such as trauma score calculation; repeat vital sign measurements and neurologic assessment every 15 minutes for patients receiving fibrinolytic therapy; or reassessment of pain score after opioids or other pain medications have been administered.

SPECIAL PATIENT POPULATIONS

Children and older adults have unique anatomic and physiologic characteristics to consider in the assessment process because of their extremes in age. Obstetric patients and patients with bariatric issues pose assessment challenges because of their change in body habitus. Attention to these variables can enhance the assessment process and optimize patient outcomes. Unit VI will address considerations for special populations

SUMMARY

This chapter describes the essential general components of the initial assessment of the ED patient. Although most patients present with conditions that are not life threatening but require resuscitation, a systematic approach to evaluation is needed to ensure that life threats are immediately identified in the primary assessment (ABCDE portion of the A-to-I mnemonic) and that all indicators of illness/injury are identified in the secondary assessment (FGHI portion of the A-to-I mnemonic). The extent of evaluation is decided by the emergency nurse based on the patient's condition at that time, the chief complaint, and environmental factors. A thorough, systematic assessment leads to priority setting for appropriate interventions throughout the patient's stay.

BIBLIOGRAPHY

Denke NJ. Nursing assessment and resuscitation. In: Sweet V, ed. *Emergency Nursing Core Curriculum*. 7th ed. St Louis, MO: Elsevier; 2018:1–22.

Emergency Nurses Association. Initial assessment. In: *Emergency Nursing Pediatric Course: Provider Manual*. 5th ed. Des Plaines, IL: Emergency Nurses Association; 2020.

Emergency Nurses Association. *Initial assessment. Trauma Nursing Core Course Provider Manual*. 7th ed. Des Plaines, IL: Emergency Nurses Association; 2014.

Emergency Nurses Association. *Position Statement: Cultural Diversity in the Emergency Setting*. 2012. https://www.ena.org/docs/default-source/resource-library/practice-resources/position-statements/culturaldiversity. Accessed April 15, 2019.

Emergency Nurses Association. *Position Statement: Weighing all Patients in Kilograms*. 2016. https://www.ena.org/docs/default-source/resource-library/practice-resources/position-statements/weighingallpatientsinkilograms. Accessed April 15, 2019.

Jarvis C. Evidence-based assessment. In: Jarvis C, ed. *Physical Examination and Health Assessment*. 7th ed. St Louis, MO: Elsevier; 2016:1–10.

10

Pain

Randy Hamm

Pain is the most frequent complaint among patients in the emergency department (ED), and traditionally pain has been inadequately treated for many patients.[1–3] More than 44 million pain-related visits to the ED occur each year in the United States.[4] In the past decade, research and efforts to improve pain management have resulted in increased attention to ED pain management. Although many strides have been made, opportunities for maximizing pain control for the individual ED patient remain great.

The ED nurse can and should play a key role in ED pain management. The ED nurse is often the patient's primary advocate for achieving optimal control of pain. Emergency nurses are usually the first to assess and identify a patient in pain. They may independently implement nonpharmacologic interventions, may request analgesic orders, are primarily responsible for assessing the adequacy of any interventions, and have an opportunity to provide patient teaching at discharge to promote optimal management of pain at home. By taking a proactive role in pain management, emergency nurses have a unique opportunity to make a meaningful difference for most patients they care for.

This chapter will discuss the pathophysiology of pain and current definitions and provide a detailed review of both adult and pediatric pain management specific to the ED.

DEFINITIONS AND CLASSIFICATIONS OF PAIN

The International Association for the Study of Pain has defined pain as "an unpleasant sensory and emotional experience associated with actual or potential tissue damage."[5] Pain has both a physiologic and an emotional component.[6] As more research has been conducted and with an additional understanding of pathophysiology, a continuum of pain has been identified.

Pain is classified as nociceptive or neuropathic. Nociceptive pain results from impulses traveling along normal nerve conduction pathways. Nociceptive pain may be stimulated by neurotransmitters contained in the soma and viscera. Neuropathic pain can result from trauma or diseases of the nerves. This causes abnormal processing of sensory impulses from the peripheral or central nervous systems. The pathophysiology of pain is discussed in the next section of this chapter.[5,7]

Acute pain is described as pain resulting from potential or actual tissue damage. Acute pain occurs suddenly and should go away when the injury has healed or the illness has resolved. Acute pain functions as a protective mechanism, warning the body of illness or injury. Defense mechanisms, such as removal of the offending cause (e.g., a bee stinger), are initiated. Acute pain has both physiologic and emotional components. Most patients are able to describe its location and intensity as well as identify what provides relief from the pain (pharmacologic and nonpharmacologic methods).[7] Acute pain continues to be one of the most common reasons why patients seek care in the ED.[3]

Chronic (cancer and noncancer) pain may be initiated by an acute event, or its source may be unknown. Chronic pain is prolonged pain lasting longer than 3 months and, in many cases, continuing for months to years. Chronic pain accounts for a large percentage of annual ED visits, and more than 100 million adults in the United States have a chronic pain condition, with related costs related reaching as much as $635 billion annually.[8]

The source of chronic pain is not always easily differentiated. It can be difficult to relate the amount of pain and the patient's response to the pain. Examples of the types of chronic pain seen in the ED are mechanical low back pain and degenerative or inflammatory joint pain. More research is necessary to understand the best methods to treat chronic pain in the ED.

A subtype of chronic pain is chronic noncancer pain. Patients with this type of pain report levels of pain weakly corresponding to identifiable levels of tissue abnormality. These patients respond poorly to standard treatments.[6]

Cancer pain is a form of chronic pain specifically related to the disease. Cancer pain may be attributed to the advance of the disease, pain associated with the treatment of the disease process (e.g., radiation or chemotherapy), or pain associated with preexisting medical problems. Cancer pain has been designated separately because treatment is generally focused on the management of the pain related to the disease process.

Pain is a multifaceted phenomenon. Table 10.1 summarizes some of the different types of pain that may be seen in the ED.[5,7,9–11] There are also multiple pain terms emergency nurses should be familiar with when evaluating pain in the ED. Table 10.2 contains descriptions of some of these terms.

TABLE 10.1 Types of Pain Seen in the Emergency Department.

Type of Pain	Characteristics	Causes
Acute	Sudden onset Warning Protective Transient in length Able to identify area of pain Specific objective signs and symptoms Anxiety	Trauma Surgery Procedures Fractures Illnesses such as pancreatitis Infections
Chronic	State of existence Less able to differentiate where the pain is Prolonged—months to years Difficult to treat Depression common	Mechanical low back pain Arthritis Migraine Pelvic pain
Cancer	State of existence May increase with treatment or changes in the disease process	Tumor HIV/AIDS Chemotherapy Radiation therapy
Neuropathic	Burning Numbness Electrical jolts	Primary lesion, dysfunction in the peripheral or central nervous system
Visceral	Squeezing Cramping Bloated feeling Stretching	Bowel obstruction Venous occlusion Ischemia
Somatic	Aching Throbbing	Bone metastasis Degenerative joint disease

HIV/AIDS, Human immunodeficiency virus/acquired immunodeficiency syndrome.

TABLE 10.2 Pain Terminology.

Terminology	Definition/Description
Allodynia	Pain due to stimulus not normally provoking pain. It involves a change in the quality of sensation. The stimulus does not normally cause pain, but the response is painful.
Analgesia	Absence of pain in response to a stimulus that should be painful.
Hyperalgesia	An increased response to a stimulus that is normally painful.
Hyperesthesia	Increased sensitivity to stimulation, excluding the special senses.
Neuralgia	Pain in the distribution of a nerve or nerves.
Neuritis	Inflammation of a nerve or nerves.
Neuropathy	A disturbance of function or pathologic change in a nerve.
Noxious stimulus	A noxious stimulus is one that is damaging to normal tissues.
Pain threshold	The least experience of pain that a patient can tolerate.
Pain tolerance level	The greatest level of pain that a patient can tolerate.
Paresthesia	An abnormal sensation, whether spontaneous or evoked.

PATHOPHYSIOLOGY OF PAIN

The pathophysiology of pain is complex, involving sensory, emotional, behavioral, and spiritual factors. The perception of pain is nociception and involves three pathways transmitting and modulating pain stimuli.[7,9] A theory explaining this phenomenon is the gate control theory. Nociceptors, or pain receptors, are located in the skin, muscles, joints, arteries, and the viscera. Nociceptors are stimulated by chemical, thermal, or mechanical stimuli. Examples of stimuli may include a laceration, heat causing tissue damage, or stretch of an abdominal muscle when there is inflammation or blood in the abdomen. Pain receptors are sensitive to multiple stimuli, but they are concentrated at various levels throughout the body. The skin has a higher concentration than the viscera, which makes sense because the skin is the first line of defense for the body.

When tissue is damaged, it releases neurotransmitters such as potassium, leukotrienes, bradykinins, serotonin, histamines, arachidonic acid, thromboxanes, substance P, and platelet activating factor. These chemicals not only play a role in acute pain but also may be a factor in chronic pain. Prostaglandins are also released but do not directly stimulate nerve endings. Instead, they make the nerve endings more sensitive.[12]

Pain Fibers

The nerve action potentials of the nociceptors are transmitted by two fiber types (Fig. 10.1). The myelinated A-delta fibers

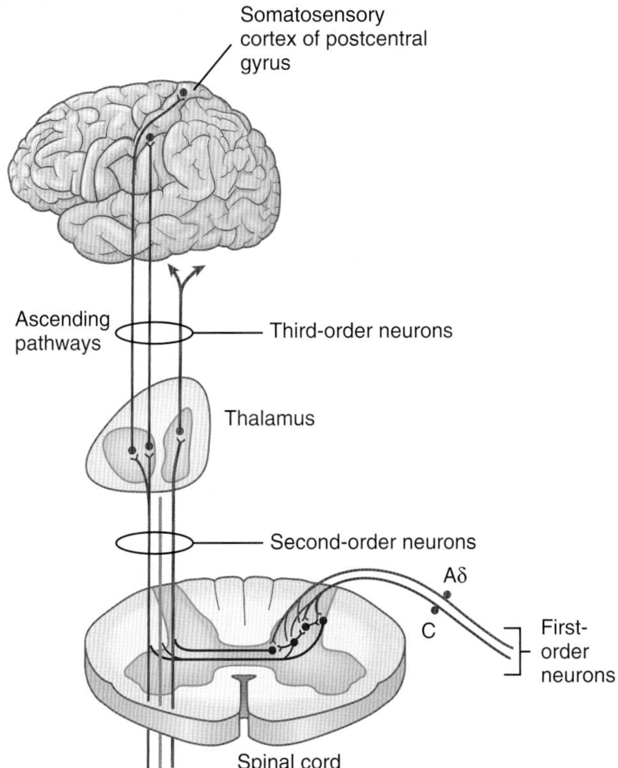

Fig. 10.1 Nociception Pathways. A-delta and C fibers constitute the primary, first-order sensory afferents coming into the gate at the posterior part of the spinal cord. Here we see second-order neurons crossing the cord (decussating) and ascending to the thalamus as part of the spinothalamic tract. Third-order afferents project to higher brain centers of the limbic system, the frontal cortex, and the primary sensory cortex of the postcentral gyrus of the parietal lobe. (From McCance KL, Huether SE: *Pathophysiology: The Biologic Basis for Disease in Adults and Children*. 8th ed. St Louis, MO: Mosby; 2019.)

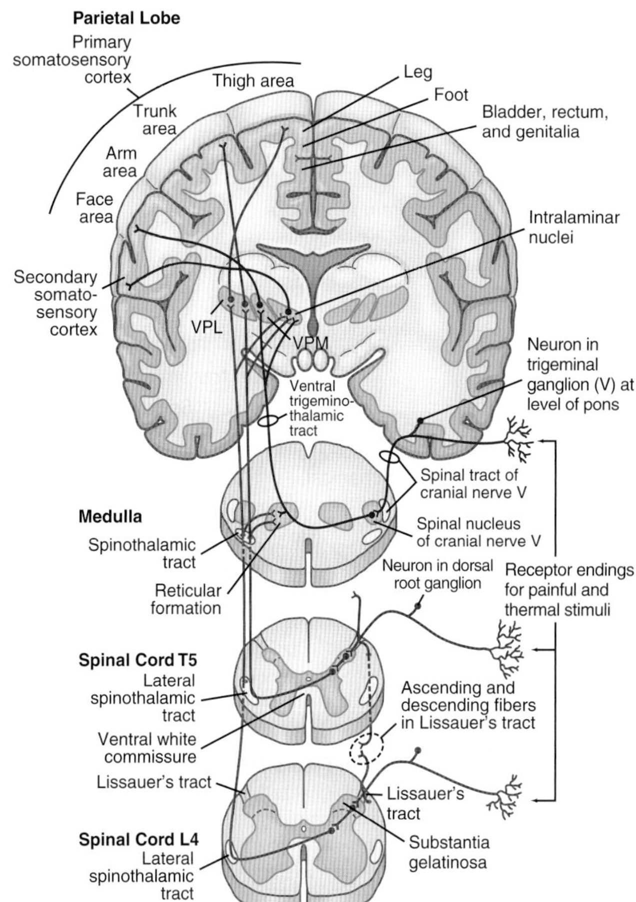

Fig. 10.2 Central Nervous System Pathways Mediating the Sensations of Pain and Temperature. *VPL,* Ventral posterior lateral thalamic nuclei; *VPM,* ventral posterior medial thalamic nuclei. (From McCance KL, Huether SE: *Pathophysiology: The Biologic Basis for Disease in Adults and Children*. 8th ed. St Louis, MO: Mosby; 2019.)

rapidly transmit the pain impulse (fast pain). This produces a sharp pain sensation. The unmyelinated C fibers are slower (slow pain) and are responsible for the diffuse burning or aching sensation of pain. C fibers also produce throbbing, deep visceral pain and the sensations associated with chronic pain. Both eventually terminate in the dorsal horn of the spinal cord. Most of these transmissions terminate in the substantia gelatinosa.[9]

Spinal Cord

Many of the afferent fibers synapse with second-order neurons in the dorsal horn. There are three classes of second-order neurons in the dorsal horn. These are projection cells relaying information to higher brain areas; excitatory interneurons, which relay nociceptive transmissions to other interneurons, other projection cells, or motor neurons involved with local reflexes; and inhibitory interneurons, which will modulate the transmission.[6,7,12] The connection between the cells of the primary- and secondary-order neurons located here compose the "pain gate." This gate postulated in the gate control theory regulates the transmission of pain impulses to the brain. It also helps explain why many nonpharmacologic methods such as acupuncture and massage can assist in pain management.[9]

There are multiple pathways through the spinal cord where a pain impulse travels to the brain, primarily, the thalamus, which functions as the relay station for pain impulses. Two of these pathways are the neospinothalamic and the paleospinothalamic. The neospinothalamic is the primary pathway for the fast pain fibers. The fibers of this tract cross to the opposite side of the spinal cord and pass upward to the thalamus. This tract transmits the discriminating aspects of pain, such as its location, intensity, and duration.[12]

The paleospinothalamic tract transmits the stimuli from the slower C fibers. Not all of these fibers cross over before ascending. The slower fibers make it more difficult to specifically localize pain sensations.[12] Substance P has been identified as the main neurotransmitter associated with slow pain sensations.

The Brain

The third-order neurons located in the thalamus, brain stem, and midbrain project to portions of the central nervous system (Fig. 10.2).[9] The sensory homunculus, located on the postcentral gyrus of the parietal lobe, is thought to be involved in the discriminative and cognitive components of pain.[9] The frontal lobe also plays a role in pain perception and interpretation.

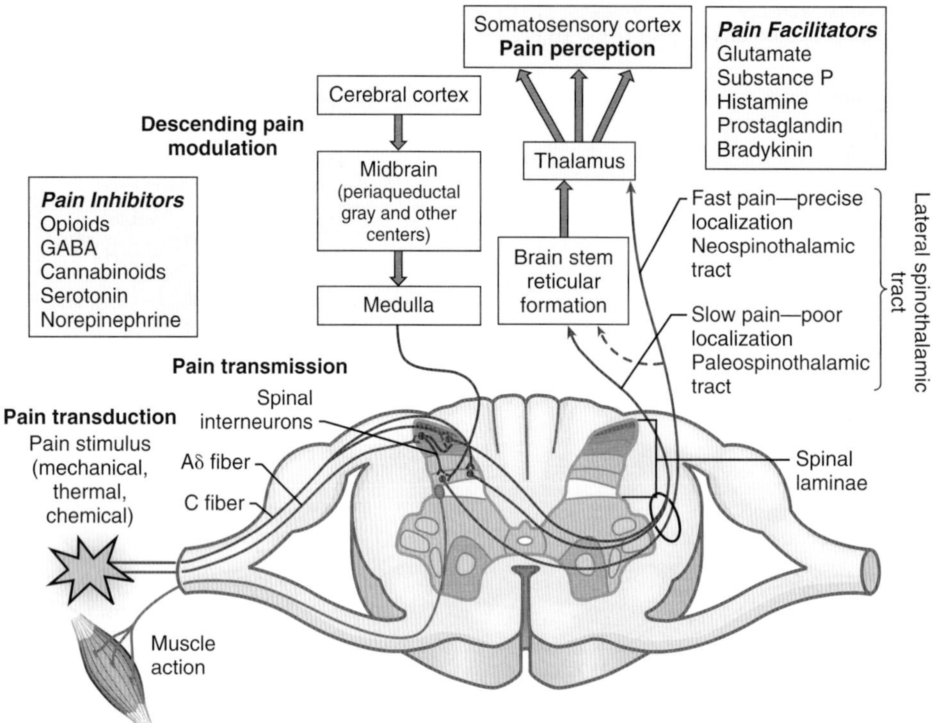

Fig. 10.3 Pain Fibers That Terminate Primarily in Laminae II and V of the Dorsal Horn. The myelinated Aδ fibers (fast localized pain) synapse on a second set of neurons that carry the signal to the thalamus via the neospinothalamic tracts. The C fibers (slow pain) synapse on laminae II and V interneurons that connect with neurons in laminae II, IV, and V and carry the pain signal to the reticular formation and midbrain via the paleospinothalamic tract. The axons of the spinothalamic tracts cross over the spinal cord to ascend in the anterior and lateral spinal cord white matter. (From McCance KL, Huether SE: *Pathophysiology: The Biologic Basis for Disease in Adults and Children*. 8th ed. St Louis, MO: Mosby; 2019.)

The limbic and the reticular tracts respond to pain signals. Stimulation of these areas of the brain will result in arousing the person to the danger, release of stress hormones, and emotional responses to pain.

Pain Modulation

The body has its own intrinsic means of managing pain. This occurs in the pain-inhibitory, or antinociceptive, response system. Afferent fibers stimulate the periaqueductal gray area, the magnus raphe nucleus, and the pain inhibitory complex in the anterior horn. This allows the body to manage debilitating pain and still survive. The gate control theory has assisted in explaining how pain can be modulated. There are sensory nerves within the dorsal horn that compete with the pain sensory fibers to "modulate" their effect. Larger A-beta fibers in the dorsal horn can decrease the amplitude of the afferent pain fibers. This again explains how using acupuncture, rubbing an injury, or using a topical medication can relieve pain.[9,12] Fig. 10.3 illustrates pain modulation.[9]

Another method of modulating pain occurs through inhibitory neurotransmitters or antinociception response. When the nociceptors are stimulated by heat, toxic chemicals, or tissue injury, there is a threshold depolarization or a direct excitation. After the tissue is injured, the inflammatory response can initiate an indirect excitation.

The spinal cord, brain, and other areas of the body produce inhibitory neurotransmitters. Neurotransmitters contributing to pain modulation, γ-aminobutyric acid (GABA) and glycine, inhibit pain impulses in the brain and spinal cord. Norepinephrine and serotonin inhibit pain impulses in the medulla and pons.

Endogenous Opioids

The human body also has its own endogenous opioids. Endogenous opioids are neuropeptides inhibiting pain impulse transmission in the brain and spinal cord. The receptor sites for these neurotransmitters are also the sites where exogenously administered opioids act. The four types of opioid neuropeptides are enkephalins, endorphins, dynorphins, and endomorphins. Until the late 1970s, with the discovery of these peptides, there was little understanding as to how pain medications work, and research and discovery still continue today. Enkephalins are weaker than endorphins but more powerful than morphine and last longer. Dynorphins will generally impede pain impulses, and endomorphins are primarily antinociceptive.[11]

The specific opioid sites where these neurotransmitters work throughout the body are the mu (μ), with subtypes μ-1 and μ-2; kappa (κ), and delta (δ). Each of these receptor sites binds differently with distinctive types of opioids.[9,12] Mu receptors inhibit the release of excitatory neurotransmitters.

Beta receptors interact with enkephalins to modulate pain impulses. Kappa receptors produce sedation and some analgesia.[11,13] Research has uncovered some other endogenous opioid peptides as well as additional subtypes to the known opioid sites. A recently discovered opioid peptide is nociception/orphanin-FQ, which resembles the dynorphins.[13]

PAIN THEORIES

Pain is a protective mechanism, and understanding its physiology has led to theories about pain. Three specific theories have been proposed. The first is the gate control theory discussed earlier. Melzack and Wall proposed in 1965 a "gate" that could be opened and closed and would manage pain impulses. This could be done by either pharmacologic (e.g., local anesthetics) or nonpharmacologic (e.g., acupuncture) means, which can "close" or slow the pain transmissions through the gate. As discussed previously, the body intrinsically "modulates" pain so the organism can survive. Research continues to demonstrate the validity of this theory.[14]

René Descartes proposed injury-activating specific pain receptors. This is known as the specificity theory and is particularly useful in explaining acute pain and acute pain management.[14] However, chronic pain and the emotional components of pain cannot be completely clarified using this theory.

Chronic pain has become a common and difficult problem in today's society and EDs. All pain management requires a holistic approach, especially chronic pain.[15] The neuromatrix theory of pain expands the gate control theory to encompass chronic pain. Chronic pain is theorized to be a multidimensional experience caused by patterns of nerve impulses known as signatures. The impulses are generated in the brain by a widely distributed network called the body-self neuromatrix. This neuromatrix includes the individual and his or her feelings, experiences, and genetic predisposition. It is composed of centers and loops of neurons whose synapses are initially genetically determined but can be modified. It can be triggered by sensory inputs from the body or independently trigged by the brain. The output of one's neuromatrix generates the neurosignature pattern of pain. This assists in explaining some forms of chronic pain, such as phantom limb pain, where there is no specific or obvious cause of the pain. It also emphasizes differences in individual pain experiences and the need for individualized management tailored to the patient. Even patients with the same complaint (i.e., acute appendicitis) will not have the same pain experience.[9,11,15,16]

PHYSIOLOGIC CONSEQUENCES OF PAIN

Even though pain plays an important role in warning and protecting humans, it can also have detrimental consequences that must be recognized by the emergency nurse. Multiple sources of pain may be experienced by the patient in the ED, such as physical pain from the illness or injury or pain produced by procedures required to manage the illness or injury. Psychosocial pain is often related to fear or anxiety, which can be caused or augmented by not understanding the ED treatment and separation from one's family. The ED environment can cause pain from such sources as noise from equipment, staff, and bright lighting. A lack of temperature control can cause or exacerbate a patient's pain. Finally, many patients have spiritual pain as victims of violence or discrimination when their symptoms are not even considered.

Pain generates many harmful effects on the body. The autonomic nervous system responds to pain by releasing "stress hormones" such as epinephrine and cortisol. These cause vasoconstriction, which may impede healing. The patient's heart rate may increase and cause an increase in cardiac output and oxygen consumption. The patient may splint his or her chest and decrease ventilations, which can lead to reduced pulmonary blood flow. This can contribute to atelectasis, pneumonia, and eventually sepsis and death. Pain can cause muscle contractions, spasms, and rigidity. Unrelieved pain will cause immune system suppression, physical changes, and psychological injury. Pain can cause suffering.[17]

Pain remains the most common complaint bringing patients to the ED. Emergency nurses must be familiar with the definitions of pain, its physiology, and its physiologic consequences. Pain must be viewed both holistically and individually so appropriate compassionate care can be provided.

MYTHS AND BARRIERS TO PAIN MANAGEMENT

Traditionally, many myths and barriers have precluded optimal pain management for all patients and include the following: (1) the perception many patients are addicted to opioids or are drug seeking, (2) disparities in treatment of minorities and women, (3) fear of negative physiologic effects of opioid administration, (4) physician and nurse lack of education regarding pain management, (5) inadequate treatment of high-risk patients (older adults, cognitively impaired patients, non–English-speaking patients, and children), and (6) the belief that physiologic signs such as tachycardia and grimacing are more reliable than patient self-report.[18,19] Myths two (2) to six (6) will be briefly addressed, and the perception that many patients are drug seeking will be elaborated on after this introduction to general myths.

Evidence shows that minorities and women receive inadequate analgesic management more frequently than whites and men. This is an important barrier to adequate analgesia in the ED, and emergency nurses can do much to avoid this barrier.[20–22] Nurses may be unjustifiably fearful of apnea and hypotension when administering opioids. Selection of the correct age-specific dose and route of analgesic combined with appropriate monitoring will allow nurses to safely administer opioids. Emergency clinicians may lack specific education in pain management. Increased knowledge will result in increased comfort when providing analgesics and optimize the ability to provide optimal pain management. Emergency nurses should also have a high index of suspicion of unrelieved pain when caring for children, older adults, cognitively impaired patients, and non–English-speaking patients. If these patients present with a chief complaint usually associated with pain, emergency nurses should advocate for appropriate analgesic management. Special attention should be paid to age when recommending the selection of analgesic agents. Nonsteroidal antiinflammatory drugs (NSAIDs) should often be avoided in older adults because of their renal and gastrointestinal side effects, and opioid doses should be reduced.[23] An additional ED-specific barrier is the commonly held belief that treatment of pain cannot begin until a diagnosis is made, in particular for patients with abdominal pain and victims of multiple trauma. This barrier will be discussed later in the chapter.

"Opiophobia" is likely the most important barrier to adequate pain management in the ED setting. With recent federal attention to the increasing incidence of prescription drug abuse, EDs have been the target of heightened concern, particularly in regard to prescription drug abuse.[24,25] Many emergency nurses and physicians are overly concerned that patients are really addicted to opioids and are drug seeking. This perception results from two facts: (1) the only valid indicator of pain is patient self-report, and nurses must believe the patient; and (2) it is nearly impossible to diagnose opioid addiction in the ED setting. An emergency nurse who assumes a patient is addicted to opioids runs the risk of not treating a patient with pain. The ethical dilemma is clear: nurses may do more harm than good when assuming many ED patients are addicted.

Despite this, some patients with back pain, migraines, and abdominal pain may have frequent visits, and treatment with opioids may or may not be appropriate.[25] Individual care plans were developed in one ED for patients with six or more visits in 1 year with the chief complaints mentioned earlier. Of the 45,000 total ED visits in the year the program initiated, only 124 (0.002%) patients met the criteria.[26] Although the number of ED visits from these patients decreased in the following years of the program, long-term effectiveness for individual patients was not measured, and the "success" of the program cannot be evaluated. However, the use of individual care plans for patients with repeat visits for analgesic management may be beneficial. Individualized plans should be developed in collaboration with the primary care provider, the patient, and the ED staff. In particular, patients with cancer, back pain, headaches, and sickle cell disease may benefit. Establishing a standard care plan that can be easily accessed by emergency clinicians will allow for standardization of care, independent of the individual nurse or physician. The goal of the plans should be to improve patient-reported pain relief, not merely to reduce ED visits.

Opioid Addiction

Opioid addiction is a growing problem both internationally and in the United States. Prescription opioids continue to be the leading cause of poisoning death in the United States.[27] In 2008 drug overdose overtook automobile accidents as the leading cause of accidental death in the United States,[28] led by more than 28,000 opioid overdose deaths in 2014.[29] The Centers for Disease Control and Prevention reports past misuse of prescription opioids ranks among the strongest risk factors for heroin abuse and overdose.[30] However, research has shown that short-term use of opioids during an ED evaluation and visit for acute painful conditions is unlikely to cause addiction,[31] although many hospital systems are now placing stricter stipulations on the prescription of opioids from the ED setting.

ADULT PAIN MANAGEMENT

Patient Expectations

Patients expect pain relief. In a study of adult ED patients with and without pain, patients reported the expectation that their pain would be reduced by 72%, and 18% of patients expected a 100% reduction in pain. There was no difference in expectation related to the severity of pain on arrival, age, or gender.[32,33] Expectations of pain relief between Hispanic and non-Hispanic white ED patients were compared, and no difference in pain-relief expectations was found. Most patients expected a decrease in pain scores between 69 and 81 mm using a 100-mm visual analog scale.[33] In another study, 48 patients with acute abdominal pain were interviewed. Forty-four percent expected complete pain relief while in the ED.[34]

Patients also expect rapid analgesic management. In a single-site study, upon arrival in the ED 620 adult patients were asked to report a "reasonable" time before receiving an analgesic. At discharge they were asked if their pain-relief needs were met and to rate their overall satisfaction with ED care. The average "reasonable" time to initial analgesic reported for the group was 23 minutes and did not vary by chief complaint. Patients who reported having their pain-relief needs met were more satisfied with their overall ED care.[35] In this era with a strong focus on patient experience, optimal pain management may help improve overall ED patient satisfaction scores. It is clear that ED patients expect rapid and aggressive pain management.

Assessment: More Than a Pain Score

It is impossible to provide optimal pain relief without conducting a thorough pain assessment. Pain assessment guides the selection of intervention (pharmacologic vs. nonpharmacologic), and reassessment is the key to ultimate pain relief or reduction of pain to meet the patient's desired goal. Pain assessment typically means obtaining a pain intensity score from the patient. The use of pain scales allows for the objective measurement of a subjective state. The numeric rating scale (0–10) is the most commonly used scale in the ED and has been validated for use with acute pain in the ED setting.[36] It is sufficient for many but not all adults.[18] Assessment tools should be age appropriate, and special consideration and scales, such as the face, legs, activity, cry, and consolability (FLACC) scale, should be given to assessing patients who are nonverbal. Although many assessment tools exist, it is not the intent of this chapter to review multiple tools, but instead to present core principles of pain assessment. Many multidimensional tools are available and assess dimensions of pain other than pain intensity. Often their use is impractical in the ED setting. However, in addition to assessing pain intensity, the ED nurse should assess the chief complaint, type of pain (acute, chronic, cancer, and end-of-life pain), location of pain, duration, prehospital interventions, patient age, and cultural expression of pain.

Merely recording a pain score in the medical record does not provide pain relief. Nurses must believe the patient and initiate appropriate interventions aimed at reducing pain. A recent study reported that ED nurses underestimate the patient's report of pain. In a single-center study of ED nurses and patients, ED nurses were asked to rate the patients' pain, and nurses scored the patients' pain an average of 2.4 points lower than the patient-reported score.[37] Minimizing the patient-reported pain score may lead to inadequate interventions.

Establishing the link between pain assessment, pain management, and patient outcomes is critical.[38] Several studies have examined the effect of a designated space in the medical record to record a pain score. The effect of recording a pain score on the actual provision of analgesics has been mixed. Nelson et al.[39] found that a significantly larger proportion of patients received analgesics during the ED visit after a documentation education intervention (25% before and 36% after). In a study of trauma patients with high pain scores, documentation of a pain assessment was associated with a higher rate of analgesic administration (60%) compared with patients without documentation of a pain score (33%).[40] In another ED, investigators implemented a chart template for nurse practitioners and physicians that was designed to improve pain assessment. Although documentation of pain assessments using the chart improved from 41% to 57% of patients, no difference in analgesic administration was noted, and the number of analgesic prescriptions provided at discharge actually decreased.[41] In summary, documentation of pain scores is important; however, nurses must take the next step and assist in the selection of the appropriate intervention and reassessment of any intervention to make sure that optimal pain management has been attained.

Management: Establishing a Pain Management Goal

Establishing the optimal and individualized pain management goal early in the ED visit is important. A pain score of 0 at discharge or reduction in pain score from admission to discharge may or may not be the right goal. Patients should be involved in determining the pain management goal whenever possible. Fosnocht et al.[35] examined this issue and recorded arrival and discharge pain scores, asking patients to report overall pain relief during the ED stay. There was no difference in change in pain scores between patients who did and did not report pain relief at discharge. These data demonstrate that a change in pain score alone cannot be used to evaluate the effectiveness of ED pain management.

Although it is critical to involve the patient in the selection of the pain management goal and plan of care, should nurses assume that patients will ask for pain medications? Recent data show that 98% of patients with abdominal pain reported pain to either the physician or nurse, but only 33% specifically requested analgesics.[34] Severity of pain intensity scores has also been found to be an unreliable indicator of whether or not patients requested analgesics.[42] These studies demonstrate that assessment cannot consist of recording a pain score alone. Emergency nurses have the opportunity to help establish a pain plan of care by actively engaging the patient in not only determining a pain management goal but also specifically inquiring whether a patient would like analgesics.

General Pain Management Principles

The policy "Pain Management in the Emergency Department" written by the American College of Emergency Physicians outlines the following basic principles: pain management should begin rapidly and not be delayed by a wait for diagnosis, opioids and nonopioids should be used, safety should be an important consideration, physician and patient education strategies should be developed, and ongoing research should be conducted.[43] These principles address fundamental points to guide pain management.

Nonpharmacologic Approaches

Nonpharmacologic interventions should be used as an adjunct when administering analgesics and, in some cases, may be sufficient in isolation. Some patients with mild pain may not require analgesic administration, and others may refuse analgesics. In one study, up to 15% of ED patients refused pain medications.[44] Many nonpharmacologic interventions are available. Some are useful, and others may not be practical for use in EDs without specialized training (e.g., hypnosis). All nurses should be able to facilitate distraction, the use of physical therapies such as positioning and elevation of extremities, and the use of heat and cold therapies. Heat may be useful for chronic pain and patients with sickle cell pain episodes. Ice should always be used for acute pain caused by musculoskeletal injuries and is often useful for pain associated with acute back injuries. Distraction techniques include music therapy, reading materials, and conversation. It is important for emergency nursing leaders to ensure distraction materials are made available and are readily accessible to promote their use. Use of distraction techniques has been found to reduce pain scores in a sample of pediatric patients with minor musculoskeletal trauma, but not for adults.[45,46] In a single-site study, adult patients reported they were satisfied with their pain management and would like to have the option of music distraction in future ED visits, despite no change in pain scores.[46] Nonpharmacologic interventions play an important role in relieving pain for many ED patients.

Pharmacologic Approaches

Pharmacologic interventions are often required to meet the patient's pain management goal. The ED nurse can help suggest the best analgesic agent, dose, and route for the individual patient. The patient's chief complaint, age, medical history, allergies, pain history, and stated pain goal should help determine analgesic interventions.

Analgesics can be administered by several routes, including oral, intravenous, subcutaneous, and patient-controlled analgesic pump. The use of intramuscular injections, especially when multiple doses will be required, is discouraged. Intramuscular injections are painful and associated with erratic absorption, tissue damage, and an increased risk for abscess development.[47] When oral analgesics are not sufficient or when the intravenous route is not available, the subcutaneous route should be used.[47] The subcutaneous route has a somewhat slower onset of action than intravenous, but it is equally effective and is commonly used with patients who have cancer or need palliative care. The intravenous route is indicated for patients with severe pain who are receiving opioids, and it has a peak effect of 15 to 30 minutes for most agents.[47] Reassessment of pain and administration of additional doses should occur if the pain goal has not been met in 15 minutes. Although multiple priorities challenge the ED nurse, all efforts should be made to reassess pain 15 minutes after administration of an intravenous or subcutaneous agent and within 60 minutes of administering an oral agent. Additional oral agents usually cannot be provided for 2 hours after the initial dose.

Finally, patient-controlled analgesia (PCA) is an excellent method of providing opioid analgesics for patients who may require multiple and frequent doses. PCA provides patients with control over their pain management. Reports of use in the ED are limited. Nurses require specific training, and the equipment and dosing cartridges should be made available in the department to promote use of PCA to provide analgesia in the ED.

It is also important to select the correct analgesic agent. Acetaminophen, NSAIDs, and opioids are the mainstays of ED pain management. Acetaminophen is useful for the relief of mild to moderate pain without inflammatory components, can be administered orally or rectally, and does not irritate the gastric mucosa.[47] It is also included in many combination oral opioid analgesics, including codeine, oxycodone (Percocet), and hydrocodone (Norco and Vicodin). The maximum daily recommended dose of acetaminophen (4000 mg for normal healthy adults) often limits the number of oral acetaminophen-opioid medications that can be administered within 24 hours. Healthy patients who exceed 4000 mg of acetaminophen within 24 hours are at an increased risk for hepatic toxicity.[47] Emergency nurses have an opportunity to educate patients about the limitations of acetaminophen when patients are discharged with analgesic prescriptions that include acetaminophen.

NSAIDs are a second analgesic category frequently used in the ED setting and are indicated for patients with mild to moderate pain, including pain with an inflammatory component (e.g., sprains and strains). Ibuprofen is most commonly used in these situations. NSAIDS can also be used as adjunct therapy to opioids for patients with severe pain associated with an inflammatory component (e.g., renal colic, acute sickle cell pain episodes, and musculoskeletal trauma). In a systematic review of patients with renal colic who received either an opioid or a NSAID, patients who received NSAIDs achieved greater reductions in pain scores.[48] However, NSAIDs alone are often not sufficient to manage renal colic pain. NSAIDs may also allow for administration of a smaller dose of opioid. When intravenous access is established, 15-mg doses of ketorolac (Toradol) may be administered intravenously every 6 hours.[47] Ketorolac can cause acute renal failure in dehydrated patients. All NSAIDs are associated with an increased risk for renal impairment, gastrointestinal bleeding due to inhibition of the enzyme cyclooxygenase (COX), and cardiovascular risks.[47] Careful consideration should be given before administering these agents to either the older adult patient or patients with a preexisting history of renal or gastrointestinal disease. At a minimum, the dose should be reduced for these patients. In 2005 the Food and Drug Administration instructed all manufacturers of NSAIDs to issue a box warning on all agents informing patients of the increased risk for gastrointestinal and cardiovascular complications, especially with long-term use.[49] Finally, NSAIDS have an analgesic ceiling effect, which means additional doses beyond a certain level will not result in any increase in analgesic affects.

Theoretically, COX-2-selective NSAIDs provide gastrointestinal protection by selectively inhibiting the COX-2 enzyme responsible for inflammation and not inhibiting the COX-1 enzyme, which is protective of the gastrointestinal system. They do not offer renal or liver protection. COX-2-selective agents have been found to be beneficial for patients with osteoarthritis. However, COX-2 inhibitors have been found to be associated with an increased risk for myocardial infarction and stroke.[49] COX-2 selective agents are very expensive and should rarely be used or prescribed in an ED setting.

Opioids are indicated for patients with severe pain, and specific agents can be administered orally (e.g., codeine, hydrocodone, morphine, and oxycodone), intravenously (morphine, fentanyl, and hydromorphone), or by using a PCA pump. Unlike NSAIDS, opioids do not have an analgesic ceiling effect. Oral agents are frequently combined with acetaminophen and are indicated for moderate pain. They are often prescribed at discharge from the ED to help manage pain after discharge. Acetaminophen with codeine is frequently prescribed. Some patients report no pain relief when taking codeine because codeine is a prodrug and not all persons are able to convert the drug to the active form.[50]

Morphine and hydromorphone (Dilaudid) are the primary options for management of severe pain in the ED setting. There is a liquid formulation of morphine sulfate (Roxanol) that can be administered sublingually or buccally when no other route is available. In a study by Chang et al.,[51] patients in the ED received either morphine 0.1 mg/kg or hydromorphone 0.015 mg/kg, equianalgesic doses. Both agents were found to be equally effective in reducing pain scores.[51] The incidence of nausea, vomiting, hypotension, and respiratory depression was similar for both agents.[51] The most frequent side effect of both agents was nausea and vomiting, with up to 19% of subjects reporting these symptoms. ED nurses should be prepared to administer antiemetics to relieve these symptoms. In this study no patients experienced a respiratory rate less than 12 breaths per minute, one patient in each group experienced an oxygen saturation less than 90%, and no patients required administration of naloxone.[51] The incidence

TABLE 10.3 Equianalgesic Dose Chart.

	EQUIANALGESIC DOSE (mg)	
Opioid	**Oral**	**Parenteral**
Morphine	30	10
Hydromorphone	7.5	1.5
Fentanyl	—	0.1
Oxycodone	20	—

From Max MB, Payne R, Edwards WT, et al. *Principles of Analgesic Use in the Treatment of Acute Pain and Cancer Pain.* 4th ed. Glenview, IL: American Pain Society; 1999.

of pruritus was reported less frequently with hydromorphone compared with morphine.[51] Data support the use of either agent for severe pain in the ED. Nurses should not be concerned about a high incidence of respiratory depression or hypotension when administering opioids. However, nurses should assist with selecting the correct agent, dose, and route when assessing individual patient characteristics (age, mental status, weight, medications, and medical history).

Selection of the appropriate starting dose for morphine and hydromorphone is important. Data from a recent study of patients in the ED randomized to receive either 0.10 mg/kg or 0.15 mg/kg of morphine sulfate demonstrate no meaningful difference in pain-relief scores and stress the importance of reassessment and individualized dosing.[52] Emergency nurses may be unaware of the dosing and equianalgesic differences between morphine sulfate and hydromorphone dosing. Table 10.3 describes these differences.[53] A typical initial dose for intravenous morphine is 0.10 mg/kg, which equals hydromorphone 0.015 mg/kg in the healthy adult who is younger than 60 years of age. For a 70-kg adult, this would roughly equal 7 mg of morphine or 1 mg of hydromorphone. Often nurses are reluctant to administer 7 mg of intravenous morphine but do not hesitant to administer 1 mg of intravenous hydromorphone.[51] This phenomenon is most likely due to lack of familiarity with equianalgesic dosing principles and the comfort of believing 1 mg of hydromorphone is much less than 7 mg of morphine. Either dose is safe and should be used as a starting point. Nurses should become familiar and comfortable with hydromorphone administration because it offers an excellent option for treatment of severe pain in the ED setting.

Fentanyl is a third opioid with specific indications for use in patients with severe pain in the ED. Fentanyl has a rapid onset (1–2 minutes) and a short duration of action, up to 60 minutes. It is useful for procedural sedation and short-term pain relief.[50] It may be particularly useful for trauma patients with an altered neurologic status or borderline hypotension because of its limited hemodynamic effect compared with other opioids and its short duration of action. Patients with the potential for altered mental status can be reevaluated in 30 to 60 minutes after the agent has worn off. Fentanyl is administered in micrograms, and 1 mcg/kg is a reasonable starting dose (70 mcg for a 70-kg adult).

No discussion of opioids is complete without mentioning meperidine (Demerol). The use of meperidine is discouraged because of its neurotoxic metabolite normeperidine, which is responsible for associated seizures and central nervous system toxicity.[47] Many other agents are available and for most patients are equally effective. However, if an individual patient receives pain relief only from meperidine, its use should not be strictly prohibited. These cases should be rare.

Selection of the correct drug, dose, and route will help promote optimal pain management. The key to effective pain management is rapid assessment, treatment, reassessment, and titration of analgesic agents until the patient's pain goal has been met.

Nurse-Initiated Analgesic Protocols

Crowded EDs are the norm and may limit the emergency nurse's ability to provide rapid analgesic management. Crowding also presents an opportunity to implement physician/nurse-developed, nurse-initiated analgesic protocols (NIAPs). Support for NIAPs is evident in the literature.[54–57] NIAPs allow nurses, in particular. Triage nurses, to administer analgesics before a physician evaluation. This can promote rapid initial analgesic management[55,56,58] and an overall increase in analgesic use.[55,56] These protocols would be most beneficial for patients with mild to moderate pain who often wait longer for initial physician evaluation because of their lower triage acuity. NIAPs are not a new concept, and emergency nurses from Australia and the United Kingdom are the leaders in this area.[54,59,60]

NIAPs typically include interventions in any of three categories: (1) nonpharmacologic, (2) nonopioid, and (3) opioid. Nonpharmacologic interventions include the use of ice, elevation, and distraction, and these interventions should be encouraged. Nonopioid protocols include ibuprofen and acetaminophen for mild pain.[55,56,58] Protocols including oral opioids most frequently allow administration of acetaminophen with codeine.[58,59] Other researchers have developed protocols allowing nurses to administer oxycodone with acetaminophen[61,62] or hydrocodone with acetaminophen.[55] Seguin[63] and colleagues developed a NIAP allowing administration of morphine, hydromorphone, and oxycodone, and Seguin reports the protocol was rarely used.

Inclusion of stronger opioids such as morphine and hydromorphone would not be appropriate for administration at triage (unless it is possible to monitor the patient's response) but would be very appropriate in the treatment areas of the ED, when a more thorough nursing assessment and adequate monitoring can occur but physician assessment may be delayed. Colleagues from Australia have implemented protocols allowing nurses to administer morphine before physician evaluation. They have developed a comprehensive training packet and monitor the effect of the protocols on analgesic management and adverse outcomes. They have reported excellent success.[64,65] Patient satisfaction with NIAP at triage has been investigated, and patients who received interventions at triage aimed at decreasing pain reported being more satisfied with their overall ED care because of the immediate attention to pain relief at triage.[46] Interventions consisted of ice and elevation and either ibuprofen or distraction.

The following barriers to implementation of NIAPs exist: (1) concern over safety, (2) reluctance to follow the protocol, (3) nurse reluctance to use NIAPs, (4) concern that patients will leave without being seen, and (5) concern about "drug-seeking" patients. Safety of analgesics, in particular opioids, before physician evaluation is a frequent concern; however, data support the safety of this practice.[59,66] Another valid concern is that nurses will not follow the protocol and will expand its use beyond the original intent. Most NIAPs exclude patients with chest or abdominal pain. Fry et al.[59] noted that nurses did administer an oral opioid to 7 patients (3%) with abdominal pain who were excluded from the protocol; no adverse events occurred. In a very small study, Seguin[63] noted the guidelines for obtaining vital signs after analgesic administration were not always followed. In the current era of medication safety, the strongest argument against NIAPs will most likely be concern over the possibility that patients may leave before physician evaluation and the "drug-seeking" patient will routinely present to the ED for oral opioids. In a prospective evaluation of 202 patients who received acetaminophen with codeine, 31 patients (15%) left before physician evaluation.[59] Although concern over liability for these patients is valid, many patients leave before physician evaluation, and the risk to patients after receiving an analgesic such as hydrocodone or codeine should be placed in the context of the many other patients who also leave before physician evaluation. All patients who leave before physician evaluation pose a potential liability. Quality monitoring procedures should be in place to track patients who leave after receiving an oral opioid, and individual patients can be managed appropriately.[61] Institutional policies can state the NIAP will not apply to patients in the future if they at any point leave before physician evaluation.

In summary, NIAPs provide an opportunity to facilitate rapid analgesic management. The development of protocols will require a collaborative approach between emergency physicians, nurses, administrators, and hospital pharmacists. Adequate training, policy development, ongoing quality improvement monitoring, and attention to medication safety will be key elements in maintaining the balance between providing optimal analgesia and preventing abuse potential and adverse outcomes.

Specific Emergency Department Pain Management Challenges

Treating Abdominal and Trauma-Related Pain

Patients with abdominal pain or those with multiple trauma are at high risk for inadequate analgesic management in the ED setting. One of the most pervasive myths and important barriers to providing analgesia in the ED setting has been the inability to provide analgesics to a patient with abdominal pain until a diagnosis was made. This myth originates from the 1987 edition of *Cope's Early Diagnosis of the Acute Abdomen,* yet the more recent 2000 edition refutes this practice.[67,68] The myth has now been refuted with data from multiple studies.[69–71] Despite the research, controversy still exists, and nurses who desire more information are referred to a 2006 editorial by Knopp and Dries.[72] Emergency nurses are encouraged to participate in developing protocols to manage abdominal pain with their emergency physician and surgical colleagues.

Patients with multiple trauma are also at risk for undertreatment of pain. Recent data report a national increase in the administration of analgesics to patients with long bone fractures.[73–75] The only absolute contraindications to analgesic administration are respiratory depression, hemodynamic instability, and coma.[76] Hypotension can be minimized by carefully selecting agents with fewer negative cardiac effects (e.g., fentanyl), administering agents very slowly, and maintaining intravascular volume.[73] Analgesics should be administered to patients who are paralyzed and intubated because they may be unable to communicate but remain able to feel pain.

Sickle Cell Acute Pain Episodes

Many ED nurses and physicians express frustration and believe patients with sickle cell disease are opioid dependent, despite data to disprove this belief.[77–79] Patients with this chronic and often debilitating disease also express frustration with ED care.[80–82] Sickle cell disease is associated with many serious pathophysiologic complications (e.g., acute stroke, acute chest syndrome, cholecystitis, chronic hemolytic anemia, iron overload, pulmonary hypertension, end-organ failure, avascular necrosis of the joints, and chronic leg ulcers) and acute pain episodes that at times require ED analgesic management. An increasing frequency of pain episodes is associated with an increased risk for death.[83]

Acute pain episodes should be treated as a high priority, and rapid analgesic management should occur.[83,84] The Emergency Severity Index, version 4, five-level triage system, specifies that patients with an acute pain episode associated with sickle cell disease should be triaged as a high-priority, level 2 patient.[85] Despite this, recent data from a multicenter project report only 27% of patients received the correct triage score and patients waited a median time of 90 minutes before receiving an analgesic. There was no difference in time to initial analgesic based on the total number of visits for an individual patient during the 12-month study period.[86]

It is possible that emergency clinicians may generalize their experiences with a few individual patients to all patients with sickle cell disease. At this time, we do not understand the reasons why some patients with sickle cell disease have more frequent visits than others. It is possible their disease is more severe, they experience more pain episodes, or other unknown sociocultural factors are responsible.

ED nurses are encouraged to initiate rapid, aggressive analgesic management for patients with an acute pain episode and sickle cell disease.[87] Guidelines recommend administration of intravenous morphine or hydromorphone within 15 minutes of ED arrival.[84] Although this may not be feasible in many cases, 90 minutes far exceeds the analgesia management recommendation. Patients with sickle cell disease represent another population at risk for inadequate analgesic management, and the ED nurse can play a crucial role in maximizing pain relief for these patients.

Health Care Worker–Induced Procedural Pain

Emergency nurses and other health care workers can cause pain by performing procedures, including insertion of urethral and intravenous catheters and nasogastric tubes. Data support the topical administration of lidocaine jelly in males, but not females, before urethral catheterization.[88,89] A variety of analgesic approaches have been evaluated to decrease the pain associated with nasogastric tube insertion. The literature supports the use of lidocaine gel administered nasally, atomized nasopharyngeal and oropharyngeal lidocaine, and lidocaine and phenylephrine for the nose and tetracaine with benzocaine spray for the oropharynx.[90–92] Finally, nurses have an opportunity to decrease the pain associated with laceration repair by applying a pharmacy-prepared mixture of lidocaine, epinephrine, and tetracaine (LET) at triage. Application of LET is associated with less pain during injection of a local anesthetic.[93] Standing orders for this or similar preparations should exist in all EDs.

Discharge Teaching

Emergency nurses play a key role in providing discharge analgesic teaching. Recent data suggest pain scores at discharge remain moderate.[3,94] Many patients continue to experience pain up to 96 hours after discharge from the ED, and up to 78% of patients reported using the analgesics prescribed at discharge from the ED.[94] Analgesic discharge teaching should include a discussion of analgesic dosing, scheduling, side effects and, when appropriate, the need to avoid additional doses of either acetaminophen or NSAIDs. Patients should always be encouraged to contact a health care provider for unrelieved pain or to return to the ED if necessary.

PEDIATRIC PAIN MANAGEMENT

Approximately one-third of all ED visits each year involve the care of children.[95] Although some of these encounters are caused by traumatic injuries such as fractures, lacerations, and blunt organ injury, chronic diseases such as cancer, bowel disorders, migraines, and acute exacerbation of diseases such as sickle cell disease and appendicitis all require developmentally appropriate pain assessment and management.[96] In addition, most of these injuries and disorders require painful and anxiety-provoking diagnostic and management procedures, such as venipuncture, heel sticks, lumbar puncture, urethral catheterization, laceration repair, diagnostic imaging, or fracture reduction. As a patient advocate, it is the emergency nurse's responsibility to be knowledgeable and skilled in the use of developmentally appropriate assessment and pain management techniques. Principles of pediatric pain assessment and management are summarized in Table 10.4.

Pediatric-Specific Pain Management Myths and Barriers

Despite research-based advances in pediatric pain management and assessment, myths and barriers continue to influence practice.[97–101] One of the most common myths is that infants and children experience less pain than adults and retain no memory of the painful event. Infants are in fact hypersensitive to painful stimuli and exhibit extreme physiologic and hormonal responses to unmanaged pain.[102] This stress response increases oxygen demands

TABLE 10.4 Procedural Pain Assessment and Management Guidelines.

GENERAL PRINCIPLES

1. All infants and children experience pain.
2. Failure to manage pain can produce negative short- and long-term effects.
3. Pain that can be predicted (procedural) should be treated prophylactically.
4. Assessment and management should be developmentally appropriate and use nonpharmacologic and pharmacologic interventions in conjunction.

Age	Assessment	Indication	Nonpharmacologic Interventions	Pharmacologic Interventions	Concerns
Newborn and infant (preverbal)	PIPP (Premature Infant Pain Profile): preterm–3 months; and FLACC (face, legs, activity, cry, and consolability): 3 months–7 years	Heel sticks, lumbar puncture (LP), venipuncture, circumcision, urethral catheterization, immunizations and injections	Parental involvement; swaddling, touching, positioning, suckling	Oral sucrose drops and pacifier, LMX4, EMLA (eutectic mixture of lidocaine and prilocaine), vapocoolants	• TAC and LET should not be applied to fingertips, toes, or penis • Sucrose not advised in unstable newborns and NPO • Do not use EMLA with history of methemoglobinemia
Preschool (verbal and nonverbal)	FLACC, Oucher Scale, visual analog scale (VAS), color analog scale (CAS), FACES Pain Scale, Poker Chip Tool	LP, venipuncture, urethral catheterization, diagnostic procedures, laceration repair, immunizations and injections	Parental involvement, blowing bubbles, distraction, play, TV/video, songs, praise, rewards, simple explanations	LMX4, EMLA, vapocoolants, TAC (tetracaine, adrenaline, and cocaine), LET (lidocaine, epinephrine, and tetracaine), S-Caine patch (lidocaine and tetracaine), lidocaine	• LMX4, EMLA for intact skin only

Continued

TABLE 10.4 Procedural Pain Assessment and Management Guidelines—cont'd

Age	Assessment	Indication	Nonpharmacologic Interventions	Pharmacologic Interventions	Concerns
Schoolage	Oucher Scale, VAS, CAS, FACES Pain Scale, Poker Chip Tool	LP, venipuncture, urethral catheterization, diagnostic procedures, laceration repair, immunizations and injections	Parental involvement (allow choice for older children), distraction, video games, trivia, deep breathing, music, praise, ice/hot pack	LMX4, EMLA, vapocoolants, TAC, LET, S-Caine patch, lidocaine	
Adolescent	Self-report, verbal numeric scale, word graphic numeric scale, VAS	LP, venipuncture, urethral catheterization, diagnostic procedures, laceration repair, immunizations and injections	Allow choice of parental involvement, distraction, video games, trivia, deep breathing, guided imagery, music, praise, ice/hot pack	LMX4, EMLA, vapocoolants, TAC, LET, S-Caine patch, lidocaine, buffered lidocaine, lidocaine iontophoresis	

NPO, Nothing by mouth.

Data from Bauman BH, McManus JG Jr. Pediatric pain management in the emergency department. *Emerg Med Clin North Am.* 2005;23(2): 393–414; Hatfield L, Messner E, Lingg K. Evidence-based strategies for the pharmacologic management of pediatric pain during minor procedures in the emergency department. *Top Emerg Med.* 2006;28(2):129; Mace S. Pain management and procedural sedation in pediatric patients. In: Mace S, Durcharme J, Murphy M, eds. *Pain Management and Sedation.* New York, NY: McGraw-Hill; 2006; Merkel S, Voepel-Lewis T, Malviya S. Pain assessment in infants and young children: the FLACC scale. *Am J Nurs.* 2002;102(10):55.

and metabolism, delays healing, and contributes to morbidity and mortality.[103] When the pain response during circumcision was evaluated, unanesthetized newborns demonstrated greater pain responses than anesthetized newborns and greater distress during subsequent immunizations 4 to 6 months later.[104,105] Severe pain can lead to posttraumatic stress disorder, affecting future health care encounters, as evidenced by avoidance behaviors, disproportionate pain and anxiety responses, nightmares, and needle phobias.[106] If pain is untreated, the ability to adequately manage subsequent painful procedures has been shown to be diminished.[107]

A second commonly held belief is that opioid administration is more dangerous in children and may interfere with physical examination and diagnosis.[108] Although opioids are used more cautiously in neonates because of immature metabolism and clearance, they are safe at smaller doses by continuous infusion.[108,109] By 3 to 6 months of age, infants metabolize and clear opioids at rates similar to those of older children, and opioid use is no more dangerous in pediatrics than it is in adults.[108] No current research or practice standards endorse the withholding of pain medication before examination and diagnosis.[98] Although myths continue to affect practice, research now clearly demonstrates that pathophysiologic findings do not substantiate these myths. Opioid administration in neonates, infants, and children is safe.

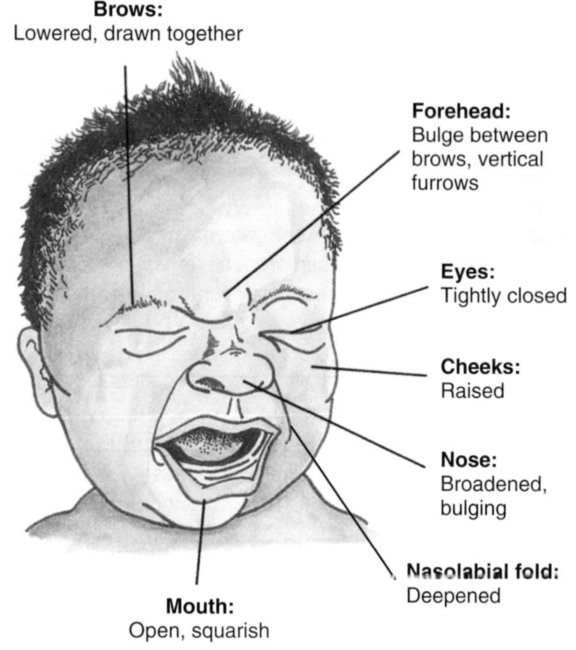

Fig. 10.4 Facial expression of physical distress is the most consistent behavioral indicator of pain in infants. (From Hockenberry MJ, Wilson D, Winkelstein ML, et al. *Wong's Nursing Care of Infants and Children.* 7th ed. St Louis, MO: Mosby; 2003.)

Pediatric Pain Assessment

Anticipating and predicting painful experiences requires the use of developmentally appropriate assessments and is paramount to successful pain management in pediatrics.[97] Because pain is a unique, individualized experience, the ED nurse must believe his or her patient's report and take into consideration age, race, gender, culture, cognition, emotions, and past experiences, all of which cannot be captured by any single assessment tool.[95] Although the clinical standard for pain assessment in children is self-report, this standard is limited to verbal, cognitively appropriate children. Fig. 10.4 illustrates facial changes

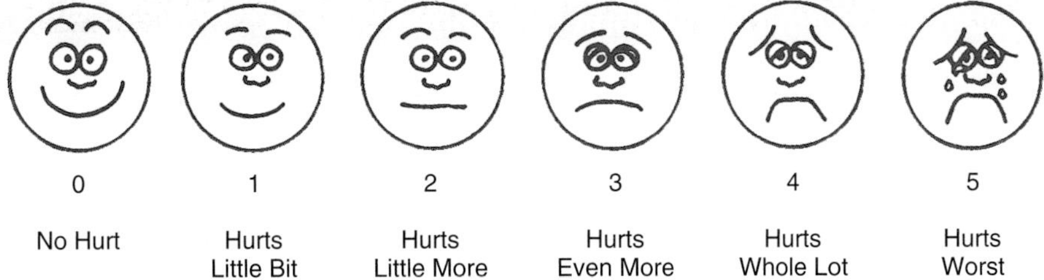

Fig. 10.5 Wong-Baker FACES Pain Rating Scale. (From Hockenberry MJ, Wilson D. *Wong's Nursing Care of Infants and Children.* 8th ed. St Louis, MO: Mosby; 2007.)

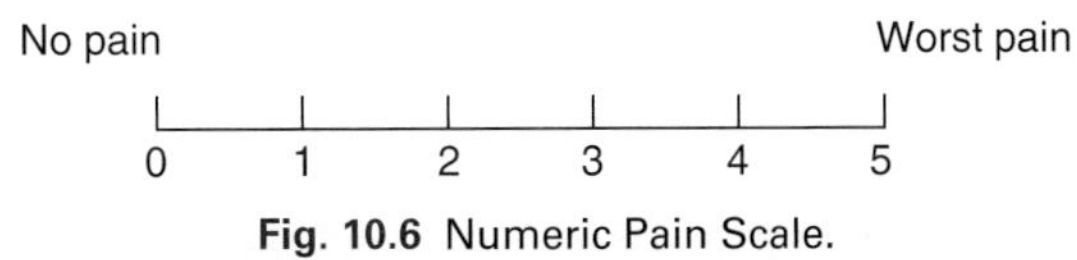

Fig. 10.6 Numeric Pain Scale.

TABLE 10.5 FLACC (Face, Legs, Activity, Cry, and Consolability): 3 Months to 7 Years.

	SCORING		
Categories	**0**	**1**	**2**
Face	No particular expression or smile	Occasional grimace or frown; withdrawn, disinterested	Frequent to constant frown, clenched jaw, quivering chin
Legs	Normal position or relaxed	Uneasy, restless, tense	Kicking or legs drawn up
Activity	Lying quietly, normal position, moves easily	Squirming, shifting back and forth, tense	Arched, rigid, or jerking
Cry	No cry (awake or asleep)	Moans or whimpers, occasional complaint	Crying steadily; screams or sobs; frequent complaints
Consolability	Content, relaxed	Reassured by occasional touching, hugging, or being talked to; distractible	Difficult to console or comfort

Each of the five categories is scored from 0 to 2, resulting in a total score between 0 and 10. Before scoring, awake children are observed for 2 minutes and asleep children are observed for 5 minutes.

From Markel S, Voepel-Lewis T, Shayevitz J, et al. The FLACC: a behavioral scale for scoring postoperative pain in young children. *Pediatr Nurs.* 1997;23(3):293–297. © 2002, The Regents of the University of Michigan. Used with permission.

that may be observed in the infant in pain. Unidimensional tools, such as the Oucher Scale, the visual analog scale, the color analog scale, the FACES Pain Rating Scale (Fig. 10.5), and the Poker Chip Tool, have all been validated in children aged 3 and older. A numeric scale (Fig. 10.6) may be used with children 5 years of age or older. Multidimensional tools, such as FLACC (Table 10.5) and the Premature Infant Pain Profile (PIPP), rely on behavioral and physiologic observations and have been validated multiculturally in nonverbal as well as cognitively impaired infants and children.[95,110]

Pediatric Pain Interventions

Appropriate initial and ongoing assessment directly contributes to successful pain management. Optimal pediatric pain management should use both nonpharmacologic and pharmacologic interventions whenever feasible. This process should always begin with preparing the child and family for the procedure. Table 10.4 identifies age-specific interventions to be used concurrently for procedural pain. Lidocaine, EMLA cream (eutectic mixture of lidocaine and prilocaine), and LMX4, when combined with distraction techniques, have been shown to be effective and safe in managing pain associated with vascular access, injections, lumbar puncture, and minor surgical procedures.[111,112] The S-Caine patch (lidocaine and tetracaine) and buffered lidocaine are effective in diminishing pain associated with vascular access when combined with distraction and music therapy in older children.[113] Vapocoolants have a rapid onset and in combination with distraction are efficient methods of reducing the pain associated with injections and immunizations.[100] Sucrose, along with swaddling, breast-feeding, maternal positioning, and touching, has been shown to be as effective in reducing pain associated with heel sticks, vascular access, injections, and urethral catheterization as other therapies for infants up to 3 months of age.[114,115]

TAC (tetracaine, adrenaline, and cocaine) and LET (lidocaine, epinephrine, and tetracaine) are topical anesthetics providing initial pain relief for open wounds requiring irrigation and suturing.[95] These agents should be applied to open wounds for approximately 15 to 20 minutes or until blanching around the edges occurs and before the use of local anesthetic blocks and suturing or irrigation to minimize the pain associated with these procedures. These agents should not be applied to fingertips, toes, or the penis or to any area with decreased circulation. More complex or lengthy procedures (e.g., diagnostic imaging, fracture reduction, and laceration

TABLE 10.6 Pediatric Procedural Sedation Recommendations.

Drug Name	Standard Dose	Maximum Dose
Midazolam	0.05–0.1 mg/kg IV over 2–3 min	Child < 5 yr: 6 mg IV/IM Child > 6 yr: 10 mg IV/IM
Ketamine	1–1.5 mg/kg IV or IM (slow titration)	Rate of administration should not exceed 0.5 mg/kg/min
Propofol	1–1.5 mg/kg IV (slow titration)	3–3.5 mg/kg
Chloral hydrate	Low dose 25–50 mg/kg PO (may repeat in 30 min) High dose 60–80 mg/kg PO (peaks 30–90 min)	Infant: 1 g Child: 2–2.5 mg/kg

IM, Intramuscular; *IV,* intravenous; *PO,* by mouth.
Data from Mace S. Pain management and procedural sedation in pediatric patients. In: Mace S, Ducharme J, Murphy M, eds. *Pain Management and Sedation.* New York, NY: McGraw-Hill; 2006; Custer JW, Rau RE, Johns Hopkins Hospital Children's Medical and Surgical Center. *The Harriet Lane Handbook: A Manual for Pediatric House Officers.* 18th ed. Philadelphia, PA: Mosby/Elsevier; 2009.

TABLE 10.7 Pediatric Pharmacologic Recommendations for Mild to Moderate Pain.

Medication	Route	Dose
Acetaminophen	PO PR	10–15 mg/kg q 4 h (75 mg/kg/day max) First dose 20–40 mg/kg, then same as PO
Ibuprofen	PO	4–10 mg/kg q 6 h
Ketorolac (age >2 yr)	IV IM	0.5 mg/kg to max 15 mg single dose 1 mg/kg to max 30 mg single dose

IM, Intramuscular; *IV,* intravenous; *max,* maximum; *PO,* by mouth; *PR,* by rectum.
Data from Bauman BH, McManus JG Jr. Pediatric pain management in the emergency department. *Emerg Med Clin North Am.* 2005;23(2):393–414.

TABLE 10.8 Pediatric Pharmacologic Recommendations for Moderate to Severe Pain.

Medication	Route	Dose for Child < 50 kg	Dose for Child > 50 kg
Codeine	PO	0.5–1 mg/kg q 3–4 h	30–60 mg q 3–4 h
Oxycodone	PO	0.1–0.2 mg/kg q 3–4 h	5–10 mg q 3–4 h
Hydrocodone	PO	0.05–0.2 mg/kg q 4–6 h	5–10 mg q 4–6 h
Morphine	IV/subcutaneous	0.1 mg/kg q 2–4 h	5–8 mg q 2–4 h
Fentanyl	IV/subcutaneous	0.5–1 mcg/kg q 1–2 h	25–50 mcg q 1–2 h
Hydromorphone	IV/subcutaneous	0.02 mg/kg q 2–4 h	1 mg q 2–4 h

IV, Intravenous; *PO,* by mouth.
Data from Bauman BH, McManus JG Jr. Pediatric pain management in the emergency department, *Emerg Med Clin North Am.* 2005;23(2):393–414.

repair) often cannot be successfully performed with distraction and topical anesthetics alone. Table 10.6 lists common anesthetic and sedative-hypnotic agents and dosages used for procedural sedation.[102]

Nonopioids, including acetaminophen and NSAIDs such as ibuprofen and ketorolac, provide excellent relief for mild to moderate pain (Table 10.7) but are often underused.[116] Oral opioids, such as codeine, oxycodone, and hydrocodone, are often required to manage moderate to severe pain.[117] Morphine and fentanyl are excellent choices for treating severe pain.[95,117] Table 10.8 suggests routes and doses for these agents.[95] Children and infants are at the same risk for respiratory depression and apnea as adults. These risks can be greatly diminished by careful dose and rate selection and appropriate ongoing assessment and monitoring.[102]

In addition to the variety of pharmacologic interventions, nonpharmacologic interventions should be combined with pharmacologic interventions to help optimize pain relief for all pediatric patients with pain in the ED setting. Table 10.4 suggests possible age-specific, nonpharmacologic techniques.

SUMMARY

From a greater understanding of pain pathophysiology specific to adults and children, to validated multidimensional assessment tools, to cutting-edge pharmacologic and nonpharmacologic interventions, the opportunity for today's emergency nurse to provide safe and effective pain relief to both adult and pediatric patients is enormous. Emergency nurses can lead a culture change and optimize excellent pain management for all of our patients. This can be facilitated by increasing and promoting education specific to pain, using current research to guide practice, serving as a patient advocate, and always maintaining an active voice.

REFERENCES

1. Cordell WH, Keene KK, Giles BK, Jones JB, Jones JH, Brizendine EJ. The high prevalence of pain in emergency medical care. *Am J Emerg Med*. 2002;20(3):165–169.
2. Hwang U, Richardson LD, Sonuyi TO, Morrison RS. The effect of emergency department crowding on the management of pain in older adults with hip fracture. *J Am Geriatr Soc*. 2006;54(2):270–275.
3. Todd KH, Ducharme J, Choiniere M, et al. Pain in the emergency department: results of the pain and emergency medicine initiative (PEMI) multicenter study. *J Pain*. 2007;8(6):460–466.
4. Pletcher MJ, Kertesz SG, Kohn MA, Gonzales R. Trends in opioid prescribing by race/ethnicity for patients seeking care in US emergency departments. *JAMA*. 2008;299(1):70–78.
5. International Association for the Study of Pain. IASP pain terminology. https://www.iasp-pain.org/terminology?navItemNumber=576. Published September 6, 2007. Accessed April 27, 2019.
6. Dunajcik L. Chronic nonmalignant pain. In: McCaffery M, Passero C, eds. *Pain Clinical Manual*. 2nd ed. St Louis, MO: Mosby; 1999.
7. Serpell M. Anatomy, physiology and pharmacology. *Surgery*. 2006;24(10):350.
8. Gaskin DJ, Richard P. The economic costs of pain in the United States. *J Pain*. 2012;13(8):715–724.
9. Huether S, Defriez C. Pain, temperature regulation, sleep and sensory function. In: McCance K, Huether S, eds. *Pathophysiology: The Biologic Basis for Disease in Adults and Children*. 5th ed. St Louis: Mosby; 2006.
10. Montgomery R, Fink R. Pain management. In: Oman K, Koziol-McLain J, eds. *Emergency Nursing Secrets*. 2nd ed. St Louis, MO: Mosby; 2007.
11. Schaffler R. Pain management. In: Hoyt S, Selfridge-Thomas J, eds. *Emergency Nursing Core Curriculum*. 6th ed. St Louis, MO: Mosby; 2007.
12. Fink WA Jr. The pathophysiology of acute pain. *Emerg Med Clin North Am*. 2005;23(2):277–284.
13. Corbett AD, Henderson G, McKnight AT, Paterson SJ. 75 years of opioid research: the exciting but vain quest for the Holy Grail. *Br J Pharmacol*. 2006;147(suppl 1):S153–S162.
14. Cutshall A, Fenske L, Kelly R, Phillips BR, Sundt TM, Bauer BA. Creation of a healing enhancement program at an academic medical center. *Complement Ther Clin Pract*. 2007;13(4):217–223.
15. Serpell M. Pharmacological treatment of chronic pain. *Anaesth Intensive Care Med*. 2005;6(2):39.
16. Melzack R. From the gate to the neuromatrix. *Pain*. 1999;(suppl 6):S121–S126.
17. Prevost S. Relieving pain and providing comfort. In: Martin P, Fontaine D, Hudack C, et al., eds. *Critical Care Nursing: A Holistic Approach*. 8th ed. Philadelphia, PA: Williams & Wilkins; 2005.
18. Jacox A, Carr D, Chapman C, et al. *Acute Pain Management: Operative or Medical Procedures and Trauma. AHCPR Clinical Practice Guidelines, No. 1. Report No. 92-0032*. Rockville, MD: US Department of Health and Human Services, Agency for Health Care Policy and Research; 1992.
19. McCaffery M, Passero C. Assessment: underlying complexities, misconceptions, and practical tools. In: McCaffery M, Passero C, eds. *Pain: Clinical Manual*. 2nd ed. St Louis, MO: Mosby; 1999.
20. Heins JK, Heins A, Grammas M, Costello M, Huang K, Mishra S. Disparities in analgesia and opioid prescribing practices for patients with musculoskeletal pain in the emergency department. *J Emerg Nurs*. 2006;32(3):219–224.
21. Raftery KA, Smith-Coggins R, Chen AH. Gender-associated differences in emergency department pain management. *Ann Emerg Med*. 1995;26(4):414–421.
22. Todd KH, Deaton C, D'Adamo AP, Goe L. Ethnicity and analgesic practice. *Ann Emerg Med*. 2000;35(1):11–16.
23. Rupp T, Delaney KA. Inadequate analgesia in emergency medicine. *Ann Emerg Med*. 2004;43(4):494–503.
24. Joranson DE, Ryan KM, Gilson AM, Dahl JL. Trends in medical use and abuse of opioid analgesics. *JAMA*. 2000;283(13):1710–1714.
25. Wilsey B, Fishman S, Rose JS, Papazian J. Pain management in the ED. *Am J Emerg Med*. 2004;22(1):51–57.
26. Brice M. Care plans for patients with frequent ED visits for such chief complaints as back pain, migraine, and abdominal pain. *J Emerg Nurs*. 2004;30(2):150–153.
27. Mowry JB, Spyker DA, Brooks DE, McMillan N, Schauben JL. 2014 annual report of the American Association of Poison Control Centers' National Poison Data System (NPDS): 32nd annual report. *Clin Toxicol*. 2015;10(53):962–1147.
28. Paulozzi LJ. Prescription drug overdoses: a review. *J Safety Res*. 2012;43(4):283–289.
29. Centers for Disease Control and Prevention. Opioid overdose fact sheet; 2016. https://www.cdc.gov/rxawareness/pdf/RxAwareness-Campaign-Overview-508.pdf. Accessed April 27, 2019.
30. Centers for Disease Control and Prevention. Data overview: injury prevention and control: prescription drug overdose. https://www.cdc.gov/drugoverdose/. Accessed April 27, 2019.
31. Butler MM, Ancona RM, Beauchamp GA. Emergency department prescription opioids as an initial exposure preceding addiction. *Ann Emerg Med*. 2016;68(2):202–208.
32. Fosnocht DE, Heaps ND, Swanson ER. Patient expectations for pain relief in the ED. *Am J Emerg Med*. 2004;22(4):286–288.
33. Lee WW, Burelbach AE, Fosnocht D. Hispanic and non-Hispanic white patient pain management expectations. *Am J Emerg Med*. 2001;19(7):549–550.
34. Yee AM, Puntillo K, Miaskowski C, Neighbor ML. What patients with abdominal pain expect about pain relief in the emergency department. *J Emerg Nurs*. 2006;32(4):281–287.
35. Fosnocht DE, Swanson ER, Bossart P. Patient expectations for pain medication delivery. *Am J Emerg Med*. 2001;19(5):399–402.
36. Bijur PE, Latimer CT, Gallagher EJ. Validation of a verbally administered numerical rating scale of acute pain for use in the emergency department. *Acad Emerg Med*. 2003;10(4):390–392.
37. Puntillo K, Neighbor M, O'Neil N, Nixon R. Accuracy of emergency nurses in assessment of patients' pain. *Pain Manag Nurs*. 2003;4(4):171–175.
38. Franck LS. A pain in the act: musings on the meaning for critical care nurses of the pain management standards of the Joint Commission on Accreditation of Healthcare Organizations. *Crit Care Nurse*. 2001;21(3):8.
39. Nelson BP, Cohen D, Lander O, et al. Mandated pain scales improve frequency of ED analgesic administration. *Am J Emerg Med*. 2004;22(7):582–585.
40. Silka PA, Roth MM, Moreno G, Merrill L, Geiderman JM. Pain scores improve analgesic administration patterns for trauma patients in the emergency department. *Acad Emerg Med*. 2004;11(3):264–270.

41. Baumann BM, Holmes JH, Chansky ME, et al. Pain assessments and the provision of analgesia: the effects of a templated chart. *Acad Emerg Med.* 2007;14(1):47–52.
42. Blumstein HA, Moore D. Visual analog pain scores do not define desire for analgesia in patients with acute pain. *Acad Emerg Med.* 2003;10(3):211–214.
43. American College of Emergency Physicians. Pain management in the emergency departments; 2007. https://www.acep.org/patient-care/policy-statements/optimizing-the-treatment-of-acute-pain-in-the-emergency-department/. Accessed April 27, 2019.
44. Tanabe P, Buschmann M. A prospective study of ED pain management practices and the patient's perspective. *J Emerg Nurs.* 1999;25(3):171–177.
45. Tanabe P, Ferket K, Thomas R, Paice J, Marcantonio R. The effect of standard care, ibuprofen, and distraction on pain relief and patient satisfaction in children with musculoskeletal trauma. *J Emerg Nurs.* 2002;28(2):118–125.
46. Tanabe P, Thomas R, Paice J, Spiller M, Marcantonio R. The effect of standard care, ibuprofen, and music on pain relief and patient satisfaction in adults with musculoskeletal trauma. *J Emerg Nurs.* 2001;27(2):124–131.
47. American Pain Society. *Principles of Analgesic Use in the Treatment of Acute Pain and Cancer Pain.* 5th ed. Glenview, IL: American Pain Society; 2003.
48. Holdgate A, Pollock T. Systematic review of the relative efficacy of non-steroidal anti-inflammatory drugs and opioids in the treatment of acute renal colic. *BMJ.* 2004;328(7453):1401.
49. US Food and Drug Administration. *FDA public health advisory: FDA announces important changes and additional warnings for COX-2 selective and non-selective non-steroidal anti-inflammatory drugs (NSAIDs).* http://www.fda.gov/Cder/drug/advisory/COX2.htm. Published September 22, 2007. Accessed
50. Berry P, Covington E, Dahl J, et al. *Pain: Current Understanding of Assessment, Management, and Treatments.* Glenview, IL: American Pain Society; 2006.
51. Chang AK, Bijur PE, Meyer RH, Kenny MK, Solorzano C, Gallagher EJ. Safety and efficacy of hydromorphone as an analgesic alternative to morphine in acute pain: a randomized clinical trial. *Ann Emerg Med.* 2006;48(2):164–172.
52. Birnbaum A, Esses D, Bijur PE, Holden L, Gallagher EJ. Randomized double-blind placebo-controlled trial of two intravenous morphine dosages (0.10 mg/kg and 0.15 mg/kg) in emergency department patients with moderate to severe acute pain. *Ann Emerg Med.* 2007;49(4):445–453.
53. Max MRP, Edwards W, et al. *Principles of Analgesic Use in the Treatment of Acute Pain and Cancer Pain.* Glenview, IL: American Pain Society; 1999.
54. Arendts G, Fry M. Factors associated with delay to opiate analgesia in emergency departments. *J Pain.* 2006;7(9):682–686.
55. Fosnocht DE, Swanson ER. Use of a triage pain protocol in the ED. *Am J Emerg Med.* 2007;25(7):791–793.
56. Stalnikowicz R, Mahamid R, Kaspi S, Brezis M. Undertreatment of acute pain in the emergency department: a challenge. *Int J Qual Health Care.* 2005;17(2):173–176.
57. Tcherny-Lessenot S, Karwowski-Soulie F, Lamarche-Vadel A, Ginsburg C, Brunet F, Vidal-Trecan G. Management and relief of pain in an emergency department from the adult patients' perspective. *J Pain Symptom Manage.* 2003;25(6):539–546.
58. Boyd RJ, Stuart P. The efficacy of structured assessment and analgesia provision in the paediatric emergency department. *Emerg Med J.* 2005;22(1):30–32.
59. Fry M, Ryan J, Alexander N. A prospective study of nurse initiated panadeine forte: expanding pain management in the ED. *Accid Emerg Nurs.* 2004;12(3):136–140.
60. Overton-Brown P, Higgins J, Bridge P. What does the triage nurse do? *Emerg Nurse.* 2001;8(10):30–36.
61. Campbell P, Dennie M, Dougherty K, Iwaskiw O, Rollo K. Implementation of an ED protocol for pain management at triage at a busy level I trauma center. *J Emerg Nurs.* 2004;30(5):431–438.
62. Musselman E, Owens I. *Pain Protocol for University ED. Indiana University Emergency Department.* Indianapolis, IN: Clarian Health Partners; 2006.
63. Seguin D. A nurse-initiated pain management advanced triage protocol for ED patients with an extremity injury at a level I trauma center. *J Emerg Nurs.* 2004;30(4):330–335.
64. Green D, Kelly A, Priestley S, et al. *Pain Management Package WH.* Australia: Emergency Departments of Western Health; 2003–2006.
65. Kelly AM. A process approach to improving pain management in the emergency department: development and evaluation. *J Accid Emerg Med.* 2000;17(3):185–187.
66. Coman M, Kelly A. Safety of a nurse-managed, titrated analgesia protocol for the management of severe pain in the emergency department. *Emerg Med Australasia.* 1999;11(3):128–132.
67. Silen W. *Cope's Early Diagnosis of the Acute Abdomen.* 17th ed. New York, NY: Oxford University Press; 1987.
68. Silen W. *Cope's Early Diagnosis of the Acute Abdomen.* 20th ed. New York, NY: Oxford University Press; 2000.
69. Mahadevan M, Graff L. Prospective randomized study of analgesic use for ED patients with right lower quadrant abdominal pain. *Am J Emerg Med.* 2000;18(7):753–756.
70. Ranji SR, Goldman LE, Simel DL, Shojania KG. Do opiates affect the clinical evaluation of patients with acute abdominal pain? *JAMA.* 2006;296(14):1764–1774.
71. Thomas SH, Silen W, Cheema F, et al. Effects of morphine analgesia on diagnostic accuracy in emergency department patients with abdominal pain: a prospective, randomized trial. *J Am Coll Surg.* 2003;196(1):18–31.
72. Knopp RK, Dries D. Analgesia in acute abdominal pain: what's next? *Ann Emerg Med.* 2006;48(2):161–163.
73. Chao A, Huang CH, Pryor JP, Reilly PM, Schwab CW. Analgesic use in intubated patients during acute resuscitation. *J Trauma.* 2006;60(3):579–582.
74. Neighbor ML, Honner S, Kohn MA. Factors affecting emergency department opioid administration to severely injured patients. *Acad Emerg Med.* 2004;11(12):1290–1296.
75. Ritsema TS, Kelen GD, Pronovost PJ, Pham JC. The national trend in quality of emergency department pain management for long bone fractures. *Acad Emerg Med.* 2007;14(2):163–169.
76. Cantees K, Yealy D. Pain management in the trauma patient. In: Peitzman A, Rhodes M, Schwab C, et al., eds. *The Trauma Manual.* Philadelphia, PA: Lippincott-Raven; 1998.
77. Pack-Mabien A, Labbe E, Herbert D, Haynes J Jr. Nurses' attitudes and practices in sickle cell pain management. *Appl Nurs Res.* 2001;14(4):187–192.
78. Shapiro BS, Benjamin LJ, Payne R, Heidrich G. Sickle cell-related pain: perceptions of medical practitioners. *J Pain Symptom Manage.* 1997;14(3):168–174.
79. Waldrop RD, Mandry C. Health professional perceptions of opioid dependence among patients with pain. *Am J Emerg Med.* 1995;13(5):529–531.

80. Maxwell K, Streetly A, Bevan D. Experiences of hospital care and treatment seeking for pain from sickle cell disease: qualitative study. *BMJ*. 1999;318(7198):1585–1590.
81. Philpott S, Mason J, Aisiku I. Patient satisfaction in the emergency department management of acute sickle cell pain. *Acad Emerg Med*. 2005;12(suppl 5):1.
82. Todd KH, Green C, Bonham VL Jr, Haywood C Jr, Ivy E. Sickle cell disease related pain: crisis and conflict. *J Pain*. 2006;7(7):453–458.
83. Platt OS, Thorington BD, Brambilla DJ, et al. Pain in sickle cell disease: rates and risk factors. *N Engl J Med*. 1991;325(1):11–16.
84. Benjamin L, Dampier C, Jacox A, et al. *Guideline for the Management of Acute Pain in Sickle-Cell Disease: Quick Reference Guide for Emergency Department Clinicians*. Glenview, IL: American Pain Society; 2001.
85. Gilboy N, Tanabe P, Travers D, Rosenau AM. *Emergency Severity Index, Version 4: Implementation Handbook*. Rockville, MD: Agency for Healthcare Research and Quality; 2005.
86. Tanabe P, Myers R, Zosel A, et al. Emergency department management of acute pain episodes in sickle cell disease. *Acad Emerg Med*. 2007;14(5):419–425.
87. Platt A, Eckman JR, Beasley J, Miller G. Treating sickle cell pain: an update from the Georgia comprehensive sickle cell center. *J Emerg Nurs*. 2002;28(4):297–303.
88. Siderias J, Guadio F, Singer AJ. Comparison of topical anesthetics and lubricants prior to urethral catheterization in males: a randomized controlled trial. *Acad Emerg Med*. 2004;11(6):703–706.
89. Tanabe P, Steinmann R, Anderson J, Johnson D, Metcalf S, Ring-Hurn E. Factors affecting pain scores during female urethral catheterization. *Acad Emerg Med*. 2004;11(6):699–702.
90. Ducharme J, Matheson K. What is the best topical anesthetic for nasogastric insertion? A comparison of lidocaine gel, lidocaine spray, and atomized cocaine. *J Emerg Nurs*. 2003;29(5):427–430.
91. Singer AJ, Konia N. Comparison of topical anesthetics and vasoconstrictors vs lubricants prior to nasogastric intubation: a randomized, controlled trial. *Acad Emerg Med*. 1999;6(3):184–190.
92. Wolfe TR, Fosnocht DE, Linscott MS. Atomized lidocaine as topical anesthesia for nasogastric tube placement: a randomized, double-blind, placebo-controlled trial. *Ann Emerg Med*. 2000;35(5):421–425.
93. Singer AJ, Stark MJ. Pretreatment of lacerations with lidocaine, epinephrine, and tetracaine at triage: a randomized double-blind trial. *Acad Emerg Med*. 2000;7(7):751–756.
94. Garbez RO, Chan GK, Neighbor M, Puntillo K. Pain after discharge: a pilot study of factors associated with pain management and functional status. *J Emerg Nurs*. 2006;32(4):288–293.
95. Bauman BH, McManus JG Jr. Pediatric pain management in the emergency department. *Emerg Med Clin North Am*. 2005;23(2):393–414.
96. Suresh S. Chronic and cancer pain management. *Curr Opin Anaesthesiol*. 2004;17(3):253–259.
97. American Academy of Pediatrics, Committee on Psychological Aspects of Child and Family Health. The assessment and management of acute pain in infants, children, and adolescents. *Pediatrics*. 2001;108(3):793.
98. Gradin M, Eriksson M, Holmqvist G, Holstein A, Schollin J. Pain reduction at venipuncture in newborns: oral glucose compared with local anesthetic cream. *Pediatrics*. 2002;110(6):1053–1057.
99. Howard RF. Current status of pain management in children. *JAMA*. 2003;290(18):2464–2469.
100. Meunier-Sham J, Ryan K. Reducing pediatric pain during ED procedures with a nurse-driven protocol: an urban pediatric emergency department's experience. *J Emerg Nurs*. 2003;29(2):127–132.
101. Probst BD, Lyons E, Leonard D, Esposito TJ. Factors affecting emergency department assessment and management of pain in children. *Pediatr Emerg Care*. 2005;21(5):298–305.
102. Mace S. Pain management and procedural sedation in pediatric patients. In: Mace S, Durcharme J, Murphy M, eds. *Pain Management and Sedation*. New York, NY: McGraw-Hill; 2006.
103. Gerik SM. Pain management in children: developmental considerations and mind-body therapies. *South Med J*. 2005;98(3):295–302.
104. Taddio A, Goldbach M, Ipp M, Stevens B, Koren G. Effect of neonatal circumcision on pain responses during vaccination in boys. *Lancet*. 1995;345(8945):291–292.
105. Taddio A, Shennan AT, Stevens B, Leeder JS, Koren G. Safety of lidocaine-prilocaine cream in the treatment of preterm neonates. *J Pediatr*. 1995;127(6):1002–1005.
106. Kharasch S, Saxe G, Zuckerman B. Pain treatment: opportunities and challenges. *Arch Pediatr Adolesc Med*. 2003;157(11):1054–1056.
107. Weisman SJ, Bernstein B, Schechter N. Consequences of inadequate analgesia during painful procedures in children. *Arch Pediatr Adolesc Med*. 1998;152(2):147–149.
108. Emergency Nurses Association. *Emergency Nursing Pediatric Course*. Des Plaines, IL: Emergency Nurses Association; 2004.
109. Siwiec J, Porzucek I, Gadzinowski J, Bhat R, Vidyasagar D. Effect of short term morphine infusion on Premature Infant Pain Profile (PIPP) and hemodynamics. *Pediatr Res*. 1999;45(5):69A.
110. Merkel S, Voepel-Lewis T, Malviya S. Pain assessment in infants and young children: the FLACC scale. *Am J Nurs*. 2002;102(10):55–58.
111. Carraccio C, Feinberg P, Hart LS, Quinn M, King J, Lichenstein R. Lidocaine for lumbar punctures: a help not a hindrance. *Arch Pediatr Adolesc Med*. 1996;150(10):1044–1066.
112. Kleiber C, Sorenson M, Whiteside K, Gronstal BA, Tannous R. Topical anesthetics for intravenous insertion in children: a randomized equivalency study. *Pediatrics*. 2002;110(4):758–761.
113. Sethna NF, Verghese ST, Hannallah RS, Solodiuk JC, Zurakowski D, Berde CB. A randomized controlled trial to evaluate S-Caine patch for reducing pain associated with vascular access in children. *Anesthesiology*. 2005;102(2):403–408.
114. Evans JC, McCartney EM, Lawhon G, Galloway J. Longitudinal comparison of preterm pain responses to repeated heelsticks. *Pediatr Nurs*. 2005;31(3):216–221.
115. Stevens B, Yamada J, Beyene J, et al. Consistent management of repeated procedural pain with sucrose in preterm neonates: is it effective and safe for repeated use over time? *Clin J Pain*. 2005;21(6):543–548.
116. Milani GP, Benini F, Dell'Era L, et al., PIERRE GROUP STUDY. Acute pain management: acetaminophen and ibuprofen are often under-dosed. *Eur J Pediatr*. 2017;176(7):979–982. https://doi.org/10.1007/s00431-017-2944-6.
117. Hatfield L, Messner E, Lingg K. Evidence-based strategies for the pharmacological management of pediatric pain during minor procedures in the emergency department. *Top Emerg Med*. 2006;28(2):129.

FURTHER READING

1. American Society of Addiction Medicine. Definitions related to the use of opioids for the treatment of pain: consensus document of the American Academy of Pain Medicine, the American Pain Society, and the American Society of Addiction Medicine. https://www.asam.org/docs/default-source/public-policy-statements/1opioid-definitions-consensus-2-011.pdf. Published 2001. Accessed (AU: Check link, add accessed date)
10. Beyer JE, Denyes MJ, Villarruel AM. The creation, validation, and continuing development of the Oucher: a measure of pain intensity in children. *J Pediatr Nurs*. 1992;7(5):335–346.
11. Bieri D, Reeve RA, Champion GD, Addicoat L, Ziegler JB. The Faces Pain Scale for the self-assessment of the severity of pain experienced by children: development, initial validation, and preliminary investigation for ratio scale properties. *Pain*. 1990;41(2):139–150.
35. Franck LS, Greenberg CS, Stevens B. Pain assessment in infants and children. *Pediatr Clin North Am*. 2000;47(3):487–512.
61. McCaig L, Nawar E. *National Hospital Ambulatory Medical Care Survey: 2004 Emergency Department Summary—Advance Data From Vital and Health Statistics*. Hyattsville, MD: National Center for Health Statistics; 2006.
62. McCormack HM, Horne DJ, Sheather S. Clinical applications of visual analogue scales: a critical review. *Psychol Med*. 1988;18(4):1007–1019.
63. McGrath PA, Seifert CE, Speechley KN, Booth JC, Stitt L, Gibson MC. A new analogue scale for assessing children's pain: an initial validation study. *Pain*. 1996;64(3):435–443.
82. Rockett IR, Putnam SL, Jia H, Smith GS. Assessing substance abuse treatment need: a statewide hospital emergency department study. *Ann Emerg Med*. 2003;41(6):802–813.
103. Tanabe P, Buschmann M. Emergency nurses' knowledge of pain management principles. *J Emerg Nurs*. 2000;26(4):299–305.
116. Weissman DE, Haddox JD. Opioid pseudoaddiction: an iatrogenic syndrome. *Pain*. 1989;36(3):363–366.
119. Wong DL, Baker CM. Pain in children: comparison of assessment scales. *Pediatr Nurs*. 1988;14(1):9–17.

11

Wound Management

Nancy J. Denke

Wounds and soft-tissue injuries are common presenting complaints seen in the emergency department (ED) annually. It is important, therefore, to understand the management of wounds depending on the type of wound, its severity, and its anatomic location. These injuries also include acute and chronic wounds. A wound can be defined as a disruption of the normal integrity and/or function of skin or tissue resulting from either direct or indirect mechanical forces applied to that skin or tissue. The goal of wound management is to restore integrity and function to damaged skin/tissue and identify risk and causative factors affecting skin integrity and wound healing. In the ED, nurses encounter many simple and straightforward wounds, but others are complex and can greatly alter the appearance and function for those individuals being cared for. Unless life-threatening bleeding or neurovascular compromise is present, individuals with wounds (surface trauma) are not considered a triage priority.

Adapting a systematic approach to wound management incorporates the basic principles of wound care: promotion of optimal healing, prevention of infection, and reduction of scar formation. This can be accomplished using the acronym **LACERATE**: **L**ook at the wound, assess it; **A**nesthetic considerations; **C**leaning the wound; **E**quipment; **R**epair; **A**ssessing results, anticipate complications; **T**etanus immunization status; and **E**ducate the patient regarding wound care.[1]

ANATOMY AND PHYSIOLOGY

The skin is the largest organ of the body and performs many vital functions such as protection and prevention of external water loss, and it even has a role in thermoregulation. Skin is a complex, dynamic, three-layered organ. Embedded within the layers of the skin are blood vessels, nerve endings, hair follicles, collagen matrixes, and glands, and all have one major job: protection of the body.[2] As part of the protection mechanism, the skin acts as a sensory organ. The layers all contain specialized sensory nerve structures that detect touch, surface temperature, and pain.

The outer layer is the epidermis, with the dermis being the underlying layer and the subcutaneous tissue being below the dermis but not always noted as part of the skin (Fig. 11.1).

The epidermis, or outer layer, contains a hard, fibrous protein known as keratin. This layer provides protection against chemicals and microorganisms, gives the skin flexibility, creates a seal preventing dehydration, and generates cells to promote wound healing. It also synthesizes vitamin D when exposed to ultraviolet radiation, which is essential for normal absorption of calcium and phosphorus, required for healthy bones. The epidermis is avascular and receives nutrients from underlying blood vessels in the dermis and subcutaneous tissues.[2] Thickness of the epidermis varies with location; it is significantly greater in the soles of the feet and palms of the hand than in the eyelids. Thickening of the epidermal layers (calluses) is caused by repeated pressure or friction, such as is seen with poorly fitted shoes, repetitive actions such as plucking guitar strings, or manual labor such as raking the yard.

The dermis (the middle layer) lies below the epidermis and is composed of collagen and elastin fibers (connective tissue) providing strength, elasticity, and protection against external forces, attaching the epidermis to the subcutaneous layers.[2] It is the thickest layer of the skin. The connective tissue of the dermis has a rich vascular supply, along with lymphatic vessels, nerves, and thermoreceptors. Collagen found in the dermis provides tensile strength, whereas elastin allows skin to resist deformation. Collagen brings numerous types of cells, including fibroblasts and keratinocytes, which become active during inflammatory conditions such as a wound, thus playing a major role in enhancing tissue growth in the wound bed.[3] Sensory receptors for pain, touch, pressure, heat, and cold are also found in the dermis, whereas hair follicles and sweat glands are found between the epidermal and dermal layers of the skin.

The subcutaneous layer lies below the dermis and above the muscle tissue, providing body contour. It stores fat below the dermis and provides insulation against heat loss. In addition, the subcutaneous tissue provides protection against injury and acts as an energy storage site. Hypoperfusion of subcutaneous tissue negatively affects wound healing. Complications of impaired healing, such as infections, often have their origin in the subcutaneous tissue.[4]

Skin regulates body temperature through sweating and evaporation. Insensible fluid loss through the skin and lungs accounts for 450 to 600 mL/day or 12 to 16 calories per hour of heat loss.[5] Skin provides innate immunity because mast cells and Langerhans cells (macrophages) in the skin respond to antigens and pathogens. The normal skin flora

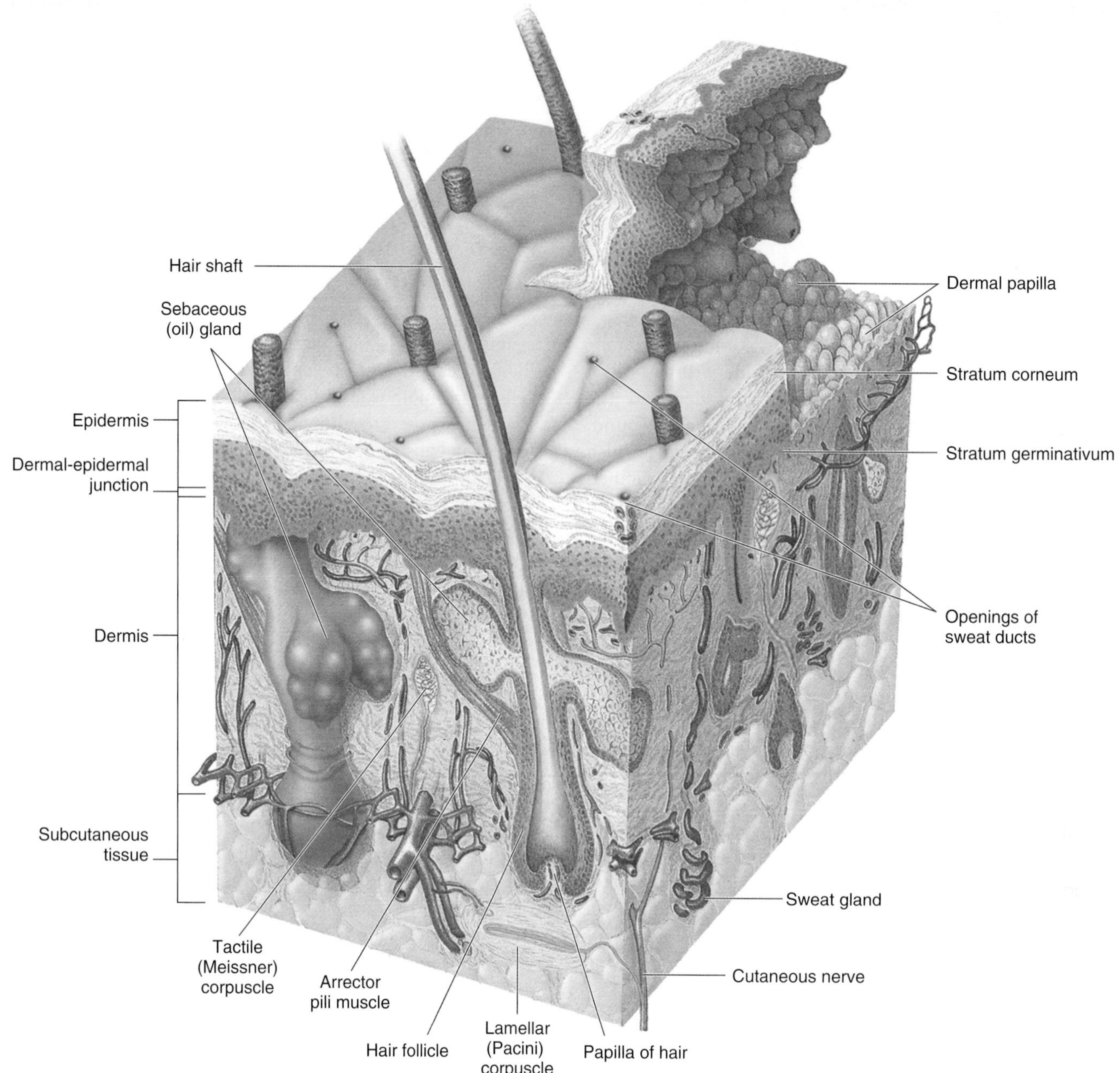

Fig. 11.1 Anatomy of the Skin. (From Patton KT, Thibodeau GA. *Structure and Function of the Body*. 15th ed. St Louis, MO: Mosby; 2016.)

(i.e., coagulase-positive and coagulase-negative staphylococci, streptococci, and diphtheroids) confer a line of defense against other microbes in the environment (Table 11.1).

SKIN CHANGES WITH AGING

The structural and functional degeneration of the skin with age is more than a merely cosmetic problem. As we age, the dermis becomes thinner and has less elasticity and resilience, therefore reducing the skin's ability to regenerate, leading to slower wound healing, which is influenced by intrinsic factors (e.g., the genetic makeup and changes in hormone levels) and extrinsic factors, such as sun exposure and tobacco smoking[6] (Table 11.2). Malnutrition, which is frequently seen in the elderly, contributes to delayed repair. When coupled with impaired mobility, an increased risk for poorly healing pressure ulcers develops.

WOUND HEALING

Normal wound healing is a systematic process that occurs in three sequential overlapping phases: the inflammatory, proliferative, and remodeling (or maturation) phases. One of the main reasons for wound healing is to restore the skin barrier to prevent further damage or infection. Each linear, dynamic phase is sequential, creating a pathway for cellular

TABLE 11.1 Cells Involved in Wound Healing.

Cell Type	Time of Action	Function
Platelets	Seconds	Thrombus formation Activation of coagulation cascade Release inflammatory mediators (PDGF, TGF-β FGF, EGF, histamine, serotonin, bradykinin, prostaglandins, thromboxane)
Neutrophils	Peak at 24 hours	Phagocytosis of bacteria Wound debridement Release of proteolytic enzymes Generation of oxygen free radicals Increase vascular permeability
Keratinocytes	8 hours	Release of inflammatory mediators Stimulate neighboring keratinocytes to migrate Neovascularization
Lymphocytes	72–120 hours	Regulates proliferative phase of wound healing, although exact mechanisms are unclear Collagen deposition
Fibroblasts	120 hours	Synthesis of granulation tissue Collagen synthesis Produce components of extracellular matrix Release of proteases Release of inflammatory mediators

Singh S, Young A, McNaugh CE. The physiology of wound healing. *Surgery*. 2017;35(9):475.

TABLE 11.2 Factors Delaying Wound Healing.

Factor	Effect on Wound Healing
Nutritional deficiencies	
• Vitamin C	Delays formation of collagen fibers and capillary development
• Protein	Decreases supply of amino acids for tissue repair
• Zinc	Impairs epithelialization
Inadequate blood supply	Decreases supply of nutrients to injured area, decreases removal of exudative debris and inflammatory response
Corticosteroid drugs	Impair phagocytosis by white blood cells, inhibit fibroblast probation and function, depress formation of granulation tissue, inhibit wound contraction
Infection	Increases inflammatory response and tissue destruction
Smoking	Nicotine, a potent vasoconstrictor, impedes blood flow of healing areas
Mechanical friction on wound	Destroys granulation tissue, prevents apposition of wound edges
Advanced age	Slows collagen synthesis by fibroblasts, impairs circulation, requires longer time for epithelialization of skin, alters phagocytic and immune responses
Obesity	Decreases blood supply in fatty tissue
Diabetes mellitus	Decreases collagen synthesis, retards early capillary growth, impairs phagocytosis (result of hyperglycemia), reduces supply of O_2 and nutrients secondary to vascular disease
Poor general health	Causes generalized absence of factors necessary to promote wound healing
Anemia	Supplies less oxygen at tissue level

Lewis SL. Inflammation and wound healing. In: Lewis SL, Bucher L, Heitkemper MH, Harding MM, Kwong J, Roberts R, eds. *Medical-Surgical Nursing: Assessment and Management in Clinical Practice*. 10th ed. St Louis, MO: Elsevier; 2017:168.

and biochemical events to occur in each of these phases. Sorg et al.[7] (2017) noted that "wound healing is a complex process, which is dependent on many cell types and mediators interacting in a highly sophisticated sequence" (p. 82). Each stage is not mutually exclusive, but rather the stages overlap over time as they create the pathway to the tissue repair process.[4] Disruption of any step in one of the wound-healing phases leads to a delay in healing by 20% to 60%, especially in patients older than 65 years of age[6] (Fig. 11.2).

Inflammatory Phase

The initial, or inflammatory, phase is a protective mechanism beginning immediately and coinciding with the key signs of inflammation, edema and erythema, at the location of the lesion, and lasting 2 to 5 days.[8] The inflammatory phase begins with the coagulation cascade (activation of fibrin and thrombin), platelets adhering to injured vessels to form a clot. It is a complex series of events consisting of cellular and histologic reactions in the affected blood vessels and adjacent tissues.[7] Neutrophils secrete proinflammatory cytokines, which amplify the inflammatory response.[7] Vasodilation occurs after the first 10 minutes, exposing the wound to increased blood flow, accompanied by inflammatory cells and macrophages (key players in this process). Macrophages then produce growth factors and cytokines, which are then recruited to the area of injury, where they fight infection and debride the wound of devitalized tissue as the body attempts to repair itself; in other words, it facilitates the cleanup of various cell debris.[4] (If macrophages are absent in this phase or the proliferation phase, there will be decreased tissue formation and even hemorrhage).[7] Beneath the clot, a network of fibrinogen strands forms to unite wound edges. Prostaglandins are powerful vasodilators, leading to increased capillary permeability, stimulating the formation of granulation tissue.[7]

After scab formation begins, the inflammatory processes begin, and the wound becomes painful and edematous. Vasodilation in injured tissues leads to protein leakage and antibody release, which creates a medium for white blood cells arriving at the site 6 hours after injury. White blood cells attack bacteria through phagocytosis by using neutrophils to surround and engulf bacteria, providing short-term defense against infection; monocytes provide long-term defense against infection. Macrophages recruit fibroblasts and create a network of collagen fibers, which in the presence of vitamin C and adequate oxygenation begin the granulation of tissue.[8]

Proliferative Phase

Transition from the inflammatory to the proliferative phase is a crucial step in the course of wound healing, beginning as early as 48 hours after injury and ending approximately 4 to 21 days later.[4,8] This complex process incorporates the simultaneous formation of granulation tissue, collagen deposition, epithelialization, and wound retraction, with the goal of reducing the area surrounding the injured tissue by contraction and closure.[4,5] The inflammatory and proliferative phases are closely interconnected, with the proliferative phase playing an important role in resolving inflammation.

During granulation, fibroblast activity peaks, forming new capillary beds, meshing with damaged tissue, and providing oxygen and proteins for tissue growth. During fibroblast activity, collagen is produced to form scar tissue. This scar tissue is initially translucent, grayish red, moist, and friable, leading it to bleed easily and become damaged with minimal force. Wound contraction begins after fibroblast formation, enhanced by collagen synthesis, which is stimulated by platelet growth factors. Angiogenesis, the restoration of the blood vessel network, begins enabling nutrients and oxygen mobilization to areas needed during wound repair. During contraction the wound matrix, which was laid down during homeostasis, is replaced by granulated tissue consisting of many fibroblasts, macrophages, and blood vessels, which attach and form collagen bundles. These bundles pull wound edges closer together, forming a scaffolding pattern.[8] This scaffolding allows wound adhesion and a decrease in the size of the wound.[8] This wound contraction and remodeling can continue for 6 to 18 months after injury, with linear wound contracting fastest and circular wounds the slowest.[5] Disturbance in this stage of healing can lead to deformity and the formation of contractures.[5]

Remodeling Phase

This third and final phase of wound healing begins about 2 to 3 weeks after injury and can last up to 2 years.[5] Initially collagen fibers develop randomly but in an organized fashion with other proteins. This involves a balance between synthesis and degradation, as they are deposited in the wound.[5] However, within 2 weeks these fibers reorganize into thick fibers along stress lines and increase in strength over weeks or months. At 2 weeks, approximately 10% to 20% of the tensile strength has returned. Despite this, wounds never achieve the same level of tissue strength, with 80% of the preinjury tensile strength returning at 3 months and remaining long term.[5] As the scar matures, the level of vascularity decreases and the scar changes from red to pink to gray with time.[5] Heredity, stress, and movement of the affected area determine the amount of scarring.

Factors Affecting Wound Healing

Wound healing is significantly affected by preexisting conditions and medication; these factors include arterial/venous insufficiency, lymphedema, morbid obesity, neuropathy, neoplasms, sickle cell disease, infection, diabetes, stress, smoking, alcohol use, malnutrition, and use of corticosteroids and chemotherapeutic drugs.[6,9] Use of nonsteroidal antiinflammatory drugs (NSAIDs) is controversial due to their decrease in the inflammatory reaction. Use of NSAIDs during wound healing should be recommended with caution. Table 11.2 describes the effects of preexisting factors on wound healing.[9] Another variable affecting wound healing is the environment of the patient at the time of the injury. Bacterial contamination

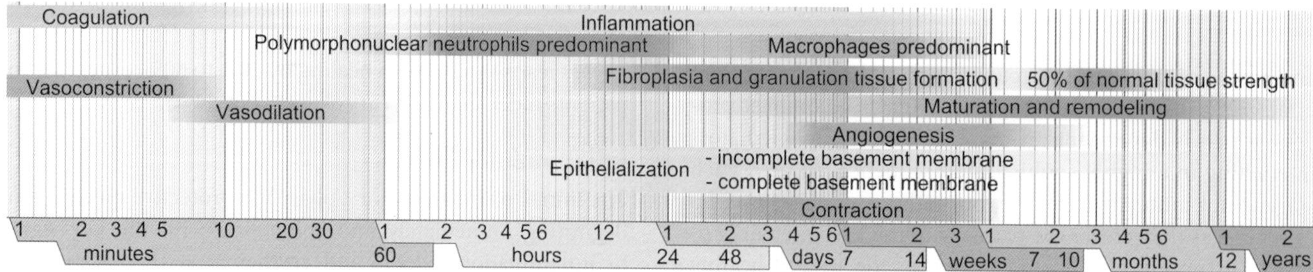

Fig. 11.2 Wound Healing Timeline. (By Mikael Häggström, used with permission.)

on the patient can increase the risk for infection, with wounds of the mouth, perineum, and web spaces of the feet hosting the highest concentration of resident flora.[10]

WOUND EVALUATION

Acute wound management varies based on the wound location and characteristics. Performing a consistent assessment is essential to providing optimal wound management. Assessment of wounds follows assessment and stabilization of the ABCs unless immediate interventions are essential because of significant hemorrhage. Mechanisms of injury can provide clues to severity of injury. Wounds caused by small objects may be superficial, whereas crush injuries as seen with a large dog's bite can cause significant deep tissue damage. Appearance of the wound provides clues to the difficulty of wound closure. Jagged edges require more skill to close and may not heal as well. The time elapsed since injury is critical because delayed care increases the risk for complications, such as infection.

Patient age, physical condition, current health status, and occupation also affect wound healing. Medical conditions such as diabetes mellitus, secondary peripheral neuropathy, morbid obesity, malnutrition, or use of medications such as corticosteroids can delay wound healing. Aspirin and NSAIDs affect coagulation and healing. The patient's occupation may influence long-term wound management and compliance with wound care. Social factors should not be overlooked. Patients who smoke often exhibit a delayed wound healing process, thus increasing their risk for infection. Allergy history and immunization status should also be evaluated during initial assessment.

The patient should be assessed for associated injuries such as fractures, dislocations, or neurovascular compromise. Tendon or ligament injuries, presence of a foreign body, and peripheral nerve damage should also be considered and managed appropriately. Wounds with contamination at the time of wounding are at an extreme risk for becoming infected. Wounds considered contaminated are those having a high inoculum of bacteria. Farming-related accidents, wounds exposed to contaminated water (ponds, lakes, coral reefs), and full-thickness human bites are representative of wounds that are usually heavily contaminated at the time of injury.[1,10]

WOUND PREPARATION

Preparation of wounds begins with the assessment of the wound in a controlled environment with good lighting. Anesthetizing the wound during preparation allows the wound to be thoroughly cleansed and examined without causing pain or discomfort to the patient. Removal of debris (foreign bodies, devitalized tissue) while controlling bleeding is necessary when exploring and evaluating any wound. Removal of hair around a wound is not absolutely necessary, especially when it comes to eyebrows. Eyebrows should never be shaved. Eyebrows may not grow back, thus leaving an obvious cosmetic defect. Leaving them intact also has them functioning as landmarks for wound alignment and closure. If hair obscures a wound, it should then be clipped or cut instead of being shaved. Shaving removes hair follicles, causing bacterial contamination during the healing process, leading to infection. Use of clean technique to remove bacteria, debris, and contamination should be performed using either high-pressure irrigation or direct contact/scrubbing. Removal of debris from a wound facilitates the inflammatory to proliferative phase of wound healing, both of which are critical steps in the healing process.[11]

Appropriate personal protective equipment should be used because of probable exposure to splashing body fluids. High-pressure irrigation, the preferred method, is excellent in removing debris and decreasing the rate of infection by preventing premature healing over an abscess pocket or infected tract.[12] Adequate pressure of the irrigating fluid is one of the most important issues when considering use of an irrigation device. Simple soaking of the wound in an antiseptic solution will not adequately remove debris and may be harmful to tissue. "Irrigating with greater than 7 pounds per square inch (psi) significantly decreases the number of bacteria and the incidence of infection" (p. 663). Using an 18-gauge needle and a 35-cc syringe with a splash protector will provide 7 to 8 psi and is as good as a commercial device in cleansing wounds.[13] Wounds with heavy contamination must be irrigated for a minimum of 5 minutes; at times lengthier irrigation may be needed. Another device found to be quick and easy to use is the "squirt bottle technique."[13] This technique uses a 500-mL bottle of sterile water or normal saline (a bottle of drinking water, not opened, could even work if out in the wilderness). This is done by wiping the cap with an alcohol wipe and then piercing the cap with an 18-gauge needle about 10 to 20 times, and then firmly squeezing the container to create a strong stream of pressurized fluid.[14] This method should be used only in low-pressurized wound cleansing, not with bites or heavily contaminated wounds. Hydrogen peroxide or concentrated povidone-iodine should not be used for irrigation because of their tissue toxicity.[1]

The ideal wound cleanser should be nontoxic to viable tissue, readily available, and cost-effective. Weiss et al.[15] (2013) found that irrigation fluid did not need to be antiseptic and there is no difference in the infection rate of wounds irrigated with either tap water or sterile saline solution. It was also noted that some antiseptic irrigants caused tissue toxicity, thus delaying wound healing. Povidone-iodine is a broad-spectrum antimicrobial solution. Hydrogen peroxide should not be used because it causes absorption of oxygen in the wound and cell destruction and gives no protection against anaerobes (Table 11.3).

Cleansing the wound by direct contact (such as using a soft brush) is effective in wound debridement but potentially destroys tissue. Soaps with strong cleaning agents or those containing alcohol may cause further tissue damage.

Puncture wounds must be irrigated vigorously because the ability to explore the wound is limited and removal of any debris that may have become buried in the wound is vitally important to proper wound healing. Be sure to ask the patient whether the object that caused the puncture wound was removed intact and if any contaminants may have been on the object. There is no evidence to suggest that soaking puncture wounds with antiseptic solutions decreases the incidence of wound infection.

TABLE 11.3 **Antiseptic Solutions.**

SUMMARY OF AGENTS USED FOR WOUND CARE					
Agent	**Biologic Activity**	**Tissue Toxicity[a]**	**Systemic Toxicity[a]**	**Potential Uses**	**Comments**
Povidone-iodine surgical scrub (Betadine 7.5%)	Virucidal; strongly bactericidal	Detergent component toxic to wound tissue	Painful in open wounds	Hand cleanser	Iodine allergy possible
Povidone-iodine solution (Betadine 10%)	Virucidal; bactericidal	Potentially toxic at full strength; 1% solution has no significant tissue toxicity	Extremely rare	Wound periphery cleanser; dilute to <1% for wound irrigation	Dilute 10:1 (saline to Betadine) if used to irrigate wounds
Chlorhexidine gluconate (Hibiclens)	Bactericidal	Toxic to tissues, including eyes	Extremely rare	Hand cleanser	Avoid in open wounds, eyes, or ears
Poloxamer 188 (Shur-Clens); Pluronic F-68	No antibacterial or antiviral activity	None known; does not inhibit wound healing	None known	Wound cleanser	Nontoxic in wounds and eyes
Hexachlorophene (pHisoHex)	Bacteriostatic against gram-positive bacteria	Potentially toxic to wound tissue	Possibly teratogenic with repeated use	Alternative hand cleanser	Systemic absorption causes neurotoxicity
Hydrogen peroxide	Very weak antibacterial agent	Toxic to tissue and red cells	Extremely rare	Wound periphery cleanser	Foaming activity removes surface debris and coagulated blood

Lammers RL, Aldy KN. Principles of wound management. In: Roberts JR, Custalow CB, Thomsen T, eds. *Robert's and Hedge's Clinical Procedures in Emergency Medicine and Acute Care.* 7th ed. Philadelphia, PA: Elsevier; 2018:627.

Nonviable injured tissue must be debrided before wound closure, and foreign bodies should be removed. Wounds may be closed by primary, secondary, or tertiary intention. The type of closure depends on age of the wound, presence of infection, and amount of contamination present.

CONTROL OF HEMORRHAGE

Control of bleeding allows for unobstructed examination, exploration, and closure of wounds. One of the most straightforward ways to achieve hemostasis is to use a tourniquet on the extremity, enabling the wound to be adequately inspected and repaired.[1,16] There are multiple forms of finger tourniquets: commercially available devices or devices modified to create a safe tourniquet such as a Penrose drain with a hemostat or donning a glove, cutting the tip of the glove over the finger of interest, and rolling the glove finger to the base of that finger[17] (Fig. 11.3). Tourniquets are frequently used and are safe for **short** durations to achieve a bloodless field. They are placed proximal to the wound, allowing bleeding vessels to be visible and easily isolated. Once the procedure is completed, the tourniquet is released. (Note: There is potential for injury if the finger tourniquet is left on longer than 30–45 minutes).[18] Another device useful for extremity wounds to establish hemostasis is a blood pressure cuff. Blood pressure cuffs are invaluable tools, often used to halt reaccumulation of pooling blood, thereby attaining a bloodless field so wounds may be effectively assessed. Each of these devices has a common factor with their use: they are only for short periods of time, and vigilance needs to be maintained in their use.[17,18]

LOCAL ANESTHESIA

Only after documentation of an appropriate neurovascular examination should any wound be anesthetized. Local anesthesia is used to block pain when cleansing, suturing, or stapling wounds to minimize discomfort during these procedures. Table 11.4 highlights anesthetic agents commonly used for local infiltration.[16]

Lidocaine is the preferred agent for local and regional anesthesia because of greater potency, decreased irritation, and long-lasting anesthetic effect in comparison with other anesthetic agents. It can be safely used at a dosing of 3 to 5 mg/kg, not exceeding 300 mg at a single injection.[13] Onset of action occurs within seconds, with effects lasting 20–60 minutes when locally infiltrating a wound.[14] If lidocaine is used as a regional nerve block, onset will occur in approximately 4–6 minutes, with effects lasting 75–120 minutes.[13] Bupivacaine (Marcaine) may be substituted for lidocaine. It provides the same anesthesia as lidocaine, but with a slightly slower onset of action and longer duration of anesthesia, up to four to eight times longer.[14,16] Other anesthetic agents include procaine, mepivacaine (Carbocaine), and tetracaine (Pontocaine). When deciding on the practical agent for local infiltration, the duration of these agents is important: procaine has a duration of 15 to 45 minutes; lidocaine has a duration of 1 to 2 hours; and bupivacaine has a duration of 4 to 8 hours.

Some pain is associated with injecting lidocaine into a wound. This pain can be minimized with the addition of sodium bicarbonate, which buffers the solution. Adding

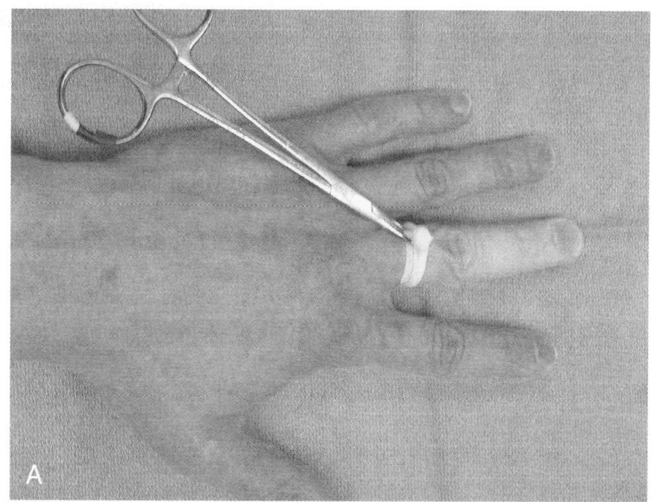

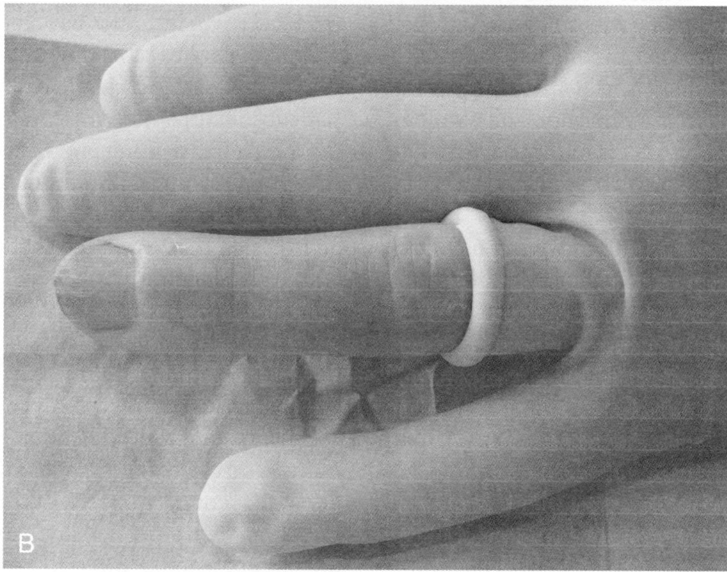

Fig. 11.3 Finger Tourniquets. ((A) From Robinson JK, Hanke CW, Siegel DM, et al. *Surgery of the Skin: Procedural Dermatology.* 2nd ed. St Louis, MO: Elsevier; 2010. (B) From Bolognia JL, Schaffer JV, Cerroni L. *Dermatology: 2-Volume Set.* 4th ed. St Louis, MO: Elsevier; 2018.)

TABLE 11.4 Anesthetic Used in Wound Closure.

Anesthetic	Class	Maximum Dosage	Duration
Lidocaine	Amide	4.5 mg/kg (not to exceed 300 mg)	1–2 hours
Lidocaine with epinephrine	Amide	7 mg/kg (not to exceed 500 mg)	2–4 hours
Bupivacaine	Amide	2.5 mg/kg (not to exceed 175 mg)	4–8 hours
Bupivacaine with epinephrine	Amide	3 mg/kg (not to exceed 225 mg)	8–16 hours
Procaine	Ester	8 mg/kg (not to exceed 1 g)	15–45 minutes
Procaine with epinephrine	Ester	10 mg/kg (not to exceed 1 g)	30–60 minutes

Moreira M. Wound management. In: Markovchick VT, Pons PT, Bakes K, Buchanan J, eds. *Emergency Medicine Secrets.* 6th ed. Philadelphia, PA: Elsevier; 2016:627.

sodium bicarbonate 8.4% with any of these agents (warmed or at room temperature) in a 1:10 ratio (1 mL bicarbonate to 10 mL lidocaine) decreases pain associated with infiltration without compromising the anesthetic effects of any of these agents.[16] Bupivacaine should be buffered with sodium bicarbonate: it precipitates as pH of the solution rises.[1]

Epinephrine is commonly added to lidocaine to prolong the duration of local anesthesia, provide hemostasis via vasoconstriction with a slower absorption of the anesthetic, and increase the level of anesthetic blockade up to 2 to 6 hours.[16,19] Lidocaine with epinephrine should only be used for lacerations in highly vascular areas. Epinephrine solutions should **never** be used in areas supplied by end arteries, including the nose, ears, digits, and penis.

Disadvantages of lidocaine are related to the dose (greater than 3–5 mL/kg) and include the possibility of an allergic reaction. Central nervous system (CNS) stimulation, seizure, myocardial depression, and cardiac conduction blocks are the toxic reactions most commonly reported. When a nurse is deciding on the practical agent for local infiltration, considering the duration of these agents is important: procaine duration is 15 to 45 minutes, lidocaine duration is 1 to 2 hours, and bupivacaine duration is 4 to 8 hours.[14]

Topical anesthetics are ideal for management of minor uncomplicated lacerations *and best limited to lacerations of 5 cm or less.* Topical anesthetics are easy to use and less painful than infiltrative anesthesia. LAT (lidocaine, adrenaline, and tetracaine) gel is a topical anesthetic that can be applied on lacerations before suturing and is an alternative to infiltrative anesthesia for laceration repair.[20] Because of the vascularity of the face and scalp, lacerations of these areas are more effectively anesthetized than the trunk or extremities. Use on the fingers, toes, nose, ear, and penis is contradicted. Available solutions include lidocaine, epinephrine (Adrenalin), and tetracaine (LET or LAT). Tetracaine, Adrenalin, and cocaine (TAC) is no longer being used because of concerns of toxicity and federal regulatory issues banning this cocaine-containing mixture.

Another topical anesthetic widely used is viscous lidocaine. This topical agent may be applied to abrasions before cleaning but is not used as an anesthetic for wound closure. Absorption of viscous lidocaine is minimal but can cause toxicity when applied to large areas (such as road rash) if enough of the medication is absorbed. Anesthetic creams such as EMLA and LMX4 are commonly used to reduce procedural pain. These agents should **only** be applied to intact skin and should **not** be used for wound repair.

Topical anesthetics may obviate the need for needle infiltration but do require a minimum of 20 minutes for adequate anesthesia. A cotton ball is saturated with 2 to 3 mL of the anesthetic solution and applied directly to the laceration. A clear dressing, such as Tegaderm, may be applied directly over the cotton ball to hold it in place while preventing absorption of the solution when tape is used. (If tape is placed over the cotton alone, be sure a glove is used while holding it in place to prevent absorption of the anesthetic.) The vasoconstrictive effect of epinephrine causes a white ring around the wound, indicating the area is anesthetized. Because of the epinephrine component, these solutions cannot be used in areas supplied by end arteries (nose, ears, digits, and penis). Infiltration of a local anesthetic agent may still be required if the desired anesthetic effect is not achieved. Anesthetic effect varies slightly with each solution because of duration of individual agents.

Local blocks can be very useful when evaluating alternative routes to wound infiltration to minimize swelling and distortion of landmarks at the wound site. Local blocks require smaller amounts of anesthetic and can be more effective by blocking afferent sensory nerves of a specific region. A local nerve block, or digital block, is accomplished by injecting the anesthetic agent along the nerve innervating the wounded area to abolish afferent and efferent impulse conduction. The syringe is aspirated before each injection to prevent inadvertent parenteral lidocaine injection.

Regional anesthesia, or Bier block (used mainly for upper extremity injuries), may be selected when a greater anesthetic effect is desired. Lacerations on the face, hands, fingers, feet, and toes and in the mouth are often well suited for regional anesthesia.

One alternative to local and regional anesthesia is nitrous oxide (N_2O). Nitrous oxide is a versatile agent that can be used in procedures that may cause anxiety and pain.[21,22] It can be safely administered in pain-provoking procedures such as reduction of fractures or suturing for pediatric patients without the need for intravenous access. Its minor amnestic effect is ideal when used in the pediatric population.[21,22] Several studies have found N_2O to be actually preferable over other sedatives (ketamine or midazolam) due to its rapid onset and clearance and fewer side effects.[22] The patient inhales a 50% mixture of nitrous oxide and oxygen during short, painful procedures such as wound debridement or suturing. Self-administration limits the amount of nitrous oxide used while providing the appropriate level of anesthesia. The patient should be continuously monitored with a pulse oximeter.

WOUND CLOSURE

Wound healing/closure occurs by one of three ways: primary, secondary, or tertiary intention. Primary intention uses various wound closure techniques to facilitate wound healing and allow the wound to heal to the best functional and esthetic condition. For other wounds, closure is enhanced when they are left open and allowed to heal either by secondary intention or by delayed primary intention.

Closure by primary intention is done immediately after the injury without complications. This type of wound healing occurs when the edges of a clean laceration or surgical incision are approximated while aligning underlying structures, producing minimal edema and eliminating dead space.

Secondary intention allows the wound to heal on its own with some scarring. Many times, there is extensive loss of tissue preventing the wound edges from being approximated. The wound is left open to heal by granulation, contraction, and epithelization.

Delayed closure, or tertiary intention, is a combination of the first two types of healing when the wound is considered "too dirty to close" with a high suspicion of infection or there is considerable edema present. These wounds are usually left open for 5 to 10 days and then are sutured to decrease the risk for infection.[16] Wounds that cannot be closed with any of the previously mentioned techniques may require a skin graft or flap closure.

A common question asked by patients is, When is it unreasonable to suture a wound? A 2013 Cochrane Review posed the same question and concluded that primary closure of wounds that are clean and with no signs of infection can be sutured within 6 to 12 hours of the injury.[23,24] The review also found that delayed primary closure has the potential to increase time to healing while potentially reducing the risk of wound infection.[23,24]

Keloids may form with any of the closures due to excess accumulation of collagen, with a thick epidermal layer developing beyond the borders of the original wound. Keloids are more common in individuals with darker pigmentation and individuals with a family history. They form frequently on earlobes, deltoids, and in the chest area.[25] Prevention focuses on tension-free closure and debridement of nonviable tissue, which in turn decreases inflammation.

Various methods are used for primary wound closure, such as wound tape, sutures, staples, and/or wound adhesive. The technique chosen depends on wound size, depth, and location, with the purpose of maintaining wound closure until the wound is resilient enough to withstand daily tensile forces and to enhance wound healing when the wound is most vulnerable.[26]

Wound tape is a set of strips of microporous nonocclusive material, used for superficial linear wounds, which are under minimal tension after proper wound preparation. Wound tape is frequently used in patients with thin, frail skin (such as older adults or steroid-dependent patients) as an adjunct after suture removal or after deeper layers are closed with sutures.[27] Tincture of benzoin is thinly applied to intact skin before application of tape to ensure adherence. Wound tapes should not be placed circumferentially on any digits. The strips are not able to expand if edema occurs during healing, thus causing constriction of the digit, leading to ischemia and possible necrosis.[27] Dressings may or may not be applied over the tape closure. An anesthetic is not necessary with simple tape closures. The advantages of wound closure with this method include ease of use, comfort to the patient, and avoidance of tissue strangulation, infection, and crosshatch marks.[26] Disadvantages include imprecise wound-edge approximation and inconsistent adhesion.[24] Tape strips remain in place until they fall off or are exposed to moisture, soap, and wound exudate.[2] Fig. 11.4 illustrates a wound managed with tape closure.

Tissue adhesives or glue, such as Dermabond and Indermil, provide simple and quick approximation of simple wound edges, especially in children and uncooperative patients. They also can be used in hairy areas. Tissue glue should not be used across areas of increased skin tension such as joints, on animal bites, on severely contaminated wounds, on mucous membranes, or on areas of high moisture content. If using around the eye, keep the patient supine and tilt the head so none of the adhesive inadvertently drips into the eye.[28] Applying a layer of petroleum around the wound can guard against the glue possibly getting into the eye. Tissue adhesive may also be used as an adjunct in full-thickness wound closure after a layer of buried sutures is placed.[28]

Application of the glue, after proper wound preparation and drying, involves manually approximating wound edges and then applying the glue to the apposed wound edges with a gentle brushing motion.[28] After applying the glue across the wound edges, hold the edges together for at least 60 seconds before releasing. Release once the area is dry and not sticky. Discharge teaching should stress not applying liquid or ointment to the closed wound. This weakens the glue, leading to improper closure of the wound. Patients should also be instructed about the adhesive sloughing off naturally, usually within 5 to 10 days.[27,28]

Staples are a fast, economical alternative for closure of linear lacerations of the scalp, trunk, and extremities (Fig. 11.5). Wounds closed with staples have a lower incidence of infection and tissue reactivity, but staples do not provide the same quality of closure as sutures. Scars are more pronounced; therefore staples are recommended only for areas where a scar will not be apparent such as the scalp (Table 11.5). Staples should not be used in areas of the scalp with permanent hair loss because of poor esthetic results. They also should not be used in delicate tissues, over bony prominences, or in highly mobile areas.[27,29] Correct placement of staples is essential. Approximating the wound is performed by pinching the skin and everting the wound edges, allowing for skin swelling during healing. Local anesthesia is optional when only one or two staples are required. Pain from infiltration of anesthetic agents is greater than pain associated with insertion of one or two staples. Staples usually remain in place 7 to 10 days. Discharge instructions consist of reminding the patient that a special staple remover is required for removal and that they cannot remove them on their own. Instructions about gentle cleansing of the wound for 24 to 48 hours should also be provided.[25] Showering is permitted immediately after staples are placed in the scalp.

Sutures approximate and attach wound edges, which decreases infection, promotes wound healing, and minimizes scar formation. The choice of sutures is dependent on depth, location, tissue reactivity, and suture characteristics (knot holding ability and tensile strength).[25] The type and size of the suture material can contribute to inflammation and cause a delay in healing.[24] Sutures may be absorbable or nonabsorbable, which means they are composed of natural or synthetic material, respectively. Essential qualities of suture material are security, strength, reaction, workability, and infectious potential. Table 11.6 describes these qualities for various suture materials.

Ideal suture material is strong, easily secured, resistant to infection, and causes minimal local reaction. Sutures cause minimal discomfort after insertion; however, they also act as a foreign body and can cause local inflammation. A thin layer of antibiotic ointment is applied after suture application and then covered by a nonadhesive dressing. Recommendations for suture removal vary with wound location. For wounds in areas of movement or increased surface tension, sutures should remain longer. Table 11.7 provides guidelines for suture removal. Aftercare instruction should include pain management, local wound care (keep the wound dry for 24 hours, and after that time it is okay to shower for a short time), and observation for signs of infection.

Wound Tape Application

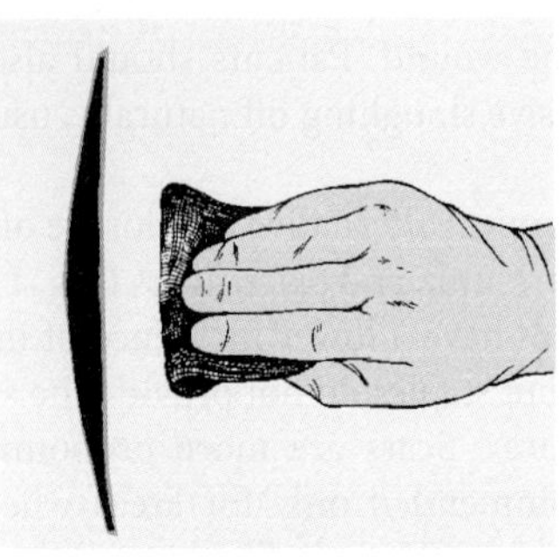

1. After wound preparation (and placement of deep closures, if needed), dry the skin thoroughly at least 2 inches around the wound. Failure to dry the skin and failure to obtain perfect hemostasis are common causes of failure of tape to stick to the skin.

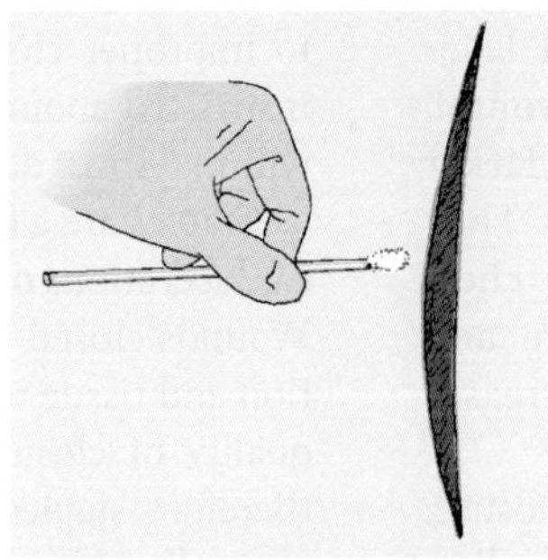

2. Apply a thin coating of tincture of benzoin around the wound to enhance tape adhesiveness. Benzoin should not enter the wound because it increases the risk of infection. Do not allow benzoin to enter the eye.

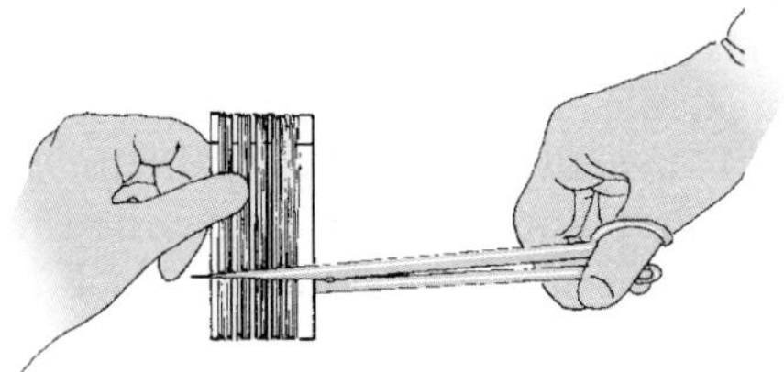

3. Cut the tape to the desired length before removing the backing.

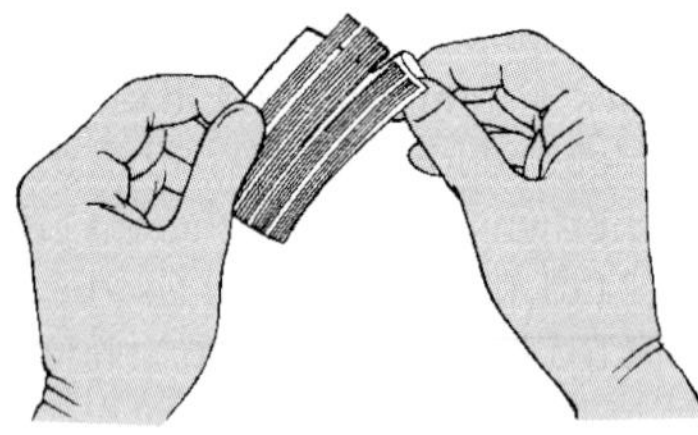

4. The tape is attached to a card with perforated tabs on both ends. Gently peel the end tab from the tape.

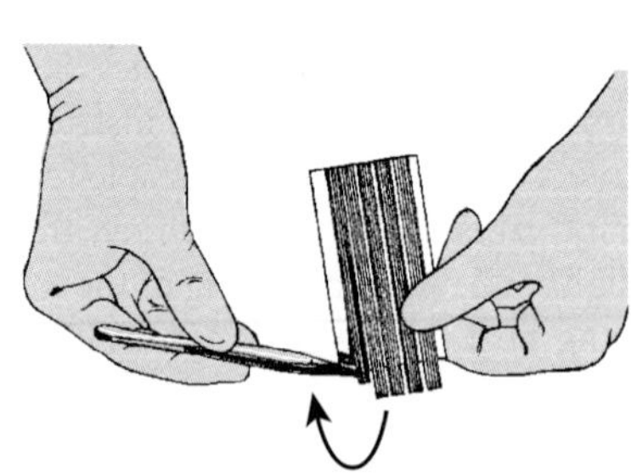

5. Use forceps to peel the tape off the card backing. Pull directly backward, not to the side.

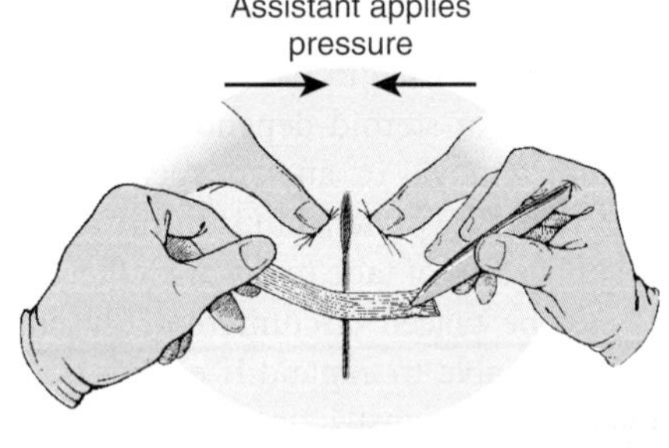

6. Place half of the first tape at the midportion of the wound; secure firmly in place.

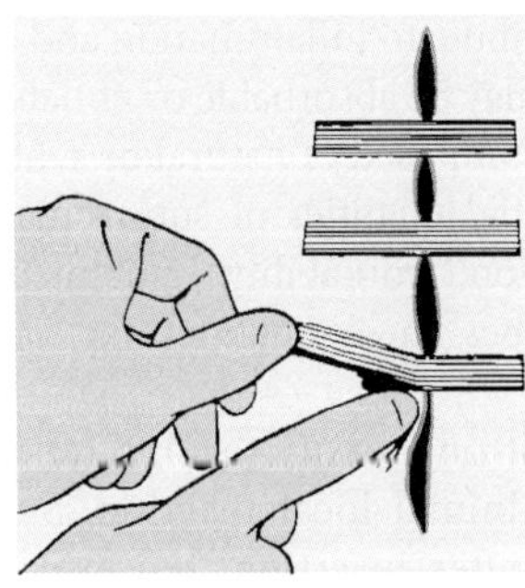

7. Gently but firmly appose the opposite side of the wound with the free hand or forceps. If an assistant is not available, the operator can approximate the wound edges. The tape should be applied by bisecting the wound until the wound is closed satisfactorily.

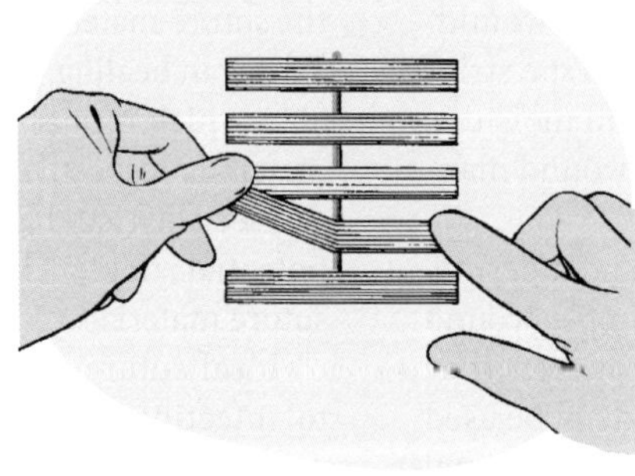

8. Wound margins are completely apposed without totally occluding the wound.

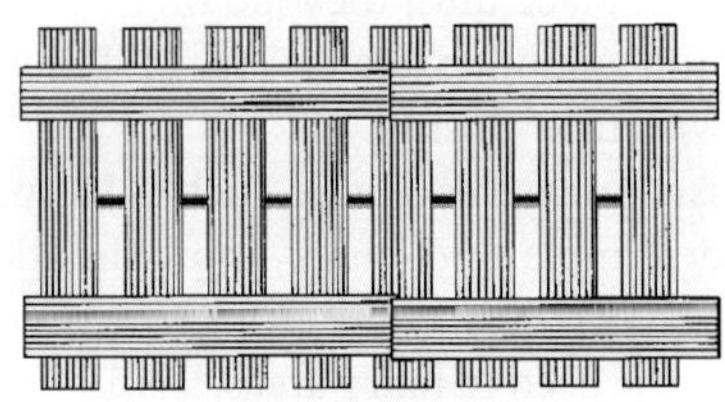

9. Only if using woven tape strips, additional supporting strips of tape are placed approximately 2.5 cm from the wound and parallel to the direction of the wound. Taping in this manner prevents the skin blistering that may occur at the ends of the tape.

Fig. 11.4 Wound Tape. (From Roberts JR, Custalow CB, Thomsen T, eds. *Robert's and Hedge's Clinical Procedures in Emergency Medicine and Acute Care.* 7th ed. Philadelphia, PA: Elsevier; 2018.)

Wound Staples

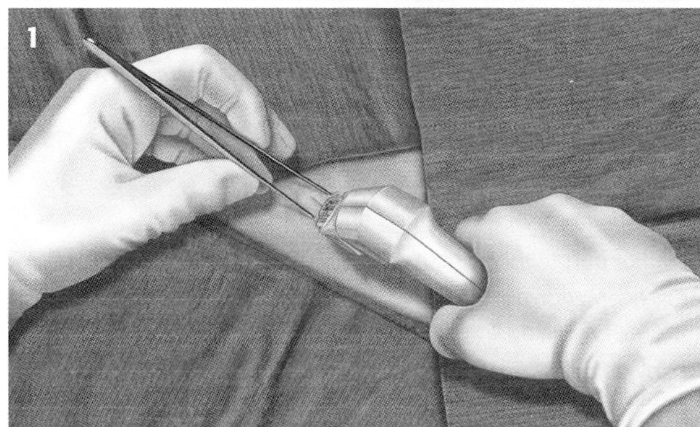

Approximate and evert the skin edges by hand or with forceps before they are secured with staples. If possible, have an assistant perform this duty. Failure to evert the wound edges is a common error that may cause an unacceptable result.

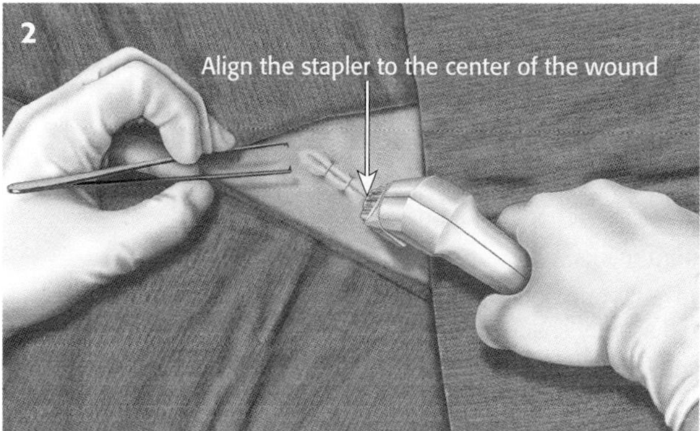

Align the center of the stapler over the center of the wound. Squeeze the stapler handle to advance one staple into the wound margins. Do not press too hard on the skin to prevent placing the staple too deeply.

3

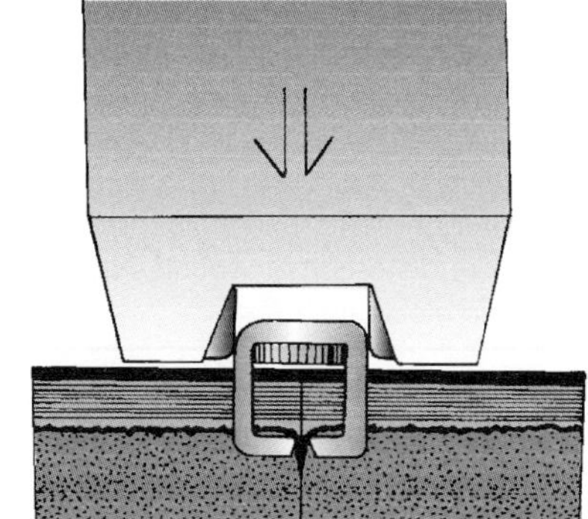

As the handle is squeezed, an anvil automatically bends the staple to the proper configuration.

4

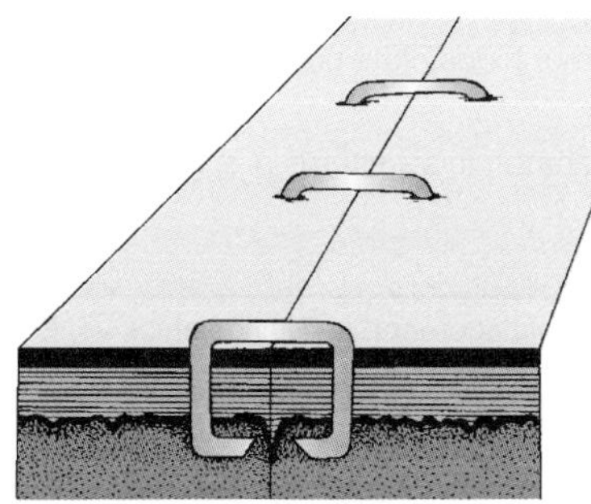

Allow a small space to remain between the skin and the crossbar of the staple. Excessive pressure created by placing the staple too deep causes wound edge ischemia, as well as pain on removal. Note that the staple bar is 2 to 3 mm above the skin line.

5

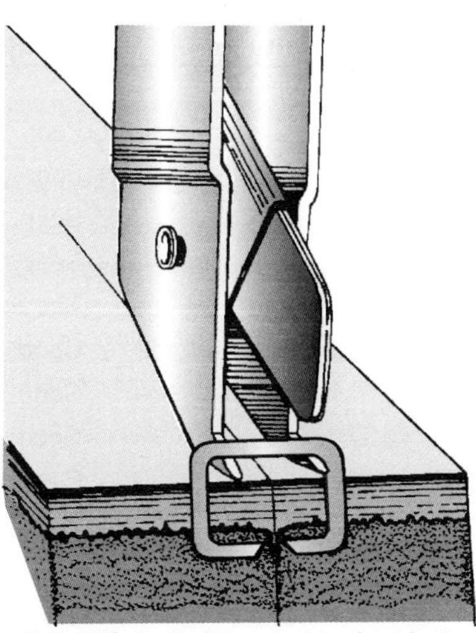

Supply the patient with a staple remover when being referred to an office for removal or for self-removal. To remove the staple, place the lower jaw of the remover under the crossbar of the staple.

6

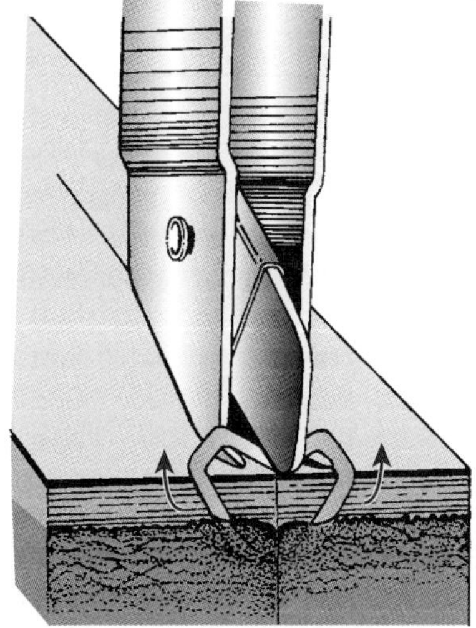

Squeeze the handle gently, and the upper jaw will compress the staple and allow it to exit the skin.

Fig. 11.5 Application of Skin Staples. (From Roberts JR, Custalow CB, Thomsen T, eds. *Robert's and Hedge's Clinical Procedures in Emergency Medicine and Acute Care.* 7th ed. Philadelphia, PA: Elsevier; 2018.)

TABLE 11.5 Minimizing Factors That Increase Visibility of Scars.

Contributing Factors	Methods to Minimize Scarring
Direction of wound (e.g., perpendicular to lines of static and dynamic tension)	Layered closure; proper direction in elective incisions of wound
Infection necessitating removal of sutures and debridement resulting in healing by secondary intention and a wide scar	Proper wound preparation: irrigation and use of delayed closure in contaminated wounds
Wide scar secondary to tension	Layered closure; proper splinting and elevation
Suture marks	Removal of percutaneous sutures within 7 days
Uneven wound edges, resulting in magnification of edges and scar by shadows	Careful, even approximation of wound top layer closure to prevent differential swelling of edges
Inversion of wound edges	Proper placement of simple sutures or use of horizontal mattress sutures
Tattooing secondary to retained dirt or foreign body	Proper wound preparation and debridement
Tissue necrosis	Use of corner sutures on flaps; splinting and elevation of wounds with marginal circulation or venous return; excision of nonviable wound edges before closure
Compromised healing secondary to hematoma	Use of properly conforming dressing and splints
Hyperpigmentation of scar or abraded skin	Use of sun protection factor 15 or greater sunblock for 6 months
Superimposition of blood clots between healing wound edges	Proper hemostasis and closure; H_2O_2 swabbing; proper application of compressive dressings
Failure to align anatomic structures properly, such as vermillion border	Meticulous closure and alignment; marking or placement of alignment suture before distortion of wound edges with local anesthesia; use of field block

Moreira M. Wound management. In: Markovchick VT, Pons PT, Bakes K, Buchanan J, eds. *Emergency Medicine Secrets*. 6th ed. Philadelphia, PA: Elsevier; 2016:627.

TABLE 11.6 Suture Materials for Wound Closure.

	CHARACTERISTICS OF SUTURE MATERIAL				
Suture Material	**Knot Security**	**Tensile Strength**	**Tissue Reactivity**	**Duration of Suture Integrity (days)**	**Tie Ability (handling)**
Absorbable					
Surgical gut	Poor	Fair	Greatest	5–7	Poor
Chromic gut	Fair	Fair	Greatest	10–14	Poor
Coated Vicryl	Good	Good	Minimal	30	Best
Dexon	Best	Good	Minimal	30	Best
PDS	Fair	Best	Least	45–60	Good
Maxon	Fair	Best	Least	45–60	Good
Biocyn	Poor	Good	Minimal	14–21	Good
Monocryl	Good	Best	Minimal	7	Good
Vicryl Rapide	Good	Good	Minimal	5	Good
Nonabsorbable					
Ethilon	Good	Good	Minimal		Good
Novafil	Good	Good	Minimal		Good
Prolene	Least	Best	Least		Fair
Silk	Best	Least	Greatest		Best

Lammers RL, Scrimshaw LE. Methods of wound closure. In: Roberts JR, Custalow CB, Thomsen T, eds. *Robert's and Hedge's Clinical Procedures in Emergency Medicine and Acute Care*. 7th ed. Philadelphia, PA: Elsevier; 2018:665.

NEW TECHNOLOGY IN WOUND CLOSURE

Closure of wounds with the use of lasers is referred to as laser welding. This process is simple. The tip of the pen moves along the surface of the wound with the water-soluble protein solder. This method has been found to increase reepithelialization, improve healing, and result in less scar formation.[24]

TABLE 11.7 Guidelines for Suture Removal.

Location	Time Frame for Removal (days)
Eyelids	3–5
Eyebrows	4–5
Ear	4–6
Lip	3–5
Face	3–5
Scalp	7–10
Trunk	7–10
Hands and feet	7–10
Arms and legs	10–14
Over joints	14

WOUND DRESSINGS

In most cases, the best dressing will depend on the wound characteristics. Covering a dry closed wound is indicated in case of wound leakage to protect against adherence of the wound to clothes.[27] A nonadhesive gauze dressing is usually used. A nonadhesive dressing should be used for skin tears or skin flap wounds.[27] Damage is generally limited to the epidermis in superficial wounds. These wounds work well with moisture-retentive dressings, which promote reepithelialization.[28] A type of moisture retentive dressing is a thin, elastic, and transparent polyurethane film dressing that provides a barrier to shield the wound from bacterial invasion.[28] These dressings should be avoided if the wound has more than scant drainage because such dressings allow fluid to collect under the film, leaving the wound to macerate. Film dressing also should not be used in individuals with fragile skin. Wounds producing excess fluids do well with foam or alginate and hydrofiber dressings and may have to be changed numerous times a day.[28–30] There are four basic principles which are often used to select the optimal dressing for a wound.

Dry wounds will require hydration.

Wounds with excessive exudates require absorbent dressings.

Wounds with necrosis or obvious debris will require debridement prior to dressing.

Infected wounds require appropriate antibacterial treatment prior to dressing (p. 513).[31]

BOX 11.1 Summary of Wound Care.

A. Stabilize the patient
B. History (be sure to include tetanus immunization status and allergies)
C. Physical examination
  1. Neurovascular examination
  2. Under sterile conditions (after the area is anesthetized, and a bloodless field is obtained) an examination of the anatomic structures, skin, nerves, tendons, vessels, muscles, and fascia should be completed
  3. Consult with specialist as indicated
D. X-rays to detect injury to bone or presence of foreign bodies
E. Wound preparation
  1. Cut—do not shave—surrounding hair to decrease the risk for microscopic injuries to the skin
  2. Prepare surrounding skin with Betadine solution
  3. Sharp debridement of foreign matter and devitalized tissue
  4. High-pressure irrigation (i.e., 18-gauge needle on a 35-mL syringe) with saline, 1% povidone-iodine (Betadine), an antibiotic solution, or a nonionic solution
F. Wound closure
  1. Adhesive tape, sutures, or staples
  2. No use of subcutaneous sutures unless wound is under high tension
G. Antibiotics
  1. Apply topical antibiotics (i.e., triple antibiotic ointment)
  2. No systemic antibiotics unless wound is at high risk
H. Dress and immobilize
I. Wound care instructions to include:
  1. Signs of infection—redness, swelling, red streaks progressing up an extremity, increased pain and fever
  2. Elevation—use of sling when appropriate
  3. Cleansing of wound daily to remove debris and crusting with use of a dilute hydrogen peroxide
  4. Immobilization, if indicated, until sutures removed
  5. Wound check—for high risk (cat bites, "fight-bites")
  6. Suture removal—may apply adhesive strips if sutures removed early

Modified from Simon B, Hern HG Jr. Wound management. In: Marx J, Hockberger R, Walls R, eds. *Rosen's Emergency Medicine*. 6th ed. St. Louis: Mosby; 2006.

Wounds to the face and ears may not require a dressing as long as the area is kept clean. Depending on the wound, a thin layer of antibiotic ointment (e.g., bacitracin or Neosporin) may be applied before the dressing. Silver-coated absorbent dressings have broad-spectrum antimicrobial actions. They are used in wounds with mild infections to reduce inflammation and promote healing.[29–31]

Wound pouching systems (e.g., KCI Wound Vac) are used for wounds draining more than 50 mL of fluid a day or are associated with fluid that is especially damaging to skin.[29,31] These wound devices are based on eliminating exudates from the wound bed, reducing edema, and increasing blood flow. This treatment is not a replacement for antibiotic use but a therapy to manage excess exudates produced by wounds that are critically colonized or infected.[29,31]

WOUND PROPHYLAXIS

Wounds are at risk for local and systemic infection from contaminants, surface organisms, tetanus, and rabies. Protection against these infectious agents begins with cleansing and irrigation.

Tetanus Prophylaxis

Tetanus is a systemic infection caused by *Clostridium tetani,* a gram-positive, spore-forming, anaerobic bacillus. Once activated, the bacillus is extremely resistant to almost anything, including sterilization. The incubation period for tetanus is 2 days to 21 days.[32] *C. tetani* spores are present in soil, garden moss, and anywhere animal or human excrement is found. Spores may contaminate wounds but remain dormant in tissue for years. After *C. tetani* enters the circulatory system, bacilli attach to cells in the CNS, causing depression of the respiratory center in the medulla. Symptoms may be mild or severe and include local joint stiffness and mild trismus or inability to open the jaw, which is where the term *lockjaw* came from. Severe tetanus is characterized by severe trismus, back pain, penile pain, tachycardia, hypertension, dysrhythmias, hyperpyrexia, opisthotonos, and seizures.[33,34] Prevention of tetanus includes immunization and scrupulous wound care, particularly for tetanus-prone wounds. For more information, visit https://www.cdc.gov/tetanus/clinicians.html.

Most patients who are not immunized are in the over-50 age-group; therefore tetanus must be considered in all patients no matter how severe the injury. Tetanus immunization is part of the childhood immunization regimen and continues with regular tetanus immunizations in adults. There are four kinds of vaccines[35] (Table 11.8).

TABLE 11.8 Types of Tetanus Prophylaxis.

Type	Use
DTaP	Diphtheria and tetanus toxoids and acellular pertussis vaccine; given to infants and children ages 6 weeks through 6 years
DT	Diphtheria and tetanus toxoids, without the pertussis component; given to infants and children ages 6 weeks through 6 years who have a contraindication to the pertussis component
Tdap	Tetanus and diphtheria toxoids with acellular pertussis vaccine; given to adolescents and adults, usually as a single dose; • Exception is **pregnant women,** who should **receive Tdap** during each pregnancy
Td	Tetanus and diphtheria toxoids; given to children and adults ages 7 years and older • **Note:** the small "d" indicates a much smaller quantity of diphtheria toxoid than in the pediatric DTaP formulation

Immunization Action Coalition. *Tetanus: questions and answers.* http://www.immunize.org/catg.d/p4220.pdf. Published 2013. Accessed April 27, 2019.

Rabies Prophylaxis

Rabies exposure can occur with bites from wild or domestic animals. Rabies is not as rare in the United States as we once thought. Rabies must be considered when an animal attack was not provoked and involved a domestic animal not immunized against rabies or a wild animal (such as a bat), with 90% of the rabies cases being from dogs.[36,37] In many cases an animal infected with rabies may not display the typical "foaming at the mouth." Instead, they display signs of rabies as an unexplained paralysis and a change in behavior[36] (see Table 11.8).

Rabies is a neurotoxic virus found in saliva of some mammals. Incubation period is 3 to 8 weeks, and this is why it is so important to seek treatment as soon as possible so the individual bitten can receive rabies postexposure prophylaxis (PEP).[38] After inoculation, the rabies virus travels by peripheral nerves to the CNS, causing encephalomyelitis. The rabies virus can be shed in saliva and tears for 2 weeks before symptoms occur and later in respiratory tract secretions or spinal fluid. Prophylaxis is always given when the animal cannot be found. PEP is administered by a series of four vaccine injections in the arm plus one dose of rabies immune globulin.

When should the rabies prophylaxis be started? This is a prophylactic treatment, not an emergency treatment. The decision to treat must be made with some urgency, especially while a patient is in the ED. Bites with a high risk for rabies transmission may warrant immediate treatment, whereas bites with a lower risk can await the 10-day observation period or laboratory results. Much depends on the offending species, the general rabies risk in the area, and the ability to quickly obtain laboratory results from public health laboratories. Consultations with local public health officials may be helpful in the decision-making process.[37,38]

One question or topic of concern for clinicians is how to approach the care of persons who awaken to find a bat in their room or their child's room even though no bite is observed. See Table 11.9. Here is what the Centers for Disease Control and Prevention recommends:

> *PEP (postexposure prophylaxis) can be considered for persons who were in the same room as the bat and who might be unaware that a bite or direct contact had occurred (e.g., a sleeping person awakens to find a bat in the room or an adult witnesses a bat in the room with a previously unattended child, mentally disabled person, or intoxicated person) and rabies cannot be ruled out by testing the bat.*[39]

TABLE 11.9 **Most Common Sources of Rabies.**

Bite Type	Aerobes	Anaerobes	Special Concerns
Dog bites	• *Pasteurella (canis)* • *Streptococcus* • *Staphylococcus* • *Neisseria*	• *Fusobacterium* • *Bacteroides* • *Prevotella* • *Propionibacterium*	• *Capnocytophaga canimorsus*
Cat bites	• *Pasteurella (multocida* and *septica)* • *Streptococcus* • *Staphylococcus* • *Neisseria* • *Moraxella*	• *Fusobacterium* • *Propionibacterium* • *Prevotella*	• *Bartonella henselae*
Human bites	• *Streptococcus (anginosus)* • *Staphylococcus (aureus)* • *Eikenella (corrodens)*	• *Fusobacterium* • *Prevotella*	

Edens MA, Michel JA, Jones N. Mammalian bites in the emergency department: recommendations for wound closure, antibiotics, and postexposure prophylaxis. *Emerg Med Pract.* 2016;18(4):16.

Use of Antibiotics for Acute Wounds

Routine use of prophylactic antibiotics in healthy individuals with uncomplicated/clean wounds has no benefit. Meticulous wound care, debridement, and proper wound closure and dressings are the most important infection control factors indicated for these minor wounds. *Topical antibiotic ointments have been found to decrease the risk of infection in minor contaminated wounds.* The use of prophylactic antibiotics is recommended in the following situations: puncture wounds, open joint or open fracture, heavily contaminated or major soft-tissue injury, bites to the hand/palm, delay in care, and in individuals who are immunocompromised or have chronic health problems (e.g., diabetes and/or cardiac valvular disease).[27]

SPECIFIC WOUNDS

Wounds can either be acute or chronic and are categorized into six basic types: abrasions, abscesses, avulsions, lacerations, puncture wounds, and bites. Their severity varies with the cause of injury and amount of tissue damaged. Wounds may be a minor inconvenience or severe, causing significant discomfort and affecting self-care, self-image, and work. In some cases, lifestyle is permanently altered. All traumatic wounds encountered in the ED must be considered contaminated.[11] Proper wound management is critical to healing and to reducing the possibility of complications such as scar formation or secondary bacterial skin infections. Without proper management, these acute wounds can become chronic wounds (Table 11.10).

Abrasions

Abrasions occur when skin is rubbed or scraped against a hard surface, usually due to friction. These friction wounds can be sustained while participating in sports or work (i.e., road rash, turf rash/burn or carpet "burns"). Superficial abrasions involve removal of the epidermis, and partial-thickness abrasions can extend into the superficial dermis. These deeper friction injuries are more painful than laceration because of the numerous nerve endings exposed. Abrasions have the same physiologic effect as a partial-thickness burn. A significant risk for infection exists from loss of skin and its protective properties.

Cleansing is critical in management of abrasions to prevent any complications. Foreign bodies left in the skin can stain the epidermis and cause permanent scars or a "tattoo." Local anesthesia by topical application or infiltration should be used for abrasions with heavy contamination. Topical antibiotic ointment and nonadherent dressings are used; however, abrasions may occasionally be left open to air. Dressings should be changed daily until eschar forms. Clothing or sunblock should be used for 6 to 12 months to prevent discoloration of fragile new tissue.

Abscesses

Localized collection of pus beneath the skin causes an abscess. Pus may eventually erupt; however, wound management does not include waiting for this to occur. The wound is cleaned, infiltrated with local anesthetic, and drained. An elliptical area of tissue may be removed to facilitate drainage, and then the wound is packed loosely with iodoform or a similar material and covered with a loose dressing. In the pediatric patient, care must be used with treating skin infections. Community-acquired methicillin-resistant *Staphylococcus aureus* (CA-MRSA) has become a common cause of skin infections. Local resistance patterns should be considered when choosing antibiotics. Follow-up with a health care provider is imperative to closely monitor the patient and wound healing.

Avulsions

An avulsion is full-thickness skin loss in which approximation of wound edges is not possible. A degloving injury is a severe avulsion injury in which skin is peeled away from the underlying fascia and muscles.[40] Degloving injuries of the fingers are more common and involve injury to tendons and ligaments. Management includes local anesthesia by injection or topical application, followed by irrigation and debridement of devitalized tissue. A split-thickness skin graft is often necessary with large avulsions. The wound should be covered with a bulky dressing to protect exposed tissue.

TABLE 11.10 Rabies Postexposure Prophylaxis Schedule.

RABIES POSTEXPOSURE PROPHYLAXIS (PEP) SCHEDULE, UNITED STATES, 2010		
Vaccination Status	**Intervention**	**Regimen[a]**
Not previously vaccinated	Wound cleansing	All PEP should begin with immediate thorough cleansing of all wounds with soap and water. If available, a virucidal agent (e.g., povidone-iodine solution) should be used to irrigate the wounds.
	Human rabies immune globulin (HRIG)	Administer 20 international unit/kg body weight. If anatomically feasible, the full dose should be infiltrated around and into the wound(s), and any remaining volume should be administered at an anatomic site (intramuscular [IM]) distant from vaccine administration. Also, HRIG should not be administered in the same syringe as vaccine. Because rabies immune globulin (human) might partially suppress active production of rabies virus antibody, no more than the recommended dose should be administered.
	Vaccine	Human diploid cell vaccine (HDCV) or purified chick embryo cell vaccine (PCECV) 1.0 mL, IM (deltoid area[b]), 1 each on days 0,[c] 3, 7, and 14.[d]
Previously vaccinated[e]	Wound cleansing	All PEP should begin with immediate thorough cleansing of all wounds with soap and water. If available, a virucidal agent such as povidone-iodine solution should be used to irrigate the wounds.
	HRIG	HRIG should not be administered.
	Vaccine	HDCV or PCECV 1.0 mL, IM (deltoid area[b]), 1 each on days 0[c] and 3.

[a]These regimens are applicable for persons in all age-groups, including children.
[b]The deltoid area is the only acceptable site of vaccination for adults and older children. For younger children, the outer aspect of the thigh may be used. Vaccine should never be administered in the gluteal area.
[c]Day 0 is the day dose 1 of vaccine is administered.
[d]For persons with immunosuppression, rabies PEP should be administered using all 5 doses of vaccine on days 0, 3, 7, 14, and 28.
[e]Any person with a history of preexposure vaccination with HDCV, PCECV, or rabies vaccine adsorbed (RVA); prior PEP with HDCV, PCECV, or RVA; or previous vaccination with any other type of rabies vaccine and a documented history of antibody response to the prior vaccination.
Rupprecht CE, Briggs D, Brown CM, et al; Centers for Disease Control. Use of a reduced (4-dose) vaccine schedule for postexposure prophylaxis to prevent human rabies: recommendations of the advisory committee on immunization practices. *MMWR*. 2010;59(RR2):6.

Contusions

Blunt trauma that does not alter skin integrity causes a contusion, or bruise. Swelling, pain, and discoloration occur with extravasation of blood into damaged tissues. After assessment of neurovascular status, therapeutic interventions include cold packs and analgesia as necessary. Large wounds or those located in an extremity should be carefully observed for cellulitis or development of compartment syndrome.

Lacerations

Lacerations are open wounds caused by shearing forces through dermal layers. Superficial lacerations involve the epidermis and dermis, whereas more severe injuries involve deeper layers, including subcutaneous tissue and muscle. Initial interventions focus on controlling bleeding and assessing neurovascular function distal to the injury. Anesthetic should be used to facilitate removal of foreign bodies and excision of necrotic or devitalized tissue. Exploration is indicated when damage to underlying structures is possible. Wound closure involves approximation of edges followed by closure with a tape closure, staples, or sutures. Deeper wounds are closed in layers. After the wound is closed, a thin layer of antibiotic ointment may be applied, followed by a nonadherent dressing.

Puncture Wounds

Puncture wounds that are uncomplicated, clean, and less than 6 hours old require only low-pressure irrigation and tetanus prophylaxis. Soaking has no proven benefit. Healthy patients do not appear to require prophylactic antibiotics. Puncture wounds do not have a dramatic appearance, and these wounds are often undertreated. Regardless of appearance, the zone of injury and the wound's proximity to underlying structures should be assessed thoroughly.

High-pressure injection injuries (such as paint gun and nail gun injuries) cause severe damage to underlying tissues. The damage may be less than what is indicated by the appearance of the surface wound. High-pressure injection injuries of the hand must be treated with tetanus prophylaxis, broad-spectrum antibiotics, and consultation with a hand surgeon because of their risk for wound contamination. Management includes removal of necrotic tissue followed by drain placement and sterile dressing application. These injuries are at great risk for becoming infected with an anaerobic organism and carry with them high morbidity and mortality rates, with delayed identification of the organisms and increased deep tissue necrosis.

Puncture wounds with a high risk of infection and poor outcomes are determined by the location of the injury, the patient's medical status, and the type of penetrating object. Poor outcomes occur when the wound is more than 6 hours old; is contaminated with foreign matter and debris; is sustained outdoors; is a penetrating injury that went through footwear; or occurred in patients with underlying disease, such as diabetes mellitus or immunosuppression.[41] Most infections from puncture wounds are caused by gram-positive organisms, with *Staphylococcus aureus* being the predominant organism.[42,43] Puncture wounds occurring through a sneaker-type shoe frequently are inoculated with *Pseudomonas aeruginosa.*[42,43] *P. aeruginosa* infections are typically treated with either ciprofloxacin (Cipro) or levofloxacin (Levaquin).[42,43]

Bites

Bites may be caused by animals or humans and involve contusions, avulsions, lacerations, and puncture wounds. Teeth can crush or tear tissue, causing extensive damage. Dog bites account for 80% to 90% of these injuries,[37,43] whereas cat bites are reported in 5% to 10%. Exotic animals such as primates, felines, alligators, and camels also cause bite injuries. Regardless of the source, bite wounds are considered contaminated. Patients often will not present until colonization by multiple microorganisms has occurred (usually 12–24 hours post bite) and the wound starts to display signs of infection such as redness, swelling, inability to move joints (flexion especially), warmth, and drainage. Infection, abscess, cellulitis, septicemia, osteomyelitis, tenosynovitis, rabies, tetanus, and loss of body parts are potential complications of bite wounds. Amoxicillin-clavulanate (Augmentin) is the drug of choice for any of these bites, with moxifloxacin used as an alternative medication in patients with penicillin allergies.[37,43] Other options for individuals who are allergic to penicillin are[43]:

- cefuroxime
- doxycycline
- erythromycin
- trimethoprim-sulfamethoxazole

Any bite must have a thorough history and examination in a bloodless field. Special attention must be paid to injuries over a joint. Along with assessment of range of motion of the joint, a neurovascular assessment must be performed. If there are signs of infection, appropriate antibiotic treatment must be initiated. Radiographs should be obtained if a joint, bony area, or foreign body is involved. Wound cultures are not usually indicated; however, blood cultures may be useful in immunosuppressed individuals. If a bite involves the hand, consider immobilizing the hand in a bulky dressing or splint to limit use. Rabies and tetanus prophylaxis should be considered for all individuals (see Table 11.10).

Human bites usually result from altercations, fights, or sexual activity, or they may even be self-inflicted, with the hands and/or upper extremities being the most common locations of injury. Infection is the greatest risk with human bites because human saliva contains 100,000,000 organisms per mL,[37,43] including *Staphylococcus aureus,* streptococci, *Corynebacterium,* and *Bacteroides* organisms.[37,43] Hepatitis B and C virus, along with the human immunodeficiency virus, may have a low risk of infection after a bite.[43]

Human bites can be divided into two categories: closed fist and occlusive bites, with most being occlusive bites. Occlusive bites occur when teeth sink into the skin with enough force to breach the integrity of the skin. This type of injury is the most common and is seen more frequently in females than in males.

Clenched/closed fist or "fight" injuries occur when a closed fist comes in contact with the teeth of the person who is hit, leaving harmless-appearing puncture marks over the dorsal aspect of the third, fourth, or fifth metacarpophalangeal joints, most classically, over the third metacarpophalangeal joint. Clenched fist injuries generally are more serious than occlusion injuries due to the involvement of the joints. Bacteria are then spread to the tendon sheath proximal to the wound, causing an inability to bend or straighten the finger or a loss of sensation over the tip of the finger. The wound should be examined thoroughly, making sure the individual has their full range of motion. This assessment will assure the provider that the extensor tendon or cartilage was not damaged when the fingers are in the flexed position.

If an injury is noted, the patient should be admitted to have a surgical exploration, irrigation, and debridement of the wound. If it has been decided that nonoperative management can pursued, the wound should then be cleaned, irrigated, and debrided. The wound should then be left open and splinted in a position of comfort.[37,43] With **the high risk for infection in human bites, antibiotics are given prophylactically whenever the wound penetrates the skin.** If the wound is grossly infected, the individual is showing systemic symptoms, or they are scheduled for irrigation and debridement in the operating room, intravenous antibiotics should be prescribed. The duration of antibiotics is 5 to 7 days.[37]

Human bites to the face should be closed by primary intention for cosmetic reasons as long as there is no overt sign of infection. Before closure, they must be irrigated and explored. Primary closure can be performed up to 24 hours after the bite.

One-half of the 4.5 million dog bites occurring in the United States each year happen in children aged 5 to 9 years, with one in five requiring medical attention.[43] The face, head, and neck are the most frequent areas involved in children; arms and extremities are the site of injury in adults. Because dogs have powerful jaws, crush injuries are common, with injury to underlying vessels, bones, and nerves. For many years, the teaching was that all dog bites should be left open. However, a 2014 study by Paschos et al.[44] revealed no increased rate of infection when dog bites were closed primarily. Timing of wound management was critical in the resultant infection rate. Primary suturing exhibited improved cosmetic appearance. Antibiotic use for dog bites is controversial because there is a very low rate of infection (Table 11.11).

Cat bites are primarily found on the arm, forearm, or hand. The long, narrow, slender teeth of cats easily penetrate skin and underlying soft tissue, creating small puncture wounds in the skin that heal quickly, thus trapping bacteria and causing infection as soon as 3 hours after inoculation. Organisms commonly found in cat bites are similar to those in dogs, but it may be difficult to appropriately copiously irrigate these small puncture wounds inflicted by cats. Cat bites are considered high risk for infection because they tend to cause deep puncture wounds.

TABLE 11.11 Risk Factors for Wound Infections.

Factor	High Risk	Low Risk
Species	Cat (domestic and wild) Human Monkey Pig Camel Bear	Dog (excluding hands and feet) Rodent
Location of wound	Hand (especially clenched fist injuries [CFIs]) Foot	Face Scalp
Wound type	Puncture Crush injury or damage to deep structures Presence of devitalized tissue Delayed presentation (more than 6 hours) Closed primarily	Laceration Superficial
Patient characteristics	Age over 50 Diabetes Renal failure Liver disease Alcoholism Immune disorder Malnutrition Use of corticosteroids or other immunosuppressive medications Peripheral vascular disease Chronic edema of the bitten area	

Eillbert WP. Mammalian bites. In: Walls RM, Hockberger RS, Gausche-Hill M, eds. *Rosen's Emergency Medicine: Concepts and Clinical Practice*. 9th ed. Philadelphia, PA: Elsevier; 2018:692.

TABLE 11.12 Recommendations for Bite Wound Closure and Prophylactic Antibiotics.

Species	Suturing	Prophylactic Antibiotics
Dogs, coyotes, wolves	The majority except hands and feet	Hand and foot wounds High-risk wounds[a]
Cat	Face only	All wounds extending through the epidermis
Human	Face only (up to 24 hours after the bite)	All wounds extending through the epidermis
Monkey	Face only (up to 24 hours after the bite)	All wounds extending through the epidermis
Rodent	All (but rarely needed)	No
Ferret, pig, horse, camel, bear, big cats	Face only	All wounds extending through the epidermis

[a]High-risk wounds: Deep puncture wounds, crush injury or damage to deep structures, delayed presentation (>6 hours), wounds closed primarily, and high-risk patients.

Eillbert WP. Mammalian bites. In: Walls RM, Hockberger RS, Gausche-Hill M, eds. *Rosen's Emergency Medicine: Concepts and Clinical Practice*. 9th ed. Philadelphia, PA: Elsevier; 2018:691.

SUMMARY

Skin is the first barrier between the body and the rest of the world. Loss of skin integrity affects the ability to resist infection, retain fluids, and regulate body temperature. Changes caused by surface trauma, such as scarring or tattooing, affect body image and can cause significant anxiety for the patient. The ED nurse plays a vital role in reducing potential wound complications through assessment, meticulous wound care, knowledge of the indications for tetanus immunization and antibiotic use, and detailed discharge teaching. The most effective intervention to decrease the risk for infection is thorough wound cleansing. Box 11.1 provides a summary of wound care management.

REFERENCES

1. Moreira M. Wound management. In: Markovchick VT, Pons PT, Bakes K, Buchanan J, eds. *Emergency Medicine Secrets*. 6th ed. Philadelphia, PA: Elsevier; 2016:625–634.
2. Thibodeau GA, Patton KT. *Anatomy and Physiology*. 9th ed. St Louis, MO: Mosby; 2016:164–171.
3. Darby IA, Laverdet B, Bonté F, Desmoulièr A. Fibroblasts and myofibroblasts in wound healing. *Clin Cosmet Investigat Dermatol*. 2015;7:301–311.
4. Gonzalez AC, Costa TF, Andrade ZA, Medrado AR. Wound healing—a literature review. *An Brasil Dermatol*. 2016;91(5):614–620.
5. Singh S, Young A, McNaugh CE. The physiology of wound healing. *Surgery*. 2017;35(9):473–477.

6. Sgonc R, Gruber J. Age-related aspects of cutaneous wound healing: a mini-review. *Gerontology*. 2013;59(2):159–164.
7. Sorg H, Tilkorn DJ, Hager S, Hauser J, Mirastschijski U. Skin wound healing: an update on the current knowledge and concepts. *Eur Surg Res*. 2017;58(1-2):81–94.
8. Landen NX, Li D, Stahle M. Transition from inflammation to proliferation: a critical step during wound healing. *Cell Mol Life Sci*. 2016;73(20):3861–3885.
9. Lewis SL. Inflammation and wound healing. In: Lewis SL, Bucher L, Heitkemper MH, Harding MM, Kwong J, Roberts R, eds. *Medical-Surgical Nursing: Assessment and Management in Clinical Practice*. 10th ed. St Louis, MO: Elsevier; 2017:172–189.
10. Adams CA, Heffernan DS, Cioffi WG. Wounds, bites, and stings. In: Moore EE, Feliciano DV, Mattox KL, eds. *Trauma*. 8th ed. New York, NY: McGraw-Hill; 2017.
11. Prevaldi C, Paolillo C, Locatelli C, et al. Management of traumatic wounds in the emergency department: position paper from the Academy of Emergency Medicine and Care (AcEMC) and the World Society of Emergency Surgery (WSES). *World J Emerg Surg*. 2016;11:30–36.
12. Gabriel A. *Wound irrigation*. https://emedicine.medscape.com/article/1895071-overview. Updated December 14, 2017. Accessed April 27, 2019.
13. Kaye A, Abubshait A. *Trick of the trade: DIY squirt bottle wound irrigation*. 2017. https://www.aliem.com/2017/07/trick-trade-diy-squirt-bottle-wound-irrigation/. Published July 31, 2017. Accessed April 27, 2019.
14. Simon BC, Hern HG. Wound management principles. In: Walls RM, Hockberger RS, Gausche-Hill M, eds. *Rosen's Emergency Medicine: Concepts and Clinical Practice*. 9th ed. Philadelphia, PA: Elsevier; 2018:659–673.
15. Weiss EA, Oldham G, Lin M, Foster T, Quinn JV. Water is a safe and effective alternative to sterile normal saline for wound irrigation prior to suturing: a prospective, double-blind, randomised, controlled clinical trial. *BMJ Open*. 2013;3:e001504. https://doi.org/10.1136/bmjopen-2012-001504.
16. Lammers RL, Aldy KN. Principles of wound management. In: Roberts JR, Custalow CB, Thomsen T, eds. *Robert's and Hedge's Clinical Procedures in Emergency Medicine and Acute Care*. 7th ed. Philadelphia, PA: Elsevier; 2018:621–654.
17. Cabrera D. *Pearls in digital wound repair*. https://emblog.mayo.edu/2014/12/07/pearls-in-digital-wound-repair/. Published December 7, 2014. Accessed April 27, 2019.
18. Wei LG, Chen CF, Chun-Yuan H, et al. Safe finger tourniquet-ideas. *Ann Plast Surg*. 2016;76(suppl 1):S130–S132.
19. Magee DL. Local and topical anesthesia. In: Roberts JR, Custalow CB, Thomsen T, eds. *Robert's and Hedge's Clinical Procedures in Emergency Medicine and Acute Care*. 7th ed. Philadelphia, PA: Elsevier; 2018:523–544.
20. Vandamme E, Lemoyne S, van der Gucht A, de Cock P, van de Voorde P. LAT gel for laceration repair in the emergency department: not only for children? *Eur J Emerg Med*. 2017;24(1):55–59.
21. Krausz A, Friedman AJ. Nitric oxide as a surgical adjuvant. *Future Sci OA*. 2015;1(1):FS O56.
22. Huang C, Johnson N. Nitrous oxide, from the operating room to the emergency department. *Curr Emerg Hospital Med Rep*. 2016;4:11–18.
23. Worster B, Zawora MQ, Hsieh C. Common questions about wound care. *Am Fam Phys*. 2015;91(2):86–92.
24. Eliya-Masamba MC, Banda GW. Primary closure versus delayed closure for non bite traumatic wounds within 24 hours post injury (Review). *Cochrane Database Syst Rev*. 2013;(10):1–21.
25. Lee HJ, Jang YJ. Recent understandings of biology, prophylaxis and treatment strategies for hypertrophic scars and keloids. *Int J Mol Sci*. 2018;19(3):711.
26. Satteson ES. *Materials for wound closure*. https://emedicine.medscape.com/article/1127693-overview. Updated August 14, 2017. Accessed April 27, 2019.
27. Lammers RL, Scrimshaw LE. Methods of wound closure. In: Roberts JR, Custalow CB, Thomsen T, eds. *Robert's and Hedge's Clinical Procedures in Emergency Medicine and Acute Care*. 7th ed. Philadelphia, PA: Elsevier; 2018:655–707.
28. Dermabond advanced. Topical skin adhesive [Video]. https://www.ethicon.com/na/products/wound-closure/skin-adhesives/dermabond-advanced-topical-skin-adhesive. Published 2017. Accessed April 27, 2019.
29. Ubbink DT, Brölmann FE, Go P, Vermeulen H. Evidence-based care of acute wounds: a perspective. *Adv Wound Care*. 2015;4(5):286–294.
30. Dabiri G, Damstetter E, Phillips T. Choosing a wound dressing based on common wound characteristics. *Adv Wound Care*. 2016;5(1):32–41.
31. Sood A, Granick MS, Tomaselli NL. Wound dressings and comparative effectiveness data. *Adv Wound Care*. 2014;3(8):511–529.
32. *Guidelines for the management of tetanus-prone*; 2017. http://www.immune.org.nz/resources/written-resources/guidelines-management-tetanus-prone-wounds. Accessed April 27, 2019.
33. Collins S, White J, Ramsay M, Amirthalingam G. The importance of tetanus risk assessment during wound management. *ID Cases*. 2015;2(1):3–5.
34. Centers for Disease Control and Prevention. *Tetanus: symptoms and complications*. https://www.cdc.gov/tetanus/about/symptoms-complications.html. Published 2017. Accessed April 27, 2019.
35. Immunization Action Coalition. *Tetanus: questions and answers*. http://www.immunize.org/catg.d/p4220.pdf. Published 2013. Accessed April 27, 2019.
36. Rupprecht CE, Briggs D, Brown CM, et al. Centers for Disease Control and Prevention. Use of a reduced (4-dose) vaccine schedule for postexposure prophylaxis to prevent human rabies: recommendations of the advisory committee on immunization practices. *MMWR*. 2010;59(RR2):1–9.
37. Edens MA, Michel JA, Jones N. Mammalian bites in the emergency department: recommendations for wound closure, antibiotics, and postexposure prophylaxis. *Emerg Med Pract*. 2016;18(4):1–20.
38. Wilson PJ, Rohde RE. *For #WorldRabiesDay: two experts share less-known facts about rabies and how to prevent it*. https://www.elsevier.com/connect/8-things-you-may-not-know-about-rabies-but-should. Published September 28, 2015. Accessed April 27, 2019.
39. Centers for Disease Control and Prevention. *Bats*. https://www.cdc.gov/rabies/exposure/animals/bats.html. Published 2017. Accessed April 27, 2019.
40. Latifi R, El-Hennawy H, El-Menyar A, Asim M, Consunji R, Al-Thani H. The therapeutic challenges of degloving soft-tissue injuries. *J Emerg Trauma Shock*. 2014;7(3):228–232.
41. James Q. Puncture wounds and bites. In: Tintinalli JE, Stapczynski JS, Ma OJ, Yealy D, Meckler GD, Cline DM, eds. *Emergency Medicine: A Comprehensive Study Guide*. 8th ed. New York, NY: McGraw-Hill; 2016:313–319.
42. Keller MC, Thun JD, Curfman AJ. How to treat puncture wounds. *Podiatry Today*. 2014;27(10):68–74.
43. Eillbert WP. Mammalian bites. In: Walls RM, Hockberger RS, Gausche-Hill M, eds. *Rosen's Emergency Medicine: Concepts and Clinical Practice*. 9th ed. Philadelphia, PA: Elsevier; 2018:690–697.
44. Paschos N, Makris EA, Gantsos A, Georgoulis AD. Primary closure versus non-closure of dog bite wounds: a randomised controlled trial. *Injury*. 2014;45(1):237–240. https://emblog.mayo.edu/files/2014/12/dig3.jpghttps://emblog.mayo.edu/files/2014/12/dig4.jpg.

12

Family Presence During Resuscitation and Invasive Procedures

Patricia Kunz Howard

Commitment to the patient and family is a primary tenet of emergency nursing.[1] The emergency nurse respects the right of the patient and family to participate in care planning decisions. Offering families the option to be present during cardiopulmonary resuscitation (family presence) has taken place for more than 25 years and is well supported by professional organizations.[2–7] Presence during invasive procedures has also been shown to be efficacious for the patient and family.[2,7–9] A care delivery model that provides support for family presence during resuscitation and invasive procedures is an essential part of providing quality care to patients and families. Current evidence reveals that patients and families believe they should have the option to be present during resuscitation and invasive procedures.[4]

Family presence is the essence of family support, allowing family members to benefit from being together during challenging situations and crises. The family has the opportunity to offer support to each other and the patient, alleviate the sense of helplessness, work through the reality of a situation, and in some cases be able to share the final moments of a loved one's life. Emergency nurses should recognize the benefits of family presence and advocate for the option of family presence as the standard of care in all emergency departments.

This chapter will provide an overview of the evidence in support of family presence and outline the benefits of family presence for patient and families as well as health care professionals. Topics presented in this chapter are the evolution of family presence during resuscitation, evidence supporting family presence during resuscitation and invasive procedures, organizational support for family presence, information on how to implement family presence, education for health care professionals, and evaluation.

EVIDENCE

The earliest reports of allowing family presence during resuscitation occurred in 1982 at Foote Hospital in Jackson, Michigan.[2] At two events, families at Foote Hospital demanded to be present.[3] Foote Hospital, like most hospitals, had a policy of "no family presence" during resuscitation and took this opportunity to examine their practice. Over a 9-year period, family members who were present during resuscitation at Foote Hospital reported positive family experiences with family presence. Specific findings revealed that 72% of families surveyed would prefer to be in the resuscitation room, and 71% of staff supported the practice of family presence. In addition, the hospital's Advanced Cardiac Life Support Committee found no difference in resuscitation events regardless of family presence.[2,3] These findings provided the framework for research delineating the benefits of family presence during resuscitation and invasive procedures. Over the next 25 years, more than 300 articles and significant research have provided substantive support for presenting the option for family presence. Although the patient and family benefits and preferences for allowing the option of family presence are clear, research continues to focus on the perceptions of the family and health care providers.

A systematic review of family presence during resuscitation and invasive procedures in pediatric critical care was performed.[9] Findings from this review illustrated that parents wanted to be present during resuscitation and invasive procedures, would want to be present again in similar circumstances, would not change their experience, and would recommend being present to other parents. Parents who were present during their child's unsuccessful resuscitation experienced better coping and adjustment to the loss of their child than those who were not present. These studies further revealed that patients (both adults and children) were comforted by the presence of family during invasive procedures and resuscitation.[9]

An investigation into nurses' perceptions of family presence revealed that most nurses had not facilitated families being present during resuscitation, yet they were confident in their ability to manage family presence. In this study, the nurses with the most confidence in their ability to facilitate family presence identified greater perceived benefits from families being present. The presence of a support person was essential, and this role was often performed by pastoral care staff. Potential barriers to family presence identified included the lack of chaplain support during the night shift.[10]

An educational intervention designed to enhance nurses' and physicians' knowledge, attitudes, and compliance with family presence during resuscitation revealed a lack of knowledge about institutional policy regarding family presence.[11] In this research, nurses were more likely than their physician colleagues to believe that family presence was a patient right. Findings from this investigation also demonstrated that the educational intervention did not alter the attitudes of nurses or physicians; however, a practice change occurred in those who received the education. Families were present 87% of the time when the health care providers had received the educational intervention compared with 23% of the time when the health care professionals did not receive the educational intervention.

Studies have focused on the perceptions of health care professionals and the impact of family presence on the health care team. Common concerns mentioned were interference with care events, disruptive family members, delayed or prolonged resuscitation events, litigation, and distress of health care professionals.[12,13] The litigation resulting from families being present during resuscitation has not been identified in the literature. In most cases, the family being present during resuscitation has resulted in the family recognizing that everything was done and resuscitation efforts have ceased sooner. Some of the concerns identified by health care professionals could truly be perceptions versus real experiences with family presence.[13]

ORGANIZATIONAL SUPPORT

In 1993 the Emergency Nurses Association (ENA) became the first major organization to endorse family presence. Since that time, ENA has developed education on family presence, supported research on the topic, and published a family presence clinical practice guideline. ENA believes that family presence is so important that education on family presence is included in the *Emergency Nursing Pediatric Course*[14] and the *Trauma Nursing Core Course.*[15] The American Heart Association has supported the option of offering family presence during resuscitation since dissemination of their 2000 Guidelines and with each subsequent revision of the guidelines for cardiopulmonary resuscitation and emergency cardiovascular care in the Advanced Cardiac Life Support course.[5] The consensus from professional health care organizations supporting family presence during resuscitation and invasive procedures is that policy and procedures should be in place to facilitate this practice, all members of the interprofessional team should be educated about family presence, and family support should be provided by a team member not directly involved in clinical care.[2–8]

IMPLEMENTATION

Positive implementation of family presence starts with a person or a group of people who have a commitment to support families. These champions are knowledgeable about the current evidence and support family presence. Department and institutional support is essential for family presence to occur in a manner that is mutually beneficial to the patient, family, and the health care team. Each facility should have a clear definition of family to include the persons designated by each patient as family. Facilitating family presence will be most successful in facilities with an established written policy, education, and interprofessional collaboration.

Roles and Responsibilities

The role of the family support person (FSP) is essential to meet the needs of the family members present during resuscitation and invasive procedures. The FSP is responsible for ensuring that the family knows what to expect while present, affirming the patient care team is aware the family wants to be present, and confirming that all team members are aware family presence is imminent. Family presence does not disrupt care when the FSP is present to provide support.

An emergency nurse or member of the pastoral care team often fulfills the role of the FSP. Other team members who possess knowledge of invasive procedures and resuscitation, such as social work or volunteers with clinical experience, may also serve in the FSP role.

EDUCATION

Education on family presence is essential for all members of the interprofessional health care team who have the potential to be involved. Education should include the following elements:

- the facility guideline or policy
- role of the family support person
- advocating for family presence
- evaluating the family presence experience

EVALUATION

Formal evaluation of family presence events will ensure that the process is achieving the desired benefit for patients and families. This evaluation should include asking the following questions of the interprofessional team, the patient (as appropriate), and the family:

- Was the process outlined in the guideline/policy followed?
- What were the perceptions of the patient (as appropriate) and/or family?
- What were the perceptions of the health care professionals providing care?
- What was the outcome of the event?

SUMMARY

Facilitating family presence is essential for the patient, family, and the health care team. The evidence is compelling regarding the benefits of family presence. It is consistent with a patient- and family-centered approach. Being present provides family members with the opportunity to provide support to the patient and each other and to make informed care decisions.

Patients' benefits from family presence parallel family benefits. Patients surviving resuscitation events report that they felt supported by their family members' presence. They felt as if someone in the room actually cared for them and helped the health care team see them as a real person. Emergency nurses and other health care professionals benefit from advocating for the patient and family. Acceptance of family presence across the health care continuum will better meet the needs of the patient and family.

REFERENCES

1. Emergency Nurses Association. *Emergency Nursing Scope and Standards of Practice*. 2nd ed. Des Plaines, IL: Emergency Nurses Association; 2017.
2. Doyle CJ, Post H, Burney RE, Maino J, Keefe M, Rhee KJ. Family participation during resuscitation: an option. *Ann Emerg Med*. 1987;16(6):673.
3. Hanson C, Strawser D. Family presence during cardiopulmonary resuscitation: Foote Hospital emergency department's nine-year perspective. *J Emerg Nurs*. 1992;18(2):104.
4. Emergency Nurses Association. *Clinical Practice Guideline: Family Presence During Invasive Procedures and Resuscitation*. In press.
5. American Heart Association. *Family presence during resuscitation*. 2015 American Heart Association Guidelines Update for Cardiopulmonary Resuscitation and Emergency Cardiovascular Care. https://eccguidelines.heart.org/index.php/circulation/cpr-ecc-guidelines-2/part-12-pediatric-advanced-life-support/intra-arrest-care-updates/family-presence-during-resuscitation/. Published 2015. Accessed April 16, 2019.
6. American College of Emergency Physicians. *Family presence fact sheet*. http://newsroom.acep.org/2009-01-04-family-presence-fact-sheet. Published 2015. Accessed April 16, 2019.
7. American Association of Critical Care Nurses. Family presence during resuscitation and invasive procedures. *Crit Care Nurse*. 2016;36(1):e11. http://ccn.aacnjournals.org/content/36/1/e11.full.pdf.
8. Twibell RS, Craig S, Siela D, Simmonds S, Thomas C. Being there: inpatients' perceptions of family presence during resuscitation and invasive cardiac procedures. *Am J Crit Care*. 2015;24(6):e108.
9. McAlvin SS, Carew-Lyons A. Family presence during resuscitation and invasive procedures in pediatric critical care: a systematic review. *Am J Crit Care*. 2014;23(6):477.
10. Tudor K, Berger J, Polivka BJ, Chlebowy R, Thomas B. Nurses' perceptions of family presence during resuscitation. *Am J Crit Care*. 2014;23(6):e88.
11. Ferrara G, Ramponi D, Cline TW. Evaluation of physicians' and nurses' knowledge, attitudes, and compliance with family presence during resuscitation in an emergency department setting after an educational intervention. *Adv Emerg Nurs J*. 2014;38(1):32.
12. Zavotsky KE, McCoy J, Bell G, et al. Resuscitation team perceptions of family presence during CPR. *Adv Emerg Nurs J*. 2014;36(4):325.
13. Porter JE, Cooper SJ, Sellick K. Family presence during resuscitation (FPDR): perceived benefits, barriers and enablers to implementation and practice. *Int Emerg Nurs*. 2014;22(2):69.
14. Emergency Nurses Association. *Emergency Nursing Pediatric Course (ENPC)*. 4th ed. Des Plaines, IL: Emergency Nurses Association; 2012.
15. Emergency Nurses Association. *Trauma Nursing Core Course (TNCC)*. 7th ed. Des Plaines, IL: Emergency Nurses Association; 2014.

13

Management of the Critical Care Patient in the Emergency Department

Renee Semonin Holleran

CRITICAL CARE IN THE EMERGENCY DEPARTMENT

Critical care patients remaining for extended periods of time in the emergency department (ED) have become increasingly more common over the past decades.[1] Multiple reasons for "boarding" of critical care patients in the ED have been identified. Some of these are a lack of inpatient critical care beds, the ongoing nursing shortage, and increasing ED visits despite a decrease in EDs. Ultimately, when hospital beds are full, patients cannot be transferred from the critical care units to floor beds, which results in critical care patients boarding in the ED. Other reasons for the increase in boarding of critical care patients in the ED are a lack of policies and procedures to facilitate patient movement from the ED to a critical care unit, lack of administrative support to improve patient flow, and lack of regionalization of health care resources to admit patients.[2]

Inpatient care of the critically ill or injured patient results in different needs than the typical initial stabilization provided in the ED. Additional education, equipment, and resources are required to ensure safe and competent critical care.

Management of the critically ill or injured patient necessitates the ED to have skilled critical care clinicians and equipment, and an area where patients can be closely monitored. Observation units have been created in EDs to alleviate some of the pressure related to limited inpatient beds. However, there are times when these units and other areas of the ED may be used to manage critical care patients. There are many unpredictable critical conditions that may occur in patients admitted to an ED observation unit, including dyspnea, shock, cardiac arrest, and death. The focus of this chapter is to discuss the common clinical conditions and interventions needed when emergency nurses care for the critically ill or injured patient boarding in the ED. Included in this chapter is the management of the artificially ventilated patient, selected invasive lines, and sepsis.

MECHANICAL VENTILATION

Mechanical ventilation of a critically ill or injured patient can be challenging in the ED. Ventilator settings, alarms, patient positioning, and oral care are just a few of the issues to be addressed.

Indications for Intubation and Mechanical Ventilation

Intubation is indicated in a variety of clinical situations but generally falls into one of three main categories: failure to maintain a patent airway, inadequate oxygenation, or ineffective ventilation.

Failure, or Anticipated Failure, to Protect or Maintain a Patent Airway

The following groups of patients are at a higher risk for airway issues:

- Obtunded or comatose patients with loss of gag reflex: traumatic brain injury (TBI), overdose, anoxia, cerebral vascular accident, cerebral aneurysm, etc.
- Patients with a partial or complete obstruction: edema due to inhalation injury, neck trauma, epiglottitis, laryngeal edema, bronchospasm, foreign object aspiration, burns
- Patients receiving some pharmacologic therapy: benzodiazepine therapy for status epilepticus, sedation/paralysis for TBI to control increased intracranial pressures (ICPs) or to obtain diagnostic imaging in combative patients

Inadequate Oxygenation

A shunt occurs when alveoli are perfused but not ventilated, as in pneumonia, acute respiratory distress syndrome (ARDS), acute lung injury (ALI), pulmonary hemorrhage or pulmonary contusion, and atelectasis. Dead space ventilation results when alveoli are ventilated but not perfused, as in pulmonary embolus, hypotension, and low cardiac output states such as cardiogenic shock.

Diffusion abnormality is caused by the obstruction or restriction of gas exchange across the capillary–alveolar membrane, as in pulmonary edema or pulmonary fibrosis. Inadequate oxygenation can also occur because of an inability of the cells to extract oxygen, such as in sepsis, carbon monoxide poisoning, or cyanide poisoning.

Inadequate Ventilation

Inadequate ventilation may result from neurologic causes such as spinal cord injury, TBI, overdose, and Guillain–Barré syndrome. Muscular abnormalities resulting from myopathies and myasthenia gravis will contribute to the failure to ventilate. Finally, anatomic causes such as pleural effusions, hemothorax, pneumothorax, flail chest, and abdominal hypertension may impair ventilation.

Definitions[3,4]

There are important definitions related to mechanical ventilation for emergency nurses to be familiar with. Box 13.1 contains a summary of these.[3–5]

Classification of Mechanical Ventilators[3]

There are two types of ventilators: positive pressure and negative pressure. It is highly unlikely that negative pressure ventilation (e.g., iron lung, cuirass) would ever be used in the ED setting. There are two types of positive pressure ventilation used in the ED. The ventilator type is named for the parameter terminating the inspiratory cycle of the ventilator: volume-controlled and pressure-controlled.

Volume-Controlled, Pressure Variable

This is the most common mode of ventilation. The tidal volume (Vt) is preset and delivered during the inspiratory phase of the ventilator cycle. Depending on the compliance and resistance of the lung, the pressure required to deliver the set Vt will vary. The advantage of this mode is the patient receives guaranteed minute ventilation volumes. The disadvantage is the potential for lung injury when high pressures are required to deliver the set Vt in patients with low lung compliance.

Modes include controlled mandatory (or controlled) ventilation, assist-control (AC) ventilation, and synchronized intermittent mandatory ventilation (SIMV).

Pressure-Controlled, Volume Variable

In this mode of ventilation, the inspiratory pressure is preset and the ventilator will deliver a breath until that pressure is reached. The Vt delivered to reach that pressure will vary depending on the compliance and resistance of the lung. The advantage of this mode is it limits the distending pressure of the lung. The mean airway pressure can be manipulated by prolonging the inspiratory time (T_i), thus reducing the potential for high peak or plateau pressures. The disadvantage is that the minute ventilation volume is not guaranteed and requires more attentive monitoring to prevent hypoventilation or hyperventilation.

Modes of Ventilation

Modes include pressure control and pressure support ventilation.

Controlled Mandatory Ventilation (CMV)

Method: Delivers a set respiratory rate at a set Vt, overriding any respiratory effort by the patient. This may cause physical discomfort for the patient and is usually used if the patient is unconscious or has received a neuromuscular blocking agent.

Set parameters: Fraction of inspired oxygen (FiO_2), Vt, ventilatory rate (VR), positive end-expiratory pressure (PEEP), ratio of inspiratory to expiratory time (I:E) or T_i

Variable parameters: Peak inspiratory pressure (PIP)

BOX 13.1 Definitions for Mechanical Ventilation.

- *Acute lung injury (ALI):* A severe form of ARDS characterized by acute hypoxemic respiratory failure, diffuse bilateral pulmonary infiltrates on chest x-ray film, pulmonary wedge pressure <18 mm Hg and PaO_2/FiO_2 ratio of <300.
- *Acute respiratory distress syndrome (ARDS):* The same definition as ALI except the PaO_2/FiO_2 ratio is <200.
- *Barotrauma:* Damage to the lung tissue due to high airway pressures. Alveolar rupture may lead to pneumothorax, pulmonary interstitial edema, and pneumomediastinum.
- *FiO_2:* Fraction of inspired oxygen ranges from 0.21 (21%) to 1.0 (100%). The normal ambient air FiO_2 is 0.21.
- *Functional residual capacity (FRC):* The volume of air remaining in the lungs at the end of normal expiration.
- *Ideal body weight (IBW):* The expected weight of a person based on sex and height.
- Males: IBW = 50 kg + 2.3 kg for each inch over 5 feet.
- Females: IBW = 45.5 kg + 2.3 kg for each inch over 5 feet.
- *I:E ratio:* The ratio of inspiratory time to expiratory time. Under normal conditions the expiratory phase is passive and is twice as long as the active inspiratory phase (1:2).
- *Inspiratory flow:* The rate at which a breath is delivered on a ventilator. It is measured in liters per minute. The higher the flow, the faster the breath is delivered.
- *Inspiratory time (T_i):* The time over which a tidal volume is delivered or a pressure maintained (depending on mode). Set as I:E ratio or inspiratory flow.
- *Mean airway pressure:* The average pressure to which the lungs are exposed over one inspiratory/expiratory cycle.
- *Minute ventilation (VE):* The volume of air moving in and out of the lungs in 1 minute. It is the product of the tidal volume and respiratory rate. V_E = Vt × rate.
- *Peak inspiratory pressure (PIP):* The measurement in the lungs at the peak of inspiration as measured on the ventilator manometer.
- *PEEP:* Positive end-expiratory pressure. A therapy used in mechanical ventilation to provide airway pressure at the end of expiration to increase the volume of gas remaining in the lungs at the end of expiration (FRC). Ideally it will increase the surface area of the alveoli to decrease the shunting of blood through the lungs and improve gas exchange.
- *Plateau pressure:* A constant pressure value that is maintained during the inspiratory phase of ventilation. It is measured by pressing the pause or hold button during mechanical inspiration.
- *Sensitivity:* A measure of the amount of negative pressure generated by a patient to trigger a mechanical ventilator into the inspiratory phase.
- *Tidal volume (Vt):* The volume of air inspired or expired in a single breath during regular respiration.
- *Volutrauma:* The volume-related overdistention injury of alveoli inflicted by mechanical ventilation.
- *V/Q:* Ventilation to perfusion ratio. Normal is 0.8. A high V/Q is indicative of dead space ventilation, and a low V/Q is indicative of shunt ventilation.
- *VR:* Ventilatory rate. Also referred to as frequency (f).

Assist-Control Ventilation

Method: The ventilator will deliver a set number of respirations at a set Vt. Sensitivity is set at a level to recognize the patient's respiratory effort with delivery of an additional full Vt with each spontaneous respiratory effort. The sensitivity can be adjusted so it takes a specific amount of respiratory effort to recognize the respiratory effort.

The patient receives a breath whenever he or she wants one without having to work hard for it. Patients can hyperventilate in this mode, and minute ventilation should be monitored and the patient adequately sedated if indicated.

Set parameters: FIO_2, Vt, VR, flow, PEEP, sensitivity

Variable parameters: PIP

Synchronized Intermittent Mandatory Ventilation (SIMV)

Method: A set Vt at a set rate is delivered every minute. This type of ventilation allows the patient to breathe spontaneously but does not provide a spontaneous breath with additional Vt support. Sensitivity is set to ensure the ventilator synchronizes the Vt breaths with the spontaneous breaths. A similar mode, intermittent mandatory ventilation (IMV), does not synchronize with the patient's spontaneous breaths.

Patients with ALI or ARDS will have a difficult time generating sufficient effort to open the demand valve and breathe through the endotracheal tube without ventilatory assistance.

SIMV can be used in combination with pressure support to allow a spontaneous breath attempt to trigger the ventilator to give a pressure-limited breath.

Set parameters: FIO_2, Vt, VR, I:E or T_i, PEEP, sensitivity

Variable parameters: PIP, sensitivity

Pressure Controlled Ventilation (PCV)

Method: There is no guaranteed minute ventilation with this mode; therefore close monitoring to prevent hypoventilation and hypoxia is required. If the VR is set too fast, auto-PEEP can develop (see discussion of complications). Sensitivity is set to recognize the patient's respiratory effort, and a full preset pressure is delivered with each ventilatory attempt (as opposed to AC, where volume is the set parameter). The sensitivity can be adjusted to require a specific amount of effort to occur for the patient's respiratory effort to be recognized.

Mean airway pressure is increased by prolonging the inspiration time. In some patients, increasing the mean airway pressure without increasing PIP may require prolonging the T_i to improve the oxygen benefit.

Set parameters: FIO_2, VR, PIP, PEEP, T_i or I:E

Variable parameters: Vt, flow

Pressure Support Ventilation (PSV)

Method: Provides inspiratory support to a spontaneously breathing patient. The patient determines the rate and with each spontaneous effort triggers the ventilator to deliver a flow to the preset pressure limit. The pressure is maintained throughout inspiration.

This is often used for ventilator weaning purposes by gradually decreasing the pressure support provided.

Set parameters: FIO_2, PIP, sensitivity, PEEP

Variable parameters: VR, Vt, T_i

Continuous Positive Airway Pressure (CPAP)

Method: No volume or pressure breaths are provided. The patient breathes spontaneously at his or her own rate and own Vt while the ventilator maintains a constant pressure throughout the respiratory cycle. This mode is used primarily to assess the patient's ability to ventilate and oxygenate before extubation. It is also used in patients who have no oxygenation or ventilation abnormalities but only need airway protection, as in patients who are alert and awake but have laryngeal edema or airway compression. This mode should be used with caution in patients who have the potential to decompensate neurologically or hemodynamically.

Set parameters: PEEP, FIO_2

Variable parameters: VR, Vt

Preventing Injury From Mechanical Ventilation

A variety of strategies have been developed to reduce ventilator-associated injuries usually caused by high plateau pressures and high inspiratory pressures. The strategy most likely to be encountered in the ED is permissive hypercapnea.

Permissive Hypercapnea

Permissive hypercapnea is a lung protective strategy decreasing alveolar ventilation to prevent lung injury due to high volumes and high pressures. It involves the use of low tidal volumes (4–6 mL/kg ideal body weight [IBW]) and pressure-limited ventilation. The arterial carbon dioxide pressure ($PaCO_2$) is allowed to rise gradually, and the pH is allowed to drop to between 7.2 and 7.25. Acidosis at this level is generally well tolerated.[20] Permissive hypercapnea is not appropriate for patients with head injuries or severe metabolic acidosis.

Inverse-Ratio Ventilation (IRV)

The normal I:E ratio is reversed so the inspiratory phase is longer than the expiratory phase. (2:1 to 4:1). It is usually done in the pressure control mode (PC/IRV).

The longer T_i lowers the PIP and plateau pressure while increasing the mean airway pressure. This prevents the potentially damaging effects of cyclical opening and closing of alveoli by maintaining a constant pressure and improving oxygenation.

This form of ventilation is extremely uncomfortable and almost always requires chemical paralysis and sedation.

Other Advanced Ventilatory Strategies

Further studies are needed to determine improved patient outcomes in the following modes.

High-frequency oscillatory ventilation. High-frequency oscillatory ventilation (HFOV) is characterized by high respiratory rates, generally between 180 and 360 breaths/min, with very low tidal volumes of 1 to 3 mL/kg. In HFOV the pressure oscillates, maintaining a constant distending pressure. Gas is pushed into the lungs during inspiration and pulled out during expiration. It is used in patients who have hypoxia refractory to normal mechanical ventilation. High-frequency ventilators for the adult population are not readily available.

Airway pressure-release ventilation (Bilevel). Airway pressure-release ventilation (APRV) is a time-cycled, pressure-limited form of ventilation maintaining a constant positive airway pressure (similar to plateau pressure) and has a regular, brief, intermittent release of airway pressure allowing for removal of carbon dioxide. This method allows the patient to breathe spontaneously so chemical paralysis is not required.

Depending on the brand of ventilator, a modified version of APRV provides pressure support during the spontaneous respiratory effort.

Vt is variable, requiring close attention to the patient's minute ventilation to prevent hypercapnea or hypocapnea.

Selecting Ventilator Settings

Ventilator mode and settings are determined by physician preference, clinical assessment, and degree of alteration in oxygenation and/or ventilation. Under the guidance of the physician, the respiratory therapist is the most skilled and knowledgeable person to set up and monitor ventilator parameters. The emergency nurse should be familiar with the concepts and therapies used and participate in collaborative discussions on the goal of ventilatory support.

Tidal Volume (Using Volume-Controlled Ventilation)

A Vt that is too high places the patient at risk for overinflation injury. Patients with ALI or ARDS should be started on a Vt of 6 mL/kg IBW. In a randomized controlled study, the ARDS Network compared patient outcomes when using 6 mL/kg IBW versus the traditional 12 mL/kg IBW. Plateau pressure was maintained at less than 30 cm H_2O, and Vt in the low-volume group was dropped as low as 4 mL/kg if necessary to meet this limitation. The low-volume group had a 22% relative reduction in mortality.[1] A Vt of 8 mL/kg IBW is appropriate for patients with chronic obstructive pulmonary disease (COPD) and asthma so fewer breaths are given at a higher Vt to allow for a longer exhalation time.

A Vt of 8 to 9 mL/kg should be adequate for people with normal lungs. Patients with neuromuscular disease may benefit from a slightly higher Vt to prevent atelectasis.

Pressure (Using Pressure-Controlled Ventilation)

Pressure must be adjusted as compliance changes (i.e., increase pressure support with decreased compliance, and decrease with increased compliance). Start with a pressure support of 20 cm H_2O, and adjust to a Vt of 6 to 8 mL/kg.

Rate

Respiratory rates set too fast place the patient at risk for inadequate expiratory time. When initially selecting the rate, consider the minute ventilation and the Vt. The desired minute ventilation is usually 5 to 10 L/min. The initial rate will generally range from 8 to 18 breaths/min depending on the Vt selected and the degree of acidosis. Draw a specimen for arterial blood gas (ABG) analysis 20 minutes after changing ventilator settings. Further adjustments of the rate depend on the clinical goal and patient response. The goal may be based on a $PaCO_2$ range (as in TBI) or a pH range (as in passive hypercarbia). In summary, increased rate equals increased pH and decreased $PaCO_2$, whereas decreased rate equals decreased pH and increased $PaCO_2$.

F_IO_2

If the patient's arterial oxygen pressure (PaO_2) is unknown, start with a F_IO_2 of 60% to 100%. The percentage of oxygen can be weaned down while monitoring oxygen saturation levels and ABGs. The F_IO_2 and PEEP should be managed to maintain the PaO_2 in the middle of the normal range for the given altitude. Patients with head injuries or heart problems should have a PaO_2 at the upper end of normal. ARDS and ALI patients can tolerate a PaO_2 in the lower end of the range so lower F_IO_2 and PEEP can be used, thereby lessening the chance of oxygen toxicity. Prolonged periods with a F_IO_2 greater than 0.6 (60%) are associated with lung injury; however, it should be used, if necessary, to prevent hypoxemia.

PEEP

PEEP exerts pressure in the patient's airway, above atmospheric level, to prevent alveolar collapse by increasing the functional residual capacity (FRC). PEEP can be used in any mode of ventilation. Most patients should receive 5 cm H_2O of PEEP to prevent atelectasis. Use PEEP with extreme caution (usually only 3 cm H_2O) in patients with COPD and asthma to prevent further air trapping. PEEP is used in conjunction with F_IO_2 to improve oxygenation. Higher levels of PEEP are helpful to decrease F_IO_2 to less than 0.6 (60%). PEEP greater than 10 cm H_2O can cause decreased venous return and hypotension. The hemodynamic effects of PEEP should be monitored closely.

I:E Ratio

The normal I:E ratio is 1:2 or 1:3. Patients with obstructive airway disease, such as asthma or COPD, should have longer expiratory times of 1:4 or longer to prevent air trapping and alveolar overdistention. In this patient population, increasing the rate, which shortens the expiratory time in an attempt to lower the $PaCO_2$, may actually increase $PaCO_2$ and worsen the clinical condition.[3-5]

Sensitivity

The sensitivity is set to recognize the patient's spontaneous respiratory effort. It is usually set at −1 to −2 cm H_2O. A setting too high will cause increased patient effort, and a setting that is too low may cause overtriggering of the ventilator and hyperventilation.

PIP

The PIP alarm should be set at 10 to 15 cm H_2O higher than baseline. This will alert staff to decreased lung compliance or conditions that do not allow full exhalation. Lung compliance will often decrease with fluid resuscitation and capillary leak associated with the inflammatory response. This will increase the PIP.

Management of the Patient on Mechanical Ventilation

Chapter 22 contains information about specific treatment of patients with pulmonary disease and ABG analysis. FiO_2 and PEEP are the settings used to improve oxygenation (PaO_2). It is often a delicate balance of increasing the PEEP to achieve a FiO_2 below 0.6 while maintaining the mean arterial blood pressure above 65 mm Hg. Vt and VR are the settings used to adjust $PaCO_2$. The emergency nurse must continuously monitor the patient's heart rate, electrocardiogram (ECG) pattern, and pulse oximetry readings. End-tidal CO_2 monitoring ($EtCO_2$) is a useful adjunct in the assessment of ongoing endotracheal tube placement in the trachea. It is of limited value in correlating to $PaCO_2$ in hemodynamically unstable patients or in patients with ventilation/perfusion (V/Q) mismatch. A self-inflating resuscitation bag should be kept at the patient's bedside at all times in the event of mechanical failure. Suction equipment should be readily available. Endotracheal tube depth should be noted on the patient's chart and assessed whenever the patient is moved or becomes agitated, air bubbles are noted in the airway, low or high PIP alarms are activated, vocal sounds are heard, or when there is any question of tube displacement. Be aware of and document the patient's baseline FiO_2, mode of ventilation, PIP, PEEP/pressure support and Vt; documentation of these should occur every 2 hours while receiving mechanical ventilation. Assess the patient for any changes. Goals of oxygenation and ventilation should be clear. If no adjustment parameters are given, the ED nurse should notify the physician when any value falls outside the desired range.

Ventilator Management

Ventilator alarms should be on at all times and set to the maximum volume. Immediately evaluate the cause of any ventilator alarm. Table 13.1 contains a summary of how to troubleshoot ventilator alarms.

Monitor for signs and symptoms of barotrauma (see complications discussed later in this chapter).

Disconnect the patient from the ventilator and ventilate with a self-inflating resuscitation bag if there is any question as to whether the patient is being adequately ventilated. Be sure the resuscitation bag has good oxygen flow, and use a PEEP valve if the patient is PEEP dependent (requires PEEP to adequately oxygenate). If it is necessary to sedate and administer a neuromuscular blocking agent to maintain adequate oxygenation, adjust the respiratory rate to the patient's premedication minute ventilation and repeat an ABG analysis.

Complications of Mechanical Ventilation[3–5]

There are multiple complications that may occur with mechanical ventilation. The following is a discussion of some complications the emergency nurse may encounter in the ED.

Hypotension. Positive pressure ventilation increases intrathoracic pressure and subsequently decreases venous return and cardiac output. In patients with marginal or low volume status, the decrease in venous return will cause hypotension. The greater the positive pressure applied, the more profound the hypotensive response. This is most apparent when the PEEP is greater than 10 cm H_2O. Hemodynamic

TABLE 13.1 Troubleshooting Ventilator Alarms.

Initial assessment:
- Airway: Is the endotracheal tube (ETT) still in? Check ETT insertion depth, check end-tidal CO_2, check breath sounds.
- Breathing: Check breath sounds, look for chest excursion, check pulse oximetry, check patient color.
- Circulation: Check the pulse, electrocardiogram (ECG), and blood pressure.

Alarm	Possible Causes	Management
Apnea	Insufficient spontaneous breathing by a patient in the CPAP or pressure support mode	• Switch ventilator mode to one which provides a set rate
High airway pressure	ETT obstruction: sputum, kink, biting Increased compliance or resistance: circumferential burns, bronchospasm, lung collapse, pneumothorax, endobronchial intubation, worsening of lung process Anxiety/fear/pain/fighting ventilator	• Suction the airway • Treat cause of resistance • Adjust mode or settings • Rule out hypoxia before treating agitation • Chest radiography analysis • Change ventilator mode to one which is better tolerated and/or provide sedation/analgesia
Low airway pressure	Ventilator disconnect Leak in ventilator system Cuff leak Inadvertent extubation	• Ensure all connections are intact and tight • Troubleshoot ETT cuff • Bag-mask device if ETT was dislodged
Oxygen pressure low	Oxygen cylinder is empty Cylinder valve is closed Unit not connected to the wall terminal	• Check wall and cylinder connections • Bag-mask ventilation until resolved

status should be monitored closely with any increase in PEEP and immediately after intubation. Optimizing fluid status will lessen the degree of hypotension.

Volutrauma. Volutrauma is the overdistention injury of alveoli inflicted by mechanical ventilation. It is most closely associated with high PIP. It is thought this damage degrades surfactant, disrupts epithelial and endothelial cell barriers, and increases cytokine levels and inflammatory cells in the lung. Lung-protective ventilatory strategies should be used in all patients with ALI or ARDS.

Barotrauma. Barotrauma is the damage caused to lung tissue because of high airway pressures and rupture of alveoli. This may lead to a pneumothorax, tension pneumothorax, subcutaneous emphysema, or pneumomediastinum. Symptoms include hypotension, tachycardia, decrease in arterial oxygen saturation (SaO_2), decrease in central venous oxygen saturation/mixed venous oxygen saturation ($ScvO_2/SvO_2$), decrease in cardiac output, decreased breath sounds, unequal chest excursion, and deviated trachea. Large tidal volumes should be avoided and PIP and plateau pressures monitored carefully.

Oxygen toxicity. A FIO_2 of greater than 0.5 for a long duration may cause the production of oxygen free radicals damaging pulmonary epithelium; inactivating surfactant; and forming intraalveolar edema, interstitial thickening, and pulmonary fibrosis.[55] The extent of injury is related to the level of FIO_2 and the duration of exposure. Using PEEP in conjunction with FIO_2, if tolerated hemodynamically, will facilitate weaning the FIO_2 to less than 0.5. With severe ARDS/ALI, it may not be possible to lower FIO_2 below 50%. However, treatment of hypoxemia and hypotension takes precedence over the possibility of oxygen toxicity.

Infection. Ventilator-associated pneumonia (VAP) is a serious and potentially life-threatening consequence of intubation and is defined as a nosocomial pneumonia developing after 48 hours of intubation and mechanical ventilatory support.[6] VAP is the most common and fatal nosocomial infection of critical care, affecting between 9% and 27% of intubated patients.[46] VAP doubles the risk for dying, prolongs the duration of ventilation, and increases the length of stay in the critical care unit, total hospital length of stay, and cost of hospitalization.[44,46] VAP may be prevented by using the following measures:

- Rigorous hand washing
- Sterile suction technique
- Avoiding the routine use of saline lavage
- Aseptic airway technique
- Bronchial hygiene
- Regular oral care
- Elevating the head of the bed 30 degrees

Summary

To provide safe and competent mechanical ventilation the emergency nurse must be familiar with the functioning and management of ventilators. Mechanical ventilation can support critically ill or injured patients, but when inappropriately managed, can cause unnecessary harm.

INVASIVE MONITORING

Every year the number of critically ill patients presenting to the ED increases, and so does their length of stay in the ED. The focus on early diagnosis and therapy for myocardial infarction, stroke, sepsis, and other time-dependent emergencies has called on ED personnel to initiate monitoring and therapy, which has traditionally fallen to the critical care units. Familiarity with the principles and management of hemodynamic monitoring, and its limitations, is essential to accurately interpreting the data obtained. The goal of hemodynamic monitoring is to initiate and guide therapy in patients at risk for tissue hypoperfusion and subsequent organ dysfunction.

General Monitoring Principles

Several general principles can be applied when preparing for and monitoring patients with invasive lines:

- A catheter is inserted into the desired location (blood vessel or brain) for direct measurement. The catheter is connected to the transducer via monitoring tubing.
- The monitoring tubing, which connects the catheter to the transducer, is stiff, low-compliance tubing preventing distortion of the signal from the blood vessel or brain to the transducer.
- The transducer system (unless using fiberoptic) is fluid filled and is maintained with a flush solution. The solution is usually normal saline, with or without heparin added depending on hospital protocol, and is flushed before connection to the catheter. The transducer senses the pressure signal from the blood vessel or brain, converts it to an electrical waveform, and displays it on the monitor.
- Air should be removed from the flush solution and drip chamber when the bag is spiked. This will prevent air from entering the system should the fluid level become low or the bag turned on its side.
- The flush bag is pressurized to 300 mm Hg to overcome the pressure of the system and prevent backflow of blood.
- The transducer system allows very low infusion rates into the catheter to prevent clotting (2–3 mL/hr). The tubing should be disabled (clamped) when connected to intracranial monitoring systems. A fast-flush on the transducer allows for bypass of the restricted flow of fluid for initial priming of the system and for clearing of blood from the system.
- The tubing should be checked and cleared of all air bubbles, including stopcock ports. Air bubbles distort the waveform and can result in inaccurate measurements.
- Open-ended (vented) stopcock caps used for zeroing should be replaced with dead-end covers. This prevents serious blood loss should the stopcock become inadvertently turned to the open position. It also helps maintain sterility.
- Connections should be tight and placed where they can be visualized regularly. Loose connections can result in serious blood loss or infection.

- Set the monitor to the appropriate scale for the pressure being measured. Generally this is a scale of 0 to 20 mm Hg or 0 to 40 mm Hg for central venous pressures (CVP) and pulmonary artery pressures (PAP), 0 to 100 mm Hg for arterial pressure readings, and 0 to 50 mm Hg for ICP monitoring.
- The transducer should be properly aligned with the reference point when zeroing. For CVP, pulmonary artery (PA) catheters, and arterial pressures this is the phlebostatic axis located at the level of the fourth intercostal space and the midway point between the anteroposterior chest walls. Transducers used for ICP monitoring are usually placed at the level of the lateral or fourth ventricle—the tragus of the ear is a good reference point. Transducers placed above the reference point will result in a falsely elevated pressure, and transducers below the reference point will result in a false low value.
- Patency of the line should be checked regularly and whenever the waveform appears dampened.
- Coagulation status should be reviewed, considered, and reversed, if necessary, before insertion of any invasive line.

Arterial Blood Pressure Monitoring

Direct arterial blood pressure monitoring is accomplished with the insertion of a catheter into an artery. Although generally inserted into the radial artery, the brachial, femoral, and dorsalis pedis arteries can also be cannulated. The catheter is attached to a fluid-filled transducer system converting the pressure to an electrical waveform and displays it on the monitor for concurrent continuous readings. The arterial waveform is pulsatile and depicts the systolic and diastolic phases of the cardiac cycle. The dicrotic notch on the waveform separates the systolic and diastolic phases (Fig. 13.1).

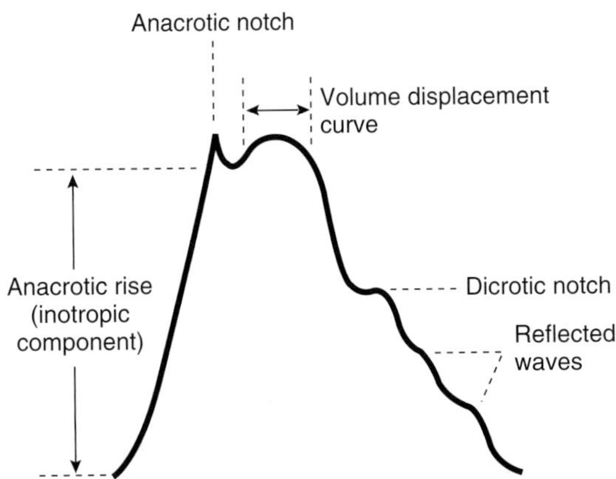

Fig. 13.1 The Arterial Waveform. Creation of the arterial pressure wave and acceleration of blood flow correlate with the inotropic upstrike. The rounded shoulder represents blood volume displacement and distention of the arterial walls. Normally the peak of both the inotropic and volume displacement phases are equal in amplitude. The descending limb represents diastolic runoff of blood; the dicrotic notch separates systole from diastole. Additional humps on the downslope relate to pulse waves reflected from the periphery. (From Davoric GO. *Handbook of Hemodynamic Monitoring.* 2nd ed. Philadelphia: Saunders; 2004.)

The arterial pressure is determined by the cardiac output and the systemic vascular resistance (volume of blood flow vs. resistance of the vessels). The relationship between pressure, flow, and volume is very complex; however, hypotension generally represents a failure of compensatory mechanisms after large-scale circulatory changes.[7] The sympathetic stress response will maintain a normal blood pressure despite declining blood volume and flow until it becomes exhausted. Blood pressure measurements are a useful screening tool and are helpful with trend assessment, but as a solitary measurement, they are of limited physiologic significance.[7]

The mean arterial pressure (MAP) represents the perfusion pressure. Diastole is longer than systole, so the MAP is not calculated by averaging the two numbers. Most monitoring systems do the math for you. The calculation is as follows:

$$\frac{\text{Systolic blood pressure [SBP]} + (2 \times \text{Diastolic blood pressure [DBP]})}{3}$$

An Allen's test is traditionally performed before radial artery cannulation. This procedure assesses for collateral blood flow to the hand by the ulnar artery in the event that the radial artery becomes occluded or damaged. The process involves having the patient clench his or her hand in a fist while the clinician applies direct pressure simultaneously to the radial and ulnar arteries, occluding flow. Ask the patient to open his or her fist, and release pressure on the ulnar artery. If collateral flow is intact, the hand will turn pink within 7 seconds. If color does not return for greater than 15 seconds, another site should be selected.

Indications for Arterial Monitoring

Arterial lines are indicated for the following:

- Close monitoring of patients who are, or have the potential to be, hemodynamically unstable
- Frequent blood gas analysis
- Guiding titration of vasoactive medications. Small changes in an infusion dose of vasoactive medications may result in a large swing in blood pressure. Direct arterial blood pressure monitoring will detect potentially harmful changes immediately so dosage adjustments can be quickly managed.
- Monitoring MAP for cerebral perfusion pressures (CPPs) in patients with neurologic injury
- Intraaortic balloon pump therapy

Complications of Arterial Monitoring

Complications of arterial lines are not common. They include ischemic tissue necrosis due to occlusion of blood flow to the insertion site, infection, thrombus formation, vasospasm, embolism, hematoma, and pseudoaneurysm. Assessment of blood flow distal to the insertion site should be performed at least every 2 hours.

Central Venous Pressure (CVP) Monitoring

Central venous catheters are traditionally placed in the superior vena cava via the internal jugular, external jugular, or subclavian vein or into the inferior vena cava via the femoral vein. The femoral site should be avoided for pressure monitoring purposes because the reliability at that distance from the right atrium is questionable. Recent studies suggest the use of ultrasound-guided central line insertion reduces complications and improves the success of insertion, particularly with less experienced operators.[7] Readings may be measured intermittently when fluids are being infused through the port, or they may be read continuously via the same fluid-filled transducer system as used in the arterial line. Multiport catheters, such as triple-lumen catheters, are particularly helpful when vasoactive medications are being infused or when continuous CVP monitoring and simultaneous port utilization is desired. The CVP is reflective of right atrial pressures caused by stretch of the muscle fibers in the heart chambers. It can represent intravascular volume status if that "stretch" is caused by blood volume in the right atria and ventricle. However, CVP values are also influenced by venous wall and right ventricle compliance, which can rapidly accommodate a wide variation in blood volume. Although there is no direct correlation of CVP to blood volume, it does provide valuable data regarding the tolerance of volume loads. Patients with fluid overload, stress, cardiac failure, and chronic renal failure are sensitive to fluid volume loads. If a titrated fluid bolus is administered and results in a large and sustained increase in CVP, then cardiac capacitance is limited. Likewise, hypovolemic and septic patients do not tolerate delayed or inadequate fluid resuscitation. In both cases, careful titration of fluids is required.[7] CVP readings are most helpful during the early stages of illness or injury when volume changes are acute. Causes of elevated CVP include increased intravascular volume, increased intrathoracic pressure, impaired right ventricular (RV) function, cardiac tamponade, pulmonary hypertension, chronic left ventricular function, or increased intraabdominal pressures. Causes of decreased CVP include hypovolemia, sudden blood or fluid loss, venodilation, or reduced intrathoracic pressures. Because CVP can be affected by position and intrathoracic pressure, readings should be taken in the supine position and read at the end of expiration at the established zero reference point (phlebostatic axis). Normal values are 6 to 10 mm Hg but are variable from patient to patient. (Water manometer systems measure in centimeters of water, instead of mercury. Normal is 6–10 cm H_2O.) Accuracy is best produced when monitoring trends rather than a single CVP measurement. Changes in CVP readings should be noted during and after fluid challenges and with the initiation and titrating of vasoactive agents. CVP is a useful adjunct to clinical assessment and should be evaluated along with the clinical presentation.

Indications for the Insertion of a Central Venous Pressure (CVP) Monitor

CVP is useful in guiding fluid resuscitation after trauma, surgery, sepsis, or other emergency conditions with suspected blood volume deficit or excess. It is especially useful when using early goal-directed therapy guidelines for sepsis in which end points in fluid resuscitation are tied to specific measurements. Infusing vasoactive medications through a central line greatly reduces the risk for irritation to peripheral veins and potential infiltration and necrosis of surrounding tissue.

Complications Related to Central Venous Pressure (CVP) Monitoring

Complications are generally associated with line insertion and include pneumothorax, hemothorax, or artery puncture. Patients with indwelling catheters are at higher risk for infection.

Pulmonary Artery (PA) Pressure Monitoring

The PA catheter can be inserted into the internal jugular, subclavian, femoral, brachial, or basilic vein. The PA catheter is usually inserted through an introducer catheter.

There are several types of PA catheters, depending on clinical indication. Catheters can provide SvO_2 measurement, transvenous pacing, and continuous cardiac output monitoring, and some have extra infusion ports. The most common catheter used is a quad-lumen catheter with a lumen containing a thermistor for measuring cardiac output. The right atrial pressure is measured through the proximal port of the catheter; the PA systolic and diastolic pressures and pulmonary wedge pressures (PWPs) are measured through the distal port. Fig. 13.2 depicts a PA catheter.

Insertion is guided by monitoring waveforms as the catheter tip passes through the right atrium, right ventricle, and PA. Once the catheter tip is in the PA, the balloon is inflated and the catheter is advanced until it lodges in a smaller branch of the PA. This is the PWP, also called PA wedge (PAW) or pulmonary capillary wedge pressure (PCWP).

When the balloon is inflated, blood flow stops and the catheter tip senses pressures indirectly from the left atrium, which is reflective of left ventricular end-diastolic pressures (LVEDP) or the "filling pressure." Pressures are reflective of stretch of the muscle fibers caused by fluid in the left ventricle and thus allow for assessment of fluid status. However, as with CVP pressure measurements, stretch is not caused solely by volume changes, but is influenced by the compliance of the ventricles and the vascular system. PEEP, pericardial tamponade, rigid chest wall, increased intraabdominal pressures, and cardiac function all reflect pressure, not volume, of the cardiopulmonary structures and will affect accuracy of the interpretation of volume status.[8] If the ventricle is stiff, small changes in volume may result in large changes in pressure measurements. A more compliant ventricle will accommodate an increase in volume with less stretch and therefore lower pressure measurement. Factors decreasing ventricle compliance (stiffness) include ischemia, left ventricular hypertrophy, restrictive cardiomyopathies, and shock states. Factors increasing ventricular compliance include afterload reduction (antihypertensive, intraaortic balloon pump therapy, etc.) cardiomyopathies (nonrestrictive), and the resolution of ischemia.

The PWP, although not a direct indicator of blood volume, will provide some indication of capacitance for additional fluids. If pressure initially increases after a fluid bolus and then

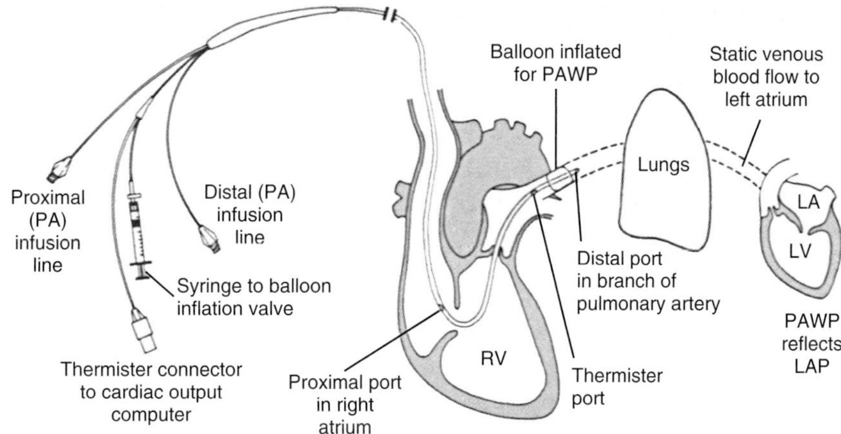

Fig. 13.2 Position of Pulmonary Artery in the Heart. *LA,; LAP,; LV,* left ventricle; *PA,* pulmonary artery; *PAWP,; RV,* right ventricle. (From Preuss T, Wiegard DL. Single pressure and multiple pressure transducer systems. In Wiegard DL, ed. *AACN Procedure Manual for Critical Care.* 4th ed. St Louis, MO: Elsevier/Saunders; 2011.)

settles within the normal range, it is probably safe to administer more fluid. However, if the PWP climbs to a higher level and remains high after 30 to 60 minutes, the capacity for additional fluids is limited.[51] Mitral valve stenosis yields elevated PWPs, which do not correlate with LVEDP. In patients without pulmonary disease, the PA diastolic pressure (PAD) can also be used to estimate the LVEDP instead of the PWP. When conditions permit and a correlation has been established in the patient, the PAD pressure is often used to decrease the frequency of balloon inflation and the associated risks, or when the balloon is not functional. PA and PWPs are affected by intrathoracic pressures and should be read at end-expiration. The appearance of the location of end-expiration on the PA waveform tracing will depend on whether or not the patient is on positive pressure ventilation. Misreading of end-expiration may result in a large discrepancy of documented and actual values. Treatment based on erroneous values can prove harmful to the patient.

The exact effect of PEEP on PWP is not fully clear. However, patients should not be removed from PEEP to take a reading. Not only does this have the potential to cause hypoxia, which may be difficult to reverse, but it will also cause an increase in venous return, and the value will be of questionable significance.

Indications for the Use of Pulmonary Artery (PA) Catheters

PA catheters provide access to direct measurements for a variety of cardiac parameters assisting in the evaluation of patients with confusing clinical presentation or with rapid hemodynamic changes. Table 13.2 discusses cardiac parameters.

The cardiac parameters and oxygen transport measurements are used to monitor patients with acute myocardial infarction, shock, trauma, or other critical illnesses in which the fluid and circulatory status is not clear.[8] In addition to its prognostic value, the PA catheter helps guide pharmacologic and fluid therapy. PA catheters take time and skill to place correctly, and potentially pose serious complications. Clinicians should weigh the risk versus benefit for each individual patient before inserting a catheter in the ED and should not proceed if it cannot be safely inserted or monitored.

Complications Related to Pulmonary Artery (PA) Catheters

In addition to the complications listed for central line access, the following complications have also been reported:

- *Balloon rupture:* Related to overinflation of the balloon and may cause air embolism and embolic balloon fragments. The balloon should be inflated slowly and should not exceed manufacturer's inflation values. If no resistance is felt when inflating the balloon, or if blood is returned through the balloon port, efforts should be discontinued and the physician notified.
- *Knotting:* Loops in the catheter usually caused by repeated withdrawal and advancement. This is problematic not only in obtaining readings, but in catheter removal as well. It may require surgical removal.
- *Pulmonary artery perforation:* Rupture may occur (1) during insertion, (2) with undetected prolonged wedging of the balloon, (3) because of shearing forces of cardiac pulsation, or (4) when catheter tip is located at a distal artery bifurcation when the balloon is inflated.[7] Perforation often presents with massive hemoptysis and can be fatal. To minimize this occurrence, do the following: (1) perform constant monitoring of pressure waveforms to detect inadvertent wedge; (2) inflate balloon slowly, and stop as soon as PWP tracing is obtained; (3) keep inflation time to a minimum; (4) use only air, not fluid, to inflate the balloon; (5) avoid high-pressure flush; and (6) never flush when the catheter is in wedge.
- *Thrombus or embolus:* Most catheters are heparin bonded to prevent thrombus formation. High-pressure system flushes can release any thrombi formation on the catheter and should be avoided.
- *Arrhythmias:* Every patient should have continuous ECG monitoring both during insertion and while the catheter is in place. Premature ventricular contractions (PVCs) frequently occur when the catheter is in the right ventricle. The PA pressure waveform should be monitored continuously and consulted for RV pressure waveform whenever increased ectopy is noted. If hospital policy permits, the nurse should

TABLE 13.2 **Cardiac Parameters.**

Parameter	Abbreviation	Calculation	Measurement	Normal Values	Evaluation
Cardiac output	CO	HR × SV	The amount of blood ejected from the ventricle in a minute	4–8 L/min	Pump effectiveness and ventricular function
Cardiac index	CI	CO/BSA		2.4–4.0 L/min	Cardiac output by body weight
Mean arterial pressure	MAP	$\frac{SBP + (DBP \times 2)}{3}$	The average pressure throughout the vascular system during systole and diastole	70–105 mm Hg	Indicates adequacy of coronary and tissue perfusion
Central venous pressure	CVP	Direct pressure reading	Indirect measurement of the right atrium filling pressures	2–6 mm Hg	RV function and volume assessment
Right atrial pressure	RA	Direct pressure reading	Filling pressure of the right atrium	2–6 mm Hg	RV function
Pulmonary artery pressures (systole/diastole)	PAP PAS PAD	Direct pressure reading	Pressures in the pulmonary artery during systole and diastole	15–25 mm Hg 0–5 mm Hg	PAS: Reflects RV pressure during systole PAD: Reflects the diastolic pressure in the pulmonary vasculature
Pulmonary wedge pressure	PWP	Direct pressure reading	Amount of myocardial fiber stretch at the end of diastole	6–12 mm Hg	Preload. The volume in the ventricle at the end of diastole. Used in fluid assessment.
Systemic vascular resistance	SVR	$\frac{(MAP - RA) \times 80}{CO}$	Resistance, impedance, or pressure the ventricle must overcome to eject blood volume	800–1200 dynes/sec/cm^2	Afterload. Resistance against the left ventricle.
Stroke volume	SV	$\frac{CO}{HR} \times 1000$ mL/L	The amount of blood ejected from the left ventricle with each contraction	60–100 mL/beat	Influenced by preload (PWP), afterload (SVR), and contractility
Stroke volume index	SVI	$\frac{SV}{BSA}$		33–47 mL/beat/m^2	Stroke volume by body weight
Pulmonary vascular resistance	PVR	$\frac{(MAP - PWP) \times 80}{CO}$	Resistance, impedance, or pressure the right ventricle must overcome to eject blood volume into the pulmonary system	<250 dynes/sec/cm^2	Resistance against the right ventricle

BSA, Body surface area; *DBP*, diastolic blood pressure; *HR*, heart rate; *RV*, right ventricle; *SBP*, systolic blood pressure.

pull the catheter back until the right atrial pressure (RA) waveform is obtained and then notify the physician.

- *Valvular damage:* Never withdraw the catheter with the balloon inflated.

Intracranial Pressure Monitoring

ICP is a measurement of the relationship between the contents of the brain: cerebrospinal fluid (CSF) (10%), blood (10%), and brain tissue (80%). The Monro–Kellie doctrine hypothesizes that when the volume of one brain component increases there is a corresponding and compensatory decrease in one of the other brain components. Under normal conditions, compliance between the three components maintains an ICP between 0 and 15 mm Hg. Once the compensatory mechanisms within the rigid confines of the brain reach capacity, the ICP will increase. At its limits, small changes in one of the components will result in a significant increase in the ICP (Fig. 13.3).

There is an inverse correlation with the magnitude and the duration of increased ICP and morbidity and mortality. Guidelines for treatment thresholds vary, but generally for adults it is 20 to 25 mm Hg, for children from 1 to 5 years it is

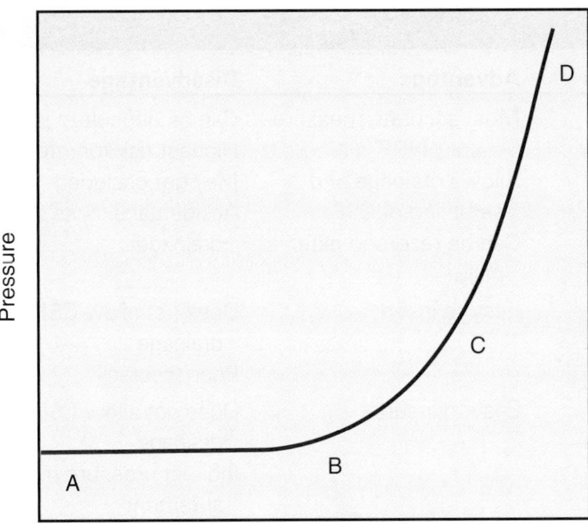

Fig. 13.3 Pressure-Volume Curve. From point *A* to point *B*, intracranial pressure (ICP) remains constant with the addition of volume and brain compliance is high. At point *B* brain compliance begins to change and ICP rises slightly. From point *B* to point *C*, compliance is low and ICP rises with increases in intracranial volume. From point *C* to point *D*, small increases in volume cause significant ICP elevations. (From McQuillan KA, Thurman PA. Traumatic brain injuries. In McQuillan KA, Makic Flynn MB, Whalen E, et al., eds. *Trauma Nursing: From Resuscitation Through Rehabilitation.* 4th ed. St. Louis: Saunders; 2009.)

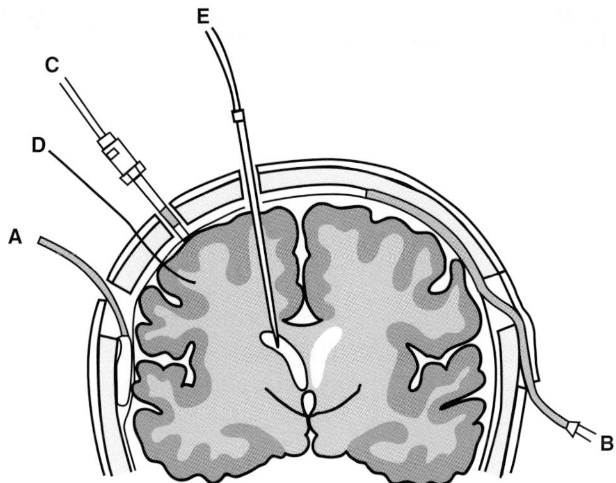

Fig. 13.4 Coronal section of the brain showing potential sites for placement of intracranial pressure monitoring devices. (A) Epidural; (B) subdural; (C) subarachnoid; (D) intraparenchymal; (E) intraventricular. (From McNair ND. Intracranial pressure monitoring. In Clochesy JM, Breu C, Cardkin S et al., eds. *Critical Care Nursing.* 2nd ed. Philadelphia: Saunders; 1996.)

15 mm Hg, and for infants it is 10 mm Hg.[7,9] The body's autoregulatory system maintains a constant cerebral blood flow (CBF) within a MAP range of 50 to 150 mm Hg. The MAP is the main driving force of blood supply to the brain. The MAP is met with resistance from the opposing force of the ICP. The difference between the two is the CPP:

$$\text{MAP} - \text{ICP} = \text{CPP}$$

Severe increases in ICP will reduce the CPP and the CBF. CPP that is too low causes ischemia, and CPP that is too high causes elevated ICP. The average CPP is 80 to 100 mm Hg; if it falls below 50 mm Hg, hypoperfusion and ischemia occur. CPP should be maintained at 60 to 70 mm Hg unless ordered otherwise.[9]

An ICP monitoring device is necessary to calculate the CPP. Multiple modalities for measuring CBF, oxygenation, temperature, and pressures are available.

ICP measurements can be obtained via intraventricular catheter, subdural, epidural, subarachnoid, or intraparenchymal transducers (Fig. 13.4). Table 13.3 contains a description of ICP monitoring devices.

The reference point for zeroing the transducer is the foramen of Monro, which corresponds externally with the external auditory meatus (tragus of the ear). Transducer systems can be external strain gauge (fluid filled) or fiberoptic. Fiberoptic transducers are zeroed before insertion and do not require further rezeroing or leveling after insertion. The cables are fragile, and care must be taken not to bend or twist the probe. The zero can drift slowly over time. Fluid-filled catheters require regular rezeroing, so any zero-drift can be corrected. Leveling with the zero reference point (external auditory meatus) must be consistent and adjusted with change in patient position. Although the ventriculostomy catheter is considered the most accurate of ICP monitoring devices, cerebral edema and collapsed ventricles often make placement difficult. This is the only device allowing for the drainage of CSF for ICP control or sampling of CSF for laboratory assessment. Accuracy of CPP calculations requires the arterial catheter (for MAP) and the ICP zero reference points be the same.[9] The foramen of Monro should be used as the reference point for both monitors. The ICP waveform is similar to arterial waveforms in that it is a pulsatile waveform. Normal ICP waveforms have three distinctive waves that become altered in pathologic conditions: P1 or percussion wave, P2 or tidal wave, and P3, known as the dicrotic wave (Fig. 13.5). The P1 wave has higher amplitude than the P2 wave, except when cerebral compliance becomes compromised and autoregulation is impaired.[9] A P2 wave equal to or greater than the P1 wave is indicative of an increase or impending increase in ICP.

Dampened waveforms call for assessment of the monitoring system for leaks or obstruction.

Indications for the Use of ICP Monitoring

Evidenced-based TBI guidelines call for the placement of an ICP monitoring device for patients with severe TBI (Glasgow Coma Scale score of less than 8) with abnormal computed tomography (CT) scan or with a normal CT scan and two or more high-risk indicators. High-risk indicators include (1) age greater than 40 years, (2) posturing motor response, and (3) SBP less than 90 mm Hg.[7,9] ICP monitoring is also used, though less frequently, with management of subarachnoid hemorrhage and stroke.

See Chapters 24 and 35 for specific conditions requiring ICP monitoring.

TABLE 13.3 ICP Monitoring Devices.

Device	Description	Transducer Options	Advantage	Disadvantage
Ventriculostomy catheter	A catheter is inserted into the lateral ventricle	Fiberoptic External strain gauge Internal strain gauge	Most accurate measurement of ICP Allows drainage and sampling of CSF Can be rezeroed externally	Can be difficult to place Highest risk for infection May get occluded Accidental excess CSF drainage
Subdural probe or catheter	A probe or catheter is placed into the subdural space	Fiberoptic External strain gauge Internal strain gauge	Easy to insert	Does not allow CSF drainage Poor accuracy
Epidural sensor	A sensor is placed in the epidural space	Fiberoptic External strain gauge	Easy to insert	Does not allow CSF drainage Indirect pressure measurement Poor accuracy
Intraparenchymal probe	A probe is placed into the brain parenchyma	Fiberoptic Internal strain gauge	Easy to insert Good accuracy	Does not allow CSF drainage Poor accuracy
Subarachnoid screw	The tip of hollow bolt is placed into the subarachnoid space	Fiberoptic External strain gauge	Easy to insert	Does not allow CSF drainage Poor accuracy

CSF, Cerebrospinal fluid; *ICP*, intracranial pressure.

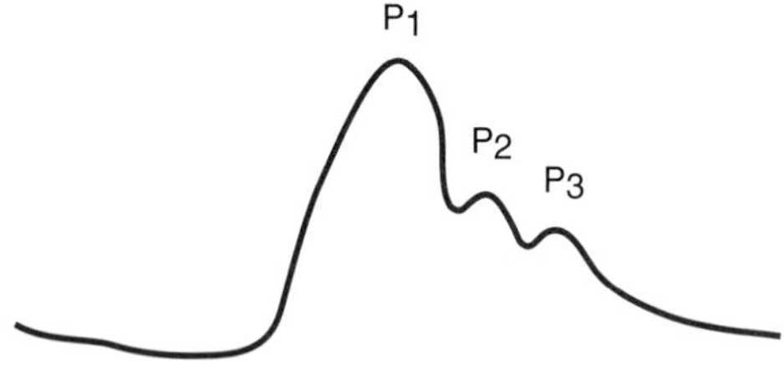

Fig. 13.5 Components of the Intracranial Pressure Wave. (From McQuillan KA, Thurman PA. Traumatic brain injuries. In McQuillan KA, Makic Flynn MB, Whalen E, et al, eds. *Trauma Nursing: From Resuscitation Through Rehabilitation*. 4th ed. St. Louis: Saunders/Elsevier; 2009.)

Complications Related to the Use of ICP Monitor

Infection: Infection is a complication related to the use of ICP monitors. Ventriculostomy catheters have a higher incidence of infection than other devices. Strict aseptic technique should be maintained on insertion and when manipulating or accessing the device. A sterile occlusive dressing should be applied and maintained.

Ventricular collapse, herniation, or hemorrhage: When draining CSF from a ventriculostomy catheter, only small amounts should be removed at a time (2–3 mL). Drainage systems can be set up to monitor continuously or to drain when a predetermined ICP is reached (using the gravity principle). Changing the level of the head without changing the level of the drainage system can cause CSF to drain beyond what is desired or to not drain at all when ICP is elevated. If CSF is drained too rapidly, brain tissue can shift into the space evacuated by the CSF, causing stretching and tearing of vessels, resulting in hemorrhage or herniation. In traumatic-brain-injured patients, the problem is not with over drainage of CSF but collapse of the ventricles. This may cause loss of waveform and pressure reading but does not damage the brain or neurologic function.[7,9] In the ED setting it is safest to keep the system on the monitor mode with the alarm on and drain CSF when the ICP reaches the treatment threshold unless otherwise ordered by the physician.

Fluid entering system: Fluid-filled transducer lines should be connected to a plain pressure tubing without a flush system. When the only available transducer system contains a flush system, it must be disabled and clamped. The line should be well marked, indicating it is an ICP line, to prevent accidental infusion of fluid into the brain.

CSF leakage or air entering the system: Make sure all connections are tightened. When using a fluid-filled transducer system, ensure it has been cleared of air and bubbles. Remove air when spiking the bag, and fill the drip chamber with fluid. Bubbles will interfere with the transmission of pressure and will give inaccurate ICP measurements.

Occlusion: Occlusion may arise from blood or brain in the system and will demonstrate as a dampened waveform. Notify the physician when unable to drain CSF from a ventriculostomy catheter. Do not directly flush the catheter unless specific guidelines and training have been established. The tubing (not the catheter) can be flushed.

Fiberoptic catheters are fragile and can break easily, which would require replacement. Handle the catheter gently, and protect from external damage. Ensure the connections are tight so that the catheter does not dislodge.

Summary

Invasive monitoring can provide important information about the patient's condition and response to selected treatments.

However, the emergency nurse must be familiar with the indications for the use of invasive monitoring, how to use the equipment, and how to recognize and manage complications related to their use in the ED.

SEPSIS

Sepsis remains one of the leading causes of death globally. In 2017 the World Health Assembly and the World Health Organization (WHO) made sepsis a global health problem. A resolution was adopted to improve the prevention, early diagnosis, and management of sepsis to improve the morbidity and mortality related to it.[10] Because the incidence of sepsis can increase with age, the number of cases will continue to rise as the population ages. The incidence of sepsis is also increased in patients who are immunocompromised, critically ill, have indwelling catheters, and are very young.

Definitions

In 1991 a consensus conference between the American College of Chest Physicians (ACCP) and the Society of Critical Care Medicine (SCCM) was assembled to clarify the definition of sepsis along the continuum of inflammatory response.[11] Before this time, terminology was poorly defined and inconsistently applied. It was the intent of this group that using universal terminology to describe the inflammatory response would improve collecting reliable epidemiologic data and outcome research. Consensus conference definitions include the following:

- *Infection:* The inflammatory response by a host to the invasion of a microorganism
- *Bacteremia:* The presence of bacteria in the bloodstream
- *Systemic inflammatory response syndrome (SIRS):* A nonspecific systemic response to a variety of insults. The causative factor is not necessarily specific to infection and can include inflammatory responses to trauma, pancreatitis, shock, burns, ischemia, or surgery.
- *Sepsis:* The systemic inflammatory response specifically attributed to an infection or a presumed infection. Two or more of the criteria for SIRS (Box 13.2) are present, and there is reasonable clinical evidence that an infection is present. Blood cultures do not need to be positive.
- *Severe sepsis:* The presence or presumed presence of an infection, single or multiple organ dysfunction, hypoperfusion, or hypotension. Hypoperfusion may present as lactic acidosis, oliguria, and/or acute change in mental status.
- *Septic shock:* A subset of severe sepsis marked by hypotension not responding to adequate volume resuscitation. Hypotension is defined as SBP less than 90 mm Hg, MAP less than 60 mm Hg, or a decrease in SBP by greater than 40 mm Hg from baseline. Normal blood pressures requiring vasopressor support to maintain those pressures are included in the septic shock definition.
- *Multiple organ dysfunction syndrome (MODS):* The potentially reversible dysfunction of at least two organs requiring medical intervention to maintain body equilibrium. Table 13.4 provides system presentation of organ ischemia and dysfunction.

BOX 13.2 SIRS Manifestations.

- Temperature <96.8°F (36°C) or >100.4°F (38°C)
- Heart rate >90 beats/min
- Respiratory rate >20 breaths/min (or $PaCO_2$ <32 mm Hg)
- Abnormal WBC counts
- *>12,000/mm³*
- *<4000/mm³*
- *>10% bands*

SIRS, Systemic inflammatory response syndrome; *WBC,* white blood cell.

TABLE 13.4 Effects of Organ Ischemia.

System	Presentation
CNS	Acute change in mental status Confusion Comatose
Respiratory	Hypoxia/hypoxemia Ventilation/perfusion mismatch Adult respiratory distress syndrome (ARDS) Acute lung injury (ALI)
Cardiovascular	Decreased ejection fraction Biventricular dilation
Renal	Oliguria Anuria Elevated creatinine level Acute renal failure
Metabolic/Endocrine	Hyperglycemia Lactic acidosis Adrenal insufficiency Hypothyroidism Catabolic
Hepatic	Elevated liver enzyme levels Hyperbilirubinemia

CNS, Central nervous system.

The treatment of sepsis requires an aggressive and time-dependent focus similar to acute myocardial infarction and stroke.[10–13] Success in reducing mortality in these studies prompted a group of international experts representing critical care and infectious disease to develop evidence-based guidelines for the management of sepsis and septic shock, with a heavy focus on early diagnosis and treatment in the initial hours of presentation.[10–13] The Surviving Sepsis Campaign is a collaborative effort by the Society of Critical Care Medicine, the European Society of Intensive Care Medicine, and the International Sepsis Forum to improve awareness and treatment of sepsis and to decrease mortality rate. These guidelines were initially presented in 2004 and include 45 recommendations for the resuscitation and management of septic patients.

In 2016 the Surviving Sepsis Campaign: International Guidelines for the Management of Sepsis and Septic Shock was revised. A 1-hour Surviving Sepsis Bundle was proposed for the diagnosis and management of suspected sepsis. This was particularly pertinent to the ED care of the patients with sepsis.[10–13]

Pathophysiology

Sepsis is the result of a series of complex events of cellular, humoral, and inflammatory interactions within a host, manifested by systemic inflammation and coagulation. Initially a localized response to a pathogen results in cellular activation of monocytes to stimulate the release of proinflammatory cytokines such as interleukin-1, interleukin-6, and tumor necrosis factor. These cytokines produce compounds causing local vasodilatation and the release of cytotoxic chemicals to fight and destroy the pathogen.[14] In normal circumstances this proinflammatory response is balanced with antiinflammatory cytokines to promote wound healing and maintain homeostasis. However, in sepsis the initial proinflammatory response spins out of control, causing damage to the endothelium and release of the cytotoxic material into the bloodstream.[14] Further damage to the endothelium leads to extravasation of cellular fluid, interstitial edema, decreased intravascular volume, and relative hypovolemia. The mass production of nitric oxide by cytokines and tumor necrosis factor causes systemic vasodilatation and hypotension. As a result, oxygen supply to tissues does not keep up with oxygen demand, and global tissue hypoxia and shock ensue. This marks the transition into sepsis and septic shock.[14] In addition, damage to the endothelium causes stimulation of the coagulation and complement cascades, causing microcirculatory coagulation, platelet aggregation, and thrombus formation.[14]

Diagnosis

Because the mortality of sepsis increases exponentially as it progresses to septic shock and organ dysfunction, early identification and treatment of sepsis is essential. However, the identification of sepsis and septic shock is not clear-cut because many of the symptoms identified in the early stages of sepsis are common in a wide variety of conditions in addition to inflammatory response. Thus diagnosis of sepsis is often determined through a combination of detailed history and assessment leading to a high degree of suspicion. Vital signs in the early stages of sepsis do not adequately reveal the level of global hypoperfusion, even though damage affecting morbidity and mortality is well under way.[10] The combination of history, symptoms associated with SIRS, and laboratory values suggestive of infection or hypoperfusion, such as elevated serum lactate, should indicate the need for immediate resuscitation.

Laboratory findings on presentation to the ED vary depending on the stage of sepsis. Early findings will be reflective of SIRS, including abnormal white blood cell (WBC) count and/or an increase in immature cells. As the inflammatory response advances, signs of hypovolemia may be evident, presenting as hemoconcentration with elevation of hematocrit and hemoglobin. Hypoperfusion of organs and tissues may present as hypoxemia, metabolic acidosis, elevated lactate, elevated liver enzymes, and hyperbilirubinemia. As the coagulation cascade is stimulated, thrombocytopenia, prolonged thrombin time, and low fibrinogen levels develop.

Imaging studies to identify the source of sepsis should be obtained as quickly as possible. The stability of the patient and the risks of transport and placement in confined areas should be considered, and the risks weighed thoughtfully.

Emergency Department Management

The landmark study by Rivers et al. compared standard therapy with early goal-directed therapy (EGDT) in the treatment of patients who presented to the ED with sepsis and serum lactate levels greater than 4 mmol/L or refractory hypotension related to infection.[15] In this study the patients were treated for 6 hours in the ED before transfer to the intensive care unit (ICU), at which point the study was discontinued. The treatment goal involved implementing a systematic process using set hemodynamic parameters to guide treatment and reverse global hypoperfusion without causing further stress on myocardial function. The in-hospital mortality rates in standard therapy and EGDT therapy were 46.5% and 30.5%, respectively. The EGDT group also had significantly shorter hospital lengths of stay, lower organ dysfunction scores, and a twofold decrease in acute respiratory failure, hypotension, and sudden episodes of cardiopulmonary complications, such as cardiac arrest. Subsequent studies have validated the results of this study.[16–17]

The Surviving Sepsis Campaign was developed to provide a focused approach to evaluating and identifying a patient at risk for sepsis. Although the principles are based on solid clinical practice, not all of the guidelines will meet every patient scenario. It is important for clinicians to use their judgment in applying the guidelines as the individual circumstance dictates. Whether intensive care is brought to the ED or the patient is delivered to the ICU, it is clear that treatment should be implemented without delay.

Surviving Sepsis Campaign Bundle: 2018

The Surviving Sepsis Campaign Bundle 2018[10] incorporates the 3-hour and 6-hour bundle into a singe hour–bundle. The goal is to begin the resuscitation and management of a patient suspected with sepsis to begin immediately. The 1-hour bundle includes the following:[10(p926)]

- Measure lactate level. Remeasure if initial lactate is >2 mmol/L.
- Obtain blood cultures prior to administration of antibiotics.
- Administer broad-spectrum antibiotics.
- Begin rapid administration of 30 mL/kg crystalloid for hypotension or lactate ≥4 mmol/L.
- Apply vasopressors if patient is hypotensive during or after fluid resuscitation to maintain MAP ≥65 mm Hg.

According to the campaign, "'Time zero' or 'time of presentation' is defined as the time of triage in the Emergency Department or, if presenting from another care venue, from the earliest chart annotation consistent with the elements of sepsis (formerly severe sepsis) or septic shock ascertained through chart review."

Assessment, Management, and Evaluation of the Patient with Sepsis in the Emergency Department

The assessment, management, and evaluation of the patient with sepsis in the ED require a focused team approach. The following is a summary of care for sepsis.

Assessment.

1. Airway, breathing, circulation, disability, and exposure (ABCDE) assessment and implementation of critical interventions
2. Obtain history of present illness to localize potential origin of infection.
   a. *Head:* ear, sinus, or throat pain; swollen lymph glands; nasal drainage
   b. *Neck:* pain, stiffness
   c. *Chest:* shortness of breath, cough, pleuritic pain, pulmonary secretions, congestion
   d. *Abdomen:* nausea, vomiting, diarrhea, abdominal pain (generalized or localized), loss of appetite
   e. *Renal/pelvic/genital:* vaginal or urethral drainage; flank, back, or pelvic pain; urinary frequency, hematuria, oliguria, or dysuria; bladder fullness; cloudy urine
   f. *Extremities:* obvious deformities, open fractures, cellulitis
   g. *Soft tissue:* erythema, pain beyond borders of erythema, localized edema, bullae, blebs
   h. *General:* headache, malaise, chills, body aches, weakness, dizziness, altered level of consciousness
   i. *Past medical and surgical history:* Immunocompromising conditions, prosthetic devices, recent exposures to communicable diseases
3. Physical assessment: signs of infection, sepsis
   a. *Fever:* core temperature greater than 101.4°F (38°C)
   b. *Hypothermia:* core temperature less than 96.8°F (36°C)
   c. *Tachypnea:* respiratory rate greater than 20 breaths/min
   d. Altered mental status
   e. Significant peripheral edema
   f. *Hypotension:* SBP less than 90 mm Hg, MAP less than 70 mm Hg, SBP decrease of more than 40 mm Hg from patient's baseline
   g. Absent bowel sounds
   h. Delayed capillary refill
   i. *Physical examination indicating localized infection:* crackles, rhonchi, or dullness to percussion on chest examination; abdominal distention, localized tenderness, rebound tenderness or guarding; erythema, crepitus, edema, tenderness; any purulent drainage; meningismus; petechial or purpuric rash
4. Diagnostic assessment associated with sepsis
   a. Hyperglycemia (greater than 120 mg/dL) not associated with diabetes
   b. WBC count greater than 12,000/mm^3, WBC count less than 4000/mm^3, WBC count normal, but with greater than 10% bands
   c. Plasma C-reactive protein greater than 2 standard deviations (SD) above the normal value
   d. *Arterial hypoxemia:* PaO_2 less than 60 mm Hg
   e. *Oliguria:* urine output less than 0.5 mL/kg/hr for more than 2 hours
   f. *Elevated creatinine:* greater than 0.5 mg/dL
   g. *Thrombocytopenia:* platelet count less than 100,000/mm
   h. *Coagulation abnormalities:* international normalized ratio (INR) greater than 1.5 baseline or greater than 4.0
   i. *Hyperbilirubinemia:* total bilirubin greater than 4 mg/dL
   j. *Hyperlactatemia:* greater than 2 mmol/L

Management. The management of a patient with sepsis and septic shock should be based on the following:[10,11]

a. Maintain/establish airway, breathing, and circulation.
b. *Obtain cultures:* Thirty to fifty percent of patients presenting with symptoms of sepsis have positive blood cultures. Cultures from all sources, including blood, urine, wounds, secretions, CSF, etc., should be drawn before initiation of antimicrobial therapy.
c. *Administer antibiotics:* Antibiotics should be administered within 1 hour of patient admission to the ED. Antibiotic selection should be sufficiently broad to cover all likely pathogens. Although the concern for antibiotic-resistant organisms is noted, the marginal physiologic reserve of patients in sepsis and septic shock warrants the use of broad-spectrum antibiotics until the pathogen and antibiotic susceptibilities are identified. Antibiotic use should be narrowed when a pathogen has been identified and sensitivities confirmed.
d. Administer fluid bolus with crystalloid or colloid solution if the patient is hypotensive (SBP less than 90 mm Hg; MAP less than 70 mm Hg; decrease in SBP of less than 40 mm from baseline or serum lactate concentration greater than 4 mmol/L).
   - Rapid bolus with crystalloid solution starting with at least 30 mL/kg over 15 to 30 minutes. (Note: for the pediatric patient the volume is 20 mL/kg)
   - Insert an indwelling urinary catheter.
   - Assess blood pressure, heart rate, urine output, and arterial oxygen saturation during the course of each fluid bolus.
   - Repeat boluses as necessary MAP is greater than 70 mm Hg, or the patient is fluid compromised (e.g., pulmonary edema).
e. *Treat ongoing hypotension as ordered:* Blood pressure goals and treatments are best monitored by the placement of an arterial catheter and continuous, ongoing measurements. Research has found it may be difficult to precisely measure the effectiveness of fluid resuscitation. Patients are also at risk for fluid overload.
f. *Vasopressor support:*[10–11] An MAP of greater than 65 mm Hg has been found to be an appropriate initial target. It is important to remember that a patient with a history of hypertension may require a higher target to maintain adequate perfusion. Norepinephrine is the preferred vasopressor because it has fewer side effects than other vasopressors.

Ongoing evaluation. Continuously monitor and record heart rate, blood pressure, and urine output. Monitor mental status. Reevaluate lactate levels intermittently throughout resuscitation to guide adequacy of resuscitation. If infusing vasoactive agents through a peripheral line, assess skin around insertion site for signs of infiltration and tissue damage. Adjust titration of vasopressor agents to maintain MAP between 65 and 85 mm Hg. Prepare for potential transport for care at another facility if necessary.

Summary

The care of the patient with sepsis has been directed at beginning resuscitation and management immediately. The Surviving Sepsis Campaign recommends an "hour-1 bundle." This includes measuring the lactate level; obtaining blood cultures before administering antibiotics; administering broad spectrum antibiotics; rapid administration of 30 mL/kg for hypotension or lactate level ≥4 mmol/L and applying vasopressors if the patient is hypotensive during or after fluid resuscitation to maintain a MAP ≥65 mm Hg.

The treatment of sepsis and septic shock is both time dependent and labor intensive. It is only with the collaboration of the emergency and critical care departments that the effect on patient care can be fully realized. The role of the emergency nurse is essential to the success of the implementation of sepsis guidelines and the continued care of the patient with sepsis and septic shock in the ED.

CARE OF THE FAMILY

The care of the critically ill patient in the ED is challenging. It requires the emergency nurse to have additional education and skills to provide safe competent care. This also includes care of the family or significant others who may accompany the patient. Many of these patients may die in the ED or may die before admission or transfer to a critical care unit.

The emergency nurse must consider ways to manage the distress of these families. This may include allowing witnessed resuscitation of the patient; providing comfort, reassurance and education about the care being provided to the patient; and keeping families informed.[18]

SUMMARY

The care of a critically ill patient presents many challenges to the ED and the emergency nurse. The need for additional skills such as the management of ventilators and invasive monitoring are required as well as ways to assure competency in these skills. Appropriate staffing so patients can be closely monitored must always be considered. As noted, the ED nursing and the critical care unit nursing staffs must work together to assure that the critically ill patient receives safe and competent care.

REFERENCES

1. Herring AA, Ginde AA, Fahimi J, et al. Increasing critical care admissions from US emergency departments, 2001–2009. *Crit Care Med.* 2013;41(5):1197–1204.
2. Siletz A, Jin K, Cohen M, et al. Emergency department length of stay in critical nonoperative trauma. *J Surg Res.* 2017;214:102–108.
3. Storzer DN. Pulmonary system. In: Hartjes TM, ed. *Core Curriculum for High Acuity, Progressive, and Critical Care Nursing.* 7th ed. St. Louis: Elsevier; 2018:34–141.
4. Bauer E. Mechanical ventilation. In: Semonin Holleran R, Wolfe A, Frakes M, eds. *Patient Transport: Principles and Practice.* 5th ed. St. Louis: Elsevier; 2018:182–197.
5. Gasowski L, Poggemeyer C. Pulmonary emergencies. In: Semonin Holleran R, Wolfe A, Frakes M, eds. *Patient Transport: Principles and Practice.* 5th ed. St. Louis: Elsevier; 2018:345–365.
6. DeLuca L, Walsh P, Davidson D, et al. Impact and feasibility of an emergency department-based ventilator-associated pneumonia bundle for patients intubated in an academic emergency department. *Amer J Infection Control.* 2017;45(2):151–157.
7. Denno J. Invasive hemodynamic monitoring. In: Sweet V, ed. *Emergency Nursing Core Curriculum.* 7th ed. St. Louis: Elsevier; 2018:70–79.
8. Goodrich C. Cardiovascular emergencies. In: Semonin Holleran R, Wolfe A, Frakes M, eds. *Patient Transport: Principles and Practice.* 5th ed. St. Louis: Elsevier; 2018:298–322.
9. Blissitt P. Neurologic system. In: Hartjes TM, ed. *Core Curriculum for High Acuity, Progressive, and Critical Care Nursing.* 7th ed. St. Louis: Elsevier; 2018:310–423.
10. Cecconi M, Evans L, Levy M, Rhodes A. Sepsis and septic shock. *Lancet.* 2018;392(10141):75–87.
11. Greenwood JC, Orloski CJ. End points of sepsis resuscitation. *Emerg Med Clin North Am.* 2017;35(1):93–107.
12. Semonin Holleran R. Shock emergencies. In: Sweet V, ed. *Emergency Nursing Core Curriculum.* 7th ed. St. Louis: Elsevier; 2018:473–482.
13. Levy MM, Evans LE, Rhodes A. The surviving sepsis Campaign bundle: 2018 update. *Intensive Care Med.* 2018;44(6):925–928.
14. Johnson A. Systemic inflammatory response syndrome and septic shock. In: Hartjes TM, ed. *Core Curriculum for High Acuity, Progressive and Critical Care Nursing.* 7th ed. St. Louis: Elsevier; 2018:602–699.
15. Rivers E, Nguyen B, Havstad S, et al. Early goal-directed therapy in the treatment of severe sepsis and septic shock. *N Engl J Med.* 2001;345:1368–1377.
16. Nguyen HB, Rivers EP, Abrahamian FM, et al. Severe sepsis and septic shock: review of the literature and emergency department management guidelines. *Ann Emerg Med.* 2006;48(1):28–54.
17. Nguyen HG, Corbett SW, Steele R, et al. Implementation of a bundle of quality indicators for the early management of severe sepsis and septic shock is associated with decreased mortality. *Crit Care Med.* 2007;35(4):1005–1112.
18. Ringer T, Moller D, Mutsaers A. Distress in caregivers accompanying patients to an emergency department: a scoping review. *J Emerg Med.* 2017;53(4):493–508.

14

Palliative and End-of-Life Care in the Emergency Department

Garrett K. Chan, Colleen Vega

OVERVIEW OF PALLIATIVE AND END-OF-LIFE CARE

Palliative care is a comprehensive and specialized way to approach patients and families who face life-threatening or severe advanced illness and focuses on alleviating physical, psychological, emotional, and spiritual suffering and promoting quality of life.[1] Palliative care emphasizes communication, advanced care planning, and symptom management using a multidisciplinary approach.[2,3] Multidisciplinary palliative care teams include professionals from nursing, medicine, chaplaincy, social services, and psychology and lay volunteers. Palliative care can coexist with disease-modifying interventions and starts with the initial diagnosis of illness or injury and continues through the time of the patient's death and beyond to the survivors, in the form of bereavement care. Palliative care is patient- and family-centered and respects personal, cultural, and spiritual values, wishes, and goals of the patient and family. The end of life is a phase in the palliative care trajectory usually focusing on the care of the person who is imminently dying. Fewer life-sustaining treatments are used or recommended during the end-of-life phase.

In the emergency department (ED), suffering and death are common. According to the Centers for Disease Control and Prevention, approximately 195,000 persons died in US EDs in 2015.[4] In addition, the ED is a fast-paced, high-stress, and high-anxiety department where staff make decisions regarding patient care with suboptimal levels of information.[5] The ED is a place of transition where patients receive initial diagnostics and stabilizing treatment and then are transferred out or discharged from the ED. This scenario may give a false impression that the sole focus of the ED is on diagnosis and initial curative treatment when, in fact, palliative care is provided to patients to help relieve pain, anxiety, and other distressing symptoms and emotions of patients and families.

Many patients who come to the ED may need palliative care. Patients who present usually have a chief complaint of a symptom such as pain, dyspnea, or nausea. Common presentations of patients who need advanced palliative or end-of-life care include patients with advanced stages of illness such as congestive heart failure, chronic obstructive pulmonary disease, dementia, and severe trauma. Other patient populations that can benefit from end-of-life care are the family of a patient with sudden infant death syndrome or the family of a woman who has miscarried.

We live in a rescue-oriented culture where cardiopulmonary resuscitation and other advanced procedures are routinely used. However, some patients may not need or benefit from these aggressive, heroic measures; instead, they may need care-and-comfort measures, especially at the end of life. It is important for the emergency nurse to recognize that some interventions nurses have at their disposal—such as intubation and chest compressions—may not be appropriate for patients near the end of life, and careful exploration regarding life goals and expectations for care will help determine what interventions may be appropriate for each situation.

Emergency nurses play a pivotal role in helping formulate an appropriate plan of care that takes into consideration the patient's and family's beliefs and desires while providing only those interventions that are beneficial and appropriate. The Emergency Nurses Association (ENA) has developed a position statement to help emergency nurses provide optimal end-of-life care.[6] The ED will continue to be a frequent setting for respite visited by patients with life-limiting illnesses. Patients with cancer, dementia, fragility, organ failure (i.e., cirrhosis, heart failure, and neuromuscular diseases) and many other life-limiting illnesses can be candidates for palliative care. Palliative care screening tools are being evaluated for the ED. One screening tool is called "P-CaRES" (Palliative care and Rapid Emergency Screening). Screening tools provide guidance to ED nurses regarding which patients would most benefit from a palliative care consult (Box 14.1).[7] Finally, it is important to ask the patient, if possible, who is considered to be family and who is their surrogate decision maker. Determining who is considered family allows the nurse to understand who should receive information, be allowed in the treatment area, and be consulted to help make care decisions.[8]

BOX 14.1 Palliative Care Screening Tool.

Consider a palliative care consultation if a patient has one item or more in each category.

1. Does the patient have a life-limiting illness?	• Advanced dementia or central nervous system disease (i.e., amyotrophic lateral sclerosis, cerebrovascular accident) • Advanced cancer • Advanced chronic obstructive pulmonary disease (i.e., 24-hour oxygen) • Advanced heart failure • End-stage renal disease (i.e., dialysis dependent, creatinine >6 mg/dL) • Septic shock along with existing severe comorbid diseases • Potential for immediate death (i.e., major trauma in older adults, advanced acquired immunodeficiency syndrome)
2. Does the patient have one or more of the following:	• Functional decline • Frequents visits to hospital or emergency department in past 6 months • Prognosis of <12 months • Caregiver distress and complex long-term needs • Uncontrolled symptoms (i.e., dyspnea, pain, nausea, and vomiting)

BOX 14.2 Common Symptoms at the End of Life.

Pulmonary	Dyspnea Cough Head/nasal congestion "Death rattle" Respiratory distress/respiratory depression
Neurologic/Functional	Pain Spinal cord compression Weakness Fatigue Immobility Insomnia Confusion/dementia/delirium Memory changes
Gastrointestinal	Nausea/vomiting Dysphagia Anorexia Weight loss Unpleasant taste Ascites Constipation/obstipation/bowel obstruction Diarrhea Incontinence of bowel Hiccups
Urinary	Incontinence of bladder Bladder spasms Changes in function or control
Integumentary	Decubitus Mucositis Candidiasis Pruritus Edema Hemorrhage Infection (e.g., herpes zoster) Diaphoresis
Psychiatric	Depression Anxiety
Other	Fever

Modified from Ferrell BR: *HOPE: Home Care Outreach for Palliative Care Education Project,* Duarte, Calif, 1998, City of Hope.

PALLIATIVE CARE PRINCIPLES IN THE EMERGENCY DEPARTMENT

There are many definitions of palliative care. However, common among the various definitions are that palliative care is multidisciplinary, is patient- and family-centered, and includes symptom management; emotional and psychological care; social care; spiritual/existential care; communication and advanced care planning; and bereavement care for the survivors.[3,6,9,10] Core palliative and end-of-life principles of symptom management, emotional, psychological, social, and spiritual care will be covered.

Symptom Management

Common symptoms at the end of life are listed in Box 14.2. It is important for emergency nurses to assess for these symptoms and intervene to reduce their severity. Although all of these symptoms are important, in this chapter the focus will be on the common symptoms seen in the ED, such as pain, dyspnea, nausea/vomiting, constipation, and delirium.[11]

Nurses must assess and reassess for the presence or improvement of symptoms before and after any intervention. Importantly, many interventions can be viewed as both palliative and therapeutic. For example, if a patient with end-stage congestive heart failure comes to the ED with a chief complaint of dyspnea, the nurse may administer furosemide (Lasix) as a palliative treatment to relieve the dyspnea from pulmonary edema. Furosemide is considered more palliative than therapeutic for end-stage congestive heart failure and pulmonary edema. Another example is if a patient with end-stage cancer comes to the ED with severe fatigue and dyspnea secondary to anemia, packed red blood cell units may be administered in an attempt to relieve the fatigue and dyspnea. In this example, the blood administration is viewed as palliative more than disease modifying because the anemia is a chronic condition that will not be reversed.

Pain

Pain is defined as an unpleasant sensory and emotional experience associated with actual or potential tissue damage or described in terms of such damage.[12] This definition reflects the multidimensional aspects of pain and takes into consideration the physiologic, emotional, and social effects of this symptom. Another commonly cited definition is "pain is whatever the person says it is, experienced whenever they say they are experiencing it."[13] It is important to recognize that pain is a subjective symptom, and self-report is a valid measure of pain. However, in patients who are not able to communicate their pain because of an altered level of consciousness, language barriers, aphasia, or other factors, the patients are considered to be in pain until it is proven otherwise. Because families may spend a significant time with the patient and understand the baseline comfort level, the patient's family may be able to determine whether the patient is in pain. The family should be asked by the nurse if they perceive that the patient is in pain or has any other symptom.

A common issue for emergency nurses is understanding the unique characteristics and differences between acute and chronic pain. Commonly, patients who have severe acute pain present with behaviors such as yelling, writhing, grimacing, and other visible signs of discomfort. However, patients who have chronic pain (i.e., pain that lasts for weeks to months beyond acute tissue injury) may lack these visible signs of discomfort, yet they experience pain nonetheless. Acute and chronic pain differ significantly, and emergency nurses should continue to believe patients who verbalize that they are in pain, regardless of the outward behaviors. It is important to note that patients may be experiencing severe pain and may be able to sleep. This phenomenon can be attributed to exhaustion and is contrary to the commonly held perceptions that pain will stop sleep. Chapter 12 explains pain pathophysiology, assessment, and management in more detail.

Patients who present with adverse side effects of opioids such as oversedation and respiratory depression (respiratory rate less than 8 breaths/min) should receive very small doses of naloxone (Narcan) to reverse the side effects without reversing the analgesic effects. Abruptly reversing both the analgesic and side effects by using naloxone may precipitate abstinence syndrome, which can cause a range of symptoms, including anxiety, myalgias, tachycardia, hypertension, pulmonary edema, and cardiopulmonary collapse. One method of administering naloxone in patients to reverse the side effects without reversing the analgesia is as follows[14]:

1. Stop opioid administration.
2. Dilute 0.4 mg naloxone (one ampule) with normal saline to a total volume of 10 mL (1 mL = 0.04 mg).
3. Remind the patient to breathe; although narcotized, patients report hearing concerned staff and being unable to open their eyes or respond.
4. Administer 1 mL intravenously (0.04 mg) every 1 minute until the patient is responsive. A typical response is noted after administering 2 to 4 mL, with deeper breathing and greater level of arousal. Gradual naloxone administration should prevent acute opioid withdrawal.
5. If the patient does not respond to a total of 0.8 mg naloxone (2 ampules), consider other causes of sedation and respiratory depression (e.g., benzodiazepines, stroke).
6. The duration of action of naloxone is considerably shorter than the duration of action of most short-acting opioids. A repeat dose of naloxone, or even a continuous naloxone infusion, may be needed.
7. Wait until there is sustained improvement in consciousness before restarting opioids at a lower dose.

BOX 14.3 Modified Borg Scale.

Scale	Severity
0	No breathlessness[a] at all
0.5	Very, very slight (just noticeable)
1	Very slight
2	Slight breathlessness
3	Moderate
4	Somewhat severe
5	Severe breathlessness
6	
7	Very severe breathlessness
8	
9	Very, very severe (almost maximum)
10	Maximum

[a]The term *breathlessness* was added for clarification of the scale.

Remember, patients may have a respiratory rate of 8 breaths/min while sleeping.

Dyspnea

Dyspnea is defined as a sense of breathlessness or shortness of breath and can be extremely distressing and frightening for both the patient and those who witness it. Many diseases cause dyspnea, including lung diseases such as chronic obstructive pulmonary disease, pneumonia, and pulmonary embolisms; heart diseases such as congestive heart failure; end-stage renal disease; anxiety; metabolic disorders; anemia; and financial, legal, family, or spiritual issues. Initial management of dyspnea is to focus on the underlying causes and intervene with any disease-modifying treatments as appropriate. However, in some cases, the underlying cause of dyspnea may not be identified. It is important to recognize that dyspnea is a subjective symptom and the treatments need to be tailored to the amount of subjective dyspnea the patient experiences. Objective data such as oxygen saturation (Sao_2) may not correlate with the amount of dyspnea a patient is experiencing.

Assessment of dyspnea can include using a numeric rating scale such as the modified Borg scale. The modified Borg scale is a scale ranging from 0 to 10 and has been validated for use in the ED (Box 14.3). Trending the modified Borg scale scores will let the nurse know whether the interventions are effective in treating the dyspnea.

There are three pharmacologic approaches used commonly for dyspnea: oxygen, opioids, and anxiolytics. Although opioids and anxiolytics have side effects that include possible respiratory depression and sedation, these medications can be administered with careful titration and monitoring to avoid the adverse side effects. In addition, nonpharmacologic interventions such as positioning the patient, providing distraction, using guided imagery, and using a fan to move air across the face (stimulating the trigeminal nerve) have been shown to be effective in managing dyspnea.

Nausea and Vomiting

There are many causes of nausea and vomiting, and these symptoms are frequently seen in the ED. Nausea and vomiting can be effectively managed if the correct medications are chosen based on an accurate assessment of the underlying pathophysiology.

Two organ systems are particularly important in nausea and vomiting: the brain and the gastrointestinal (GI) tract.[1] In the brain, the chemoreceptor trigger zone at the base of the fourth ventricle, the cortex, and the vestibular apparatus are areas involved in stimulating nausea and vomiting. In the GI tract, the gastric and small intestine linings have chemoreceptors that are responsible for nausea and vomiting.

If stimulated, the neurotransmitters serotonin, dopamine, acetylcholine, and histamine can cause nausea and vomiting. These four neurotransmitters are found in the chemoreceptor trigger zone; however, in the vestibular apparatus, acetylcholine and histamine are predominant. In the GI tract, serotonin is the major neurotransmitter responsible for nausea and vomiting. The cortex is more complex and is not associated with specific neurotransmitters. Knowing the physiology of nausea and vomiting will help the emergency nurse understand which antiemetic might be most helpful in managing the nausea and vomiting. Using the acronym VOMIT (vestibular, obstruction of bowel, dysmotility of upper gut, infection/inflammation, toxins stimulating the chemoreceptor trigger zone) can also help emergency nurses remember the causes of nausea.[15]

Dopamine-mediated nausea is the most common form of nausea. Dopamine antagonists are classified into two categories: phenothiazines and butyrophenone neuroleptics. The phenothiazines include medications such as prochlorperazine (Compazine), promethazine (Phenergan), and metoclopramide (Reglan). The butyrophenone neuroleptics include haloperidol (Haldol) and droperidol (Inapsine). Both the phenothiazines and butyrophenone neuroleptics have the potential to cause drowsiness and extrapyramidal side effects.

Serotonin antagonists are commonly used in the ED. Often these medications are very effective, especially with chemotherapy-induced nausea or nausea from GI distention, or with nausea that is refractory to other therapies. They are expensive and should be stopped if a short trial does not control the nausea. Medications in this drug category include ondansetron (Zofran) and granisetron (Kytril).[16]

Histamine antagonists may also be used in nausea that may be due to medications such as opioids or chemotherapeutic agents. The histamine antagonists may also have anticholinergic properties as well. Medications in this category include diphenhydramine (Benadryl), meclizine (Antivert), or hydroxyzine (Vistaril or Atarax).

Anticholinergic agents are effective if the nausea is caused by a disturbance in the vestibular apparatus. Medications in this class may be combined with other classes of antiemetics. An example of an anticholinergic medication is scopolamine.

Adjunctive agents that may also be used in combination with the previously mentioned medications include dexamethasone, tetrahydrocannabinol (THC), and lorazepam (Ativan). The mechanisms of action are unclear but have been proved to be effective in clinical trials.[15]

Constipation

Constipation can be a very painful and distressing symptom with many causes. With opioid use, many symptoms decrease with long-term use except for constipation. Therefore a bowel regimen should be in place for all patients receiving opioids. Prevention of constipation is the best strategy in managing constipation.

The most helpful class of medications for constipation is the stimulant laxatives. Stimulant laxatives increase the peristaltic activity of the GI tract. Agents in this class include prune juice, senna preparations, and bisacodyl. Osmotic laxatives draw water into the bowel lumen, thereby increasing the stool volume and the moisture content in the stool. Medications in this class include milk of magnesia, magnesium citrate, and lactulose. Detergent laxatives, also known as stool softeners, increase the water content in the stool and facilitate the dissolution of fat in water, increasing the stool volume. Medications in this class include sodium docusate and a Phospho-Soda enema. Lubricant stimulants lubricate the stool and irritate the bowel, thus increasing the peristaltic activity. Glycerin suppositories and mineral oil are two examples of lubricant stimulants. Large-volume enemas, such as warm water or soapsuds, may be used to distend the colon and increase peristalsis.

BOX 14.4 Causes of Terminal Delirium.

Opioid toxicity	High doses of opioids or prolonged opioid administration can cause somnolence, agitation, or mixed subtype.
Uncontrolled pain	Severe pain can lead to agitation. Communicating pain may be difficult for some patients.
Fever or sepsis	Fever can reduce cerebral oxidative metabolism, leading to delirium.
Drug interactions	Hypnotics, steroids, anticonvulsants, alcohol, or antimuscarinics can cause agitation.
Elevated intracranial pressure	Increased intracranial pressure from brain tumors, stroke, or cerebral metastasis can lead to agitation.
Hypercalcemia	Hypercalcemia is most commonly seen in patients with cancer. From 10% to 30% of patients with cancer are affected by hypercalcemia.

Delirium

Delirium is a common symptom seen in the last weeks or days of life. It can be very disturbing and overwhelming for families to witness. Managing delirium is paramount to diminishing the suffering that can be present at the end of life. Delirium is characterized as an abrupt onset of confusion, a reduced awareness of events, a disruption in the sleep/awake cycle, and inattention. There are three types of delirium: hyperactive (agitation and restless behavior), hypoactive (inactivity, somnolence), and mixed (hypoactive and hyperactive). Unfortunately, delirium has been associated with short-term survival rates.[9]

There are multiple causes of delirium (Box 14.4). A new onset of delirium should be treated immediately if the causes are reversible (i.e., hypoglycemia, hypoxia, sepsis, meningitis, thiamine deficiency, and overdoses of medications/toxins). In the ED, assessing vital signs and glucose can be appropriate for certain patients whose prognosis is longer than a few days.

Antipsychotics, like haloperidol, are commonly used to treat hyperactive delirium. At the end of life, refractory delirium may require sedating medications, like lorazepam or diazepam, when standard interventions have failed.[9] Although medications are frequently used to treat delirium, changing a patient's environment can also be done to reduce delirium. Decreasing excessive lights or darkness, maintaining a sleep/awake cycle, or reducing noise and frequent room changes can diminish the symptoms of delirium. Glasses, hearing aids, and dentures should be offered to patients who use them, and physical restraints should be avoided. Providing a safe environment for patients, families, and staff is key to a successful management of delirium.[9,17]

Emotional, Psychological, Social, and Spiritual Care

Emergency nurses are experts at delivering aggressive, heroic measures to patients in distress. However, another aspect of good emergency nursing practice is taking care of the patient's and family's emotional, psychological, social, and spiritual needs. Patients and families come to the ED in crisis, and their coping skills are challenged. Patients and families may exhibit taxing behaviors because they have distressing symptoms and feel out of control. In addition, patients' existential distress may amplify their symptom experience and affect their ability to retain information they are provided. Patients and families may require frequent repetition of information.

Simple interventions that emergency nurses may use to address these concerns are to communicate clearly and often to the patient and family about the plan of care and what to expect during their stay in the ED and to encourage them to seek support from trusted members of their social network, such as calling their chaplain, family, or friends. Anticipating their needs may help avert an escalation of distress. Family presence during resuscitation is an important method of providing care to survivors and is another way to provide family-centered care (see Chapter 13). The ENA accepted a resolution in 1993 allowing the option of family presence during a resuscitation (FPDR). Although FPDR is still controversial, there is growing evidence showing psychological benefits of FPDR in the hospital and out-of-hospital settings.[18,19] The arrival of the emergency care team often triggers families' understanding of the severity and reality of the death of their loved one. There are some situations when the presence of family might not be in the best interest of a patient or staff (i.e., for overly aggressive behavior, intoxicated family members, or emotionally unstable individuals). In general, it is up to each institution to adopt policies that address FDPR especially because resuscitation is often unsuccessful.

Spirituality

Spiritual suffering can exist when a patient's beliefs are not met. Characteristics of spiritual suffering can manifest as pain, insomnia, depression, despair, anger, self-harm, or guilt.[17,20,21] Facing a severe illness can challenge a patient's beliefs. Patients may feel betrayed or abandoned. Addressing patients' beliefs may help them relieve their spiritual suffering. Over time, a patient's spiritual or religious views may change as they face their mortality. Identifying a patient's belief system may assist health care professionals with addressing goals of care, treatment options, or building trust and rapport. Additionally, addressing a patient's belief system may provide an effective source to help them cope with their illnesses.

COMMUNICATION ISSUES IN PALLIATIVE AND END-OF-LIFE CARE

Emergency nurses witness suffering and death frequently in the ED. Caring for patients in distress may become routine, and staff may become desensitized to the suffering around them.[22] This desensitization can have a profound effect on the nurse's ability to communicate effectively and respectfully with patients, families, and colleagues. At the same time, patients and families are often unfamiliar with death and dying. They come to the ED in crisis with unexpected injuries or illnesses, chronic disease exacerbations, or perhaps with terminal illnesses, seeking symptom management and life-saving or life-prolonging treatment.[5] The patients and families are in crisis and seek help and answers from emergency clinicians.

To avoid feeling unprepared to handle these situations, it is important that the emergency clinician work with other disciplines such as social services, chaplaincy services, and trained volunteers to role-play these scenarios and to create policies and procedures surrounding issues such as death notification, bereavement services, follow-up contact, and written information about what to do after a death.[23,24]

The following areas of communication are essential in delivering quality end-of-life care: deciding on a plan of care and death notification/delivering serious news.

Deciding on a Plan of Care

There are seven trajectories to approaching death in the ED: (1) dead on arrival; (2) prehospital resuscitation with subsequent death in the ED; (3) prehospital resuscitation with survival to admission; (4) terminally ill and comes to the ED; (5) frail and hovering near death; (6) alive and interacting on arrival, but arrests in the ED; and (7) potentially preventable death by omission or commission.[1,25] Although emergency clinicians are skilled at resuscitation, there are dying trajectories that require different care interventions than resuscitative measures. Some dying trajectories benefit from aggressive symptom management and humanistic care, whereas others call for more aggressive heroic interventions such as chest compressions, defibrillation, and intubation.

Recognition of poor prognoses and framing beneficial interventions as best for the patient will determine the plan of care.[26] Although resuscitative measures are the standard of care, they may not be appropriate for all patients near the end of life. Taking the time to discuss with the survivors and surrogate decision makers which interventions are appropriate to the situation may help establish the best treatment goals. Fear of liability may be a concern of emergency clinicians.[5,27]

However, expanding the definition of a "success" from the traditional concept of the patient being resuscitated back with a pulse to aggressive palliative care management will ease clinicians' feelings of abandoning the patient.[27]

Death Notification/Delivering Serious News

Notifying survivors about sudden and unexpected deaths or giving serious news can be stressful for clinicians.[23] Death notification can be done in person or over the telephone, or it may include assistance from other agencies such as police departments. Dr. Kenneth Iserson[23] has written an excellent resource to improve death notification. Dr. Iserson strongly recommends developing policies and procedures related to death notification. Death notification can be divided into four stages: prepare, inform, support, and afterward (PISA). An introductory review of PISA follows.

In the prepare stage, there are four activities to prepare to give serious news: anticipate, identify, notify, and organize. Nurses should anticipate the needs of bereaved survivors, such as arranging a quiet room to include comfortable places to sit, provide tissues, provide a telephone for the survivors to notify others and a "panic button" to summon help if needed, and think of members of other disciplines that will be helpful, such as a chaplain or a child-life specialist. Nurses should also have a list of agencies that survivors may need to contact, such as the medical examiner/coroner's office, funeral homes, and bereavement services.

The health care team should also positively identify the individual who has died and identify the name and relationship of the person who will be notified. The health care team should have the complete information about the circumstances surrounding the death and any details that may be comforting to the survivors. Notification of the death to the key survivors should be done by the most experienced individual with support from other staff members. Sit at the same level as the survivors. If multiple fatalities occurred in one incident, attempt to notify all the primary survivors at the same time. Notification of the primary care provider is important as well.

Organization of the health care team allows for smoother communication with difficult news. If there is more than one victim, assign one staff member to each group of survivors. Escort the survivors to a more comfortable and quiet room. Be sure that all clinicians are wearing identification badges, are presentable, and do not have blood or other body fluids on their clothing when giving the serious news. Accurately identify which family is in which room if multiple casualties were involved. If a staff member such as a social worker or chaplain has already interacted with the family, be sure to have that staff member present when giving the serious news. Before you enter the room, give yourself a moment to think about what you are going to say and perhaps practice with another staff member if you feel uncomfortable. Be sure to let the health care team know that you are going to give serious news and are not to be interrupted.

In the inform stage, two activities are central: introductions and delivering the news. Before the serious news is given, identify the persons in the room and ask them to explain their relationship to the patient. Introduce yourself and the other health care team members with you and their role in the patient's care. Always refer to the patient by his or her name, and avoid terms such as "the victim," "the decedent," or "our patient."

When giving the news, first ask the survivors what they know about the events to get an understanding about what is known and not known. Then briefly describe the prehospital and hospital events that led up to the serious condition or death, including any resuscitative efforts. Use clear, nontechnical language and avoid jargon. If the survivor asks you if the person is dead, he or she is giving you two pieces of information: (1) the survivor is ready for the news, and (2) he or she may be ready to cope with the answer that the person is dead.

The hardest part about death notification is using a "D" word—"dead," "died," or "death." Avoid using euphemisms such as "passed away," "no longer with us," "did not make it," "gone," or other confusing term. Using these ambiguous terms can create confusion for the survivors, and they may not understand the very important point that the patient is dead. If the survivors do not seem to understand, use another "D" word. After giving the serious or bad news, pause for a couple of moments to let the news sink in and for the survivors to react. Be prepared for any type of reaction to the news, including, but not limited to, disbelief, denial, anger, guilt, or exacerbation of a medical condition.

In the support stage the activities by the health care team are designed to support the survivors who are grieving. Not all survivors may need these activities in this stage; however, the emergency nurse should be prepared to provide support based on his or her assessment of the survivors. Reassure the survivors that everything that could be done was done and that any cultural or religious customs will be honored to the best of the health care team's ability. Ensure that information is collected in a respectful manner—it is not possible to honor cultural or religious customs unless the team is aware of them. Spiritual care is often an excellent resource for this process. Emergency nurses should also assuage the family's guilt and mental anguish. Often survivors question their role and sometimes blame themselves for not seeking help sooner. Relieve this guilt by reassuring them that the event was not their fault, unless it is very obvious that this is not true.

Reassure the survivors that the patient did not suffer. Useful phrases such as "most people with a bad head injury never have a memory of the accident" or "[the patient's name] was not conscious, and we do not believe that he [or she] was in pain."

In pediatric death, challenge any unrealistic expectations parents may have about their roles. Remind the parents that there was no way to protect their child from this death, unless this is not the case. Also, in pediatric deaths nurses should help the parents and other family members realize that they are grieving not only for the child but also for the hopes, dreams, and expectations they had for the child. Parents may also experience anxiety, depression, stress disorder, and grief when they have a miscarriage (pregnancy loss before 20 weeks). ED nurses should acknowledge the grief that can accompany miscarriages and offer emotional support to the bereaved families.[6,21]

Assist the survivors by being available to answer questions, and provide comfort measures such as giving water or tissues, calling other family members, listening to their stories and concerns, facilitating cultural or spiritual rituals, and allowing the survivors time to view the patient. In addition, protecting the families and survivors from the media or graphic footage is important to providing privacy in this distressing time.

Finally, in the support stage, emergency nurses should provide a written list of local contacts for funeral arrangements, medical examiner/coroner's office, and support groups such as those for sudden infant death syndrome, murder victims, older adult survivors, and pediatric death. Conclude the encounter with the survivors by asking if they have any other questions and provide them with a contact phone number at the hospital if they have additional questions. Advise the survivors that everything they need to do in the hospital is complete and they may leave whenever they feel ready. Accompany the survivors to the exit or to their transportation to provide them support.

BIOETHICAL CONSIDERATIONS

There are several ethical and legal issues that are specific to end-of-life care. Many of these issues are governed by local, state, or national laws and regulations. However, it is important to note that we should not confuse that which is legal with what is the most ethical thing to do. Common bioethical considerations in the ED include advance directives, organ and tissue donation, postmortem procedures, autopsy, withholding or withdrawing life-sustaining measures, the principle of double effect, assisted suicide, and euthanasia.[6]

Advance Directives

Since the landmark court case of Karen Ann Quinlan more than 30 years ago, patients have been encouraged to express their thoughts and feelings on end-of-life decisions with an advance directive. Because of this court case, the Patient Self-Determination Act was passed in 1991 to alleviate this fear. This act states that at the time of a patient's admission to the hospital, patients (or parents or guardians of children) must be presented with information about advance directives and their rights in making medical care decisions. These wishes then become a part of the patient's permanent record. Many people fear being kept alive by medical technology beyond what they feel is a meaningful existence. No one should have the power to overrule the decisions of the individual, particularly when it comes to choosing the manner of death. The advance directive should be a guide to the individual's wishes and is based on the concept that the patient is competent and has a right to refuse treatment. These documents become effective only when the patient loses decision-making capacity. Decision-making capacity can be determined with a few questions focusing on a patient's ability to understand and evaluate the consequences of their decisions (Box 14.5).

But what if there is no advance directive? Medical ethicists have been trying to answer that question despite considerable legal uncertainty in this area.

BOX 14.5 Decision-Making Capacity.

1. Patient's ability to understand	• Does the patient have the ability to understand the basic information needed to make a decision?
2. Patient's ability to evaluate	• Can the patient reason and weigh the consequences of their decisions? • Does the patient make a decision? • Is the decision reasonably consistent over time?
3. Patient's ability to communicate	• Can the patient communicate the decision?

Advance directives come in three forms: living will, durable power of attorney for health care, and do not resuscitate (DNR)/do not attempt resuscitation (DNAR)/allow natural death (AND). A living will is a legal document in which an individual can direct treatment modalities against extraordinary measures in the event of irreversible coma and terminal illness. The legality of this document varies from state to state and from country to country; however, it does not ensure a patient's right to die regardless of geographic location. The durable power of attorney for health care designates a surrogate decision maker when a patient is unable to make decisions. The patient can specify limits or parameters for the type of medical treatment that must be followed by the designated surrogate.

The DNR/DNAR/AND is an order that should be documented on the chart. A witness may be required in some areas. The DNR order addresses what lifesaving measures should be initiated, specifying limits such as cardiopulmonary resuscitation only, medications only, or no defibrillation. Despite the presence of a DNR order, every effort is made in these situations to ease pain and make the patient comfortable. Advance directives vary from state to state, so health care professionals must be familiar with stipulations in their respective states. Allow natural death recognizes that death is a natural course of illness and that no interventions will be attempted to alter the course of the disease.

POLST/MOLST

There are many valuable tools used by palliative care teams to document a patient's goals of care. The Physician Orders for Life-Sustaining Treatment (POLST) or Medical Orders for Life Sustaining Treatment (MOLST) are commonly used to identify patients' goals of care. These forms can clarify what kind of medical treatments patients prefer as they near the end of their life. Physicians and/or medical clinicians (physician assistants, advanced practice nurses) complete these forms with patients or their designated decision maker. It is recommended that POLSTs are completed if a patient is diagnosed with a terminal illness or for individuals who have less than 1 year to live. For information about your state's POLST, visit http://polst.org/programs-in-your-state.[21,28,29]

In most states, prehospital DNR orders are recognized as valid in the ED.[1] A pitfall in emergency nursing and medicine is the failure to determine whether a DNR order or an advance directive exists or to ignore these documents. It is important to have discussions after reading these documents to determine what the goals of care are for the patient and proxy decision maker to provide the care that is consistent with their wishes.

Society has obviously done its part by passing this act, forcing health care providers to confront questions the individual may shy away from and may not want to address with patients. Despite written evidence of the patient's wishes, it is still difficult for many caregivers to let go. Most health care providers are as uncomfortable with the idea of death as the families are. Health care professionals have been trained to preserve life, not to practice death care. Establishing a good relationship between patients and their families and health care providers in the ED may be difficult in a crisis situation. Unfortunately, it may be difficult if not impossible to identify the patient's wishes in the ED. Living wills, advance directives, and other documents may not be immediately available in the ED. Families in crisis may not be able to make a decision. It is critical for the emergency nurse to maintain ongoing contact with the patient and family throughout a crisis event. Families may find it easier to ask for information and advice from the nurse. Making yourself available to assist families with these difficult issues as they arise is a vital nursing function.

Organ and Tissue Donation

Federal law (Public Law 99-5-9; Section 9318) and Medicare regulations require that hospitals give the surviving family members the chance to authorize donation of their family member's tissues and organs.[27] Initiating the conversation about organ and tissue procurement can be difficult. However, some families have asked to donate organs or tissues. An important aspect surrounding organ or tissue procurement is respecting the family's grieving process and giving them all the information they need to make a decision with which they will be comfortable. See Chapter 14 for more information on organ donation.

Postmortem Procedures

The practicing of certain skills such as endotracheal intubation, cricothyrotomy, central line placement, and other procedures on the newly deceased patient is a sensitive topic. There is a balance between the need for health care providers to master these skills to be prepared for future situations calling for these high-risk, low-frequency skills and the respect for the patient and the wishes of the survivors. The ENA, the American College of Emergency Physicians (ACEP), and the American Academy of Pediatrics (AAP) have developed position statements clearly defining their positions.[6,30] ENA's position includes some of the following issues:

- ENA believes providers should have specific education regarding the difficulties raised by the death of a patient. The critical, life-threatening nature of the situations requiring these procedures demands competence and confidence on the part of the provider.
- The practitioner should be prepared, through a structured learning process, to maximize the educational experience.
- ENA believes in protocols regarding family presence, end-of-life care and death, and best practice-outlining procedures after a patient's death should be established:
  - communicating the news of a patient's death to family,
  - completion of death certification,
  - an addition to the consent for autopsy or donation,
  - optimal collaboration and documentation with local and state death review teams,
  - clear process for autopsy and organ donation.

Autopsy

The decision to perform an autopsy is usually made by the medical examiner or coroner's office in the county in which the patient died. EDs should develop policies and procedures delineating when to contact the medical examiner or coroner. Regulations vary from state to state and even within states. ED clinicians should consult with their local medical examiner, coroner, and other agencies to determine the local regulations, preferences, and procedures.

Several factors are taken into account to determine whether an autopsy is warranted.[2] First is the cause of death. Any death associated with a known or suspected criminal activity is cause for an autopsy. Second, autopsies are performed to determine the cause of any sudden, traumatic, or unexpected death. Finally, family members may request an autopsy. In the last case, the autopsy may be performed by any pathologist rather than the medical examiner.

Withholding or Withdrawing Life-Sustaining Measures

Withholding or withdrawing treatments is challenging to emergency clinicians because we are trained and commonly are called upon to institute resuscitation interventions. However, morally and legally, withholding or withdrawing treatments is justified and has strong roots in the common law that reflects the American regard for self-determination and is supported by the ethical principles of autonomy, beneficence, and nonmaleficence.[10] Patients and surrogate decision makers may be allowed to refuse or withdraw a treatment at any time according to hospitals' patients' bill of rights. Refer to your hospital's policy on the patients' bill of rights. Withholding treatment is considered morally equivalent to withdrawing treatment—the end result is the patient is without the treatment; however, it is more difficult for emergency clinicians to withhold a treatment than it is to withdraw a treatment.

Principle of Double Effect

The ethical principle of double effect distinguishes between the intended and unintended consequences of a particular action. In certain cases, an action has two effects: one good and one bad.[16] In a situation where there is no alternative but to cause harm in trying to fulfill one's duty to bring about good for a patient, the action is still permissible.[31]

The principle of double effect is most commonly applied when pain medication is being administered to a dying patient. Opioids are used to relieve pain and other symptoms of suffering. The relief of suffering is the good effect. However, opioids also have the potential adverse, or bad, effect of causing respiratory and cardiovascular depression, which may, if left untreated, lead to death. If the nurse's intention is to relieve pain and suffering, yet the nurse incidentally foresees that the patient may die, it is morally and legally permissible to administer the opioid if the intention is to relieve suffering. If the primary intention is to have the patient die, then it is not morally or legally permissible to administer the opioid. In end-of-life cases, it is important to note that the patient will eventually die as a result of the natural disease progression, regardless of the opioid administration. The main issue is whether the nurse will allow the suffering to continue until the patient dies or the nurse will attempt to relieve the suffering. It is good nursing practice to relieve the suffering of patients.

Assisted Suicide and Euthanasia

Distinguishing between the two concepts of assisted suicide and euthanasia is important both ethically and legally. Assisted suicide is defined as the act of providing the means to commit suicide knowing that the recipient plans to use the means to end his or her life. Provider-assisted suicide specifically refers to a provider making available medications or other interventions with the understanding that a patient plans to use them to commit suicide and subsequently does so.[32] Euthanasia is defined as someone other than the patient committing an act with the intent to end the person's life. Euthanasia is further divided into (1) voluntary euthanasia, in which an action is taken by another to end the patient's life at the patient's request; and (2) nonvoluntary euthanasia, in which an action is taken by another to end the person's life without the patient's knowledge or consent.[32]

In some states, patients may have the right to request physician aid in dying (PAD). Approximately 18% of all US citizens live in a state that has a legal pathway to PAD.[32] A lethal dose of medications is prescribed to a competent, terminally ill patient to use to end their life. Four states have laws (End of Life Option Act) allowing PAD: California, Oregon, Washington, and Vermont. Additionally, Montana offers PAD as a result of a Supreme Court decision. There are safeguards built into most PAD laws: a patient must have capacity to make decisions, and a second, independent consultant physician must verify the terminal diagnosis.[32]

Because of these moral choices, palliative care and subsequent management of a patient's dying process is often the responsibility of nurses. Ethicists, physicians, and nurses play an active role in the decision-making preceding withdrawal of life support. Ethicists concern themselves with the ethics of the decision-making process, the definition of death, and even considerations about giving pain medications that may be thought to shorten the patient's life. Numerous professional organizations have issued guidelines to assist in this decision-making process and give us an avenue to explore with patients and their families when death becomes imminent. But after the decision is made and goals to a good death are obtained, the ethicists leave, and care of the dying patient is left up to the nurse. A clear understanding of the goals must be specified for this dying patient so a "good death" can be achieved. Many times, the major and only goal is comfort care with family support.

CARE FOR THE CAREGIVER

Some deaths will affect individuals on a significant level, perhaps because the death of the patient may remind us of a death of someone close to us. Death of children, fetal demise, a mass casualty, death of someone the clinician knows, or a particularly horrific, traumatic death can have a profound effect on the clinician. It is important for the clinician to recognize that a death was meaningful to manage the stress of the event. Colleagues must be supportive and discover ways to support each other rather than dismissing the effect the death has on a clinician.

Many strategies can be used to cope with the event. Some strategies can be used immediately after the incident; other strategies are more long term. Examples of strategies include asking to be relieved from care responsibilities and taking a break, if possible; asking for reassignment to another part of the ED, if possible; finding a colleague or friend with whom you can discuss the event—consider speaking with your manager about stress debriefing; self-reflection—taking a moment to reflect on how you feel after exposure to the event. What do you think? How do you behave? Pay attention to any physical symptoms and to thoughts and feelings; use self-monitoring—assess your responses to traumatic situations, and compare them with your normal responses. Minimize the effect of negative thoughts; focus on what you did right. Include therapies that follow basic health principles such as incorporating physical exercise, meditation, humor, music, relaxation (e.g., acupressure, reflexology, therapeutic massage), guided imagery, proper nutrition, and getting adequate rest.[33]

It is important to recognize symptoms and signs of compassion fatigue (burnout) and posttraumatic stress. Working in the ED is hard work with many demands on clinicians' time, resources, and physical and emotional abilities. Recognition of symptoms and signs of traumatic stress is important in maintaining a healthy home and work life. Dealing with death on a constant basis can take its toll on our well-being. Therefore it is imperative to monitor ourselves and each other. Symptoms of compassion fatigue and posttraumatic stress may include increase in the number of sick days, indecision, difficulty with problem solving, isolation or withdrawal, behavioral outbursts, and other distressing symptoms.[33] Signs of burnout or posttraumatic stress may include tachycardia, increased respiratory rate, or elevated blood pressure.[33]

The role of a caregiver can also include family members and friends. Caregivers are defined as any individual who provides formal or informal support and assistance, to individuals with disabilities or long-term conditions. The tasks of caregiving can take a heavy toll on the caregiver. Depression, diminished quality of life, impaired immunity, anxiety, and early death have been linked to caregiving.[5] Additionally, there can be a significant financial burden to family caregivers who have to quit their jobs to care for their loved one. Caring for the family and caregiver is an important component to include in the care provided to a patient in the ED.[5]

SUMMARY

Palliative and end-of-life care are cornerstones of good emergency nursing care and supplement other therapies initiated by nurses in the ED. Technological advances that have brought about improved health care and greater choices in medical services have also resulted in questions concerning not how, but when, to make use of these choices and improvements. People still want to die with dignity, and we as health care providers should enable them to do just that. The manner in which these issues are handled will influence not only the medical outcome but also the quality of patient and family care.

REFERENCES

1. Emanuel L, Quest T, eds. *Education in Palliative and End-of-Life Care for Emergency Medicine*. Chicago, IL: The EPEC Project; 2007.
2. Kelly CT. Death and dying in the emergency department. In: Oman KS, Koziol-McLain J, Scheetz LJ, eds. *Emergency Nursing Secrets*. Philadelphia, PA: Hanley & Belfus; 2001.
3. Puntillo KA, Benner P, Drought T, et al. End-of-life issues in intensive care units: a national random survey of nurses' knowledge and beliefs. *Am J Crit Care*. 2001;10(4):216–229.
4. Rui P, Kang K, National Hospital Ambulatory Medical Care Survey. 2015 *Emergency Department Summary Tables*. http://www.cdc.gov/nchs/data/ahcd/nhamcs_emergency/2015_ed_web_tables.pdf. Published 2015. Accessed April 27, 2019.
5. Chan GK. End-of-life care models and emergency department care. *Acad Emerg Med*. 2004;11(1):79–86.
6. Emergency Nurses Association, American Academy of Pediatrics, American College of Emergency Physicians. *Death of a child in the emergency department [Joint Technical Report]*. Des Plaines, IL: Emergency Nurses Association; 2013:1–24. https://www.ena.org/docs/default-source/resource-library/practice-resources/white-papers/deathofachildined-jointtechnicalreport.pdf?sfvrsn=b78f4ea3_4. Accessed May 22, 2018.
7. George N, Barrett N, McPeake L, Goett R, Anderson K, Baird J. Content validation of a novel screening tool to identify emergency department patients with significant palliative care needs. *Acad Emerg Med*. 2015;22(7):823–837.
8. Institute of Medicine (US). Committee on care at the end of life. In: Field MJ, Cassel CK, eds. *Approaching Death: Improving Care at the End of Life*. Washington, DC: National Academies Press; 1997.
9. Hosker CM, Bennett MI. Delirium and agitation at the end of life. *BMJ*. 2016;353:i3085.
10. Luce JM, Alpers A. End-of-life care: what do the American courts say? *Crit Care Med*. 2001;29(suppl 2):N40–N45.
11. McClain K, Perkins P. Terminally ill patients in the emergency department: a practical overview of end-of-life issues. *J Emerg Nurs*. 2002;28(6):515–522.
12. International Association for the Study of Pain. IASP Terminology. https://www.iasp-pain.org/Education/Content.aspx?ItemNumber=1698. Published 2017. Accessed June 8, 2018.
13. McCaffery M, Pasero C. *Pain: Clinical Manual*. 2nd ed. St Louis, MO: Mosby; 1999.
14. Dunwoody CJ, Arnold R. Fast facts and concepts #39: using naloxone. https://mypcnow.org/blank-fnbfg. Published 2015. Accessed June 25, 2018.
15. Hallenback J. Fast facts and concept #5: The causes of nausea and vomiting (V.O.M.I.T.). https://www.mypcnow.org/blank-ggr79. Published 2015. Accessed June 25, 2018.
16. Weissman DE. Fast facts and concepts #25: opioids and nausea. https://www.mypcnow.org/blank-f0hxt. Published 2015. Accessed May 12, 2018.
17. Mierendorf S, Gidvani V. Palliative care in the emergency department. *Perm J*. 2014;18(2):77–85.
18. Baren JM. Family presence during invasive medical procedures: the struggle for an option. *Acad Emerg Med*. 2005;12(5):463–466.
19. Helmer SD, Smith RS, Dort JM, Shapiro WM, Katan BS. Family presence during trauma resuscitation: a survey of AAST and ENA members. *J Trauma*. 2000;48(6):1015–1024.
20. Long C. Cultural and spiritual considerations in palliative care. *J Pediatr Hematol Oncol*. 2011;33:S96–S101.
21. Wang D. Beyond code status: palliative care begins in the emergency department. *Ann Emerg Med*. 2017;69(4):437–443.
22. Walters DT, Tupin JP. Family grief in the emergency department. *Emerg Med Clin North Am*. 1991;9(1):189–206.
23. Iserson KV. The gravest words: sudden-death notifications and emergency care. *Ann Emerg Med*. 2000;36(1):75–77.
24. Li SP, Chan CW, Lee DT. Helpfulness of nursing actions to suddenly bereaved family members in an accident and emergency setting in Hong Kong. *J Adv Nurs*. 2002;40(2):170–180.
25. Chan GK. *Trajectories of Approaching Death in The Emergency Department*. Nice, France: Paper presented at: 3rd Mediterranean Emergency Medicine Congress; 2005:1–5.
26. Chan GK. End-of-life issues in the emergency department. In: Hoyt KS, Selfridge-Thomas J, eds. *Emergency Nursing Core Curriculum*. St Louis, MO: Saunders; 2007.
27. Campbell M, Zalenski R. The emergency department. In: Ferrell BR, Coyle N, eds. *Textbook of Palliative Care*. 2nd ed. New York, NY: Oxford University Press; 2006.
28. Emergency Nurses Association. *Position statement: Palliative and end-of-life care in the emergency setting*. Des Plaines, IL: Emergency Nurses Association; 2013:1–4. https://www.ena.org/docs/default-source/resource-library/practice-resources/position-statements/palliativeendoflifecare.pdf?sfvrsn=1777bb45_6. Accessed May 12, 2018.
29. National Consensus Project. National Consensus Project. https://www.nationalcoalitionhpc.org/ncp/. Accessed April 27, 2019.
30. American College of Emergency Physicians. Ethical issues at the end of life. https://www.acep.org/patient-care/policy-statements/ethical-issues-at-the-end-of-life/#sm.0012vrsdx1dw2cyb11sp8n274un75. Updated April 2014. Accessed June 29, 2018.
31. Sulmasy DP. Commentary: double effect—intention is the solution, not the problem. *J Law Med Ethics*. 2000;28(1):26–29.
32. Strouse T. End-of-life options and the legal pathways to physician aid in dying. *J Community Support Oncol*. 2017;15(1):1–3.
33. Badger JM. Understanding secondary traumatic stress. *Am J Nurs*. 2001;101(7):26–32.

15

Organ and Tissue Donation

Nancy Bonalumi

Twenty people die in the United States each day because of the lack of an organ to provide a lifesaving transplant. In 2017 more than 114,000 people were on the organ donor waiting list in the United States, but only 34,770 transplants were performed.[1] Two out of every three people on the waiting list are over the age of 60, almost 2000 children under age 18 are listed, and approximately 58% of the people on this list are ethnic minorioties.[1] The lack of organs is the result of a lack of organ donors. Ninety-five percent of US adults support organ donation; however, only 54% are signed up as organ donors.[1] Four of five donations come from deceased donors. Living donors, primarily of kidneys, contributed more than 6100 organs[1] in 2017.

Everyone who is near death or dies in the hospital should be considered a potential candidate for organ donation. Hospitals are required to give families of the deceased an opportunity to authorize donation of a family member's tissue and/or organ according to federal law.[2] There are very few absolute exclusion criteria (Table 15.1) and no firm upper or lower age limits.[3] Yet, despite the increased public awareness and expressed willingness to support organ donation, the number of people waiting for transplants outpaces potential donors by more than three to one.[4]

Barriers to donation include failure of hospitals to identify potential donors and notify an organ procurement organization (OPO), failure to discuss donation with families, use of requestors who are not knowledgeable about the donation process, and cultural barriers between potential donor families and the medical staff who are discussing donation. Identifying potential donors and improving the authorization process are needed to give families wanting to donate that opportunity.[5]

In the emergency department (ED) setting it is imperative to determine the potential for donation from patients who have died or whose death is imminent. Emergency nurses have a unique and vital role to play in supporting the decision-making and organ procurement processes. The emergency nurse's presence with patients and families during critical moments provides an opportunity to disseminate information, ascertain the patient's or family's wishes, and safeguard that those wishes are followed. The emergency nurse should ensure that the local OPO is contacted so that trained designated requestors approach families about donation. If the ED staff are involved in the request process, families may get the impression that the people caring for their loved one may not be providing appropriate lifesaving care if they are anticipating organ donation.

OVERVIEW AND HISTORY

The first reported medical transplant occurred in the third century. Significant advances in medical transplantation began early in the 20th century with the first successful transplant of a cornea (Table 15.2).

Improved surgical techniques and a sequence of three events resulted in transplants becoming a viable option to save and meaningfully extend lives. The first event was the development in the late 1960s of neurologic criteria for determining death. This criterion allowed a person to be declared dead upon the cessation of all brain activity. The second event, occurring shortly after Dr. Christiaan Barnard's successful transplant of a heart in November 1967, was the adoption of the Uniform Anatomical Gift Act in 1968. An important feature of the act created the right to donate organs, eyes, and tissue, allowing individuals to donate their or their loved one's organs or tissues. The Uniform Anatomical Gift Act was revised in 1987, 2006, and again in 2013 to address changes in circumstances and in practice.[6] The third event was the development of immunosuppressive drugs that prevented organ recipients from rejecting transplanted organs. This permitted many more successful organ transplants, thus contributing to the rapid growth in the demand for organs.

In 1984 the US Congress passed the National Organ Transplant Act to address the nation's critical organ donation shortage and improve the organ matching and placement process. This act established the Organ Procurement and Transplantation Network (OPTN) (https://optn.transplant.hrsa.gov) to maintain a national registry for organ matching. The OPTN seeks to ensure the success and efficiency of the US organ transplant system.[7] The goals of the OPTN are to increase the number of and access to transplants, improve survival rates after transplantation, and promote patient safety and efficient management of the system. OPTN has contracted with the United Network for Organ Sharing (UNOS) since 1986 to implement the National Organ Transplant Act. Responsibilities overseen by UNOS include facilitating the organ matching and placement process through its Organ Center operating 24

TABLE 15.1 Absolute and Relative Contraindications for Organ Donation.

Absolute Contraindications	Relative Contraindications
• Age older than 80 yr • Human immunodeficiency infection • Active metastatic cancer • Prolonged hypotension or hypothermia • Disseminated intravascular coagulation • Sickle cell anemia or other hemoglobinopathy	• Malignancy other than in the central nervous system or skin that is in remission (>5 yr) • Hypertension • Diabetes mellitus • Physiologic age older than 70 yr • Hepatitis B or C • History of smoking

Sweet V. *Emergency Nursing: Core Curriculum*. 7th ed. St Louis, MO: Elsevier; 2018:80–89.

hours a day; developing consensus-based policies and procedures for organ recovery, distribution (allocation) and transportation; collecting and managing scientific data about organ donation and transplantation; maintaining a secure computer system containing the nation's organ transplant waiting list and recipient/donor organ characteristics; and providing professional and public education about donation and transplantation and the critical need for donation. Under federal law, all US transplant centers and OPOs must be members of the OPTN to receive any funds through Medicare[8] (Table 15.3).

Hospitals are required to work collaboratively with their local OPO to contact them in a timely manner about individuals whose death is imminent or who die in the hospital. Only OPO staff or trained hospital staff referred to as designated requestors should approach families about organ donation. A designated requestor is defined in the rule as an individual who has completed a course offered or approved by the OPO.[7–9]

ORGAN DONATION BEST PRACTICES

Organizational Structure

Hospitals should have a strong culture of accountability, with hospital leadership across many levels and disciplines (administrators, physicians, nurses, etc.) participating in organ donation initiatives. A collaborative and integrated relationship between hospitals, local OPOs, transplant centers, and medical examiners' offices is desired. Benchmarking donation rates against local and national levels is encouraged.[1]

Early Referral

Initial identification of potential donors often occurs in the ED setting. The hospital is required to notify the OPO of patients who have died or who are mechanically ventilated and whose death is imminent. This is mandated by the Centers for Medicare and Medicaid Services[8] and is a Joint Commission standard.[9] Developing "triggers," such as a low Glasgow Coma Scale score, may assist ED providers with identifying patients at risk for progression to death. Early notification of a potential donor gives the local OPO representative adequate time to determine the suitability of the donor and to prepare the family for the request to donate a loved one's organs or tissue.

Cultural Competence

Information about organ donation and the request for donation must be delivered in the most culturally sensitive and efficacious manner.[5] One successful strategy has been to train requestors who mirror the community population, which reduces cultural and language barriers. Historically, minorities donate at a significantly lower rate. Research has identified that donor registration has a positive effect on increasing authorization rates of potential donors. Public education efforts targeted at minority communities to increase donor registration is a strategy that OPOs and health care systems should consider in addition to in-hospital assessment and approach techniques.[10]

First Person Authorization

Under the regulations of the Uniform Anatomical Gift Act, a person may authorize organ donation after death. The legal basis upon which human organs and tissues can be donated for transplantation is based on the principles of the Uniform Anatomical Gift Act, not informed consent, which applies to health care treatment decisions. The Uniform Anatomical Gift Act requires three elements: intent, transfer, and acceptance. As such, donating an organ is a voluntary, legally binding, uncompensated transfer from one individual to another. The donor's autonomous decision should be considered final and cannot be overruled by family[11] (Box 15.1).

In-House Coordinators

Donor referrals and organ donation are increased when a local OPO assigns an in-house coordinator to large trauma centers.[12] The role of the in-house coordinator is to be a member of the acute care team and to represent the local OPO. Being onsite improves communications, increases the use of standards and audits as tools to improve performance, and allows the coordinator to serve as a liaison between clinical teams, local OPOs, and donor families.[12]

OTHER STRATEGIES TO INCREASE ORGAN DONATION

Living Donor Donation

Although most organ and tissue donations occur after the donor has died, some organs and tissues can be donated while the donor is alive. The first successful transplant in the United States was made possible by a living donor and took place in 1954. A man donated a kidney to his identical twin brother. As a result of the growing need for organs for transplantation, living donations have increased as an alternative to deceased donation, with more than 6000 living donations taking place each year. Most living donations occur between family members or close friends. Single kidney donation is the most frequent living donor procedure. Living individuals can donate one of their two kidneys, and the remaining kidney provides the donor with the necessary function needed to remove waste from his or her body. A living

TABLE 15.2 **Milestones in Organ and Tissue Transplantation.**

Date	Event
1682	Meekran attempted to replace a portion of a soldier's cranium with the skull bone from a dog.
1800	Corneal graft surgery was performed by Wolfe.
1860s	Grahm developed and used a wooden hoop dialyzer to treat renal failure patients.
1881	Skin grafting was tried as a temporary means for treating a severe burn.
1893	Williams attempted transplanting a sheep's pancreas into a human.
1902	Ullman attempted transplanting kidneys in a goat model.
1940s	Sir Peter Medawar treated skin grafts with cold refrigeration; he also worked on immune response and rejection phenomenon.
1940s	Kolft designed the dialysis machine that is the basis for machines used today.
1954	Merrill and colleagues implemented dialysis therapy.
1954	Murray and Harrison performed the first kidney transplantation between living identical twins.
1963	Starzl performed the first liver transplantation.
1963	Hardy performed the first lung transplantation.
1967	Lillehei performed the first kidney and pancreas transplantation.
1967	Barnard performed the first heart transplantation.
1968	Uniform Anatomical Gift Act of 1968 was adopted as law in all 50 states. The law allows the individual to decide to become an organ or tissue donor and introduces the option of donor cards to identify the person's wishes.
1968	*Harvard Criteria for Determination of Brain Death* was published.
1981	Shumway performed the first heart-lung transplantation.
1984	Organ Transplant Act (PL 98-507) was passed.
1986	Report of Organ Transplantation Task Force was published, which led to the development of the United Network for Organ Sharing (UNOS), a private, nonprofit agency that serves as a clearinghouse for organs and tissues.
1986	The United States was divided into 11 UNOS regions with a single organ procurement organization (OPO) designated for each region. Visit https://optn.transplant.hrsa.gov/members/regions/ for more information.
1987	Consolidated Omnibus Reconciliation Act of 1986 (PL 99-272) was revised so hospitals receiving Medicare funding must meet standards for education of patients and staff.
Late 1980s	Uniform Anatomical Gift Act was passed on a state-by-state basis.
1996	Congress authorized mailing organ and tissue donation information with income tax refunds (sent to approximately 70 million households).
1997	National Organ and Tissue Donation Initiative was launched by the US Department of Health and Human Services to increase the number of organs and tissues available for donation. The final rule for organ, tissue, and eye donation for hospitals to participate in Medicare and Medicaid was published.
1998	Final rule for donation took effect, which requires each hospital to contact their OPO in a timely manner about those whose death is imminent or those who die in the hospital. Provisions limit discussion of donation to OPO staff or trained hospital staff.
2002	Up-to-the-minute data on the number of people waiting for organ transplants in the United States became available online through the Organ Procurement and Transplantation Network (OPTN).
2003	Secretary of the US Department of Health and Human Services, Tommy G. Thompson, designated April as National Donate Life Month.
2003	The Organ Donation Breakthrough Collaborative was launched by the US Department of Health and Human Services to increase donation in the nation's largest hospitals by implementing an intensive and highly focused program to promote widespread use of best practices. In 2005 transplant centers joined the initiative with the goal of increasing the number of organs per donor. A revised version of the program continues today as the Donation and Transplantation Community of Practice.
2004	Organ Donation and Recovery Improvement Act (PL 108-216) expanded authorities of the National Organ Transplant Act to, among other things, provide reimbursement of travel and subsistence expenses for living organ donors, and grants to states and public entities.
2005	The first successful partial face transplant was performed in France.
2006	Institute of Medicine (IOM) released a new report, Organ Donation: Opportunities for Action. The IOM examined the ethical and societal implications of numerous strategies to increase deceased donation and considered several ethical issues regarding living donation, resulting in the presentation of 17 recommendations for action.
2010	The first successful full-face transplant was conducted at Vall d'Hebron Hospital, Spain.
2014	Vascularized composite allographs (VCAs) is added to the definition of organs covered by federal regulation (the OPTN Final Rule) and legislation (the National Organ Transplant Act). The designation went into effect on July 3, 2014.

TABLE 15.3 Conditions of Participation: Organ, Tissue, and Eye Procurement.

Organ Procurement Responsibilities	Organ Transplantation Responsibilities
The hospital must have and implement written protocols which: • Incorporate an agreement with an OPO which it must notify, in a timely manner of individuals whose death is imminent or who have died in the hospital; • The OPO determines medical suitability for organ donation and medical suitability for tissue and eye donation • Incorporate an agreement with at least one tissue bank and at least one eye bank to cooperate in the retrieval, processing, preservation, storage and distribution of tissues and eyes, as may be appropriate to assure all usable tissues and eyes are obtained from potential donors, insofar as such an agreement does not interfere with organ procurement; • Ensure, in collaboration with the designated OPO, that the family of each potential donor is informed of its options to donate organs, tissues, or eyes or to decline to donate. The individual designated by the hospital to initiate the request to the family must be an organ procurement representative or a designated requestor; • A designated requestor is an individual who has completed a course offered or approved by the OPO and designed in conjunction with the tissue and eye bank community in the methodology for approaching potential donor families and requesting organ or tissue donation; • Encourage discretion and sensitivity with respect to the circumstances, views, and beliefs of the families of potential donors; • Ensure the hospital works cooperatively with the designated OPO, tissue bank and eye bank in educating staff on donation issues, reviewing death records to improve identification of potential donors, and maintaining potential donors while necessary testing and placement of potential donated organs, tissues, and eyes take place.	• A hospital in which organ transplants are performed must be a member of the Organ Procurement and Transplantation Network (OPTN). • If a hospital performs any type of transplants, it must provide organ-transplant-related data, as requested by the OPTN, the Scientific Registry, and the OPOs.

OPO, Organ procurement organization.
42CFR 482.45. Condition of participation: Organ, tissue, and eye procurement. (n.d.). https://www.law.cornell.edu/cfr/text/42/482.45. Accessed April 27, 2019.

BOX 15.1 First Person Authorization.

(Individuals have the right to make a legally binding anatomical gift prior to death.)

FPA must be honored and decision is final *(UAGA Section 8)*	Permission from family is not warranted	Law states: donor's decision is not subject to change by others	Family does not have power, right or authority to consent to, amend or revoke decision	Hospital team's obligation: to respect and honor autonomy rights of the donor *(UAGA C.26:6–89)*

FPA, First person authorization; *UAGA,* Uniform Anatomical Gift Act.
Organ Donation and Transplantation Alliance. First person authorization [table]. In: Legal aspects of a registered donor: what you need to know. Hospital C-Suite Snapshot Series. https://organdonationalliance.org/wp-content/uploads/2017/10/CSuite-Snapshot-Fall-2017-FINAL.pdf. Published Fall 2017. Accessed April 27, 2019.

donor can donate one of two lobes of his or her liver. This is possible because liver cells in the remaining lobe of the liver grow or regenerate until the liver is almost back to its original size. This regrowth of the liver occurs in a short time in both the liver donor and the liver recipient. It is also possible for living donors to donate a lung or part of a lung, part of the pancreas, or part of the intestines. Although these organs do not regenerate, both the donated portion of the organ and the portion remaining with the donor are fully functioning.[13]

Each potential living donor is evaluated to determine his or her suitability to donate. The evaluation examines the expected psychological and physical responses to the donation process. This is done to minimize the risk that an adverse outcome will occur before, during, or after the donation. Generally, living donors should be physically fit, in good health, between the ages of 18 and 60, and be screened for the presence of absolute and relative contraindications to be an organ donor.[2] The decision to be a living donor must be weighed carefully as to the benefits versus the risks for both the donor and the recipient. Often the recipient has very little risk because the transplant will be lifesaving. However, the healthy donor does face the risk of an unnecessary major surgical procedure and recovery. Living donors may also face other risks. A small percentage of donors have had problems with maintaining life, disability, or medical insurance coverage at the same level and rate once donation has occurred. Living donors may also have financial concerns because of possible delays in returning to work due to unforeseen medical problems.[13]

Donation After Circulatory Death

Approximately three out of every four organs that are transplanted are recovered from deceased donors. The most rapid increase in organ recovery from deceased donors is in the category of donation after circulatory death (DCD). This is defined as death declared on the basis of cardiopulmonary criteria (irreversible cessation of circulatory and respiratory function) rather than the neurologic criteria used to declare "brain death" (irreversible loss of all functions of the entire brain).[14] A DCD donor may be called a nonheartbeating, asystolic, or donation after cardiac death donor.

The process of obtaining organs from donors after cardiac death was common until the development of brain-death criteria. Organ procurement and preservation techniques were primitive, and the physiologic functions of organs from brain-dead, heart-beating donors were superior.[1] Given the critical shortage of organs and improved preservation techniques, organ recovery from nonheart-beating donors has reemerged.[15]

The Organ Procurement and Transplantation Network/United Network for Organ Sharing (OPTN/UNOS) has developed rules for DCD.[14] These rules describe the organ recovery process after death by irreversible cessation of circulatory and respiratory functions. Potential DCD donors are patients who have died or for whom death is imminent. They also include patients when the decision is made that medical interventions no longer offer a benefit to them, as determined by the patient, the patient's authorized surrogate, or the patient's advance directive, and there is a decision to withdraw care. Life-sustaining measures are withdrawn under controlled circumstances in the surgical setting. Once the donor is pronounced dead, the organs are then recovered. To avoid obvious conflicts of interest, neither the surgeon nor others involved in the organ procurement can participate in the end-of-life care or declaration of death.[6]

The Joint Commission Transplant Safety accreditation standard requires hospitals to have a written donation policy that addresses organ donation after cardiac death. The hospital, medical staff, and OPO must document how they will approach asystolic recovery.[9]

Presumptive Consent

Refusal by families to consent to donation is a major barrier to organ donation. Presumptive consent, or an "opt-in" approach to organ donation, switches the donation authorization from having donors specifically sign up, such as through a designation on a driver's license, to assuming everyone is a donor unless stated otherwise. Some version of opt-out organ donation exists in about 30 European nations, including Spain, Belgium, France, and Wales.[16] Historically, requestors use a "value-neutral" approach in which organ donation is described in an unbiased manner. Consent is achieved by overcoming all the objections a family has to the organ donation concept. The traditional request for consent often has led to a negative reply simply because the family is unable to make one more decision in an overwhelmingly stressful time. Presumptive consent assumes the donor has a desire to help others and save lives. The benefits of donation are emphasized, and the clinical aspects of donation, which often generate a visceral response in the family, are avoided. Ongoing research on this method of obtaining consent will determine whether this method is successful in increasing the rate of organ donation.[17,18]

THE DONATION PROCESS

When a patient dies, the local OPO representative determines whether the patient is a potential organ or tissue donor. Four key steps must be completed before the retrieval of organs or tissue:

1. determination and declaration of death
2. medical examiner's approval (as required by state law)
3. notification of the local OPO
4. consent from the next of kin

Determination of Death

A patient must be declared dead for the donation process to begin. Traditionally, death was believed to occur when a person's heart stopped beating. As technology evolved, a patient could be maintained on mechanical support devices. Consequently, determination of death by brain-death criteria became a recognized practice. The 1981 Uniform Determination of Death Act defines brain death in the following manner: an individual who has sustained either (1) irreversible cessation of circulatory or respiratory functions or (2) irreversible cessation of all functions of the entire brain, including the brainstem.[19] A determination of death must be made in accordance with accepted medical standards. After death has been determined, it must be documented in the patient's medical record, including the time of death. If the local OPO has not evaluated the patient for suitability as a donor, then required notification is undertaken at this time, before a designated requestor discusses donation with the family.

Medical Examiner's Approval

It is estimated that as many as 70% of potential organ donors fall under medical examiner/coroner (ME/C) jurisdiction.[20] OPOs must have approval from the ME/C before proceeding to organ and tissue procurement in these cases, regardless of patient or family consent or donation wishes. The national Association of Medical Examiners position statement on organ and tissue donation states that ME/Cs should permit organs and tissue procurement in cases falling under their jurisdiction, providing that there are cooperative agreements in place to ensure that ME/Cs are able to fulfill their legal mandates regarding determination of cause and manner of death and of appropriate collection and preservation of evidence.[20]

Although medical examiner regulations vary from state to state, in general, a medical examiner must be notified when death takes place under certain circumstances, including the following:

1. homicide
2. suicide
3. accidental death
4. death within 24 hours of admission
5. when the patient is admitted in a coma-like state and dies
6. for the death of a person 18 years of age or younger

Notation of communication with the medical examiner should be included in the patient's medical record.

Obtaining Consent for Donation

Emergency nurses are often the first to interact with and provide support to families of potential donors. Supporting the family or next of kin in the donation process is one of the more difficult yet potentially rewarding responsibilities that emergency nurses assume in their professional careers. Assisting a family through the donation process offers the family a measure of comfort and consolation. The comfort is not necessarily experienced at the time of the death, but later, when the death has been realized. Knowing that their loved one has been able to help another often helps families cope with the loss and continue their lives.

The best person to support the family through donation is a professional who has developed a rapport with the family. The person designated to carry out this responsibility should be familiar with the donation process and comfortable with his or her own feelings about death and the donation of tissues and organs. Emergency nurses are in an ideal position to support the family during the process of donation. They have been working with the family and patient throughout the admission and have in most situations developed the greatest rapport with the family.

Physicians, emergency nurses, social workers, and pastoral care providers are all examples of team members that contribute to the donation process. The local OPO representative, designated requestor, and family supporter are key roles in the process. Each hospital, in collaboration with the local OPO, will determine who fills these roles. The person who approaches the family about donation and who provides information about donation to the family must be a trained designated requestor or local OPO representative. The emergency nurse may participate as a supporter or designated requestor in the process, dependent on training and hospital protocols. Emergency nurses in supporter roles may need less intense training than individuals in requestor roles. Each institution may have an established protocol for offering donation to a family, and this protocol should be given consideration before proceeding.

Some institutions may have a program in collaboration with the local OPO to train staff members as designated requestors. These requestors, along with the local OPO staff, are the only people who can approach families about their options for donation. The emergency nurse caring for the patient who has just died may not be familiar with the process of donation. The requestor can be a great resource and can assist with the process. The nurse can also talk to the local OPO for support in this matter; a coordinator from the agency can obtain consent from the family in person or over the telephone. Telephone consent requires two witnesses on the phone to confirm donation. An ED education program can be requested concerning the donation process.

The Effect of Family Presence During Resuscitation on Organ Donation

Many EDs across the United States are offering the option of family presence during resuscitation. (See Chapter 12.) Family presence is most commonly defined as "the presence of family in the patient care area, in a location that affords visual or physical contact with the patient during invasive procedures or resuscitation events."[21] Studies have found that family members who remained with relatives during resuscitation reported that the experience removed doubt about what was happening and reinforced that everything possible was done. Family members who do not choose the option to be present during resuscitation may be more likely to suffer psychological difficulties during bereavement. The option to be present during a resuscitation should be given to families when the patient's clinical condition indicates the patient may not survive.[22]

Notification of Death

Before the family is made aware of the opportunity to donate organs or tissue, they must be told the patient has died. The family must be comfortable with the knowledge that everything possible was done to prevent death and all available treatments were implemented. The family's sense of devastation may be extreme; members are grieving and unlikely to believe that death has occurred. Discussion of anything immediately after the discussion of death may be impossible. The family needs time to grieve and to grasp what has happened before they are asked to consider another critical decision.

Patients who survive a critical event may be admitted to a critical care setting, where a series of tests is administered to determine that the criteria for brain death have been met. When death is to be declared by brain-death criteria, the family has more time to adjust to the death. Helping the family understand that death has occurred is difficult. Information must be provided for the family by the primary physician in terms they can understand and must be educationally reinforced by the primary nurse and other available health care professionals.

When the patient in the ED is declared dead by the criterion of cardiac asystole, death is physically more obvious to the family. Grasping the reality of the event is poignant. Death as a result of cardiac arrest is recognized as a tangible end point. Family members have less time to consider possible options or treatments and to adjust to their loss. Donation after cardiac death is an option that can be offered to families in this circumstance.

Emotions can be labile. The family may be in shock, engulfed by many different emotions and feelings. Before the option of donation is presented, family members should be given time to gain control of their thoughts and adjust, if possible, to the reality that a family member has died and is not going to return.

Family Assessment and Support

Family members in the ED should be provided a private room or a comfortable, quiet location that allows those present an opportunity to share feelings of loss and grief. Realizing that the family member is dead is the greatest hurdle the family must overcome. Viewing the body of the person who has just died can be a critical step in this process. A support person such as a chaplain or social worker should be available if the family chooses to view the deceased. Being culturally competent in the beliefs and practices of various religious, racial, and ethnic groups surrounding death is crucial to successfully caring for the family of the deceased.

Assessment of what the family knows or what they have been told is of great importance before offering the option of donation. Until the family can accept that death has occurred, donation should not be discussed. The family must hear the words *death* and *dead* when references are made to the status of its family member. A common error in health care is to refer to the death euphemistically, for example, saying the patient "has expired," "passed on," "will no longer be with us," or "it is over." Saying the word *dead* when talking to the family is straightforward and prevents misinterpretation. Because of shock and denial, the family may not comprehend the effect of the message that there is "no hope" for their loved one. This understanding is critical in the case of the family of a patient considered dead by brain-death criteria.

Other goals when assessing the family should include assessment of the family's cultural and religious background and its effect on donation. A decision not to offer donation because of religious and cultural biases based on assumptions about the family's last name and background is inappropriate. The choice belongs to the family.

If a family says no to donation, the response is perfectly reasonable. Donation is not an option for every family or every person. Whatever the decision about donation, it is the right one for that family or person and should be accepted. The emergency nurse's role is to support the family as they make the decision.

Family Education

The family needs information about donation to decide what is right for the family and what the family member would have wished. Detailed, understandable information is essential. The family should not be coerced into a decision about donation and its benefits, even if using a presumptive approach to consent.

The family should know that if they authorize donation, the donation will be carried out promptly. A slight chance exists of changes in physical appearance related to incisions required for different donations. The family should know that this causes no disfigurement that would prevent an open casket or alter funeral arrangements. Although it is important to address the topic of disfigurement, it is also very important to discuss the benefits of organ donation, as discussed in the section on presumptive consent.

Because there are so few absolute exclusion criteria today, the screening questions families must answer are minimal. Tissue and organ retrieval occur after authorization is given by the family and when recovery teams can be arranged to recover the tissue.

Procurement of internal organs and some tissue takes place in an operating suite. Multitissue, multiorgan procurement procedures are usually completed in 4 to 5 hours from the time the procurement begins. The local OPO provides technical staff to recover the eyes, valves, and skin. If the family made special funeral arrangements, they should inform the emergency nurse or donation coordinator of those plans. Eyes may be recovered in the morgue.

A donation coordinator from the local OPO is available for support during any donation process. For most donations of internal organs, the coordinator comes to the hospital to evaluate the patient and meet the family, obtains consent from the family, and coordinates the donation procurement process. In the case of tissue donation only, the coordinator is less likely to be at the hospital but is available for consultation and the availability of necessary support. The coordinator works with the emergency nurse, other contact staff at the hospital, and the respective procurement teams.

THE PROCUREMENT PROCESS

Tissue and organ donors are managed differently. The potential organ donor declared brain dead still has a beating heart. Patients who are donors after cardiac death or who are tissue donors have been declared dead and have a nonbeating heart. Management of the tissue or organ donor is discussed in the next sections. These patients must be managed carefully to ensure viable tissues and/or organs for transplant. Tissues and organs that can be transplanted are listed in Box 15.2.

Tissue Procurement

Tissue procurement is less complex than internal organ procurement. The coordinator from the procurement agency arranges for the services of a recovery team and works with nursing staff in the operating suite to set up surgery times and conditions convenient for all parties involved.

Maximum time allowed for recovery of tissue after asystole is approximately 10 hours for bone, 6 to 10 hours for heart valves, and 24 hours for corneas and skin. These time limits may vary, depending on the procurement agency and availability of refrigeration. The preferred time of recovery is the time closest to asystole.

After death, the eye donor should be maintained in a refrigerated room if available, with the head elevated at 20 degrees and the eyes taped closed with paper tape. Artificial

BOX 15.2 Transplantable Organs and Tissues.

Tissue	Organ
Cornea	Liver
Bone	Kidney
Pancreatic islet cell	Heart
Bone marrow	Pancreas
Ligaments	Intestines
Tendons	
Heart valves	
Skin	
Veins	
Middle ear	

tears may be instilled in each eye before taping, but this is not mandatory. Cool compresses can be placed over the eyes to prevent swelling and ease the procurement process. Recovery of eyes is a clean procedure using sterile technique and requires only 20 to 30 minutes. The eye tissue is packed in preservative solution; the container is placed on ice and dispatched to the respective eye recovery center for processing. Corneas are generally transplanted within 24 to 48 hours.

For recovery of heart valves, the entire heart is removed from the donor. The valves are dissected from the heart, their integrity examined, and the entire heart examined for pathologic conditions. Serologic examinations are performed, and after a brief quarantine, usually 40 days, valves are released for homograft transplant according to size and need. The donor has a single incision on the chest, which does not prevent an open casket if the family so wishes.

Skin recovery can also take place in the morgue. A clean room and sterile technique are required. A dermatome is used to recover skin from the buttocks, thighs, back, and abdomen. A split-thickness graft, removed from the top surface of the body, is barely visible unless the donor has a dark tan or is of high pigment. After skin is recovered, it is treated with antibiotics, prepared surgically for grafting, and stored at 70°F. The recovered skin is used for temporary grafts in severely burned patients to provide protection from infection, fluid shifts, and other complications of burns.

Solid-Organ Procurement

Recovery of solid organs for transplant is complex and requires the cooperation of a multidisciplinary team. The OPO coordinator will oversee the clinical management of the donor, ensuring adherence to the following interventions, including monitoring vital signs and fluid intake and output, maintaining blood pressure for perfusion of vital organs, and using IV therapy and medications, including antibiotics.[14]

After the patient has been accepted as a donor and all organs to be recovered have been assigned to receiving patients, recovery teams convene. The donor is transported to the operating room fully supported by mechanical means and is hemodynamically maintained in the operating room according to goals outlined previously. The donor is maintained throughout the organ dissection and mobilization of the respective tissues until organs and tissues are freed for immediate removal and preservation. Organs are removed from the donor, examined individually in a sterile basin, flushed with preservative solution, and packed in a sterile container for transport or immediate transplant (in the case of the heart, heart and lung, and single lung). For kidneys, approximately 24 hours may elapse before transplantation takes place. For the pancreas and liver, time to transplant ranges from 6 to 20 hours. Tissue typing is primarily carried out between kidney donor and recipient and in some cases between heart, heart and lung, and single-lung donor and recipient.

FINANCIAL CONSIDERATIONS

The donor's family does not pay for any costs associated with patient management or donation from the time the patient has brain death criteria established through organ procurement. The recipient, third-party insurance, Medicare, or Medicaid pays all costs related to the donation. All charges related to the donation process should be removed from the deceased donor's bill. The local OPO coordinator should inform the family of this during the discussion about consent.

The average cost of transplantation in 2017 ranged from $414,000 for a single kidney to more than $2.5 million for multiorgan transplants such as heart-lung or kidney-heart.[23] Health insurance may cover some or most of these costs, but insurance policies vary widely. Medicare and Medicaid are publicly funded health insurance programs that can help eligible people pay for the costs of transplantation.[6]

SUMMARY

The emergency nurse has significant responsibility related to tissue and organ donation. By contacting the local OPO, emergency nurses provide the family with the opportunity to donate tissue and/or organs when a patient meets the criteria for brain death or dies in the ED. It is important for emergency nurses to be knowledgeable about the identification of potential donors, life support of potential donors, and accessing resource personnel from state or local transplant teams. It is within the role of the emergency nurse to facilitate, coordinate, and intervene with families of potential organ donors.

For too long, the concept of donation has been associated solely with trauma victims: patients maintained and declared dead by brain-death criteria in the critical care setting. Almost any person who dies can be a donor of some tissue or organ for transplantation. This is an integral part of the emergency nursing care for patients and families in crisis.

REFERENCES

1. US Department of Health and Human Services. Organ Donation Statistics. https://www.organdonor.gov/statistics-stories/statistics.html. Updated January 2019. Accessed April 27, 2019.
2. Sweet V. *Emergency Nursing: Core Curriculum*. 7th ed. St Louis, MO: Elsevier; 2018:80–89.
3. Finge EB. Organ procurement considerations in trauma [overview, organ distribution, criteria for organ donors]. Medscape website. https://emedicine.medscape.com/article/434643-overview. Updated January 4, 2016. Accessed April 27, 2019.
4. US Department of Health and Human Services. Organ Procurement and Transplantation Network. https://optn.transplant.hrsa.gov/. (n.d.). Accessed April 27, 2019.

5. Shemie SD, Robertson A, Beitel J, et al. End-of-life conversations with families of potential donors. *Transplantation*. 2017;101(5S suppl 1):S17–S26. https://doi.org/10.1097/tp.0000000000001696.
6. Anatomical Gift Act Summary. (n.d.). https://www.uniformlaws.org/committees/community-home?CommunityKey=155faf5d-03c2-4027-99ba-ee4c99019d6c. Accessed April 27, 2019.
7. Organ Procurement and Transplantation Network. [USC03] 42 USC 274 (n.d.). http://uscode.house.gov/view.xhtml?hl=-false&edition=prelim&req=granuleid:USC-2014-title42-section274&num=0.
8. Condition of participation: Organ, tissue, and eye procurement. 42 CFR 482.45. (n.d.). Cornell Law School Legal Information Institute website. https://www.law.cornell.edu/cfr/text/42/482.45.
9. Transplant safety. The Joint Commission website. https://www.jointcommission.org/. (n.d.).
10. Shah MB, Vilchez V, Goble A, et al. Socioeconomic factors as predictors of organ donation. *J Surg Res*. 2018;221:88–94. https://doi.org/10.1016/j.jss.2017.08.020.
11. Samuel L. To solve organ shortage, states consider 'opt-out' organ donation laws. STAT website. https://www.statnews.com/2017/07/06/opt-solution-organ-shortage/. Published July 6, 2017. Accessed April 12, 2018.
12. Sarlo R, Pereira G, Surica M, et al. Impact of introducing full-time in-house coordinators on referral and organ donation rates in Rio de Janeiro public hospitals: a health care innovation practice. *Transplant Proc*. 2016;48(7):2396–2398. https://doi.org/10.1016/j.transproceed.2015.11.044.
13. US Department of Health and Human Services. The Living Donation Process. https://www.organdonor.gov/about/process/living-donation.html. (n.d.).
14. Organ Procurement and Transplantation Network policies. https://optn.transplant.hrsa.gov/media/1200/optn_policies.pdf. (n.d.).
15. Overby KJ, Weinstein MS, Fiester A. Addressing consent issues in donation after circulatory determination of death. *Am J Bioeth*. 2015;15(8):3–9. https://doi.org/10.1080/15265161.2015.1047999.
16. Organ Donation and Transplantation Alliance. First Person Authorization [table]. In: Legal aspects of a registered donor: what you Need to Know. Hospital C-Suite Snapshot Series. https://organdonationalliance.org/wp-content/uploads/2017/10/CSuite-Snapshot-Fall-2017-FINAL.pdf. Published Fall 2017.
17. Willis BH, Quigley M. Opt-out organ donation: on evidence and public policy. *J R Soc Med*. 2013;107(2):56–60. https://doi.org/10.1177/0141076813507707.
18. Kirby J. Beyond influence and autonomy: expanding the scope of ethical considerations in organ donation registration. *Am J Bioeth*. 2016;16(11):31–33. https://doi.org/10.1080/15265161.2016.1222015.
19. Determination of Death Act Summary. http://www.uniformlaws.org/ActSummary.aspx?title=Determination of Death Act. (n.d.). Accessed April 27, 2019.
20. Pinckard JK, Geiselhart RJ, Moffatt E, et al. National Association of medical examiners position paper: medical examiner release of organs and tissues for Transplantation. *Acad Forensic Pathol*. 2013;4(4):497–504.
21. Powers KA, Candela L. Nursing practices and policies related to family presence during resuscitation. *Dimens Crit Care Nurs*. 2017;36(1):53–59. https://doi.org/10.1097/dcc.0000000000000218.
22. Emergency Nurses Association. Clinical Practice Guideline: Family Presence During Invasive Procedures and Resuscitation. Schaumburg, IL: Emergency Nurses Association. https://ena.org/docs/default-source/resource-library/practice-resources/cpg/familypresencecpg3eaabb7cf0414584ac2291feba3be481.pdf?sfvrsn=9c167fc6_12. Published December 2012.
23. Bentley TS, Phillips SJ. 2017 *US Organ and Tissue Transplant Cost Estimates and Discussion*. Milliman Research Report. http://us.milliman.com/uploadedFiles/insight/2017/2017-Transplant-Report.pdf, Published August 2017. Accessed June 20, 2018.

16

Air and Surface Patient Transport

Reneé Semonin Holleran

Patient transport is an integral part of all emergency departments (EDs). Whether a patient must be transferred to another care facility, moved from the ED for diagnostic testing, or transported within the hospital for admission, patients will be moved. Transport nursing has evolved into a specialty involving detailed education and training.[1] Emergency nurses are frequently involved with patient preparation and stabilization before transport. This requires that the emergency nurse be familiar with indications for transport, how the practice of nursing and medicine differ in the transport environment, preparation for transfer and transport, how transport can affect the patient, and the legal issues related to patient transport.

Transport teams may be staffed with a variety of personnel, including nurses, advanced practice nurses, physicians, physician assistants, paramedics, respiratory therapists, and emergency medical technicians (EMTs). Patient transport levels can vary from basic life support (BLS) to critical care. The condition and needs of the patient must dictate the type of team needed.

Transport vehicles include modular and van types of ground ambulances, fixed-wing aircraft, and helicopters (Fig. 16.1). The condition of the patient, the timely need for further care, the location of the patient, the weather, and the availability of specific transport services may influence the type of vehicle used to transport the patient.

The overriding concept of patient transport should always be safety. This includes patient safety, transport team safety, and the safety of anyone who interacts with the transport team and the vehicle used.

The quality and competency of the transport team, the vehicles, the equipment, and the training of the personnel should always be considered when choosing a transport team. The Commission on Accreditation of Medical Transport Systems (CAMTS) (http://www.camts.org) accreditation provides documentation that the transport program has met a set of standards, ensuring the patient will receive organized, safe, and expert care before and during the transport process.

HISTORICAL PERSPECTIVE

Transferring patients from one location to another is not a new concept, and nurses have played a role in many of the historical landmarks related to transport. Florence Nightingale assisted in the transport of injured soldiers during the Crimean War.[2] Throughout the ages, soldiers on the battlefield have been transported in all types of moving conveyances. Dominique Larrey, Napoleon's private physician, developed an organized system to triage and transport injured soldiers from the battlefield in carts.

The first hospital-based ambulance service was started in Cincinnati, Ohio, in 1865. Unfortunately, patient transport continued to develop in parallel with war. In 1945, the first helicopter rescue was recorded in the jungles of Burma.[3] In the 20th century, the use of air medical transport expanded.

The Korean War, the Vietnam conflict, and the wars in the Middle East have demonstrated the effectiveness of helicopter transport in the care of the injured from the battlefield. The first hospital-based helicopter programs began in the early 1970s in Colorado and California. Today there are more than 270 civilian-based helicopters transporting patients all over the United States and the world, including Europe, Africa, Australia, and New Zealand.[4]

During the 1960s and 1970s, Congress enacted numerous pieces of legislation addressing emergency medical care and transport. The Emergency Medical Treatment and Active Labor Act (EMTALA) was established to clarify guidelines for transfer and transport of patients. The discussion about legal regulations related to emergency nursing practice and patient transport is in Chapter 2.

TYPES OF TRANSPORT

Patient transport occurs in two distinct environments: on the surface by ambulance or in the air by a rotor-wing vehicle (helicopter) or fixed-wing vehicle (airplane). Air and surface transport have advantages and disadvantages. Therefore an informed decision to use air or surface transport must be made on the basis of many factors, such as patient condition, out-of-hospital time, weather, terrain, work space, equipment, personnel, and proximity of a landing site.

Surface Transport

Surface transport is most often accomplished using a modular type of vehicle (Fig. 16.2). Patient access is generally easier in most surface vehicles. These vehicles can also accommodate

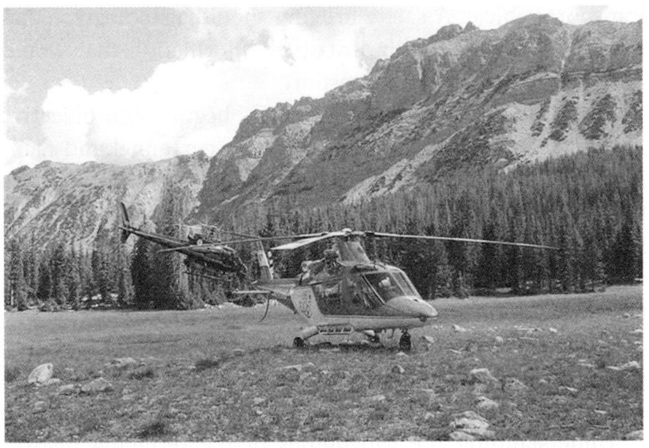

Fig. 16.1 Helicopter Transport. (© Arlene Jean Gee.)

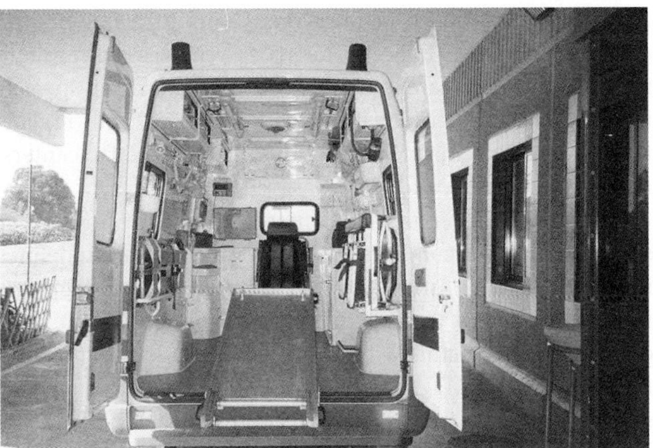

Fig. 16.2 An Example of a Ground Transport Vehicle. (© Marek Pawluczuk.)

larger pieces of equipment such as isolettes, ventilators, and intraaortic balloon pumps. The level of care during transport varies with the education and training of the transport personnel, from BLS to critical care transport. Critical care transport teams and vehicles available in many parts of the United States also provide transport of critically ill and injured patients who require complex physiologic support. In choosing a transport vehicle, the referring center must remember that, legally, the quality and level of care cannot diminish during the transport. In addition, the sending/transferring physician maintains accountability for the level of care provided during the transfer of the patient.

Adverse weather conditions influence the transport decision. When roads are impassable, air transport is usually the only alternative. When weather has grounded air transport vehicles, surface transport is the only option. Another important transport consideration is transit time. For many critically ill or injured patients, the shorter the out-of-hospital time, the better the patient's chance for survival. Finally, choice of a transport vehicle depends on the needs of the community. Some isolated rural areas have only one surface ambulance for a largely scattered population base. If this vehicle is taken out of service for an interfacility transport, the community is left without coverage for the duration of the transport.

Air Transport

Air transport should not be chosen indiscriminately. In many parts of the United States, air medical transport should be considered an adjunct to, and not a replacement for, surface-based services. However, in rural and frontier areas of the country, it may be the most cost-effective and safest way to transport patients. Research remains inconclusive as to the advantage of rotor-wing transport over surface transport. Some of the reasons that a helicopter may be chosen over a surface vehicle include time or length of transport and the critical care capabilities of the medical crew. However, there are critical care teams available in some areas of the country that only perform ground transport.

Rotor-wing aircraft, or helicopters, provide rapid point-to-point transport. Helicopters can reach most areas, bypassing difficult terrain. Landing zones can be made at or near the patient to prevent lengthy surface transport time. Most helicopters operate within 150 miles of their base station to allow routine flights without refueling. One disadvantage of helicopters is that their use depends on minimum weather conditions, without which flights can be delayed or canceled. Helicopter cabin size and configuration can restrict access to the patient and limit in-flight interventions. Weight limitations restrict the number of passengers and amount of equipment on board. When transferring by helicopters, comprehensive patient stabilization may be required before transport.

The advantage of fixed-wing transport is the ability to travel long distances. Care is provided in a pressurized cabin with sophisticated on-board medical equipment. Many fixed-wing aircraft can transport multiple patients. All-weather navigational equipment allows for transfer during inclement weather. Fixed-wing transport requires suitable airfields to ensure safety of the crew and patient. Accessibility to such fields may be a problem in isolated areas.

Transport Process

Patient transport today requires an organized process. There are multiple elements to the transport process, and to make it smooth and time-effective, these components should be put in place before a transport is required.

This process continues to vary throughout the United States and throughout the world. Multiple organizations, including prehospital, emergency, and critical specialties, have published recommendations on how to perform patient transport. EDs must be familiar with indications for patient transport of ill and injured patients from their facilities as well as what resources are available to them.

Prehospital Transport

In most parts of the country, prehospital transport can be initiated by laypersons through the 9-1-1 and enhanced 9-1-1 emergency access numbers. Sophisticated prehospital emergency medical services (EMS) provide patient transport to the nearest appropriate medical care facility. Emergency nurses possess the knowledge to function as prehospital care providers, but their ability to function in this role varies from

BOX 16.1 Indications for the Use of Air Medical Transport From the Out-of-Hospital Setting.

Timely need for specific interventions, for example, bleeding control in an operating suite
Injuries resulting in unstable vital signs requiring transport to the most appropriate center for care
Need to be transported by a team with more advanced intervention skills, for example, chest tube insertion
Location of the patient makes air medical transport a more reasonable mode of transportation
Distance of the patient to definitive care
Significant trauma in patients <12 years of age and >55 years of age
Pregnant patient with trauma or prenatal complications
Multisystem injuries
Ejection from a vehicle
Pedestrian or a cyclist struck by a vehicle
Crush injury to the head, chest, or abdomen
Glasgow Coma Scale score <13
Spinal cord injury
Significant abdominal pain
Presence of a "seat belt" sign
Flail chest
Amputations (specialty hospital need)
Major burns based on the American Burn Association criteria
Emergency medical services provider judgment

state to state. Surface transport can also be initiated for interfacility transport of patients with medical needs that exceed the capabilities of the local hospital.

The use of helicopters in the prehospital transport environment (scene responses) may be governed by local EMS or other state agencies. The National Association of EMS Physicians[5] and the American College of Emergency Physicians[6] have proposed guidelines and policies for the use of air medical transport from the field. Some of these indications are summarized in Box 16.1.

Interfacility Transfers

Every emergency nurse has the potential to become involved with organizing and implementing an interfacility transfer. Effective organization includes assessment and understanding of the referring facility's capabilities and an in-depth knowledge of available EMS and transport systems. Implementation of the transport process is expedited if this knowledge is part of a proactive referral strategy developed well in advance.

Emergency nurses must be aware of the potential role they may be asked to play in patient transport. Today there are few places in the United States where a transport team may not be available. If an emergency nurse or any other nurse is asked to accompany a transport team on a patient transfer, he or she must be aware of the type of equipment accessible in the transport vehicle, how to operate it, and the skill level of the team that is accompanying the patient. The safety of the nurse is also an important component of the transfer process. Appropriate restraint devices should be present in the transport vehicle. A safety briefing should also be given and the nurse provided with any other information that would assist in providing a safe transport.

Development of transfer strategies begins with objective assessment of the referring institution's personnel and facilities. Qualifications and availability of physicians and nurses to care for all patients who come to the ED must be examined. Specific areas that should be considered include the critical care unit; the operating suites; and pediatric, obstetric, neonatal, and psychiatric units. Ability to perform advanced diagnostic testing and to provide adequate blood and blood products must also be analyzed. All these factors influence the level of care available to sick or injured patients.

Understanding the capabilities of the receiving institution is an inherent responsibility of the referring institution. Trauma patients are best cared for in facilities designated by the American College of Surgeons Committee on Trauma as trauma centers. High-risk neonates benefit from care in a neonatal intensive care unit. Other areas of advanced specialized care include stroke centers, burn centers, limb replantation centers, pediatric centers, high-risk obstetric centers, open-heart centers, and hyperbaric centers.

The act of transferring a patient from one facility to another should be well documented and fall within legal guidelines identified by each institution. Determining the appropriate mode and type of team is one of the most important roles of the referring facility. Choices must be made using federal mandates (e.g., EMTALA). If a patient is unable to give consent because of his or her medical condition, and no family is located, a patient may be transferred under the implied consent law. The patient, a family member, or a representative of the referring facility should sign a consent form for the transport. Box 16.2 contains some questions that may assist the referring center with determining what type of patient should be transferred and the appropriate transport mode.[5,7–9]

Communication

There should be nurse-to-nurse communication from the referring facility to the receiving facility. If this cannot be accomplished, a member of the transport team may provide a report. A copy of the medical record and relevant laboratory and radiographic studies must accompany the patient. When possible, this information should be provided to the receiving facility as soon as possible. Telehealth has made this much easier. Policies and procedures should exist within transport programs that assist in directing how communication will be initiated and followed up between the referring and receiving facilities. Health Insurance Portability and Accountability Act (HIPAA) guidelines must be followed when communicating protected health care information.

Transport Team Members

The team members who accompany a patient will be determined by the condition and level of care that the patient requires. CAMTS standards[10] outline the required team members for BLS, advanced life support (ALS), and critical care transport. Two team members at a minimum, along with

BOX 16.2 Determining Whether a Patient Should Be Transferred and the Most Appropriate Mode of Transport.

- Does the patient's condition require minimal time out of the hospital during transport?
- Does the patient require time-sensitive evaluation or treatment not available at the referring facility?
- Is the patient located in a place where surface transport may pose a problem?
- What is the current and predicted weather along the transport route?
- Is there a helipad or an airport available to the referring facility?
- What is the weight and size of the patient?
- What type of equipment must accompany the patient?
- What type of team does the patient require? For example, critical care, pediatric, neonatal?
- Would the use of a surface vehicle leave the referring facility or community without adequate emergency services?
- Is there a specialty ground service available to the referring facility?
- Is rotor- or fixed-wing service available to the patient?
- If the patient requires international transport, is there a service available for the patient's medical needs?

Modified from Thomson D, Thomas S: Guidelines for air medical dispatch, *Prehosp Emerg Care* 7(2):265, 2003.

the vehicle operator, should accompany the patient. Teams should reflect the scope of service of the transport service. Specialty teams should be used when indicated. For example, a neonatal team may be required for a critically ill neonate. All team members should be competent in the transport process.

Most transport teams operate using patient care protocols. They should have the ability to communicate with a physician to provide medical direction if there is a variation from protocol or a problem develops.

Transport team configurations are many and varied. Transport nursing has developed into its own specialty. Transport nurses now go through specific and rigorous training before joining a transport team. The Air and Surface Transport Nurses Association (ASTNA), formerly the National Flight Nurses Association, has developed a flight and ground transport nursing core curriculum to provide standardized education and training in such areas as flight physiology, stabilization, communications, and medicolegal issues.[1] Initial training should include classroom and clinical experiences, including advanced airway management, invasive skills, and critical and emergency care. Preceptor programs are frequently used to allow the new transport nurse exposure to the transport environment. Recurrent training is required to maintain skills, update information regarding current therapies, and review policies and procedures. Monthly transport reviews provide performance improvement opportunities and promote shared learning experiences among staff. Continuous performance improvement should be one of the guiding principles of transport nursing practice.

Nurses should have advanced cardiac life support (ACLS) or its equivalent verified with training and continuous evaluation of advanced airway management skills and other invasive skills such as chest tube insertion, needle thoracostomy techniques, and intraosseous needle insertion. Depending on the scope of service of the transport program, additional education may include invasive line intraaortic balloon pump management.

If the transport program's scope of service includes trauma patients, the team may require ATLS (Advanced Trauma Life Support); TPATC (Transport Professional Advanced Trauma Course, or TNCC (Trauma Nursing Core Course) with invasive skills.

Transport nurses should obtain certification, which may include the CFRN (Certified Flight Registered Nurse) or the CTRN (Certified Transport Registered Nurse). Many transport nurses may also choose to be certified in the area of specialty, such as critical or emergency care.

Some states require additional credentials for nurses who work in the prehospital environment. These may include the need to become an EMT or an EMT-paramedic (EMT-P). It is the professional responsibility of transport nurses to be aware of the regulations that may dictate their practice within the states in which they perform transports.

Specialty teams should be used for the transport of the obstetric, pediatric, or neonatal patient. These teams undergo specific training to provide care for these patients. The American Academy of Pediatrics offers guidelines for the education, training, and specific equipment required to stabilize, manage, and transport pediatric and neonatal patients.[11]

Transport team members work under a unique set of circumstances. Interactions with the patient are short and often rushed. The patients who are transported are at an increased risk for further injury or death because of circumstances necessitating transport. Transport personnel must remember that they are often the only contact the family has with the receiving hospital. The team should try to make contact with the family, explaining interventions and other procedures that may be needed for transport. Maintaining contact and follow-up with referring personnel also provides the transport team with opportunities to communicate patient status. Fostering collegial relationships instills a sense of commitment and pride in the transport nurse role as well as providing an opportunity to improve patient care.

Transport Equipment

State and local regulations generally dictate what equipment should be on both surface and air transport vehicles. However, there are some general guidelines recommended by CAMTS, the National Association of Emergency Medical Services Physicians (NAEMSP), the American College of Emergency Physicians (ACEP), the American Academy of Pediatrics, and the American College of Surgeons for equipment that should be available for transport.[5,6,10,11]

The mission, size of the transport vehicle, and patient clinical condition are factors that influence the equipment carried during transport. General equipment should include equipment used to monitor and manage airway, oxygenation, and vital signs as well as devices necessary for resuscitation and

BOX 16.3 Recommended Equipment for Patient Transport.[a]

Airway and Ventilation

Portable and fixed suction device
Large-bore suction catheter
Suction catheters (varied sizes depending on the patients transported)
Laryngoscope handles with extra batteries and bulbs (age-related handles)
Laryngoscope blades (sizes depending on the types of patients transported)
Endotracheal tubes (cuffed and uncuffed depending on age of patients transported)
Syringes
Magill forceps (size dependent on ages of patient transported)
Lubricating jelly
Gastric tubes (depending on ages transported)
End-tidal CO_2 devices
Bag-mask device
  Hand-operated, self-inflating (age-appropriate sizes)
Alternative airways as approved for use by medical direction or state or local regulations
Nebulizer
Pulse oximeter with age-appropriate probes
Portable ventilator

Cardiac

Portable, battery-operated monitor, defibrillator, and external pacemaker

Vascular Access

Intravenous catheters (age-appropriate)
Intravenous access equipment either in packets or separate components
Crystalloid solutions
Intravenous administration sets
Intravenous pumps or solution monitors
Intraosseous access equipment

Medications

Cardiovascular medications
Antidysrhythmics
Epinephrine
Nitroglycerin
Aspirin
Vasopressors
Respiratory medications
Albuterol
Analgesics
Narcotic
Nonnarcotic
Antiepileptics
Sedation or other intubation adjuncts
Neuromuscular blocking agents
Glucometer and glucagon or D50W

Immobilization Devices

Rigid cervical collars (appropriate for patient age and size)
Head immobilization device
Lower extremity traction device
Splints
Radiolucent backboard

Bandages

Burn pack
Triangular bandages
Dressing supplies
Gauze rolls
Elastic bandages
Occlusive dressing
Tape (various sizes)
Large dressing

Communication

Two-way radio communication
Cell phone

Obstetric

Delivery pack
Bulb suctions
Thermal absorbent and head cover
Appropriate heat source

Miscellaneous

Depends on local protocols, state regulations, or mission of the transport team

[a]Note that this is a suggested list and may vary as noted.

stabilization, such as a defibrillator and external pacemaker. Medications for advanced life support and pain management should also be included.

All equipment should be routinely evaluated to ensure proper functioning. Annual preventive maintenance checks should be dated and visible for team members to view. Medications must be checked for expiration and stored at the appropriate temperature. Policies and procedures must be in place to ensure that team members receive the proper education and training regarding how to use the equipment. There should be an established method of removing and replacing malfunctioning equipment. Documentation of this process is imperative.

As technology continues to advance, many pieces of equipment are becoming multifunctional and longer lasting. In addition, advanced procedures such as extracorporeal perfusion can now be continued during transport. Box 16.3 contains a summary of some of the equipment that may be used during transport.

Preparation for Transport

Preparation for transfer of an ill or injured patient depends on the specific illness, injury, and age of the patient. The mode of transport and the size and capabilities of the transport vehicle will also assist in determining how to prepare the patient for transport. Potential problems during transport must be identified before departure, and proper interventions must be undertaken at the scene or the referring hospital.

The referring EMS agency (scene transports) and the referring hospital (interfacility) can help in reducing the time it may take to prepare the patient by beginning the appropriate evaluation and stabilization within their resources and personnel available. Unnecessary procedures and diagnostic tests should be avoided so that once the transport team arrives, the patient can be quickly and safely packaged and moved.

AIRWAY AND BREATHING

Airway patency during transport is of the greatest importance. Potential airway compromise must be anticipated before transport so that proper interventions can be accomplished under controlled circumstances rather than during transport. Endotracheal intubation should be considered in patients who might aspirate, have difficulty with chest expansion, or need ventilatory support (e.g., patients with altered level of consciousness, facial fractures, airway obstruction, or inhalation burns). The interior size of the transport vehicle and location of the transport team within the vehicle may also contribute to the decision to stabilize the airway before transport.

Patients with chest wall injury, spinal cord injury, or neurologic dysfunction may also require ventilatory assistance. Chest tube placement for a possible pneumothorax or hemothorax should be done before transport. A closed drainage system or flutter valve should be in place to avoid recurrence of a pneumothorax.

HEMODYNAMIC STABILIZATION

Interventions to maintain an adequate pulse rate and blood pressure should be initiated before transport. These include control of bleeding, correction of hypovolemia, insertion of a urinary catheter, and institution of cardiac monitoring. Control of external bleeding sites with pressure dressings or wound closure may be necessary. Splints for long-bone fractures and pelvic stabilization devices for pelvic injuries stabilize fractures and control bleeding.

Proper intravenous (IV) access is needed to replace fluid loss. Large-bore IV catheters with blood tubing provide rapid fluid resuscitation routes. Blood replacement products prepared for transport and placed in a proper container may accompany the patient.

Patients requiring fluid management should have a urinary catheter (if not contraindicated) attached to a device to properly measure urinary output. In addition to measuring output, bladder drainage decreases patient discomfort during a long transport.

All IV access lines should be checked for patency and secured. When there are multiple lines, labeling can decrease the risk for using the wrong line to administer medications during transport. If a subclavian or internal jugular line has been inserted, a chest radiograph should be obtained to rule out the presence of a pneumothorax before air transport.

Medications should be placed on infusion pumps or monitoring devices based on transport protocols. Most transport teams at a minimum will place all vasoactive medications on a pump or infuser. Medications not on monitors require careful observation during transport.

NEUROLOGICAL STABILIZATION

All attempts should be made to stabilize the patient's neurologic condition (i.e., maintain normal intracranial pressure, control seizure activity, and preserve integrity of the spinal cord).

Maintenance of cerebral perfusion pressure in the head-injured patient includes measures to control increased intracranial pressure. The receiving neurologist or neurosurgeon should be consulted to decide what therapeutics, such as medications (i.e., mannitol, sedation, and neuromuscular blocking agents), fluid resuscitation, patient position, and ventilation settings, must continue during transport.

Whether prophylactic medications are needed to reduce the risk for seizures during transport should be determined during the physician-to-physician consultation. Any patient at risk for seizure activity who has received neuromuscular blocking agents should receive antiseizure prophylaxis as directed by medical control.

A patient with a suspected or documented spinal cord injury should be appropriately immobilized. This should be done if the patient has an altered mental status with blunt trauma; spinal pain or tenderness; a specific neurologic complaint such as extremity numbness or tingling; anatomic deformity of the spine; high mechanism of injury; or drug or alcohol intoxication. Long transport times are not uncommon, and preventive measures should be undertaken to reduce risk for pressure sore development. Padding of bony areas or the use of a vacuum splint may better serve the patient.[12]

MUSCULOSKELETAL STABILIZATION

Care of the patient with musculoskeletal injuries should include prevention of blood loss, fracture immobilization, wound care, and administration of analgesia.

Splints should permit assessment of distal pulses as well as observation of increased swelling or bleeding during transport. Air splints respond to pressure changes during air transport and should not be used in this environment. Pelvic fractures should be stabilized with a pelvic binder. Traction splints for femur fractures may be used in transport.

Patients transferred for limb replantation require special care. Wrapping the amputated part in saline-moistened gauze and placing it in a plastic bag should preserve the affected part. The plastic bag should be placed in a sealed container on ice inside a cooler. The part should not be allowed to freeze—this causes tissue destruction and prevents replantation.

Wound care before transport may be limited to control of bleeding, initial cleansing, and the application of a sterile dressing. The transport team member should note if tetanus prophylaxis has been administered, if known.

Burn care includes calculation of the percentage of body surface area burned and fluid resuscitation (see Chapter 41). Fluid resuscitation must be continued throughout transport. The transport team must ensure that an adequate supply of fluid is available in the transport vehicle. The patient must be kept warm, which may require running a heater in the transport vehicle even during the summertime. Constricting rings, necklaces, and clothing should be removed. If circulation impairment is present, escharotomy must be performed before transport under the direction of medical control.

EMOTIONAL AND PSYCHOSOCIAL SUPPORT OF THE PATIENT AND FAMILY

The patient and the family of the patient who requires transport will have many physical, emotional, and psychosocial needs. Emergency and transport nurses can address these needs by recognizing the patient's fears and answering any questions.

Removing patients from their homes, family, and a familiar environment increases patient stress. Patients that must be transported by air may have a fear of flying. The patient and the family may be angry, with their anger directed at the referring hospital for being unable to care for them. The need for transport is often translated in patients' or family's minds to mean the patient is dying. The stresses of transport may produce anxiety, causing increased heart rate and respiratory rate, diaphoresis, nausea, vomiting, and a general worsening of condition.

Personnel from the referring hospital and the transport team can work together to alleviate the patient's fears by thoroughly explaining all procedures, noises, and reasons for the transport. Transport personnel should work to instill confidence in the patient concerning the referring hospital. This confidence is important because, if the patient survives, he or she will be returning to the home community and may be cared for by the referring hospital in the future.

Research has shown that families have specific needs when a patient is to be transported to another hospital.[13–17] Families want to feel that the transport team truly cares for their loved ones. They want to know specific facts about the patient's condition, including the prognosis, especially whether the patient will live or die; have procedures and treatments explained in terms that they can understand; have questions answered honestly; and at a minimum feel there is some hope as to a positive outcome. This information should always be given so that the family's reaction can be evaluated. Working with a family may appear to be a time-consuming activity, but it is an important part of transport care.

The patient's family also has tremendous fears. If the patient is acutely ill or injured, this interaction may be the last one they have with their loved one. The family may not understand the need for the transport. Time must be taken to explain the necessity for immediate transfer. The family may also have what is called the "Mecca syndrome," an inflated idea of what can be done for the patient at the receiving facility. The family may believe the receiving hospital will save the life of a patient, when in fact that may not happen.

A family member may want to accompany the patient. In helicopter transports, this option may not be possible because of space and weight limitations.[3,8] However, depending on the type of surface ambulance or fixed-wing aircraft, room may be available for a family member. Transport personnel should make the decision whether to allow the family member to come with the patient during a surface transport, but the final decision in air transport is the responsibility of the pilot in command. The family member's presence may alleviate some of the patient's anxiety, especially when the patient is a child. The decision should not be made until the time of the transport because the patient's condition may change and promises cannot always be kept.

To alleviate family anxiety, provide as much information as possible about the receiving hospital. Maps, plans for patient admission, and a telephone contact give them some direction after the patient departs. The family should be informed of the estimated length of transport and expected time of arrival at the receiving hospital. This time should be calculated taking into consideration weather, unexpected delays, changes in time zone, and other factors. Overestimation of time is always best—if the transport is completed sooner than anticipated, the family will feel relief. On the other hand, if the transport takes longer than expected, the family may fear the outcome of the transport itself.

One of the last things that should be done, whenever possible, before departure is to allow the family time with the patient. The last remarks and the last kiss goodbye may be the most important few minutes of the transport.

Documentation

Documentation of the transfer is essential. It confirms adherence to legal mandates, ensures compliance with established standards of care, and protects the caregiver in potential litigious situations. Documentation of prehospital care includes mechanism of injury, time of injury, time of EMS arrival, care provided in the field and during transport, and protocols or orders used during transfer. Documentation related to interfacility transfer includes the prehospital record, the ED record, and documentation of care during the transfer. A consent for transport form and an indication for transport form should be included with the documentation. The content of these forms may vary from one health care system to another.

Care During Transport

Transport personnel must be prepared to implement interventions to maintain patient stability. Protocols and physician orders regarding specific interventions clarify expectations for the transporting team. Interventions that may be needed during transport include securing the airway, suctioning, administering fluids, performing emergency thoracotomy, administering medications, and performing ALS measures. In unforeseen emergencies when sophisticated medical equipment and personnel are critical, diversion to a closer facility may be necessary. The location of these facilities should be identified before transport to prevent unnecessary delays.

Appropriately trained personnel should manage any equipment that is not usually used by the transport team, such as a left ventricular assist device or an intraaortic balloon pump. Any additional persons who accompany the transport team must receive an orientation to the transport environment that includes safety and operational issues. They should also be clothed in uniforms and helmets if going by air.

All care during transport should be documented. A copy of the transport form should be inserted in the patient's chart at the receiving facility. Documentation should include patient assessment, interventions, and the patient's response to these interventions. Unusual events or effects of the transport on the patient's condition should also be noted.

Communication

Effective communication is an essential component of the entire transport process. When a request for transport is placed to an emergency operations center, the dispatcher notifies appropriate units to respond. Radio communication is established, and pertinent information is transmitted. Depending on severity and local protocols, the mobile unit can be directly linked to the medical command center or the base station at the receiving hospital. Transmission of pertinent data is necessary so the transport team can receive specific protocols for intervention.

Successful communication includes a complete loop in which all parties are notified and aware of the patient's status. This begins with the physician-to-physician contact that establishes the transport process. Communication is ongoing and should focus on essential information for the transporting and receiving personnel.

Communication techniques, radio codes, and communication technology are too extensive to be included here. Emergency and transport nurses must be familiar with the communication centers and methods used in their area of service. Regardless of technology used, every effort should be made to protect patient confidentiality during any communication. Use of patient names or other identifying factors must be avoided. A standard reporting format may be developed by the transport program to ensure quality assurance for each communication.

Medical Control

Organization of medical control varies from system to system. Online medical control is direct communication between transport personnel and the physician (or physician-surrogate) via radio or telephone for the purpose of providing orders for patient care. Offline medical control includes those administrative functions necessary to ensure quality of care. Each medical control officer is a physician who is directly responsible for care provided in transport. It is the medical control officer's responsibility to ensure proper training, orientation, and continuing education for those people working under his or her control.[18]

Transfer of Care

While the patient is in transit, the referring and receiving facilities share responsibility for care of the patient. Only after arrival at the receiving facility is the referring hospital's legal responsibility terminated.

STRESSES OF TRANSPORT

Exposure to environmental factors occurs during transport of patients. Problems encountered depend on changes in atmospheric conditions, vehicle configurations, motion of the aircraft, and the patient's condition. Some of these can be detrimental to the patient, but with proper nursing care before and during transport, these harmful effects can be minimized or eliminated. It is also important to keep in mind that these factors can cause stress to both the patient and the transfer team, and interventions may be required for both the patient and the team members to complete a safe transport.

Effects of Altitude

Atmospheric changes occur when the aircraft's altitude changes. Ascending into the atmosphere from sea level causes a decrease in atmospheric pressure, which in turn causes a decrease in the partial pressure of gases, temperature, and expansion of gases. The opposite occurs during descent.

According to Boyle's law, the volume of gas is inversely proportional to its pressure. As an aircraft ascends, atmospheric pressure decreases and gas expands. One hundred milliliters of gas at sea level expands to 130 mL at an altitude of 6000 feet, 200 mL at 18,000 feet, and 400 mL at 34,000 feet. Gas expansion is a potential problem in all transports in which the aircraft ascends.

Patients with a pneumothorax, pneumopericardium, pneumomediastinum, abdominal distention, or trapped gas or any equipment that may be affected by gas expansion, such as some mechanical ventilators, must be closely monitored for the effects of changes in barometric pressure. Interventions such as chest thoracotomy or insertion of a gastric tube must be done before transport.[19]

Fixed-wing and rotary-wing vehicles are designed according to different principles. Fixed-wing aircraft used in patient transport are pressurized, which allows for a comfortable cabin atmosphere when flying at high attitudes. Pressurization differentials allow for different cabin pressures at different atmospheres. Generally, the lower the altitude at which a plane is flying, the lower the cabin pressure that can be achieved. This ability to maintain a physiologically comfortable environment within the aircraft is a benefit when transporting patients who may be affected by atmospheric changes. Although pressurization allows for flights at high altitudes, even subtle changes in the environment may be harmful to a person whose condition is severely compromised.

If the pressurization system fails, pressurization within the cabin might be lost, causing a sudden change in atmospheric pressure. This rapid decompression causes the interior of the cabin to equalize with the pressures outside the cabin, resulting in sudden and often detrimental effects on the human body: rapid loss of oxygen, sudden drop in temperature, and expansion of gas. A healthy person may be able to withstand these changes, but the person in poor health may deteriorate rapidly. Those transporting patients should be aware of these effects and do everything possible before departure to minimize complications.

Helicopters are not pressurized; therefore these atmospheric changes are felt whenever the helicopter ascends and descends. As a result, patients transported by helicopter may be at greater risk than those transported by fixed-wing aircraft. If a higher altitude may be a problem for the patient, the transport nurse should ask the helicopter pilot to fly as low as safely possible.

Hypoxia

Many patients transported by air are hypoxic as a result of their condition. This hypoxic state is potentiated when changes in atmospheric pressure occur. There are four major types of hypoxia[19]:

- *Hypoxic hypoxia:* results from insufficient oxygen in the air breathed or when oxygen is prevented from diffusing from the lungs to the bloodstream
- *Hypemic hypoxia:* results from reduction in oxygen-carrying capacity in the blood
- *Stagnant hypoxia:* results from inadequate circulation
- *Histotoxic hypoxia:* results from interference with the use of oxygen by the body's tissues

When an aircraft ascends in altitude, the partial pressure of oxygen (Po_2) decreases and causes a decreased diffusion gradient for the oxygen molecule to cross the alveolar membrane.

Room air is 21% oxygen. If the patient is receiving oxygen, the fraction of inspired oxygen is used for the patient's oxygen therapy. Assuming that water pressure is equal to 47 mm Hg, the Po_2 at sea level is 150 mm Hg: (760 mm Hg atmospheric pressure − 47 mm Hg) × (0.21) = 150 mm Hg. At an altitude of 6000 feet, the calculated Po_2 is 118 mm Hg: (609 mm Hg − 47 mm Hg) × (0.21) = 118 mm Hg.

The decrease in Po_2 that occurs in the respiratory tree is approximately 45 mm Hg; therefore at the alveolar level, the PaO_2 at sea level is approximately 105 mm Hg and the PaO_2 at 6000 feet is about 73 mm Hg. The Po_2 of venous blood is approximately 40 mm Hg; therefore the diffusion gradient at sea level is 65 mm Hg (105 − 40) and at 6000 feet it is 22 mm Hg. Patients with disease-induced hypoxia are severely affected by this drop in diffusion gradient and are at increased risk for compromise during air medical transport. Patients at risk include those with heart failure, respiratory distress syndrome, carbon monoxide poisoning, hypovolemic shock, an inadequate amount of circulating hemoglobin, and stagnant hypoxia induced by low-flow states such as hypothermia. Altitude-induced reduction in Po_2 causes further deterioration in these patients if interventions are not performed to correct the problems related to hypoxia. Risk for hypoxia is even greater when the patient smokes.

Signs and symptoms of hypoxia include changes in vital signs, tachycardia, pupillary constriction, confusion, disorientation, and lethargy. All of these signs may be caused by a number of other illnesses and injuries, making the diagnosis of hypoxia more difficult. Astute observation of the patient is necessary to detect and correct the problems related to hypoxia. Transporting patients by pressurized fixed-wing aircraft can limit complications secondary to this drop in Po_2. Most aircraft used for air transport are able to maintain a sea level cabin pressure when flying below 7000 to 10,000 feet. At higher altitudes, the cabin can be pressurized. Maximum cabin pressure altitude is generally maintained well below 9000 feet. When cabin pressures are controlled, atmospheric changes that occur are limited, controlled, and within a tolerable range.

Before the patient is transported, stabilization measures can be taken to reduce effects of atmospheric changes in oxygenation. Supplemental oxygen can be provided, and if the patient has previously required oxygen, the percentage of oxygen may need to be increased. This increase in oxygen delivery is prophylactic, a temporary measure during transport. When the patient arrives at the receiving institution, oxygen can be decreased or terminated pending outcome of arterial blood gas analysis.

Proper positioning of the patient combats the effects of hypoxia. Ensuring proper chest excursion by loosening chest restraints on the stretcher allows the patient to breathe easier. Elevation of the patient's head when not contraindicated may also assist with ventilation and oxygenation.

The hypovolemic patient may receive transfusions to increase hematocrit and oxygen-carrying capacity of the blood. Patients who are alert are generally anxious regarding their outcome, which increases respiratory rate and decreases oxygenation. Providing a calm environment and thoroughly explaining all procedures, noises, and equipment can reduce the patient's feeling of helplessness.

Level of consciousness, continuous pulse oximetry readings, and vital sign monitoring provide the best indicators of how a patient is tolerating the transport. Oxygen use should be considered during transport based on the patient's illness or injury.

Dehydration

Another problem encountered during an increase in altitude is a drop in ambient humidity. Loss of humidification is magnified in a pressurized fixed-wing aircraft, because recycling air and removing moisture from it achieve system pressurization. Patients who are dehydrated or diaphoretic are at increased risk for dehydration and possible fluid volume deficits. Supplemental IV fluids should be administered to prevent dehydration.

Other patients affected by dehydration include mouth breathers and those who are intubated. These patients have lost the natural respiratory humidification mechanisms, so secretions become tenacious and difficult to mobilize. Suction should be available to ensure that the airway remains patent.

Decreased Temperature

As altitude increases, temperature decreases. For each 1000-foot gain in altitude, temperature drops 2°C until it reaches −55°C. During ascent, this temperature drop cools the aircraft. Although transport vehicles are heated, the fuselage becomes quite cold and radiates cold into the cabin interior. Outside temperature changes will also affect the patient being transported by ground. The coldest area of all transport vehicles is against the outside walls. This cooling, although most significant during cold-weather months, is noticeable at all times of the year.

In addition to altitude-induced and outside temperature changes, a number of environmental conditions affect transport of patients. Of particular importance is a drop in environmental temperature. Interhospital transports require patient movement outside the hospital, transport outside to the helipad or into an ambulance for transfer to the airfield, and subsequent transfer into the transport vehicle. The opposite occurs at the receiving end of the transfer. These multiple transfers expose the patient to changing environmental conditions, including cold weather. A patient requiring transport, especially an infant or older adult patient, is less able to tolerate these stresses and can exhibit signs and symptoms of cold stress, including decreased level of consciousness, increased heart rate, and shivering. These symptoms increase the patient's oxygen demands, causing mild hypoxia to worsen significantly.

Awareness of an environmental drop in temperature allows adequate stabilization before the transport. Minimizing exposure to environmental conditions is of utmost importance. The interior temperature of the transport vehicle can be controlled in accordance with the patient's needs rather than needs of the transport crew. Maintaining an adequate supply of linen, and wrapping the patient in a rescue blanket is useful in cold environments. A cap can be put on the patient's head to reduce radiated heat losses.[19]

Cold can also affect transport equipment. Transport teams should be aware of the temperature ranges that affect their equipment. Policies and procedures should be in place to monitor and replace anything that may become damaged.

Other problems that develop with cold environments include cooling IV solutions and crystallization of medications, most notably mannitol. A patient with cold stress resulting from changes in the environment requires warm IV fluids. Solutions stored in the aircraft or solutions exposed to the environment are quite cold and must be warmed before administration. If possible, solutions should be stored in the warmest spot in the cabin. Some transport vehicles have environmental drawers to manage medications.

Remember that medications such as neuromuscular blocking agents can interfere with the patient's ability to maintain his or her body temperature. The use of these types of medications dictates that the patient be closely monitored during transport. The patient should be covered at all times, even when the transport team feels that the environment is comfortable for them.

Acceleration and Deceleration Forces

Acceleration forces occur during takeoff and "climb-out." Blood pools in dependent areas, most commonly the lower extremities, causing fluid shifts that may not be tolerated by the severely compromised patient. Restoration of intravascular volume and proper positioning of the patient can minimize the effects of these forces.

Deceleration forces occur during slowing, stopping, or rapid descent. For the patient lying head forward in an aircraft, deceleration forces cause blood to pool in the head and upper body. Pooling produces what is known as "red-out" as blood rushes to the head, causing an increase in blood within the ocular cavity. Deceleration forces are most harmful to a patient with increased intracranial pressure. The phenomenon may also adversely affect a patient with congestive heart failure.

Effects of acceleration and deceleration forces vary with speed, angle, and duration. These forces are much more pronounced in a fixed-wing aircraft. In certain instances, pilots can control these effects as long as safety measures and regulations are met. If a patient is known to be severely ill or injured, transport personnel should discuss this problem with their flight crew. A slow descent is often an option. If the airfield is long enough, a longer landing roll can decrease some deceleration forces that occur as the aircraft is slowed to a stop.

Positioning of the patient is crucial to counter these forces. In many aircraft, stretcher restraints are not interchangeable; therefore the patient must be loaded headfirst into the cabin. If the patient can tolerate a head-elevated position, effects of these forces can be minimized, because fluid shifts would be centered at the core of the body rather than in the head.

Helicopters are also subject to acceleration and deceleration forces but to a lesser magnitude than fixed-wing aircraft. In addition to forward and rearward movement, helicopters are capable of lateral movement. Forces resulting from these movements are of little consequence. Because of confined space within the helicopter, positioning the patient to counteract these forces is usually more difficult, if not impossible. Fortunately, pilot control is much greater in the helicopter.

Motion Sickness

Changes in equilibrium caused by excessive motion can cause motion sickness either by air or ground transport. Nausea and vomiting may develop in the patient and transport personnel. Prophylactic premedication is the best intervention available to limit these complications.

Other causes of motion sickness include hypoxia; excessive visual stimuli, such as blinking lights on the aircraft control panel; stress; fear; unpleasant odors; heat; and poor diet. Gastric gas expansion occurring during ascent can worsen the problem. To prevent or limit these symptoms, transport personnel should provide adequate oxygenation, stare at a fixed visual reference, cool the cabin interior, attempt to limit stressors and fear, and have the patient lie in the supine position.

For transport team members with motion sickness, premedication may be needed. Medications should be selected that do not cause drowsiness or interfere with the transport team member's ability to provide patient care and remain safe during the transport. Other preventive measures include eating ginger cookies and using acupressure bracelets. Crew members often "recover" from motion sickness when they focus their attention on the patient; however, residual symptoms may occur after the transport.

Noise

Transport vehicles are inherently noisy. Engine noises create a constant loud hum that not only is distracting but also increases stress. Reducing extraneous noise is often impossible, but limiting sound input can be accomplished by application of earplugs, headphones, or helmets. Unfortunately, use of noise reduction devices by the patient reduces communication so he or she is not able to hear. The patient may become increasingly agitated, believing the team is talking about him or her. It is essential to include the conscious patient in as much conversation as possible.

Noise also interferes with ability to hear breath sounds, heart sounds, and blood pressure. Doppler devices are available to assist with detecting blood pressure but are of little use for hearing breath or heart sounds. Other assessment techniques to ascertain adequate ventilation include observing for bilateral chest wall movement, using pulse oximetry, and placing the stethoscope over the trachea to listen for air movement.

The transport team may be familiar with noises of the aircraft or ground transport vehicle, but the patient should be warned ahead of time. Many aircraft have audible warning signals to prevent accidents, but to the patient these alarms may indicate the aircraft is in danger of crashing. Continual reminders to alleviate these fears should follow a preflight and transport briefing with the patient.

Long-term noise exposure is also a problem for the transport team. Protective earplugs or helmets should be used to minimize the deleterious effects of noise over time. Periodic hearing tests are recommended to monitor changes in hearing.

Vibration

As a result of vehicle design, aircraft vibrate. The effects of vibration are much more noticeable in a helicopter, especially during takeoff and landing. This constant motion can cause equipment to loosen and become a danger during flight. Federal Aviation Administration (FAA) regulations require that all equipment be secured during takeoff and landing. Equipment should be secured at all times in anticipation of unexpected turbulence.

The patient should be secured to the stretcher at all times. Before loading and unloading, stretcher restraints should be checked for proper fit. During transport, straps may be loosened to allow the patient to move; however, restraints should never be fully released.

Vibrations may affect equipment. Again, equipment should be routinely inspected to prevent any problems.

Immobilization

Long transport times combined with prolonged immobilization of the patient can lead to pressure sores and venous stasis. Space limitations and the inability to change the patient's position exacerbate these problems. The patient at greatest risk is one with a suspected spinal injury who is secured to a backboard.

Before departure, all splints, casts, and pressure areas should be padded. A small towel or pad can be placed under the coccyx area of a patient with a suspected cervical spine injury who is secured to a backboard. In transport, proper positioning and assessment of range of motion should be performed within the space constraints. Assessing for areas of decreased perfusion should be part of assessment of vital signs.

Length of transport includes not only the time it takes to fly from the referring location to the receiving hospital, but also surface transport times, unexpected delays, and transfer times. For example, a patient injured in a motor vehicle crash at a remote site is secured to a backboard to protect the cervical spine. This patient is then transported by surface ambulance to the nearest hospital. After evaluation of injuries, it is determined that the patient requires care in a major trauma center. Radiographs of the cervical spine are inconclusive, so the patient must remain on the backboard during transport. Subsequently the patient is taken by surface ambulance to the nearest airport, flown to the receiving airfield, and again transferred by surface ambulance to the trauma center.

Consideration of injuries must take precedence during stabilization of the patient, but using padded splints, traction devices, and protecting bony prominences are a necessary follow-up, limiting preventable problems associated with immobilization.

TRANSPORT OF THE PEDIATRIC PATIENT

Pediatric transport teams should be considered for the transport of the ill or injured pediatric patient. If a pediatric team is not available, the team performing the transport should have received additional education and training to ensure that they can safely and competently manage the ill or injured child during transport.

Many of the problems associated with transport of children are similar to those for adults. However, interventions must take into account the unique anatomic and physiologic features of children. Because equipment of the appropriate size varies with age and weight of the child, the appropriate equipment must be available.

Pediatric patients are more prone to the effects of hypoxia. Children may not be able to tolerate or cooperate with application of an oxygen mask. In these cases, the oxygen mask can be placed in front of the child's face, and oxygen can be blown at the child. A family member accompanying the child can assist with administration of oxygen by holding the mask and encouraging the child to cooperate.

Because the gastric cavity of a child is small, the child has a greater tendency to develop complications from gastric gas expansion. Many gastric tubes for children do not have a sump port and should not be used because absence of the sump port makes emptying the stomach more difficult.

The greater ratio of surface area to body mass in children makes them more susceptible to evaporative heat losses. The proportionally larger surface area of the head and neck also enhances radiated heat loss, which puts the child at great risk for hypothermia. A stocking cap and extra linen help keep the child warm.

Children should be secured and transported in age-appropriate equipment. Providing familiar items such as toys and security blankets helps alleviate the child's fear of the unknown.

If the child's condition is stable, including a family member in the transport may be advantageous. The family member can comfort the child, help explain procedures, and provide diversionary activities as warranted to keep the child occupied.

SAFETY

Safety before, during, and after transport must always be the primary concern of all persons involved. There are inherent risks with patient transport whether by air or ground, and all involved in the transport process should be aware of how to keep themselves and their patients safe.

Transport team members require recurrent training in handling the emergencies that may occur during transport. In addition, a safety program that includes education of the personnel who use the transport service should be in place.

Safety education must include how to assist the vehicle operator during an emergency (based on the type of vehicle), emergency oxygen shutoff, and how to prepare the patient. Communication should occur as to what to do after an emergency has occurred. The safety plan should include where the team would assemble, how to contact help, and basic survival skills. ASTNA's position statement, Critical Care Transport Nurse Safety in the Transport Environment, contains pertinent and useful information about safety related to transport. It can be accessed from https://cdn.ymaws.com/astna.site-ym.com/resource/collection/4392B20B-D0DB-4E76-959C-6989214920E9/ASTNA_Safety_Position_Paper_2018_FINAL.pdf.

Transport team members must always feel comfortable and be supported in refusing to participate in or tolerate unsafe practices. Each transport service must have a safety program that continuously evaluates the transport environment and provides a way to communicate safety.

Fixed-Wing Transports

All equipment must be secured in accordance with FAA regulations. Meeting stringent requirements ensures that flying objects do not injure passengers and crew during turbulence or if a crash occurs. Equipment not secured to the airframe itself should be kept in soft packs and placed on the floor during takeoff and landing. Equipment or extraneous items should never block emergency exits.

Ground personnel must be trained and briefed regarding aircraft safety. This briefing should include information on loading and unloading the patient. For instance, weight distribution is critical in the aircraft, but ground personnel may not be aware of these requirements. Also, ground personnel should be trained to avoid hazardous areas, such as propellers and the exhaust cowling on a jet engine. No one should approach the aircraft until the pilot in command or a designated member of the transport team has given approval to do so.

The pilot in command is responsible for safety of the aircraft at all times and may determine whether to cancel a flight because of weather conditions; however, all members of the team are responsible for safety. Most flight programs do not discuss the severity of the patient's condition with the pilot until a decision has been made regarding weather. This relieves the pilot of undue stress when a life-or-death mission is being considered; the pilot should be able to make this decision without feelings of guilt or doubt affecting his or her judgment.

Everyone involved in the transport should be briefed before departure. Pilots should be informed of the patient's condition and specific needs related to takeoff and landing. For example, a short landing that results in shifts in internal organs and fluids adversely affects some patients. Family members should be briefed on the length of the flight, in-flight expectations, and the location and operation of emergency exits. Smoking is prohibited. Seat belts are required on landing and takeoff, although their use is preferred throughout the flight.

Fire extinguishers should be clearly marked, and all personnel must be trained in their use. Emergency procedures for rapid egress should be practiced on a regular basis.

Rotor-Wing (Helicopter) Transports

Helicopter transports create a sense of drama. Many people assemble to watch a helicopter land and take off. Bystanders must be kept away from danger. A safe landing zone (LZ) should be established in a clearing that measures 100 feet × 100 feet up to 200 feet × 200 feet, depending on the size of the helicopter. All wires, trees, and possible hazards should be marked and described over the radio to the pilot. Smoke flares can be ignited to assist the pilot in locating the LZ. Flares are blown away from the helicopter during landing, which could ignite a fire. The patient, ground personnel, and bystanders should be at least 500 feet from the LZ and should turn their backs to the helicopter while it is landing. The rotor wash (wind created by the rotor blades) causes swirling dust, dirt, and gravel, which pose hazards to people on the ground.

Ground personnel should not approach the helicopter until the pilot or a designated transport team member gives the signal it is safe to do so and from the direction (front or side) as directed by the transport team. The helicopter should be approached from the downhill side, never the uphill side. Many injuries occur because people approach the helicopter while the blades are still rotating. When blade rotation slows down, the blades drop, which may cause unexpected injury. Each aircraft is different, so it is a good idea to be familiar with those that provide service to the ED. A "hot" loading or unloading is one that is performed with rotor blades

BOX 16.4 Guidelines for Helicopter Landing Safety.

Landing zone (LZ) size ranges from 100 to 200 square feet, depending on size of the helicopter.
Select an easily identifiable LZ, as level as possible, and free of debris and overhead obstructions.
Mark one corner of the LZ with a smoke flare, so the pilot can estimate wind speed and direction.
Flashing emergency lights are difficult to see in daylight. Landmarks such as intersections, waterways, distinctive buildings, or baseball or football fields are much easier to find from the air.
Turn off unnecessary lights and white lights such as strobe lights or headlights at night. These lights interfere with the pilot's night vision. Never direct a spotlight at an approaching helicopter.
Flags, cones, safety tapes, ambulance mattresses, poles used for intravenous infusion, other loose equipment, sticks, stones, and broken glass can be drawn into rotor blades or thrown during landing and liftoff.
Only people such as firefighters with proper personal protection, including safety goggles, should be permitted in the vicinity of the LZ.
Assign personnel to guard the area. Prohibit smoking, and keep spectators at a safe distance.
Never approach the helicopter unless signaled to do so by the pilot or another air medical crew member. Keep low if the main rotor is still spinning.
Always approach the helicopter within the crew's line of sight and never from the rear or sloped side. If the aircraft is rear loading, approach cautiously with head down after being signaled by the pilot or crew.
Only transport team members should lock, unlock, or otherwise handle aircraft doors.
Assist the transport team only as requested. Never attempt to contact the pilot by radio during the helicopter's final approach unless an extreme emergency jeopardizes safety.

turning at idle power. Only in extreme circumstances and only by experienced personnel should this procedure be used. Additional guidelines for helicopter landing safety are listed in Box 16.4. This information should be reviewed frequently and be readily available for review when a helicopter transport is expected. Most transport programs are very happy to provide ongoing education to the departments that use them.

Surface Transports

Surface vehicles should be inspected and licensed by their local or state regulatory agencies. The location of the emergency oxygen shutoff valves and fire extinguishers should be known. Restraints should be available for all who ride in a surface vehicle and must be used. Equipment should be secured so that it does not injure transport team members or patients.

A policy for the use of lights and sirens should be in place. Just as with air transport, surface team members must feel comfortable and be supported in refusing a transport that may put themselves and their patients at risk.

Vehicle Crashes

Because many EDs are involved with both surface and air transport programs, they should be aware of the postaccident/incident plan (PAIP) that a program has in place and what role they may play in its implementation. Unfortunately, crashes, injuries, and deaths do occur, and in many areas the ED will be the place where the victims are brought. Some hospitals have specific codes that indicate that a crash may have occurred so that emergency personnel can prepare.

The PAIP should contain notification procedures, resources for staff and family, and how to manage the inevitable publicity and community concerns that are a part of any incident. For some EDs, vehicle accidents are incorporated within their disaster plans.

SUMMARY

Air and surface patient transport has improved outcomes for many patients. Proper stabilization procedures anticipate and plan for potential problems that may be encountered during transport. Using specialized equipment and personnel trained in transporting patients ensures the patient is provided with safe and competent care during the transport process.

Patient transport is a nursing specialty requiring specific education and training. Transfer and accepting patients requiring transport for specialty care is also an intricate part of emergency nursing practice. Intertwining the concepts of patient care along with safety will allow the emergency nurse to provide the competent care for the patient who requires transport.

REFERENCES

1. Clark D, Stocking J, Johnson J, Treadwell D, Corbett P. *Critical Care Transport Core Curriculum*. Aurora, CO: Air and Surface Transport Nurses Association; 2017.
2. Donahue P. *Nursing, The Finest Art*. St Louis, MO: Mosby Elsevier; 2011.
3. Carter G, Couch R, O'Brien M. The evolution of air transport systems. *J Emerg Med*. 1988;6(6):499.
4. Hankins D. Air versus ground transport studies. *Air Med J*. 2010;29(3):102–103.
5. Floccare DJ, Stuhlmiller D, Braithwaite SA, et al. Appropriate and safe utilization of helicopter emergency medical services: a joint position statement with resource document. *Prehospit Emerg Care*. 2013;17(4):521–525.
6. American College of Emergency Physicians. Appropriate and safe utilization of helicopter emergency medical services. Approved 2011. https://www.acep.org/globalassets/new-pdfs/policy-statements/appropriate-and-safe-utilization-of-helicopter-ems.pdf?_t_id=1B2M2Y8AsgTpgAmY7PhCfg==&_t_q=helicopter&_t_tags=andquerymatch,language:en|language:7D2DA0A9FC754533B091FA6886A51C0D,

siteid:3f8e28e9-ff05-45b3-977a-68a85dcc834a|siteid:84BFAF-5C52A349A0BC61A9FFB6983A66&_t_ip=&_t_hit.id=ACP_Website_Application_Models_Media_DocumentMedia/_1e274bb4-1fa7-4b65-b344-e32a13b9b9f2&_t_hit.pos=1&_t_id=1B2M2Y8AsgTpgAmY7PhCfg==&_t_q=helicopter&_t_tags=andquerymatch,language:en|language:7D2DA0A9FC754533B091FA6886A51C0D,siteid:3f8e28e9-ff05-45b3-977a-68a85dcc834a|siteid:84BFAF5C52A349A0BC61A9FF-B6983A66&_t_ip=&_t_hit.id=ACP_Website_Application_Models_Media_DocumentMedia/_1e274bb4-1fa7-4b65-b344-e32a13b9b9f2&_t_hit.pos=1. Accessed July 22, 2018.

7. Hunt D. Transfer of the critically ill adult. *Surgery (Oxford)*. 2018;36(4):166–170.
8. Lyphout C, Bergs J, Stockman W, et al. Patient safety incidents during interhospital transport of patients: a prospective analysis. *Int Emerg Nurs*. 2018;36:22–26.
9. Swickand S, Winkelmann C, Huky F, Kerr M, Reimer A. Patient safety events during critical care transport. *Air Med J*. 2018;37(4):253–258.
10. Commission on Accreditation of Medical Transport Systems. *Standards*. 11th ed. Anderson, SC: Commission on Accreditation of Medical Transport Systems; 2018.
11. Insoft R, Schwartz H, Romito J. In: *Guidelines for Air and Ground Transport of Neonatal and Pediatric Patients Manual*. Elk Grove Village, IL: American Academy of Pediatrics; 2015.
12. Grabowski RL, Wolfe A. Neurologic trauma. In: Semonin Holleran R, Wolfe A, Frakes M, eds. *Patient Transport: Principles and Practice*. St Louis, MO: Mosby/Elsevier; 2018:231–249.
13. Brown J, Tompkins K, Chaney F, Donovan R. Family member ride-along during interfacility transport. *Air Med J*. 1998;17(4):169–173.
14. Macnab A, Gagnon F, George S, Sun C. The cost of family-oriented communication before air medical interfacility transport. *Air Med J*. 2001;20(4):20–22.
15. Perez L, Alexander D, Wise L. Interfacility transport of patients admitted to the ICU: perceived needs of family members. *Air Med J*. 2003;22(5):44–48.
16. Joyce C, Libertin R, Bigham M. Family-centered care in pediatric critical care transport. *Air Med J*. 2015;34(1):32–26.
17. Hansen M, Hansen E. Left behind: caring for children in families experiencing patient transport. *Air Med J*. 2014;33(2):69–70.
18. Carubba C. Role of the medical director in air medical transport. In: Blumen I, Lemkin D, eds. *Principles and Directions of Air Medical Transport*. Salt Lake City, UT: Air Medical Physicians Association; 2006.
19. Swearingen C. Transport physiology. In: Semonin Holleran R, Wolfe A, Frakes M, eds. *Patient Transport: Principles and Practice*. St Louis, MO: Mosby/Elsevier; 2018:27–43.

17

Health Emergency Management

Michael De Laby

To understand the objectives of Emergency Management or Disaster Preparedness programs, it is first important to define what constitutes a disaster. Disasters, both natural and man-made, can dramatically affect life and property within communities—leaving ongoing destruction lasting from days to months or even years. The term disaster itself can be difficult to define because disasters are largely unpredictable and effects vary depending on the event and community affected. An event leading to as few as 10 casualties may be considered a disaster for a rural community with limited resources or geographic areas that prevent adequate resource deployment without outside assistance. In these terms, disaster is best defined as an incident or event that overwhelms the infrastructure of a community in which it occurred.[1] The United Nations International Strategy for Disaster Reduction (UNISDR) defines disaster as "a serious disruption of the functioning of a community or a society involving widespread human, material, economic, or environmental losses and effects, which exceeds the ability of the affected community or society to cope using its own resources."[1]

The United States Department of Homeland Security's National Response Framework describes a disaster as "any natural or man-made incident, including terrorism, which results in extraordinary levels of mass casualties, damage, or disruption severely affecting the population, infrastructure, environment, economy, national morale, or government functions."[2], p. 1.

Historic events such as the attack on the World Trade Center in 2001, the Tohoku Japan Earthquake and tsunami in 2011, and Hurricanes Katrina in 2005, Irma in 2017, and Harvey in 2018 reinforce the need for a national coordinated emergency response. Emergency responders, including nurses, are compelled by a sense of duty as the magnitude of any disaster unfolds and graphic images of human suffering are replayed over various media outlets. However, responding to human need is not as simple as grabbing a few supplies and jumping on the next bus to help.

In 1995 a nurse was killed by falling debris in Oklahoma City in the aftermath of the explosion at the Alfred P. Murrah Building, illustrating the need for protective equipment and proper training. Hundreds of rescue and medical personnel who showed up via public transportation and private vehicles had to be turned away in the Gulf Coast region after Hurricane Katrina. Although professional skills were needed in specific locations, local officials did not have the means to feed or shelter unexpected personnel, verify professional credentials, or spare the resources to identify and coordinate proper work assignments in the midst of the actual event. Stockpiles of unrequested, unused supplies received were unable to be distributed due to the inability to coordinate efforts to sort and distribute donated items. The lack of a coordinated effort in dealing with these complex issues makes it challenging and sometimes impossible to use these resources in a time of need. Planning and preparation about the roles, responsibilities, and resource management strategies are essential to matching personnel, equipment, and supplies with the people and communities who need them most. The development of Emergency Management programs assists in providing the infrastructure to coordinate resources and meet community demands during disasters.

The need to prepare at the local level is critical to coordinate emergency management functions for communities affected. Many mistakenly view the federal government (and in particular, the Federal Emergency Management Agency [FEMA]) in a lead and primary role in this regard. In reality, local emergency managers make intrastate and interstate requests for assistance long before a federal disaster response is activated by the governor of an affected state.[3] These activations typically occur when local and state resources are exhausted or insufficient to meet the demands of the incident. FEMA is just one of many federal departments or agencies that may be called upon to assist in rescue and recovery efforts.

EVOLUTION OF EMERGENCY MANAGEMENT

As a function of public health and safety, emergency management is an essential role of the government. During the Cold War era, the principal disaster risk in the United States was believed to be a nuclear attack by the Soviet Union. Individuals and communities were encouraged to build bomb shelters, and every community had a civil defense director. Preceded by a string of natural disasters in the 1960s, a national focus on emergency management in the 1970s resulted in the formation of FEMA during the Carter administration. In the 1970s, new categories of catastrophes also became evident—those caused by human error or malfeasance and involving chemicals or other toxic agents.[4]

Several federal legislative milestones have been identified over the past decade making federal assistance available at the

TABLE 17.1 Major Federal Legislative Milestones.

Year	Milestone or Legislative Action	Key Elements
1803	Congressional Act	One of the first federal actions to provide local financial assistance (Portsmouth, NH, devastated by fire)
1934	Flood Control Act	Authorized US Army Corps of Engineers to design and build flood control projects
1950	Civil Defense Act	Created shelter, evacuation, and training programs to be implemented by state and local governments
1950s	Ad hoc legislation	Provided disaster assistance funds after a series of hurricanes
1968	National Flood Insurance Act	Created the National Flood Insurance Program (NFIP)
1974	Disaster Relief Act	Coordinated federal response and recovery efforts through the NFIP
1979	Executive order by President Carter	Federal Emergency Management Agency (FEMA) created
1988	Robert T. Stafford Disaster Relief and Emergency Assistance Act	Amended Disaster Relief Act—constituted statutory authority for most federal disaster response activities, encourages hazard mitigation measures to reduce losses from disasters, authorized creation of the Federal Response Plan, required all states to prepare their own Emergency Operations Plans
1994	Stafford Act amended	Incorporated most of the former Civil Defense Act of 1950
1995	Nunn-Lugar Act	Core purpose was to reduce the nuclear threat to the United States domestically and abroad; it became the first federal legislation reflecting the government's concern for domestic disaster management resulting from terrorism
1996	Emergency Management Assistance Compact	Provided form and structure to interstate mutual aid
2001	Patriot Act	Significantly increased the surveillance and investigative powers of law enforcement agencies in the United States
2002	Homeland Security Act	Established Department of Homeland Security and refocused the country on terrorism
2002	Public Health Security and Bioterrorism Preparedness and Response Act	Related to public health preparedness and improvements; controls on biologic agents; protecting food, drug, and drinking water supplies; created state bioterrorism preparedness block grant program
2006	Pandemic and All-Hazards Preparedness Act	Transferred the National Bioterrorism Hospital Preparedness Program (NBHPP) from the Health Resources and Services Administration (HRSA) to the assistant secretary for preparedness and response (ASPR); ASPR is the principal advisor to the secretary of health and human services on public health and medical preparedness and response

local level (Table 17.1). One of the most significant pieces of emergency management legislation was enacted by Congress in 1988. The key provision of the Robert T. Stafford Disaster Relief and Emergency Assistance Act included authorization (statutory authority) for most federal disaster response activities. The Stafford Act also encouraged hazard mitigation measures to reduce losses from disasters, authorized creation of the Federal Response Plan, and required all states to prepare their own Emergency Operations Plans. The Federal Response Plan, a landmark federal document when it was released in 1992, identified and organized Emergency Support Functions (ESFs) as a mechanism for grouping activities most frequently used to provide federal support, both for declared disasters and emergencies under the Stafford Act and for non–Stafford Act incidents. ESF #8, the Public Health and Medical Services Annex,[5] was revised in 2008 and is categorized into the following core functional areas:

- assessment of public health/medical needs
- health surveillance
- medical care personnel
- health/medical/veterinary equipment and supplies
- patient evacuation
- patient care
- safety and security of drugs, biologics, and medical devices
- safety of blood and blood products
- food safety and security
- agriculture safety and security
- worker safety and health
- all-hazard public health and medical consultation
- technical assistance and support
- behavioral health care
- public health and medical information
- vector control
- potable water/wastewater and solid waste disposal
- fatality management
- veterinary medical support
- human services coordination

In the months after the 2001 attack on the World Trade Center, President George W. Bush created the Homeland Security Council within the executive branch of the federal government and began issuing a series of executive orders commonly known as "Homeland Security Presidential Directives," or HSPDs, which record and communicate presidential decisions about the homeland security policies of the

United States. Among them, in February 2003 President Bush issued Homeland Security Presidential Directive (HSPD)-5, *Management of Domestic Incidents,*[6] which directs the secretary of homeland security to develop and administer a National Incident Management System (NIMS). This system is intended to provide a nationwide template to enable federal, state, local, and tribal governments to work effectively together to manage a range of domestic incidents.

Under NIMS, agencies can take a comprehensive approach to incident management that can apply to emergencies of all types and sizes, allowing for flexible, coordinated, and efficient responses to each incident. Under the NIMS structure, the secretary of homeland security is the principal federal official for domestic incident management. HSPD-5 requires all federal departments and agencies to adopt NIMS and to implement it across all programs. The directive also requires federal departments and agencies to mandate compliance with NIMS as a condition for federal preparedness assistance (i.e., grants, contracts, and other activities). As a result, NIMS became an essential component of the US health care system through the National Bioterrorism Hospital Preparedness Program.[7] Originally administered by the Health Resources and Services Administration (HRSA), the National Bioterrorism Hospital Preparedness program is now located in the US Department of Health and Human Services (DHHS) under the assistant secretary for preparedness and response (ASPR). The focus of the program has become all-hazards preparedness and not solely bioterrorism. The NIMS model for incident management is the Incident Command System (ICS). ICS is a standardized on-scene emergency management system designed to aid in the management of resources during incidents. When organizations use the ICS model as the basis for their disaster planning, they adopt predefined management hierarchy, processes, and protocols that come into play in an emergency, allowing for integration with other organizations during a response.

EMERGENCY MANAGEMENT PROGRAMS

Emergency management programs aim to strengthen a jurisdiction's capacity and capability to prepare, respond and recover from all types of emergencies. Disasters differ in scope, size, and scale and often require integrated coordination across multiple agencies and, at times, across multiple jurisdictions. Emergency management programs exist at many different levels and within many different types of organizations, including federal, state, local, nongovernment organizations, such as the American Red Cross, faith and university-based programs, and private sectors, such as hospital and business programs.[8]

With the goal of saving lives, preventing injury, and protecting the environment and property, emergency management programs focus on the four phases within the disaster cycle. Current thinking defines these four phases as mitigation, preparedness, response, and recovery. Mitigation includes efforts to limit the effects from hazards by improving the ability to return to a normal state.[9] Preparedness includes planning efforts to respond to hazards, and response includes reducing or eliminating the hazard effects.[9] Recovery is restoration from the impact to its preincident level of functioning.[9] Emergency management programs use the disaster-cycle model to shape public policy and planning efforts to improve preparedness, warning systems, and response coordination and reduce vulnerabilities to limit the effects on people, property, and infrastructures.

Health Emergency Management

Health emergency management programs also aim to strengthen a jurisdiction's capacity and capabilities with a focus on health care sectors. Examples of health emergency management program sectors include public, behavioral and environmental health, health laboratory, epidemiology and infectious disease, emergency medical services, nursing, and emergency medicine.[10] Objectives for health emergency management and health care preparedness efforts are structured to preserve life, minimize health impacts, and protect responders.[11] In times of emergencies, health care sectors are faced with unique challenges involving an increase in the number of patients seeking care and the availability of supplies, equipment, pharmaceuticals, and staff to meet increased demand. Many health care sectors are also challenged by the availability of physical space to provide patient care. Emergency management can address impacts to health care by supporting development of preparedness activities for health care facilities and staff and facilitating training in incident command systems.

Health Care Facilities

Hospitals are an essential participant in the event of a disaster and will be considered a response component for the community when incidents occur. Emergency departments may receive a large number of patients via the emergency medical services system, or patients may arrive by private auto.[2] It is essential for emergency nurses to maintain awareness of and screen for potential hazards or exposures that may increase risks for the patient or the nurse themselves.[2] Recognizing this, many accrediting bodies, such as The Joint Commission, have strengthened standards to improve patient management and ensure hospitals are better prepared to care for patients during disasters.

Although hospitals are a significant part of the health care system, many other types of health care facilities and providers should be considered and included in health emergency management planning and preparedness. This need has prompted the Centers for Medicare and Medicaid Services (CMS) to publish Emergency Preparedness Requirements for Medicare and Medicaid Participating Providers and Suppliers[12] in 2016. This rule affects inpatient providers such as long-term care and skilled nursing facilitates and outpatient care providers such as surgical and dialysis centers, clinics, home health agencies, and hospice providers. The new CMS rule requires licensed health care providers to develop an emergency plan, policies to address patient care during a disaster, a communications plan, and training and exercise programs to test the facilities' disaster preparedness capabilities.[13] Including these facilities in health care preparedness activities helps ensure the needs of vulnerable populations with specific health issues will be cared for during a disaster.

Health care coalitions (HCCs) are one prominent model to bring health care facilities together to address health care disaster preparedness and response activities for all levels of providers within the community. These groups of individual health care and response organizations play a critical role in providing and linking health care and public health preparedness and response capabilities. Serving as hubs to facilitate the sharing of information, resources, policies, and practices, HCCs are able to support health care infrastructures before, during, and after events. DHHS has developed objectives to assist in driving preparedness, response and recovery efforts to maximize care capacity and capabilities in the setting of disasters. HCC partners can engage in emergency preparedness planning and activities to meet their own needs as well as serve the health care needs of the jurisdiction as a whole.[14]

Disaster Nursing

The role of the nurse in disasters is integral as nursing is the largest component of the health care team. The use of nurses in disasters dates back to Florence Nightingale and the Crimean War in the 1850s. Wartime health care is similar to disaster health care in that the needs far outweigh the resources. During the flu pandemic of 1918 to 1919, the health care system was overwhelmed and required alternative care sites. It was the adaptability and flexibility of nurses that allowed for patient care to be provided with limited resources and outside normal duties. The day to day roles of nurses make them exceptional providers in disaster settings.

But emergency preparedness is more than being prepared and knowing what to expect. The nurse should understand the core nursing-related principles that prepare the nurse to function in a disaster setting. Currently, there is a lack of overall education related to disaster and preparedness activities. Additionally, nurses and other health care providers are not always included in planning and disaster drills. Compared with the increasing number of threats, the level of preparedness activities targeting the nursing profession is largely inadequate.[1] Nurses and other health care professionals should ensure a personal preparedness plan and should seek out disaster education and training to address the needs of the communities in which they live.[1]

Compounding the problem, despite the effect of disasters on the health care system infrastructure and ability to respond during emergencies, many nurses do not view themselves as emergency responders and do not invest the time to educate themselves on disaster nursing. In actuality, during an emergency, nurses will be on the front lines helping those in need. Nurses were deployed to provide care for the Ebola crisis in West Africa. Unfortunately, some nurses did not have the proper personal protective equipment or the ability to "don and doff" the personal protective equipment correctly, and they were subsequently exposed to the virus. This illustrates the need for nurses to educate themselves in emergency management concepts, prepare themselves, and understand their role and any limitations they may have as well as understand the response to different types of events.[15]

Emergency nurses routinely plan, assess, adapt, and respond, and they can easily transition to unpredictable and chaotic environments while caring for patients. To serve as active participants in a disaster response, emergency nurses should gain additional skills and knowledge through an understanding of the ICS and of the various disciplines of emergency management—mitigation, preparedness, response, recovery, and communications[8]—before a disaster occurs.

Nurses who educate themselves and who are involved in disaster play an important role and are able to meet the goals of obtaining the best possible level of health for people, making sure people are able to first meet basic survival needs. Nurses are an ideal resource for the community in the setting of disaster as they are able to assess available resources, correct inequalities in access to care, and ensure cultural, linguistic, and religious diversity is respected. Establishing priorities, identifying health needs of affected groups, determining actual and potential public health problems, and collaborating to obtain and maintain access to care are other important roles the nurse fills in a disaster. Nurses communicate, triage, prioritize, teach, lead, and meet the physical and emotional needs of their patients daily, which are all qualities needed in response and recovery. The Emergency Nurses Association (ENA) has written a position statement regarding the nurse's role in emergency preparedness.

Nurses who educate themselves are able to become disaster responders within their own communities, or they may be able to serve other communities in need. Whether part of a hospital staff, medical reserve corps (MRC), disaster medical assistance team (DMAT), or other community groups organizing to assist during a disaster, emergency nurses can play leadership roles in personal and community domestic preparedness. Using the Homeland Security All-Hazards Taxonomy, as well as a full range of publications available from national organizations and federal agencies on disaster preparedness as a guide, emergency nurses can perform on a personal and professional basis through the four mission stages related to homeland security.

Training and Education Overview of ICS and NIMS

The concept of ICS was developed more than 30 years ago, in the aftermath of a devastating wildfire in California. During 13 days in 1970, 16 people died, 700 structures were destroyed, and more than a half million acres burned. The cost and loss associated with these fires totaled $18 million per day. Although all of the responding agencies cooperated to the best of their ability, numerous problems with communication and coordination hampered their effectiveness. As a result, Congress mandated the US Forest Service to design a system to effectively coordinate interagency actions and to allocate resources that would be applicable to multiple-fire situations. This system became known as Firefighting Resources of California Organized for Potential Emergencies

(FIRESCOPE). FIRESCOPE ICS is primarily a command and control system delineating job responsibilities and organizational structure for the purpose of managing day-to-day operations for all types of emergency incidents.

By 1981, ICS was widely used throughout southern California by the major fire agencies. It was quickly recognized that ICS could help public safety responders provide effective and coordinated incident management for a wide range of situations: floods, hazardous materials incidents, earthquakes, and aircraft crashes.[7] This system was flexible enough to manage catastrophic incidents involving thousands of emergency response and management personnel. By introducing relatively minor terminology and organizational and procedural modifications to FIRESCOPE ICS, ICS became adaptable to an all-hazards environment.

ICS Requirements for Hospitals and Practitioners

NIMS requires all federal, state, local, tribal, private sector, and nongovernmental personnel with a direct role in emergency management and response to be NIMS and ICS trained.[16] This includes all emergency services–related disciplines such as emergency medical services (EMS), hospitals, public health, fire service, law enforcement, public works/utilities, skilled support personnel, and other emergency management response, support, and volunteer personnel. Emergency nurse managers involved or interested in hospital preparedness should enroll in FEMA Training IC 100 and 200 HCA for hospitals and health care systems. The Hospital Incident Command System (HICS, formerly HEICS) is an important foundation for the more than 6000 hospitals in the United States in their efforts to prepare for and respond to various types of disasters.

Credentialing of Emergency Responders

Three principal efforts among FEMA's HSPD-5 initiatives are directed at supporting NIMS' policies to improve mutual aid processes. These include establishment of common performance standards for training emergency responders, use of common definitions for typical response resources (National Mutual Aid and Resource Management Initiative or "Resource Typing"), and implementing a national system for credentialing emergency responders that can be used to easily support mutual aid through the verification of the identity and qualifications of emergency response personnel. The credentialing system, currently referred to as the National Emergency Responder Credentialing System (NERCS) can help prevent unauthorized (i.e., self-dispatched or unqualified) personnel access to an incident site. Most homeland security experts agree that once the system is fully operational, access to a disaster scene will be restricted to those with a documented mission assignment and authorization to provide assistance through interstate mutual aid agreements.

National Bioterrorism Hospital Preparedness legislation in 2002 mandated that a state-based national system be implemented to meet the needs of hospital workforce emergency surge capacity. The Emergency System for Advance Registration of Health Professional Volunteers (ESAR-VHP) was developed and is currently operational in several states. The system comprises four levels based on the types of credentials required of a given health profession and what can be verified. Information about ESAR-VHP is available at https://www.phe.gov/esarvhp/Pages/about.aspx.

BOX 17.1 National Planning Scenarios.

- Nuclear Detonation: 10-kiloton Improvised Nuclear Device
- Biological Attack: Aerosol Anthrax
- Biological Disease Outbreak: Pandemic Influenza
- Biological Attack: Plague
- Chemical Attack: Blister Agent
- Chemical Attack: Toxic Industrial Chemicals
- Chemical Attack: Nerve Agent
- Chemical Attack: Chlorine Tank Explosion
- Natural Disaster: Major Earthquake
- Natural Disaster: Major Hurricane
- Radiologic Attack: Radiologic Dispersal Device
- Explosives Attack: Bombing Using Improvised Explosive Device
- Biological Attack: Food Contamination
- Biological Attack: Foreign Animal Disease
- Cyber Attack

From Homeland Security Council. *The National Planning Scenarios.* Washington, DC, 2006.

SUMMARY

Emergency preparedness is every citizen's responsibility; health care professionals carry a greater responsibility in ensuring preparedness efforts are addressed for all phases of the disaster cycle. Emergency nurses interested in deployment opportunities during disasters must receive proper ICS and disaster-related safety training and participate in state credentialing programs in advance of a disaster. Some hospitals and health systems have established and equipped medical teams who could provide emergency response during a disaster. Most jurisdictions will not accept self-deployed responders during a disaster because of the challenges created by on-site logistics, credentialing, and liability. Individual responders are generally not requested; however, individuals who organize and train together as a team (such as a local or state ENA chapter, Community Emergency Response Team [CERT], or Medical Reserve Corps) could be eligible for funding and grants and could be requested and deployed through the EMAC process to support a mutual aid response. Opportunities for individuals may also exist through the National Disaster Medical System.[7] Most important, emergency preparedness begins at home. Personal preparedness assists us with being ready to support ourselves and our families when affected and to respond as health care professionals when needed.

REFERENCES

1. Ciottone GR. *Ciottone's Disaster Medicine*. 2nd ed. Philadelphia, PA: Elsevier; 2016.
2. Emergency Nurses Association. Position statement: Disaster and emergency preparedness for all hazards. https://www.ena.org/docs/default-source/resource-library/practice-resources/position-statements/allhazardspreparedness.pdf?sfvrsn=ea0879a4_10. Published 2014. Accessed May 3, 2019.
3. Centers for Disease Control and Prevention. Section I: systems approach to planning. In: *Medical Management Guidelines. Volume II: Hospital Emergency Departments*. http://www.atsdr.cdc.gov/MHMI/mhmi-v2-1.pdf. Published 2011. Accessed May 3, 2019.
4. Rubin CB, ed. *Emergency Management: The American Experience 1900-2005*. Fairfax, VA: Public Entity Risk Institute; 2007.
5. US Department of Homeland Security. Federal response framework ESF #8—Public Health and Medical Services Annex. https://www.fema.gov/media-library-data/20130726-1825-25045-8027/emergency_support_function_8_public_health___medical_services_annex_2008.pdf. Published January 2008. Accessed June 15, 2018.
6. White House The. Homeland Security Presidential Directive/HSPD-5. https://www.hsdl.org/?view&did=439105. Published 2003. Accessed June 15, 2018.
7. US Department of Health and Human Services. National Disaster Medical System. https://www.phe.gov/Preparedness/responders/ndms/Pages/default.aspx. Published 2018. Accessed July 5, 2018.
8. Haddow GD, Bullock JA. *Introduction to Emergency Management*. 5th ed. Burlington, MA: Elsevier Butterworth-Heinemann; 2014.
9. Koenig KL, Schultz CH, eds. *Koenig and Schultz's Disaster Medicine, Comprehensive Principles and Practices*. 2nd ed. New York, NY: Cambridge University Press; 2016.
10. Office of the Assistant Secretary for Preparedness and Response Hospital Preparedness Program. Healthcare preparedness capabilities: National guidance for healthcare system preparedness. http://www.phe.gov/Preparedness/planning/hpp/reports/Documents/capabilities.pdf. Published January 2012. Accessed.
11. Fagel MJ. *Principles of Emergency Management and Emergency Operations Centers*. Boca Raton, FL: Taylor & Francis Group; 2011.
12. Lord E, Camidge C. The CMS rule and healthcare coalitions. Healthcare Ready website. https://www.healthcareready.org/system/cms/files/1491/files/original/Healthcare_Coalition_Conference_Session_on_CMS_Rule.pdf. Accessed June 15, 2018.
13. Centers for Medicare and Medicaid. Center for Clinical Standards and Quality/Survey & Certification Group [memorandum summary and *Fed Reg*. 78(249):79082, December 27, 2013. September 2016. https://www.cms.gov/Medicare/Provider-Enrollment-and-Certification/SurveyCertificationGenInfo/Downloads/Survey-and-Cert-Letter-14-09.pdf. Accessed May 3, 2019.
14. US Department of Health and Human Services. Public health emergency. In: *MSCC Handbook*. www.phe.gov/Preparedness/planning/mscc/healthcarecoalition/chapter1/Pages/default.aspx. Published Feb 14, 2012. Accessed May 3, 2019.
15. Sellwood C, Wapling, eds. *Health Emergency Preparedness and Response*. Boston, MA: CAB International; 2016.
16. Federal Emergency Management Agency. National Incident Management System Training Program. https://www.fema.gov/pdf/emergency/nims/nims_training_program.pdf. Published September 2011. Accessed June 15, 2018.

18

Chemical, Biological, Radiologic, Nuclear (CBRN) Threats

Michael De Laby

WEAPONS OF MASS DESTRUCTION: THE THREAT

Emergency nursing requires preparation for many types of disasters and mass casualty incidents (MCIs), including those caused by Chemical, Biological, Radiologic, and Nuclear (CBRN) agents, collectively referred to as potential weapons of mass destruction (WMD). The United States Code, Title 50, defines WMD as "any weapon or device that is intended or has the capacity to cause death or serious bodily injury to a significant number of people through the release, dissemination, or impact of (a) toxic or poisonous chemicals or their precursors; (b) a disease organism; or (c) radiation or radioactivity." WMD are used or stockpiled by both terrorists (domestic and foreign) and military agencies because their primary purpose is to kill, injure, sicken, threaten, or strike fear in a target population. Because of the potential for such a widespread psychological effect, WMD have also been termed weapons of mass effect (WME).[1] This chapter outlines the characteristics and medical response considerations for CBRN agents of mass destruction.

Who Threatens

Both domestic and foreign terrorist threats could involve CBRN agents. These threats include lone individuals, political and special-interest groups, nonaligned groups, doomsday or religious cults, and insurgents.[2] Domestic terrorists are those from the United States. They may be individuals such as Ted Kaczynski (i.e., the "Unabomber"); Timothy McVeigh, who was convicted of the Murrah Federal Building bombing; or Eric Rudolph (Olympic Park Bomber). Domestic terrorists may also belong to hate-associated organizations such as the Ku Klux Klan (KKK); ecology "special interest" groups like the Earth Liberation Front (ELF), which was responsible for multiple acts of arson to vehicles and buildings; religious cults such as the Aum Shinrikyo, which was responsible for the sarin gas attacks in Japan; and/or followers of the Bhagwan Shree Rajneesh, who were responsible for sickening hundreds of residents in (the city of) The Dalles, Oregon. Foreign terrorists may belong to organizations such as al Qaeda, Hamas, and/or may be state sponsored.[3] Terrorists seek to injure, kill, cause destruction, and instill fear for their personal or political agenda. The use or threatened use of WMD agents is a federal crime, with the Federal Bureau of Investigation having jurisdictional authority.

Why Chemical, Biological, Radiologic, and Nuclear Agents

CBRN agents are practical tools for terrorism. CBRN weapons require only small quantities of an agent or pathogen to achieve a high impact. CBRN agents are easy to conceal and transport and can be hard to detect. Many of these small, potent agents do not have a characteristic odor or other obvious physical characteristics. CBRN components are widely available within the community, are readily made, and are relatively inexpensive. Bioweapons have been cited as "the poor man's atomic bomb" because of their potentially high impact and relatively low cost.[4] Materials can be found in local factories, hardware stores, industrial settings, school laboratories, universities, and hospitals.

Mass Casualty Differences

There are differences between the mass casualties arising from a natural disaster and those resulting from terrorism involving CBRN components. MCIs occur every day, resulting in injured persons presenting to the emergency department (ED). MCIs may result from manmade events such as a transportation crash or mass shootings or from natural events such as an earthquake, hurricane, tornado, or epidemic. Natural disasters are not premeditated, whereas terrorism is a planned and perpetrated event. Terrorism or threats of terrorism are federal crimes and require collaboration with multiple organizations, which includes following chain of custody when collecting the victim's personal belongings. Responders must be aware of possible secondary terrorism devices intended for the rescuers.[5] There is a greater potential for death and destruction with CBRN agents. Many natural disasters come with some sort of warning beforehand; however, there is usually little to no preparation for an act of terrorism. MCIs involving CBRN agents, whether accidental (e.g., Chernobyl, Russia) or intentional (e.g., Tokyo, Japan), will result in reactions of anxiety and increased fear of possible exposure or contamination. Persons with exacerbations of preexisting psychogenic illnesses may also present to the ED.[6]

Hospital and emergency medical services (EMS) systems could easily become overwhelmed.

NUCLEAR-RADIOLOGIC THREATS

Most people are exposed to some level of environmental radiation every day. Ionizing radiation sources are used in commercial food sterilization processors, smoke detectors, medical therapy devices, radiopharmaceuticals, and radiography devices, to name a few. A nuclear threat may be the result of an accident or malfunction, or it may involve a terrorist's use of a radioactive source either alone, in combination with an explosive, or in a nuclear detonation. A nuclear detonation is considered the least likely threat-scenario because of its complexity and the security processes in place; however, it may create the greatest destructive impact.[7] The nuclear detonations at Hiroshima and Nagasaki, Japan, during World War II were some of the first accounts of overt nuclear-radiologic threats against man. Current nuclear threats are considered to come from nations such as North Korea and Iran and from both domestic and foreign terrorist elements.

Types of Nuclear-Radiologic Devices

Potential radiologic and nuclear threats include the following:

- *Radiologic exposure device (RED):* A radioactive source is placed where numerous individuals can be unknowingly irradiated. A RED could be placed in a common public location, or radioactive material could be placed in food or drink, causing internal irradiation, as experienced by the Soviet dissident Alexander Litvinenko.[8]
- *Radiologic dispersal device, or RDD (dirty bomb):* A radioactive source is combined with/in a traditional explosive device. The bomb explodes and spreads radioactive particulate and aerosolized radiation sources. Geographic areas and people within the plume incur varying levels of contamination. Injuries can arise from explosion burns, blast, radioactive contaminates, contaminate inhalation, and shrapnel injuries.
- *Nuclear installation or reactor:* Intentional (sabotage) or unintentional (cracks or meltdown) damage to a reactor can release high levels of radiation via contaminated steam and smoke.
- *Improvised nuclear device:* A fabricated or crude nuclear bomb that could result in a 10- to 20-kiloton blast similar to the explosion that destroyed Nagasaki, Japan. Fissile materials could be acquired by terrorists to create this WMD.[9,10]
- *Thermonuclear weapon:* A weapons-grade, atomic or hydrogen bomb. This device creates energy from atomic fission or fusion. The effects of a 1-kiloton blast (equivalent to 1000 tons of TNT) over 1 minute would be as follows:
  - Blast range of approximately 400 yards
  - Thermal radiation burns approximately 400 yards out
  - High rates of radioactive fallout up to ½ mile from blast
  - Gamma and neutron radiation up to ½ mile from blast
  - Electromagnetic pulse (EMP) that would destroy or damage computer microchips and circuits (an aerial burst would increase the effects of an EMP)

All of these nuclear threats have the potential to release ionizing radiation in the form of alpha, beta, and gamma rays; neutrons; and x-rays in either a particulate matter or "wave-like" form.

Radiation Basics

Radiation is energy emitted from a source and is a constant occurrence in our natural environment. We are surrounded by low-level, background radiation coming from the soil, sun, and certain products within our living space and workplace.[11] There are two principal radiation forms, nonionizing and ionizing, and the ionizing radiation poses the potential health risks addressed here. Ionizing radiation has enough energy to break chemical bonds of impacted atoms, creating energized or ionized, particles. There are two forms of ionizing radiation: waves (electromagnetic) and particles. Types of ionizing radiation include alpha, beta, gamma, neutron, and x-rays. Under the correct conditions and amounts, the ionized particles can interact with living cells, creating free radicals that cause chemical changes within those cells. Biologic damage can occur to cellular DNA bonds, proteins, and membranes, and can be expressed later as tissue alterations, mutations, tumors, or cancers.

Types of Radiation

Ionizing radiation may be emitted directly in the forms of alpha or beta particles along with gamma and or x-rays. Neutrons are indirectly ionizing particles because they do not carry an electrical charge.

- Alpha particle radiation is composed of two neutrons and two protons and is very energetic and highly ionizing. Alpha is the least penetrating, traveling several centimeters in air, and particles can be blocked by a sheet of paper, clothing, or the outer layer of dead human skin. There is a minimal external-exposure threat, but inhalation or absorption/internalization can be a serious hazard.
- Beta radiation is emitted from the nucleus. It is a smaller particle than alpha and penetrates moderately, moving up to a few meters in air and a few millimeters through tissue. Beta particles can be blocked with glass, wood, or plastic. Beta particles and energy can cause skin injury known as "beta burns" over time.
- Gamma rays and x-rays are high-energy, wavelike forms of radiation that can penetrate deeply and are difficult to shield. Gamma rays travel farther and require special shielding, such as appropriate amounts of lead or concrete.
- Neutrons are highly penetrating and energetic particles emitted from the nucleus. Neutrons, like gamma rays and x-rays, require special shielding.[12]

Dose

To understand exposure, one must study or measure the dose of radiation. Radiation measurement factors include the activity (A), absorbed dose (D), and the dose-equivalent (H).

Activity is a measurement of ionized particles discharged and is measured in a unit called a curie (Ci). More curies present means more radioactivity. The time it takes for a quantity of radioactive material to decay by half of its original amount is its "half-life." A Geiger counter is used to detect and measure radioactive decay. Absorbed dose (D), or rad, is energy deposited in the tissue per unit mass of irradiated tissue. The rad is the US standard unit of measurement, whereas the International System (SI) of units for the absorbed dose is the gray (Gy). Dose-equivalent (H) is measured in rems, comprises the absorbed dose (D), and is weighted for the effectiveness of causing biologic damage.[11] The Sievert is the SI unit used to measure dose-equivalent. Dose-equivalent assists by providing a common scale for all types of radiation tissue damage.

Everyone receives natural, background radiation exposure from his or her living and working environment. The annual natural background radiation dose a person receives from sun, soil, building materials, and the like is approximately 300 millirem (300 mrem). Airline passengers flying from Los Angeles to New York might receive 2.5 mrem of cosmic radiation, whereas an unprotected ED nurse potentially receives 5 mrem during a portable chest x-ray examination. Other typical patient radiation doses include the following: bone scan, 400 mrem; abdominal computerized tomography scan, 760 mrem; barium enema, 870 mrem; and cardiac catheterization, 45,000 mrem. The goal is to keep radiation exposure and contamination levels as low as reasonably achievable (ALARA).

The hospital radiation safety officer or health physicist can assist with calculating dose exposures and monitoring the effectiveness of decontamination actions.

Protection Principles: Time, Distance, and Shielding

Principles for protection from the effects of ionizing radiation include factors of time, distance, and attenuation, or shielding. Limiting time spent near a radioactive source limits its dosage and possible effects. Remain as far away from a source as possible. The intensity of ionizing radiation is minimized by the inverse of the distance squared (i.e., the greater the distance, the less of a dose received). Radiation attenuation or shielding with proper materials can reduce radiation exposure and dose received. Proper shielding materials are a factor of the type of radiation emitted, with alpha particles being blocked by clothing or paper and beta particles by a thicker plastic or wood material, which can impede absorption. Gamma rays, neutrons, and x-rays require substantially more shielding with appropriate amounts of lead (aprons or lead-lined rooms), concrete (radiation bunkers), or earth (berms).

Exposure, Contamination, and Incorporation

Radiation injury begins after external or internal exposure (contamination) or irradiation occurring from exposure to a penetrating radioactive source. The body's incorporation or uptake of radioactive contaminants results in systemic injury. Contamination occurs after internal or external exposure to radioactive materials by inhalation, ingestion, or when deposited on the body or clothing. Patients considered potentially contaminated should be surveyed and appropriately decontaminated.

External irradiation exposure does not make the victim radioactive or pose a threat to caregivers. A person contaminated with radioactive isotopes should be medically stabilized, appropriately decontaminated, and referred for further treatment and evaluation.[13]

Internal contamination results when radioactive contaminants are blast embedded, inhaled, or ingested. This might occur to victims near a detonated RDD when radioactive fragments and bomb particulates become imbedded or nuclear material is aerosolized and inhaled. Incorporation begins when the cells and tissues of the body's radiosensitive system cells, such as bone marrow stem cells, gastrointestinal (GI) villi, liver cells, and thyroid cells, begin uptake of the radioactive contamination.[12]

Acute Radiation Syndrome

The acute illness arising from a significant and penetrating, partial- or whole-body irradiation is referred to as acute radiation syndrome (ARS). Ionizing radiation affects the most radiosensitive cells first, which include those involving hematopoiesis, digestion, and the central nervous system (CNS).[7] ARS is subdivided into three syndromes that are based on the body's affected system and includes potential cutaneous radiation injury.

Body Systems Affected

The order of syndrome appearance is based on cell radiosensitivity and the absorbed dose. Syndromes include the hematopoietic syndrome, the GI syndrome, CNS or neurovascular syndrome, and cutaneous radiation injuries.

Hematopoietic syndrome. Bone marrow stem cells and accessory cells are most notably radiosensitive, and their irradiation results in increasingly rapid cellular death and alterations in blood component formation. The destruction of bone marrow stem cells and similar systems results in lymphopenia, pancytopenia, sepsis, and hemorrhage. Radiation doses resulting in a hematopoietic syndrome may be seen in an exposure of 0.3 to 0.7 Gy (30–70 rads).[14] The rate of decline in absolute lymphocytes over a 2-day period is used to help predict radiation level exposure.

Gastrointestinal syndrome. Destruction of microvilli and GI tract lining occurs with absorbed doses of 6 to 10 Gy (600–1000 rads). Mucosal lining breakdown and sloughing of the intestinal wall results in diarrhea, severe nausea, vomiting, abdominal pain, and subsequent systemic effects that could include fever, GI bleeding, dehydration, and anemia. The LD_{100}, or lethal dose for 100% of the population, is approximately 10 Gy (1000 rads).

Central nervous system syndrome. CNS syndrome is equated with an expectant or fatal outcome. CNS syndrome may be noted after absorbed doses of 20 to 50 Gy (2000–5000 rads) and is indicated by nervousness, confusion, altered level of consciousness, convulsions, and death. Symptoms can begin minutes after exposure to this intense irradiation.

Cutaneous radiation injury. Radiation injury to the skin and tissues can occur with doses as low as 2 Gy (200 rads). Because minimal energy is required, injury can occur without other ARS symptoms. An example would be the beta burns resulting from beta radiation. Dermal and underlying tissue damage increases as dose is increased. Radiation burn injuries can present over weeks or months and are staged and graded. Symptoms can include itching, tingling, edema, erythema, and ulcerations, and the injuries may result in dry or moist desquamation and necrosis. Pain management and infection control are important for care.

Acute Radiation Syndrome Stages

ARS symptoms are also classified into a sequence of four phases or stages. Stage development is dependent on cell radiosensitivity and dose and type of radiation received. The four stages of ARS are prodromal, latent, manifest illness, and recovery or death. The prodromal, or nausea-vomiting-diarrhea stage, is dose dependent. It usually begins minutes to days after exposure, and symptoms may last for days. The latent phase occurs hours to weeks after the prodromal stage and is marked as a period when the patient feels and may look healthy. In the manifest illness stage, symptoms due to the particular syndrome appear and may last from hours to months. The recovery or death stage lasts from days to years, again depending on the syndrome.[14]

Diagnosis and Treatment

ARS follows a predictable course of illness after substantial irradiation. Complete blood count (CBC) analysis can be correlated to exposure level. ARS should be evaluated with serial CBC analysis with a focus on lymphocyte count every 2 to 3 hours for the first 8 to 12 hours after exposure, and then every 4 to 6 hours for the subsequent 2 to 3 days.[15] Dosimetry for exposure dose levels can also be quantified via genetic assay with dicentric chromosome analysis considered the gold standard. Record all symptoms, including nausea, vomiting, diarrhea, skin erythema, and any blistering, as well as their time of onset. The onset time of vomiting has been correlated to prognosis and exposure level. Treatment considerations will be largely supportive based on ARS symptoms and include antiemetics and fluids. Other possible treatments include stem cell replacement, cytokines, and if internalized or incorporated, cathartics, chelators, and binding agents, some of which may be implemented in the ED.

Planning

- Stabilize the patient first. Ensure airway, breathing, and circulation.
- If contamination is suspected, decontaminate appropriately and survey for effectiveness.
- An exposure without contamination does not require decontamination.
- Treat any traumas, burns, or other injury symptoms. Provide supportive care.
- Notify public health and law enforcement.
- Obtain laboratory specimens, including serial CBC, human leukocyte antigen (HLA), and serum amylase. Other specimens collected might include swab samples from body orifices and urine specimens if contamination or a substantial dose was internalized. Consider dicentric chromosomal assay.
- Consult specialists, including the hospital radiation safety officer, health physicist, Radiation Emergency Assistance Center Training Site (REAC/TS), and/or the Armed Forces Radiobiology Research Institute (AFRRI).[14]

BIOLOGIC AGENTS

Biologic pathogens have been researched, weaponized, and used by armies against their opponents for hundreds of centuries. Pathogens were used in the Middle Ages, during the French and Indian War, and by Germany in World War I and Japan in World War II. In 1984 The Dalles, Oregon, was the scene for the first known biologic attack in the United States. There the Rajneeshee, a religious cult, attempted to gain control of the local county government by spraying *Salmonella* on salad bars and throughout public venues before a county election. More than 500 persons became ill.[16] The September 2001 anthrax attacks on various US news media offices and two US Senate offices resulted in 22 infections, including 5 deaths.

Today both domestic and foreign terrorists have developed and deployed bioweapons. Countries with offensive biologic weapons programs have included South Africa, United States, Soviet Union, Great Britain, Iraq, Syria, North Korea, and Iran. The signing of the 1972 Biological Weapons Convention Treaty by a majority of nations, including the United States, ended offensive biologic weapons development for the signing countries. Although it also signed, the Soviet Union reportedly continued clandestine research, development, and production of genetically altered "super pathogens" well into the 1990s. Production activities were curtailed and facilities closed after defecting Soviet microbiologists revealed ongoing bioweapons activities and facility locations.[17]

Biologic Threats: Bacteria, Viruses, and Toxins

Biologic threat agents include bacteria, viruses, and toxins. Bacteria are single-celled microorganisms that may form spores and produce a tissue inflammatory reaction. Viruses are the simplest pathogen, consisting of protein-coated RNA or DNA. Viruses require a host cell and can cause a variety of cell-specific diseases. Viral diseases may end in vascular damage and multiple system organ failure. Toxins are nature's poisons and are more deadly than comparable amounts of any manmade chemical agent.[18] Toxins or their precursors may be found in the outside garden (ricin) or may exist in the kitchen pantry (botulinum).

The infection methods or delivery routes include inhalation, ingestion, injection, and dermal contact. Examples include inhalation of respiratory droplets infected with a virus such as smallpox, ingestion of *Salmonella,* or dermal contact with anthrax spores. Many biologic agents are contagious from person to person.

The Centers for Disease Control and Prevention (CDC) has categorized certain bacterial, viral, and toxin biologic threats into Category A, B, and C diseases or agents. Categorization factors include ease of dissemination; transmissibility; potential for high morbidity and mortality; potential for social disruption; surveillance needs, and ease of production, among others. The CDC Category A agents are anthrax, botulism, plague, smallpox, tularemia, and viral hemorrhagic fevers (VHFs), including Ebola, Marburg, Lassa, and Machupo.[19] All suspected biologic agent cases should result in notification of the infection control practitioner, appropriate hospital personnel, and public health officials.

Epidemiology: The Clues

A biologic attack or infectious outbreak will be insidious, yet there will be clues. Clues include infections unusual for a geographic region; increased deaths among the immunocompromised; multiple, similar outbreaks of disease; multiple, drug-resistant pathogens; increased or many sick and dying animals; physical evidence; or agent delivery device. Disease surveillance factors during triage and medical history might include travel history, infectious contacts, activities over the previous 3 to 5 days, and employment history.[18] The hospital infection control practitioner along with local and state public health officials should be notified for any suspected Category A patient.

CDC Category A Bacteria

Anthrax. *Bacillus anthracis* is a rod-shaped, gram-positive, spore-forming bacteria endemic within certain agricultural regions and livestock populations and may cause woolsorter's disease from handling contaminated hides or fluids. Spore inoculation may result in cutaneous anthrax; spore ingestion may result in GI anthrax, whereas spore inhalation may result in respiratory or inhalational anthrax. Infection results in bacterial migration to regional lymph nodes, producing an edema-factor toxin or a lethal-factor toxin.[20] Inhalational anthrax is the most lethal variation and may result in mediastinitis, as opposed to pneumonia, as evidenced by a widened mediastinum on chest x-ray films.

Manifestations. Cutaneous anthrax results in itching skin and papular lesions that become vesicular and ulcerative. Ulcerative areas may develop moderate to severe edema. The lesions develop a black eschar within 1 to 2 weeks. There is a slight possibility that cutaneous anthrax could be transmitted by contact with another person.

GI anthrax arises from spore germination within the upper or lower intestinal tract. Upper GI tract involvement results in edema, lymphadenopathy, and sepsis. Lower GI tract involvement includes symptoms of bloody diarrhea, ascites, abdominal pain, and sepsis associated with a partially necrotic lower intestine.

Inhalational anthrax victims may initially feel like the seasonal flu victim. Those infected may experience a 2- to 6-day incubation period followed by a dry cough, myalgias, fatigue, and fever. Victims may experience a short period of improvement followed by a sudden onset of high fever, respiratory distress, shock, and death, possibly with 24 to 36 hours. Patients may develop a mediastinitis, and approximately 50% will have hemorrhagic meningitis.

Treatments. Standard precautions are needed when caring for anthrax or potentially anthrax-exposed patients.[5] Avoid any contact with wound drainage. Anthrax victims will require specimen cultures and then antibiotics. Treatments approved by the Food and Drug Administration (FDA) include ciprofloxacin, levofloxacin, doxycycline, and penicillin. Other care includes supplemental oxygen, managing respiratory compromise, and supportive care. A vaccination regimen involving six courses is available to the Department of Defense, whereas a new civilian anthrax vaccination protocol is being developed by the CDC.

Planning

- Hospitals, including EDs, should have a protocol and/or plan to deal with potentially contaminated mail and "white powder" events.
- Report suspected cases to the infection control practitioner and public health officials.
- Use standard precautions, and avoid wound drainage contact.

Plague. Plague, or *Yersinia pestis,* is a non–spore-forming, gram-negative bacillus responsible for pandemics in AD 541 and 1346, the latter known as the "Black Death" or "great pestilence." Found in certain rodents, including some rats, ground squirrels, and prairie dogs, *Y. pestis* is endemic to the western United States and every continent except Australia. *Y. pestis* is transmitted to humans by bites from fleas that have been feeding and living on infected rodents, including rats and mice.[21]

This disease has several variations, including bubonic, septicemic, and pneumonic plague. The bubonic version is transmitted to the human's regional lymph nodes, causing adenitis or bubos (large, painful, inflamed lymph nodes), hence its name—bubonic plague. *Y. pestis* can progress from a bubonic to septicemic plague; however, neither is contagious person to person. A few individuals may develop a secondary pneumonic plague, which is highly contagious and spread via respiratory droplets.[22] Pneumonic plague probably represents the most significant biowarfare or terrorism threat. Techniques to aerosolize and induce pneumonic plague were developed in the later years of US and Soviet Union biowarfare production. The World Health Organization (WHO) reported that if 50 kg of *Y. pestis* were released over a city of 5 million inhabitants, approximately 150,000 would develop pneumonic plague and 36,000 would die. Other contagious inhabitants would flee the city, and the infection would spread.[23]

Manifestations. Bubonic plague symptoms, including chills, fever, weakness, and the development of painful bubos, begin 2 to 8 days after a bite from an infected flea. Bubos tend to form in the axilla, groin, or cervical region, and their pain restricts movement of the affected areas.[24] Untreated, the disease will progress into a fatal septicemic or possible pneumonic plague.

Pneumonic plague symptoms should start with a 1- to 6-day incubation period followed by high fever, myalgias, chills, headache, chest pain, and cough with bloody sputum. If untreated, dyspnea, cyanosis, and shock may result in death. Other complications for pneumonic and septicemic plague may include acral gangrene, which can affect the fingers, toes, earlobes, nose, and/or penis.

The diagnosis of plague is made by history, Gram stain and cultures of lymph node aspirates, and sputum and cerebrospinal fluid samples. Bipolar, "safety-pin" staining may be present with a Wright, Giemsa, or Wayson stain.[5]

Treatment. Patients with confirmed bubonic plague require standard precautions. Those patients being ruled out for bubonic versus pneumonic plague or diagnosed probable pneumonic plague require strict respiratory droplet precautions. Antibiotics are required as soon as possible after culture specimens are collected. Antibiotic therapy considerations for active disease and postexposure prophylaxis include streptomycin, gentamicin, doxycycline, ciprofloxacin, and chloramphenicol.[21]

Planning

- The hospital laboratory/microbiology should be notified when plague is suspected.
- Report suspected cases to the infection control practitioner and public health officials.
- Cohort patients if large numbers of suspected pneumonic plague victims make isolation impractical.

Tularemia. Tularemia, caused by the bacterium *Francisella tularensis,* is a potentially fatal illness that occurs naturally in the United States, North America, and Eurasia. It is commonly called "rabbit fever" because it is found in small animals, especially rodents, rabbits, squirrels, and hares. Tularemia is one of the most pathogenic diseases known, requiring as few as 10 organisms via inoculation or inhalation to cause infection.[18] It has been studied as a potential bioweapon for years. The Japanese investigated *F. tularensis* as a weapon in Manchurian research units between 1932 and 1945. Russia, the United States, and other countries have previously experimented and stockpiled *F. tularensis* as an offensive weapon. By 1973, the United States had destroyed its offensive arsenal.[25] Because of its ease of infection, dissemination, and capacity to cause illness and death, *F. tularensis* is considered a dangerous potential biologic weapon. Although human tularemia infections may occur with ingestion, contact, or aerosol inhalation, it is not transmissible from person to person.

Manifestations. Infection takes place through bacilli contact with mucous membranes, GI tract, and the lungs. Symptoms of tularemia appear 3 to 5 days after exposure but can take up to 14 days. Like other flulike illnesses, symptoms can include sudden fever, chills, headaches, sore throat, dry cough, diarrhea, muscle aches, and progressive weakness.[26] Manifestations can include pleuritic chest pain, shortness of breath with pneumonias, hemoptysis, hilar lymphadenopathy, and sepsis.

Treatment. Standard precautions are warranted for suspected tularemia patients. Diagnosis will be made by sputum Gram stain and blood cultures. Designated national reference laboratories can aid in rapid diagnostic testing and identification. Immediate antimicrobial treatments, with streptomycin as drug of choice or gentamicin, are usually indicated for adults and children. A tularemia vaccine is available as an investigational new drug (IND) and under review by the FDA.

Planning

- After an aerosol delivery, expect multiple victim presentations with similar symptoms.
- Report suspected cases to the infection control practitioner and public health officials.
- Implement standard precautions for patients with suspected tularemia.

CDC Category A Viruses

Smallpox. Smallpox is caused by one of two species of poxvirus, variola minor or variola major. Variola major, hereafter called smallpox, is a highly virulent and contagious disease that spreads from person to person by aerosols or droplet nuclei via cough, sneeze, and direct contact. It results in a fever, characteristic rash, and death rate of 30%. Smallpox had been a significant cause of illness and death in developing countries until the 1970s, when the last outbreak occurred in Somalia[27] in 1977. By 1980, WHO certified the eradication of smallpox among the world's populations. The only specimens known to exist are in the CDC Laboratory in Atlanta, Georgia, and the Vector Laboratory in Moscow, Russia.

Smallpox has been a consistent choice for biologic warfare using contagious pathogens. Variola was probably first used as a weapon between 1754 and 1767, during the French and Indian War, when British soldiers distributed infected blankets to the American Indians.[18] The Indian death rate from this contagious disease was approximately 50%. In 1796 Edward Jenner's cowpox vaccination prevented the spread of smallpox. Dr. Ken Alibek, a microbiologist and former director of the Soviet biologic weapons program, reported Soviet efforts to further weaponize smallpox in a variety of munitions. This included developing industrial quantities of genetically altered smallpox and other pathogens that would be more virulent and resistant to possible drug therapies.[17]

Manifestations. Smallpox inoculation occurs via face-to-face encounter or contact with infected body fluids, contaminated objects, and bedding. The incubation period ranges from 7 to 17 days, after which the virus spreads to lymph nodes and multiplies. The first symptoms include high fever and may include malaise, headache, body aches, and sometimes nausea and vomiting. During the next 2 to 4 days, the most contagious phase, a rash develops on the tongue and in the mouth. The rash then spreads to the face, arms, legs, and distally to the hands and feet. Fever may fall. The rash evolves into fluid-filled, painful bumps that later thicken and develop a characteristic central depression or umbilicus. Fever rises, and the bumps turn into sharply raised pustules that crust over and scab. The person is considered contagious until the scabs fall off.[28]

Treatment. Smallpox is very contagious. Evaluation and care should be in a negative-pressure environment using strict airborne and contact infection control precautions. Diagnosis is made by clinical presentation, positive tissue cultures, and/or positive virus identified with electron microscopy.

Smallpox treatment is supportive. Antivirals and immune globulin may aid treatment, although vaccination remains the most effective prevention tool.

Planning

- Any case of smallpox indicates bioterrorism and is considered a federal crime; therefore criminal investigation should be anticipated.
- Identify a response team within the ED whose members are protected by recent smallpox vaccination.
- Report suspected cases to the infection control practitioner and public health officials.

Viral hemorrhagic fevers. VHF refers to an illness characterized by fever and bleeding disorders caused by one of four virus families. VHF illnesses are caused by distinct families of RNA viruses that cause high fevers, vascular abnormalities, sepsis, hemorrhaging, and multisystem organ failure. The four VHF virus families are Filoviridae (Marburg and Ebola), Arenaviridae (Lassa fever), Flaviviridae (yellow fever), and Bunyaviridae (Rift Valley fever).[29] These pathogens are endemic to parts of Africa, Central and South America, and the Middle East, with infections usually transmitted during insect bites or contact with infected body fluids. Other diseases that belong to this group include hantaviruses, Crimean-Congo fever, and others. Several countries have investigated weaponizing VHFs because of contagiousness along with high morbidity and mortality rates.[30] The VHFs are limited in treatment and vaccine options.

Manifestations. VHF symptoms include fever, myalgias, rash, weakness, hypotension, prostration, jaundice, and bleeding complications, including conjunctival injection, petechiae, disseminated intravascular coagulation, and shock. Laboratory findings will likely indicate thrombocytopenia and may indicate renal or liver failure.

Treatment. Most VHF viruses are very contagious. Patients should be placed in a private room with standard, droplet, and contact precautions. Airborne precautions including negative pressure might also be chosen for patients with respiratory involvement or those undergoing pulmonary procedures or treatments that stimulate coughing.[18] Most VHFs do not have a vaccine; however, yellow fever is the exception. Arenaviruses, bunyaviruses, and those VHFs of unknown causes may be effectively treated with ribavirin.[30] The majority of VHF treatment will be supportive, including intravenous fluids, hemodynamic monitoring, ventilation, dialysis, and antibiotics for secondary infections. Needle punctures and anticoagulant therapies are contraindicated.

Planning

- Additional barriers might be necessary to prevent contact with large amounts of body fluids and/or secretions.
- Fever and hemorrhaging from any site are characteristic for VHF.
- Report suspected cases to the infection control practitioner and public health officials.

CDC Category A Toxin

Toxins are harmful substances naturally produced by living organisms and can be more toxic per unit measure than any manmade chemical or synthetic poison. Toxins tend not to cause illness via contact (except trichothecene mycotoxins [T2 mycotoxins]) or spread from person to person.[31] Toxins are usually ingested, but their aerosol versions can be inhaled. Examples of toxins include botulinum, the most potent neurotoxin; ricin, a deadly cytotoxin; staphylococcal enterotoxin B (SEB), which causes incapacitating gastroenteritis; and the T2 mycotoxins, the only dermally active toxin. Of these, botulinum is the only CDC Category A toxin.[19]

Botulinum. *Clostridium botulinum* is the spore-forming, anaerobe bacillus that produces botulinum toxin and is the most poisonous substance by weight known.[32] Botulism is a neuroparalytic disease occurring naturally in three forms: foodborne, infant botulism, and wound botulism. Inhalational botulism would be an unnatural occurrence and a result of a biologic attack. Properly manufactured, dispersed, and inhaled, a single gram of botulinum would kill more than 1 million people. Botulism has been an agent for bioterrorism and bioweapons development for years. During the 1930s, the Japanese Unit 731 fed botulinum cultures to prisoners in biologic warfare experiments. Countries that have developed and stockpiled, or are thought to be developing, botulism weapons include the United States, Soviet Union, Iraq, Iran, North Korea, and Syria. As an agent of bioterrorism, the doomsday cult Aum Shinrikyo unsuccessfully attempted aerosolized botulism attacks on multiple Japanese locations[33] between 1990 and 1995.

Manifestations. Signs and symptoms begin 6 hours to 2 weeks after exposure and are the same for all forms of botulism, including inhalational. Disease symptoms depend on the rate and amount of toxin absorbed. Neurologic symptoms include symmetric, descending flaccid paralysis with bulbar palsies including ptosis, blurred vision, diplopia, dysphagia, and dysphonia.[5] Patients may appear comatose, requiring months of mechanical ventilation before recovery. Clinical diagnosis is made by bulbar palsy with descending paralysis. Positive *C. botulinum* specimen cultures and mouse neutralization assay can confirm diagnosis.

Treatment. Standard precautions are appropriate when caring for botulism victims. Therapy for botulism includes early use of type-specific botulinum antitoxin after rapid diagnosis. Supportive care may include extended mechanical ventilation and enteral or parenteral tube feeding.

Planning

- Report suspected cases to the infection control practitioner and public health officials.
- The ED or hospital encountering botulism should consider foodborne substances, including home-canned products and potential contaminated illegal drug use.
- There is no person-to-person spread of botulism.

CHEMICAL AGENTS

Chemical agents can be used as weapons of mass destruction and have been deployed by various nations' military and by terrorists. Many chemical components of a terrorism attack are readily available in the community. These threats can be found in local hardware stores, schools, laboratories, and in tankers transiting community highways and railroads. Depending on their primary effect, most chemical agents can be classified as nerve agents, vesicants, blood agents, or pulmonary/choking agents. Chemical agent response will require coordination with EMS, poison control, and planning for effective decontamination and appropriate personal protective equipment use by hospital first receivers and decontamination team.

Some of the first uses of chemical weapons included toxic smoke directed by Spartan allies in 423 BC; the use of poisons in hollow, explosive mortar shells during the 15th and 16th centuries, and the deployment of chlorine gas[34] in World War I. Chemical weapons used during recent military engagements have included mustard agents, phosgene, cyanide, and probably sarin. Many nations, including the United States and Soviet Union, signed the 1972 Biological Weapons Convention Treaty indicating they would eliminate biologic and chemical weapons, but intelligence sources have indicated continued offensive chemical weapons operations by some signatory nations.

Nerve Agents

Nerve agents were developed specifically for warfare. As the most toxic of chemicals, they are likened to very powerful organophosphates. These agents are acetylcholinesterase (AChE) inhibitors, disrupting and blocking the effects of the enzyme acetylcholinesterase. The result is accumulated acetylcholine at the receptor sites, causing repeated stimulation of the nerve. Nerve agents were discovered while a German scientist was trying to develop an insecticide during the late 1930s and have been called "bug poison for people."[35] Since that time, nerve agents such as tabun (GA), sarin (GB), soman (GD), cyclosarin (GF), and VX have been developed and stockpiled by various countries for military deployment. The G (German) agents are volatile and soluble in water. VX is not nearly as volatile or soluble. VX is persistent in the environment with an oilylike nature and therefore presents a greater contact hazard.

The United States began destruction of its stockpiles of nerve agents with the signing of the 1972 Biological Weapons Convention Treaty.[36] In 1988 Iraqi military reportedly bombed a Kurdish community of 80,000 with a cocktail of chemical agents, including sarin, soman, mustard gas, and other agents. Although nerve agents have been historically developed and controlled by the military, they have also been used by terrorists. A "low-potency" sarin was made and released by the doomsday cult Aum Shinrikyo in Matsumoto, Japan, and on Tokyo, Japan, subways in 1995. The Tokyo subway release killed 12 people and sent more than 5000 to area hospitals seeking evaluation and treatment.[37,38]

Manifestations

Nerve agents disrupt nerve impulse transmission and result in overstimulation of nerves, producing nicotinic effects (skeletal muscle twitching, cramping, weakness, flaccid paralysis, tachycardia, and high blood pressure) and muscarinic effects (pinpoint pupils; miosis; hypersecretion by salivary, lacrimal, sweat, and bronchial glands; nausea, vomiting, and diarrhea). CNS effects can include behavioral changes, irritability, seizures, and apnea. Mild/moderate exposure symptoms may include localized sweating, fasciculations, nausea, vomiting, weakness, and dyspnea. Severe exposure symptoms include unconsciousness, seizures, convulsions, apnea, and flaccid paralysis.[39] Exposure is toxic in all amounts, with little difference between a lethal and survivable dose. Exposure can occur through inhalation, dermal/eye contact, ingestion, or injection. Exposure signs and symptoms are remembered with the mnemonic SLUDGEM:

S Salivation and increased secretions
L Lacrimation
U Urinary incontinence
D Defecation, incontinence
G Gastrointestinal distress
E Emesis
M Miosis

Treatment

Decontamination and antidote delivery for the nerve agent exposure are critical. After exposure, clothing should be removed and the patient properly decontaminated as quickly as possible. Up to 75% to 90% of the chemical contamination can be stopped by removing the victim's clothing. Respiratory support, including supplemental oxygen, suctioning of secretions, and possible intubation, may be necessary. Diazepam may be necessary for seizure activity.

Nerve agent antidotes include atropine and pralidoxime chloride (2-PAM Cl). The US military has developed Mark 1 antidote kits that comprise two autoinjectors: one autoinjector delivers 2 mg atropine in 0.7 mL diluent IM, and the other contains 600 mg of 2-PAM Cl in 2 mL diluent. ED management includes administration of the antidotes with dosage based on age and degree (mild, moderate, or severe) of symptom presentation. The antidotes are given until the symptoms begin to subside; therefore large doses may be required. Seizures are treated with diazepam.[40]

Planning

- Nerve agents are extremely toxic and can cause death within minutes to hours after exposure.
- Patients presenting to the ED are a potential threat from vapor off-gassing or contaminant contact.
- First receivers need to be adequately protected and trained for the chemical casualty decontamination response.
- Report suspected cases to the infection control practitioner, public health officials, and law enforcement.

Vesicants

The vesicants, or blister agents, are manmade chemicals that cause vesicles or skin blisters with potential systemic effects and include sulfur, three variations of nitrogen mustard (H1, H2, and H3), lewisite, and phosgene oxime. Vesicants have been used in warfare since World War I, during the 1980s Iran-Iraq war, and reportedly by Iraq against the Kurds[41] in 1988. Vesicants can cause dermal burns and represent a contact and inhalation threat. The mustard gases are named because of their distinctive garlicky or mustard odor. Sulfur mustard is a terrorist threat because it is inexpensive and can be dispersed as a droplet or vapor. Mustards are oily and stable, persist in the environment, and attack the skin, mucous membranes, lungs, and blood-forming organs.[42] Mustard exposure is not immediately painful on contact and has a latent reaction period, whereas lewisite produces immediate pain and discomfort. The mustard agents and phosgene oxime do not have an antidote, but lewisite does—British antilewisite (BAL).

Manifestations

Exposure to vesicants will most likely occur via contact or inhalation, but ingestion of contaminated food or water is possible. Symptoms can include eye tearing and conjunctivitis, eyelid swelling, blepharospasms, itching, redness, ophthalmic injury, and burning and blisters especially in warm, moist areas (axilla, groin, etc.). Other symptoms include throat and mucous membrane burning, hoarseness, shortness of breath, cough, abdominal pain, emesis, and diarrhea. Inhalation of a vesicant can lead to systemic effects, pulmonary edema, and death. Substantial mustard gas exposures can induce bone marrow stem cell suppression, leucopenia, and subsequent decreased immunity.[34,43]

Treatment

Treatment for exposure to vesicants is mostly supportive but begins with immediate decontamination because injury begins within 2 minutes of exposure. Eye exposures receive copious irrigations, topical mydriatics, and antibiotics. Bronchodilators may be helpful. Supportive care objectives are to relieve symptoms, promote healing, and prevent secondary infection and may take months.

Planning

- Sulfur mustard victims may complain of a mustard, garlic, or onion odor. Ocular exposures may produce a sensation of grittiness in the eyes.
- Antibiotic therapy should be guided by laboratory and culture sensitivity findings.
- Report suspected cases to the infection control practitioner and public health officials.

Blood Agents: Cyanides

Blood agent is an antiquated term for a chemical category that includes mostly cyanides, powerful chemicals that kill quickly by interfering with the blood's ability to transport oxygen to tissues. Although not an ideal weapon for war, due to its rapid evaporation and dispersion, hydrogen cyanide (HCN) was used as a weapon by France in World War I, allegedly by Japan in World War II, and by the Iraqi government in the 1980s against the Kurds. Cyanide (as Zyklon B) was used as an agent of genocide during World War II to kill gas chamber victims in concentration camps.

In recent history, various individuals and groups have used cyanide as an agent in murder and mass suicide. The range of settings and modes of delivery illustrate the versatility and ease of use of cyanide in intentional poisonings. Some of these recent events include the following:

- In July 2004, a 19-year-old from Maryland was sentenced to life in prison after being convicted of poisoning his best friend's soda with cyanide.
- In 1982 seven Chicagoans were killed after ingesting cyanide-laced Extra-Strength Tylenol capsules.
- In 1978 in Jonestown, Guyana, 913 followers of Rev. Jim Jones committed suicide with cyanide-laced Kool-Aid.

Because cyanide possesses many of the characteristics of an "ideal" terrorist weapon, the CDC and the Department of Homeland Security consider it to be among the most likely agents of chemical terrorism.

- Cyanide is used in many industries and is transported throughout the country via rail and highway, and is therefore plentiful, readily available, and can be easily accessed by terrorists via theft or hijacking attempts.
- Unlike many biologic or nuclear weapons, cyanide does not require special scientific or technical knowledge to use.
- Because of its rapidly lethal mechanism of action, cyanide is capable of causing mass incapacitation and casualties, as well as mass confusion and panic created by the difficulty in identifying the source.
- Cyanide requires large quantities of a specific resource (antidote) to combat—a major public health readiness obstacle in most countries.

Exposure to cyanide can occur through several methods. Because it is absorbable into the body through inhalation, contact, or ingestion, the ease of dispersal is of grave concern. Most often discussed is the release of hydrogen cyanide gas into an enclosed space such as an office building, subway, or stadium. But cyanide salts also could be introduced into pharmaceuticals or the food and water supply. Terrorists are likely to initiate an explosion and fire as a secondary component of the act of terrorism. The resulting fire and burning contents including plastics could become a source of cyanide exposure, especially if in an enclosed area such as a tunnel.[44]

Manifestations

Cyanide effectively blocks aerobic metabolism and energy production, resulting in cellular hypoxia and cellular death. No amount of supplemental oxygen can overcome the deficit in affected cells, and anaerobic metabolism causes high levels of lactic acid to accumulate. At moderate to high exposure concentrations, cyanide can kill very quickly—within minutes to hours, depending on the route of exposure. A cellular asphyxiate, cyanides can cause severe respiratory distress and death. However, if recognized and diagnosed in a timely manner, cyanide poisoning can be effectively treated.

Cyanide is reported to have a smell like bitter almonds; however, 60% of the population is genetically unable to detect this odor. Symptoms of exposure include anxiety, tachypnea, agitation, vertigo, weakness, nausea, confusion, lethargy, convulsions, bradypnea, apnea, cardiac dysrhythmias, and death.

Occasionally, excessive venous saturation may result in a rose-colored or cherry-red skin.[34] Other effects may include headache and significant eye, nose, and throat irritation. Elevated plasma lactate levels are also useful as a surrogate marker for elevated cyanide levels.[44,45]

Treatment

Exposure treatment includes immediate movement into a well-ventilated area or into fresh air and supplemental oxygen. Cyanide gas is lighter than air, making decontamination by immediate clothing removal in a clean air environment very effective. Several therapeutic treatments exist for acute cyanide poisoning: an antidote kit including sodium nitrite, sodium thiosulfate, amyl nitrite components and more recently, hydroxocobalamin, which counteract the effects of cyanide; buffer agents such as sodium bicarbonate to counteract the effects of severe metabolic acidosis that accumulates in the bloodstream after HCN exposure; sympathomimetics such as epinephrine to augment coronary and cerebral blood flow during the low flow states associated with HCN poisoning; and anticonvulsants such as diazepam, lorazepam, midazolam, and phenobarbital for the treatment of repeated or prolonged generalized seizures.

Planning

- Victims may report smelling bitter almonds, or caregivers might smell bitter almonds on patient's breath.
- Victims may appear with rose-colored or cherry-red skin.
- Report suspected cases to law enforcement and public health officials.
- Provide antidote kit(s) for EMS units.

Pulmonary and Choking Agents

Used as weapons during World War I, pulmonary and choking agents are found in great quantities within the community and are transported daily on highways and railways. These agents include chlorine, phosgene, ammonia, and those chemicals that cause stress to the respiratory tract and irritate and damage lung tissue. Inhalation of pulmonary or choking agents can create noncardiac pulmonary edema, leading to asphyxiation.[46] When these chemicals come in contact with moisture, they begin forming acids or alkalis, causing inflammation, irritation, burns, or delayed tissue injury. Although primarily an inhalation threat, these chemical exposures may also occur via skin contact, ingestion, or ocular exposure.

Manifestations

Patients may take on the smell of the product to which they were exposed. Patients may report an acrid, pungent odor with chlorine exposure or the scent of new-mown hay, which is a characteristic odor of phosgene.[3] Exposure to these agents can result in eye irritation, conjunctivitis, coughing, wheezing, chest tightness, headaches, nausea, choking sensation, dyspnea, cyanosis, respiratory distress, and symptoms of pulmonary edema, including copious frothy sputum. Moderate to significant exposures to some agents, including phosgene, may result in a relatively asymptomatic or latent period that may last for hours. The latent period is usually followed by dyspnea, hypoxia, and pulmonary edema brought about by simple exertion.

There are no diagnostic laboratory findings or tests for pulmonary or choking agent exposure.

Treatment

Care is supportive. There are no antidotes for the choking/pulmonary agents. Actions include removal from the agent source and thorough decontamination. Medical therapies may include airway maintenance, including possible intubation; respiratory support with supplemental oxygen and possible mechanical ventilation; and administration of inhaled bronchodilators. Dermal exposures should be decontaminated with large volumes of tap water. Ocular exposures should receive large volumes of saline irrigation and thorough evaluation. Patients should be in a high-Fowler's position to promote chest excursion and respiratory ease.[38] Patients exposed to phosgene should also be forced to rest and not be allowed to exert themselves because of the potential latent period effects.

Planning

- First receivers need to be adequately protected and trained for the chemical casualty decontamination response.
- Decontaminate with copious amounts of water, paying particular attention to warm, moist areas, including axillae and groin.
- Report suspected cases to the infection control practitioner and public health officials.
- Plan for victim forced rest after exposure.

SUMMARY

Emergency nursing requires knowledge and preparation for many kinds of MCIs. Terrorism and disasters involving CBRN agents are a documented source of MCI victims throughout history. CBRN agents are relatively inexpensive, widely available, and offer a potential for high impact and terror by causing dramatic death and illness. The increase in domestic and foreign terrorism, along with geopolitical instability in many countries, indicates the potential for more CBRN events. Effective emergency nurse response planning begins with potential threat awareness and appropriate medical treatments.

REFERENCES

1. Homeland Security Advisory Council Weapons of Mass Effect Task Force. Preventing the entry of weapons of mass effect into the United States. http://www.dhs.gov/xlibrary/assets/hsac_wme-report_20060110.pdf. Published January 10, 2006. Accessed June 15, 2018.
2. Bowman S. Weapons of mass destruction: the terrorist threat. CRS Report for Congress. http://www.fas.org/irp/crs/RL31831.pdf. Accessed May 4, 2019.
3. US Department of State. Patterns of global terrorism. Report. https://www.state.gov/j/ct/rls/crt/2003/31644.htm. Published April 29, 2004. Accessed June 15, 2018.
4. Lyell L. Chemical and biological weapons: the poor man's bomb. North Atlantic Assembly. https://fas.org/irp/threat/an253stc.htm. Accessed May 4, 2019.
5. Bartlett J, Greenburg M. *PDR Guide to Terrorist Response.* Montvale, NJ: Thompson PDR; 2005.
6. DiGiovanni C. Domestic terrorism with chemical or biological agents: psychiatric aspects. *Am J Psychiatry.* 1999;156(10):1500.
7. *Medical Management of Radiological Casualties: Handbook.* Bethesda, MD: Armed Forces Radiobiology Research Institute; 2013. Accessed June 15, 2018.
8. Doctors seek poisoning clues during autopsy. CNN website. http://edition.cnn.com/2006/WORLD/europe/12/02/uk.spy.autopsy/index.html. Published December 2, 2006. Accessed June 15, 2018.
9. Ferguson C, Potter W. Improvised nuclear devices and nuclear terrorism. The Weapons of Mass Destruction Commission, No. 2. http://www.wmdcommission.org/files/No2.pdf. Published 2005. Accessed June 22, 2018.
10. Centers for Disease Control and Prevention. Radiological and nuclear terrorism: medical response to mass casualties. https://emergency.cdc.gov/radiation/masscasualties/training.asp. Published 2006. Accessed June 23, 2018.
11. Eckhardt R. "Ionizing radiation: it's everywhere". *Los Alamos Science.* 1995;(23):23–27. http://library.lanl.gov/cgi-bin/getfile?23-01.pdf. Accessed June 15, 2018.
12. Dainiak N. Medical management of acute radiation syndrome and associated infections in a high casualty incident. *J Radiation Res.* 2018;59(suppl 2):ii54–ii64.
13. Davari F, Zahed A. A management plan for hospitals and medical centers facing radiation incidents. *J Res Med Sci.* 2015;20(9):871–878.
14. Centers for Disease Control and Prevention. Acute radiation syndrome: a fact sheet for physicians. Homeland Security Digital library website. https://www.hsdl.org/?abstract&did=3883. Published 2005. Accessed June 26, 2015.
15. Radiation Emergency Assistance Center/Training Site. The medical aspects of radiation incidents. https://orise.orau.gov/reacts/documents/medical-aspects-of-radiation-incidents.pdf. Published 2017. Accessed June 23, 2018.
16. Tucker J. Historical trends related to bioterrorism: an empirical analysis. *Emerg Infect Dis.* 1999;5(4):6. https://www.ncbi.nlm.nih.gov/pmc/articles/PMC2627752/. Accessed June 12, 2018.
17. Alibek K. *Biohazard.* New York, NY: Random House; 1999. https://www.nlm.nih.gov/nichsr/esmallpox/biohazard_alibek.pdf. Accessed May 4, 2019.
18. US Army Medical Research, Institute of Infectious Diseases. *U.S. Army Medical Research Institute of Infectious Diseases Handbook.* 5th ed. Fort Detrick, Frederick, MD: US Army Medical Research, Institute of Infectious Diseases; 2004.
19. Centers for Disease Control and Prevention. Centers for Disease Control and Prevention website. Bioterrorism agents/diseases. https://emergency.cdc.gov/agent/agentlist-category.asp. Accessed June 11, 2018.
20. Friedlander A. Anthrax. In: *Textbook of Military Medicine, Medical Aspects of Chemical and Biological Warfare. Office of the Surgeon General, Department of the Army.* Washington, DC: Borden Institute; 1997.
21. Inglesby T, Dennis D, Henderson D, et al. Plague as a biological weapon: medical and public health management. *JAMA.* 2000;283(17):2281–2290.
22. Centers for Disease Control and Prevention. Plague. Centers for Disease Control and Prevention website. https://www.cdc.gov/plague/index.html. Accessed June 12, 2018.
23. Center for Biosecurity, University of Pittsburgh Medical Center. Yersinia pestis (plague). http://www.centerforhealthsecurity.org/our-work/pubs_archive/pubs-pdfs/fact_sheets/plague.pdf. Accessed June 20, 2018.
24. McGovern T, Friedlander A. Plague. In: *Textbook of Military Medicine, Part 1.* Falls Church, VA: Office of the Surgeon General; 1997.
25. Department of Homeland Security Working. Group on Radiological Dispersal Device (RDD) Preparedness, Medical Preparedness and Response Sub-Group. https://www.hsdl.org/?view&did=437718. Published 2003. Accessed June 22, 2018.
26. Centers for Disease Control and Prevention. Tularemia. Centers for Disease Control and Prevention website. https://www.cdc.gov/tularemia. Accessed June 18, 2018.
27. Centers for Disease Control and Prevention. Smallpox fact sheet. Centers for Disease Control and Prevention website. http://www.cdc.gov/smallpox. Accessed June 22, 2018.
28. Henderson D, Inglesby T, Bartlett J, et al. Smallpox as a biological weapon: medical and public health management. *JAMA.* 1999;281(22):2127–2137.
29. San Francisco Department of Public Health. Infectious disease emergencies: viral hemorrhagic fevers. https://www.sfcdcp.org/wp-content/uploads/2018/01/VHF-Binder-Chapter.2008.FINAL-id316.pdf. Accessed June 30, 2018.
30. Centers for Disease Control and Prevention. Viral hemorrhagic fevers. Centers for Disease Control and Prevention website. https://www.cdc.gov/vhf/index.html. Accessed June 12, 2018.
31. Franz D. Defense against toxin weapons. In: *Textbook of Military Medicine, Medical Aspects of Chemical and Biological Warfare. Office of the Surgeon General, Department of the Army.* Washington, DC: Borden Institute; 1997.
32. *U.S. Army Medical Management of Biological Casualties Handbook.* 5th ed. Fort Detrick, Frederick, MD: US Army Medical Research Institute of Infectious Diseases; 2004.
33. Arnon S, Schechter R, Inglesby T, et al. Botulinum toxin as a biological weapon: medical and public health management. *JAMA.* 2001;285(8):1059–1070.
34. US Army Medical Research Institute of Chemical Defense. *Medical Management of Chemical Casualties Handbook.* 3rd ed. Aberdeen Proving Ground, MD: Chemical Casualty Care Division, USAMRICD; 2000.
35. Centers for Disease Control and Prevention. Chemical Emergencies: Facts About Sarin. Centers for Disease Control and Prevention website. https://emergency.cdc.gov/agent/sarin/basics/facts.asp. Accessed June 12, 2018.

36. Geldblat J. The biological weapons convention—an overview. *International Review of the Red Cross*. 1997:251–265. (No. 318) http://www.icrc.org/Web/Eng/siteeng0.nsf/html/57JNPA. Accessed June 18, 2018.
37. Olson K. Aum Shinrikyo: once and future threat? *Emerg Infect Dis*. 1999;5(4):513.
38. Urbanetti J. Toxic inhalational injury. In: *Textbook of Military Medicine: Medical Aspects of Chemical and Biological Warfare. Office of the Surgeon General, Department of the Army*. Washington, DC: Borden Institute; 1997.
39. Agency for Toxic Substances and Disease Registry. Nerve agents tabun (GA) CAS 77-81-6, sarin (GB) CAS 107-44-8, soman (GD) CAS 96-64-0, and VX CAS 5078269-9. https://www.atsdr.cdc.gov/toxfaqs/tfacts166.pdf. Accessed June 18, 2018.
40. Ciottone GR. *Ciottone's Disaster Medicine*. 2nd ed. Philadelphia, PA: Elsevier; 2016.
41. Sidell F, Urbanetti J, Smith W, et al. Vesicants. In: *Textbook of Military Medicine, Medical Aspects of Chemical and Biological Warfare. Office of the Surgeon General, Department of the Army*. Washington, DC: Borden Institute; 1997.
42. Dennis D, Inglesby T, Henderson D, et al. Tularemia as a biological weapon: medical and public health management. *JAMA*. 2001;285(21). 2763-1273.
43. Chemical casualty treatment. In: *Jane's Chem-Bio Handbook*. 6th ed. Alexandria, VA: Jane's Information Group; 2000.
44. Baskin ST, Brewer TG. *Medical Aspects of Chemical and Biological Warfare*. Washington, DC: Office of the Surgeon General, Department of Army; 1997.
45. Flomenbaum NE, et al. *Goldfrank's Toxicologic Emergencies*. New York, NY: McGraw-Hill; 2006.
46. Sidell F, Patrick W, Dashiell T. Pulmonary agent effect. In: *Jane's Chem-Bio Handbook*. 6th ed. Alexandria, VA: Jane's Information Group; 2000.

UNIT IV

Medical and Surgical Emergencies

19

Communicable Diseases and Organisms in the Health Care Setting

Sherri-Lynne Almeida

An infection is the detrimental colonization of a host organism by a foreign species. Three factors form the chain of infection: agent, host, and mode of transmission.[1] In an infection, the infecting organism seeks to use the host's resources to multiply, usually at the expense of the host. The infecting organism, or pathogen, interferes with the normal functioning of the host and can lead to chronic wounds, gangrene, loss of an infected limb, and even death. The host's response to infection is inflammation.

A pathogen is usually considered a microscopic organism, although the definition is broader and includes bacteria, parasites, fungi, and viruses. The property of an infectious agent that determines the extent to which overt disease is produced or the power of an organism to produce disease is called pathogenicity. Some agents are highly pathogenic and routinely cause disease, whereas other agents cause disease only when normal host defenses are impaired.

A susceptible host is one who lacks effective anatomic and physiologic resistance to a pathogenic agent. Characteristics influencing susceptibility include nutritional and immunization status, hormonal influences, age, medical and medication history, underlying pathologic condition, and specific insult to the body such as trauma. The severity with which a pathogen causes disease in a specific host, the severity of the resulting diseases, the efficiency with which the organism is transmitted to or from the host, or a combination of these factors is known as the virulence of the pathogen.

Transmission of pathogens is essential to their ultimate survival. Major modes of transmission are contact (direct and indirect), airborne, and droplet. Direct transmission occurs when person-to-person contact occurs between an infected source and a susceptible host with a receptive portal through which human or animal infection can enter. Examples of direct contact include biting; sexual intercourse; direct inoculation with contaminated blood (needlestick injury); or direct projection of droplet spray onto conjunctiva of the eye, nose, or mouth during sneezing, coughing, spitting, or vomiting. Indirect transmission occurs when a susceptible host contacts an inanimate object contaminated with an infectious agent and the agent is transported and introduced into the host through a suitable portal of entry.

Vehicle-borne agents are contaminated, inanimate materials such as patient care equipment, soiled linen, surgical instruments, dressings, food, water, milk, and biologic products such as blood, serum, plasma, tissues, or organs. *Vector-borne* transmission occurs with injection of saliva during biting, regurgitation, or dermal exposure to feces or other material capable of penetrating nonintact skin. And finally, *airborne* transmission is defined as dissemination of microbial aerosols through a portal, usually the respiratory tract. Close contact with an infected source who is coughing or sneezing can transmit large infectious particles through the air. Factors influencing airborne transmission include ambient airflow, proximity, and spatial orientation to the infected person.

INFECTION PREVENTION IN THE ACUTE CARE SETTING

In the hospital environment, transmission of an infectious agent to a susceptible host occurs by contact and inhalation exposure. Health care-associated infections (HAIs) are infections acquired during hospital care that were not present or incubating at admission. HAIs infections are those occurring more than 48 hours after admission, up to 3 days after discharge, up to 30 days after surgery, and in a health care facility when a patient was admitted with a diagnosis that is unrelated to infection.

Many factors contribute to HAIs. Hospitalized patients are often immunocompromised, or they undergo invasive examinations and treatments. Patient-care practices and the hospital environment may facilitate the transmission of microorganisms among patients. The selective pressure of intense antibiotic use promotes antibiotic resistance. Although progress in the prevention of HAIs has been made, changes in medical practice continually present new opportunities for development of infection. The most common types of infections are central line associated (CLABSI), surgical site (SSI), catheter-associated urinary tract infection (CAUTI), and ventilator-associated pneumonia (VAP), which are all caused by various organisms.

Inappropriate hand hygiene or lack of hand hygiene is the most significant factor for development of HAIs, and compliance with hand hygiene recommendations is poor. According to the Centers for Disease Control and Prevention (CDC), health care providers wash their hands less than half of the time required. This situation is due to a variety of reasons, such as noncompliance, lack of appropriate accessible equipment, high staff-to-patient ratios, allergies to hand-washing products, insufficient knowledge of staff about risks and procedures, and the duration of time recommended for washing.

When hands or other skin surfaces are contaminated with blood or other body substances, the area should be cleaned as soon as possible. Hands should be washed before and after every patient contact regardless of whether gloves are worn; if hands will be moving from a contaminated body site to a clean site during an examination; after contact with inanimate objects such as medical equipment or hospital room furniture; and before eating.

In addition to the protection of patients from infectious agents, clinical and nonclinical health care personnel need to protect themselves as well. Health care personnel are at risk for occupational exposure to pathogens, such as hepatitis B virus (HBV) and human immunodeficiency virus (HIV), *Clostridium difficile,* methicillin-resistant *Staphylococcus aureus* (MRSA), and tuberculosis (TB). Exposures occur through needlesticks or cuts from other sharp instruments contaminated with an infected patient's blood or through contact of the eyes, nose, mouth, or skin with a patient's blood, or through close contact with a patient with a respiratory illness.

Standard precautions should be applied to all patient-care and transmission-based precautions when appropriate (Table 19.1).[2]

Many needlesticks and other penetrating exposures can be prevented by using safer techniques (needleless systems), disposing of used needles in appropriate sharps disposal containers, and using medical devices with safety features designed to prevent injuries. Using appropriate barriers such as gloves, eye and face protection, or gowns when contact with blood is expected can prevent many exposures to the eyes, nose, mouth, or skin.

Exposure to pathogens is of concern in health care settings. The emergency nurse will encounter transmittable diseases, depending on where he or she works and the mobility of the patient population. Any infectious agent presents a potential risk under the right circumstances.

PATHOGENS OF CONCERN

Clostridium difficile

C. difficile is a gram-positive bacillus causing an inflammation of the colon. The most common symptoms of *C. difficile* infection (CDI) are watery diarrhea and fever. Patients at an increased risk for CDI are those with exposure to antibiotics, proton pump inhibitors, gastrointestinal surgery, a long length of stay in a health care facility, immunocompromising conditions, underlying illnesses, and advanced age.

TABLE 19.1 Standard Precautions and Transmission-Based Precautions.[2]

Standard Precautions	Transmission-Based Precautions
Perform hand hygiene.	Contact Precautions: • Ensure appropriate patient placement. • Use personal protective equipment (PPE) appropriately. • Limit transport and movement of patients. • Use disposable and dedicated patient care equipment. • Prioritize cleaning and disinfection of rooms.
Use PPE when there is a possibility of exposure to infectious material.	Droplet Precautions: • Source control. • Ensure appropriate patient placement. • Use PPE appropriately. • Limit transport and movement of patients. • Prioritize cleaning and disinfection of rooms.
Follow respiratory hygiene/cough etiquette.	Airborne Precautions: • Source control • Ensure appropriate patient placement in an airborne infection isolation room (AIIR). • Restrict susceptible health care workers from entering the room. • Limit transport and movement of patients. • Immunize susceptible persons as soon as possible after unprotected contact with vaccine-preventable infection.
Ensure appropriate patient placement.	
Properly handle/clean/disinfect patient care equipment and the environment.	
Handle textiles and laundry with care.	
Follow safe needle-handling practices and ensure health care workers' safety.	

Adapted from CDC: Infection Control Basics (2016).

CDC data estimate *C. difficile* caused approximately 500,000 infections in the United States in 2011, and 29,000 people died within 30 days of the initial diagnosis.[3]

C. difficile is shed in feces. Any surface, device, or material contaminated with infected feces may serve as a reservoir for the spores. The spores can be transferred to patients via the hands of health care providers who have touched a contaminated surface and failed to wash their hands appropriately. The length of *C. difficile* incubation is not known but generally is less than 7 days; however, the spores can survive in the environment up to 70 days and can be transmitted via hands through contact with contaminated surfaces.[3]

Patients presenting to the emergency department with fever and a history of three or more unformed stools (watery diarrhea) within 24 hours should be tested for *C. difficile.* A stool culture should be ordered. This is the most sensitive test available; however, it is frequently associated with false-positive results. Because the *C. difficile* toxin is unstable and degrades at room temperature, it is important to promptly test or refrigerate the specimen to prevent false-negative results.

According to the CDC, approximately 20% of patients with CDI will have their condition resolve within 2 to 3 days of discontinuing the antibiotic. The infection can usually be treated with an appropriate course (about 10 days) of antibiotics, including metronidazole, vancomycin (administered orally), or recently approved fidaxomicin. After treatment, repeat *C. difficile* testing is not recommended if the patient's symptoms have resolved, as patients may remain colonized. In about 20% of the patients with CDI, the infection will return and can be very debilitating.[3]

Fecal microbiota transplants (fecal transplants) appear to be the most effective method for helping patients with recurring *C. difficile* infections. The purpose is to replace bacteria that has been killed or suppressed and overpopulate the colon with "good" bacteria.

Hepatitis

Hepatitis is an acute or chronic viral infection of the liver that may be mild or life-threatening. Acute viral hepatitis is caused by five agents, the hepatitis A, B, C, D, and E viruses. Of the hepatitis viruses, only HBV, hepatitis C virus (HCV), and hepatitis D virus (HDV) can cause chronic hepatitis.

Hepatitis B Virus

HBV is an infection attacking the liver that causes acute and chronic infection. Chronically infected people represent the major source of patients with HBV. Individuals have an increased risk for mortality and morbidity associated with chronic liver disease and primary hepatocellular carcinoma. Prevalence of HBV infection varies widely. The World Health Organization (WHO) estimates 257 million people are living with HBV (defined as being hepatitis B surface antigen [HBsAg] positive). In 2015 hepatitis B resulted in 887,00 deaths, most commonly from complications of the diseases.[4] These chronically infected persons are at high risk for death from cirrhosis of the liver and liver cancer. In 2016 the United States reported a total of 3218 acute cases of hepatitis B. The incidence rate was 1.0 cases per 100,000 population.[5] The rate of new HBV infections has increased, which is most likely related to increasing use of drugs by injection.[6]

HBV is transmitted by contact with blood or body fluids (saliva; cerebrospinal fluid; peritoneal, pleural, pericardial, and synovial fluid; amniotic fluid; semen and vaginal secretions, and any other body fluid containing blood; and unfixed tissues and organs) of an infected person. Transmission occurs by exposure to infected body fluids via the percutaneous or per mucosal route.

Worldwide, the major modes of HBV transmission include sexual or close household contact with an infected person, mother-to-infant transmission, the reuse of unsterilized needles and syringes, needlesticks or sharp instrument exposure or the sharing of razors or toothbrushes with an infected person. In addition, HBV is an infectious occupational hazard of health care and public safety workers.

The incubation period for HBV averages 90 days, with a range of 60 to 150 days.[6] The surface antigen (HBsAg) can be detected from 1 to 9 weeks after exposure.[6] Variation in the incubation period is related in part to the amount of virus in the inoculum, mode of transmission, alteration of viral pathogenicity by chemical or physical means, administration of a specific antibody, and unusual virus-host interactions.[6]

Diagnosis of HBV is based on clinical, serologic, and epidemiologic findings. Detection of HBV infection serologic markers—HBsAg—confirms hepatitis B infection. Infection may present with a variety of symptomatology: acute illness with jaundice followed by recovery, subclinical infection followed by recovery, acute illness that progresses to chronic active hepatitis, subclinical infection followed by chronic active hepatitis, and fulminant disease.[7] A short prodromal phase, varying from several days to more than a week, may precede the onset of jaundice. Typical symptoms include anorexia, weakness, and fatigue. Nausea, vomiting, and diarrhea may also occur. Many patients complain of right upper quadrant abdominal pain. In the icteric phase, the urine darkens, followed by jaundice. The appearance of dark urine results from bilirubinuria, followed by light or gray stools and yellowish discoloration of mucous membranes, sclera, conjunctivae, and skin. Jaundice becomes apparent when total bilirubin levels exceed 2.0 to 3.0 mg/dL. Hepatic tenderness and hepatomegaly are also present.[4]

Recovery begins with the disappearance of jaundice and other symptoms. HBsAg and hepatitis E surface antigen also disappear. The appearance of hepatitis B surface antibodies (anti-HBs) indicates the infection is subsiding. This potentially fatal disease is characterized by mental confusion, emotional instability, bleeding manifestations, and coma.

The most effective prevention against hepatitis B is the hepatitis B vaccine. The hepatitis B vaccine prevents hepatitis B disease and its consequences, such as hepatocellular carcinoma. Three single-antigen vaccines and three combination vaccines are available in the United States. The vaccination schedule most often used for children and adults is three intramuscular injections, with the second and third doses administered 1 and 6 months, respectively, after the first dose.

Studies indicate immunologic memory remains intact for at least 30 years among healthy vaccinated individuals who initiated hepatitis B vaccination after 6 months of age. The vaccine confers long-term protection against clinical illness and chronic HBV infection. Cellular immunity appears to persist even though antibody levels might become low or decline below detectable levels. Among vaccinated cohorts who initiated hepatitis B vaccination at birth, long-term follow-up studies are ongoing to determine the duration of vaccine-induced immunity.[5]

Postvaccination testing for adequate antibody response is not necessary after routine vaccination of infants, children, adolescents, or adults. It is recommended only for individuals whose clinical management is dependent on knowledge of their immune status (infants born to HBs-AG positive mothers, health care and public safety workers at high risk for percutaneous or mucosal exposure to blood or body fluids, patients receiving chronic hemodialysis, patients infected with HIV and other immunocompromised patients, and sex partners of individuals with chronic HBV).[5]

A combination of active and passive immunization is used for nonimmunized persons who have sustained a percutaneous or mucous membrane exposure to blood potentially containing HBsAg. If the decision is made to provide postexposure prophylaxis, then a single dose of hepatitis B immune globulin (HBIG) at 0.06 mL/kg should be given as soon as possible, or at least within 24 hours of a high-risk needlestick, and the hepatitis B vaccine series should be started. If the vaccine cannot be given, a second dose of HBIG should be provided 1 month after the first.[5]

Hepatitis C Virus

HCV has been found in every part of the world. The prevalence is directly related to poor parenteral practices in the health care setting and to persons who share injection equipment. The WHO estimates that 71 million people globally have chronic hepatitis C infection and approximately 399,000 people die each year of this disease.[8]

HCV is a bloodborne virus and can be transmitted through direct contact with human blood. Transmission through blood transfusions that are not screened for HCV infection, through the reuse of inadequately sterilized needles, syringes, or other medical equipment, or through needle sharing among drug users, is well documented. Sexual and perinatal transmission may also occur, although less frequently. Other modes of transmission such as social, cultural, and behavioral practices using percutaneous procedures (e.g., ear and body piercing, circumcision, tattooing) can occur if inadequately sterilized equipment is used.

The incubation period ranges from 2 weeks to 6 months, with the average between 6 and 9 weeks. Eighty percent of people do not exhibit any symptoms after the initial infection.[8] HCV infection is usually asymptomatic; therefore few people are diagnosed in the acute phase. Those who are symptomatic may present with fever, fatigue, decreased appetite, nausea, vomiting, abdominal pain, dark urine, gray-colored stool, joint pain, and jaundice. The disease is usually less severe in the acute stage, but chronicity is common. Chronic infection may be symptomatic or asymptomatic. Persons with chronic hepatitis C may develop cirrhosis or hepatocellular carcinoma.

Diagnosis depends on detecting antibodies (anti-HCV) to HCV. Infection can be detected 4 to 10 weeks after infection. Assays of HCV RNA by polymerase chain reaction can detect infection approximately 2 to 3 weeks post infection.

There is no vaccine against HCV. In the absence of a vaccine, all precautions to prevent infection must be taken, including screening and testing of blood and organ donors; virus inactivation of plasma-derived products; implementation and maintenance of infection control practices in health care settings, including appropriate sterilization of medical and dental equipment; promotion of behavior change among the general public and health care workers to reduce overuse of injections and to use safe injection practices, and risk reduction counseling for persons with high-risk drug and sexual practices.

Treatment guidelines recommend no treatment for acute hepatitis C. Patients should be followed and treatment should be considered only if HCV RNA persists after 6 months.[7]

HUMAN IMMUNODEFICIENCY VIRUS/AIDS

HIV targets and weakens the immune system. The virus destroys CD4+T cells, which are critical to fighting disease. The advanced stage of HIV infection is acquired immunodeficiency syndrome (AIDS). In 2016 the WHO reported approximately 37 million people living with HIV, with 1.8 million people becoming newly infected globally. HIV has claimed more than 35 million lives and continues to be a global public health issue.[9]

The course of HIV disease is variable and dictated by the severity of the individual's immune deficiency and any resulting complications. The primary causative viral agent is the virus HIV-1, and it is the infectious agent that has led to the worldwide AIDs epidemic. In 1986 a less common, less virulent type of HIV, HIV-2, was isolated from AIDS patients in West Africa. Both HIV-1 and HIV-2 have the same modes of transmission and are associated with similar opportunistic infections and AIDS. In persons infected with HIV-2, immunodeficiency seems to develop more slowly and to be milder. Compared with persons infected with HIV-1, those with HIV-2 are less infectious early in the infection.

The primary mode of HIV transmission is person to person through unprotected intercourse; contact of abraded skin or mucosa with body secretions such as blood, cerebrospinal fluid, or semen; the use of HIV-contaminated needles and syringes; transfusion of infected blood or its components; and the transplantation of HIV-infected tissues or organs. HIV can also be transmitted from mother to child. Breastfeeding by HIV-infected women can transmit infection to the infant.

The risk of transmission of HIV infection related to percutaneous exposure to infected blood is estimated at about 0.3% for each exposure.[10] The CDC estimates one HIV seroconversion for every 200 contaminated needlesticks. From the literature, we can also find that the probability of infection of

HIV by needle injury is in the range of 0.03% to 0.3%, which increases with the depth of injuries, volume of inoculated blood, and hollow needle injuries.[11] Wyzgowski et al.[11] noted that most of the people diagnosed with AIDS exhibited high-risk behaviors that led to HIV infection. This also applies to health care workers, whose risky behaviors are the cause of about 95% of HIV infections.

The HIV incubation period is variable. The CDC suggests everyone between the ages of 13 and 64 years be tested for HIV at least once as part of a routine physical.[12] High-risk populations should be tested more frequently. Three types of tests are available: nucleic acid tests (NAT), antigen/antibody tests, and antibody tests. HIV tests are typically performed on blood or oral fluid. They may also be performed on urine. No test can detect HIV immediately after infection. The NAT can usually detect infection within 10 to 33 days postexposure. An antigen/antibody test on serum can usually detect infection within 18 to 45 days postexposure, and antibody tests can take 23 to 90 days.[12]

CD4 lymphocytes are the major cellular target for HIV. The CD4 count and the rate of decline have prognostic predictive value and are used to determine the need for antiretroviral therapy and for opportunistic infection prophylaxis. HIV infection can produce a variety of clinical syndromes. These syndromes correlate with the duration of the illness and severity of immunosuppression. More than a dozen opportunistic infections are considered AIDS infections, including several cancers, pulmonary and extrapulmonary TB, recurrent pneumonia, wasting syndrome, neurologic disease (HIV dementia or sensory neuropathy), and invasive cervical cancer. AIDS is a severe, life-threatening clinical condition. This syndrome represents the late clinical stage of infection with HIV and is most often the result of progressive damage to the immune and other organ systems.

Currently, no vaccine prevents HIV. Prevention of infection relies on controlling transmission of the virus. Control includes both prevention counseling, preexposure prophylaxis (PrEP) and postexposure prophylaxis (PEP). Precautions to minimize the risk for transmission in the health care setting must be implemented. Prevention of occupational exposures should involve education and reinforcement of the use of barrier precautions. In addition, the implementation of safety devices and the appropriate disposal of contaminated materials are essential.

High-risk populations for HIV can take medicine daily to lower the chances of becoming infected (known as PrEP). This therapy combines two medications (tenofovir and emtricitabine). Studies have shown combination therapy to be a highly effective in preventing HIV if used consistently. This therapy can lower the risk of HIV infection from sex by more than 90% and from IV drug use by 70%.[12]

PEP is widely accepted after a high-risk occupational exposure. PEP must be started within 72 hours after an exposure to HIV. Research has shown PEP has little or no effect in preventing HIV infection if it is started longer than 72 hours after HIV exposure. The course of treatment lasts for 28 days, with medication being taken once or twice daily.

Health care providers with occupational exposure to HIV should receive follow-up postexposure testing, medical evaluation, and counseling regardless of whether they receive PEP.

Influenza (Flu) Virus

Influenza is a contagious respiratory illness. Historically, influenza has caused outbreaks of respiratory illness for centuries, including three pandemics (worldwide outbreaks of disease) in the 20th century. The four types of influenza viruses are A, B, C, and D. Influenza type A viruses have the potential to cause pandemics. Seasonal influenza outbreaks can be caused by either influenza type A or type B viruses. Influenza type C viruses are detected less frequently and can cause a mild illness in humans.

Of the four types of influenza viruses, only type A is divided into subtypes. Subtype designations are based on the presence of two viral surface proteins (antigens): hemagglutinin (H) and neuraminidase (N). To date, 18 different hemagglutinin and 11 different neuraminidase surface proteins have been identified in influenza A viruses.[13] Subtypes are designated as the H protein type (H1–H18) solely or followed by the N protein type (N1–N11). Influenza A subtypes found in humans are H1N1 and H3N2. Influenza A viruses vary in virulence, infectivity to specific hosts, modes of transmission, and the clinical presentation of infection.[13]

Influenza viruses are normally highly species-specific, meaning viruses infect an individual species and stay true to the specific species, only rarely spilling over to cause infection in other species. Influenza type D is not known to infect or cause illness in humans.

Seasonal (or common) flu is a respiratory illness caused by influenza (A or B) viruses. Individuals may present with sudden onset of fever, cough, headache, muscle and joint pain, severe malaise, sore throat, or runny nose. The incubation period is about 1 to 4 days after exposure to the virus.

The virus can be transmitted when infected people cough, sneeze, or talk. Tiny droplets containing the virus are dispersed into the air, and persons in close proximity can breathe in these droplets and become infected. People are most contagious in the first 3 to 4 days after the illness begins. Some may be able to infect others beginning 1 day before symptoms and up to 5 to 7 days after becoming ill.[13]

Influenza can cause severe illness and/or death in certain high-risk populations, such as people older than 65 years of age, those with chronic medical conditions, pregnant women, and young children. Complications of the influenza virus range from an ear infection to bacterial pneumonia or congestive heart failure.

Most cases of influenza are clinically diagnosed. However, when influenza activity is low, the collection of respiratory samples and diagnostic testing may be required to differentiate between influenza and other respiratory viruses (rhinovirus, respiratory syncytial virus, and adenovirus).

Individuals diagnosed with influenza who are not at high risk can be managed with symptomatic treatment. This treatment focuses on relieving symptoms. Those with severe or progressive illness due to the influenza virus infection should be

TABLE 19.2 Strategies to Prevent Seasonal Influenza in a Health Care Setting.[13]

Promote and administer seasonal influenza vaccine.	Manage visitor access and movement within the facility.
Minimize potential exposure: • Screening and triage for symptomatic patients • Implementation of respiratory hygiene and cough etiquette	Monitor influenza activity.
Monitor and manage ill health care personnel.	Implement environmental and engineering controls.
Adhere to standard precautions: • Hand hygiene • Gloves • Gowns	Train and educate health care personnel.
Adhere to droplet precautions.	Administer antiviral treatment and chemoprophylaxis of patients and health care personnel (when appropriate).
Use caution when performing aerosol-generating procedures.	

Adapted from CDC: Influenza (flu). (2019).

treated with antiviral medication. Antiviral treatment should begin within 48 hours after the onset of symptoms. It can decrease the symptoms and shorten the duration of the illness. In addition, it may reduce complications in children and adults.

Although influenza is primarily community based, HAIs can occur when there is a high prevalence in the community. Strategies to prevent seasonal influenza in a health care setting[13] are listed in Table 19.2.

The CDC and the WHO recommend a yearly flu vaccine and note vaccination as the most crucial step in preventing influenza infection.[13,14]

Pandemic flu is virulent human flu causing a global outbreak, or pandemic, of serious illness. This happens when a new influenza A virus emerges. Because there is little natural immunity, the disease can spread easily from person to person and can sweep across the country and around the world in very short time.

Pandemic influenza viruses can result from direct infection of humans with a nonhuman influenza A virus or when a nonhuman influenza A virus exchanges genetic information with other influenza A viruses.

In 2009 a novel influenza A virus (H1N1) emerged. It was first identified in the United States and spread across the world. The CDC estimated there were 60.8 million cases (range, 43.3–89.3 million), 274,304 hospitalizations (range, 195,086–402,719), and 12,469 deaths (range, 8868–18,306) in the United States due to the (H1N1)pdm09 virus. The CDC also estimated between 151,700 and 575,400 people worldwide died of the 2009 H1N1 virus infection during the first year the virus was in circulation. Globally, an estimate of 80% of (H1N1)pdm09 virus-associated deaths were in people younger than 65 years of age.[13]

On August 10, 2009 the WHO stated the H1N1 pandemic had ended. However, the (H1N1)pdm09 virus continues to circulate as a seasonal influenza virus causing illness and deaths worldwide annually.[13]

Methicillin-Resistant *Staphylococcus aureus*

S. aureus bacteria are generally harmless unless they enter the body through a cut or other wound, and even then, they often cause only minor skin problems in healthy people. Decades ago, a strain of staphylococcus emerged in hospitals that was resistant to the broad-spectrum antibiotics commonly used to treat it. This strain became known as methicillin-resistant *Staphylococcus aureus* (MRSA). It is resistant to antibiotics called β-lactams. β-Lactam antibiotics include methicillin, oxacillin, penicillin, and amoxicillin.

An estimated one in three people are colonized with *S. aureus* at any given time and are without illness. Two in 100 people are colonized with MRSA.[15] A 2014 CDC study showed life-threatening MRSA infections are declining in the health care setting. There was a 54% decline in invasive infection[15] between 2005 and 2011.

Colonization is the presence of the bacteria on or in a person's body without observable clinical symptoms. MRSA colonization can also occur in the nose, pharynx, axilla, rectum, and perineum.

Infection refers to the invasion of bacteria into tissue with growth of the organism. Infection may occur when the bacteria enter a break in the skin. *S. aureus* infections, including MRSA, generally start as small red bumps resembling pimples, boils, or spider bites but can quickly turn into deep, painful abscesses that may require surgical draining. Sometimes the bacteria remain confined to the skin. But they can also burrow deep into the body, causing potentially life-threatening infections in bones, joints, heart valves, and lungs. MRSA infection can be fatal.

MRSA is a prevalent nosocomial pathogen in the United States. *S. aureus* infections, including MRSA, occur most frequently among persons in hospitals and health care facilities (such as nursing homes and dialysis centers) who have weakened immune systems. Health-care associated MRSA infections include surgical wound infections, urinary tract infections, bloodstream infections, and pneumonia.

In hospitals, the most important reservoirs of MRSA are infected or colonized patients. Although hospital personnel can serve as reservoirs for MRSA and may harbor the organism for many months, they have been more commonly identified as a link for transmission between colonized or infected patients.

The primary route of transmission of MRSA has been well documented as the hands of health care workers, which may become contaminated by contact with colonized or infected patients; colonized or infected body sites of the personnel themselves; or devices, items, or environmental surfaces contaminated with body fluids containing MRSA.

The ability of MRSA to contaminate a large variety of hospital items (e.g., chairs, bed frames, and mattresses) has been demonstrated in several studies. Studies have also shown that *S. aureus* has the potential to survive for extended periods and is resistant to desiccation. Although there is no evidence demonstrating the direct transmission of MRSA from the environment to patients, evidence suggests that contamination of the environment with MRSA is sufficient to contaminate the gloves of health care providers and thus lead to transmission to patients.

MRSA is diagnosed by checking a tissue sample or nasal secretions for signs of drug-resistant bacteria. In the hospital, patients may be tested for MRSA if they show signs of infection or if they are transferred into a hospital from another health care setting where MRSA is known to be present. Patients may also be tested if they have a previous history of MRSA.

Along with *S. aureus,* many significant infection-causing bacteria are becoming resistant to the most commonly prescribed antimicrobial treatments. Antimicrobial resistance occurs when bacteria change or adapt in a way that allows them to survive in the presence of antibiotics designed to kill them. In some cases, bacteria become so resistant no available antibiotics are effective against them. The following are leading causes of antibiotic resistance:

- *Unnecessary antibiotic use in humans:* Like other resistant bacteria, MRSA is the result of decades of excessive and unnecessary antibiotic use. For years, antibiotics have been prescribed for viral infections that do not respond to these drugs, as well as for simple bacterial infections normally clearing on their own.
- *Antibiotics in food and water:* Prescription drugs are not the only source of antibiotics. In the United States, antibiotics can be found in cattle, pigs, and chickens. Antibiotics given in the proper doses to sick animals do not appear to produce resistant bacteria.
- *Germ mutation:* Even when antibiotics are used appropriately, they contribute to the rise of drug-resistant bacteria because they do not destroy every targeted germ. Bacteria live on an evolutionary fast track, so germs surviving treatment with one antibiotic soon learn to resist others. And because bacteria mutate much more quickly than new drugs can be produced, some germs end up resistant to most available treatments.

People infected with antibiotic-resistant organisms like MRSA are more likely to have longer and more expensive hospital stays and may be more likely to die because of the infection. When the drug of choice for treating an infection is not effective, treatment with second- or third-choice medicines may be less efficacious, more toxic, and more expensive.

According to the CDC, standard precautions and contact precautions should be used for all patients who present with open or draining skin or soft-tissue infections and all patients known to be infected with MRSA or at high risk (Box 19.1)[16] for being infected with MRSA. The following conditions should apply:

- Examine the patient in a private room.
- Wear gloves (clean nonsterile gloves are adequate) when providing care for patients. Change gloves after having contact with infective material that may contain high concentrations of microorganisms (e.g., wound drainage or dressings). Remove the gloves before leaving the patient's room and wash the hands immediately with an antimicrobial agent. After glove removal and hand washing, do not touch potentially contaminated environmental surfaces or items in the patient's room to avoid transfer of microorganisms to other patients and environments.
- Wear an isolation gown when providing care if there will be substantial contact with the patient's wound. This will protect skin and prevent soiling of clothes during procedures and patient-care activities that are likely to generate splashes or sprays of blood, body fluids, secretions, and excretions or cause soiling of clothing. Remove the gown before leaving the examination room.
- Wear a mask and eye protection or a face shield to protect mucous membranes of the eyes, nose, and mouth during procedures and patient-care activities likely to generate splashes or sprays of blood, body fluids, secretions, and excretions.
- Transport or move the patient from the examination room for essential purposes only.
- Handle patient-care equipment soiled with blood, body fluids, secretions, and excretions in a manner preventing skin and mucous membrane exposures, contamination of clothing, and transfer of microorganisms to other patients and environments. Ensure that reusable equipment is not used for the care of another patient until it has been appropriately cleaned and reprocessed, and ensure that single-use items are properly discarded.
- Handle, transport, and process used linen soiled with blood, body fluids, secretions, and excretions in a manner preventing skin and mucous membrane exposures, contamination of clothing, and transfer of microorganisms to other patients and environments. Any unused linen in the room should be discarded as if it were soiled.
- Ensure patient-care items and potentially contaminated surfaces are cleaned and disinfected after use.
- Clean noncritical medical equipment surfaces with a detergent/disinfectant.
- Do not use alcohol to disinfect large environmental surfaces.
- Use barrier-protective coverings as appropriate for noncritical surfaces that are (1) touched frequently with

BOX 19.1 Risk Factors Associated With MRSA.[16]

- History of MRSA infection, colonization
- History of (within past 12 months) hospitalization, dialysis or renal failure, diabetes, surgery, long-term care residence, indwelling catheter or medical device
- Injection drug use, incarceration
- Close contact with someone known to be infected or colonized with MRSA
- High prevalence of MRSA in community or population
- Local risk factors: consult local public health department

MRSA, Methicillin-resistant *Staphylococcus aureus.*
Adapted from CDC: *Staphylococcus aureus* in Healthcare Settings. (2019).

gloved hands during the delivery of patient care, (2) likely to become contaminated with blood or body substances, or (3) difficult to clean.

- Select Environmental Protection Agency (EPA)-registered disinfectants, if available, and use them in accordance with the manufacturer's instructions.
- Keep housekeeping surfaces (e.g., floors, walls, tabletops) visibly clean on a regular basis and clean up spills promptly.
- Use an EPA-registered hospital detergent/disinfectant designed for general housekeeping purposes in patient-care areas when uncertainty exists regarding the presence of multidrug-resistant organisms.

Tuberculosis

Tuberculosis is the top infectious killer and one of the top 10 causes of death worldwide.[17] In 2016 the WHO estimated 10.4 million new TB cases globally and 1.7 million deaths. Globally, the TB mortality rate[17] fell by 37% between 2000 and 2016. Prevalence of TB is not distributed evenly throughout the world or the US population. Some subgroups or individuals have a higher risk for TB because they are more likely than others to be exposed and infected or because their exposure is more likely to progress to active TB. The overall incidence of TB in the United States is very low, at 2.9 cases per 100,000 population[18] as of June 2017; however, case rates are high among specific populations, such as HIV-infected patients, the homeless, recent immigrants from countries with a high prevalence of TB, intravenous drug users, inner-city dwellers, and minorities.

A total of 9272 TB cases were reported in the United States in 2016. These data[18] reflect a decrease of 2.9% from 2015 and a 65.2% decrease from 1992. Per the WHO, the largest number of new TB cases in 2016 occurred in India, Indonesia, China, the Philippines, Pakistan, Nigeria, and South Africa, which accounted for 64% of incident cases globally.

TB is caused by *Mycobacterium tuberculosis* and usually infects the lungs (pulmonary TB) or respiratory system. However, infection can occur in the kidneys, spine, and brain. There are two TB-related conditions: latent TB infection and TB disease. If not treated properly, both can potentially be life-threatening. Latent TB can exist without making the individual ill. The body is able to fight the bacteria and prevent acute illness. Individuals have no symptoms and do not feel sick. They are not infectious and cannot spread the bacteria to others. They will normally have a positive TB skin test or TB blood test. TB disease can develop if the latent infection is not treated. For those who may be immunocompromised, the bacteria can become active and cause TB disease.

When the immune system can longer prevent TB bacteria from multiplying, TB disease develops. People are symptomatic and are capable of infecting other individuals. Symptoms[18] of TB disease may include a cough lasting 3 weeks or longer, chest pain, coughing up of blood or sputum, weakness or fatigue, weight loss, loss of appetite, chills, fever, and night sweats.

Until 50 years ago, there were no medications to cure TB. Now, strains resistant to a single drug have been documented in every country surveyed; what is more, strains of TB resistant to all major anti-TB drugs have emerged. Drug-resistant TB is caused by inconsistent or partial treatment, when patients do not take all their medications regularly for the required period because they start to feel better, because doctors and health care workers prescribe the wrong treatment regimens, or because the drug supply is unreliable. A particularly dangerous form of drug-resistant TB is multidrug-resistant TB (MDR-TB), which is defined as the disease caused by TB bacilli resistant to at least isoniazid and rifampicin (rifampin), the two most powerful anti-TB drugs available.

Although drug-resistant TB is generally treatable, it can be treated by taking multiple drugs for 6 to 9 months. The emergence of extensively drug-resistant (XDR) TB, particularly in settings where many patients with TB are also infected with HIV, poses a serious threat to TB control and confirms the urgent need to strengthen basic TB control and apply the WHO guidelines for the management of drug-resistant TB.

TB spreads when a person is exposed to tubercle bacilli carried in airborne particles or droplet nuclei. The droplet nuclei are produced by people with pulmonary or respiratory tract TB during expiratory efforts such as coughing, singing, or sneezing. The nuclei are then inhaled into the pulmonary alveoli by a vulnerable contact, where they are taken up by the alveolar macrophages. Some macrophages can kill the bacillus; others cannot. The bacilli multiply within the cells and produce infection. Factors influencing the progression of infection to disease include the intensity of exposure, interval since infection, age, and other coexisting or comorbid diseases. Extrapulmonary TB develops when the bacillus travels to other organs by way of the bloodstream.

The incubation period, the time from infection to demonstrable primary lesion or significant tuberculin reaction, is about 2 to 10 weeks. Theoretically, if viable tubercle bacilli are discharged in the sputum, the person may be infectious.

The degree of communicability is dependent on the number of bacilli discharged; virulence of the bacilli; adequacy of ventilation; exposure of bacilli to sun or ultraviolet light; and opportunities for aerosolization through coughing, sneezing, talking, or singing, or during procedures.

Nosocomial transmission of TB has been associated with close contact with people who have infectious TB and performance of procedures such as bronchoscopy, endotracheal intubation, suctioning, open abscess irrigation, and autopsy. Sputum induction and aerosol treatments that induce coughing may also increase the potential for transmission.

Two tests are available to diagnose TB infection: the TB skin test and the TB blood test. The TB skin test is performed by injecting a small amount of fluid (called tuberculin) into the skin on the lower part of the arm. A person given the tuberculin skin test must return within 48 to 72 hours to have a trained health care worker look for a reaction on the arm. The result depends on the size of the raised, hard area or swelling.[18] Results can as follows:

Positive skin test: The person's body was infected with TB bacteria. Additional tests are needed to determine whether the person has latent TB infection or TB disease.

BOX 19.2 Triage Assessment for Possible Tuberculosis.[19]

Historical and social information:
- Recently moved from or traveled to a high-risk country
- Previous history of tuberculosis with no treatment or poor compliance with treatment regimen
- Resident of long-term care facility, nursing home, correctional institution, mental hospital, or homeless shelter
- Close contact with an infected person
- Intravenous drug abuse or alcohol abuse
- Health care worker

Objective clinical information:
- Weight loss, anorexia, malaise
- Cough worsening over weeks or months
- Productive cough with mucopurulent or blood-streaked sputum
- Night sweats, chills, low-grade fevers
- Malnourished
- Coinfection with human immunodeficiency virus
- Preexisting medical conditions (e.g., diabetes mellitus, hematologic disorders, end-stage renal disease)
- Prolonged steroid or immunosuppressive therapy
- History of positive skin test or radiograph

Adapted from Jensen PA, Lambert LA, Iademarco MF, Ridzon R. Guidelines for preventing the transmission of *Mycobacterium tuberculosis* in health-care settings. *MMWR*. 2005;54/No. RR–17.

Negative skin test: The person's body did not react to the test, and latent TB infection or TB disease is not likely.

Two TB blood tests are available in the United States: the QuantiFERON–TB Gold In-Tube test (QFT-GIT) and the T-SPOT.TB test (T-Spot).[18]

Positive TB blood test: The person has been infected with TB bacteria. Additional tests are needed to determine whether the person has latent TB infection or TB disease.

Negative TB blood test: The person's blood did not react to the test, and latent TB infection or TB disease is not likely.

TB prevention and control programs should be established in all countries and health care settings. Triage guidelines should include identification of potential TB patients (Box 19.2).[19] If a patient is diagnosed with active TB disease, the following therapeutic interventions should be considered: airborne precautions to prevent spread, administration of antituberculin drugs, and supportive care. For pulmonary TB, control of infectivity is best achieved through prompt, specific drug treatment, usually leading to sputum conversion in 4 to 8 weeks. Hospitalization is necessary for patients with severe disease requiring hospital-level care and for those who are unable to care for themselves due to medical or social circumstances. Negative-pressure ventilation rooms are recommended for isolation of patients with TB. Patients who have bacteriologically negative sputum, who do not cough, or are known to be on appropriate chemotherapy do not require isolation.

For patients with latent disease, preventive chemotherapy is recommended for persons who are or have been in contact with TB infection and TB disease has been ruled out. Treatment is also recommended for high-risk individuals.

In nonindustrialized countries, the bacille Calmette-Guérin (BCG) vaccine is administered to prevent TB disease. BCG is used in many countries with a high prevalence of TB to prevent childhood tuberculous meningitis and miliary TB. However, BCG is not generally recommended for preventive use in the United States because of the low risk for infection with *M. tuberculosis,* the variable effectiveness of the vaccine against adult pulmonary TB, and the vaccine's potential interference with tuberculin skin test reactivity.

SUMMARY

Recognition of the potential for infectious disease is paramount in the care of any patient in the emergency department. With the prevalence of life-threatening infectious diseases, one must assume any patient may be a potential source of infection and use standard precautions whenever a potential for exposure exists. Careful attention to the risk associated with infectious diseases reduces the spread of infection and contamination.

REFERENCES

1. Mandell G, Douglas R, Bennett J, eds. *Principles and Practices of Infectious Diseases*. 8th ed. Philadelphia, PA: Elsevier; 2015.
2. Centers for Disease Control and Prevention. Infection Control. Centers for Disease Control and Prevention Website. https://www.cdc.gov/infectioncontrol/basics/index.html. Updated January 2016. Accessed May 12, 2019.
3. Centers for Disease Control and Prevention. *Clostridioides Difficile* Infection. Centers for Disease Control and Prevention website. https://www.cdc.gov/hai/organisms/cdiff/cdiff_infect.html. Updated January 9, 2019. Accessed May 9, 2019.
4. World Health Organization. Hepatitis B. World Health Organization website. http://www.who.int/en/news-room/fact-sheets/detail/hepatitis-b. Published July 18, 2018. Accessed May 9, 2019.
5. Centers for Disease Control and Prevention. Hepatitis B questions and answers for health professionals. Centers for Disease Control and Prevention website. https://www.cdc.gov/hepatitis/hbv/hbvfaq.htm#overview. Updated October 31, 2018. Accessed May 9, 2019.
6. Harris AM, Iqbal K, Schillie S, Britton J, Kainer MA, Tressler S, et al. Increases in acute hepatitis B virus infections—Kentucky, Tennessee, and West Virginia, 2006–2013. *MMWR Morb Mortal Wkly Rep*. 2016;65(3):47–50.

7. American Association for the Study of Liver Diseases, Infectious Diseases Society of America. HCV guidance: recommendations for testing, managing, and treating hepatitis C. https://www.hcvguidelines.org/. Accessed May 9, 2019.
8. World Health Organization. Hepatitis C. World Health Organization website. http://www.who.int/en/news-room/fact-sheets/detail/hepatitis-c. Published July 18, 2018. Accessed May 9, 2019.
9. World Health Organization. HIV/AIDS. World Health Organization website. http://www.who.int/en/news-room/fact-sheets/detail/hiv-aids. Published July 19, 2018. Accessed May 9, 2019.
10. Centers for Disease Control and Prevention. Occupational HIV Transmission and Prevention Among Health Care Workers. Centers for Disease Control and Prevention Website. https://www.cdc.gov/hiv/workplace/healthcareworkers.html. Updated April 17, 2019. Accessed May 10, 2019.
11. Wyzgowski P, Rosiek A, Grzela T, Leksowski K. Occupational HIV risk for health care workers: risk factor and the risk of infection in the course of professional activities. *Ther Clin Risk Manag*. 2016;12:989–994.
12. Centers for Disease Control and Prevention. HIV basics. Centers for Disease Control and Prevention website. https://www.cdc.gov/hiv/basics/index.html. Updated July 23, 2018. Accessed May 9, 2019.
13. Centers for Disease Control and Prevention. Influenza (flu). Centers for Disease Control and Prevention website. https://www.cdc.gov/flu/index.htm. Updated March 29, 2019. Accessed May 9, 2019.
14. World Health Organization. Influenza (seasonal). World Health Organization website. http://www.who.int/en/news-room/fact-sheets/detail/influenza-(seasonal). Published November 6, 2018. Accessed May 9, 2019.
15. Centers for Disease Control and Prevention. Methicillin-resistant *Staphylococcus aureus* (MRSA). Centers for Disease Control and Prevention website. https://www.cdc.gov/mrsa/. Updated February 5, 2019. Accessed May 9, 2019.
16. Centers for Disease Control and Prevention. *Staphylococcus aureus* in Healthcare Settings. Centers for Disease Control and Prevention Website. https://www.cdc.gov/hai/organisms/staph.html. Updated 1 March 2019. Access May 10, 2019.
17. World Health Organization. Tuberculosis: global tuberculosis report 2018. World Health Organization website. http://www.who.int/tb/publications/factsheet_global.pdf?ua=1. Published 2018. Accessed May 9, 2019.
18. Centers for Disease Control and Prevention. Tuberculosis (TB). Centers for Disease Control and Prevention website. https://www.cdc.gov/tb/. Updated December 31, 2018. Accessed May 9, 2019.
19. Jensen PA, Lambert LA, Iademarco MF, Ridzon R. Guidelines for preventing the transmission of *Mycobacterium tuberculosis* in health-care settings. *MMWR*. 2005;54:RR–17. https://www.cdc.gov/mmwr/pdf/rr/rr5417.pdf. Accessed May 10, 2019.

Fluids, Fluid Replacement, Electrolytes, and Vascular Access

Betty Kuiper

Water is the most abundant fluid medium in the body, composing 65% of total body weight for the average adult, 75% in a full-term infant, and as little as 45% in an older adult.[1] In a healthy physiologic state, this fluid medium has a constant balance of electrolytes controlled by a unique system of checks and balances. Effects of fluid and electrolyte disturbances are often a primary or secondary reason for many emergency department (ED) visits. Fluid and electrolyte abnormalities may be caused by gastrointestinal (GI), urologic, cardiac, respiratory, and endocrine diseases, as well as many forms of traumatic injury.

Assessment of circulatory status and manipulation of the variables involved is a cornerstone of patient management in the ED, regardless of the presenting complaint or symptoms. Fluid replacement is used for patients with subtle and overt volume losses. Solution, rate, and amount are determined by patient condition, underlying pathologic condition, and current fluid imbalance. Maintenance fluids are used for patients with little or no oral intake, whereas aggressive fluid replacement is indicated for patients with significant volume depletion. Patients with hematologic disorders, cancer, or hemorrhage may also require blood or blood product replacement.

Vascular access may be necessary for medication administration, fluid and electrolyte replacement, or transfusion of blood or blood products. Routine access involves inserting catheters into peripheral veins of hands and arms. Site selection depends on the urgency of the situation, the condition of the patient's veins, and the characteristics of the solution administered. Central veins may be used for invasive hemodynamic monitoring, to infuse certain concentrated solutions, or when peripheral veins are not easily accessed. Needle insertion into bone marrow (intraosseous insertion) is also used for emergency vascular access. Patients may have catheters or implanted ports for long-term therapies.

This chapter describes the interrelationship of water, water metabolism, aspects of fluid replacement, electrolyte composition, and vascular access options.

PATHOPHYSIOLOGY

Water and electrolytes are interdependent. The pathophysiology of one affects the function and value of the other. Normal fluid and electrolyte levels are the result of structural, physiologic, and environmental factors.

WATER

Water has many important metabolic functions, including transport of nutrients and other essential substances, removal of metabolic waste products, normal cellular metabolism, and maintenance of normal body temperature. Age, weight, body fat, gender, and environmental factors such as ambient temperature determine individual fluid requirements.[2] Fat is virtually water free; therefore increases in body fat are associated with decreases in the percentage of body water. The average adult ingests 2300 mL of water per day from food and drink.[1] The most common areas of the body for fluid excretion are bowels, skin, lungs, and kidneys. The kidneys are the primary regulators of fluid and electrolyte balance, and approximately 1500 mL of urine is excreted daily.[1]

Total body water (TBW) is distributed between extracellular and intracellular compartments. Extracellular fluid (ECF) constitutes one-third of TBW, or approximately 15 L.[2] Plasma, interstitial fluid, cerebrospinal fluid, intraocular fluid, fluids of the GI tract, and fluids of potential spaces (i.e., pleural space, peritoneal space) are examples of ECF.[2] Intracellular fluid (ICF) accounts for two-thirds of TBW and represents the sum of fluid content for all the cells in the body, approximately 25 L.[2]

Two regulatory mechanisms influential in maintaining normal water volume and tonicity, or osmotic pressure, are thirst and renal function. Thirst is the primary regulator for intake of water. It is triggered by receptors in the anterolateral hypothalamus that respond to increased plasma osmolality (as little as 2%) or decreased body fluid volume.[1] Thirst ensures adequate replacement of fluid losses and is stimulated by ECF hypertonicity and decreased ICF volume.[3] Similarly, thirst is depressed by ECF hypotonicity and increased ICF volume. Because the thirst mechanism is triggered by increased osmolality, thirst is not effective in hypotonic or hyponatremic dehydration in which water and sodium losses are equal. Hypothalamic dysfunction also decreases the capacity for thirst.[3] Other factors adversely affecting the thirst mechanism include brain injury and psychosocial factors such as depression, confusion, and fear of incontinence.

Renal regulation of water balance is twofold, affecting both tonicity and body water. When the glomerular filtrate is hypertonic, osmoreceptors in the hypothalamus are stimulated and antidiuretic hormone (ADH) is released by the pituitary gland.[3] ADH makes renal collecting tubules more permeable to water so water is reabsorbed into the body, diluting blood and concentrating urine. If plasma or glomerular filtrate is hypotonic, ADH secretion is inhibited and collecting tubules reabsorb less water. Blood becomes concentrated and the urine is diluted as more water exits the kidneys.[3]

The kidneys, through the renin-angiotensin-aldosterone system, regulate the volume of body water. When ECF volume, specifically blood volume, is low, receptors in the kidneys secrete an enzyme called renin. Renin stimulates angiotensinogen (a normal plasma protein) to release angiotensin I, which is then converted to angiotensin II by another enzyme, primarily in the lungs.[3] Angiotensin II stimulates the adrenal cortex to secrete aldosterone, which increases sodium reabsorption from glomerular filtrate in exchange for potassium and hydrogen ions.[3] This exchange increases plasma tonicity, which leads to ADH secretion, water retention, and increased volume. With excessive ECF volume (blood volume), aldosterone secretion is depressed, so tubular reabsorption of sodium and water decreases.

FLUID REPLACEMENT

Intravenous (IV) fluids may be given to maintain fluid requirements or to replace fluid losses. Isotonic, hypotonic, and hypertonic crystalloid solutions may be used as initial and therapeutic fluids.[4] Isotonic fluids (lactated Ringer's and 0.9% normal saline (NS) are similar in composition to body fluids and provide greater intravascular volume because more fluid remains in the vascular space.[4] Hypotonic fluids (NS 0.45%, NS 0.2%, and dextrose 5% in water) shift fluid into intracellular spaces and are more useful for preventing cellular dehydration.[4] They deplete circulatory volume, and blood pressure may drop with their administration. Hypertonic fluids (dextrose 5% in NS, dextrose 10% in NS, dextrose 10% in water, dextrose 5% in 0.45 NS, and dextrose 20%) move fluid from cells to the extravascular space and may be used to replace electrolytes and promote diuresis.[4]

Crystalloid and colloid solutions are used for volume replacement. Crystalloid solutions increase intravascular volume through actual volume administered, whereas colloids pull fluid into the vascular space through osmosis (Table 20.1).[4] Synthetic and natural colloid solutions are available.

Blood and Blood Products

Blood loss depletes the body of blood cells and clotting factors; whole blood replacement is ideal in frank blood loss. However, whole blood is expensive and not readily available, and it has risk for transmission of infectious diseases.[4] Blood may be separated, and only those components needed are administered. This process preserves valuable components for other potential patients. Packed red blood cells (RBCs) are used most often for blood replacement.[4] Other blood products used for component replacement include platelets, fresh frozen plasma, and albumin.[4] Blood products are always administered using normal saline. A blood warmer is recommended for multiple trauma/massive blood loss and cold agglutinin disease.[4] In pediatrics, blood warming should be used for exchanged transfusions in infants and for blood infusion rates exceeding 15 mL/kg per hour in children.[4]

Before blood administration, a blood sample should be obtained for type and crossmatch. Ideally, complete type and crossmatch should be done on all blood before administration; however, this procedure can take a prolonged time. Additional time may be required if antibodies are found. Table 20.2 summarizes compatible types of plasma and RBCs for different donor types. Type-specific blood or blood that is not completely crossmatched may be given to patients with critical blood loss. The physician must acknowledge responsibility for potential adverse effects. Type O blood may be given for patients with extreme blood loss who cannot wait for type-specific blood. Type O-negative blood is given to female patients, and type O-positive blood is given to male patients.[5]

TABLE 20.1 Crystalloids/Colloids.

Crystalloids (Increase Intravascular Volume)	Colloids (Pull Fluids into The Vascular Space)
0.9% Normal saline	Dextran (synthetic)
0.45% Normal saline	Hetastarch (synthetic)
5% Dextrose	Fresh frozen plasma
Lactated Ringer's	Plasmanate
Hypertonic saline (7.5%)	Albumin
	Whole blood and packed red blood cells
	Whole blood and packed red blood cells

Data from Alexander M, Corrigan A, Gorski L, Hankins J, Perucca R. *Infusion Nursing: An Evidence-Based Approach.* 3rd ed. St Louis, MO: Saunders Elsevier; 2010.

TABLE 20.2 Blood Type Identification.

Patient	Compatible Transfusion
Type A	A or AB plasma
	A or O RBCs
Type B	B or AB plasma
	B or O RBCs
Type AB	AB plasma
	A, B, AB, or O RBCs
Type O	A, B, AB, or O plasma
	O RBCs
Rh–	Must receive Rh– blood
Rh+	Can receive Rh– or Rh+ blood
O–	Universal donor for RBCs
AB+	Universal donor for plasma

RBCs, Red blood cells.
Data from Elkin MK, Perry AG, Potter PA: *Nursing Interventions and Clinical Skills.* 3rd ed. St Louis, MO: Mosby; 2004.

However, many facilities give type O-negative blood to both females and male patients.

Blood administration is not without risk. Blood-processing procedures have reduced risk for transmission of infectious diseases; however, transfusion reactions can occur because of transfusion of incompatible blood, patient allergy, or depletion of clotting factors.[4] Unrecognized transfusion reactions represent a significant threat to the patient's life. Before transfusion, blood and patient identification should be checked carefully according to institutional policies. During the transfusion, the patient should be carefully monitored for signs of reaction, including fever, chills, urticaria, breathing difficulty, back pain, and hematuria.[4] IV medications cannot be added to a blood transfusion. If the ordered medications cannot be delayed for the duration of the transfusion, an additional access site is required.

ELECTROLYTES

An electrolyte is a substance capable of carrying an electrical charge. An electrolyte with a positive charge is called a cation, whereas an electrolyte with a negative charge is an anion.[3] Electrolytes are found in varying concentrations in ECF and ICF (Fig. 20.1).

For the purposes of this chapter, serum electrolyte measurements are equivalent to extracellular electrolyte values (Table 20.3). Direct measurement of intracellular electrolyte concentrations in the clinical setting is not yet feasible, so ICF electrolyte concentrations must be inferred from serum electrolyte values.

All fluids outside the cells are collectively referred to as ECF. Electrolytes in ECF, from greatest to least concentration, are sodium, chloride, potassium, bicarbonate, and hydrogen. ECF also contains oxygen, carbon dioxide, proteins, and a few miscellaneous anions.

ICF represents fluid found in cells in the body, about 25 L.[2] Electrolytes in the ICF, from greatest to least concentration, are potassium, phosphate, and sulfate combined; magnesium; and finally sodium, hydrogen, and bicarbonate in equal concentrations. The ICF also contains several proteins.

The delicate balance of water and electrolytes between intracellular and extracellular compartments is an ongoing process of checks and balances easily disturbed by disease or injury. Regulatory processes and the role of each electrolyte are described in the following sections.

Sodium

Sodium, the principal cation in ECF, is primarily responsible for osmotic pressure.[1] Sodium is exchangeable across cell membranes to maintain sodium and water balance and normal arterial pressure. Sodium and chloride play an important role in maintaining body water; movement of glucose, insulin, and amino acids across cell membranes; and maintaining muscle strength, neural function, and urinary output.[1,3] Sodium is essential for the sodium-potassium pump, which moves sodium and potassium across the cell membrane during repolarization (Fig. 20.2). As sodium diffuses into the cell and potassium out of the cell, an active transport system supplied with energy delivers sodium back to the extracellular compartment and potassium to the intracellular compartment.[1]

Sodium levels are maintained through the renin-angiotensin-aldosterone system, the sympathetic nervous system, and a less well-defined system mediated by atrial natriuretic factor.[1,3] Decreased fluid volume decreases blood flow and arterial pressure, which stimulate baroreceptors in the kidneys (Fig. 20.3). Baroreceptors stimulate the sympathetic nervous system, which leads to vasoconstriction of renal arterioles,

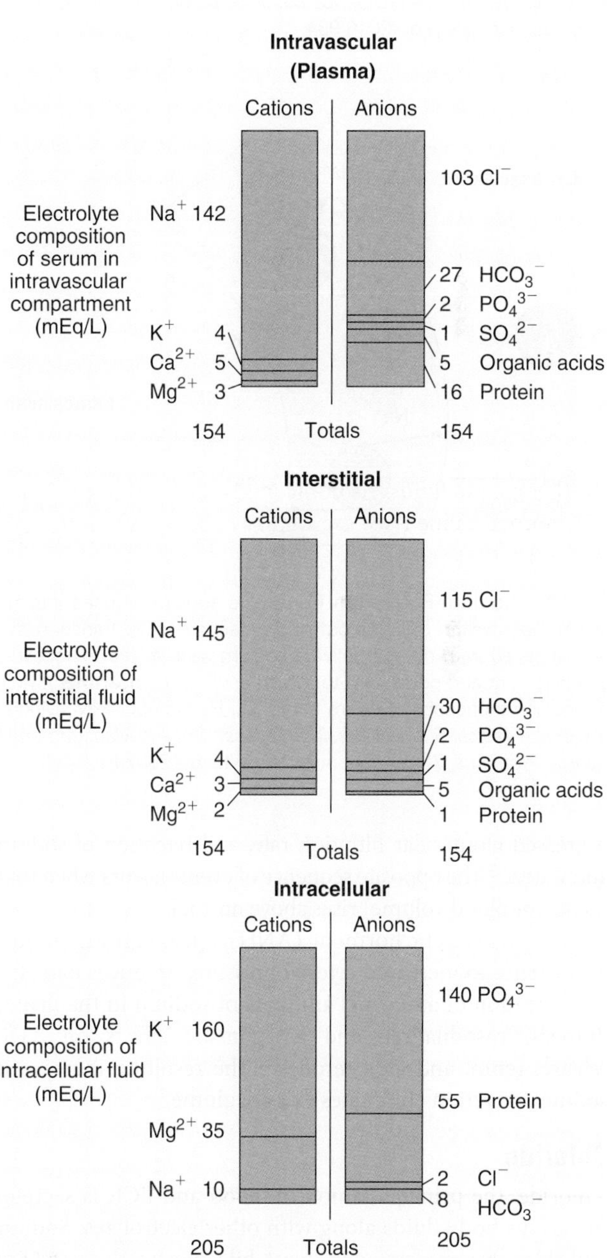

Fig. 20.1 Electrolyte Content of Fluid Compartments. (From Lewis SL, Heitkemper MM, Dirksen SR, et al: *Medical-Surgical Nursing: Assessment and Management of Clinical Problems.* 7th ed. St Louis, MO: Mosby, 2007.)

TABLE 20.3 Laboratory Normal Values for Adults.

Item Measured	Normal Value in Serum of Blood
Electrolytes	
Sodium (Na^+)	136–145 mEq/L (136–145 mmol/L
Potassium (K^+)	3.5–5.0 mEq/L (3.5–5.0 mmol/L)
Chloride (Cl^-)	98–106 mEq/L (98–106 mmol/L)
Total Calcium (Ca^{2+})	8.4–10.5 mg/dL (2.1–2.6 mmol/L)
Magnesium (Mg^{2+})	1.5–2.5 mEq/L (0.75–1.25 mmol/L)
Phosphate	2.7–4.5 mg/dL (0.87–1.45 mmol/L)

Data from Alexander M, Corrigan A, Gorski L, Hankins J, Perucca R. *Infusion Nursing: An Evidence-Based Approach.* 3rd ed. St Louis, MO: Saunders Elsevier; 2010:934.

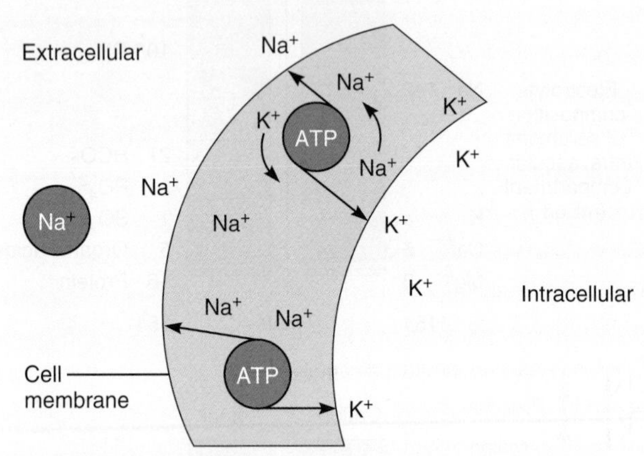

Fig. 20.2 Sodium-Potassium Pump. As sodium diffuses into the cell and potassium diffuses out of the cell, an active transport system supplied with energy delivers sodium back to the extracellular compartment and potassium to the intracellular compartment. *ATP,* Adenosine triphosphate. (From Lewis SL, Heitkemper MM, Dirksen SR, et al: *Medical-Surgical Nursing: Assessment and Management of Clinical Problems.* 7th ed. St Louis, MO: Mosby, 2007.)

decreased glomerular filtration rate, and retention of sodium and water.[1,3] The opposite sequence of events occurs when fluid intake (or blood volume) rises above normal.

Atrial natriuretic hormone (ANH), released from the atria in response to increased arterial pressure, produces natriuresis (excretion of abnormal amounts of sodium in the urine), diuresis, vasodilation, and antagonistic effects on ADH release, renin, and aldosterone.[1,3] The resulting increase in sodium excretion eliminates excess volume.

Chloride

Chloride, the principal anion of blood and ECF, is secreted in various body fluids along with other electrolytes. Sodium and chloride are excreted in sweat, bile, pancreatic fluids, and intestinal fluids. Gastric juice contains chloride and hydrogen. As with sodium, chloride plays a cooperative role in maintaining acid-base balance and takes part in the exchange of oxygen and carbon dioxide in red blood cells.[1,3] Serum chloride levels are passively regulated by serum sodium levels. When serum sodium increases, serum chloride also increases. However, chloride levels are inversely related to bicarbonate levels because chloride is sacrificed in the kidneys to produce more bicarbonate.

Potassium

Potassium is the most abundant cation in the body, with 98% in the ICF and 2% in the ECF.[6] Potassium is primarily responsible for cell membrane potential and is the counterpart to sodium in the sodium-potassium pump. Potassium governs cell osmolality and volume and is secreted in sweat, gastric juice, pancreatic juice, bile, and fluids of the small intestine.

Potassium level is primarily controlled through secretion of potassium by the distal and collecting tubules in the kidney.[6] Potassium secretion increases in response to increased ECF potassium concentration, aldosterone levels, and distal tubular flow. A rise in ECF potassium stimulates the sodium-potassium pump located in the renal tubules. This pump maintains a low intracellular sodium concentration through exchange of potassium across the cell membrane. Increased extracellular potassium also triggers aldosterone secretion by the adrenal cortex. Aldosterone increases the rate at which tubular cells secrete potassium and the permeability of the renal tubular lumen for potassium. This is a negative feedback system regulated by the serum potassium level. Finally, increased distal tubular flow causes rapid secretion of potassium into the urine.[1]

Alkalosis temporarily decreases serum potassium by driving potassium into the cells in exchange for hydrogen ions.[6] Conversely, acute acidosis is the major factor that decreases potassium secretion and increases serum potassium.[6] Acute acidosis increases hydrogen ion concentration in the ECF, causing potassium to move out of the cell in exchange for excess hydrogen ions.[6]

Calcium

Approximately 99% of the body's calcium is found in bone; however, 1% is found in ICF and 0.1% in ECF.[1] Bone acts as a large reservoir for calcium when ECF calcium levels fall. Calcium is transported in the blood in two forms. Half is bound to plasma proteins, usually albumin, and a small amount of nonionized calcium forms complexes with anions such as phosphate, citrate, and sulfate. The rest exists as an ionized form that is free and metabolically active.[1] Most ionized calcium is found in the ECF. Due to the large amount of calcium bound to plasma proteins, assessment of total serum calcium without simultaneous measurement of serum proteins has limited value in determining hypocalcemia or hypercalcemia.

Calcium has many important functions—smooth and skeletal muscle contraction, bone and brain metabolism, blood clotting, and as a primary ingredient in lung surfactant.[1] Calcium is essential for membrane polarization and depolarization, action potential generation, neurotransmission, and muscle contraction.[1] Calcium channels in myocardial cells allow transmembrane calcium transport.

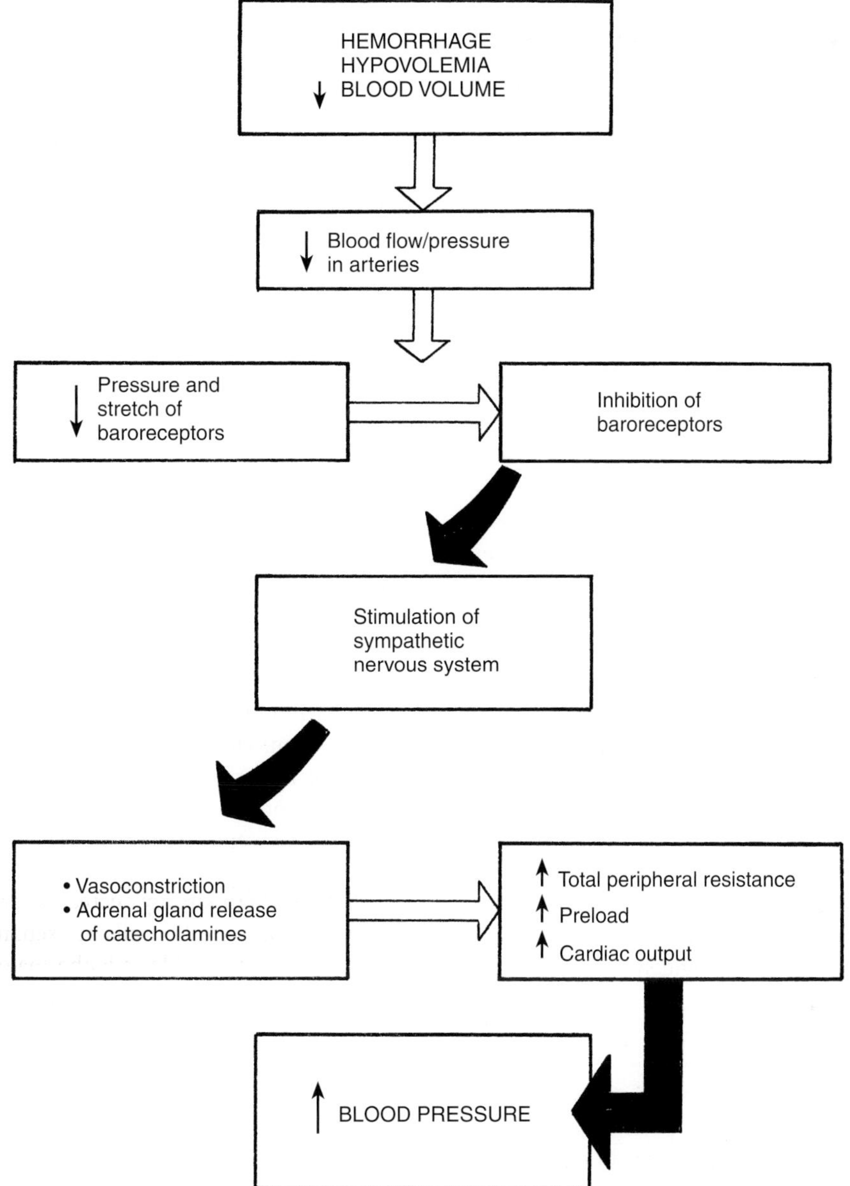

Fig. 20.3 Baroreceptor Response.

The most important regulatory factors for calcium homeostasis are parathyroid hormone (PTH), calcitonin, and vitamin D.[6] When ECF calcium falls below normal levels, parathyroid glands release PTH, which acts directly on bones to stimulate the release of large amounts of calcium into ECF. When calcium ion concentration is elevated, PTH secretion decreases, causing excess calcium to deposit in the bones.

Bones rely on proper intake and absorption of calcium to maintain calcium stores. Calcium absorption in the kidneys and GI tract is regulated by PTH levels. In hypocalcemic states, PTH activates vitamin D_3, the form of vitamin D necessary to increase intestinal calcium reabsorption. PTH also directly stimulates the kidneys to increase renal tubular calcium reabsorption, which prevents loss of calcium in the urine.[6]

Another factor influencing calcium reabsorption is plasma concentration of phosphate. Serum calcium levels are inversely related to serum phosphate levels. Increases in plasma phosphate may indirectly stimulate PTH, which increases calcium reabsorption by renal tubules and reduces calcium loss in the urine.[6]

In response to elevated calcium levels, the thyroid gland secretes a hormone called calcitonin. The effect of calcitonin on plasma calcium levels is directly opposite that of PTH. Calcitonin decreases plasma calcium levels by increasing calcium deposits in bone and decreasing formation of new osteoclasts, the cells responsible for breakdown and removal of bone.[6] Calcitonin also has minor effects on calcium absorption in the renal tubules and GI tract.

Phosphate and Phosphorus

Phosphorus, the major anion in the ICF, is essential for metabolism of carbohydrates, lipids, and proteins. Phosphate also plays a role in hormonal activities and acid-base balance and has a close relationship to calcium in maintaining homeostasis.[1]

Renal tubules maintain a normal phosphate level by an "overflow" mechanism. When the phosphate level in the glomerular filtrate falls below the normal level, essentially all filtered phosphate is reabsorbed. When extra phosphate is present in the glomerular filtrate, excess phosphate is excreted in the urine.

Magnesium

Magnesium is the second most important intracellular cation.[6] More than half the body's magnesium is stored in bones, with the rest in cells, particularly muscle. Only a small fraction of the body's magnesium is found in the ECF. Magnesium plays an essential role in cellular metabolism.[6]

FLUID AND ELECTROLYTE ABNORMALITIES

Imbalances in fluid and electrolytes may be due to physiologic abnormalities, injury, or stress. Fluid and electrolyte levels are closely related. For example, sodium losses are almost always associated with water losses, just as sodium retention is associated with water excess.

Fluid and electrolyte therapy has three objectives—maintain daily requirements, restore previous losses or excesses, and prevent further losses or excesses. Oral electrolyte replacement is preferred. However, most patients who present to the ED with vomiting, diarrhea, or other fluid losses can no longer be treated orally for such losses. Treatment of electrolyte abnormalities focuses on slowly restoring previous balance and carefully correcting the underlying cause. Electrolyte levels, hydration, and function of cardiovascular, renal, and neurologic systems should be carefully monitored.

Water Abnormalities

Water abnormalities may be due to underlying disease, iatrogenic causes, environmental factors, or psychological abnormalities. ECF imbalances may be caused by an extracellular volume deficit, which includes an increase in insensible water loss or perspiration (high fever, heatstroke), diabetes insipidus, osmotic diuresis, hemorrhage, GI losses (vomiting, gastric suction, diarrhea, fistula drainage), overuse of diuretics, inadequate fluid intake, and third-space fluid shifts (burns and intestinal obstruction).[2] An extracellular volume excess may be caused by an extreme intake of isotonic or hypotonic IV fluids, heart failure, renal failure, primary polydipsia, syndrome of inappropriate antidiuretic hormone (SIADH), Cushing syndrome, and the long-term use of corticosteroids.[2] Determining the cause should occur concurrently with fluid replacement.

Water Depletion

Water depletion may be due to reduced water consumption, diarrhea, vomiting, excessive sweating, excessive respiration, renal disease, ADH deficiency (i.e., diabetes insipidus), excessive diuretic use, and diabetic ketoacidosis (DKA). Water deficiency is almost always associated with loss of sodium.

Signs and symptoms of water deficiency include thirst, loss of eyeball and skin turgor, dry mucous membranes, flushed skin, decreased urinary output, increased urine specific gravity, increased temperature, tachycardia, delirium, and coma. Most patients with water deficiency are also deficient in sodium and other electrolytes, so oral or parenteral fluid replacement must be determined on an individual basis. Frequently selected fluids to replenish water and sodium loss include normal saline (0.9%).[3] Serial electrolyte and plasma osmolarity levels are required to determine appropriate fluid replacement.

Water Excess

Water excess is characterized by weight gain, muscle twitching and cramps, pulmonary or peripheral edema, hyperventilation, confusion, hallucination, coma, and convulsions. Water excess may be due to increased water ingestion, excessive IV therapy, renal disease, excess ADH, and inadequate water transport to the kidney (e.g., shock, heart failure).[3]

The aim of treatment for fluid volume excess is to identify the cause, and the treatment goal is to remove fluid volume excess without producing abnormal changes in electrolyte composition. Diuretics and fluid restriction are the primary forms of treatment.[1,3,6,7] Other possible treatments include restriction of sodium intake, abdominal paracentesis for ascites, and thoracentesis for a pleural effusion.

Electrolyte Abnormalities

Electrolyte abnormalities may be caused by an underlying disease or may be the result of starvation, therapeutic drugs, drug overdose, or other iatrogenic causes. Electrolyte abnormalities are almost always associated with some degree of neuromuscular dysfunction (e.g., weakness, paralysis, cramps, restless legs, tetany, areflexia, hyperreflexia, and myotonia).[2] Cardiac abnormalities are another common occurrence with many electrolyte abnormalities. Ventricular dysrhythmias may be seen with hypokalemia and hypercalcemia, and cardiac arrest may be seen with hyperkalemia; torsades de pointes has been seen with hypocalcemia. Dysrhythmias associated with hypomagnesemia include ventricular ectopy, torsades de pointes, and atrial fibrillation. Hypermagnesemia may cause atrioventricular block.

Anion Gap

The balance between positive and negative electrolytes is measured by calculating the anion gap: $Na^+ - (Cl^- - HCO_3^-)$.[6] Some formulas may include potassium with the sodium. This measurement is particularly useful in determining whether metabolic acidosis is due to acid excess or bicarbonate loss. The reference range for the anion gap in adults is 10 to 14 mmol/L.[3,6] Abnormalities in the anion gap may be due to a change in unmeasured anions or cations or an error in measurement of sodium, chloride, or bicarbonate.

Causes of high-anion-gap metabolic acidosis are lactic acidosis, ketoacidosis (diabetic, alcoholic, starvation), toxins (ethylene glycol, methanol, salicylates), and renal failure (acute and chronic).[6,7]

Sodium Abnormalities

Sodium and chloride travel together across most membranes, so sodium abnormalities are usually associated with chloride abnormalities. For the purpose of this discussion, abnormalities are described separately.

Hyponatremia

Hyponatremia is probably the most common electrolyte imbalance seen in the clinical arena. Hyponatremia is characterized by vague signs and symptoms, so diagnosis can rarely be made from clinical evaluation. Clinical manifestations are due to decreased osmolarity and cerebral edema and include nausea, weakness, confusion, agitation, and disorientation. When serum sodium levels become very low, seizures, coma, or death can occur.[2,6,7]

Mild hyponatremia does not require treatment. If the primary cause of hyponatremia is fluid imbalance, normal saline is the treatment of choice. In severe symptomatic hyponatremia, hypertonic (3%) saline solution may be cautiously administered with an infusion pump.[2] The patient should be carefully monitored for fluid overload secondary to sodium replacement.

Hypernatremia

Hypernatremia is a significant risk for infants, older adults, and the debilitated because of their inability to independently replace fluid losses. Clinical signs and symptoms are similar to those seen with hyponatremia but are secondary to hyperosmolarity and cellular dehydration. The patient will be thirsty and appear dehydrated. Early symptoms include anorexia, nausea, and vomiting. As serum sodium levels rise above 145 mEq/L, neurologic symptoms such as agitation, irritability, lethargy, coma, muscle twitching, and hyperreflexia may occur.[1,6] Intracranial hemorrhages can result from shrunken brain tissue or engorged vasculature.[1,6]

Treatment of sodium excess focuses on restoring normal fluid volume and osmolarity. Fluid replacement is the first step when hypovolemia is the cause of sodium excess. If oral fluids cannot be ingested, IV solutions of 5% dextrose in water or hypotonic saline may be given initially.[4,6] Rapid overcorrection of hypernatremia can result in cerebral edema and seizures.

Chloride Abnormalities

Chloride abnormalities rarely occur independently but usually occur in conjunction with sodium or potassium abnormalities.

Hypochloremia. Hypochloremia occurs in conjunction with hyponatremia and may also be seen with hyperkalemia caused by excretion of potassium chloride. Symptoms of chloride deficiency are basically the same as hyponatremia with the additional problems of profound muscle weakness; twitching; tetany; slow, shallow respirations; and respiratory arrest.[1] Treatment includes chloride and sodium replacement with careful monitoring of serum levels to determine effectiveness.

Hyperchloremia

Hyperchloremia not only produces all the signs and symptoms seen with hypernatremia but also causes deep, labored breathing. Causes of hyperchloremia are the same as those causing hypernatremia, with one exception: ammonium chloride ingestion. Treatment of hyperchloremia is essentially the same as for hypernatremia.

Potassium Abnormalities

Potassium is subject to multiple influences within the body. Alkalosis, aldosterone, insulin, and β_2-agonists drive potassium into the cell, whereas acidosis and hyperosmolarity cause potassium to leave the cell.[8] Potassium abnormalities are almost always associated with ECG changes, which may or may not correlate with severity.

Hypokalemia

Hypokalemia is characterized by muscle weakness, cramps, paralysis, hyporeflexia, paralytic ileus, paresthesia, latent tetany, cardiac dysrhythmias, hyposthenuria (inability to form urine with a high specific gravity), and a serum potassium level of less than 3.5 mEq/L [mmol/L].[2,3,6] Muscle weakness is usually more pronounced in the lower extremities and proximal muscle groups. Respiratory muscle weakness may lead to respiratory failure and arrest. Rhabdomyolysis may also occur.[3] ECG changes such as flattened or inverted T waves and U waves do not correlate well with clinical severity. The ECG may demonstrate ST-segment depression, presence of U wave, and bradycardia. Ventricular ectopy is the most common dysrhythmia.

Hypokalemia is the result of decreased potassium intake or shifts of potassium from the ECF to the cells. Vomiting, diarrhea, intestinal obstruction, fistulas, GI suctioning, renal insufficiency, and renal losses such as the use of diuretics, hyperaldosteronism, and magnesium depletion are associated with hypokalemia.[2,3,8] Nephritis, dialysis, DKA, diuretics, Cushing syndrome, and steroid therapy are also associated with hypokalemia.[2,3,8]

Treatment is recommended when potassium level is lower than 3.5 mEq/L. Potassium supplements added to IV solutions should never exceed 40 mEq/L.[3] Administer potassium through a large-bore peripheral site or through a central line at a rate of 5 to 10 mEq/hour; this rate is never to exceed 20 mEq/hour under any circumstances, to prevent hyperkalemia and cardiac arrest.[2] An infusion pump is always recommended. Cardiac monitoring and serial evaluation of potassium levels are recommended to prevent inadvertent hyperkalemia secondary to potassium replacement. In less acute situations, oral potassium may be used, or potassium may be added to enteral feedings. Serum magnesium levels should be checked because both electrolytes can be depleted with persistent hypokalemia.

Hyperkalemia

Hyperkalemia is characterized by prominent cardiac changes and neuromuscular effects, such as paresthesia and muscle weakness leading to flaccid paralysis, and a serum potassium level greater than 5.0 mEq/L [mmol/L]. Various ECG changes correlate well with severity in hyperkalemia.[2,6,8] Elevated T waves occur when serum potassium reaches 5.5 to 6.5 mEq/L, whereas prolonged PR interval and widened QRS complexes are evident when the level reaches 6.5 to

8.0 mEq/L.[6] Dysrhythmias include sinus bradycardia, sinus arrest, first-degree heart block, nodal rhythm, idioventricular rhythm, and ventricular fibrillation.[2,3,8] Asystole may also occur.[2,9] Hyperkalemia may be due to increased oral or IV intake, acute renal disease, potassium-sparing diuretics, potassium-containing salt substitute, crush injuries, tumor lysis syndrome, renal disease, angiotensin-converting enzyme (ACE) inhibitors, adrenal insufficiency, acidosis, anoxia, and hyponatremia.[2,3,6]

IV calcium chloride or calcium gluconate is the most rapid method for neutralizing neuromuscular effects of hyperkalemia. Serum potassium is rapidly reduced by administration of glucose, insulin, and sodium bicarbonate (controversial), which drives potassium into the cell in exchange for sodium.[3] However, this intervention provides only a temporary reduction in serum potassium. Urinary potassium excretion is promoted with loop or osmotic diuretics.[2] If these efforts fail, renal dialysis may be needed for significant hyperkalemia. Ion exchange resins such as sodium polystyrene sulfonate (Kayexalate, oral or rectal) may be used in nonemergency situations.[2] Continuous cardiac monitoring and serial potassium levels are essential for the patient with hyperkalemia.

Calcium Abnormalities

Calcium abnormalities may be due to diet, medications, injury, or disease.[3] Bones provide a large reservoir of calcium; however, adequate dietary intake is necessary to maintain stores. Calcium abnormalities are often associated with phosphorus and magnesium abnormalities.[3,6]

Hypocalcemia

Hypocalcemia makes the nervous system more excitable, which can lead to cardiac dysrhythmias, constipation, and lack of appetite.[1,2] In skeletal muscle, excitability can lead to tetanic muscle contractions. Seizures are occasionally seen as a result of increased excitability of brain tissue.[3] Clinical signs include a positive Trousseau sign (carpal spasms induced by inflating a blood pressure cuff on the upper arm) and a positive Chvostek sign (abnormal facial spasms elicited by light taps on the facial nerve).[3]

Other manifestations include muscle twitching and cramping; facial grimacing; numbness and tingling of fingers, toes, nose, lips, and earlobes; hyperactive deep tendon reflexes; and abdominal pain.[2,3] The ECG may show a prolonged QT interval, and the patient may appear anxious, irritable, and even psychotic.[2,3]

Calcium abnormalities occur with hypoparathyroidism, hypovitaminosis D, malabsorption syndrome, malnutrition, kidney disease, Cushing syndrome, and metastatic carcinoma of the bone.[1–3,6] Overdose of calcium channel blockers can also cause hypocalcemia. Multiple blood transfusions, usually more than 10 units, are associated with hypocalcemia because citrate in banked blood binds with calcium, making it inactive.[3]

Before treatment for hypocalcemia is started, hypomagnesemia should be excluded because patients with low serum magnesium levels respond poorly to calcium replacement. Hypocalcemia is easily managed with IV calcium. For adults, one to two ampules of 10% calcium gluconate (each containing 93 mg of elemental calcium) mixed in 5% dextrose in water (D_5W) is administered over 10 to 20 minutes.[6] In severe deficits, a continuous infusion may be necessary after the initial bolus. Calcium levels, cardiac rhythm, and blood pressure should be carefully monitored during calcium administration.

Hypercalcemia

Hypercalcemia is characterized by vague symptoms such as headache, irritability, fatigue, malaise, difficulty concentrating, anorexia, nausea, vomiting, and constipation.[6] Neurologic effects are often the primary symptoms. Patients may be lethargic or confused and have a depressed level of consciousness.[6] Deep tendon reflexes may be depressed, the QT interval may be shortened, and the patient may have polyuria, polydipsia, or an ileus. Chronic hypercalcemia is associated with renal lithiasis, peptic ulcer, and pancreatitis.[3,6]

Correction of hypercalcemia includes treating the underlying cause and increasing renal excretion of calcium with IV hydration and loop or osmotic diuretics.[3] Other therapeutic options depend on the specific clinical situation and include corticosteroid administration to decrease intestinal calcium absorption and increase urinary calcium excretion.[3] Administration of calcitonin or phosphate inhibits bone reabsorption.[3]

Phosphate Abnormalities

Phosphate abnormalities are associated with a reciprocal calcium abnormality. Phosphate elevations occur with calcium losses, whereas phosphate depletion occurs with calcium excess. The patient with a phosphate abnormality should be carefully monitored for the effects of calcium abnormality.

Hypophosphatemia

Hypophosphatemia has a variable clinical presentation ranging from no symptoms to anorexia, muscle weakness, rhabdomyolysis, respiratory failure, hemolysis, and altered mental status.[6] Causes include hyperparathyroidism, vitamin D deficiency, intestinal malabsorption, and kidney failure, starvation, alcohol abuse, and malignancy.[2,6]

Management of a mild phosphorus deficiency may involve oral supplements and ingestion of foods high in phosphorus.[2] Severe hypophosphatemia can be serious and may require IV administration of sodium phosphate or potassium phosphate.[3] Frequent monitoring of serum phosphate levels is necessary to guide the therapy.[3] Sudden symptomatic hypocalcemia, secondary to increased calcium phosphorus binding, is a potential complication of IV phosphorus administration.[3]

Hyperphosphatemia

Hyperphosphatemia is associated with a reciprocal fall in serum calcium and the resultant clinical effects of hypocalcemia. The most serious effect of excess phosphate relates to precipitation of calcium phosphate crystals in soft tissues such as the cornea, lung, kidney, and blood vessels. Causes include hypoparathyroidism, acute and chronic renal disease, Addison disease, leukemia, sarcoidosis, osteolytic metastatic bone tumor, and milk-alkali syndrome.[2,6]

Treatment includes limiting phosphate intake, using oral phosphate-binding agents such as aluminum hydroxide, and increasing excretion.[6] IV hydration with saline is followed by diuretics to enhance excretion.

Magnesium Abnormalities

Magnesium abnormalities are frequently associated with other electrolyte abnormalities. Clinically, hypomagnesemia and hypermagnesemia have the same effect on release of PTH and calcitonin as hypocalcemia and hypercalcemia. Calcium and magnesium excretion are interdependent.

Hypomagnesemia

Hypomagnesemia may result from malabsorption syndrome, ulcerative colitis, small bowel bypass, cirrhosis, alcoholism, chronic renal disease, DKA, diuretic therapy, hyperthyroidism, nephrotoxins, and malnutrition.[2,3,6] Symptoms include nausea, vomiting, sedation, increased deep tendon reflexes, and muscle weakness.[1,2] With significant hypomagnesemia, hypotension, bradycardia, coma, respiratory paralysis, and cardiac arrest may occur.[2] Generalized weakness, muscle fasciculations, and positive Trousseau and Chvostek signs may also be seen.[1,2,6] Dysrhythmias such as prolonged QT, torsades de pointes, ventricular tachycardia, and ventricular fibrillation have been associated with hypomagnesemia.

Treatment depends on severity of symptoms. Mild magnesium deficiencies can be treated with oral supplements and increased dietary intake of foods high in magnesium.[6] If the condition is severe, IV or intramuscular magnesium sulfate should be administered.[6] Vital signs, deep tendon reflexes, fluid intake, urinary output, and magnesium levels should be carefully monitored, because too-rapid administration of magnesium can lead to cardiac or respiratory arrest.

Hypermagnesemia

Hypermagnesemia may result from reduced excretion secondary to advanced renal failure, adrenocortical insufficiency, overdose of therapeutic magnesium, or routine doses of magnesium in the patient with renal compromise. Symptoms that may be seen are hypotension, respiratory depression, and cardiac arrest.[3,6] Treatment of hypermagnesemia depends on severity of symptoms. Treatment may include the administration of calcium gluconate, diuresis, or dialysis.[3] Serial magnesium levels, vital signs, and deep tendon reflexes should be closely monitored.

VASULAR ACCESS AND PATHOPHYSIOLOGY

Low-pressure vessels located throughout the body receive blood from capillary beds and return it to the heart. Small venules flow into increasingly larger veins, which eventually flow into the inferior and superior vena cava. Vessel diameter varies among patients and with location in the body. Surface vessels in hands and arms are primary peripheral access points; however, vessels in the neck, legs, feet, and head may be used. Valves located within veins prevent backflow; therefore IV catheters must be inserted in the same direction as venous flow. Older adult patients lose collagen in vessel walls, which causes significant thinning over time. Peripheral veins of the neck flow into the subclavian vein and can be used for vascular access. The external jugular vein is visible in most patients on the lateral aspect of the neck. The internal jugular vein is located beneath and medial to the external jugular. Subclavian veins are used for access to central circulation.

Peripheral Venous Access

Inserting peripheral IV catheters is a routine skill for emergency nurses. Some agencies also allow nurses to insert central catheters, depending on training and state regulations. Catheters are usually inserted into peripheral veins of the hand, arm, or the external jugular veins of the neck. Vessels in the dorsal venous network of the foot and the saphenous vein are rarely used for routine vascular access in adults because of increased incidence of embolism and phlebitis; however, these veins are commonly used in infants.

Vascular access is obtained using aseptic technique. Initial insertion attempts should begin with distal veins and progress up the extremity. Proximal veins are not routinely used unless patients require immediate fluid replacement, such as patients with trauma or patients in hypovolemic shock. During cardiac compressions, peripheral veins are used to avoid interruption in compressions, which upper-body central line insertion would require. To minimize the slower delivery of medications via this route, drug doses are followed by a rapid fluid bolus. Proximal peripheral veins are also used for patients receiving drugs with an extremely short half-life, which could become metabolized before reaching their target organ (e.g., adenosine), and also for rapid boluses of contrast media required for specific imaging studies (e.g., spiral chest computed tomography). Scalp veins have no valves, so fluid can be infused in either direction; they are also easily visualized, making them an ideal alternative in infants.

Insertion of IV catheters is not without risk to the patient and the emergency nurse. Potential complications for the patient include infiltration of fluid/medications; phlebitis; embolism of blood, air, or catheter fragments; infection; and cellulitis. Catheters that are inserted under emergent conditions should be assessed to determine whether an appropriate aseptic technique was used. If it was not, the catheter must be replaced as soon as possible. It is important for the ED nurse to frequently review the Centers for Disease Control and Prevention's Guidelines for the Prevention of Intravascular Catheter-Related Infections (https://www.cdc.gov/infectioncontrol/guidelines/bsi/). The emergency nurse risks exposure to potentially infectious blood through a needlestick or direct contact with blood or body fluids. Extreme care should be taken to minimize risks through use of standard precautions and appropriate disposal of needles.

Catheter Selection

The size and type of catheter are determined by urgency of need and patient size, age, and vasculature. Larger-diameter catheters are used for administering significant volume, colloid solutions, or blood or blood products, whereas smaller-diameter catheters are used for routine vascular access. The smallest size and shortest length of catheter that will deliver the prescribed therapy should be selected to decrease the potential for developing phlebitis. Catheters too large for a vessel can impede flow around the catheter and cause damage to the surrounding vessel wall. Catheters over needles are ideal for aggressive fluid replacement but can present problems with stabilization, particularly in distal veins of the hand. Winged catheters are easily inserted and can be stabilized with minimal effort; however, these catheters are not ideal for rapid fluid replacement. Their availability in smaller sizes increases their usefulness for pediatric and older adult patients. Unfortunately, they may be more uncomfortable than other catheters. Dual-lumen peripheral catheters must be flushed before insertion to activate a hydrolytic lubricant on the outside of the catheter. IV catheters with safety features such as self-capping needles and retracting needles are readily available to decrease the health care worker's potential exposure to bloodborne pathogens.

Insertion

Aseptic technique is essential to protect the patient from infection during IV catheter insertion. Gloves should be worn for site preparation and catheter insertion; additional precautions are required for central line insertion. The selected insertion site should have adequate circulation and be free of infection. Peripheral veins in hands and arms are the first choice for IV access. Other sites include veins of the lower extremities or the external jugular veins. The external jugular vein is accessible in most patients but requires turning the patient's neck for access. Lowering the patient's head distends the vein and decreases risk for air embolism during insertion. Use of the external jugular vein is not recommended for patients with suspected neck injury. Use of the internal jugular vein is contraindicated in these patients.

After an extremity site is selected, a tourniquet is placed proximally to distend vessels for easy insertion. Because veins may be more prominent in older adult patients, a tourniquet may not be required. Tourniquets may actually rupture vessels because of increased pressure in fragile veins. Gently tapping or rubbing vessels below the tourniquet increases vessel size by dilation. When vessels are not easily visualized or palpated, applying warm towels over the vein for 5 minutes causes vasodilation and can facilitate catheter insertion.

Local anesthesia is not routinely used for catheter insertion when time is an issue. However, after site preparation, lidocaine 1% may be injected at the insertion site for immediate anesthetic effect. A topical anesthetic (EMLA, LMX-4, Ametop) can be applied over the insertion site as an alternative to injection if time allows—depending on the agent used, 30 to 60 minutes is required to achieve an anesthetic effect.

Central Venous Access

The subclavian, internal jugular, and cephalic veins are used for short- and long-term vascular access. Short-term central venous access is indicated when peripheral access cannot be obtained or when the patient's condition requires hemodynamic monitoring. Long-term vascular access is indicated for prolonged IV therapy, total parenteral nutrition, extended antibiotic therapy, or therapy with caustic drugs such as vancomycin, and in patients with debilitating diseases such as cancer or acquired immunodeficiency syndrome. To decrease the patient's risk for developing a catheter-related infection, sterile surgical technique should be used to insert these devices: the person inserting the line and the nurse assisting should be wearing sterile gloves and gown, mask, and cap, and the patient should be draped from head to toe. In the ED, establishing central venous access is usually an emergent procedure using the subclavian or jugular veins. Complications related to initial insertion include infection, hematoma, pneumothorax, and air embolism.

The femoral vein located medial to the femoral artery may also be used for access to central circulation in some patients. The femoral vein is an excellent choice in cardiac arrest because cardiac compressions can continue during insertion. Access via the femoral vein also provides an opportunity for hemodynamic pressure monitoring. Complications associated with femoral vein access include hematoma and infection. Femoral sites should always be considered contaminated and replaced as soon as adequate alternative access can be obtained.

Single-lumen and multiple-lumen catheters are available. Awareness of access sites and indications for each lumen is critical for appropriate management. The proximal lumen, which can be used for medication and blood component administration, can also be accessed for blood collection after infusions have been stopped according to hospital policy. The distal port, which is generally larger, can be used to administer high-volume or viscous fluids, colloids, and medications. Some catheters have additional ports, which should be used according to manufacturer recommendations.

Patients may come to the ED with nonemergent, long-term access central lines in place. These include catheters that are peripherally inserted, tunneled externally, or totally implanted. Long catheters inserted peripherally in the cephalic or basilic vein can be left in place for several weeks.[9] The safe length of time to leave these catheters in place is steadily increasing. The midline catheter (MLC) ends just inside the subclavian vein, whereas a peripherally inserted central catheter (PICC) extends as far as the superior vena cava. Complications include infection and catheter migration. Tunneled external lines and implanted ports are used for long-term access, usually over months or even years. Implanted infusion ports are placed in the subcutaneous tissue, usually below the right clavicle or inner aspect of the upper arm. A catheter is threaded from the port through a large vein and into the superior vena cava. Only noncoring (e.g., Huber) needles are used to access the port.

Groshong catheters are a type of tunneled catheter with a unique slit that remains closed unless blood is withdrawn or fluid or medications are given. The slit collapses during blood withdrawal but opens during fluid or medication administration. Because of this unique feature, heparin flush is not required for Groshong catheters.[9] However, the catheter is still flushed with saline solution after each use. Hospital guidelines should always be consulted for appropriate volumes and concentrations of flush solutions for a specific catheter.

Venous access devices should be used according to manufacturer recommendations whenever these lines are available and patent. Many of these devices can be used for blood collection and fluid replacement. Aseptic technique, masks, and gloves are essential when accessing central catheters to minimize risk for infection. Introduction of contaminants into the central circulation represents significant risk for patients with central venous access devices. Central venous catheters must be flushed appropriately after use to ensure patency. Inadequate flushing jeopardizes patency and leads to painful device replacement.

Problems related to central lines include venous occlusion from a lodged catheter tip, mural thrombus (found on or against the wall of the vessel), and fibrin sleeve formation.[9] Symptoms of occlusion include pain in the insertion area or path of the catheter, facial edema, or edema at the insertion site. Superficial veins may become more pronounced as vascular workload increases around the occluded vessel. The catheter tip can also migrate or become lodged against the endocardium or vessel wall. This problem is usually identified when blood cannot be withdrawn or when the external marker is not in the appropriate location. Turning the patient to the side, raising the arm, or asking the patient to cough may help move the catheter back into proper position.

A fibrin sleeve can develop on the tip of the catheter and prevent blood withdrawal. The fibrin sleeve is confirmed with a chest radiograph. Treatment includes fibrinolytic administration with tissue plasminogen activator, also known as alteplase, or Cathflo Activase.[9] Other conditions such as mechanical failure and deposits of lipids or medication precipitates can also cause catheter malfunction and should be ruled out before considering this therapy. Specific protocols, including drug dose and catheter dwell times, are described in the drug package insert and hospital protocols.

Irritation of the intimal lining of the vessel wall by medications, friction from the catheter tip, or bacteria can lead to a mural thrombus in the vessel in which the catheter is inserted. When this occurs, blood cannot be withdrawn from the device.

Intraosseous Infusion

This method is used for rapid access in both adults and children. An intraosseous needle, bone marrow aspiration needle, or spinal needle is inserted into the marrow cavity of the anterior tibia, medial malleolus, sternum, distal femur, humerus, radius, ulna, clavicle, or iliac crest.[10] The needle size for a neonate weighing less than 3 kg is 18 gauge, and a 15- to 16-gauge needle is used for adults.[10] Immediately after insertion, marrow may be withdrawn and used for some diagnostic studies. Fluids, blood and blood products, and medications can be safely infused into the intraosseous site. Manual pressure or an infusion device may be necessary for rapid fluid administration. The tibia is the preferred insertion site in children; the thin sternum should not be used. Fig. 20.4 shows preferred sites. A needle should not be inserted through infected or burned tissue. Intraosseous infusion is contraindicated in a fractured extremity, cellulitis, and osteoporosis.[10] Complications related to this technique include air or fat emboli, bone fracture, osteomyelitis, compartment syndrome, and subcutaneous abscess.[10] Alternative vascular access should be obtained as rapidly as possible because an intraosseous site is a bridge to more definitive access and should be removed within 24 hours.[10]

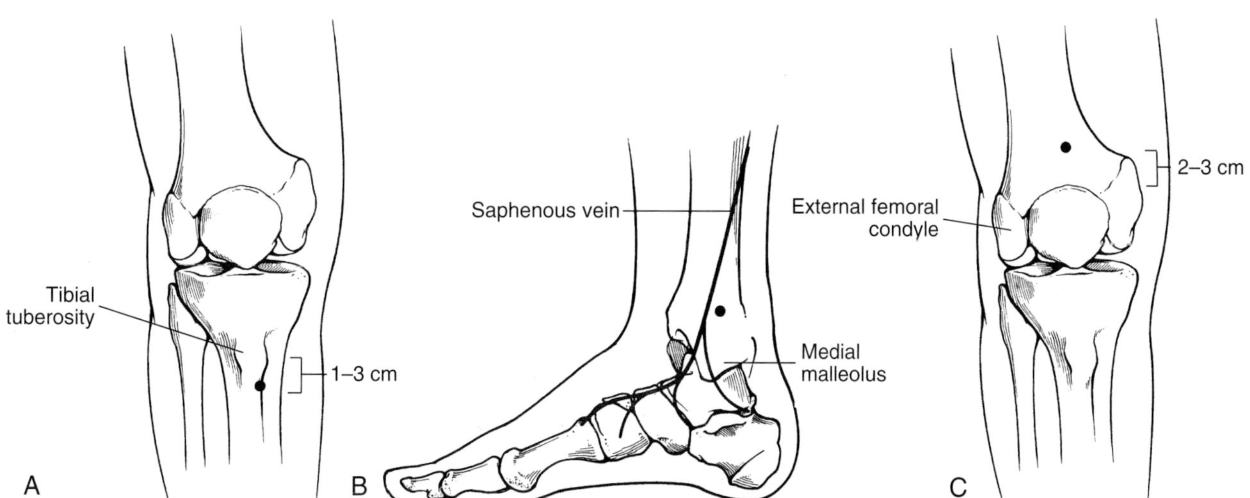

Fig. 20.4 **Schematic Diagram Demonstrating IO Insertion Sites.** (A) The proximal tibia. The IO needle is inserted 1 to 2 cm distal to the tibial tuberosity and over the medial aspect of the tibia. The bevel of the needle is directed away from the joint space. (B) The distal tibia. The IO needle is inserted on the medial surface of the distal tibia at the junction of the medial malleolus and the shaft of the tibia, posterior to the greater saphenous vein. The needle is directed cephalad, away from the growth plate. (C) The distal femur. The IO needle is inserted 2 to 3 cm above the external condyles in the midline and directed cephalad, away from the growth plate. *IO,* Intraosseous.

SUMMARY

Whether caring for a patient with trauma, a chronically ill geriatric patient, or a previously healthy person with acute simple gastroenteritis, an assessment of the circulatory system should not be overlooked. The ED nurse should anticipate abnormalities of fluids and electrolytes and the need for vascular access. The recognition of abnormalities and potential adverse events is essential for effective treatment and prevention of complications.

REFERENCES

1. McKinley MP, O'Loughlin VD, Bidle TS. Fluids and electrolytes. In: *Anatomy & Physiology*. New York, NY: McGraw-Hill; 2013:982–1013.
2. Workman ML. Assessment and care of patients with fluid and electrolyte imbalances. In: Ignatavicius DD, Workman ML, eds. *Medical-Surgical Nursing: Patient-Centered Collaborative Care*. 8th ed. Vol. 1. St Louis, MO: Elsevier; 2016:148–173.
3. Porter RS, Kaplan JL, Lynn RB. *The Merck Manual*. 20th ed. Rahway, NJ: Merck Sharpe & Dohme Corp; 2018.
4. Alexander M, Corrigan A, Gorski L, Hankins J, Perucca R. *Infusion Nursing: An Evidence-Based Approach*. 3rd ed. St Louis, MO: Saunders Elsevier; 2010.
5. Fung MK, Eder AF, Spitalnik SL, Westhoff CM. *AABB Technical Manual*. 19th ed. Bethesda, MD: AABB; 2017.
6. Reddi AS. *Fluid, Electrolyte and Acid-Base Disorders*. 2nd ed. Cham, Switzerland: Springer; 2018.
7. Braun MM, Barstow CH, Pyzocha NJ. Diagnosis and management of sodium disorders: hyponatremia and hypernatremia. *Am Fam Physician*. 2015;91(5):299–307.
8. Viera AJ, Wouk N. Potassium disorders: hypokalemia and hyperkalemia. *Am Fam Physician*. 2015;92(6):487–495. https://www.aafp.org/afp/2015/0915/p487-s1.html.
9. Weinstein SM, Hagle ME. *Plumer's Principles and Practice of Infusion Therapy*. 9th ed. Philadelphia, PA: Wolters-Kluwer; 2014.
10. Parker M, Henderson K. Alternative infusion access devices. In: Alexander M, Corrigan A, Gorski L, Hankins J, Perucca R, eds. *Infusion Nursing: An Evidence-Based Approach*. 3rd ed. St Louis, MO: Saunders-Elsevier; 2010:516–524.

21

Shock Emergencies

Gina Carbino

Shock is the clinical manifestation of inadequate tissue perfusion. It results from a dysfunction of oxygen delivery, transfer, or utilization occurring when the body's demand for oxygen is greater than its supply. In early stages, complex compensatory mechanisms help alleviate hypoperfused cells. As delivery of oxygen continues to be insufficient, cells will deviate from aerobic to anaerobic metabolism in an attempt to meet the body's metabolic demands. This can rapidly progress to death if unrecognized and without intervention in the early stages.[1,2] This chapter will discuss the pathophysiology, the categories, and management of shock in the emergency department (ED) and the effects of shock on selected patient populations.

PATHOPHYSIOLOGY

Shock results from inadequate tissue perfusion that leads to failure of the delivery and/or use of oxygen, causing tissue dysfunction.[1] In the presence of hypoxia and inadequate tissue perfusion, cells do not receive oxygen and nutrients, particularly glucose, and are unable to remove metabolic waste products. Cellular damage and eventual death ensues when cellular oxygen demands exceed the tissue's oxygen supply for a sustained time.

Normal cell metabolism requires an aerobic environment to break down glucose and oxidize substrates. During this process, enzyme-mediated chemical reactions transfer energy into adenosine triphosphate (ATP). Oxidative energy synthesis of ATP is necessary for cell survival and is a fundamental characteristic of life. This process is also referred to as cellular respiration.

Cellular respiration occurs within organelles known as mitochondria, which are located in the cell's cytoplasm. Within the mitochondria, ATP synthesis and energy production occurs. Lysosomes in the cytoplasm store hydrolytic or digestive enzymes that mediate chemical reactions within the cell.

The production of cellular energy and synthesis of ATP is dependent on a continuous oxygen supply. Oxygen delivery (DO_2) is influenced by many factors, such as blood flow, oxygen saturation, factors affecting hemoglobin's affinity to oxygen, and factors that affect oxygen transfer to tissues. Oxygen consumption (VO_2) is the amount of oxygen removed from the blood by the tissues for metabolism. Oxygen debt refers to the difference between cellular demand for oxygen and cellular consumption of available oxygen. A continuous oxygen debt creates an anaerobic environment, forcing the cell to switch to less efficient way to produce energy: anaerobic metabolism.

Anaerobic metabolism leads to the accumulation of lactate, hydrogen ions, and inorganic phosphates within the cell. ATP production is diminished and protein production is compromised. This results in damage to the mitochondria of the cell. Damage to the mitochondria triggers problems with electron transport and the activation of apoptosis, or cell death. Intracellular enzymes activated by these changes release enzymes that further deplete ATP stores and damage cellular membranes, including uninjured cells.

Sodium shifts into the cell to increase cellular volume, causing potassium to be displaced outside the cell. From here, cells begin to swell from the absorption of interstitial fluid. This swelling narrows capillary lumens and further decreases the supply of oxygen and nutrients to the cells. The shift in potassium interferes with nervous, cardiovascular, and muscular cell function. Eventually, energy-dependent potassium channels fail, causing arterioles to dilate, leading to uncompensated shock.

The tissue damage results in the body initiating an immune response releasing proinflammatory cytokines and phospholipids. This sets off a cascade of changes that assist in protecting the body. Proinflammatory cytokines activate the immune system, which results in a hyperinflammatory response, or SIRS (systemic inflammatory response syndrome). One function of the immune system is to stop the apoptosis that occurs with SIRS. If the cause of shock is not recognized and managed early, SIRS will continue and result in the production of arachidonic acids, prostaglandins, thromboxanes, and other metabolites that continue the inflammatory response cascade.[3]

In an effort to maintain homeostasis, antiinflammatory mediators are produced. Unfortunately, these mediators are responsible for immunosuppression, leaving the patient at greater risk for infection. The body's ability to successfully balance proinflammatory and antiinflammatory responses depends on early and appropriate interventions to manage and treat the cause of the shock state, in hopes of fighting and healing the infection.

The activation of cytokines, arachidonic acid metabolites, and other toxins instigates the plasmatic cascade system. This system plays a role in endothelial and parenchymal cell death and coagulation. This can result in an inability of cell repair and the development of disseminated intravascular coagulation (DIC).[3] This condition develops into a vicious cycle that can ultimately lead to death.

Gluconeogenesis is triggered to provide fuel for the struggling cells. In addition, the liver and kidneys produce more glucose in response to the secretion of epinephrine, norepinephrine, glucagon, and cortisol. This results in elevated serum glucose. Insulin resistance occurs due to increased production of serum cytokines.[4] An increased production of glucose and insulin resistance further impair cellular growth and metabolism. This has led to the development of protocols to use insulin therapy in the care of patients in shock, particularly for sepsis.[4,5]

Fig. 21.1 provides a summary of impaired cellular metabolism occurring as a result of inadequate tissue perfusion, impaired oxygen, and glucose use.

Stages of Shock

Regardless of the cause of the shock state, the body mobilizes a series of compensatory responses. These mechanisms are stimulated by decreasing tissue perfusion. Ideally, the outcome of these compensatory mechanisms is to increase the delivery of oxygen to the tissues. To accomplish this, blood is shunted from the kidneys, gastrointestinal (GI) tract, liver, and skin to vital organs. Key compensatory responses include the baroreceptors, sympathetic nervous system, fluid shifts, and the endocrine system. Without these compensatory mechanisms, shock progresses to multiorgan system failure (MOF), and ultimately death.

In Stage I of shock, also known as compensatory shock, mechanisms are working to maintain systolic blood pressure within normal limits. Peripheral vasoconstriction will cause an elevated diastolic blood pressure and a narrowed pulse pressure. During this stage, the patient may seem anxious or restless. As the kidneys retain water, decreased urinary output may become evident. Increased respiratory rate occurs to increase oxygen delivery and blow off carbon dioxide.

In Stage II of shock, known as decompensated or progressive shock, compensatory mechanisms can no longer keep up with the degree of hypoperfusion. The systolic blood pressure will decrease, furthering the already narrowed pulse pressure. The patient will become tachycardic, appear cool and clammy, and exhibit an altered level of consciousness and/or unconsciousness. During this stage, serum lactate levels begin to rise and there is a base excess dysfunction. Reversal may still be possible during this stage.

Stage III, or irreversible shock, is the final stage of shock. Even with aggressive and extraordinary efforts, it is rare that this stage does not result in DIC, MOF, and ultimately death. During Stage III, the patient is generally comatose, presenting with severe hypotension and global acidosis. An ominous sign is bradycardia. Coagulopathies, such as DIC, purpura, or petechiae, are often present.

Table 21.1 summarizes the progression of the shock state.

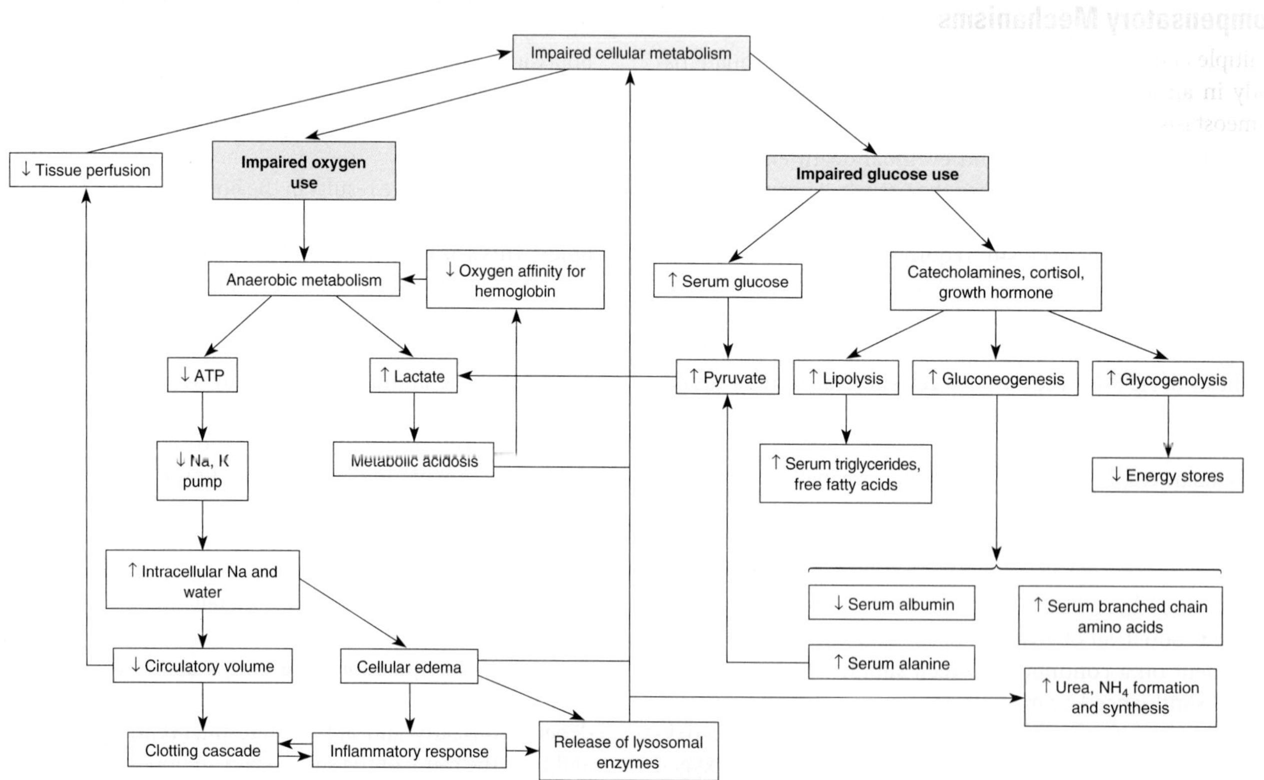

Fig. 21.1 Impairment of Cellular Metabolism by Shock. *ATP*, Adenosine triphosphate. (From Baldwin KM, Morris SE. Shock, multiple organ dysfunction syndrome, and burns in adults. In: McCance KL, Huether SE. *Pathophysiology: The Biologic Basis for Disease in Adults and Children*. 5th ed. St Louis, MO: Mosby; 2006.)

TABLE 21.1 Stages of Shock.

Stage	Pathophysiology
Compensated (nonprogressive) stage	Various receptors sense the drop in systemic pressure and initiate a cascade of physiologic changes. Homeostatic compensatory mechanisms, mediated by the sympathetic nervous system, increase end-organ perfusion. Aerobic metabolism changes to anaerobic metabolism and lactic acid is produced.
Uncompensated (progressive) stage	Compensatory mechanisms begin to fail. Mechanisms that were initially helpful now cause more injury. Cellular derangement occurs, which causes organ death. Severe lactic acidosis and inflammatory/immune system activation contribute to this.
Irreversible (refractory) stage	In refractory shock, no treatment can reverse the shock process. The cause of the shock is indistinguishable. The clinical progression of the shock state is unique to the patient and is influenced by factors such as the cause of the shock, the age of the patient, the severity and duration of the hypoperfused state, and the presence of preexisting diseases.

Modified from Holleran RS. Shock emergencies. In: Hoyt KS, Selfridge TJ, eds. *Emergency Nursing Core Curriculum.* 6th ed. St Louis, MO: Mosby; 2007.

Compensatory Mechanisms

Multiple compensatory mechanisms are triggered within the body in an attempt to compensate and maintain a state of homeostasis during a shock state. The following is a discussion of these.

Baroreceptors

Baroreceptors are a collection of specialized neural tissues located in the aortic arch and the right and left carotid sinuses, proximal to the bifurcation of the common carotid arteries. Baroreceptor reflexes respond to the stretch in these vessels by sending signals to the medulla oblongata. This causes an autonomic nervous system response based on the degree of stretch. If the vessel is stretched less than normal, as in a hypovolemic state, inhibition or reduction of baroreceptors stimulation occurs. This results in activation of the sympathetic nervous system response. Conversely, an increase in stretch, such as in fluid overload, causes an increase in baroreceptors and results in a parasympathetic response. These responses occur very rapidly, most often within seconds to minutes.[2]

Chemoreceptors

Chemoreceptors are situated in same location as baroreceptors. They are stimulated in response to changes in pH, oxygen, and carbon dioxide in the blood. When pH and oxygen are low and carbon dioxide is high, chemoreceptors stimulate the respiratory center to increase the rate and depth of respirations.

Sympathetic Nervous System

A decrease in circulating volume and cardiac output will stimulate the sympathetic nervous system. This results in release of epinephrine, norepinephrine, and other endogenous catecholamines stimulating α- and β-receptors. Stimulation of α-receptors is followed by arteriolar and venous vasoconstriction, shunting blood to organs. Other effects include stimulation of the adrenal glands, which ultimately leads to fluid retention by the kidneys. This also has a cardiac chronotropic effect, or tachycardia. β-Receptor stimulation has a positive inotropic effect, increasing myocardial contractility and improving coronary artery blood flow. The α- and β-adrenergic effects augment venous return, increasing ventricular filling, heart rate, and myocardial contractility. This facilitates ventricular emptying and improves cardiac output and blood pressure.[6]

Shift of Interstitial Fluid

Normal distribution of body fluid is 75% intracellular and 25% extracellular. Of the extracellular fluid, one-third is located intravascular and two-thirds are located interstitially. Hydrostatic pressure and plasma colloid oncotic pressure (COP) are forces that maintain normal fluid distribution between the intravascular and interstitial compartments. Hydrostatic pressure pushes fluid from the arterial end of the capillary bed into the interstitial space. COP pulls fluid into the venous capillary bed due to plasma proteins such as albumin.

Renin-Angiotensin-Aldosterone System

Renal hypoperfusion and mediation of β-receptors by the sympathetic nervous system secondary to shock cause release of renin. Renin activates conversion of angiotensinogen to angiotensin I. Angiotensin I is converted by angiotensin-converting enzyme (ACE) in the vascular endothelium of the lungs. This causes vasoconstriction and production of aldosterone. Aldosterone promotes sodium and water reabsorption within the distal renal tubules. Angiotensin also causes the posterior pituitary to release antidiuretic hormone (ADH), increasing water retention. The net effect is water movement from the interstitial space into the intravascular space. Ideally, circulating volume and cardiac output increases. There is a corresponding decrease in urinary output and increase in urine specific gravity as a result of these responses. As shock progresses, oliguria and renal failure will occur.

Adrenal Gland Response

The adrenal glands are stimulated by the sympathetic nervous system when a patient is in shock, which causes the release of epinephrine and norepinephrine. The release of these endogenous catecholamines causes tachycardia and increased contractility, resulting in improved cardiac output to aid in end-organ perfusion. Both epinephrine and norepinephrine cause peripheral vasoconstriction to increase peripheral vascular resistance and increase blood return to the heart.

The triggering of the stress response stimulates the hypothalamus to secrete corticotropin-releasing hormone, which stimulates the pituitary to release adrenocorticotropic hormone (ACTH). This causes the release of cortisol (another stress-response hormone) from the adrenal glands, elevating blood glucose and causing renal retention of water and sodium.[6]

CATEGORIES OF SHOCK

Shock has been categorized in multiple ways. The most commonly used method is based on the cause of the tissue hypoxia or shock. This method separates shock into four categories: hypovolemic, cardiogenic, obstructive, and distributive. The type of shock most frequently seen by the emergency nurse will depend on the population served by the affiliated ED.[7] The following sections describe the categories of shock based on the cause.

Hypovolemic Shock

Hypovolemic shock results from loss or reduction in intravascular volume. It can be defined as an inadequate amount of circulating volume. Decreased circulating volume can be caused by loss or redistribution of whole blood, plasma, or other body fluids. Hemorrhagic shock is a type of hypovolemic shock resulting from blood loss. This can result from blunt force or penetrating trauma, upper or lower GI bleeding, posterior nosebleeds, intraabdominal hemorrhage from coagulopathies, or perioperative bleeding. Nonhemorrhagic causes include heatstroke, burns, diarrhea, vomiting, hypoaldosteronism, diuresis, and third spacing. Redistribution, or third-space sequestration, occurs when fluid shifts from the intravascular compartment to the interstitial space. This can occur with changes in capillary permeability or capillary fluid pressures, as in burn injuries or sepsis. Loss of volume in the intravascular space causes a reduction in preload. Preload lowers stroke volume, which in turn lowers cardiac output. Table 21.2 illustrates the physiologic response to hemorrhage based on a 70-kg male patient.

Cardiogenic Shock

Cardiogenic shock occurs when the heart fails as a pump, causing a significant reduction in cardiac output. Injury to the myocardium impairs contractility, which decreases ventricular emptying. This increases ventricular end diastolic pressure and decreases tissue perfusion. Cardiogenic shock carries a high mortality rate and can be the result of many different pump failure issues. These include, but are not limited to, myocardial infarction with damage to more than 40% of the left ventricle, severe myocardial contusion, valvular heart disease, cardiomyopathies, ruptured papillary muscle, ruptured ventricular septum, and stunned myocardium after cardiac arrest. This also includes any hypotension-causing dysrhythmias.

When pump failure occurs, the myocardium cannot forcibly eject blood. Stroke volume decreases because of decreased contractility, which decreases cardiac output and blood pressure. Subsequent alterations in tissue perfusion precipitate myocardial ischemia and extend the region of injury, further compromising cardiac contractility. Myocardial contractility is also affected by hypoxemia, metabolic acidosis, ventricular diastolic volume, and sympathetic nervous system stimulation.

Incomplete emptying of the left ventricle during diastole elevates pressures in the left ventricle, left atrium, and pulmonary vessels. There is a corresponding increase in pulmonary pressures as pulmonary capillaries leak fluid into the alveolar spaces, causing pulmonary edema. Elevated pulmonary pressures increase right ventricular and atrial pressures, which can lead to right-sided heart failure.

Increased myocardial performance as a compensatory response to shock translates to increased myocardial oxygen demand and increased myocardial ischemia. This further compromises cardiac output and eventually progresses to cardiovascular collapse.

Obstructive Shock

Obstructive shock occurs from mechanical obstruction or compression of the pulmonary vasculature that prevents adequate cardiac output. Inadequate cardiac output and tissue hypoperfusion occur when the obstruction prevents adequate emptying of the myocardium during systole or filling during diastole. A pulmonary embolus prevents right ventricular emptying when a large portion of the pulmonary artery lumen is obstructed. Pulmonary hypertension causes the right ventricle to fail as it struggles to pump against the high pressure in the pulmonary vessels. An air embolus obstructs

TABLE 21.2 Physiologic Responses to Hemorrhage (Based on 70-kg Male).

Class % Blood Loss	Pulse	Blood Pressure	Pulse Pressure	Level of Consciousness	Respiratory Rate	Urinary Output
Class One (I) Up to 15% (up to 750 mL)	<100	Normal	Normal or increased	Slightly anxious	14–20	>30 mL/h
Class Two (II) 15%–30% (750–1500 mL)	>100	Normal	Decreased	Mildly anxious	20–30	20–30 mL/h
Class Three (III) 30%–40% (1500–2000 mL)	>120	Decreased	Decreased	Anxious, confused	30–40	5–15 mL/h
Class Four (IV) >40% (>2000 mL)	>140	Decreased	Decreased	Anxious, confused	30–40	5–15 mL/h

From Emergency Nurses Association. *Trauma Nursing Core Course (TNCC)*. 8th ed. Des Plaines, IL: Emergency Nurses Association; 2020.

flow from the right atrium to the pulmonary outflow tract, preventing emptying of the right ventricle during systole. Pericardial tamponade compresses the heart and prevents filling of the atria and ventricles, leading to a reduction in cardiac output. Tension pneumothorax, constrictive pericarditis, and restrictive cardiomyopathy are additional causes of obstructive shock.

Distributive Shock

Distributive shock is a type of shock that results from release of mediators that produce peripheral vasodilation. It can be further divided into three types: neurogenic, anaphylactic, and septic shock.

Neurogenic Distributive Shock

Neurogenic shock is most often associated with acute spinal cord disruption from trauma or spinal anesthesia. Other causes of neurogenic shock are brain injury, hypoxia, drug actions, and hypoglycemia associated with insulin shock. In neurogenic shock, outflow from the vasomotor center in the medulla is inhibited or depressed, causing loss of sympathetic vasomotor regulation. Uncontested parasympathetic responses cause vasodilation and loss of sympathetic tone. Inhibition of sympathetic innervation impedes release of norepinephrine and interferes with the body's ability to vasoconstrict. Consequently, venous return (preload) and cardiac output are decreased.

Anaphylactic Distributive Shock

Anaphylactic shock is a profound hypersensitivity reaction with a systemic, life-threatening antigen-antibody response. Antibodies develop after an initial exposure to a foreign protein or antigen. An acute immune and inflammatory response caused by a rapid release in histamine or other mediators form mast cells. These are most commonly from immunoglobin E (IgE)–mediated reactions to insect venom, pollens, shellfish, food, and medications. Current research suggests that the pathophysiology of anaphylactic shock results from a profound reduction in venous tone and extravasation of fluid, which causes reduced venous return and depressed myocardial function.[3] Clinical manifestations are usually acute and sudden and include hypotension, altered mental status, hives, urticaria, angioedema, shortness of breath, nausea, diarrhea, and in some cases, cardiac arrest.

Septic Distributive Shock

Septic shock is defined as the presence of sepsis with hypotension despite fluid resuscitation. This often requires vasopressors to maintain a mean arterial pressure (MAP) greater than or equal to 65 mm Hg and an elevated lactate level (>2 mmol/L).[7] However, the emergency nurses should be aware that the definitions of sepsis and septic shock are not unanimously accepted. Septic shock is the most common type of distributive shock and can be associated with a mortality of 40% to 50%.[7] Septic shock is caused by an infectious agent or infection-induced mediators that produce a systemic inflammatory response. As a result, there is widespread cellular dysfunction that brings about acute respiratory distress syndrome (ARDS), DIC, MOF, and eventually death. This is the most common type of shock in patients admitted to the intensive care unit.[7]

CLINICAL MANIFESTATIONS OF SHOCK

Although shock occurs at the cellular level, manifestations of the shock state are evident at the systemic level. A thorough physical examination is needed to identify clinical findings such as hypotension, tachycardia, altered mental status, delayed capillary refill, decreased urinary output, and pale, cool skin. These have been found to be some of the most reliable physical signs of shock.[1] The following is a discussion of some of the other clinical findings of shock.

Respiratory

During shock, respiratory effectiveness is affected by hypoxia. Evaluation of respiratory rate, rhythm, and work of breathing should be performed. Tachypnea is a common finding and occurs in an effort to decrease carbon dioxide, increase oxygen, and compensate for cellular acidosis. Adequate oxygenation may be indicated by pulse oximetry, but in reality, inadequate circulating volume perpetuates cellular hypoxia and anaerobic cellular metabolism. Therefore gradual increases in depth and rate of respiration may be early signs of impending shock. There may also be absent, unequal, or diminished breath sounds. Wheezes, crackles, or coarse breath sounds indicate pulmonary congestion, which often occurs with cardiogenic shock.

Circulatory

Cardiac output is determined by stroke volume and heart rate. Stroke volume is affected by preload, afterload, and contractility. Preload is the volume in the right and left ventricles at the end of diastole. It is affected by circulating volume, right arterial pressure, and intrathoracic pressure. Preload affects myocardial stretch and the force of myocardial contractility. Afterload is the arterial pressure or resistance the ventricles must overcome with each contraction, which is the amount of pressure necessary for the left ventricle to contract. Afterload is affected by aortic pressure, pulmonary arterial pressure, and systemic vascular resistance. An increase in afterload decreases stroke volume and subsequently decreases cardiac output. Contractility refers to the heart's contractile force.

The pulse rate increases when the sympathetic nervous system responds to decreased cardiac output in shock. A corresponding decrease in stroke volume results in weak, thready pulses. Evaluate and compare peripheral pulses with central pulses for presence, rate, equality, and quality. A drop in systolic blood pressure occurs from decreased cardiac output or decreased venous return. In early stages of shock, the diastolic blood pressure rises because of a sympathetic effect on peripheral vascular resistance, causing vasoconstriction. Consequently, pulse pressure narrows in the presence of decreased systolic blood pressure. As shock progresses, sympathetic activity becomes less effective and diastolic blood pressure begins to fall.

A reduction in arterial distention caused by decreased cardiac output and a proportionate decrease in stroke volume causes flattened jugular veins when the patient is supine. Flat neck veins are an indication of decreased systemic volume, or hypovolemia. Conversely, the patient in obstructive shock or cardiogenic shock may demonstrate jugular vein distention as a result of right-sided ventricular failure or increased pulmonary pressures.

Auscultate heart sounds to evaluate rate, quality, and the presence of abnormal sounds such as S_3 or S_4 and to identify irregularities such as murmurs, friction rubs, or a gallop. Distant heart tones may indicate cardiac tamponade. Cardiac dysrhythmias develop frequently as a result of injury to the myocardium or from metabolic acidosis. Stimulation of the sympathetic nervous system causes tachycardia. Progression of shock and depletion of epinephrine stores lead to bradycardia, heart blocks, and ventricular dysrhythmias, such as ventricular fibrillation.

Level of consciousness is a sensitive assessment of shock and its progression. Decreased cerebral perfusion and hypoxia are initially manifested by restlessness, anxiety, or confusion. Continued progression of shock with significant cerebral hypoperfusion and hypoxia leads to an obtunded, unresponsive patient.

Other Organ Systems

When tissue perfusion decreases, the body shunts blood to three organs that are essential: the brain, heart, and lungs. Blood is shunted away from "nonessential" organs in an attempt to maintain cardiac output and cerebral perfusion. Sympathetic nervous system activity and peripheral vasoconstriction shunt blood from the skin, causing cool skin, pallor, cyanosis, and diaphoresis. Capillary refill greater than 2 seconds is seen. Skin perfusion and capillary refill may be altered by hypothermia or preexisting peripheral vascular disease.

Normal urinary output is 0.5 to 1 mL/kg per hour. In shock, urinary output falls secondary to renal hypoperfusion and release of ADH. Urine specific gravity increases with reabsorption of water and sodium in the renal distal tubules. Potassium is excreted in the urine. Blood urea nitrogen (BUN) and creatinine levels increase as renal perfusion decreases.

Vasoconstriction leads to hypoperfusion of the GI tract, or gut ischemia. Clinical manifestations include hypoactive or absent bowel sounds, leakage of pancreatic enzymes with an elevated serum amylase level, and inability of the liver to metabolize substrates such as lactic acid. In addition, peristalsis ceases and increases the risk for a paralytic ileus or necrosis of the GI tract. This can transpose gut bacteria, leading to infection and septic shock. Concurrently, there is hypoperfusion of the liver and alteration of hepatic function that result in decreased conversion of lactate to bicarbonate and mobilization of glycogen stores, resulting in increased blood glucose levels. These effects worsen the metabolic acidosis found in the patient in shock.

MANAGEMENT OF THE PATIENT IN SHOCK

Patient Assessment

The assessment of a patient who is in shock is composed of clinical, historical, and laboratory findings. The emergency nurse must maintain a high index of suspicion for the patient to be at risk for developing shock based on a significant history or if the patient is exhibiting one or more of the following clinical findings: hypotension, tachycardia, altered mental status, delayed capillary refill, decreased urinary output, and pale, cool skin or extremities.

HISTORY

A history related to the patient's illness or injury needs to be rapidly collected. The emergency nurse should consider factors that would place the patient at risk for shock, including mechanisms that may cause injuries to organs such as the liver, spleen, or long bones that can cause blood loss; recent exposure to an infectious agent; or the presence of an invasive device such as a urinary catheter, peripherally inserted central catheter, or feeding tube. Immunosuppressed patients, such as patients with human immunodeficiency virus or those who have had an organ transplant or are receiving chemotherapy, are at risk for sepsis and septic shock. A history of diabetes, cardiovascular disease, or hematologic disorders are a few of the medical conditions that can place a patient at greater risk for complications from inadequate tissue perfusion.

Medications such as corticosteroids, antibiotics, and immunosuppressants may produce additional risk factors for shock complications. Anticoagulants such as warfarin sodium may cause excessive blood loss, even from minor injuries, which can lead to hemorrhagic shock. Finally, recent surgery or immobility can be risk factors for obstructive shock from a pulmonary embolus or septic shock from skin breakdown. The more information that can be gathered from the patient, family, or significant others, the more likely the cause of shock can be identified and appropriate interventions started.

Box 21.1 contains a summary of some of the pertinent pieces of history related to shock.

Resuscitation

The resuscitation of any patient begins with the primary assessment and implementation of the critical and correct interventions. Early recognition of the cause of the shock and goal-directed therapies are critical for a positive patient outcome. Adequate oxygenation and circulatory support to correct hypoxia and inadequate tissue perfusion are essential. A stable airway should be obtained or maintained along with support of effective ventilation. This may require endotracheal intubation and mechanical ventilation. Positive pressure ventilation can assist with ventilations. Supplemental oxygen should be applied to the patient to increase oxygen delivery.

Resuscitation End Points

Over the past two decades, shock resuscitation has been extensively evaluated. Using evidence-based methods, resuscitation end points have been identified to manage patients

BOX 21.1 Pertinent Historical Data.

Chief complaint
Pain, pressure (PQRST)
- Provocation
- Quality
- Radiation/region
- Severity (scale 0–10)
- Time (time of onset)

Level of consciousness
Dizziness, syncope
Weakness, fatigue
Difficulty breathing
Edema: location and type
Vomiting, hematemesis
Diarrhea, melena
Vaginal bleeding
Fever, chills
Rash, urticaria
Polyuria, thirst
Injury, location, mechanism, force, protective device
Bleeding, site, estimated blood loss
Medical-surgical history
Allergies

with specific shock syndromes, including hemorrhagic and septic shock.[8] The objectives for the use of resuscitation end points are the following:

- identification of the severity of the physiologic derangement of the shock state
- the ability to predict the risk for developing MOF or death
- to determine end points that would predict whether the patient may or may not survive without multiple-organ dysfunction
- to improve patient survival by using the appropriate resuscitation end points

Suggested resuscitation end points include oxygen delivery measured by the monitoring of mixed venous oxygen saturation (SVO_2), hemodynamic profiles measured by central venous pressure (CVP) and pulmonary capillary wedge pressure, and acid-base status measured by monitoring base deficits and lactate levels.

Management of Circulation and Perfusion

Management of circulation is directed toward identification of fluid or blood loss in hypovolemic/hemorrhagic shock. Active bleeding must be controlled through direct pressure, embolization, or operative management. The emergency care team must recognize what capabilities are available for patient management and appropriately transfer a patient if resources are not offered at the current care facility. Peripheral veins should be cannulated with a large-caliber intravenous (IV) catheter. Central venous access may be necessary, but careful consideration must be given to the risk for infection and delay in care. Intraosseous access is a rapid alternative for volume and drug administration.

There is limited evidence to guide fluid resuscitation.[1] Aggressive fluid resuscitation should be avoided in a patient with penetrating trauma until the bleeding can be surgically controlled. Evidence-based guidelines recommend target blood pressures during shock resuscitation should be maintained in the following ways[8]

- for uncontrolled hemorrhage due to trauma: mean arterial pressure (MAP) of 40 mm Hg until bleeding is controlled
- for traumatic brain injury without systemic hemorrhage: MAP of 90 mm Hg
- for all other shock states: MAP greater than 65 mm Hg

Circulation and Perfusion in Hemorrhagic Shock

There is controversy about resuscitation of the patient in hemorrhagic shock.[2,6,9] The major themes are related to fluid type, amount of fluid, the use of blood, and the role of permissive hypotension. As previously discussed, research continues to demonstrate that during active hemorrhage, the blood pressure should be managed based on the patient's response, not on a specific number. Aggressive fluid resuscitation has been associated with dislodgement of blood clots, dilation of the venous system, dilution of clotting factors, exacerbation of coagulopathies, and hypothermia.[6,10]

Massive blood product use has been associated with coagulopathies, the development of ARDS, MOF, and death. In addition, blood supplies are limited and expensive. Triggers for blood transfusions for hemorrhagic shock need to be in place in all institutions that use blood as part of the resuscitation of hemorrhagic shock.[11] Future control of hemorrhage may include the administration of recombinant factor VIIa, hemoglobin-based oxygen carriers, and blood substitutes.[1] Tranexamic acid has been shown to reduce mortality in adult patients with trauma and significant risk of ongoing hemorrhage and has been added to the World Health Organization's Model List of Essential Medicines.[12]

Circulation and Perfusion in Cardiogenic Shock

Options to enhance cardiac output and myocardial contractility include administration of sympathomimetic agents, or vasopressors. They should be used only after hypovolemia has been corrected and preload optimized. Vasopressors include dopamine, dobutamine, norepinephrine, epinephrine, and phenylephrine. Mechanical support may be initiated to provide support for a failing heart. Devices for mechanical support may include intraaortic balloon pumps, right ventricular assist devices, and left ventricular assist devices.

Circulation and Perfusion in Neurogenic Shock

Spinal cord injuries may be managed initially by fluid resuscitation. If there is no response and other sources of hypotension have been ruled out, vasopressors may be used to maintain an adequate MAP.

Circulation and Perfusion in Septic Shock

The management of sepsis and septic shock has received a great deal of attention over the past 10 years.[13] The ED plays a key role in the initiation of goal-directed therapy for the management of severe sepsis and septic shock. Research has demonstrated better outcomes when there is a seamless and organized continuum of care from the ED to the critical care unit.[14] Hypotension should be managed through crystalloid or colloid-equivalent fluid at a rate of 30 mL/kg, although some researchers question the appropriateness of a set volume amount to infuse. If the patient's hypotension does not respond to fluid resuscitation, norepinephrine should be initiated to maintain a MAP greater than 65 mm Hg.

Circulation and Perfusion in Anaphylactic Shock

Profound hypotension and cardiovascular collapse can be sudden and rapid in the patient with anaphylaxis. This situation requires aggressive fluid resuscitation to restore volume to the heart. It is important to remember that a quick and simple intervention to augment preload or test for fluid responsiveness is a passive leg raise. It is accomplished by placing the patient in a supine position and raising both legs of the patient. Epinephrine is administered to increase cardiac output through its direct β-effect on the heart. When the patient is in profound shock, only the IV infusion of epinephrine is found to be effective.[9]

Circulation and Perfusion in Obstructive Shock

To restore circulation and adequate perfusion in obstructive shock, the source of the obstruction must be identified and proper critical interventions performed. For example, for a tension pneumothorax, an emergent needle thoracentesis should be performed, followed by insertion of a chest tube.

Acid-Base Balance

Inadequate tissue perfusion and hypoxia lead to acidosis. The body will attempt to compensate for acidosis in multiple ways. The lungs and the kidneys play a key role in acid-base balance for the patient who is in shock. The major body buffer systems are found in the interstitial fluids, the blood, intracellular fluid, urine, and bones.

In early shock, respiratory alkalosis occurs because of tachypnea. This is the body's attempt to increase oxygen levels and decrease carbon dioxide levels in the body's tissues. Increased carbon dioxide and hydrogen ions in chemoreceptors stimulate respiratory centers in the brain and increase the rate and depth of the patient's respirations. Anaerobic metabolism increases serum lactic acid, causing metabolic acidosis. Importantly, lactate levels and base deficit can also be influenced by other factors, such as liver and renal diseases. A persistently high base deficit and low pH may be an early indicator of complications. Metabolic acidosis is corrected by providing adequate oxygenation and perfusion through ventilation, fluids, and medications. The cause of the shock state needs to be quickly identified and appropriate management initiated to correct the origin of the anaerobic process. If the pH is less than 7.1, administration of sodium bicarbonate may be needed to correct the pH. However, sodium bicarbonate should not be administered before adequate ventilation and fluids have been established.

HEMODYNAMIC MONITORING

The need for hemodynamic monitoring in the ED is a controversial topic. As with any invasive modality, the risk versus benefit to the patient must be considered. These monitoring avenues, such as continuous hemodynamic values and immediate feedback on interventions, can play a role in caring for the patient in shock. Risks include infection, bleeding, vessel dissection, and misuse of time and resources.

Pulse Oximetry

Pulse oximetry is a noninvasive method of determining hypoxia through measurement of arterial hemoglobin saturation. Light is transmitted through tissue to a light detector via a probe attached to the patient. The light absorption abilities of oxyhemoglobin and deoxyhemoglobin are calculated by the monitor to determine the percentage of arterial saturation. Changes in peripheral circulation, use of vasoactive medications, hypothermia, anemia, hemodilution, and ambient light will affect the validity of pulse oximetry.

Central Venous Pressure

Central venous pressure (CVP) is used to indirectly measure preload or blood volume returning to the right side of the heart. Normal CVP measurements range from 2 to 8 L/min pressure. CVP measurements lower than 2 L/min indicate decreased circulating volume. A measurement greater than 8 L/min signifies higher than normal pressure. This can often be a result of pulmonary edema, fluid overload, pericardial tamponade, or tension pneumothorax. CVP monitoring has been suggested to be a useful tool to measure the effectiveness of early goal-directed therapies in shock management,[1] although this research, too, is contested.

Arterial Lines

Arterial pressure may be measured directly using an invasive arterial line or indirectly using noninvasive blood pressure monitoring (NIBP). The accuracy of NIBP in a critically ill patient in shock is widely debated.[7,12] Arterial lines have superior precision and can provide continuous monitoring when titration of vasoactive drugs is necessary. They also decrease the number of punctures required for the measurement of laboratory values, which is particularly important for a patient with coagulopathies. Normal MAP is between 70 and 90 mm Hg. A MAP of less than 65 mm Hg is generally accepted as inadequate to perfuse vital organs, such as the brain, kidneys, and coronary arteries.

Mixed Venous Oxygen and Central Venous Oxygen Saturation Monitoring

The measurement of mixed venous oxygen (SVO_2) and central venous oxygen saturation ($ScvO_2$) is used as an indirect measure of tissue oxygenation.[15] SVO_2 is monitored by using a fiberoptic, pulmonary artery catheter to measure oxygen in the blood that has been mixed from both the inferior and superior vena cava in the pulmonary artery. $ScvO_2$ is monitored with a specialized central line measuring the oxygen content in the superior vena cava only. Because $ScvO_2$ represents blood from the upper part of the body, specifically the brain and coronary vessels, SVO_2 is thought to be more predictive of global tissue oxygenation.[16] The normal range for SVO_2 and $ScvO_2$ is 65% to 70%. SVO_2 is generally higher than $ScvO_2$, as $ScvO_2$ measures blood returning from the brain and coronary vessels, where oxygen extraction is greatest. Low values may be obtained in hemorrhage, anemia, hemodilution, and shock states. High values are obtained in late septic and anaphylactic shock, hypothermia, and increased FiO_2. $SvcO_2$ and SVO_2 monitoring can be used to monitor the effectiveness of goal-directed therapy for various types of shock.[16]

LABORATORY AND DIAGNOSTIC TESTING FOR SHOCK EMERGENCIES

Diagnostic and laboratory testing is targeted at finding the cause of shock. A complete blood count; type and screen or crossmatch; serum chemistry panel, including glucose, BUN, and creatinine; liver function tests; and a coagulation profile should all be considered. If the source of the shock is cardiac, a cardiac profile should also be evaluated. Serum lactate levels, arterial blood gas values, and base deficit levels provide an estimate of the severity of the oxygen debt in hypoperfused patients.

On the basis of the patient's history, specific radiographic studies may be ordered. All patients should have a chest radiograph. If the patient had a traumatic injury, radiographs of affected areas where blood loss may have occurred, such as the pelvis or long bones, should be obtained. The focused assessment sonography for trauma (FAST) can assist in rapidly identifying abdominal bleeding. A computed tomography or magnetic resonance imaging scan may also aid in identifying areas of blood loss or possible sources of infection.

Other diagnostic procedures may include a 12- to 18-lead ECG, diagnostic peritoneal lavage, bronchoscopy, paracentesis, gastroscopy, and/or endoscopy.[17]

EMERGENCY NURSING MANAGEMENT

The emergency nursing care for a patient with a shock emergency begins with a history and physical examination. Any potential source for shock needs to be quickly identified from the patient's history and chief complaint. The general appearance of the patient should be evaluated. This includes the patient's level of consciousness and behaviors, as anxiety and confusion are signs of inadequate tissue perfusion and hypoxia. Color and temperature of the patient's skin should also be assessed. Skin can be described as pink, pale, mottled, warm, cool, or moist, and these terms are descriptors for skin perfusion. Purpuric lesions and petechiae may be hidden under clothing or mistaken for bruising.

A primary assessment should be performed and critical interventions initiated. Any signs of obvious bleeding must be controlled.[8] The appropriate use of a tourniquet or pressure dressing is recommended for selected serious bleeding. Several steps can be taken to avoid injury from a tourniquet. These include the following steps[18,19]

- placing the tourniquet as distally as possible, but at least 5 cm proximal to the wound
- avoiding application over a joint
- applying the tourniquet directly to exposed skin, which can prevent unnecessary movement or slipping
- releasing the tourniquet as soon as it is medically safe (generally, if the tourniquet is in place less than 2 hours, there should be little damage)
- never applying a tourniquet directly over a foreign object

Ensuring an airway in an obtunded patient or a patient with a decreased level of consciousness is a priority. Applying supplemental oxygen can help increase oxygen delivery DO_2 to tissues. Obtaining a blood pressure can be difficult because of vasoconstriction and low cardiac output. Central and peripheral pulses should be palpated, but they should never be used to estimate a blood pressure value, as this method is highly inaccurate.[20] Capillary refill has been found to be of particular value in the pediatric patient to assess perfusion. However, the influence of temperature should always be considered. Breath sounds, heart tones, and bowel sounds should be auscultated.

Fluids, blood, and blood products may be required for volume replacement. If large amounts of blood and blood products are needed for resuscitation, massive transfusion protocols should be instituted to ensure that the patient receives the appropriate ratio of volume replacement to prevent adverse outcomes such as hemodilution. O-negative packed red blood cells may be used before a patient is typed and screened. O-positive packed red blood cells are sometimes used for male patients when O-negative blood is limited. If blood needs to be administered to a premenopausal female whose blood type is unknown, Rh_O(D) immune globulin should be considered.[15]

Pharmacologic management of shock may include vasopressors. The choice of vasopressor is based on the type of shock. These medications require close monitoring for effect and the possibility of tissue infiltration. Short-term administration of vasopressors through peripheral lines has been shown to be safe.[21] Providing comfort and pain management should not be ignored, as patients may be anxious and fearful. Allowing the presence of family members may also facilitate recovery.

COMPLICATIONS ASSOCIATED WITH SHOCK

Multiple complications occur with shock states. The most deadly is MOF, which ranges from multiple-organ impairment to organ failure to death.[22] The sequential organ failure assessment score (SOFA) was developed to describe the degree of organ failure and how it progresses. Included in the assessment are respirations, coagulation (platelets), liver function (bilirubin), cardiovascular (inotrope use), central nervous system, and renal function (creatinine).

DIC is a widespread microvascular coagulation followed by depletion of clotting factors. Microthrombi form and are distributed to the microvasculature of various organs, producing infarction, tissue ischemia, and hemorrhagic necrosis when secondary fibrinolysis fails to lyse the fibrin quickly. Secondary fibrinolysis reduces clotting factors and impairs the release of fibrin degradation products that act as anticoagulants. These processes contribute to serious bleeding tendencies. DIC may occur after a massive transfusion of blood products or in association with acute lung injury. Other factors that place the patient at risk for the development of DIC include polytrauma, neurotrauma, and fat emboli. Severe toxic or immunologic reactions to snakebites may also initiate DIC. The primary intervention for DIC is early identification and interventions to correct or manage the primary cause. For the patient with a shock emergency, that would include detection of the source of bleeding or infection. Continuous bleeding from IV sites or wounds serves as an important signal of DIC. Patients should be observed for obvious or occult bleeding, hematuria, petechiae, and ecchymosis.

SPECIAL POPULATIONS

It is important for the emergency nurse to recognize that pediatric, older adult, and pregnant patients respond differently to volume depletion and other causes of shock. Young children can only increase their cardiac output by increasing their pulse rate. This also leads to increased oxygen consumption by the heart. If allowed to continue, this compensatory mechanism will eventually fail. Bradycardia is an ominous sign of impending arrest in the child. Normal physiologic differences or changes associated with the very young and the very old may interfere with the body's ability to cope with some of the causes of shock, such as volume loss. The older adult patient may have limited ability because of preexisting cardiac disease or failure to maintain an increased heart rate. Medications such as β-blockers will impede the heart's ability to increase its rate.

Table 21.3 highlights some of these differences. Emergent conditions in these populations are covered in greater detail in other chapters of this text.

TABLE 21.3 Shock in the Pediatric, Older Adult, or Pregnant Patient.

Patient	Description
Pediatric	Increases cardiac output by increasing heart rate; fixed stroke volume; sustains arterial pressure despite significant volume loss; loses 25% of circulating volume before signs of shock occur; hypotension and lethargy are ominous signs: early clinical manifestations are tachycardia, tachypnea, pallor, cool mottled skin, and delayed capillary refill; volume replaced with 20 mL/kg bolus of crystalloid
Older adult	Shock progression often rapid; normal physiologic changes of aging reduce compensatory mechanisms; predisposed to hypothermia; preexisting disease states contribute comorbidities
Pregnant	Hypervolemia of pregnancy means patient can remain normotensive with up to a 1500-mL blood loss; compression of inferior vena cava by gravid uterus reduces circulating volume by 30%; place patient on left side, manually displace uterus to the left, or elevate right hip with towel; risk for aspiration resulting from decreased gastric motility and decreased gastric emptying; treat suspected hypovolemia to prevent placental vasoconstriction associated with catecholamine release; potential for fetal distress exists despite maternal stability

SUMMARY

Shock is a progressive, dynamic process caused by inadequate tissue perfusion and oxygenation. Regardless of the etiology, the cellular effects of shock are the same. Nursing assessment, early recognition, and appropriate interventions are essential to prevent or reverse the shock process and to ensure a positive patient outcome.

REFERENCES

1. Antonelli M, Levy M, Andrews PJ, et al. Hemodynamic monitoring in shock and implications for management. *Intensive Care Med*. 2007;33(4):575–590.
2. McCance KL, Huether S. *Pathophysiology: The Biologic Basis for Disease in Adults and Children*. 5th ed. St Louis, MO: Mosby; 2006.
3. Keel M, Trentz O. Pathophysiology of polytrauma. *Injury*. 2005;36(6):691–709.
4. Zauner A, Nimmerrichter P, Anderwald C, et al. Severity of insulin resistance in critically ill medical patients. *Metabolism*. 2007;56(1):1–5.
5. Van den Berghe G. Insulin therapy for the critically ill patient. *Clin Cornerstone*. 2003;5(2):56–63.
6. Emergency Nurses Association. *Trauma Nursing Core Course (TNCC)*. 8th ed. Des Plaines, IL: Emergency Nurses Association; 2014.
7. Shankar-Hari M, Phillips GS, Levy ML, et al. Developing a new definition and assessing new clinical criteria for septic shock: for the Third International Consensus Definitions for Sepsis and Septic Shock (Sepsis-3). *JAMA*. 2016;315(8):775–787.
8. Tisherman S, Barie P, Bokhari F, et al. Clinical practice guideline: endpoints of resuscitation. *National Clearinghouse*. 2007.
9. Brown SG. The pathophysiology of shock in anaphylaxis. *Immunol Allergy Clin North Am*. 2007;27(2):165–175.
10. Berry R. Management of shock in trauma. *Anaesth Intensive Care Med*. 2005;6(9):308.
11. Mitra B, Mori A, Cameron P, et al. Massive blood transfusion and trauma resuscitation. *Injury*. 2007;38(9):1023–1029.
12. Vincent JL, De Backer D. Circulatory shock. *N Engl J Med*. 2013;369(19):1726–1734.
13. Nguyen HB, Rivers EP, Abrahamian FM, et al. Severe sepsis and septic shock: review of the literature and emergency department management guidelines. *Ann Emerg Med*. 2006;48(1):28–54.

14. Rivers E. Early goal directed therapy in severe sepsis and septic shock: converting science to reality. *Chest*. 2006;129(2):217–218.
15. Dickens JJ. Central venous oxygenation saturation monitoring: a role for critical care? *Curr Anaesth Crit Care*. 2004;15:378–382.
16. Goodrich C. Continuous central venous oximetry monitoring. *Crit Care Nurs Clin North Am*. 2006;18(2):203–209.
17. Holleran RS. Shock emergencies. In: Hoyt KS, Selfridge TJ, eds. *Emergency Nursing Core Curriculum*. 6th ed. St Louis, MO: Mosby; 2007.
18. Langley D, Criddle L. The tourniquet debate. *J Emerg Nurs*. 2006;32(4):354–356.
19. Schreiber MA, Tieu B. Hemostasis in operation Iraqi freedom iii. *Surgery*. 2007;142(suppl 4):S61–S66.
20. Deakin CD, Low JL. Accuracy of the advanced trauma life support guidelines for predicting systolic blood pressure using carotid, femoral, and radial pulses: observational study. *BMJ*. 2000;321(7262):673–674.
21. Kheng CP, Rahman NH. The use of end-tidal carbon dioxide monitoring in patients with hypotension in the emergency department. *Int J Emerg Med*. 2012;5(1):31.
22. Gupta S, Jonas M. Sepsis, septic shock and multiple organ failure. *Anesth Intensive Care Med*. 2006;7(5):143.

22

Respiratory Emergencies

Andi Foley and Vicki Sweet

Patients present to the emergency department (ED) with a variety of respiratory complaints that can range from mild to life-threatening. It is crucial to recognize early warning signs of respiratory compromise and rapidly intervene to prevent decompensation.

This chapter will discuss the basic anatomy and physiology of the respiratory system and frequent respiratory emergencies, including asthma, bronchitis, emphysema, pulmonary edema, pulmonary embolus, near-drowning, and spontaneous pneumothorax.

ANATOMY AND PHYSIOLOGY

The respiratory system includes the upper and the lower airway structures. The upper airway includes the nasopharynx, oropharynx, and laryngopharynx. The structures within the upper airway are supported by cartilaginous rings preventing collapse during respiration. Cartilaginous rings are replaced with smooth muscle fibers in the lower airways for stability and support. Connecting the upper and lower airways is the larynx, which acts as a gate to prevent aspiration. The lower airway comprises the larynx, trachea, bronchi, bronchioles, and alveoli. The functional unit of the pulmonary system is the alveolus, which interacts with adjacent capillaries to ensure oxygen transport from alveolus into blood.[1]

Within the pleural cavity there is negative intrathoracic pressure, which causes a vacuum effect, pulling air into the lungs during inspiration. During expiration, this negative pressure decreases and the air is passively expelled. During inspiration, air is filtered, warmed, and humidified as it travels through the upper and lower airways. Cilia are hairlike structures within the passageways to help move air toward the alveoli. The cilia help move mucus and debris out of the pulmonary system, keeping the lower airways from being contaminated. The sterility of the lower airway is achieved with the help of mucus-secreting goblet cells. Mucus traps debris and keeps the airway moist. During expiration, the negative pressure decreases, the lungs recoil, and the air is passively expelled. Oxygen and carbon dioxide (CO_2) are exchanged in the respiratory bronchioles, alveolar ducts, alveolar sacs, alveoli, and pulmonary capillaries.

The major function of the respiratory system is to supply the body with oxygen and expel carbon dioxide. Cellular oxygenation is dependent on several factors: (1) an adequate supply of oxygen carried to the cell, (2) the affinity of hemoglobin for oxygen, and (3) the ease with which hemoglobin releases oxygen to cells. The affinity of hemoglobin for oxygen is described by the oxygen-hemoglobin dissociation curve. If the curve shifts to the left, hemoglobin picks up oxygen more easily in the lungs but does not easily release oxygen to tissues. Conditions shifting the curve to the left include acidosis, hypothermia, increased carbon monoxide, increased methemoglobinemia, and decreased levels of 2,3-diphosphoglycerate (2,3-**DPG**).[2] When the curve shifts to the right, oxygen uptake by hemoglobin is less rapid, but oxygen delivery to cells is easier. Oxygen dissociation is affected by temperature, acid-base balance, and carbon dioxide pressure (Pco_2) levels.

Normal gas exchange depends on adequate ventilation and perfusion. Respiration is divided into pulmonary ventilation, diffusion of oxygen and carbon dioxide across the alveolar capillary membrane, transport of oxygen and carbon dioxide to and from the cells, and regulation of ventilation.[1] Ventilation refers to the mechanical flow of air into and out of the lungs. Respiration is the actual exchange of oxygen and carbon dioxide at the cellular level. Diffusion is a process in which particles in a fluid move from an area of higher concentration to an area of lower concentration, resulting in an even distribution of particles in the fluid. Perfusion relates to the transport of blood to the tissues. Ventilation/perfusion (V/Q) mismatch occurs when either ventilation or perfusion is inadequate. When there is an extreme imbalance, inadequately oxygenated blood is shunted into the arterial system.

PATIENT ASSESSMENT

The respiratory assessment should begin with an across-the-room assessment. Quickly assess the patient's skin color and work of breathing. Complete the respiratory assessment in a systematic fashion, beginning with airway patency. Anytime there is an intervention, stop and reassess. The patient must first have a patent airway. Once patency has been established, assess the patient's work of breathing, looking for nasal flaring, retractions, accessory muscle use, tracheal tugging, or dyspnea.[3,4] Be alert to other signs of distress, including abnormal color such as pallor or cyanosis, grunting, difficulty speaking in complete sentences, tripod positioning, or decreased mental status. Changes in the patient's mental status can be an early warning sign of deterioration. Once airway, breathing, and circulation have been assessed, then perform a quick head-to-toe assessment. Listen for adventitious breath sounds, and obtain a full set of vital signs. While performing the assessment, pay attention to the patient's body language and physical characteristics. For instance, patients with chronic obstructive pulmonary disease (COPD) may have a barrel chest and/or club fingers. Although these can be normal in some patients, they can be indicative of cardiovascular abnormalities, valvular heart disease, or congenital defects. Palpate the chest for any crepitus or tenderness. Auscultate all lung fields for any adventitious breath sounds (wheezes, rhonchi, or crackles) and obtain a full set of vital signs.

The patient history should include onset of symptoms, any history of recent trauma or injury, pain on inspiration or expiration, type of cough (if present), hemoptysis, fever and/or chills, smoking history, work history, environmental history, any recent travel, human immunodeficiency virus (HIV) status, orthopnea, nocturnal dyspnea, and past medical history including heart disease, emphysema, asthma, history of deep vein thrombosis (DVT), or allergies. If the onset of respiratory symptoms was rapid, the ED nurse should consider pneumothorax, pulmonary embolism, aspiration, or a cardiac event as possible diagnoses. Asthma, pneumonia, and pulmonary edema can progress over hours to days.[3,4] If the symptoms have been progressive in nature, consideration should be given to COPD, pleural effusion, anemia, left ventricular heart failure, pulmonary hypertension, or a chronic lung disease. Make note of any associated symptoms the patient is experiencing. It is important to determine what, if any, treatment was used before arrival to the ED. While obtaining the history, inquire about occupational hazards the patient may have been exposed to, such as asbestos, beryllium dust, bird droppings, coal dust, iron oxide, or silica dust. These agents are associated with the following lung diseases, respectively: asbestosis, berylliosis, bird handler's lung, black lung, siderosis, and silicosis.

If the patient smokes, determine how much the patient smokes and how long he or she has been smoking. Smoking decreases lung compliance because it damages the elastin and collagen fibers. Patients who smoke usually have a decreased sense of taste and smell along with increased secretions and cough. Cigarette smoke negatively affects the functions used to clear the pulmonary system. Smoking increases the likelihood of cancer, chronic bronchitis, emphysema, and the incidence of infection.

Patients presenting with respiratory emergencies should be placed on a bedside monitor for continuous monitoring of oxygen saturation, cardiac rhythm, and vital signs. The patient's oxygen saturation will often be decreased in respiratory emergencies. Always treat the patient—do not rely simply on a number on the bedside monitor. Factors such as artificial fingernails, nail polish, and cold extremities can skew the oximetry readings displayed on the bedside monitor. If the patient is having difficulty breathing, administer oxygen using the device most appropriate for the situation, such as nasal cannula, nonrebreather, or bag-mask device.

Imaging may be necessary to diagnose and treat the patient in the ED. At a minimum, the patient should have a two-view chest x-ray. If there is concern for pulmonary embolus (PE), lung mass, or pleural effusion, a computed tomography (CT) scan is indicated. Specimen testing, including complete blood count (CBC), comprehensive metabolic panel (CMP), and arterial blood gas (ABG) should be obtained on all patients with respiratory emergencies.[3,4]

SPECIFIC PULMONARY EMERGENCIES

Acute Bronchitis

Acute bronchitis is an inflammatory process usually caused by a virus. Some of the common offenders include influenza virus A or B, parainfluenza virus, respiratory syncytial virus, rhinovirus, Coxsackie virus, and adenovirus.[5] Acute bronchitis is more common during cold and flu season and does not have age boundaries. Secondary infections are possible from organisms such as *Mycoplasma pneumoniae, Haemophilus influenzae,* pneumococci, and streptococci. The highest incidence of acute bronchitis occurs in smokers, older adults, and young children and during the winter months. Patients complain of sore throat, stuffy nose, and cough. Initially, the cough will be dry and nonproductive and may worsen at night. Aggravating factors include exposure to cold, talking, deep breathing, and laughing. After a few days, the patient's cough usually becomes productive. Other symptoms can include low-grade fever, chest discomfort, and fatigue.[5]

Diagnosis is based on the clinical presentation. Chest radiograph distinguishes between acute bronchitis and pneumonia. Treatment of acute bronchitis includes increasing fluid intake, avoiding smoke or other irritants, using cough preparations, and using a vaporizer to add moisture to the air. Antibiotics are not helpful other than for secondary infections.

Pneumonia

Pneumonia is an inflammatory reaction caused by a viral, bacterial, or fungal infection, which can occur on either one or both sides of the lungs. It may be preceded by an upper respiratory tract infection, ear infection, or eye infection. Pneumonia can occur at any age, but those younger than 2 years and older than age 65 are at the greatest risk.[6] Patients who are immunocompromised or smoke or have an underlying chronic disease are also at risk of developing pneumonia.[6] Some underlying chronic conditions that could increase a patient's risk of pneumonia include cystic fibrosis, COPD, diabetes, heart failure, and being immunocompromised because of HIV or acquired immunodeficiency syndrome (AIDS), chemotherapy, or history of a transplant.[6] Patients who are immobile or bedridden and those with rib fractures are at an increased risk.

Patients typically present with fever, chills, malaise, productive cough, hemoptysis, dyspnea, and pleuritic chest pain. Occasionally, patients will have headache, nausea, vomiting, and diarrhea. In the older adult population, there may be mental status changes instead of the typical symptoms.[6] On physical examination, the patient will have crackles that do not clear with coughing, as well as lung consolidation. There are different types of pneumonia based on the causative factors. These include community-acquired pneumonia (CAP), hospital-acquired pneumonia (HAP), ventilator-associated pneumonia (VAP), atypical pneumonia, and aspiration pneumonia.[1] CAP is the most common type of pneumonia caused by pneumococcus bacteria. Typically, it occurs during the winter months. HAP is more serious than CAP, as the patient is already hospitalized for another illness and then develops pneumonia during the hospital stay. VAP is when a patient is on a ventilator and develops pneumonia. Atypical pneumonias are caused by *Legionella pneumophila, Mycoplasma pneumoniae,* or *Chlamydia pneumoniae.*[6] Aspiration pneumonia can occur in patients who have dysphagia or brain injury.[6]

Treatment for patients with pneumonia will be based on the type but typically includes humidified oxygen, antibiotics, and monitoring of fluid and electrolyte balance. The diagnosis is based on clinic presentation, sputum culture and Gram stain, chest radiograph, and CBC. Pulse oximetry is obtained initially and monitored over time to determine any changes in the patient's oxygenation. ABG values may be obtained as a baseline.

Pneumococcal pneumonia vaccines are recommended for those patients younger than 2 years and older than 65 years. Vaccines are also recommended for those between this age range who smoke or have underlying medical conditions.[6,7] When obtaining the patient's history, be sure to ask about immunizations such as influenza and pneumococcal vaccines. Education should include the importance of pneumococcal vaccines, influenza vaccines, and smoking cessation, if the patient smokes or is frequently around smokers.[7]

Asthma

Asthma is an obstructive disease of the lungs characterized by airway inflammation and hyperreactivity. Symptoms can range from mild to severe. Asthma can be controlled, not cured, and has an unpredictable course with increasing prevalence and hospitalizations. Most patients with asthma are children, and males are affected more than females. Thirty percent of those diagnosed with asthma during childhood will have it as adults. There is a positive family history in more than one-third of patients with asthma.[8]

Airway inflammation and hyperresponsiveness occur in response to certain triggers (Box 22.1). Immunologic triggers cause a humoral immune response with complex multicellular activation, including mast cells, eosinophils, and immunoglobulin E (IgE) antibodies (Fig. 22.1). Inflammatory mediators cause smooth muscle contraction, vasodilation, mucosal edema, increased mucus secretion, and macrophage eosinophil infiltration. Acetylcholine directly increases airway resistance and bronchial secretions. This cholinergic response further stimulates histamine and inflammatory mediator release, with the exception of IgE.

Nonimmunologic triggers stimulate the autonomic nervous system and cause mast cell and inflammatory mediator response. The pathway of emotional triggers is through the

BOX 22.1 Triggers of Acute Asthma Attacks.

- Allergen inhalation
  - Animal dander
  - House dust mite
  - Pollens
  - Molds
- Air pollutants
  - Exhaust fumes
  - Perfumes
  - Oxidants
  - Sulfur dioxides
  - Cigarette smoke
  - Aerosol sprays
- Viral upper respiratory infection
- Sinusitis
- Exercise and cold, dry air
- Stress
- Drugs
  - Aspirin
  - Nonsteroidal antiinflammatory drugs
  - β-Adrenergic blockers
- Occupational exposure
  - Metal salts
  - Wood and vegetable dusts
  - Industrial chemicals and plastics
  - Pharmaceutical agents
- Food additives
  - Sulfites (bisulfites and metabisulfites)
  - Beer, wine, dried fruit, shrimp, processed potatoes
  - Monosodium glutamate
  - Tartrazine
- Hormones/menses
- Gastroesophageal reflux
- Emotional stress

From Lewis SL, Heitkemper MM, Dirksen SR et al. *Medical-Surgical Nursing: Assessment and Management of Clinical Problems.* 7th ed. St Louis: Mosby; 2007.

parasympathetic nervous system and stimulation of the hypothalamus. Aspirin sensitivity exacerbates asthma through reaction to prostaglandin synthesis. Exercise-induced asthma occurs after 10 to 20 minutes of vigorous exercise because of airway cooling secondary to decreased warming, reduced humidification, and increased respiratory rates. Exercise may be the only trigger for some patients and is usually limited to the early phase. Gastroesophageal (GE) reflux, a common condition associated with asthma, involves esophageal spasm, with reflux of gastric acid causing spasm of nearby bronchial and esophageal structures.[8]

Immunologic and nonimmunologic triggers cause increased mucus production, airway hyperresponsiveness, airway narrowing, and chronic inflammatory airway changes. These triggers can cause either an early or late response in patients with asthma. Early-phase reactions involve rapid bronchospasms, whereas late-phase reactions involve inflammatory epithelial lesions, increased mucosal edema, and increased secretions. Complex interactions among lung cells cause a chronic inflammatory process irritating airways. An

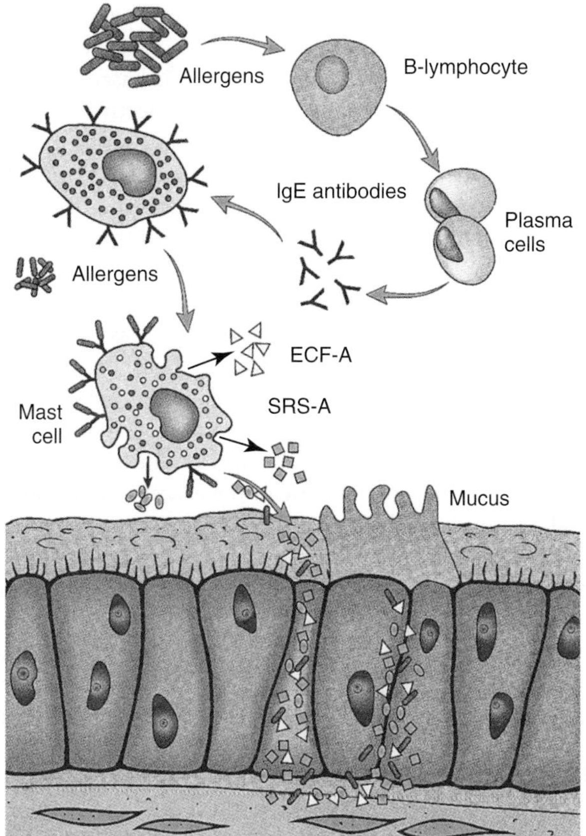

Fig. 22.1 Early-phase response in asthma is triggered when an allergen or irritant cross-links immunoglobulin E receptors on mast cells, which are then activated to release histamine and other inflammatory mediators. *ECF-A,* Eosinophil chemotactic factor of anaphylaxis; *IgE,* immunoglobulin E; *SRS-A,* slow-reacting substance of anaphylaxis. (From Lewis SL, Heitkemper MM, Dirksen SR, et al. *Medical-Surgical Nursing: Assessment and Management of Clinical Problems.* 7th ed. St Louis, MO: Mosby; 2007.)

acute exacerbation involves airway obstruction caused by spasms, inflammation, and mucus plugging.

There are no definitive tests to diagnose asthma. The diagnosis should be based on careful history, examination, and laboratory studies.[8] The history should include symptoms, patterns, usual triggers, family history, and allergies the patient may have. Physical examination may reveal upper airway rhinitis, sinusitis, or nasal polyps, as well as wheezes and a prolonged expiratory phase. Laboratory studies should include CBC with differential, nasal smears, and sputum specimen. The CBC may have elevated eosinophils. There may be increased hilar or basilar infiltrates or areas of atelectasis secondary to mucus plugging and alveolar collapse on chest radiographs. To aid in the diagnosis of asthma, patients older than 5 years should have spirometry, which evaluates the air capacity of the lungs using a spirometer and measures the volume of air inhaled and exhaled. Spirometry can demonstrate obstruction and assess reversibility of airway narrowing. Peak expiratory flow rate (PEFR) is the greatest flow velocity produced during forced expiration after fully expanding lungs during inspiration.[8] It is measured using a peak flowmeter. PEFR is used to monitor response to therapy in acute episodes but is not designed as a diagnostic tool.[8] PEFR measurement is effort dependent, so measurement duplication provides most accurate results.

The 2012 *Expert Panel Report 3: Guidelines for the Diagnosis and Management of Asthma* expanded previous guidelines and recommended updates based on new evidence.[8] Focus areas include prevention, risk reduction, and reduction of impairment associated with exacerbations. The panel recommended a stepwise approach to long-term asthma management focusing on different age-groups, with emphasis on patient education and control of environmental factors or comorbid conditions affecting asthma. There are also modifications to treatment strategies for managing asthma exacerbations, which include

- simplifying the classification of severity of exacerbations;
- encouraging the development of prehospital protocols to allow administration of albuterol, oxygen and, with medical oversight, anticholinergics and oral systemic corticosteroids;
- adding levalbuterol;
- adding magnesium sulfate or heliox (a medical gas mixture of helium and oxygen) for severe exacerbations unresponsive to initial treatment;
- emphasizing oral corticosteroids;
- emphasizing that anticholinergics are used in emergency care, not hospital care; and
- considering initiation of inhaled corticosteroids at discharge.

Inhaled allergens are common triggers, particularly for patients younger than 30 years of age. For patients who have persistent asthma, skin testing to assess sensitivity to indoor allergens is recommended. Although patients may have positive skin reactions to food allergens, these usually do not lead to acute exacerbations. In addition to inhaled allergens, other triggers such as occupational exposures, viral illnesses, and GE reflux can stimulate an asthma attack. GERD is associated with nocturnal exacerbations nonresponsive to inhaled nebulizers. When GERD is suspected, a thorough gastrointestinal workup is indicated.

Occupational asthma initially presents with rhinitis or eye irritation along with evening or nocturnal cough. With prolonged exposure the patient will note increased symptoms, such as coughing, wheezing, and dyspnea. These symptoms will diminish with time away from exposure to irritants. Smokers have a higher incidence of occupational asthma because of increased airway irritation.

Clinical manifestations of asthma include cough, wheezing, prolonged expiratory time, and reduced peak expiratory flow.[8] Patients may also experience increased work of breathing and accessory muscle use. When a patient presents to the ED with decreased air movement, low oxygen saturation, altered level of consciousness, and increased work of breathing, immediate interventions are required. These patients require high-flow oxygen and continuous pulse oximetry, along with nebulizer therapy, in an effort to provide some relief of symptoms. Close observation is required because their symptoms can lead to respiratory failure if rapid interventions are not provided. Severity can be assessed by determining type and frequency of home medications required to control symptoms, prior intubation, recent hospitalizations, spirometric indexes of airflow obstruction, nocturnal symptoms, and number of prior ED visits.[8] ABG values initially indicate reduced arterial oxygen pressure (PaO_2) and arterial carbon dioxide pressure ($Paco_2$) from hyperventilation. $Paco_2$ eventually rises, which creates further V/Q (ventilation/perfusion) mismatching.

Management goals are to maintain near-normal pulmonary function and exercise levels, to prevent chronic symptoms and acute exacerbations, and to avoid adverse effects of medications. Therapy includes objective measurement of lung function, environmental control, avoidance of triggers, select drugs, and comprehensive patient education.

PEFR provides objective data for management, documents personal best and daily variations, detects impending exacerbation, guides medicine therapy, and helps identify triggers. To correctly obtain peak expiratory flow measurements, the patient should stand, if able, take a deep breath, and forcefully blow out all inspired air. The highest of three readings is recorded. A diary of peak expiratory flow measurements, along with documentation of viral infections, weather, medicine changes, environments, and other possible triggers, aids in management of asthma.

Avoidance and environmental control of allergens such as dust mite antigens, animal dander, pollens, and molds can greatly reduce symptoms. Encasing pillows and mattresses in dust mite–proof covers, washing bedding every week in water temperatures greater than 130°F, and carpet removal or mite treatment aid in the reduction of dust mites. Keep pets outside the house to decrease dander allergens, outdoor pollens, and mold. Patients with asthma should remain inside with air-conditioning during early morning and midday hours to further reduce exposure.

Drugs for asthma reduce bronchial spasms, airway inflammation, mucosal edema, and airway hyperreactivity. These medications can be given orally, intravenously, or subcutaneously or be inhaled. There are several forms of inhaled therapy, such as nebulizers and inhalers. Advantages of inhaled therapy include smaller drug amounts, rapid onset of action, direct delivery to respiratory system, fewer side effects, and painless, convenient administration.

Asthma exacerbation can be defined as an episode of progressively worsening shortness of breath, cough, wheezing, and chest tightness. The most severe exacerbations require admission to the intensive care unit for optimal monitoring and treatment. Special attention should be given to infants and those who are at increased risk for death associated with asthma.[7] Patients with a history of recent (within the past year) intubation or admission to the intensive care unit, two or more admissions to the hospital because of asthma exacerbation, three or more visits to the ED, or those who have been to the ED within the past month for asthma exacerbation are at an increased risk for death.[8] Patients who use more than two canisters of short-acting β_2-agonists (SABAs) per month are also at increased risk.[8]

In the ED, patients with moderate to severe exacerbations will present with a variety of symptoms. The best way to determine the extent of the exacerbation is based on objective measures such as lung function. Objective measurements are a more reliable indicator of the severity than the symptoms alone. Treatment options in the ED are aimed at relieving hypoxemia and airflow obstruction and decreasing airway inflammation. Some of these treatments include oxygen therapy, SABAs, and the addition of inhaled ipratropium bromide and systemic corticosteroids. In addition, treatment options should look at adjunct therapy such as intravenous (IV) magnesium sulfate or heliox in those patients with severe exacerbation who are not responding to other treatment options. Successfully relieving the exacerbation is the goal in the ED, but good follow-up care must be provided in an effort to prevent a relapse of the exacerbation. Patients should be instructed to have follow-up asthma care within 1 to 4 weeks and be given specific instructions about any medications prescribed while in the ED. Teaching should be done with regard to increasing medication or seeking medical care if the patient's symptoms become worse. Current guidelines also encourage that the inhaler technique be reviewed, and initiating inhaled corticosteroids should also be considered.

Chronic Obstructive Pulmonary Disease

COPD is a progressive and irreversible syndrome characterized by diminished inspiratory and expiratory capacity of the lungs. COPD includes emphysema and chronic bronchitis.[9] Almost every case of COPD is associated with a history of smoking, both active and passive. Cessation of smoking may prevent the development of COPD. There are four stages of COPD. Stage I is mild COPD. With stage I COPD, the patient may not even realize he or she has abnormal lung functioning. Stage II is considered moderate COPD. At this point the patient may seek treatment because of chronic respiratory symptoms and exertional dyspnea. With stage III, the patient will have increased shortness of breath and reduced exercise capacity, and the quality of life may be affected because of repeated exacerbations. Stage IV is very severe COPD,[9] which involves serious airway limitations. The quality of life is greatly affected, and exacerbations of COPD may be life-threatening.

When patients present to the ED, it is important to differentiate between other possible causes of respiratory difficulty. Differential diagnoses for COPD include asthma, congestive heart failure, bronchiectasis, tuberculosis, obliterative bronchiolitis, or diffuse panbronchiolitis. Patients with an acute exacerbation of COPD will complain of worsening dyspnea, an increase in sputum production, and an increase in sputum purulence. Typically, patients with COPD will have a barrel chest, chronic cough, distant breath sounds, and tachypnea. During times of acute exacerbation, these patients may also have an upper respiratory infection, fever, wheezing, tachycardia, and tachypnea.[9]

On physical examination, rhonchi and/or wheezes may be noted. If the patient has an acute infection, crackles may be present. Note the patient's respiratory pattern and work of breathing. Signs of distress include pursed lips, nostril flaring, and use of accessory muscles. The patient may want to lean or sit forward to help his or her work of breathing.

Patients with COPD fall into two primary categories: chronic bronchitis as primary disease and others with COPD. With the chronic bronchitis COPD, patients appear edematous and cyanotic. They have increased mucus production and inflammation from bronchitis and panlobular emphysema. Decrease in ventilation and increase in cardiac output cause a V/Q mismatch, which leads to polycythemia and hypoxemia. Others with COPD are markedly dyspneic and have a pink skin color. Alveolar cell destruction decreases oxygen exchange; however, the body compensates with hyperventilation and decreased cardiac output. Patients with nonprimary bronchitis COPD have highly oxygenated blood with decreased cardiac output.

Patients with COPD are taught how to manage their disease at home. These patients must avoid irritants and practice good bronchial hygiene, which includes adequate hydration, humidification, and postural drainage. These patients routinely use bronchodilators, expectorants, and mucolytics to control their symptoms.[9] Anticholinergic bronchodilators may have better results than intermittent nebulizer treatments for these patients. Corticosteroids are used sparingly, although infections should be treated aggressively. Viral and bacterial infections play a major role in exacerbations of COPD and contribute to disability. Patients should receive influenza and pneumococcal vaccines. Changes in cough and sputum production and characteristics require prompt antibiotic therapy. Proper education, patient compliance, adequate nutrition, and exercise are important parts of therapy.

In advanced disease, chronic respiratory failure with severe hypoxemia and hypercapnia are present; serum carbon dioxide levels no longer provide the drive for respiration. Hypoxia, or low serum oxygen, becomes the drive for respiration. Chronic oxygen delivery is necessary if PaO_2 falls below 55 mm Hg. Management in the ED includes oxygen therapy, nebulized medications, bronchodilators, and steroids.[9] Low-flow oxygen may be administered with nasal cannula or Venturi mask. High-flow oxygen should not be withheld when the patient is in respiratory failure.

Emphysema

Emphysema is the permanent abnormal enlargement of the respiratory tract distal to the terminal bronchioles and associated destructive changes of the alveolar wall. The pathologic changes leading to alveolar destruction are associated with the release of proteolytic enzymes from inflammatory cells.[9] Alveolar damage results from inflammation of the parenchyma and the inactivation of α_1-antitrypsin. α_1-Antitrypsin protects the lung parenchyma. With the loss of alveolar walls, there is also a marked reduction in the pulmonary capillary bed, which is essential for exchange of oxygen and carbon dioxide between the alveolar air and capillary blood. The loss of elastic tissue within the lung leads to diminished smaller bronchioles. Increased pressure around the outside of the airway lumen leads to increased airway resistance and decreased airflow.

Within a person's lungs there are 25,000 acini, airways distal to the terminal bronchiole, and 3 million alveoli. The three categories of emphysema, which are dependent on the area of lung tissue involved, are centrilobular, panlobular, and bullous. Centrilobular emphysema involves the upper lung fields and occurs in the center of lobules, corresponding to the enlargement of the respiratory bronchioles. It is associated with chronic bronchitis. Centrilobular emphysema rarely occurs in nonsmokers. Panlobular emphysema is less common, associated more with familial α_1-antiprotease deficiency.[1] Panlobular emphysema occurs primarily in lower and anterior fields and is not directly associated with cigarette smoking. Entire acini and many bullae (airspaces less than 1 mm in diameter in distended state) are involved. Bullous emphysema is characterized by isolated emphysemic changes within the bullae without generalized emphysema.

There is a direct correlation between smoking, chronic bronchitis, and emphysema, but not all smokers develop emphysema. Genetic or familial traits may predispose patients to this disease process. A small minority of patients have a genetic deficiency of serum α_1-antiprotease or α_1-antitrypsin, in which protease digestion of elastin and collagen lung fibers is inhibited. Protease is found in macrophages and polymorphonuclear leukocytes during inflammatory processes. The inhibitors are inactivated by irritants such as smoke and pollutants.

The end result is destruction of elastic properties of the lung and loss of natural recoil and support. During expiration, increased intrathoracic pressure causes collapse with premature closure of airways, whereas decreased support of the lung causes large residual volumes and decreased flow rates. Inspiratory rates are normal unless there is airway obstruction from chronic bronchitis, air trapping, and overdistended airspaces. Eventually, the area for gas exchange at the alveolar capillary membrane decreases because of destruction of the alveolar wall, causing V/Q mismatch with patchy emphysemic changes, increased physiologic dead space, and abnormal ABG values.

Patients may exhibit signs of chronic bronchitis in the beginning of the disease process. There will be exertional dyspnea slowly progressing to dyspnea at rest. Primary emphysema presents with dyspnea. There is no associated cough or sputum production. The severity of dyspnea does not correlate with the severity of destructive changes within the lung. Increasing dyspnea indicates increasing airway obstruction. As the disease progresses, there may be structural changes evident such as an increased anteroposterior diameter of the chest, dorsal kyphosis, elevated ribs, flare at the costal margin, and widening of the costal angle. Upon auscultation, diminished breath sounds and expiratory wheezes will be noted, as well as hyperresonance. Radiography will reveal hyperinflation of the lungs. Other evidence of emphysema includes decreased vascular markings, hyperlucency, and deeper space between the sternum and heart. Pulmonary function tests reveal hyperinflation, increased residual volume, reduced vital capacity, and increased total lung capacity with decreased expiratory flow rates.[1] Emphysema may be differentiated from asthma or bronchitis because of the reduction in diffusion capacity. ABG values may be normal in mild cases of emphysema with the exception of decreased PaO_2. As the disease progresses, $Paco_2$ becomes elevated.

Treatment regimens for patients with emphysema include the use of bronchodilators. Inhaled sympathomimetics and ipratropium bromide are the treatments of choice. Patients must practice good bronchial hygiene to mobilize secretions. All patients should be encouraged to stop smoking. Smoking cessation programs should be offered to patients at each visit. In addition, at each visit, question the patient about smoking habits and evaluate his or her readiness to stop. Patients should be encouraged to participate in graded aerobic exercise. Abdominal diaphragmatic breathing exercises with pursed-lip breathing will improve muscle conditioning for breathing and promote exhalation of more air from the lungs. All patients with emphysema should avoid pollution and irritants—especially cigarette smoke. As the disease progresses, the patient may require home oxygen therapy during exercise, only at nighttime, or for continuous use. During times of exacerbation, the patient should be managed in the ED with continuous pulse oximetry, oxygen therapy, bronchodilators, and steroids. Any patient with decreased oxygen saturation should receive a high triage priority and have treatment initiated immediately.

Chronic Bronchitis

Chronic bronchitis is a COPD of the larger airways. It is most often associated with cigarette smoking but has been associated with other environmental pollutants. Inflammation of the bronchial mucous membranes causes increased mucus production and is a direct result of various irritants such as cigarette smoke, fumes, and dust. This increased mucus production leads to swelling and enlargement of the submucosal glands and may result in obstruction of the airways.[10]

Chronic bronchitis is diagnosed when the patient has a productive cough lasting at least 3 consecutive months annually for at least 2 years.[11] This disease is most often diagnosed in patients from 40 to 55 years of age.[11] Patients with chronic bronchitis will often have a hacking cough, rhonchi that clear with coughing, barrel chest, and prolonged expiration. As the disease progresses, patients will exhibit wheezing and dyspnea at rest. Patients generally will not seek treatment until they have difficulty breathing or notice increased sputum production, which can vary in color.

When assessing patients with chronic bronchitis, elicit a history from them regarding how they function at home and whether they have issues with fatigue, sleep patterns, and sleep positions. Patients may sleep in an upright position for comfort. On examination, patients may be using accessory muscles and appear cyanotic. As the disease progresses, patients will retain carbon dioxide. If their $Paco_2$ levels are too high, patients may be confused and complain of a headache and light sensitivity. Patients with chronic bronchitis may have peripheral edema and jugular vein distention. Adventitious lung sounds such as scattered crackles and wheezing will be present, as well as a prolonged expiration. In the late stages, chest radiography will reveal hyperinflation of the lungs.

Interventions include low-flow oxygen therapy, bronchodilators, and possibly steroids.[1] If patients are receiving home oxygen therapy, remind them of the dangers of smoking near oxygen. Antibiotics may be given if there is an infection present. It is important to discuss smoking cessation with these patients.

Pulmonary Embolus

A PE is an undissolved piece of material occluding a vessel and obstructing the circulation distally. Early assessment and intervention have reduced mortality from 10% of patients with a fatal PE dying within 1 hour after symptoms begin to a report of median time to death after presentation of 6 days.[12] Approximately 100,000 patients will die of PE annually.[13] PE is commonly underdiagnosed.

Generally, the presenting symptoms may be nonspecific, depending on the size of the blockage, which can lead the emergency nurse to initially consider other causes. The most common symptom is dyspnea. Patients may also exhibit tachycardia, tachypnea, signs of restlessness, apprehension, and anxiety.[1] Patients may complain of sudden shortness of breath and severe chest pain. The pain may worsen with inspiration. On examination, the patient may be diaphoretic and have crackles on auscultation. The patient may also complain of cough, hemoptysis, fever, or syncope. Petechiae may be seen on the patient's chest wall; this is most likely associated with fat emboli (commonly associated with long-bone fractures).[1] If the embolism occludes a large vessel, symptoms may be more severe and include hypotension and signs of right ventricular failure. The diagnosis of PE can be very challenging because the clinical presentation is often nonspecific.

Pulmonary thromboemboli frequently originate in the deep veins of the legs. The most common risk factors for a venous thromboembolus include immobility, trauma, surgery, long-bone fractures, pregnancy, cancer, heart failure, and estrogen use.[13] Venous thromboembolus is also seen with obesity, decreased peripheral circulation, congestive heart failure, and thrombophlebitis. Sometimes congestive heart failure or myocardial infarction can lead to pulmonary emboli.

Stasis of blood, damage to epithelium of the vessel wall, and alterations in coagulation, known as Virchow triad, can lead to formation of venous thrombi. An embolus becomes dislodged and travels through the venous system and through the right side of the heart, finally lodging in a pulmonary vessel, obstructing blood flow, and decreasing perfusion to a portion of the lungs. If the embolism lodges in a large pulmonary vessel, pulmonary vascular resistance increases and cardiac output is decreased. The embolism causes the body to respond by releasing serotonin, histamine, prostaglandins, and catecholamines, which trigger bronchospasms and vasoconstriction. The production of surfactant ceases, and alveoli collapse.

There are no simple diagnostic tests for a PE. To determine whether there is a V/Q mismatch, a V/Q scan or spiral (also called helical) CT scan will be performed. A diagnosis of PE is confirmed if there is adequate ventilation with impaired blood flow to the pulmonary vasculature on the V/Q scan or if there is a filling defect in the pulmonary arterial tree on the spiral CT scan. Additional tests include ABG measurement, 12-lead ECG, chest radiograph, and cardiac enzymes. Laboratory studies are completed to rule out other possible causes. The chest radiograph may be normal. The 12-lead ECG will have nonspecific T-wave and ST-segment changes along with T-wave inversion. Additional ECG changes include new-onset right bundle branch block and right axis deviation with peaked P waves in limb leads and depressed T waves in right precordial leads (V_1 to V_3). The ABG values will have decreased PaO_2 and $Paco_2$. The only conclusive test for PE is pulmonary arteriography. This invasive procedure is usually reserved for last.[13] Duplex ultrasonography of both lower extremities should be completed.

Patients presenting to the ED with these clinical symptoms should have continuous cardiac monitoring and supplemental oxygen therapy. Analgesics may be given for patient comfort. IV fluids and vasopressors should be used to maintain pressure. Once a diagnosis is made, IV anticoagulants are initiated to prevent further clot formation. Weight-based heparin protocols or home therapy with low-molecular-weight heparin are the preferred anticoagulant options for these patients. If there are no contraindications, fibrinolytic therapy, such as tissue plasminogen activator, should be started immediately in the unstable patient and may be considered in the ED for any patient with a diagnosed pulmonary embolus. Surgical intervention may be necessary and may include an embolectomy or placement of an inferior vena caval umbrella filter.

Pulmonary Edema

Pulmonary edema is not a primary disease process, but rather the result of an acute event. Pulmonary edema is a life-threatening complication manifested by severe dyspnea, diaphoresis, hypertension, tachycardia, anxiety, and tachypnea. Many times, the patient will have pink, frothy sputum production.

The two types of pulmonary edema are cardiogenic and noncardiogenic. Cardiogenic pulmonary edema occurs when there is inadequate left ventricular pumping, which leads to increased fluid pressure. Increased left ventricular pressure inhibits left atrial emptying, blood backs up into alveolar-capillary membranes, and pulmonary capillary filtration increases. Fluid from the pulmonary circulation floods the alveolar-capillary membrane and fills alveolar spaces normally containing air. The end result is increased fluid in the lungs. Potential causes of cardiogenic pulmonary edema include acute coronary syndromes and heart failure.

Noncardiogenic pulmonary edema is the result of primary damage to the alveolar-capillary membrane. Loss of integrity increases membrane permeability, which causes fluid and protein accumulation in interstitial spaces and eventually floods the alveoli, causing significant fluid accumulation in the lungs.

Acute respiratory distress syndrome (ARDS) is a cause of noncardiogenic pulmonary edema resulting from acute lung injury. Damage to the alveolar epithelium and pulmonary vasculature leads to edema from an increased capillary permeability.[5] The patient with ARDS will have decreased lung compliance, refractory hypoxemia, severe acute respiratory distress, and pulmonary parenchymal consolidations. During the period shortly after initial pulmonary injury, there will be pulmonary capillary congestion, endothelial cell swelling, and extensive microatelectasis. During days 1 through 5 after initial injury, airspace ossification begins and progresses to a uniform appearance on chest radiograph. Late stages of ARDS are characterized by hyperplasia of type II alveolar cells and collagen deposition. The overall mortality rate associated with ARDS is approximately 40% to 70%.[1] Many conditions, such as trauma, sepsis, and fluid overload, predispose patients to ARDS.

Excessive extracellular fluid volume can result in pulmonary edema as increased pressure at the arterial capillary membranes pushes fluid into surrounding tissues. Fluid shifts across the alveolar-capillary membrane into the alveoli, resulting in pulmonary edema. Fluid overload inhibits left ventricular pumping, and excess fluid backs up into the left atrium with the same effect as cardiogenic pulmonary edema. Excessive fluid volume may be caused by increased sodium intake such as with packaged foods, abuse of tap water enemas, or overload of IV fluids high in sodium. Renal disorders and cirrhosis can also cause fluid overload.

Patients with pulmonary edema have cardiovascular and respiratory symptoms. Cardiovascular symptoms result from generalized fluid overload. Poor left ventricular function is generally followed by poor right ventricular function, leading to heart failure with engorged neck veins, sacral edema when the patient is sitting with legs not in a dependent position, lower extremity pitting edema, weight gain, rapid and bounding pulse, and S_3 and S_4 heart sounds. If the condition is left untreated, the pulse will become weak and thready. The skin is cool, pale, and moist and may appear cyanotic or mottled in some patients. Blood pressure initially increases in an attempt to pump the excess fluid but decreases as the condition worsens.

Respiratory symptoms occur because increased alveolar fluid impairs oxygen exchange across the alveolar-capillary membrane. The patient develops dyspnea, and respiratory rate increases in an effort to increase oxygenation. Increased respiratory rate decreases Pco_2, causing respiratory alkalosis. As the condition worsens, metabolic acidosis occurs in an effort to rid the body of metabolic waste products. Respiratory effort becomes labored as the patient tires from the effort of breathing. Fluid in the lungs causes crackles and productive cough with frothy, white sputum. Sputum can have a pink tinge in fulminate pulmonary edema. Cyanosis may be present, and oxygen saturation decreases as hypoxia increases. Bronchospasms may develop, causing wheezing, crackles, and rhonchi.[1] Chest radiographs usually show bilateral interstitial and alveolar infiltrates.

Treatment focuses on improving oxygenation by administering high-flow oxygen, improving cardiac function, and decreasing cardiac workload.[1] Bronchodilators may be given via aerosol inhalation treatments to decrease bronchospasms. Positive end-expiratory pressure is indicated when hypoxia continues despite aggressive oxygen therapy. Most patients with hypoxemia refractory to maximum ventilation have a poor prognosis because of secondary multiple-system organ failure.

Heart rate increases in an attempt to manage excess fluid; however, this leads to decreased filling time and decreased contractility. Digoxin is given via IV push to increase contractility and decrease heart rate. IV dobutamine is given to increase contractility and reduce peripheral vascular resistance. Dopamine is indicated for hemodynamically significant hypotension, whereas nitroprusside is used to decrease afterload by vasodilation. Cardiac workload is also decreased through diuretic therapy (e.g., furosemide, bumetanide) and by positioning the patient in the high-Fowler's position with legs dependent. The dependent-leg position results in venous distention in the lower extremities or pooling of blood, which decreases circulatory volume. IV morphine causes vasodilation, which increases venous pooling and decreases preload. Preload is the result of blood volume in the left ventricle. In pulmonary edema, treatment is given to decrease volume so backflow into the atria is decreased and to increase strength of contraction by preventing overstretch of muscle fibers (Starling law). Nitroglycerin may be administered to increase venous distention and venous pooling, which decreases blood return to the heart. Other interventions include using a urinary catheter to monitor urine output and the effects of diuretics.

Lung Transplants

Lung transplants are a last resort treatment for irreversible lung failure. Lung failure occurs when the lungs are no longer able to exchange oxygen and carbon dioxide. Patients with transplanted lungs now have longer survival rates and are more likely to seek emergency care. The most common complications include pleural space complications, pulmonary parenchymal complications, opportunistic infections, and immunosuppression-induced complications. Early postoperative complications of the pleural space include pneumothorax or hemothorax. Other complications include chylothorax and empyema. At any time, the patient may present with an episode of acute rejection or a pulmonary embolism. Opportunistic infections can be caused by bacterial, viral, mycotic, or parasitic organisms, and antibiotics should be started as soon as possible in the ED. Other complications may be related to the patient's chronic medication regimen. Patients with transplants who present to the ED have an increased risk for infection because of their immunocompromised state and should be placed in protective precautions (a positive-pressure-flow environment is essential) while in the ED.

Spontaneous Pneumothorax

Spontaneous pneumothorax may occur with or without an underlying pulmonary condition. Primary spontaneous pneumothorax occurs in individuals who do not have known pulmonary disease, whereas a secondary spontaneous pneumothorax occurs in those with a history of pulmonary conditions, such as COPD or pulmonary fibrosis. Generally, primary spontaneous pneumothorax occurs in males 20 to 40 years of age who are tall and thin. Older males will more likely experience a secondary spontaneous pneumothorax. Smokers have an increased risk for developing a spontaneous pneumothorax. With spontaneous pneumothorax the cause is usually rupture of an apical, subpleural emphysematous bleb. Iatrogenic pneumothorax can result from invasive procedures, such as insertion of a subclavian catheter or transthoracic needle aspiration, or from trauma secondary to mechanical ventilation and cardiopulmonary resuscitation.

Patients with a pneumothorax experience dyspnea and chest pain on the affected side. The larger the pneumothorax, the more acute the symptoms will be. With a larger pneumothorax, there may be subcutaneous emphysema noted, as well as cyanosis, hypotension, and severe dyspnea. Monitor the patient's oxygen saturation closely. Interventions are based on the clinical presentation and the degree of collapse. Asymptomatic patients with less than 15% pneumothorax may be observed on an inpatient or outpatient basis. Other treatment options include needle aspiration and tube thoracostomy. These patients are more likely to return to the ED for the same complaint.

Inhalation Injury

Three factors to be considered when evaluating a patient who has had an inhalation injury are exposure to asphyxiants (or asphyxiation), thermal or heat injury, and smoke inhalation injury/exposure (or pulmonary irritation). Exposure to asphyxiants is the most frequent cause of early mortality. Carbon monoxide (CO) is the most frequent asphyxiant from a fire.

Carbon Monoxide Poisoning

Hemoglobin has a greater affinity for CO than for oxygen, resulting in oxygen being displaced from the hemoglobin. This displacement leads to hypoxia within the tissues. Carboxyhemoglobin (COHb) levels greater than 10% indicate CO exposure. Smokers or individuals exposed to automobile exhaust can have baseline COHb levels of 10%.[1] Fetal hemoglobin binds even more quickly with CO, so a fetus is at greater risk for injury from CO poisoning. As the COHb levels increase, symptoms worsen. Patients may complain of a headache, vertigo, nausea, vomiting, loss of coordination, or dyspnea, and the patient may appear "cherry red," flushed, confused, and lethargic.[1] Patients may also complain of visual disturbances. Cardiac complications include ST depression due to profound myocardial hypoxia. With higher COHb levels, the patient may be comatose or have seizures, or ectopy may be noted on the cardiac monitor. Pulse oximetry readings may be deceiving because the oximeter cannot distinguish between oxygenated hemoglobin and carboxyhemoglobin. Hyperbaric oxygen therapy may be considered for patients with COHb levels above 25% to 30%.

An additional consideration with CO poisoning is the potential for exposure to other asphyxiants. For example, cyanide can be produced with combustion of wool, silk, paper products, rubber, plastics, and polyurethane; the risk for exposure to these increases when in a confined space. Cyanide impedes cellular metabolism, causing anaerobic metabolism and resulting in lactic acidosis and decreased oxygen consumption. The clinical presentation of cyanide poisoning may include multiple symptoms because cyanide inhalation affects the respiratory, cardiovascular, and central nervous systems. Treatment in the ED will include administration of a cyanide antidote containing amyl nitrate, sodium nitrate, and thiosulfate or use of a Cyanokit.

Thermal or Heat Injury

Unless the cause of heat injury is from steam, explosive or volatile gases, or hot liquid aspiration, it is rare to have heat injury below the oropharyngeal airway. The respiratory tract's ability to efficiently exchange heat, combined with closure of the glottis, protects lower airways from extreme heat. Extreme heat on the upper airway initially causes erythema, edema, and blisters of the mucosa. These patients should be closely monitored for the first 24 to 48 hours after injury because the airway can become obstructed from increasing mucosal edema.

Smoke Inhalation Injury

Inhalation of toxic gases, such as hydrogen chloride, phosgene, ammonia, and sulfur dioxide, define smoke poisoning. These toxins damage pulmonary endothelial cells and destroy epithelial cilia, leading to mucosal edema. Surfactant production decreases, followed by atelectasis. Pulmonary edema can develop within 24 to 48 hours of the initial injury. Interventions for these patients include humidified oxygen, vigorous pulmonary toilet, and bronchodilators. Intubation and mechanical ventilation may be necessary to maintain airway patency should severe pulmonary edema occur.

When assessing patients with a potential inhalation injury, it is crucial to obtain a detailed history. Determine whether the patient was in an enclosed space, how long the patient was exposed to toxic gases, and what was the general environment where the incident occurred. Mortality increases with age and physical and cognitive disabilities, so it is crucial to obtain a detailed medical history. Initial interventions include protecting and maintaining a patent airway while supporting the patient's hemodynamic status. Patients with carbonaceous sputum, singed facial or nasal hair, or burns of the neck or face should be carefully evaluated for inhalation injury. Hoarseness, wheezing, dyspnea, and restlessness may also be present. These patients may require early intubation to maintain the airway before excessive edema occurs. Patients with smoke poisoning should be placed on 100% oxygen. COHb half-life is 4 to 5 hours on room air. This time can be shortened with the administration of 100% oxygen and even shorter in a hyperbaric chamber.[1]

Foreign Body Aspiration

Foreign body aspiration can have a variety of presentations. It most often occurs in children aged 6 months to 4 years.[1] Foreign body aspiration in the upper airway will present with obvious clinical symptoms and may be immediately life-threatening. When a foreign body is aspirated into the lower airways, the presentation can vary. A new onset of sudden coughing, gagging, and choking commonly occurs. Unless the airway is completely obstructed, the patient may become asymptomatic for some time.

The treatment depends on the severity of the case. If there is foreign body occlusion of the upper airway, follow basic life support measures in an attempt to clear the airway. If basic life support measures fail to clear the airway, direct visualization laryngoscopy should be performed. If all attempts fail to clear the airway, needle or surgical cricothyroidotomy should be performed.[3] Chest and/or neck radiography may reveal the foreign body. The foreign body will have to be removed via direct visualization. Lower airway obstruction usually requires bronchoscopy to relieve the airway obstruction.

Submersion Injury

Submersion injuries are most common in water but can occur in chemicals or dry substances, such as grain.[1] Submersion deaths are more common in children younger than 5 years and in young adult males.[1] Risk factors can include lack of supervision, poor swimming skills, poor judgment, and alcohol or substance abuse.

The cause of death in all drowning victims, whether freshwater or saltwater, is profound hypoxia. Aspiration of water floods the alveoli, causing a loss of surfactant, which leads to impaired gas exchange. Contaminants such as chlorine, algae, sand, and mud worsen the pulmonary injury. The most significant physiologic effect of drowning is hypoxemia from laryngospasms. In some individuals, asphyxiation results in relaxation of the airways, allowing water to enter the lungs. In a small number of patients, aspiration of water does not occur because the airway does not relax until cardiac arrest and cessation of respiratory attempts.[14]

Clinically, patients may present with respiratory distress, bronchospasm, loss of consciousness, pulmonary edema, hypothermia, poor perfusion, hypotension, dysrhythmias, metabolic acidosis, electrolyte abnormalities, and associated injuries such as spinal cord damage. Spinal cord injuries are more common in adolescents and young adults injured when diving or falling headfirst into water. The outcome of submersion injuries is determined by age, length of submersion, type of liquid medium, fluid temperature, and associated injuries.[14] Submersion injury in cold, icy waters is associated with better neurologic recovery. Bradycardia, apnea, and vasoconstriction occur during cold water submersion, causing shunting of blood and oxygen to the coronary and cerebral vasculature.

Care for the patient with a submersion injury includes maintaining a patent airway and stabilizing the cervical spine. Assess the patient's ventilatory status. Administer supplemental oxygen to maintain adequate oxygen saturation levels. If oxygen saturation cannot be maintained with supplemental oxygen, then proceed with intubation and mechanical ventilation. If hypothermia occurs, rewarm the patient slowly. Begin fluid resuscitation with an isotonic crystalloid solution, if appropriate. Obtain laboratory studies (CBC, electrolytes, and ABG) and chest radiograph.[1] Other nursing interventions include placement of a gastric tube to decompress the stomach and minimize risk for aspiration and a urinary catheter to monitor output and volume status. Early recognition of associated injuries is important. Additional treatments such as diuretic therapy, intracranial pressure monitoring, and neuromuscular blocking agents may be indicated for some patients. Prophylactic antibiotics and steroids are not recommended.[1]

SUMMARY

Respiratory emergencies can result in rapid clinical deterioration. Accurate assessment skills and knowledge of signs and symptoms associated with respiratory compromise are both vital in the role of the ED nurse. Without rapid intervention, respiratory compromise can lead to respiratory failure and death.

REFERENCES

1. Emergency Nurses Association. *Emergency Nursing Core Curriculum (ENCC)*. 7th ed. St Louis, MO: Elsevier; 2017.
2. Varjavand N, Kaye JM, Wang S, Primiano Jr FP. The interactive oxyhemoglobin dissociation curve. http://www.ventworld.com/resources/oxydisso/dissoc.html. Published June 1, 2000. Accessed May 11, 2019.
3. Emergency Nurses Association. *Trauma Nursing Core Course Provider Manual (TNCC)*. 8th ed. Des Plaines, IL: Emergency Nurses Association; 2020.
4. Emergency Nurses Association. *Emergency Nursing Pediatric Course Provider Manual. (ENPC)*. 5th ed. Des Plaines, IL: Emergency Nurses Association; 2020.
5. Kinkade S, Long NA. Acute bronchitis. *Am Fam Physician*. 2016;94(7):560–565. https://www.aafp.org/afp/2016/1001/p560.html. Accessed May 11, 2019.
6. National heart, lung, and blood institute. pneumonia. https://www.nhlbi.nih.gov/health-topics/pneumonia. (n.d.) Accessed May 11, 2019.
7. Centers for Disease Control and Prevention. Vaccines and preventable diseases. Pneumococcal vaccination. Centers for Disease Control and Prevention website. https://www.cdc.gov/vaccines/vpd/pneumo/index.html. Updated December 6, 2017. Accessed May 11, 2019.
8. National Heart, Lung, and Blood Institute. *Expert Panel Report 3: Guidelines for the Diagnosis and Management of Asthma*. https://www.nhlbi.nih.gov/sites/default/files/media/docs/asthma_qrg_0_0.pdf. Updated September 2012. Accessed May 11, 2019.
9. Global Initiative for Chronic Obstructive Lung Disease (GOLD). Global strategy for the diagnosis, management and prevention of COPD. In: *Pocket Guide to COPD Diagnosis, Management, and Prevention: A Guide for Health Care Professionals*. 2018. report. https://goldcopd.org/wp-content/uploads/2018/02/WMS-GOLD-2018-Feb-Final-to-print-v2.pdf. Published 2018. Accessed May 11, 2019.
10. Cheng Y, Tu X, Pan L, et al. Clinical characteristics of chronic bronchitic, emphysematous and ACOS phenotypes in COPD patients with frequent exacerbations. *Int J Chron Obstruct Pulmon Dis*. 2017;12:2069–2074.
11. Lahousse L, Seys LJ, Joos GF, Franco OH, Stricker BH, Brusselle GG. Epidemiology and impact of chronic bronchitis in chronic obstructive pulmonary disease. *Eur Respir J*. 2017;50(2):1602470.
12. Omar HR, Mirsaeidi M, Abraham B, Enten G, Mangar D, Camporesi EM. A portrait of patients who die in-hospital from acute pulmonary embolism. *Am J Emerg Med*. 2018;36(10):1914–1916. https://doi.org/10.1016/j.ajem.2018.02.035.
13. Aggarwal V, Nicolais CD, Lee A, Bashir R. Acute management of pulmonary embolism. American College of Cardiology website. https://www.acc.org/latest-in-cardiology/articles/2017/10/23/12/12/acute-management-of-pulmonary-embolism. Published 10 24, 2017. Accessed May 11, 2019.
14. World Health Organization. Water-related diseases: drowning. https://www.who.int/water_sanitation_health/diseases-risks/diseases/drowning/en/. Accessed May 11, 2019.

23

Cardiovascular Emergencies

Andi Foley, Vicki Sweet

The American Heart Association (AHA) estimates 6.3% of Americans age 20 and older have some form of coronary heart disease (CHD).[1] Many men and women who die suddenly of CHD do so without having had or recognizing any early warning signs. The AHA calculates that an American will die of a myocardial infarction (MI) every 40 seconds.[1] The generally accepted risk factors contributing to the development of CHD include elevated blood cholesterol levels; untreated hypertension; tobacco use; diabetes; obesity; lack of regular physical activity; poor dietary intake, including low intake of daily fruits and vegetables; and overindulgence in alcohol.

Evidence suggests prevention is the key to reducing complications associated with heart disease. In CHD, time really is muscle. The earlier interventions begin, the greater the opportunity for the patient to experience a positive outcome and return to a productive life. Regulatory agencies and third-party payers are focused on ensuring that appropriate, timely care is delivered.

Core measures have been identified by the Centers for Medicare and Medicaid Services to ensure that patients with acute coronary syndrome (ACS) receive appropriate evidence-based standards of care. Health care facilities must meet the standards associated with the core measures or face serious sanctions and loss of financial reimbursement. Although evidence-based practice is the gold standard for care, challenges continue to arise and facilities struggle to change their policies, procedures, and practices to meet the increasing complex requirements. Data associated with core measure compliance are available for review online.

Patients affected by cardiovascular diseases do not always have obvious signs and symptoms before presenting or even during their evaluation in the emergency department (ED). Understanding basic anatomy and physiology, along with disease development and its effect, is imperative in providing emergency care. The focus of this chapter is on cardiovascular emergencies related to disease processes and their progression.

ANATOMY AND PHYSIOLOGY

The heart is a muscular, four-chambered organ with valves separating each chamber. The primary function of these valves is to prevent backflow of blood. Despite being a two-pump system, the heart works in synchrony. Deoxygenated blood from the venous system enters the right atrium through the inferior and superior vena cavae. Blood is then pumped from the right ventricle into the pulmonary vasculature, where it becomes oxygenated in the lungs. After the exchange of carbon dioxide and oxygen occurs, the oxygenated blood moves to the left atrium via the pulmonary veins. The left ventricle then pumps this blood, via the arterial system, to the body. Fig. 23.1 illustrates cardiac anatomy and blood flow through the heart. The left ventricle is stronger than the right and has the ability to pump 4 to 8 L of blood per minute. Oxygenation of the heart muscle is provided by blood from the right and left coronary arteries. The coronary arteries lie on the surface of the heart and are filled during ventricular diastole.[2]

The heart is divided into three distinct layers: epicardium, myocardium, and endocardium. The epicardium, also known as the visceral pericardium, serves as the outer layer of the heart, including the coronary arteries. Next is the myocardium, the thick and muscular portion of the heart. It is composed of concentric muscular fiber rings. The contraction of these concentric rings facilitates blood flow into and out of the ventricles. Finally, the endocardial layer is the innermost portion of both the atria and ventricles and is made of smooth tissue. The endocardial layer also includes the surface for the heart valves. The entire heart is surrounded by a fibrous sac called the pericardium. This sac holds the heart in place and has fluid inside to lubricate the heart and prevent friction during contractions.

One of the most unique characteristics of cardiac tissue is automaticity, which means the ability to initiate electrical activity. Fig. 23.2 shows the heart's electrical conduction system. The sinoatrial (SA) node has the highest rate of automaticity, spontaneously depolarizing between 60 and 100 times per minute. The impulses generated by the SA node are carried to the atrioventricular (AV) node by intraatrial tracts (i.e., Bachmann bundle, Wenckebach and Thorel tracts). Electrical stimulation of heart muscle begins in the atria and causes the mechanical event of atrial contraction. At the AV node, there is a slight delay in impulse transmission, which allows for atrial contraction to be completed before ventricular stimulation begins. From the AV node, the electrical impulse is carried to the ventricles by the bundle of His, which includes the right and left bundle branches. The bundles terminate at

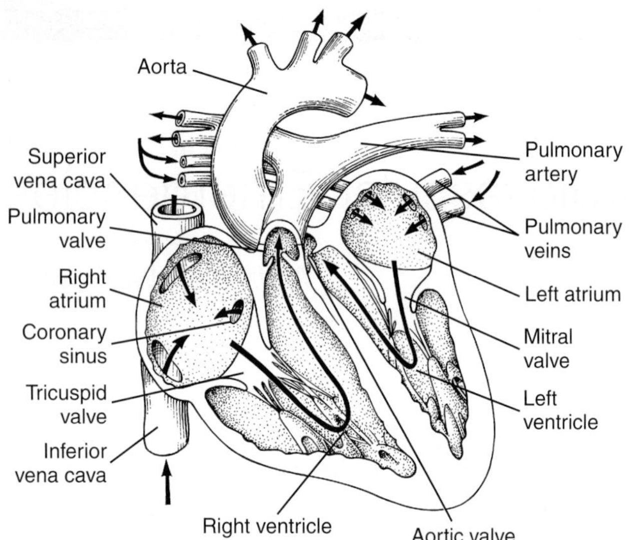

Fig. 23.1 Circulation of Blood Through the Heart. *Arrows* indicate direction of flow. (From Atkinson LJ, Fortunato NM. *Berry and Kohn's Operating Room Technique*. 8th ed. St Louis, MO: Mosby; 1996.)

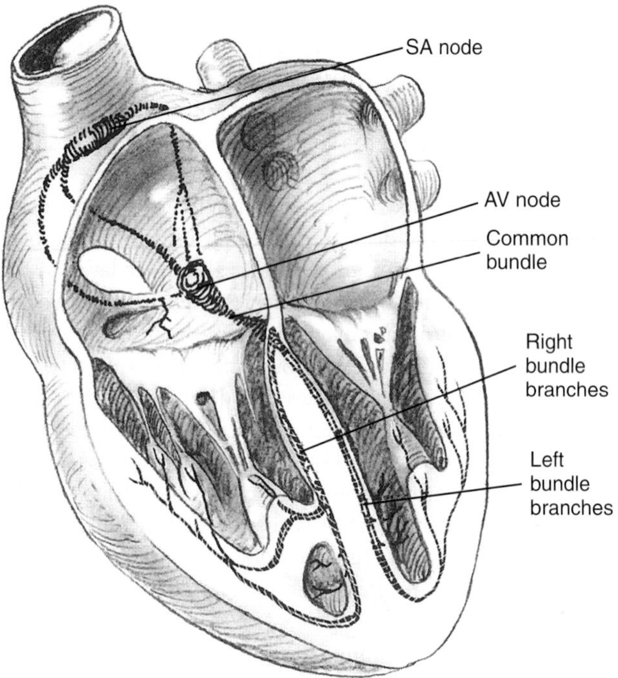

Fig 23.2 Conduction System of the Heart. *AV*, Atrioventricular; *SA*, sinoatrial. (From Davis JH, Drucker WR, et al. *Clinical Surgery*. Vol 1. St Louis, MO: Mosby; 1987.)

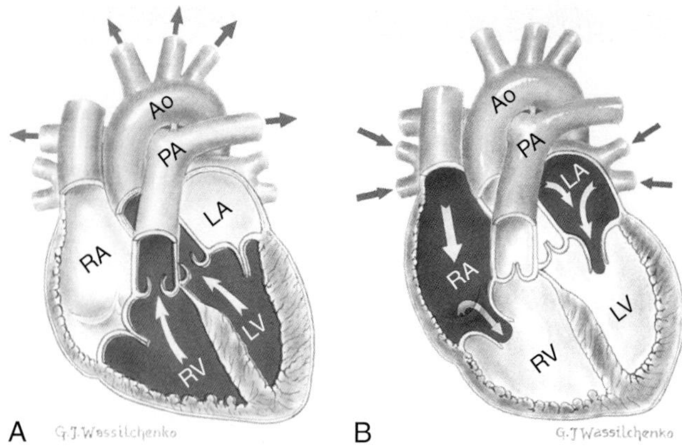

Fig. 23.3 Blood flow during (A) systole and (B) diastole. *Ao*, Aorta; *LA*, left atrium; *LV*, left ventricle; *PA*, pulmonary artery; *RA*, right atrium; *RV*, right ventricle. (From Canobbio MM. *Mosby's Clinical Nursing Series. Cardiovascular Disorders*. Vol 1. St Louis, MO: Mosby; 1990.)

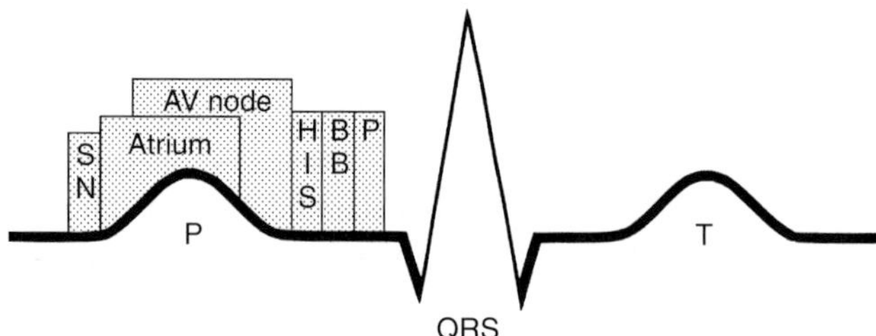

Fig. 23.4 Schematic Drawing of Cardiac Activation Related to the Surface ECG. The timing of activation of the components of the conduction system is superimposed on the surface ECG. *AV*, Atrioventricular; *BB*, bundle branches; *HIS*, common bundle of His; *P*, Purkinje network; *SN*, sinus node. (From Lounsberry P, Frye SJ. *Cardiac Rhythm Disorders: A Nursing Process Approach*. 2nd ed. St Louis, MO: Mosby; 1992.)

the Purkinje fibers, where the impulses are delivered to the ventricular muscle, resulting in ventricular contraction.

The mechanical events of the cardiac cycle are called diastole and systole. Approximately 60% of the cardiac cycle is diastole, the time when the ventricles are filling.[2] During diastole, the aortic and pulmonic valves close while the mitral and tricuspid valves open. Electrically, this corresponds to electrical stimulation and mechanical contraction of the atria. As the atria contract, the pressure in the atria becomes greater than in the ventricles, causing the AV valves to open and allowing blood to flow from an area of greater pressure to an area of lower pressure (Fig. 23.3). The systolic phase of the cardiac cycle corresponds with ventricular contraction and opening of pulmonic and aortic valves. During contraction, AV valves close and chordae tendineae contract to prevent any regurgitation of blood. Fig. 23.4 depicts the relationship between electrical and mechanical components of the cardiac cycle.

The pressures within the cardiovascular system are affected by both preload and afterload, which greatly affect cardiac output. Preload refers to the *volume* of blood entering the right side of the heart. Afterload refers to *pressure* in the arterial system the heart must overcome to pump out its ventricular blood volume.

Cardiac activity is regulated by branches of the autonomic nervous system, and the specific effects of each branch are described in Table 23.1. Receptors in the heart and great vessels respond to signals from the sympathetic nervous system (Table 23.2). Their stimulation affects heart rate, contractility, automaticity, conduction, and vascular smooth muscle. These receptors help prepare the body for the fight-or-flight response to either perceived threats or actual physiologic changes, including blood volume loss.

TABLE 23.1 Parasympathetic and Sympathetic Stimulation of the Heart.

Nerve Activation	Cardiac Effect	Clinical Manifestations
Parasympathetic	Slows SA node discharge Slows AV node conduction and increases refractoriness	Symptomatic bradycardia Transient heart block
Sympathetic	Heart rate increases Enhances AV node function Shortens His-Purkinje and ventricular muscle refractoriness Increased ventricular contraction Increased peripheral vascular resistance	Tachycardia Hypertension Increased cardiac output

AV, Atrioventricular; *SA*, sinoatrial.

TABLE 23.2 Sympathetic Nervous System Receptors.

Sympathetic Receptor	Location	Clinical Response
α	Vascular smooth muscle	Vasoconstriction
β_1	Myocardium	Increased heart rate, contraction, automaticity, and conduction
β_2	Peripheral vasculature and lungs	Vasodilation of peripheral vasculature and bronchodilation
Dopaminergic	Renal, mesenteric, cerebral, and coronary arteries	Vasodilation

SPECIFIC CARDIOVASCULAR EMERGENCIES

Cardiac Arrest

Sudden cardiac arrest occurs when cardiac electrical impulses are disrupted, causing cardiac pump failure.[3] A common cause of sudden cardiac arrest in adults is ventricular tachycardia (VT), which, if left untreated, deteriorates into ventricular fibrillation (VF). These lethal dysrhythmias are usually the end result of an evolving myocardial infarction; however, these dysrhythmias and resulting cardiac arrest may also be associated with aneurysm rupture, cardiomyopathies, rheumatic heart disease, mitral valve prolapse, and cardiac surgery. Sudden cardiac arrest can also be associated with many other conditions or events. Table 23.3 reviews some of the other potential causes of cardiopulmonary arrest and their causes, signs, symptoms, and therapeutic interventions. In addition, the health care team should gather information related to the events of the arrest. Determining the cause of the cardiac arrest event may assist the health care team in preventing a recurrence.

In a cardiac arrest situation, immediate interventions begin with initiation of basic life support.[4] Effective cardiopulmonary resuscitation, focused on effective compressions, is essential for a positive outcome to occur. Advanced life support measures should not be initiated until the basics have been addressed. The steps involved in both basic and advanced life support evolve based on ongoing research; therefore all health care providers must stay abreast of the changes to provide patients with the best evidence-based care possible.

Basic life support begins with the primary survey and appropriate interventions. After establishing poor responsiveness, initial basic life support concepts of compressions, airway, breathing (C-A-B) are followed. Properly performed chest compressions produce approximately 30% of normal cardiac output, which is enough blood flow through the heart and brain to sustain tissue viability for a short time. Chest compressions are best accomplished with the pulseless patient supine on a firm surface. This positioning allows for even compression of the chest cavity. Compressions should be smooth, even, and strong enough to generate a central pulse—either carotid or femoral. Defibrillation is another critical step in the initial resuscitation effort. Evidence has clearly shown the need for early defibrillation in an effort to restore a viable heart rhythm. The use of electricity in resuscitation, both defibrillation and synchronous cardioversion, will be discussed in more detail later in this chapter.

Mechanical cardiopulmonary resuscitation devices have been available for years. Many versions are available; some devices simply provide chest compressions, whereas others are capable of providing both chest compressions and synchronous ventilations for the patient. Recording devices are available for resuscitation activities, including the patient's rhythm, compressions being performed, and any attempts at defibrillation or cardioversion provided. Advantages of using a recording device or a feedback device are to assist in providing consistent chest compressions and reduce or prevent rescuer fatigue during long resuscitation events or extended transport times for rural emergency medical services units. In addition, in the absence of multiple staff to participate in the resuscitation, using a chest compression device may allow the rescuer to begin providing advanced life support measures while the basics are fulfilled using the mechanical device. Use of these devices should be restricted to specially trained and experienced personnel only.

TABLE 23.3 Differential Diagnosis of Cardiopulmonary Arrest.[a]

Causes	Specific Cause	Signs and Symptoms	Therapeutic Interventio	Notes
Metabolic	Hypoglycemia	Loss of consciousness, Physical signs of insulin or oral hypoglycemic agent usage; tachydysrhythmias; seizures; aspiration	Dextrose, 50% IVP or if unable to obtain an IV, give glucagon IM	Consider hypoglycemia a strong possibility in patients who have a history of diabetes
	Hyperkalemia	ECG: Prolonged QT interval; peaked T waves; loss of P waves; wide QRS complexes	IV calcium chloride or calcium gluconate, sodium bicarbonate, insulin, and glucose	Often seen in patients having hemodialysis and renal failure; also seen in patients taking potassium-sparing diuretics and patients with rhabdomyolysis
Drug-induced	Tricyclic antidepressants, amitriptyline (Elavil), amitriptyline and perphenazine (Etrafon, Triavil), imipramine (Tofranil), doxepin (Sinequan), protriptyline (Vivactil)	Tachydysrhythmias Prolonged QT/torsade de pointes	Sodium bicarbonate IV	Causes direct cardiac toxicity; often delayed toxicity in adults
	Opiates	Bradydysrhythmias; heart blocks	Naloxone IV	Street drugs may be mixed with multiple substances
	β-Blockers	Cardiac: Heart blocks; bradydysrhythmias; PVCs	Atropine	PVCs may be caused by slow rate
		Respiratory: Bronchospasm	Aminophylline	
Pulmonary (any disease causing severe hypoxia)	Asthma	Severe bronchospasm causing hypoxia and respiratory acidosis ECG: Tachydysrhythmias (especially ventricular fibrillation)	Endotracheal intubation and ventilatory support	Abuse of sympathomimetic inhalants
	Pulmonary embolus	Pleuritic chest pain; shortness of breath in high-risk patients (postoperative, those taking birth control pills); syncope (recent study shows 60% have syncope as part of initial complaint); tachydysrhythmias	Good ventilatory support; consider fibrinolytic agents	Pathophysiology; acute hypoxia and cor pulmonale leading to tachydysrhythmias
	Tension pneumothorax	Distended neck veins; tracheal deviation; asymmetric chest expansion ECG: Often PEA	Needle thoracostomy; chest tube	Often seen in patients with blunt chest trauma; often occurs during CPR because of chest compressions (especially in patients with COPD)
Neurogenic	Increased intracranial pressure from any cause (e.g., subarachnoid hemorrhage, subdural hematoma)	Central neurogenic breathing; dilated pupil(s); abnormal posturing (decerebrate/decorticate) ECG: Wide range of dysrhythmias, especially heart blocks	Central neurogenic hyperventilation (causes respiratory alkalosis, which results in cerebral vasoconstriction); steroids; diuretic agents; surgery	Damage to brain stem and autonomic centers

Continued

TABLE 23.3 **Differential Diagnosis of Cardiopulmonary Arrest.[a]—cont'd**

Causes	Specific Cause	Signs and Symptoms	Therapeutic Interventio	Notes
Hypovolemic	Anything that causes volume loss, such as gastrointestinal bleeding, severe trauma with organ damage, ruptured ectopic pregnancy, dissecting or leaking aneurysm	Tachycardia; decreasing blood pressure; skin cool, clammy, pale; obvious signs of external blood loss	IV fluids; shock; position; surgery	A major unrecognized cause of cardiopulmonary arrest
Other cardiac causes	Pericardial tamponade	Distended neck veins; decreasing blood pressure; distant heart sounds; widening pulse pressure ECG: PEA; bradydysrhythmias	IV fluids: Atropine; isoproterenol; pericardiocentesis; thoracotomy	Look for this especially in patients with blunt chest trauma or prolonged CPR

COPD, Chronic obstructive pulmonary disease; *CPR,* cardiopulmonary resuscitation; *IM,* intramuscular; *IV,* intravenous; *IVP,* intravenous push; *PEA,* pulseless electrical activity; *PVC,* premature ventricular contraction.

[a]There are many causes of cardiopulmonary arrest other than primary cardiac abnormalities, and therefore the health care provider must be very familiar with potential causes and their associated signs and symptoms. Timely, accurate identification of the cause of the patient's problem via the use of diagnostic testing in conjunction with assessment findings will determine the definitive therapeutic interventions needed. This table lists some of these nonprimary cardiac abnormalities that may result in cardiopulmonary arrest. Also listed in the table are therapeutic interventions for each condition and basic to advanced cardiac life support measures possibly necessary with these patients.

Special note: Receiving accurate, rapid assessment and interventions provide the patient's best chance for having a good outcome.

Indications for an open thoracotomy and cardiac massage in the ED are limited to patients who are in full cardiopulmonary arrest secondary to penetrating chest trauma.[5] Generally, patients who have sustained blunt trauma have very poor outcomes after open thoracotomy during resuscitative efforts. Open thoracotomy and cardiac massage are rarely performed and should be attempted only when the facility has the appropriate resources available to manage the patient if a pulse returns after open thoracotomy is performed.

Family Presence During Resuscitation

Allowing a family member to be present during resuscitation is not only a common occurrence but is also supported by many organizations, including the Emergency Nurses Association and the American Association of Critical-Care Nurses. Providing the option for family presence during resuscitation is discussed in detail in Chapter 12.

Therapeutic Electrical Interventions

The use of electricity in the treatment of patients with heart disease is a common therapeutic intervention. Whether it is pacing, defibrillation, or cardioversion, electricity is frequently a lifesaving intervention. The goal is to restore normal electrical conduction within the heart, which in turn should initiate contractions and restore essential cardiac output. Patients who are in cardiopulmonary arrest require a prompt and accurate assessment to determine their current cardiac rhythm, followed by implementation of the appropriate evidence-based algorithm and emergency care. Health care providers should be aware of basic defibrillator safety concepts to avoid injury to both the patient and staff. Some noteworthy safety points to be aware of before any therapeutic electrical intervention use include the following[4]:

- Remove all medication patches; if left on, they can cause arcing during shock delivery and burn the patient.
- When hands-free adhesive pads/patches are being used, carefully inspect wires regularly for any fraying or cracking.
- Do not place hands-free patches directly over implanted devices.
- Always loudly announce, "I'm clear, everybody clear" before delivering each shock, and physically look to ensure everyone is clear of the patient.

Defibrillation. For practical purposes, defibrillation is a definitive way the rescuer uses electricity in an attempt to convert a patient's lethal rhythm into a viable one. In addition to being able to recognize dysrhythmias, the emergency nurse must be knowledgeable of current evidence-based interventions for each abnormal rhythm. The first step is to be familiar with the equipment used at your facility. Is the defibrillator monophasic or biphasic? Can it pace, defibrillate, and synchronize cardiovert, or is it only an automated external defibrillator (AED)? Before using the defibrillator, it is important to be sure the machine is either plugged in or has a fully charged battery. This maintenance procedure should be performed daily to ensure the defibrillator will be fully functional in the event of an emergency.

Previously, the standard monophasic defibrillators allowed electrical current to flow in only one direction. With the advancement of technology, biphasic defibrillators have evolved, which allow the energy to flow in both directions. With biphasic energy delivery, the amount of energy required to convert a lethal rhythm is significantly reduced. When deciding on the energy needed for defibrillation or synchronized cardioversion, confirm whether the defibrillator is monophasic or biphasic and be aware of the manufacturer's recommendations for energy delivery.

After confirming that the patient's rhythm requires defibrillation, place the adhesive electrode pads on the patient's bare chest. One pad goes to the upper chest just right of the sternum and the other at the apex of the heart on the patient's left lateral chest, under the left breast. An alternative option is for one pad to be placed anteriorly slightly left of the sternum and the other posteriorly on the back. Both options are shown in Fig. 23.5. If paddles are used, they are held firmly in the same locations after being covered with conduction gel or placed on commercially prepared defibrillator pads. If the patient has any implanted devices, pad/paddle placement may need to be slightly altered. Do not place the pad/paddle directly over the implanted device. External devices should be at least 1 inch away.

To deliver the defibrillation, the machine must be turned on and the desired mode selected. Ensure the "defib" mode is engaged. Next, the energy level must be selected/programmed in and the machine charged. When fully charged, the machine will sound an alert. At this time, the rescuer must loudly announce that a shock is going to be delivered ("I'm clear, everybody clear") and physically look to verify all personnel are free from contact with the patient. To deliver the energy, press and hold the appropriate button on the device until the shock is delivered. In the defibrillation mode, the shock will be delivered immediately; rescuers should resume chest compressions immediately after the shock is delivered.

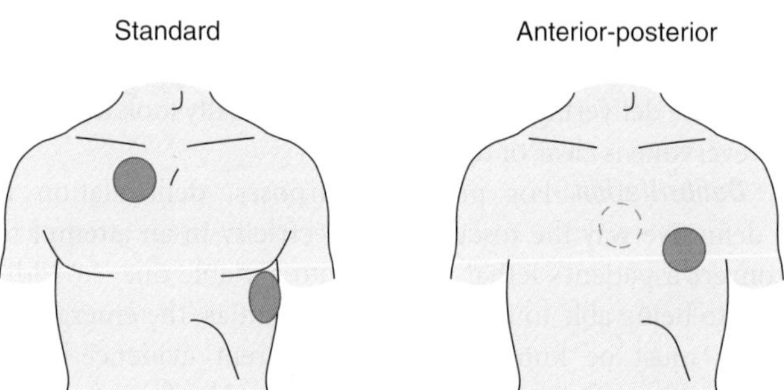

Fig. 23.5 Standard and Anterior-Posterior Electrode Placement for Defibrillation. (From Rosen R, Barkin R; *Emergency Medicine: Concepts and Clinical Practice*. 4th ed. St Louis, MO: Mosby, 1998.)

Successful defibrillation depends on multiple factors. The reason the patient arrested is important. Determining the cause will be instrumental in correcting the issue and preventing reoccurrence. Using the AHA advanced cardiac life support (ACLS) guidelines,[4] health care providers should consider reasons for the initial arrest (see Table 23.3) and perhaps identify the reason for an unsuccessful defibrillation.

Cardioversion. Synchronized cardioversion is used when either the patient has become hemodynamically unstable or pharmacologic interventions have been unsuccessful in managing sustained ventricular tachycardia, supraventricular tachycardia, atrial fibrillation, or atrial flutter. In synchronized cardioversion, energy is timed with the cardiac R wave and avoids shock delivery during the relative refractory period, which could produce ventricular fibrillation.[4] Synchronized cardioversion decreases potential energy delivery during the vulnerable period of repolarization, the T wave of the electrocardiogram (ECG) (Fig. 23.6). Required energy levels for synchronized cardioversion may be higher for irregular tachyarrhythmias.

The procedure for cardioversion is the same as for defibrillation, with four important distinctions:

1. The procedure should be explained to the patient and informed consent obtained whenever possible.
2. The machine must be set to synchronous mode.
3. Sedation should be given for the conscious patient if time allows.
4. When the delivery button is pushed, there will be a slight delay in firing because the machine is sensing the R wave to deliver the energy at the appropriate moment.

As has been previously discussed, it is important to determine the cause of the patient's current condition. Potential treatable "Hs & Ts" causes of cardiac arrest are found in Table 23.4. When possible, a baseline 12-lead ECG should be obtained before and after the attempted cardioversion. Immediately after the procedure, the patient's cardiac rhythm, vital signs, and level of consciousness should be assessed and closely monitored until the patient is hemodynamically stable and returns to an acceptable rhythm. Complications of cardioversion include asystole, junctional rhythms, premature ventricular contractions (PVCs), ventricular tachycardia, ventricular fibrillation, embolization, and return to the original dysrhythmia.

Another method to convert a patient's rhythm is through stimulation of the vagus nerve using a Valsalva maneuver: forceful blowing into a syringe as if to blow the plunger out of the

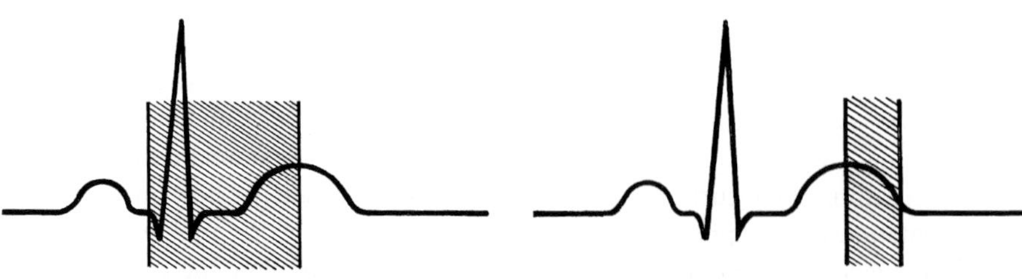

Fig. 23.6 Absolute and Relative Refractory Periods on the ECG.

TABLE 23.4 Potential Causes to Consider for Cardiac Arrest.

Hs	Ts
Hypovolemia (bleeding or dehydration)	Thrombosis (coronary or pulmonary)
Hypoxia	Tension pneumothorax
Hypokalemia/hyperkalemia	Tamponade (cardiac)
Hypothermia	Tablets (overdose or ingestion)
Hydrogen ion (acidosis)	Toxins
Hypoglycemia	Trauma

barrel. Stimulation of the vagus nerve may slow the heart rate and may terminate the dysrhythmia. In the past, ocular pressure and application of ice water to the patient's face have been used; however, these methods are no longer recommended.

The physician may try carotid sinus massage to convert the rhythm. This is accomplished by placing pressure on the carotid bodies, which stimulates the baroreceptors and therefore the parasympathetic branch of the autonomic nervous system. This stimulation decreases blood pressure and heart rate. Only one side should be done at a time. If any of this plaque were dislodged during the procedure, the patient would be at risk for a stroke.

Before, during, and after the attempt, the patient should be closely monitored. In more than 75% of the population, preferential massage of the right carotid body affects the SA node, whereas left carotid body massage affects the AV node. If the SA node is completely shut down, the AV node can provide pacemaker activity. If the left side is massaged first, complete block of the AV node could occur and lead to a slow ventricular rate. Even when properly performed, carotid massage may cause asystole for 15 to 30 seconds, followed by a few idioventricular complexes before a new pacemaker site becomes active. Emergency resuscitation equipment and medications should be readily available whenever carotid massage is performed. Complications of carotid massage include further dysrhythmias (e.g., ventricular tachycardia, ventricular fibrillation, asystole), stroke, cerebral anoxia, and seizures.

Pacemakers. A pacemaker is an electrical device used to restore an adequate heart rate and cardiac output. It can be used either via the transvenous or transcutaneous routes. A transcutaneous pacemaker (TCP) is a temporary intervention for patients experiencing symptomatic, unstable bradycardia and second- or third-degree heart blocks because it is easily applied and managed until the patient can receive definitive treatment. The TCP can be applied by following these steps[4]:

1. Place the pacing electrodes on the patient's bare chest as recommended by the manufacturer.
2. Turn the pacemaker on, and set the demand rate as ordered by the physician (usually between 60 and 70 beats/min).
3. Turn up the milliamperes (mA) current slowly, increasing the dose until capture occurs, with pacer spikes noted on the patient's monitored rhythm.

Keep the pacer's mA at the lowest level possible to maintain electrical capture (pacer spikes) and mechanical capture (patient's pulse) and at a rate to keep the patient clinically stable. Continuous pacing can be uncomfortable; therefore analgesia or anxiolytics should be considered.

Patients with complete heart block may be unable to electrically or mechanically respond to the pacemaker stimulus. Successful pacing depends on the condition of the myocardium. Mechanical capture is evaluated by the presence of a pulse consistent with paced beats. Both types of capture (electrical and mechanical) must be present for pacing to be considered effective. Two major reasons for lack of capture are acidosis and hypoxemia. Evaluate the patient's oxygen saturation and acid-base levels to determine whether further airway or ventilatory interventions are needed. If there is a lack of pacer spikes, begin by checking the TCP electrodes followed by inspecting all the wires and connections. If necessary, replace electrodes to ensure that contact between external pacing electrodes and skin surface is adequate. Skin should be clean and dry before electrode application.

Implantable cardioverter-defibrillator. The implantable cardioverter-defibrillator (ICD) is a small generator used in patients at risk for life-threatening dysrhythmias—especially ventricular dysrhythmias. The ICD device is surgically placed under the skin in the chest wall just below the clavicle or in the abdominal cavity. This minigenerator monitors the patient's rhythm, providing pacing, cardioversion, or defibrillation based on the patient's needs, device capability, and programming.

When a patient with an ICD requires external defibrillation because the implanted device has malfunctioned or failed, it is important to know how to perform this intervention in a safe and effective manner. Defibrillator paddles or hands-free adhesive patches must not be placed directly over the ICD device. If standard paddle/patch placement and defibrillation attempts are unsuccessful, the resuscitation team should try the anterior-posterior placement for defibrillation. Health care professionals who have direct physical contact with the patient may experience a slight harmless tingling sensation when the ICD device fires. If the ICD fires inappropriately, the device can be deactivated by placing a magnet over the ICD generator. If the ICD may be malfunctioning, manufacturers have a variety of methods for device "interrogation," and some hospitals have device interrogation machines within the ED.

Resuscitation Interventions

Fluid resuscitation. The use of intravenous (IV) fluids during resuscitation is determined on an individual patient basis. Some patients may require crystalloid fluid boluses secondary to volume loss, whereas others may be in a fluid overload state requiring strictly limited intake. In addition to determining the patient's current status, it is important to gather as much of the health history as possible because this information will influence the amount, rate, and type of IV fluids administered. After every intervention, it is necessary to reassess and evaluate the patient's response.[6,7] Because of adverse effects on cerebral tissue, dextrose-containing solutions are not recommended during resuscitation; instead, the fluids of choice are normal saline or lactated Ringer's solution.

Pharmacologic therapy. Emergency drug therapy depends on the patient's cardiac rhythm, 12-lead ECG, and hemodynamic status. Emergency nurses should be familiar with emergency medications commonly used in their facility and by their local emergency medical services teams. The first-line drug in management of cardiac arrest, specifically asystole, pulseless electrical activity (PEA), VF, and pulseless VT is epinephrine.[4] It is important to remember that the management of VF and pulseless VT requires immediate defibrillation followed by chest compressions before the administration of medications.[4]

Patients with ventricular dysrhythmias associated with cardiopulmonary arrest may benefit from amiodarone administration. Other antidysrhythmic agents considered for management of patients with VF or pulseless VT include lidocaine or magnesium. After the ventricular dysrhythmia is controlled, an infusion of the converting agent is necessary to maintain therapeutic drug levels. Antidysrhythmics should not be given to patients with third-degree AV block, with an escape rhythm, or with bradycardia and PVCs. Ectopic beats may contribute to the patient's cardiac output; therefore antidysrhythmics could effectively reduce output and cause further decompensation or asystole.

Bradycardic dysrhythmias, *if stable,* are initially managed with atropine, which blocks stimulation of the vagus nerve. Atropine may not be effective for high-degree AV block dysrhythmias. Isoproterenol is a β-adrenergic agonist and may be used to increase cardiac output in bradydysrhythmias. Routine use of isoproterenol is not recommended because of effects on ventricular irritability; however, it is considered a first-line drug for the heart transplant patient with symptomatic bradycardia. Atropine is not used for patients with heart transplants because the vagus nerve is not reattached during the transplant. Bradycardic rhythms affecting hemodynamic stability require cardiac pacing.

Supraventricular rhythms impair effective cardiac output by decreasing cardiac filling time and may decrease the patient's hemodynamic stability.[8] Adenosine is used to treat reentry dysrhythmias. It is an extremely fast-acting drug, with a half-life of less than 10 seconds. For this reason, it must be given rapidly and in a proximal vein, immediately followed by a saline bolus.[4] Side effects include flushing, dyspnea, hypotension, chest pain, transient bradycardia, transient asystole, and ventricular ectopy. These side effects usually terminate spontaneously without further medical or nursing interventions. Other pharmacologic agents such as ibutilide, β-adrenergic blocking drugs (e.g., metoprolol), and calcium channel blocking agents (e.g., verapamil and diltiazem) can be used for controlling the ventricular response rate in patients with supraventricular tachycardia (e.g., atrial fibrillation, atrial flutter, supraventricular tachycardia, atrial tachycardia). Monitor for bradycardia and hypotension when administering these medications. Tachycardic rhythms creating a pulse but affecting hemodynamic stability require synchronized cardioversion.

Other miscellaneous drugs used during cardiac arrest include sodium bicarbonate, calcium, and magnesium sulfate. Sodium bicarbonate is reserved for specific clinical situations including hyperkalemia, preexisting bicarbonate-responsive acidosis, and tricyclic antidepressant overdose. Magnesium is considered useful in the treatment of torsades de pointes, suspected hypomagnesaemia, and refractory ventricular fibrillation. Calcium, an ion essential for myocardial contractions and impulse formation, is recommended for hyperkalemia, hypocalcemia, and calcium channel blocker toxicity.

During cardiopulmonary arrest, hemodynamic status is unstable and requires intervention to stabilize not only the patient's cardiac rhythm but also the cardiovascular system. Refer to Table 23.5 for an overview of cardiovascular drugs to give via the intraosseous route or endotracheal tube when IV access cannot be established.[1,4,9]

Post–Cardiac Arrest Targeted Temperature Management

Recent evidence has demonstrated that patients postarrest may benefit from controlled hypothermia. The AHA has endorsed the use of targeted temperature management in the unresponsive patient after cardiac arrest for 24 hours after resuscitation.[4] This support is based on research results demonstrating improved neurologic status for survivors in whom cooling has been used. If cooling is used, the postarrest patient's body temperature should be closely monitored and cooled to 33°C or 36°C, depending on facility protocol. Regardless of the cooling method used, great care should be taken to prevent unintentional overcooling.[4]

Acute Coronary Syndrome

Acute coronary syndrome (ACS) is a general term used to describe a group of coronary artery diseases and their clinical symptoms. These include unstable angina; ST elevation myocardial infarction (STEMI), also called a Q-wave myocardial infarction; and non-STEMI, also referred to as the non–Q-wave myocardial infarction. Initial presenting symptoms are very similar and require prompt, thorough assessments and diagnostic testing to determine the most appropriate treatment. Mortality from the infarction can be reduced significantly if the patient receives prompt and definitive care in the early phases of the infarction.[10] ACS evolves from inflammation, rupture, or erosion of atheromatous plaque within the coronary arteries. The resulting platelet activation changes the membranes, allowing aggregation of the platelets, resulting in interruption of coronary blood flow.

Pathogenesis of atherosclerosis includes accumulation of lipids on the intimal lining of the arteries, calcification and sclerosis of the medial layer of arteries, and thickening of the walls of the arteries. Generally, atherosclerosis affects the aorta and the coronary, cerebral, femoral, and other large or middle-size arteries. Risk factors for atherosclerosis include smoking, hyperlipidemia, hypertension, diabetes mellitus,

TABLE 23.5 Alternate Routes for Medication Administration in Cardiovascular Emergencies.

Route	Nursing Management
Intraosseous (IO)	
May be used in patients of any age:	Use aseptic technique to insert an IO needle.
• Patients under 3 kg should receive an 18-gauge needle.	Be sure to follow the manufacturer's guidelines when using devices to insert IO (e.g., EZ-IO).
• All other ages/weights receive a 15-gauge needle. Length is dependent on location of insertion.	Confirm placement by aspiration of bone marrow, and freely flowing fluid without evidence of infiltration.
Can be placed in any portion of the tibia excluding the epiphyseal plates (e.g., distal tibia, midanterior distal one-third of the femur, iliac crest, humerus); the sternum can be used as a site in patients age 3 years or older.	Secure firmly with dressing to prevent dislodgement. Monitor for extravasation of IV fluids at, below, or distal to the site; confirm patency before giving any fluids or medications. Flush with saline to maintain patency. Dilute hypertonic-alkaline solutions before administration.
Use for medications, fluids, and blood and blood products.	
Endotracheal (ET)	
When IV access is not available, can administer selected emergency drugs: Epinephrine Atropine Lidocaine Naloxone	Dilute drug in sterile saline or sterile water (i.e., 10 mL for adults and 1–2 mL for children). Administer medications as far down ET tube as possible; consider inserting intracatheter in ET tube and advancing to give medication. Administer drug quickly down ET tube, follow with three to four rapid insufflations of bag-mask device to aerosolize medication in tracheobronchial tree.
Consider dose 2.0–2.5 times recommended IV dose.	
Vasopressin (ET dose same as IV dose)	

IV, Intravenous.

stress, lack of exercise, aging, diet high in fat and cholesterol, gender, and family history.[1] Multiple existing risk factors increase the individual's chance of developing ACS.

Overview of Acute Coronary Syndrome

As discussed earlier, the major cause of acute myocardial infarction (AMI) is thrombosis formation in a narrowed coronary artery from a ruptured or fissured atherosclerotic plaque and platelet activation. Subsequent vessel occlusion and thrombosis cause myocardial hypoxia and necrosis. Myocardial hypoxia may also be caused by coronary artery spasm or a dissecting aortic aneurysm. Complete necrosis occurs over several hours. The area surrounding the zone of necrosis is ischemic. Damage to the myocardium predisposes the patient to pump failure and various dysrhythmias secondary to conduction defects and irritability of myocardial tissue. Location and size of the infarct depend on which coronary artery is affected and where the occlusion occurs. AMI often results from blockage of the left anterior descending coronary artery, which causes involvement of the anterior wall of the myocardium.

Non-STEMI is usually related to intermittent occlusive thrombosis causing distal myocyte necrosis in the region supplied by the related coronary artery. As the clot enlarges around the thrombus, it may embolize and eventually occlude the coronary microvasculature, resulting in small elevations of cardiac enzymes. The underlying pathologic change for unstable angina is partial occlusion by a thrombus of atherosclerotic plaque. Patients with either non-STEMI or unstable angina are at high risk for progression to transmural myocardial infarction.

When the coronary artery or arteries becomes narrowed or occluded, the myocardium becomes hypoxic, often resulting in classic retrosternal chest discomfort or angina pectoris. Pain is frequently described as crushing, burning, sharp, or heavy. Not all patients will present with classic signs and symptoms. Some have vague complaints not readily associated with cardiac disease; therefore it is imperative to perform a rapid assessment and health history. Additional information will be invaluable in performing risk stratification and appropriately treating the patient in a timely manner. Pain, when present, can last several minutes to several weeks and may vary in location. Local hypoxia, lactate buildup, and sensory response of the hypoxic myocardium contribute to the amount of pain experienced. The pain may localize in the substernal area or radiate to the jaw or down the left arm. Associated symptoms include nausea, vomiting, diaphoresis, and hiccups if the phrenic nerve is stimulated.

With AMI, the patient's blood pressure may decrease because of poor pump action, which decreases cardiac output. Sodium and water retention may also occur as a result of decreased cardiac output and increased venous pressures. When AMI occurs, ventricular failure can occur. Severe ventricular failure causes stroke volume to decrease and ventricular diastolic pressure to increase, whereas the sympathetic response decreases blood flow to the periphery. Decreased blood flow to the kidneys slows glomerular filtration rate (GFR). Decreased GFR stimulates renal cells to produce renin, causing angiotensin levels to rise and aldosterone to be secreted. Increased aldosterone and decreased GFR cause sodium and water retention and formation of interstitial edema.[2]

Patient Assessment for Acute Coronary Syndrome

Immediate assessment of patients experiencing symptoms of ACS is crucial because of the increased incidence of ventricular fibrillation during the first hour after onset of symptoms. It is common for patients to delay seeking treatment secondary to denial of a serious condition. Most patients are resting or engaged in only moderate activity when their symptoms begin. Chest pain indicative of AMI is usually severe, lasts longer than 30 minutes, and is not relieved with rest or vasodilators such as nitroglycerin.[4] Ironically, up to 20% of patients with AMI do not feel chest pain.[1] Patients with diabetes mellitus are more prone to neuropathy and may not experience any pain. Among patients older than 85 years, the classic symptom of AMI is shortness of breath.[1] Patients with heart transplants also do not experience chest pain because pain receptors are denervated during their transplant procedure.

Doing risk stratification after obtaining a brief but accurate history of the patient's chest pain is crucial; the PQRST mnemonic is an organized and systematic way to get all the necessary information. In addition, patients suspected of having angina should have a differential diagnosis made between angina pectoris and AMI.[1,5,10] The two types of angina are stable and unstable (Table 23.6). Stable angina, known as typical angina, occurs as a predictable occurrence during or after exercise or straining activities. The two categories of unstable angina are typical unstable angina and Prinzmetal angina. Attacks of typical unstable angina, also called preinfarction angina, are usually prolonged, occur more frequently, and worsen with each episode. Typical unstable angina is associated with a higher incidence of left main and proximal left anterior descending coronary arterial disease. In patients with typical unstable angina, 50% have total or near-total occlusion (70%–100% stenosis) of a coronary artery (Fig. 23.7). Prinzmetal angina, or variant angina, occurs when the patient is at rest and usually occurs at the same time each day.

In addition to assessing the patient's pain, determine whether there are any associated symptoms such as diaphoresis, nausea, vomiting, indigestion, dyspnea, palpitations, or dizziness.[5] Obtaining a pertinent medical history and an accurate list of all medications (prescription, nonprescription, vitamins, and herbal preparations) is very important. Knowing all the medications the patient may be taking can provide valuable information when considering other possible causes for the chest pain (differential diagnosis). For example, drugs such as H_2 blockers, antacids, sucralfate, and nonsteroidal antiinflammatory medications can assist in differentiating cardiac pain from gastrointestinal problems such as hiatal hernia, gastric or peptic ulcers, pancreatitis, esophageal spasms, Mallory-Weiss syndrome, Boerhaave syndrome, and/or musculoskeletal discomfort secondary to trauma, degenerative disk disease, xiphoidalgia, costochondritis, Mondor disease, and postherpetic syndrome. Table 23.7 lists common etiologic factors frequently associated with chest pain.

Assessment findings associated with AMI are usually consistent with a patient who is acutely ill. Because of the hemodynamic effects of AMI, the patient may have a variable heart rate and multiple dysrhythmias.[5] These patients may be hypertensive secondary to low cardiac output and

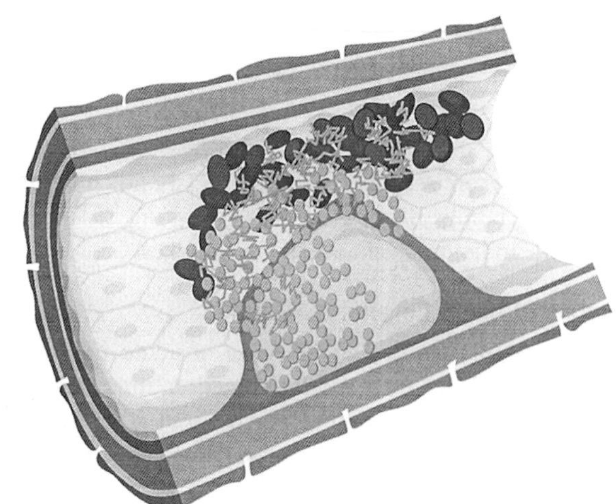

Fig. 23.7 Thrombus Formation. (From Roetting M, Tanabe P. Emergency management of acute coronary-syndromes. *J Emerg Nurs.* 2000;26(6 suppl.):S1–S42.

TABLE 23.6 Differential Diagnosis of Angina.

Characteristic	Stable Angina	Unstable Angina
Location of pain	Substernal; may radiate to jaws, neck, and down arms and back	Substernal; may radiate to jaws, neck, and down arms and back
Duration of pain	1–5 min	5 min; occurring more frequently
Characteristic of pain	Aching, squeezing, choking, heavy burning	Same as stable angina but more intense
Other symptoms	Usually none	Diaphoresis; weakness
Pain worsened by	Exercise; activity; eating; cold weather; reclining	Exercise; activity; eating; cold weather; reclining
Pain relieved by	Rest; nitroglycerin; isosorbide	Nitroglycerin; isosorbide may give only partial relief
ECG findings	Transient ST-segment depression; disappears with pain relief	ST-segment depression; often T-wave inversion; ECG may be normal

ECG, electrocardiogram.

TABLE 23.7 **Etiologic Factors to Be Considered in the Differential Diagnosis of Chest Pain.**[1,5,10]

Etiologic Factors	P *Precipitating/ Palliating*	Q *Quality*	R *Radiating/Region*	S *Severity/ Symptoms*	T *Time/Temporal*
Ischemic/Anginal	Precipitating factors: Effort-related activity, large meals, emotional stress Palliation: Ceases with activity abatement, relief with nitroglycerin, relief with rest	Tightness, burning, deep, constrictive	Retrosternal, area affected the size of the palm of the hand Pain may radiate to left shoulder, left hand (e.g., especially the fourth and fifth fingers), epigastrium, trachea, larynx Never involves region above the level of the eye	Associated symptoms: Profuse diaphoresis, weakness, shortness of breath, nausea, vomiting	Gradual onset of pain builds up to maximum pain intensity; usually anginal pain lasts 1–5 min
Myocardial infarction	Precipitating factors: Effort-related activity, large meals, emotional stress	Severe chest pain	Chest pain; may have radiation of pain to back, jaw, or left arm	Associated symptoms: Palpitations, dyspnea, diaphoresis, nausea, vomiting, dizziness, weakness, sense of impending doom	Usually pain has lasted 30 min or more
Pericarditis	Precipitating factors: May occur after AMI, may also be related to viral, collagen, or vascular disorders	Chest pain may be dull to severe and crushing type of pain	Anterior chest pain with radiation to the neck, arms, or shoulders; pain may be intensified by deep inspiration	Associated symptoms: Fever (i.e., 101°–102°F or 38.3°–38.9°C); pericardial friction rub; ECG: ST-segment elevation in all leads except V_1 and aV_R	May be hours to days
Dissecting aortic aneurysm	Sudden onset	Severe, ripping, tearing type pain	Anterior and posterior chest Often radiates from anterior chest to intrascapular region or to abdomen Pain may move with progression of aortic dissection	Associated symptoms: Dyspnea, tachypnea, CHF (i.e., secondary to aortic regurgitation caused by dissection); also CVA, syncope, paraplegia, and pulse loss associated with dissecting aneurysm	Sudden onset
Esophageal disorders (esophageal reflux, esophageal spasm)	Precipitating factors: Often triggered by exercise, or by food (large meal, spicy foods, acidic foods, cold foods) or ethanol intake	Burning or pressure-like pain May be severe	May radiate to neck, ear, jaw, or lower abdomen	Associated symptoms: Dysphagia, aspiration	Minutes to days
Cocaine induced	Precipitating factors: Cocaine use Palliation: Relieved with nitroglycerin	Sharp, heaviness, pressure of the chest Severe type of pain	Substernal location, with radiation to both arms	Associated symptoms: Tachycardia, palpitations, diaphoresis, nausea, dizziness, syncope, dyspnea	Occurs 1–6 hours after cocaine use

Continued

TABLE 23.7 **Etiologic Factors to Be Considered in the Differential Diagnosis of Chest Pain.[1,5,10]—cont'd**

	P	Q	R	S	T
Etiologic Factors	***Precipitating/ Palliating***	***Quality***	***Radiating/Region***	***Severity/ Symptoms***	***Time/Temporal***
Postoperative coronary artery bypass graft (CABG) due to harvest of internal mammary artery (IMA)	Precipitating factors: Use of IMA for graft of CABG patient	Mild to severe chest pain, burning, prickling, and dull type of sensations	Anterior chest, may radiate over entire chest wall and particularly over the site of the graft, may radiate to neck or axilla	Associated symptoms: Numbness, tenderness on palpation of the sternum, hyperesthesia along the incision line, delayed healing of the sternum	Persistent type of pain Shooting type of pain may last for several seconds and occur several times per day
Mitral valve prolapse	Palliation: Relief in recumbent position, no relief with nitroglycerin	Dull and aching, although may also be sharp	Nonretrosternal chest pain	Associated symptoms: Systolic murmur, unexplained dyspnea, weakness, midsystolic (apical) click	Onset may be sudden or recurrent May last for a few seconds or be persistent for days
5-Fluorouracil (5-FU) therapy	Precipitating factors: After infusion of 5-FU Palliation: relief with nitroglycerin	Mild to severe pain	Central chest pain; radiates to left shoulder and left arm	Associated symptoms: Nausea, vomiting, tachycardia, hypertension	Occurs several hours after IV bolus or infusion of 5-FU No chest pain between treatment
Spontaneous pneumothorax	COPD, chronic asthma	Sharp or stabbing; described as moderate to severe	Usually pain of entire lung region (hemithorax), may radiate to back and neck	Associated symptoms: Decreased or absent breath sounds; pneumothorax per chest radiograph	Continuous pain until treated
Tachydysrhythmias	Precipitating factors: anxiety, digitalis toxicity, exercise, organic heart disease Palliation: terminated by antiarrhythmics, direct current shock, vagal maneuvers	Sharp, stabbing type of chest pain May have palpitations, "skipped beats"	Precordial chest pain	Associated symptoms: Weakness, fatigue, lethargy, palpitations, dizziness, vertigo	Paroxysmal in onset Lasts briefly to hours
Anxiety disorders	May have history of depression or anxiety	Pain may be vague, diffuse; may be further described as disabling	Anterior chest and abdomen	Associated symptoms: Dyspnea, fatigue, anorexia	Variable; often continuous for hours to days
Monosodium glutamate	Occurs with food ingestion high in monosodium glutamate	Burning type of chest pain	Retrosternal chest pain	Associated symptoms: Facial pain, nausea, vomiting	Occurs shortly after meals or up to several hours after meal
Musculoskeletal	Precipitating factors: pain with inspiration or with musculoskeletal movement	Generalized aching, stiffness with point tenderness, swelling	Tenderness of the anterior chest wall	Persistent chest pain without relief with rest	Duration of pain is longer than pain generally associated with angina

AMI, Acute myocardial infarction; *CHF,* congestive heart failure; *COPD,* chronic obstructive pulmonary disease; *CVA,* cerebrovascular accident; *ECG,* electrocardiogram.

sympathetic stimulation or as a result of pump failure. The first heart sound may be decreased because of decreased myocardial contractility, whereas the second heart sound may be increased because of increased pulmonary artery pressure. An S_3 sound (gallop) may be present as the result of ventricular dilation and increased ventricular fluid pressure. The presence of a new systolic murmur indicates ischemic mitral regurgitation or a ventricular septal defect.

A transient pericardial friction rub may occur secondary to the inflammatory response of an evolving necrosis. There may also be an alternating pulse rate caused by left-sided heart failure (HF). Jugular vein distention can also develop as pressures increase from congestion, causing backflow of blood into jugular veins. This can be seen when the patient is sitting at a 45-degree angle. These patients may also have an elevated temperature caused by inflammation and necrosis of the myocardial tissue.

The patient is often diaphoretic and anxious. Diaphoresis is related to the autonomic nervous system response, whereas anxiety may be due to pain, fever, or fear. It is not uncommon for patients to have an intense sense of doom or dread. Cyanosis may be present and is caused by decreased oxyhemoglobin concentration and reduced blood supply to the peripheral vascular system.

Electrocardiogram. Changes in the ECG provide information regarding the location of coronary artery occlusion, myocardial ischemia, and the presence of tissue necrosis. Lead placement of the ECG determines which area of the heart the ECG signal is representing (Figs. 23.8 and 23.9). Changes in the ECG occur when alterations in electrical current flow are seen secondary to myocardial injury or ischemia (Fig. 23.10). When current flows toward a lead, an upward ECG deflection occurs; when the current flows away from a lead, a downward deflection occurs. If the current flows perpendicular to a lead, a biphasic ECG deflection occurs.[8] Figs. 23.11 through 23.14 illustrate ECG changes with myocardial infarction. Serial ECGs are an important tool used in conjunction with patient assessment, history, and other diagnostic measures to confirm the diagnosis of AMI. A single ECG cannot be used exclusively. ECG findings are sensitive only 50% of the time, and ECG changes can occur with other conditions.

Elevation of the segment between the end of the S wave and the beginning of the T wave (ST segment) is indicative of myocardial injury and occurs minutes after occlusion of a coronary

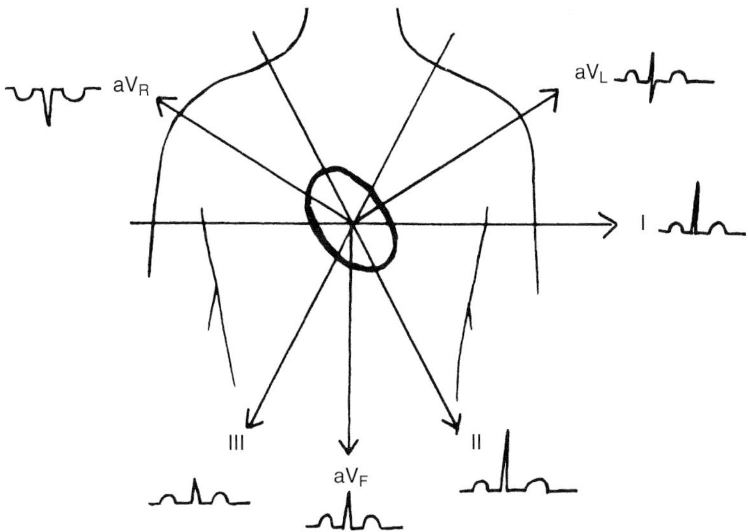

Fig. 23.8 Six limb leads (leads I, II, III, aV_R, aV_L, and aV_F) normally appear as shown.

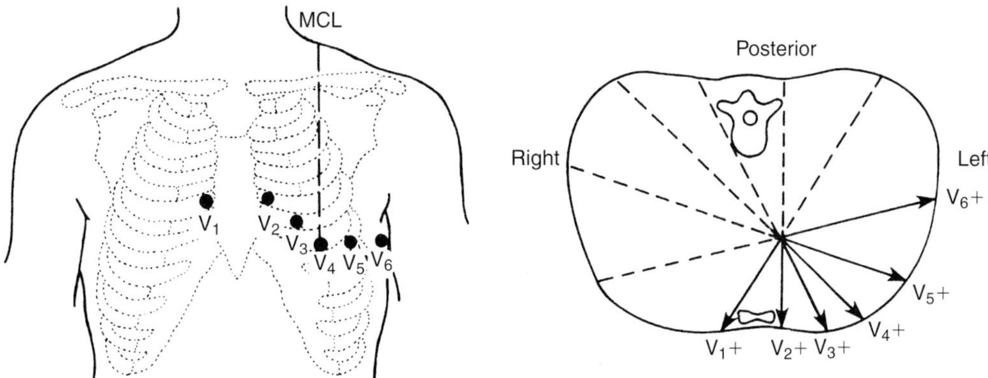

Fig. 23.9 Precordial or Chest (V_1 Through V_6) Leads. *MCL,* Modified chest lead.

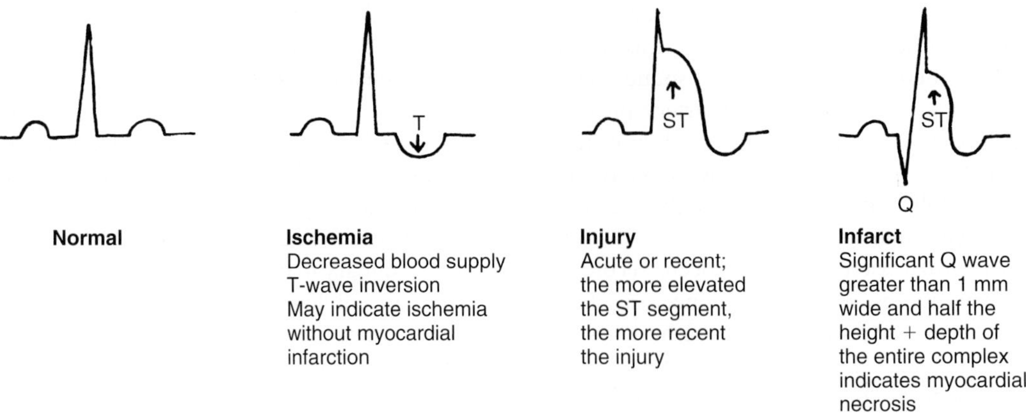

Fig. 23.10 Electrocardiogram Changes.

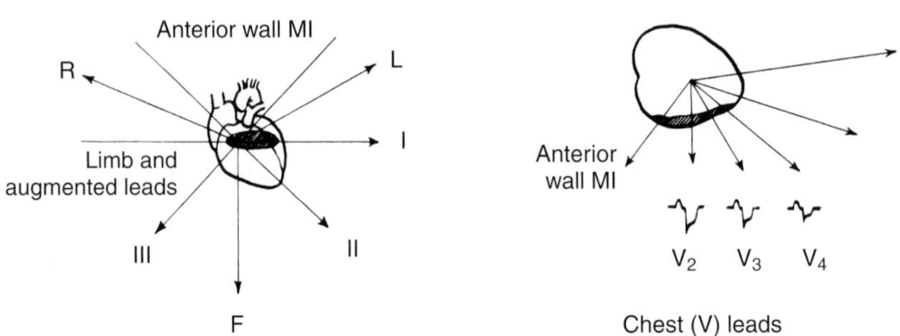

Fig. 23.11 Anterior Myocardial Infarction (V_2, V_3, and V_4).

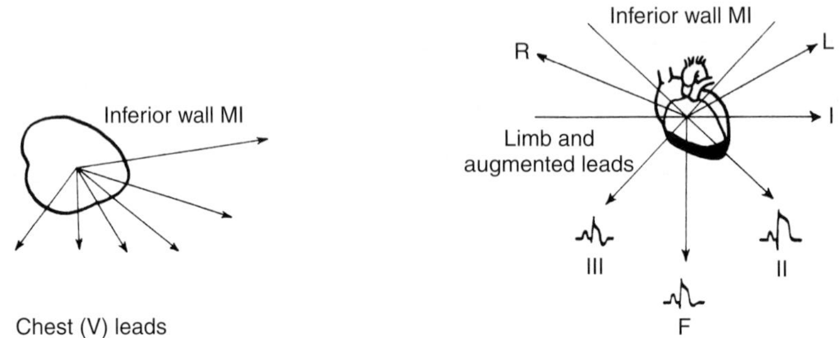

Fig. 23.12 Inferior Myocardial Infarction (II, III, and aV_F).

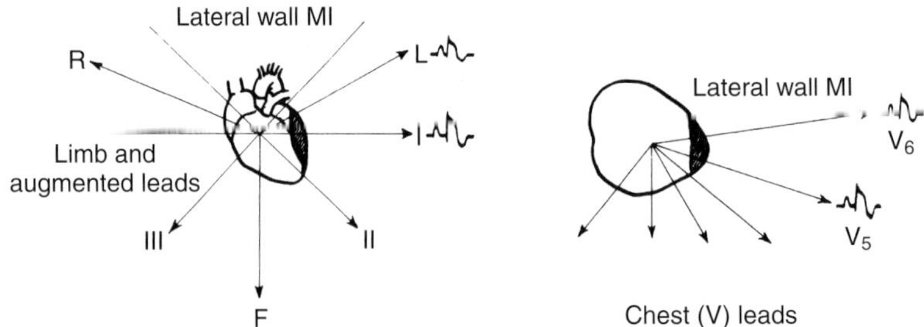

Fig. 23.13 Lateral Myocardial Infarction (I, aV_l, V_5, and V_6).

artery. ECG signs of a myocardial infarction are noted in Table 23.8. A probable new transmural AMI has occurred if there is 1 mm or greater elevation of the ST segment in at least two leads or if there are abnormal Q waves noted in two or more leads. The ST segment can remain elevated for 24 hours after the event. Pathologic Q waves, measuring more than 0.04 second in width and at least 25% or more of overall QRS height, occur within 24 hours and indicate irreversible myocardial cell death. T-wave inversion occurs 6 to 24 hours after an ischemic event and can persist for months to years. Hypoxia should also

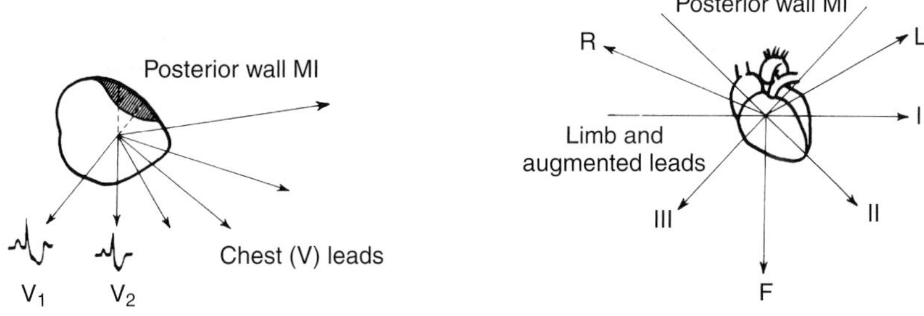

Fig. 23.14 Posterior Myocardial Infarction (V_1 and V_2).

TABLE 23.8 Electrocardiographic Signs of Myocardial Infarction.

ECG Signs	Onset/Appearance	Area of Injury	Indicates
Tall, peaked T waves	Very early (hyperacute) sign	Subendocardium	Ischemia; will disappear if ischemia resolves
T-wave inversion	T wave appears deep and symmetric	Myocardium	Ischemia; will disappear if ischemia resolves
ST-segment elevation	Elevation above the isoelectric line indicates acuteness of injury	Epicardium	Injury: the ST segment returns to the isoelectric line within hours or days
Significant Q waves	Appear within 24 hours of infarct Q waves are (1) at or greater than 0.04 seconds in duration, (2) greater than 25% of the R wave in depth, (3) or both	Myocardium	Infarct; may remain permanently

From Emergency Nurses Association. *Emergency Nursing Core Curriculum*. 7th ed. St Louis, MO: Elsevier; 2017.

BOX 23.1 Criteria for Significant ECG Changes.

Probable New Transmural AMI
≥1 mm ST-segment elevation in ≥ two leads
OR
Abnormal Q waves in ≥ two leads

New Strain or Ischemia
≥1 mm ST-segment depression in ≥ two leads

New ST OR T-Wave Changes of Ischemia or Strain
ST depression <1 mm and T-wave inversions (can represent ischemia or strain)

AMI, Acute myocardial infarction; *ECG*, electrocardiogram.

be considered when T-wave inversion is present. ST-segment depression 1 mm or greater may also be associated with an AMI. Reciprocal changes (ST-segment depression and peaked T wave) may be seen in ECG leads viewing regions opposite the damaged area. Hyperkalemia should be eliminated as a cause of tall, peaked T waves (Box 23.1).

Patients with stable angina can have ST-segment depression, whereas ST-segment elevation can occur with unstable angina and Prinzmetal angina. Pericarditis may cause ST-segment elevation in many leads, hemorrhagic stroke is associated with T-wave inversion, and ventricular aneurysms may be associated with ST elevation.[1,5,8]

Presence of a Q wave has been associated with transmural AMI; however, studies now demonstrate that both Q-wave (STEMI) and non–Q-wave (non-STEMI) infarcts can be transmural or subendocardial. In general, Q-wave infarctions are associated with a larger region of myocardial necrosis, higher enzyme levels, fresh coronary thrombosis, frequent vomiting, congestive HF, conduction defects, dysrhythmias, and less collateral circulation. When ST-segment depression occurs in the inferior (II, III, aV_F), lateral (I, aV_L, V_5, V_6), or anterior (V_1 through V_6) leads and cardiac enzymes are elevated, diagnosis of non-STEMI is supported. ST elevation is most frequently associated with Q-wave infarctions.[1,10,11]

All patients with suspected inferior or lateral AMI should be evaluated for right ventricular infarction. Right ventricular infarct is present in up to 40% of patients with inferior myocardial infarctions resulting from occlusion of the right coronary artery.[1,11] Changes noted on the ECG may include isolated ST-segment elevation in V_1 or ST elevation in V_1 through V_4. A more reliable method of determining right ventricular infarct is the use of right ventricular leads (V_{3R} through V_{6R}). Fig. 23.15a and Box 23.2 illustrate right ventricular lead placement. Use of lead V_{4R} has a high degree of sensitivity for right coronary artery occlusion.[8]

ECG changes in a posterior infarct (ST depression in V_1 to V_4) represent reciprocal changes of the anterior wall, the

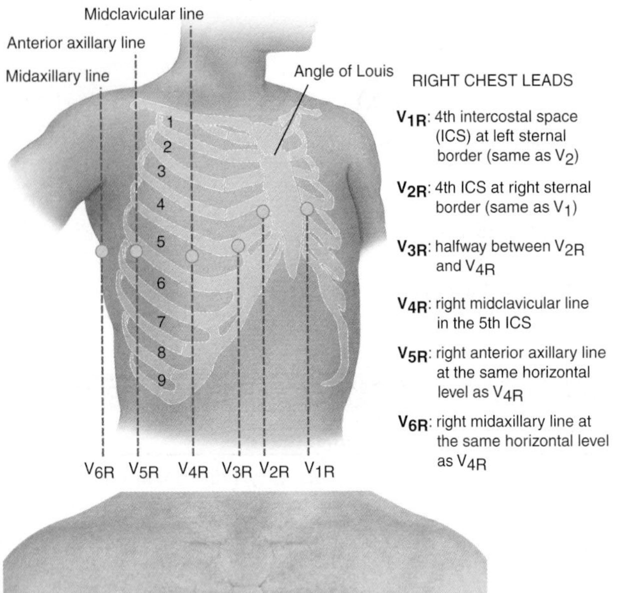

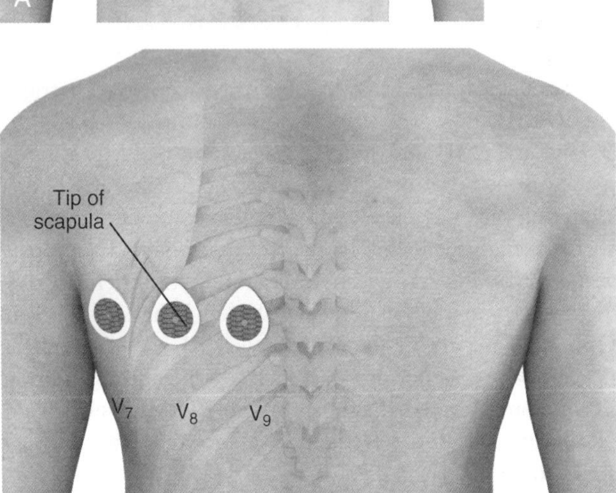

Fig. 23.15 Right ventricular (a) and posterior wall (b) electrocardiogram lead placement.

portion of the heart opposite the posterior portion. Other changes include R waves longer than 0.04 second in V_1 and V_2 and R wave to S wave ratio[8] larger in V_1 and V_2. Further evaluation may include posterior ECG leads (V_7 to V_9; see Fig. 23.15b and Box 23.2).

Continuous ECG monitoring in one or more leads is essential for the patient with AMI. Dual-lead or continuous ST-segment monitoring is available to detect changes in the ECG and identify dysrhythmias. The best leads to use for diagnosing wide-complex QRS rhythms are MCL_1 and MCL_6. This combination of a limb lead and a precordial lead is valuable both in detecting ST-segment changes associated with further blockage of coronary arteries and for dysrhythmia detection. If bedside monitoring permits, the combination of leads V_1, I, and aV_F allows quick evaluation of ECG axis. Fig. 23.16 provides an overview of axis based on leads I and aV_F. Evaluation of axis during wide-complex QRS rhythms or dysrhythmias assists in differentiating supraventricular from ventricular dysrhythmias. Leads III, V_3, and V_5 reflect the left anterior descending artery.[4,8] Leads II, III, and aV_F reflect the right coronary artery. Leads V_1 to V_6 reflect the left anterior descending artery. Leads V_5 and V_6 reflect the left anterior descending or the left circumflex artery. Leads I and aV_L reflect the left circumflex artery and the left anterior descending artery. Multilead ECG monitoring and continuous ST-segment monitoring have become more common, and it is essential that the emergency nurse be able to accurately interpret these readings.

BOX 23.2 Lead Placement for Right Ventricular and Posterior Leads.

Right Ventricular Leads

V_{3R} = Between V_1 and V_{4R}
V_{4R} = Fifth intercostal space right midclavicular line
V_{5R} = Fifth intercostal space right anterior axillary line
V_{6R} = Fifth intercostal space right midaxillary line

Posterior Leads

V_7 = Fifth intercostal space posterior axillary line
V_8 = Fifth intercostal space between V_7 and V_9
V_9 = Fifth intercostal space next to vertebral column

Cardiac biomarkers. In addition to ECG monitoring, cardiac biomarkers are measured as part of the diagnostic workup for ACS. Cardiac-specific troponin is a protein found in the myofibrils of muscle. There are two subforms of cardiac-specific troponin: troponin I and troponin T. Both are very specific for the cardiac muscle because of their role in myocardial muscle contractions. Troponin T is detectable 3 to 12 hours after an AMI, peaks at 12 to 48 hours, and returns to baseline in 10 to 14 days. Troponin I can be measured as early as 3 to 12 hours as well, peaking at 10 to 24 hours after AMI and returning to baseline in 3 to 7 days.[11]

Additional cardiac biomarkers released from necrotic myocardium include CK and CK-MB. These once were the gold standard for a definitive diagnosis of AMI; however, CK-MB can take 4 to 12 hours to elevate. Because of the cardiac-specific nature of available troponin I and T testing, CK-MB, along with myoglobin testing, is no longer recommended for AMI or NSTEMI diagnosis.[11] Emergency nurses should be familiar with the applicable reference ranges for cardiac biomarkers measured in their facility.

Further evaluation of the patient with ACS includes a chest radiograph to rule out other causes of chest pain such as pneumonia, pneumothorax, trauma, and malignancy. A chest radiograph is also valuable in determining the presence of cardiomegaly and pulmonary congestion.[5] In some situations, an echocardiogram may be used to evaluate myocardial wall motion, valve abnormalities, and septal wall

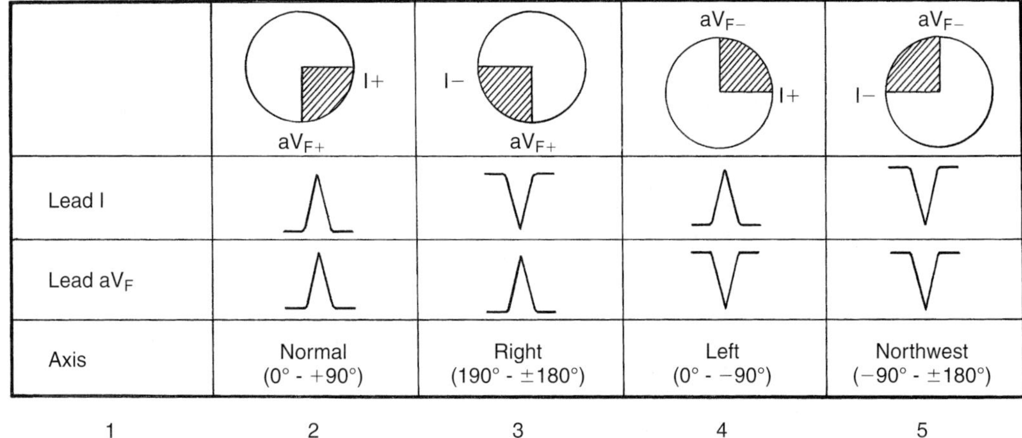

Fig. 23.16 Determination of QRS axis. *(1)* Note predominant QRS polarity in leads I and aVF. *(2)* If QRS during tachycardia is primarily positive in I and aVF, axis falls within normal quadrant from 0 degrees to 90 degrees. *(3)* If complex is primarily negative in I and positive in aVF, right axis deviation is present. *(4)* If complex is predominantly positive in I and negative in aVF, left axis deviation is present. *(5)* If QRS is primarily negative in both I and aVF, markedly abnormal "northwest" axis is present that is diagnostic of ventricular tachycardia. (Modified from Drew BJ: Bedside electrocardiographic monitoring. *Heart Lung.* 20:610, 1991.)

defect. Although not diagnostic of AMI, an echocardiogram is useful in determining the extent of damage to the myocardium. Extensive myocardial damage puts the patient at risk for complications such as HF and cardiogenic shock. Coronary computed tomography angiography may be more efficient and less costly than stress test imaging in evaluating patients with symptoms of ACS. The goal of this diagnostic procedure is to rule out acute coronary artery atherosclerosis in patients who have normal ECGs and negative biomarkers.

Patient Management

The approach to the patient suspected of having an AMI should be one of professional efficiency. Obtaining the patient's history while simultaneously assessing the patient's current status and beginning basic interventions and diagnostic procedures is imperative if definitive care is to be initiated in a timely manner; remember, time is muscle.

Ongoing assessments include frequent blood pressure measurements, continuous ECG, and pulse oximetry monitoring. In addition, assessment and reassessments of pain and its intensity, location, and radiation are important components of the patient's care. After every intervention, it is important to assess the patient's response to determine whether the desired outcome has been achieved.

Patients with respiratory difficulties or an oxygen saturation under 90% should receive supplemental oxygen.[11] If oxygenation cannot be maintained or the patient is acidotic, intubation and mechanical ventilation are indicated.

After the initial evaluation, aspirin should be given orally (to be chewed) unless contraindicated (e.g., allergy, active gastrointestinal bleeding). If the patient is unable to tolerate oral aspirin, one rectal aspirin suppository may be administered. The recommended oral dose of aspirin ranges from 160 to 325 mg of nonenteric-coated tablets. If the patient is "allergic" to aspirin, other oral antiplatelet agents such as ticagrelor, clopidogrel, or prasugrel can be considered.[1,11,12] Further treatment options for anticoagulation to be considered are IV administration of standard heparin or low-molecular-weight heparin, such as enoxaparin.

Nitroglycerin is highly recommended medication for the treatment of chest pain related to angina pectoris and AMI in patients without contraindications. Nitroglycerin can be administered sublingually in 0.3- or 0.4-mg tablets or in a metered-dose spray.[1,11,12] One tablet or spray is administered every 5 minutes, up to three doses. Nitroglycerin dilates coronary arteries, reduces afterload by dilating peripheral venous circulation, and reduces preload by decreasing venous return to the heart. Nitroglycerin is not usually given unless systolic blood pressure (SBP) is at least 100 mm Hg because of potential decreased blood pressure. If sublingual nitroglycerin is not effective, IV nitroglycerin can be used.

Another medication for the treatment of chest pain is morphine sulfate. Opiates, such as morphine or fentanyl, may reduce pain when nitrates have been ineffective. As an opioid analgesic, morphine relieves both chest pain and anxiety, thereby decreasing myocardial oxygen consumption.[1,11,12] Monitor respiratory status and hemodynamic response carefully after each morphine administration.

Percutaneous coronary intervention. Percutaneous coronary intervention (PCI) is a general term used to describe a host of invasive procedures performed in the cardiac catheterization laboratory to reestablish blood flow in the occluded coronary artery or arteries in the patient experiencing an AMI. Evidence has demonstrated that the use of PCI has improved outcomes for patients over the previous standard of fibrinolytic therapy.[1,11,12] Current standard time from arrival in the ED to intervention is 90 minutes for patients with diagnosed STEMI.

The emergency nurse should be knowledgeable about the PCI procedure and the placement of stents. Patients may return to the ED after stent placement with symptoms of ACS from stent occlusion if they do not comply with the pharmacologic regimen to maintain stent patency. Most patients will receive an IV glycoprotein IIb/IIIa inhibitor before the procedure and for 24 hours after the procedure. This therapy will be followed by a course of oral antiplatelet agents.

Fibrinolytic therapy. The frequency of fibrinolytic therapy for the patient with AMI is decreasing because evidence is now supporting improved patient outcomes with the use of early PCI. The goal of fibrinolytic therapy is to lyse coronary thrombi, restore blood flow to a hypoperfused myocardium, and abort or prevent complete evolution of the infarction process. Treatment with fibrinolytics is recommended to be initiated within 12 hours of onset of symptoms or when door-to-device time for PCI may exceed 120 minutes.[12]

Fibrinolytic therapy targets elements of the clotting process to cause fibrinolysis, the process of clot degradation. Lysis of the clot begins with activation of plasminogen, which converts to plasmin. Plasmin degrades or breaks down fibrin in the clot, circulating fibrinogen, factor V, and factor VIII. Fibrinolytic agents are an exogenous source of plasminogen.

Fibrinolytic agents greatly increase the risk for bleeding complications; therefore it is crucial that a thorough assessment and accurate health history be obtained before administration. Absolute contraindications for fibrinolytic therapy include any history of previous cerebrovascular accident or intracerebral hemorrhage within the past year. Complications occurring in the patient receiving fibrinolytic therapy include reperfusion dysrhythmias, bleeding from puncture sites, reocclusion/reinfarction, and hemorrhagic stroke. Patients can be considered for rescue PCI or emergency coronary bypass surgery if they have not improved after the administration of fibrinolytic therapy.[12]

During and after infusion, it is important to monitor the patient closely for hypotension, decreased hemoglobin and hematocrit, and tachycardia. Monitor for respiratory distress, rash, or urticaria. Minimize tissue trauma by keeping the patient on bed rest, limiting arterial and venous punctures, and limiting use of noninvasive blood pressure cuffs. Reperfusion cannot be absolutely determined without benefit of cardiac angiography; however, markers of reperfusion assessed by the emergency nurse include resolution of chest pain, normalizing of ST changes, and occurrence of reperfusion dysrhythmias such as accelerated idioventricular rhythms.

Additional pharmacologic therapy. A heparin infusion is recommended in conjunction with fibrinolytic therapy to prevent formation of a new clot and reocclusion of the coronary vessel. The recommended bolus is administered at the same time as initiating fibrinolytic therapy. Heparin is also indicated for use in patients with non–ST-elevation ACS. Options for heparin include IV heparin, subcutaneous unfractionated heparin, or low-molecular-weight heparin (e.g., enoxaparin).[10–12]

Angiotensin-converting enzyme (ACE) inhibitor agents for patients with AMI (e.g., enalapril, captopril, lisinopril) should be started within 24 hours of AMI. Use of ACE inhibitors has been associated with reduced mortality. Known contraindications to ACE inhibitor therapy include allergies, history of renal failure, or bilateral renal artery stenosis.[11–13]

β-Blockers are recommended within 24 hours of an AMI because they help decrease mortality and morbidity by decreasing myocardial oxygen demands and reducing the possibility of ventricular fibrillation. Use of β-blockers is contraindicated in patients who are bradycardic or hypotensive with an SBP less than 100 mm Hg. In addition, patients with chronic obstructive pulmonary disease and those who have symptoms of heart blocks or HF should not be given β-blockers.[12] Once it is decided to administer β-blockers, the emergency nurse must monitor the patient closely for side effects, including hypotension, bradycardia, and heart blocks.

Glycoprotein IIb/IIIa inhibitors are another potential option to manage non–ST-elevation ACS. Platelet adhesion, activation, and aggregation play major roles in development of thrombus, which can potentiate evolution of this ACS into an AMI. Glycoprotein IIb/IIIa inhibitors antagonize or inhibit the receptor sites, which inhibits platelet aggregation. IIb/IIIa medications reduce the risk for development of thrombus independent of aspirin and heparin therapies.

Dysrhythmias

Blood flow deprivation to the myocardium as a result of CHD can affect the heart's electrical conduction system, causing various dysrhythmias. Table 23.9 summarizes dysrhythmias and categories of antidysrhythmics according to the modified Vaughan-Williams classification schema. By understanding drug classifications, the emergency nurse can anticipate expected actions of the drug and nursing implications for drug administration and patient assessment.[8,9]

Bradycardia

Bradycardia is defined as a heart rate less than 60 beats/min and frequently occurs in patients with AMI, particularly those with inferior wall infarctions. Bradycardic dysrhythmias include AV blocks. Four different types of blocks occur, depending on the area and degree of damage to the conduction system. These AV blocks are referred to as first-degree; second-degree Mobitz type I (Wenckebach); second-degree Mobitz type II; and third-degree, or complete heart block. Blocks in conduction may be caused by myocardial infarction, infection, degenerative changes in the conduction system, rheumatic heart disease, or medications such as β-blockers, calcium channel blockers, and cardiac glycosides. Management of symptomatic bradycardia and heart blocks includes drugs such as atropine and epinephrine. An external, transcutaneous pacemaker or internal transvenous pacemaker may also be used. Second-degree Mobitz type I heart block is associated with a conduction defect through the AV node and is usually benign and transient. This rhythm is commonly associated with inferior infarctions because the right coronary artery supplies the inferior area of the heart and AV node. Second-degree Mobitz type II AV block occurs when conduction through the bundle branches is impaired, usually secondary to blockage of the left coronary artery, which supplies the anterior wall and bundle branches.[2,8] This form of second-degree block is more likely than the other form to progress to third-degree block.

Other Dysrhythmias

Long QT syndrome is a disorder affecting the mechanisms of ion channels within the heart and causing slowed ventricular repolarization. With the alteration of ion movement, polymorphic ventricular tachycardia, also known as torsades de

TABLE 23.9 Antidysrhythmic Pharmacologic Agents as Classified by Modified Vaughan-Williams Classification Schema.

Class	Pharmacologic Action	Electrophysiologic Effects	Indications	Drug Examples	Comments
I	Sodium channel blockade (stabilizes cell membrane)	Decreases conduction velocity; prolongs PR and QRS intervals	Ventricular dysrhythmias	Moricizine (Ethmozine)	Risk for proarrhythmia potential
IA		Blocks and delays repolarization, thereby lengthening the action potential duration and the effective refractory period	Atrial and ventricular dysrhythmias	Quinidine sulfate (Quinidex) Procainamide HCL (Pronestyl) Disopyramide (Norpace)	Observe for heart block, hypotension, prolonged PR/ QRS/QT intervals
IB		Shortens the action of potential duration	Ventricular dysrhythmias	Lidocaine HCL (Xylocaine) Tocainide HCL (Tonocard) Mexiletine HCL (Mexitil)	Potential toxicity: Dizziness, vertigo, confusion, seizures
IC		Slows conduction of electrical impulses in atria, AV node, and ventricular/ His-Purkinje fibers	Ventricular dysrhythmias	Flecainide acetate (Tambocor) Propafenone (Rythmol)	Risk for proarrhythmia potential
II	β-Adrenergic blockade	Inhibition of the sympathetic stimulation—reduces heart rate, decreases myocardial irritability, and shortens action potential	Supraventricular and ventricular dysrhythmias	Propranolol HCL (Inderal) Esmolol HCL (Brevibloc) Acebutolol (Sectral)	Observe for hypotension, bradycardia, heart block
III	Potassium channel blockade	Delayed repolarization and prolongation of the action potential, thus decreasing myocardial irritability	Ventricular tachycardia and ventricular fibrillation	Amiodarone HCL (Cordarone) Dofetilide (Tikosyn) Ibutilide fumarate (Corvert)	Observe for exacerbation of dysrhythmias, hypotension Pulmonary fibrosis may occur with amiodarone use
IV	Calcium channel blockade	Slows conduction of electrical impulses and decreases rate of impulse initiation	SVT and atrial dysrhythmias	Verapamil (Calan) Diltiazem (Cardizem) Nifedipine (Procardia)	Observe for hypotension, bradycardia, heart block
Unclassified	Potassium channel opener	Slows conduction through AV node and increases refractory period in AV node	SVT	Adenosine (Adenocard)	Has very rapid effect, short half-life

AV, Atrioventricular; *HCL*, hydrochloride; *SVT*, supraventricular tachycardia.

pointes, can occur. This disorder can develop after using any medications that prolong the QT interval, such as particular diuretics, antibiotics, antihistamines, antifungals, antidepressants or heart, cholesterol-lowering, or diabetic medications. This syndrome can also be a congenital abnormality of the heart's electrical conduction system and is now found in at least nine genes. Treatment for long QT syndrome depends on the severity of the patient's symptoms. It can be as simple as lifestyle modifications or medications such as β-blockers or include invasive implanted devices such as ICDs and pacemakers. The main goals are to prevent any severe symptoms or sudden death.

Another commonly occurring dysrhythmia is supraventricular tachycardia, which may be indicative of myocardial ischemia or anterior wall infarct. Often associated with chest pain, tachycardias are dangerous because they increase myocardial oxygen consumption and may extend an infarct. Treatment depends on clinical findings from initial and frequently repeated assessments. For hemodynamically unstable patients, therapy may include pharmacologic agents such as adenosine, verapamil, and procainamide. Vagal maneuvers or synchronized cardioversion may also be used. Evaluation of dysrhythmias requires a systematic approach (Box 23.3).

BOX 23.3 Systematic Evaluation of Cardiac Rhythms.

Rate
Bradycardia: Under 60 beats/min
Normal rate: 60–100 beats/min
Tachycardia: Over 100 beats/min

Rhythm
Is the rhythm regular or irregular?

P Waves
Are P waves present? Does one P wave appear before each QRS? Is P wave deflection normal?

QRS Complex
Normal is 0.06–0.12 second. Are the QRS complexes normal shape and configuration?

P/QRS Relationship
Does QRS complex follow every P wave?

PR Interval
Normal is 0.12–0.2 second. Is the interval prolonged? Shortened?

Heart Failure

HF occurs when the myocardium (one or both ventricles) fails to function adequately as a pump. This inadequacy can also be classified as systolic (impaired pumping) or diastolic (impaired filling of the ventricles), resulting in venous congestion, decreased stroke volume, decreased cardiac output, and increased peripheral systemic pressure.[2] Onset may be gradual or sudden. The primary precipitating event for HF is some type of myocardial damage that activates many compensatory mechanisms, which, over time, are exhausted and result in the occurrence of symptoms. HF can be seen alone or in conjunction with pulmonary edema. HF is a symptom of underlying damage from ACS or a problem such as hypertension, fluid overload, valvular heart disease, dysrhythmias, cardiomyopathy, hyperthyroidism, fever, and adult respiratory distress syndrome. HF may also occur with oxygen toxicity syndrome, pneumothorax, and drugs such as methotrexate, busulfan, and nitrofurantoin.

Symptoms of HF are severe dyspnea, orthopnea, fatigue, weakness, abdominal discomfort (secondary to ascites or hepatic engorgement), dependent edema, distended neck veins, bilateral rales, and a third heart sound (gallop). Assessment and reassessments of the patient should be organized and systematic, beginning with airway, breathing, and circulation, to ensure the patient has a patent airway, breathing is effective, and circulation is adequate. The patient's vital signs must be watched closely and the ECG rhythm monitored for potential dysrhythmias. Monitoring oxygen saturation, auscultating lung and heart sounds, and observing for distended neck veins and peripheral edema are also important components of nursing care for patients with this condition.[5]

Interventions include diagnostic tests such as a serum B-type natriuretic peptide (BNP). This is a cardiac hormone secreted in response to ventricular wall stretch. Measurement of BNP assists the health care team in determining the severity of the patient's HF and treating causes as they are identified. Interventions and diagnostics should be simultaneously coordinated. Initial interventions include having the patient in a high-Fowler's position, applying oxygen, and administering medications as appropriate (e.g., ACE inhibitors to decrease systemic vascular resistance, dobutamine) to increase cardiac output. Left ventricular assistive devices may also be used in these patients as a temporary measure. It is also very important to maintain IV access, with strict control of infused fluids, and accurate documentation of intake and output.

Pericarditis

Pericarditis is inflammation of the pericardial sac and can be caused by AMI, trauma, infection, or neoplasms. Among younger patients, causes of pericarditis include infectious processes such as Coxsackie virus, streptococci, staphylococci, tuberculosis, and *Haemophilus influenzae.* An early pericardial friction rub may be auscultated with pericarditis in conjunction with AMI. Friction rub occurs when the inflamed area over a transmural infarction causes the pericardial surface to lose its lubricating fluid. Pericarditis is most evident 2 to 3 days after an AMI.

Patients with pericarditis experience fever, chills, dyspnea, and severe chest pain increasing during inspiration and increased activity.[5] Tachycardia or other dysrhythmias may also be present. Pericardial friction rub increases in intensity when the patient leans forward. The patient may complain of general malaise, and ST-segment elevation 1 to 3 mm will be seen in all ECG leads except aV_R and V_1. Therapeutic interventions include oxygen via nasal cannula, sedation, analgesia, and bed rest. Antiinflammatory agents and steroids may also be indicated.[5]

Aortic Aneurysm

An aneurysm is a dilated area of the artery (at least 1.5 times its normal size) caused by weakness of the arterial wall. Aneurysms can occur anywhere along the aorta and are generally caused by atherosclerosis and related factors such as infection, smoking, hypertension, trauma, hyperlipidemia, diabetes, syphilis, and heredity. Abdominal aortic aneurysms occur more often than thoracic aneurysms and are seen more often in men than women.[14]

The atherosclerotic process contributes to weakening and eventual destruction of the medial wall of the artery. Over time, the hemodynamic forces of blood flow cause thickening of the wall and replacement of muscle fibers with fibrous tissue and calcium deposits. The aneurysm enlarges over time, and the wall tension of the aneurysm increases. Dilation of the aneurysm allows development of a thrombus, which may be dislodged and cause thromboembolism distally in the patient's circulation; for example, in the lower extremities.

Three types of aneurysms are fusiform, saccular, and dissecting. Fusiform aneurysms are characterized by a segment of artery dilated around the entire circumference of the artery,

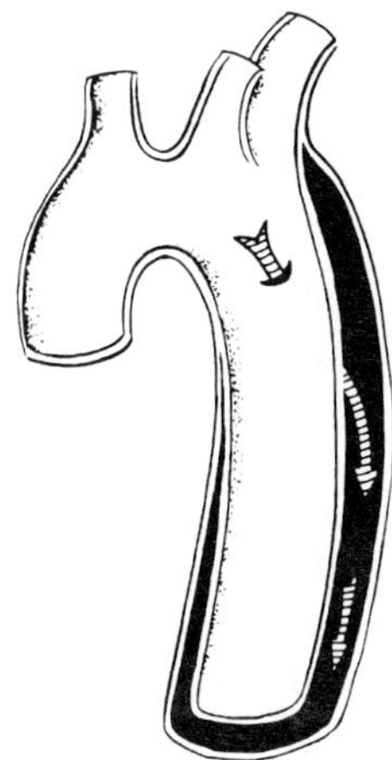

Fig. 23.17 Dissecting Aortic Aneurysm.

whereas a saccular aneurysm dilates only a portion of the artery.[2] A dissecting aneurysm actually results in a tear of the artery's intimal layer, which allows blood to flow between the intimal and medial layers (Fig. 23.17). Dissecting aneurysms are further classified by the extent of the tear and location. Type 1 dissection occurs in the ascending aorta and extends beyond the aortic arch. Type 2 dissection occurs only in the ascending aorta, and a type 3 dissection begins distal to the left subclavian artery.

As the aorta dissects, major vessels (e.g., myocardial, cerebral, mesenteric, and renal) branching off the aorta may be occluded. Rupture of the dissection can cause pericardial tamponade or hemorrhage into the thoracic cavity, resulting in exsanguination, shock, and imminent death.

Patient Assessment

Signs and symptoms depend on the location and size of the aneurysm; it is very uncommon for patients to have early symptoms, and some may be totally asymptomatic until a rupture occurs. An abdominal aortic aneurysm may be discovered during the physical examination when a pulsating mass is felt while palpating the abdomen[5]; this may be difficult to feel in the obese patient. Patients who present to the ED with a leaking or rupturing abdominal aortic aneurysm may have a classic presentation characterized by extreme back pain accompanied by abdominal pain and tenderness with palpation. Back pain may radiate to the legs, groin, or lower back secondary to stretching of the anterior spinal ligament. Patients with a dissecting thoracic aneurysm may complain of excruciating, "ripping," substernal chest pain with radiation to the back, dyspnea, and stridor or cough secondary to pressure on the trachea.[5] Rupture of the aneurysm compromises hemodynamic stability and blood flow distal to the aneurysm. Regardless of aneurysm location, patients may have severe apprehension, tachycardia, unilateral absence of major pulses, bilateral blood pressure differences, hypertension, hemiplegia, or paraplegia. Accurate initial and reassessments of vital signs, including comparing blood pressures and pulses bilaterally, can give the health care provider valuable information regarding the aneurysm status.

Diagnostic tests can include a portable chest radiograph, magnetic resonance imaging, computed tomography scan with contrast of the suspected area (chest or abdomen), sonogram, transesophageal echocardiogram, and angiogram.

Patient Management

All patients should be placed in a high-Fowler's position (if hemodynamically stable), given high-flow oxygen, and have two large-caliber IV catheters initiated. The main goals in treating these patients are control of pain, anxiety, and blood pressure. Close monitoring of blood pressure is critical; if hypertension is present, drugs such as nitroprusside sodium can be used to maintain blood pressure at the desired level. Dissecting aneurysms are often managed with a β-blocker to control heart rate and blood pressure as low as possible (systolic 90–120 mm Hg). If the patient has signs of hypovolemic shock, interventions then focus on maintaining ABCs, fluid resuscitation, and preparing for emergency surgery.

Hypertensive Crisis

Blood pressure ranges are evidence based and have the following categories and ranges[15]:

- Normal: systolic pressure under 120 mm Hg and/or diastolic pressure under 80 mm Hg
- Elevated: systolic pressure of 120 to 129 mm Hg and/or diastolic pressure under 80 mm Hg
- Stage I hypertension: systolic pressure of 130 to 139 mm Hg and/or a diastolic pressure of 80 to 89 mm Hg
- Stage II hypertension: systolic pressure greater than 140 mm Hg and/or diastolic pressure greater than 90 mm Hg

When blood pressure becomes abruptly elevated to extreme levels, the patient has a life-threatening situation. Hypertensive crisis is categorized by the degree of acute-target end-organ damage and the rapidity with which the blood pressure must be lowered. Hypertensive crisis has been further categorized into hypertensive emergencies and hypertensive urgencies. Hypertensive emergencies are clinical situations in which excessively high blood pressure must be lowered quickly, within 1 to 2 hours, to prevent new or worsening organ damage. Hypertensive urgencies may develop over days to weeks and generally demonstrate an elevated diastolic blood pressure (DBP) without signs of end-organ damage; treatment should occur within 24 to 48 hours after identification.

Regardless of the underlying mechanism of hypertension, elevated blood pressure increases systemic or peripheral vascular resistance and cardiac output. These increases perpetuate the cycle by stimulating the release of catecholamines, which increases sympathetic activity and activates the renin-angiotensin system. The net result is continued increases in blood pressure. Hypertensive crisis usually occurs in patients with a history of hypertension. Other conditions causing or precipitating hypertensive crisis include renal parenchymal disease (e.g., acute glomerulonephritis, vasculitis), endocrine problems (e.g., pheochromocytoma, Cushing syndrome), use of sympathomimetic drugs (cocaine, amphetamines, phencyclidine, lysergic acid diethylamide, diet pills), and food-drug interactions (e.g., monoamine oxidase inhibitors and tyramine interaction).[5,15]

Patient Assessment

Patients with hypertensive crisis usually have an SBP greater than 180 mm Hg or a DBP greater than 120 mm Hg.[15] Primary symptoms are consistent with new or evolving end-organ damage. Increase in systemic peripheral vascular resistance and sympathetic stimulation imposed by the significant hypertension causes an increase in myocardial workload and myocardial oxygen consumption. Cardiovascular manifestations include congestive heart failure, chest pain, angina, and AMI. Neurologic changes include headache, nausea, vomiting, dizziness, visual disturbances (e.g., blurred vision, temporary visual loss, decreased visual acuity, photophobia), altered mental states (e.g., agitation, confusion, lethargy, coma), and seizures.[1] Other neurologic symptoms include focal cranial nerve palsy, sensory deficits, motor deficits, aphasia, and hemiparesis. Funduscopic evaluation may reveal papilledema from the effects of hypertension on the retina.

Patient Management

In addition to closely monitoring for any ECG changes and dysrhythmias, frequent and accurate vital sign measurements must be performed. IV access should be established, and if possible an arterial line should be initiated for the most accurate blood pressure readings. If insertion of an arterial line is not possible, a noninvasive blood pressure device can also be used for continuous blood pressure monitoring. Caution must be taken to ensure the right cuff size is used and applied correctly for the readings to be accurate. The goal of management is to lower DBP to parameters appropriate for the patient. Data suggest the SBP should be lowered to between 140 mm Hg to 160 mm Hg, depending on patient comorbidity risks, because lower pressures may compromise cerebral blood flow. IV pharmacologic agents such as nitroprusside sodium, nitroglycerin, clevidipine, fenoldopam mesylate, enalapril and enalaprilat, labetalol hydrochloride, nicardipine hydrochloride, and esmolol hydrochloride are used because they can be titrated for safe, effective reduction of SBP. Assess the patient's response to these agents (i.e., whether presenting symptoms have improved or new symptoms are not present).

SUMMARY

Cardiac disease is a major health threat to American society. Emergency nurses are challenged to stay current not only with research and the evidence-based practice changes it brings, but also with the rapid advancements in technology affecting the diagnostic and interventional tools available to care for this patient population.

REFERENCES

1. Benjamin EJ, Virani SS, Callaway CW, et al. Heart disease and stroke statistics—2018 update: a report from the American Heart Association. *Circulation.* 2018;137(12):e67–e492. https://www.ahajournals.org/doi/10.1161/CIR.0000000000000558. Accessed May 20, 2019.
2. Scanlon VC, Sanders T. *Essentials of Anatomy and Physiology.* Philadelphia, PA: FA Davis; 2014.
3. American Heart Association. Heart Attack or Sudden Cardiac Arrest: how are they Different? American Heart Association Website. https://www.heart.org/en/health-topics/heart-attack/about-heart-attacks/heart-attack-or-sudden-cardiac-arrest-how-are-they-different. Updated July 31, 2015. Accessed May 20, 2019.
4. Neumar RW, Shuster M, Callaway CW, et al. Part 1: executive summary: 2015 American Heart Association guidelines update for cardiopulmonary resuscitation and emergency cardiovascular care. *Circulation.* 2015;132(18 suppl 2):S315–S367.
5. Emergency Nurses Association. *Emergency Nursing Core Curriculum (ENCC).* 7th ed. St Louis, MO: Elsevier; 2017.
6. Emergency Nurses Association. *Trauma Nursing Core Course: Provider Manual (TNCC).* 8th ed. Des Plaines, IL: Emergency Nurses Association; 2020.
7. Emergency Nurses Association. *Emergency Nursing Pediatric Course: Provider Manual (ENPC).* 5th ed. Des Plaines, IL: Emergency Nurses Association; 2020.
8. Dubin D. *Rapid Interpretation of EKG's: An Interactive Course.* Tampa, FL: Cover Publishing Company; 2000.
9. American Heart Association. *Advanced Cardiovascular Life Support: Provider Manual.* American Heart Association; 2015.
10. Jneid H, Addison D, Bhatt DL, et al. 2017 AHA/ACC clinical performance and quality measures for adults with ST-elevation and non-ST-elevation myocardial infarction: a report of the American College of Cardiology/American Heart Association Task Force on performance measures. *J Am Coll Cardiol.* 2017;70(16):2048–2090.
11. Amsterdam EA, Wenger NK, Brindis RG, et al. 2014 AHA/ACC guideline for the management of patients with non–ST-elevation acute coronary syndromes: a report of the American College of Cardiology/American Heart Association Task Force on practice guidelines. *J Am Coll Cardiol.* 2014;64(24):e139–e228.
12. O'Gara PT, Kushner FG, Ascheim DD, et al. 2013 ACCF/AHA guideline for the management of ST-elevation myocardial infarction. *J Am Coll Cardiol.* 2013;61(4):e78–e140.
13. Ibanez B, James S, Agewall S, et al. 2017 ESC Guidelines for the management of acute myocardial infarction in patients presenting with ST-segment elevation: the task force for the management of acute myocardial infarction in patients presenting with ST-segment elevation of the European Society of Cardiology (ESC). *Eur Heart J.* 2017;39(2):119–177.
14. Zucker EJ, Prabhakar AM. Abdominal aortic aneurysm screening: concepts and controversies. *Cardiovasc Diagn Ther.* 2018;8(suppl 1):S108–S117. https://www.ncbi.nlm.nih.gov/pmc/articles/PMC5949596/. Accessed May 20, 2019.
15. Carey RM, Whelton PK. Prevention, detection, evaluation, and management of high blood pressure in adults: synopsis of the 2017 American College of Cardiology/American Heart Association Hypertension Guideline. *Ann Inter Med.* 2018;168(5):351–358. doi:10.7326/M17-3203.

24

Neurologic Emergencies

Lorie Ledford

Patients present to the emergency department (ED) with a diverse array of neurologic symptoms caused by primary neurologic pathologies such as stroke, meningitis, and seizures or by secondary disease processes such as sepsis, toxic encephalopathy, or cardiorespiratory compromise. Neurologic symptoms may be acute, subacute, or chronic. Regardless of cause, a neurologic emergency is one with the potential to cause severe disability or that presents an immediate threat to the patient's life. This chapter will review neuroanatomy and physiology followed by the focused neurologic patient assessment. Some commonly seen neuropathologies will be discussed. Neurologic trauma will be discussed in Chapters 35–37.

ANATOMY AND PHYSIOLOGY

The nervous system is the command center of the body, controlling all body functions as well as thought, intellect, and emotion.[1] It receives sensory input from the body and the environment. Sensory input is then interpreted to control the body's physiologic response via the somatic and autonomic nervous systems. The nervous system is composed of the central nervous system (CNS) and the peripheral nervous system (PNS). The CNS consists of the brain and spinal cord. The PNS contains the spinal nerves and all nerves outside the CNS, including the cranial nerves.

At the cellular level, the nervous system is composed of two types of cells: neurons and glial cells. Neurons are the information-processing cells. Glial cells nourish, provide support, and protect the neurons. Sensory (afferent) fibers transmit information from the body and environment to the CNS. Motor (efferent) fibers transmit excitatory or inhibitory signals from the CNS to the body that result in muscle, glandular activity, or smooth muscle response.

Functionally, the CNS connects to skeletal muscle and the skin via the somatic nervous system, which allow for voluntary movement. The CNS affects smooth muscle, the internal organs, and glands through the autonomic nervous system, which controls involuntary action. The autonomic nervous system is further divided into the sympathetic and the parasympathetic systems. The sympathetic system regulates "fight-or-flight" functions. The parasympathetic system controls "rest-and-relax" responses.

Central Nervous System

More than *300 billion neurons* are at work controlling the human body.[1,2] Neurons communicate at junctions called synapses. *Most synapses are chemical, using neurotransmitters to* relay information from one neuron to the next. Examples of neurotransmitters include acetylcholine, dopamine, serotonin, and histamine. Electrical synapses propagate depolarization from one neuron to the next.

Protective Layers

The delicate tissues of the CNS provide layers of protection from outside insults. The brain is protected by the hair, scalp, cranial bones, meninges, and cerebrospinal fluid (CSF). The cranium is composed of eight fused bones (frontal, two parietal, two temporal, occipital, sphenoid, and ethmoid). Beneath the bones are the three layers of the meninges: dura mater, arachnoid mater, and pia mater. Extensions of the dura mater form supporting structures for the brain, including the tentorium cerebelli, which separates the cerebrum from the brain stem and the cerebellum. Finally, CSF circulates through the ventricular system, around the brain and the spinal cord in the subarachnoid space, creating a cushion. The spinal cord is protected by skin, muscle, 33 vertebrae (7 cervical, 12 thoracic, 5 lumbar, 5 fused sacral, and 4 fused coccygeal), the meninges, and CSF. Twenty-four intervertebral discs strengthen the vertebral joint, allowing for limited movement of the vertebral column and serving as a shock absorber.

Brain

The adult brain weighs approximately 3 pounds, or 2% of total body weight. At rest, the brain receives 750 to 900 mL of blood per minute, approximately 15% to 20% of the cardiac output. Autoregulation mechanisms can maintain a consistent cerebral blood flow with a mean arterial pressure (MAP) ranging from 60 mm Hg to 140 mm Hg.[3] Cerebral blood flow is autoregulated based on carbon dioxide, hydrogen ion, and oxygen concentration. The brain has no stores of oxygen and does not have the capacity for anaerobic metabolism. Just a few seconds without blood flow causes cerebral hypoxia. The brain responds to cerebral hypoxia with cerebral vasodilation, rapidly increasing blood flow. The brain is capable of storing about 2 minutes of glucose. The brain does not require insulin to move glucose into the cell and is thus capable of glucose metabolism despite insulin dysfunction, but it is sensitive to hypoglycemia.

Structurally, the brain consists of the cerebrum, the cerebellum, and the brain stem. Each of these components has a unique function, working synergistically to control all body functions. The cerebrum is divided into the left and right cerebral hemispheres. Each hemisphere is further divided into four lobes: frontal, parietal, temporal, and occipital. The cerebral cortex is responsible for sensory, motor, and intellectual functions. The cerebellum is responsible for integrating spatial orientation and equilibrium to maintain balance and coordination. The brain stem, consisting of the midbrain, pons, and medulla oblongata, relays messages between the brain and the spinal cord. Control of many involuntary, vital body functions comes from the brain stem, such as heart rate, blood pressure, respirations, body temperature, and wakefulness. Within the brain is a system of ventricles: one large lateral ventricle in each cerebral hemisphere, the third ventricle above the midbrain, and the fourth ventricle between the brain stem and the cerebellum. CSF is produced in and flows through the ventricles. Blockage of CSF flow through the ventricular system results in a noncommunicating hydrocephalus. Overproduction or altered reabsorption of CSF creates communicating hydrocephalus.

Cranial Nerves

There are 12 pairs of cranial nerves (CN). CN I and II are attached to the cerebrum. CN III through XII are attached to the brain stem. The names of the nerves (Table 24.1) describe their distribution (i.e., facial) or their function (i.e., optic). Cranial nerves may be purely motor, purely sensory, or mixed.

TABLE 24.1 Cranial Nerves and Their Functions.

Number	Name	Function
I	Olfactory	Smell
II	Optic	Vision
III	Oculomotor	Elevate upper lid, pupillary constriction, most extraocular movements
IV	Trochlear	Downward, inward movement of the eye
V	Trigeminal	Chewing, clenching the jaw, lateral jaw movement, corneal reflexes, face sensation
VI	Abducens	Lateral eye deviation
VII	Facial	Facial motor, taste, lacrimation, and salivation
VIII	Acoustic	Equilibrium, hearing
IX	Glossopharyngeal	Swallowing, gag reflex, taste on posterior tongue
X	Vagus	Swallowing, gag reflex, abdominal viscera, phonation
XI	Spinal accessory	Head and shoulder movement
XII	Hypoglossal	Tongue movement

Many cranial nerves have both somatic and autonomic functions. Because of their location along the brain stem, cranial nerve function is particularly useful in monitoring increased intracranial pressure (ICP).

Cerebral Blood Flow

The internal carotid arteries supply anterior cerebral blood flow, and the vertebral arteries supply posterior blood flow. The internal carotids branch into bilateral anterior cerebral arteries (ACA), a single anterior communicating artery (AcoA), and bilateral posterior communicating arteries (PcoA). The vertebral arteries branch into bilateral posterior cerebral arteries (PCA). The ACA, AcoA, PcoA, and PCA anastomose to create the circle of Willis. The communication of vessels facilitates continued blood flow despite narrowing of one of the vessels. However, only about 50% of the population has a completely functional circle of Willis. Other arterial branches from the internal carotids further supply blood flow to the anterior brain, and branches from the vertebral arteries provide flow to the posterior brain.

Venous drainage occurs through venous sinuses located in the dura. Flow continues into the cerebral veins and ultimately empties into the internal jugular vein.

The blood-brain barrier (BBB) is a highly specialized mechanism to protect the brain. Selective permeability controls the passage of substances into the brain. Oxygen and glucose pass through readily while toxins are blocked. While providing a necessary protection for the brain tissue, the BBB can also inhibit the passage of therapeutic substances, such as antibiotics needed for disease treatment. Insults to the brain, such as trauma, hypoxia, radiation, and infection, can alter the BBB, exposing delicate cells to substances that are toxic to brain tissue.

Cerebral Perfusion

The average adult skull is capable of containing approximately 1500 mL of total volume. Normally this is distributed as 80% brain tissue, 10% blood, and 10% CSF. The body will compensate brief increases in ICP by reducing the volume of CSF. However, continued increases in ICP will result in the shunting of blood, which reduces oxygen and glucose delivery. Normal ICP is 0 to 15 mm Hg. Sustained ICP elevations above 20 mm Hg lead to the destruction of brain tissue. Monitoring the cerebral perfusion pressure (CPP) guides the treatment of increased ICP. CPP is defined as the MAP – ICP. CPP needs to be maintained in the 50- to 60-mm Hg range for adequate cerebral perfusion. Vasopressors may be used to increase the MAP. Osmotic diuresis or external ventricular drainage of CSF are used to lower the ICP. Individually or combined, these therapies are used to maintain the CPP. If autoregulation and therapeutic treatment fail to decrease the ICP, cerebral herniation can occur, causing brain death (Fig. 24.1).

Cerebrospinal Fluid

CSF is produced by the choroid plexus, which is located in the lateral ventricles. Approximately 500 mL of CSF is produced

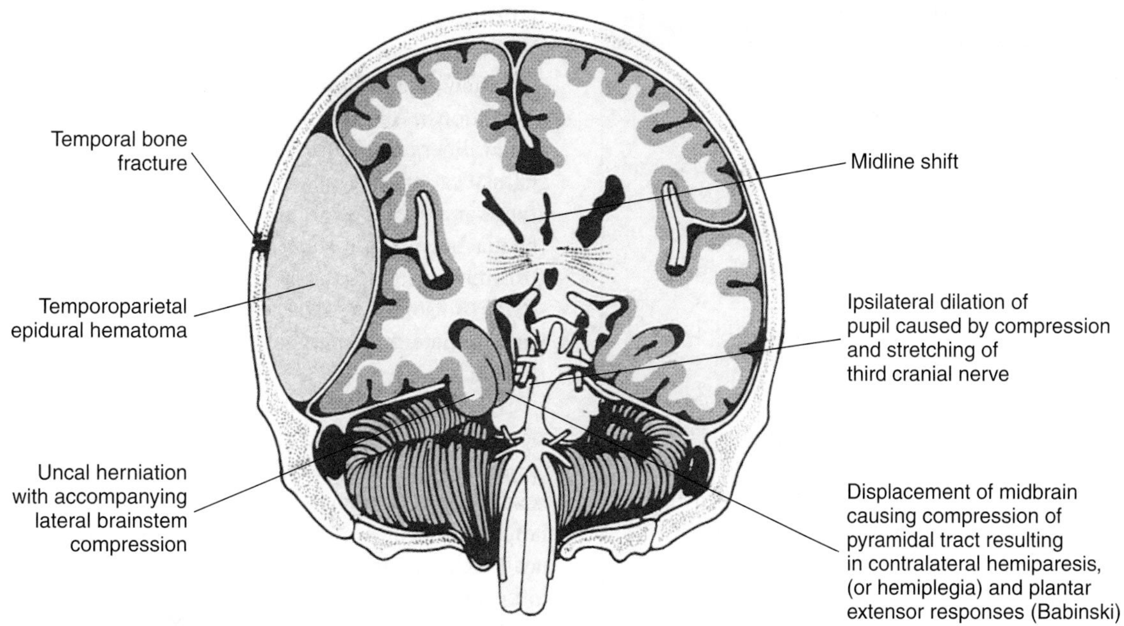

Fig. 24.1 Cross-section showing herniation of lower portion of temporal lobe (uncus) through tentorium caused by temporoparietal epidural hematoma. Herniation may occur also in the cerebellum. Note mass effect and midline shift. (From Meeker MH, Rothrock JC. *Alexander's Care of the Patient in Surgery*. 10th ed. St Louis, MO: Mosby; 1995.)

TABLE 24.2 Normal Cerebrospinal Fluid.

Quality	Value/Description
Appearance	Clear, colorless, odorless
Cell count	WBC count 5/mm^3
	RBC count 0/mm^3
Pressure	80–180 mm H_2O
Glucose	60–80 mg/100 mL (two-thirds serum glucose value)
Protein	15–45 mg/100 mL (lumbar)
pH	7.35–7.40
Sodium	140–142 mEq/L
Chloride	120–130 mEq/L
Volume	125–150 mL

RBC, red blood cell; *WBC*, White blood cell.

daily, with 135 to 150 mL of circulating volume at any one time. CSF is reabsorbed by the arachnoid villi within the subarachnoid space. Blood or pus in the arachnoid space can hamper reabsorption by the arachnoid villi, causing hydrocephalus. Normal supine CSF pressure is 136 mm of water (10 mm Hg). Elevated CSF pressure creates increased ICP. Low CSF pressure causes a spinal headache. Table 24.2 summarizes normal CSF characteristics.

Spinal Cord

The spinal cord begins at the medulla and extends to L1 or L2. The dura sack containing CSF extends to S2. Extending from the base of the spinal cord is a bundle of long nerve fibers named the cauda equine. The spinal cord is situated in the spinal canal of the vertebral bodies. It transmits sensory and motor signals back and forth from the brain via various tracts. Exiting through the intervertebral foramina are 31 pairs of spinal nerves. The sensory components of spinal nerves are distributed in predictable dermatomes across the body. Spinal reflexes, such as the patellar reflex, function in an arc independent of any brain activity. Therefore spinal reflexes are not a good indicator of brain function.

PATIENT ASSESSMENT

A good baseline neurologic assessment is important for patients presenting with primary and secondary neurologic conditions. Only with a reliable baseline assessment can the nurse evaluate improvement or deterioration in the patient's neurologic status. The first indication of neurologic dysfunction is an altered level of consciousness (LOC). Patients with confusion, dementia, delirium, or encephalopathy may not be the most reliable source of information. In addition, subtle changes in LOC, such as mild anxiety, may not be apparent to the nurse but are readily recognized by the family. Thus the first step of a neurologic assessment is determining who is the best historian of the current event.

Assessment begins with obtaining a history of the current event, including preceding events, onset, symptoms, history of similar events, and relevant past medical history. Physical assessment begins with the Glasgow Coma Scale (GCS) score. It is the most widely known score used in the neurologic assessment (Box 24.1). However, the GCS has a level of subjectivity and does not identify lateralized signs or consider pupillary function. Other scoring systems such as FOUR Score Coma Scale are being researched but are not globally recognized.

Motor function, pupillary examination, cranial nerve function, and vital signs round out the neurologic examination.

BOX 24.1 Glasgow Coma Scale.

Eye Opening	
Spontaneous	4
To verbal command	3
To pain	2
No response	1
Best Motor Response	
Obeys commands	6
Localizes pain	5
Withdraws from pain	4
Abnormal flexion (decorticate)	3
Abnormal extension (decerebrate)	2
No response	1
Best Verbal Response	
Oriented	5
Confused conversation, able to answer questions	4
Inappropriate speech, discernable words	3
Incomprehensible sounds or speech	2
No response	1
TOTAL	3–15

Motor function assessment is limited to evaluating strength and comparing the two sides. Pupillary examination includes estimating the size of each pupil and its reaction to light. The pupillary examination can be subjective. Use of a pupilometer will provide a more consistent and accurate pupillary examination. Anisocoria, a difference of up to 1 mm between the two pupils, is present in up to 20% of the population.[1] Knowing whether the patient has anisocoria at baseline is critical for a reliable baseline neurologic assessment. Cranial nerve assessment provides information about cerebral and brain stem function. Finally, vital signs are considered in the neurologic examination. Heart rate and rhythm, respiratory rate and rhythm, blood pressure, and temperature are regulated by the brain stem. Changes in vital signs may be a signal of a deteriorating neurologic status.

EMERGENCY NURSE MANAGEMENT OF THE PATIENT WITH NEUROLOGIC CONDITIONS

Regardless of the underlying condition, emergency care of patients with neurologic conditions begins with assuring an intact airway, adequate breathing, and effective circulation (ABCs). As a rule of thumb, a patient with a GCS of 8 or less requires intubation to manage the airway. Intubation should be considered in a vomiting patient with severely altered mentation. Depressed respiratory drive resulting from drugs or toxins or irregular respirations resulting from increased ICP require intubation to mechanically manage ventilation. Hypertension and tachycardia can be seen with elevated ICP. Immediate intervention is necessary to avoid brain herniation. After stabilization of ABCs, patient comfort is addressed, including managing pain, nausea, and other symptoms. Diagnostic testing may rule out other conditions. Definitive management of patients with neurologic emergencies is dependent on the specific condition.

Headache

Headache is a common complaint seen in the ED; however, very few headaches are associated with emergent medical conditions.[4] A headache is not a disease, but rather a symptom of an illness or injury. The third edition of the International Classification of Headache Disorders classifies more than 250 types and subtypes of headaches.[5] Life-threatening causes of headaches include subarachnoid hemorrhage, venous sinus thrombosis, temporal arteritis, meningitis, and carbon monoxide poisoning. An accurate history and assessment can differentiate an emergent headache from a less emergent headache.

Headache assessment should include onset of symptoms, location of headache, intensity, pain description, duration, preceding events, and associated symptoms.[4] Preceding events, such as exercise or trauma, and associated symptoms, such as dizziness, nausea, vomiting, or visual disturbances, will help guide diagnostic examination. Sudden onset of "the worst headache of my life," which was sudden at onset and maximal at onset, is a red flag signaling a possible subarachnoid hemorrhage (SAH). A focused past medical history should seek injuries or diseases to aid in determining an underlying cause of the headache, such as prior history of headache, hypertension, ventriculoperitoneal shunt, seizures, recent infection, or prior cranial surgery.

Headaches may be caused by an extracranial or intracranial condition. Extracranial causes include dental problems, temporomandibular joint (TMJ) issues, visual refraction problems, glaucoma, sinusitis, cervical strain, fever, hypoxia, anemia, hypertensive crisis, allergies, heat-related illnesses, and dehydration.[4] Trigeminal neuralgia, lumbar puncture, concussion, medications, disrupted sleep patterns, and psychosis are other extracranial, nonemergent headache causes. Intracranial causes of headache include migraine headache, tension headache, cluster headache, and temporal arteritis. Trauma is also an intracranial cause of headache (see Chapter 35). The diagnostic evaluation focuses on confirming the cause of the headache, which will guide effective treatment. Laboratory studies may aid in diagnosis, but radiologic studies have limited benefit in diagnosing extracranial causes of headache.

Migraine Headache

More than14% of the US population reports having migraine or severe headaches.[6] These disorders affect adult women twice as often as men. Roughly 1.2 million ED visits per year in the United States are for migraine headaches.[7] There are no diagnostic tests to confirm the diagnosis of migraine. Diagnosis is based on the patient's history and symptoms. Laboratory tests and radiologic studies provide no benefit in the management of migraine in the ED. Treatment goals in the ED are to rule out other causes of the headache and alleviate pain so that the patient can be discharged to outpatient management.

Migraine may be triggered by foods, dieting, emotion, menses, medications, weather changes, sleep disturbances, and bright lights.[8] Patients should be encouraged to keep a headache journal in an attempt to identify triggers.

Historically, migraine headache was thought to be vascular in origin. More recent evidence indicates migraines are the result of impaired nociceptive processing.[7,8] The overactive sensory pathways turn benign stimuli into a headache and other symptoms frequently associated with migraine. Migraine symptoms include moderate to severe pain lasting 4 to 72 hours, usually at a unilateral location and described as pulsating or stabbing, and they may include nausea, vomiting, photophobia, and phonophobia made worse by activity.

Current recommendations for the treatment of acute migraine in the ED are metoclopramide or prochlorperazine and subcutaneous sumatriptan.[7] Diphenhydramine or midazolam may be given to prevent or treat akathisia.[9] Other medications that may provide benefit in migraine are intravenous (IV) acetaminophen, aspirin, chlorpromazine, ketorolac, and valproate.[7]

Opioids continue to be administered in nearly 50% of all ED visits for migraine headache.[7] Studies have shown opioids to be ineffective in treating migraine and associated with higher levels of return ED visits. Dexamethasone, on the other hand, has been shown to potentially reduce the incidence of recurrence of migraine and should be included in treatment. IV fluid administration is not necessary unless the patient has symptoms of dehydration.

Patients with chronic migraine should be managed as outpatients and have preventative treatment.[10] Certain triptans, β-blockers, antiepileptic drugs, and antidepressants have been shown to help decrease the frequency, duration, and severity of migraine headaches. Antihistamines and angiotensin-converting enzyme (ACE) inhibitors are possibly effective, although research continues. Evidence is equivocal for the use of calcium channel blockers and diuretics in migraine prevention. Onabotulinum toxin A is effective to reduce headache in chronic migraine but offers no benefit for episodic migraine.[11] Excessive use of caffeine-containing over-the-counter medications and medications containing butalbital should not be routinely used for headache because these medications may induce medication overuse headaches.[12]

Temporal Arteritis

Temporal arteritis is an immune-mediated inflammation of vessels.[13] The cranial branches of the carotid artery are frequently involved. The condition is more common in women, rarely occurs before 50 years of age, and is found almost exclusively in Caucasians.[14] Symptoms of temporal arteritis include headache, abrupt onset of visual disturbances, fever, elevated erythrocyte sedimentation rate, and elevated C-reactive protein. ED management of the patient with suspected temporal arteritis is emergent administration of corticosteroids to avoid permanent vision loss, pain management, and discharge referral to a rheumatologist for outpatient care. Definitive diagnosis is made by performing a temporal artery biopsy.

Seizures

A seizure is caused by abnormal excessive electrical activity in the brain. All seizures are a symptom of a disease process, not a disease entity in itself. Not all seizures can be attributed to epilepsy. Causes of epilepsy include traumatic brain injury, brain tumor, encephalitis, and congenital or genetic malformations. Causes of nonepileptic seizures include hyponatremia, head trauma, fever, pregnancy-induced hypertension, hyperglycemia, benzodiazepine withdrawal, alcohol withdrawal, and metabolic encephalopathy. Psychogenic nonepileptic seizures present with symptoms mimicking a seizure; however, they lack abnormal electrical activity within the brain.[13] More than 60% of seizures are idiopathic.[15]

Approximately 2.2 to 3 million Americans are living with a diagnosis of epilepsy. Seizures have historically been classified as grand mal and petit mal. In 2017 the International League Against Epilepsy published a new seizure classification system based on three features of the seizure: where the seizure is in the brain (focal, unilateral, or bilateral), level of awareness during a seizure (aware or impaired awareness), and other seizure features (motor and nonmotor behaviors)[16] (Box 24.2). Psychogenic seizures may present with a mixed symptomology and ictal phase. Recent studies have identified elevated prolactin and creatine kinase (CK) levels in some seizure types but normal levels in psychogenic seizure.[17] These biomarkers do not appear to differentiate between seizure types but are useful to rule out epileptic seizure.

Treatment varies depending on the type of seizure. Patients present to the ED with first-time seizures, breakthrough seizures, and status epilepticus. Goals of ED care are to abort seizure activity, treat seizure sequelae, and rule out emergent causes of the seizure. Current recommendations for seizure management include patient safety measures, such as padding side rails and performing frequent blood glucose checks and medication management, as ordered.

Status Epilepticus

Status epilepticus is a seizure lasting longer than 5 minutes or repeat seizures without return of baseline neurologic status between seizures. Status epilepticus is a medical emergency with the potential for significant morbidity and mortality if not managed promptly.[4] Prolonged seizure can cause hypoxia, fever, cardiac dysthymia, aspiration, rhabdomyolysis, renal failure, acidosis, cerebral edema, increased ICP, hypoglycemia, and death.

Treatment of status epilepticus begins the same as single seizures. Intubation may be necessary to maintain a patent airway. Paralytics should be avoided during rapid sequence intubation (RSI) to avoid masking underlying seizure activity. Midazolam or propofol are safer alternatives for RSI. Anesthetic levels of propofol, pentobarbital, or midazolam are indicated to reduce cerebral electrical activity. Continuous electroencephalography (EEG) is useful to monitor for sufficient burst suppression when drugs are used at anesthetic levels. Frequent assessment is imperative to avoid or quickly identify seizure sequelae with immediate intervention.

Stroke

Stroke is the sudden onset of neurologic dysfunction caused by a disruption to blood flow and lasting more than 24 hours. Stroke is the fifth leading cause of death in the United States,

BOX 24.2 Seizure Types.

Focal Seizure With Retained Awareness (Previously Called Simple Partial Seizure)

Symptoms
- Dependent upon region of the brain affected
  - Occipital region may cause flashing lights
  - Motor cortex may cause jerking movements

Postictal Period
- May have period of neurologic dysfunction in affected area
- May mimic transient ischemic attacks or stroke

Focal Seizure With Impaired Awareness (Previously Called Complex Partial Seizure)

Symptoms
- May appear awake but not respond to commands or interact with the environment
- Repetitive behaviors such as lip smacking, grimacing, or repetitive speech

Postictal Period
- May appear awake but does not respond to commands or interact with the environment
- Somnolence, confusion, amnesic to the event

Generalized Seizures (Previously Called Grand Mal or Tonic-Clonic Seizure)

Symptoms
- Sudden loss of consciousness
- Tonic phase followed by clonic phase

Postictal Period
- Deeply sleeping with relaxed breathing

Generalized Seizure Subtypes
- Absence seizures
  Assessment: Brief impaired consciousness
- Clonic
  Assessment: Rhythmic muscle jerking
- Myoclonic
  Assessment: Brief muscle contractions
- Tonic
  Assessment: Muscle stiffening
- Atonic
  Assessment: Loss of muscle control

Adapted from Brodie M. The 2017 ILAE classification of seizure types and the epilepsies: what do people with epilepsy and their caregivers need to know? *Epileptic Disord.* 2018;20(2):77–87.

and almost 800,000 people have a stroke and 130,000 people die of a stroke annually. Stroke is the most common disabling neurologic disorder in the United States.[13]

Disrupted blood flow deprives tissues of oxygen, leading to cellular ischemia and death. Eighty-seven percent of strokes are ischemic and occur as the result of vessel occlusion from a thrombus or an embolus. The other 13% are hemorrhagic from intracerebral hemorrhage (ICH), cerebral aneurysm, and arteriovenous malformation (AVM). A transient ischemic attack (TIA) is the sudden onset of neurologic dysfunction resolving within 24 hours. Up to 10% of patients experiencing a TIA will have a stroke within 2 days, and up to 20% experience a stroke within 90 days.[8] Up to 80% of strokes are preventable by managing risk factors. Modifiable risk factors include hypertension, diabetes mellitus, obesity, substance abuse, smoking, atherosclerosis, cardiac valve disease, atrial fibrillation, and carotid artery occlusion. Nonmodifiable factors include age, gender, race/ethnicity, and family history of stroke.

Stroke care begins in the community and prehospital settings.[18] Public education on the signs of a stroke conveyed by using a simple tool such as the FAST (face, arms, speech, time) can aid in the early recognition of stroke. Delays in stroke symptom recognition vastly reduce the time to treatment, eligibility for thrombolytics, and endovascular treatment, which increase the burden of disability on the patient. If stroke symptoms are suspected, emergency care should be expedited emergently.

Research activity is ongoing to determine faster, yet effective, methods to streamline stroke care. A systemic review completed in 2018 failed to identify a stroke scale that would accurately predict a large vessel occlusion with sufficient specificity and sensitivity to recommend the patient being taken directly for embolectomy upon arrival.[19]

Thrombotic ischemic strokes are the result of atherosclerotic plaque buildup in vessels.[1] Bifurcations and curves in the vessels are particularly vulnerable. When occlusion causes diminished blood flow that is unable to meet the demands of the cerebral tissues, ischemia results. The center core of ischemic cells is surrounded by hypoperfused tissue known as the penumbra. The penumbra may be rescued with early reperfusion. As time passes, anoxic insult will result in death of the penumbra. Embolic stroke occurs when an embolus travels to the brain, occluding blood flow. Atrial fibrillation is responsible for more than 50% of cardioembolic strokes. Other sources are vegetation or clots on heart valves, endocarditis, air, and fat. The neurologic deficits observed in stroke depend on the area affected. Predictable deficits are seen with occlusion of major cerebral vessels. Table 24.3 outlines a few of these patterns.

The initial management of a patient with an ischemic stroke begins with managing ABCs. Oxygen is administered as needed to maintain the oxygen saturation at or over 94%.[20] Measure the blood glucose and administer $D_{50}W$ for glucose under 60 mg/dL. Complete a National Institutes of Health Stroke Scale assessment. Establish IV access. Draw blood for a complete blood count (CBC), PT/PTT, international normalized ratio (INR), and troponin. Obtain a 12-lead ECG and a chest x-ray. Obtain a noncontrast head computed tomography (CT) scan. Do not delay the head CT scan to obtain blood for the laboratory, or the 12 ECG.

If the patient is a candidate for endovascular thrombectomy or intraarterial tPA, obtain a cerebral vascular CT scan. The goal is to administer tissue plasminogen activator (tPA), which is currently the only thrombolytic for stroke treatment approved by the US Food and Drug Administration, within 60 minutes of ED arrival for patients

TABLE 24.3 Stroke Symptoms by Vessel or Region.

Anterior cerebral artery	Contralateral paralysis of foot and leg Impaired gait Sensory loss of foot, toes, and legs Loss of willpower Flat affect Perseveration
Posterior cerebral artery	Memory impairment Visual deficits: homonymous hemianopsia, color blindness, loss of depth perception Inability to recognize objects
Middle cerebral artery	Hemiplegia Sensory impairment Homonymous hemianopia Global aphasia if dominant hemisphere affected
Vertebral artery	Dizziness Nystagmus Dysphagia Facial pain Ipsilateral facial numbness and weakness Ataxia Clumsiness
Basilar artery	Tetraplegia
Anterior inferior cerebellar artery	Vertigo Nausea Vomiting Nystagmus Ipsilateral paresis of lateral conjugate gaze Contralateral impaired pain and temperature sensation in trunk and limbs
Left sided	Right side hemiplegia Receptive, expressive, or global aphasia Intellectual impairment Slow and cautious behavior Defects in right visual fields
Right sided	Left side hemiplegia Impulsive behavior Poor judgment Defects in left visual fields

meeting eligibility, but this medication should be started as soon as possible. See Box 24.3 for tPA dosing and contraindications. Nearly 2 million brain cells die each minute ischemia persists.[21] Do not delay tPA administration for laboratory results. The tPA can be stopped if laboratory results make the patient ineligible for tPA. If the patient is eligible for tPA, the medication is given regardless of plans for endovascular treatment.[20]

Blood pressure management is necessary for patients who have had a stroke. Blood pressure must be below 185/110 mm Hg before tPA administration. IV labetalol or nicardipine are recommended to control blood pressure. Sodium nitroprusside may be considered for a diastolic blood pressure higher than 140 mm Hg. If the patient is not a candidate for tPA, permissive hypertension is necessary to maintain cerebral perfusion. IV labetalol or nicardipine is indicated for a blood pressure higher than 220/120 mm Hg, with the goal of decreasing the blood pressure by no more than 10% to 15% over 24 hours.

Avoidance of insertion of IV or monitoring lines in noncompressible areas is mandatory for patients receiving tPA.[20] Indwelling urinary catheters should be inserted before tPA administration and only if necessary or delayed until at least 30 minutes after tPA bolus is completed. All patients diagnosed with a stroke must remain nil by mouth (NPO) until a dysphagia screening is completed by a trained individual. Safe patient handoff is necessary between hospital staff or receiving facility for transfer patients. If possible, a jointly conducted National Institutes of Health Stroke Scale assessment is indicated.

Timeliness to administration of tPA is crucial to improve the outcome of a patient with ischemic stroke. The drive to improve the use of tPA in eligible patients also increases the incidence of patients receiving thrombolytic therapy for a condition that may mimic a stroke. One study found that the overall risk of intracerebral hemorrhage for a patient definitively diagnosed with a stroke mimic is minimal.[22]

A hemorrhagic stroke is the result of bleeding into the subarachnoid space or intracerebral tissues.[1] Mortality from hemorrhagic strokes approaches 50%, and only a small percentage of patients regain full function.

Intracerebral hemorrhage (ICH) is most commonly caused by hypertension. Stimulant abuse, rupture of an aneurysm or AVM, brain tumor, coagulation disorders, and anticoagulation use are other causes. ICH accounts for 10% of all strokes. Typical symptoms include sudden onset of neurologic function, headache, vomiting, and rapidly deteriorating level of consciousness.

The other 3% of strokes are the result of cerebral aneurysm or AVM rupture resulting in a subarachnoid hemorrhage (SAH) in most cases. The patient will complain of sudden onset of "the worst headache of my life" that was maximal at its sudden onset and frequently followed by nausea, vomiting, and a deteriorating level of consciousness. A noncontrast head CT scan will show blood in the brain parenchyma or subarachnoid space. Lumbar puncture of a patient with SAH will reveal bloody CSF. Cerebral angiography may be completed to identify the source of the bleeding.

Initial management of the patient with a hemorrhagic stroke begins with securing ABCs. With little spare room in the cranial vault, the collection of blood will quickly increase ICP, and the brain will begin to shift. Rapid intervention to stop the bleeding and reduce ICP is required to prevent brain herniation and brain death.

Emergent reversal of the antithrombotic may be necessary. Selection of a reversal strategy is dependent on the antithrombotic agent[23] (Table 24.4). Blood pressure management is needed with a goal of reducing the blood pressure to decrease bleeding while maintaining adequate CPP.

Blood pressure management is a balancing act. Elevated blood pressure is managed with labetalol or nicardipine to reduce pressure in the vessel while maintaining a MAP sufficient to sustain CPP above 60 mm Hg. Vasopressors are initiated if the CPP cannot be sustained above 60 mm Hg.

BOX 24.3 Tissue Plasminogen Activator Criteria and Infusion.

Dose: 0.9 mg/kg
Maximum dose 90 mg
Bolus dose: 10% of total dose
Infusion: remainder of dose over 1 hour

Safe medication administration practice requires removal of the waste before administration of the tissue plasminogen activator.

Intravenous tubing priming volumes may approach 20 mL. The line should be cleared of tissue plasminogen activator at the end of the infusion by infusing normal saline through the line to ensure the patient receives the full dose.

Inclusion Criteria:

Age ≥18 years old
4.5 hours or less since last known normal for patient <80 years of age
3 hours or less since last known normal if over 80 years of age
Disabling neurologic symptoms with no upper or lower limit of National Institutes of Health Stroke Scale (NIHSS) score
Over 80 years of age:
3 hours or less since last known normal if history of both diabetes mellitus and prior stroke,
NIHSS score >25, taking anticoagulants
4.5 hours since last known normal if none of the above are present

Contraindications:

Intracranial hemorrhage on computed tomography scan
Systolic blood pressure >185 or diastolic blood pressure >110 despite treatment
Platelets <100,000/mm^3
International normalized ratio >1.7, activated partial thromboplastin time >40 seconds, prothrombin time >15
Low-molecular-weight heparin within 24 hours
Direct thrombin inhibitor, direct factor Xa inhibitors within 48 hours, unless laboratory test demonstrates normalized coagulation
Major surgery within 14 days
Severe head trauma within 3 months
Endocarditis
Intracranial or spinal surgery within prior 3 days
Prior ischemic stroke in the previous 3 months
Gastrointestinal bleed within 21 days
Prior intracranial hemorrhage
Intracranial neoplasm
Blood glucose <50 mg/dL

Relative contraindications: consideration of benefit outweighing risks

Pregnancy
Postpartum ≤14 days
Bleeding diathesis or coagulopathy history
Coumadin use with international normalized ratio ≤1.7
Major trauma within 14 days
Recent myocardial infarction
Pericarditis
Left-sided heart thrombus
Arterial puncture in noncompressible site within 7 days
Unruptured, unsecured cerebral aneurysm or arteriovenous malformation
Hyperglycemia
Seizure – must ensure symptoms are not postictal

Adapted from Demaerschalk B, Kleindorfer D, Adeoye O, et al. Scientific rationale for the inclusion and exclusion criteria for intravenous alteplase in acute ischemic stroke. *Stroke.* 2016;47:581–641.

TABLE 24.4 Antithrombotic Reversal Agents.

Antithrombotic	Reversal Agent
Vitamin K antagonists	Vitamin K, FFP, prothrombin complex concentrate
Direct factor Xa inhibitors	Prothrombin complex concentrate
Direct thrombin inhibitor	Dabigatran–Praxbind All others—prothrombin complex concentrate
Unfractionated heparin	Protamine
Low-molecular-weight heparin	Protamine, rFVIIa
Thrombolytic agents	Cryoprecipitate, tranexamic acid, aminocaproic acid
Antiplatelet agents	DDAVP, platelets

DDAVP, Trade name for desmopressin; *FFP,* fresh frozen plasma; *rFVIIA,* recombinant factor VIIa.
Adapted from Frontera JA, Lewin JJ III, Rabinstein AA, et al. Guideline for Reversal of Antithrombotics in Intracranial Hemorrhage: A Statement for Healthcare Professionals from the Neurocritical Care Society and Society of Critical Care Medicine. *Neurocrit Care.* 2016;24(1):6-46.

In addition, measures may be taken to reduce ICP. Insertion of an external ventricular drain permits measurement of the ICP as well as drainage of CSF to reduce intracranial volume, thereby reducing ICP.

Other measures include keeping the head of bed elevated, keeping the head maintained in the midline position, administering pain or sedation medications, reducing stimuli, and providing osmotic diuresis with mannitol or hypertonic saline. Monitoring and intervention are indicated to normalize blood glucose and core body temperature. End-tidal CO_2 monitoring is indicated to maintain eucapnia. Hyperventilation causes cerebral vasoconstriction, which reduces blood flow to the brain. Hyperventilation should be reserved for pending herniation while definitive treatment is completed. Anticonvulsant medications are not administered prophylactically but are added if seizure occurs. Patients are maintained NPO until a dysphagia screening is completed.

Definitive treatment of ICH is poorly defined.[24] Ongoing research seeks to define the mortality and outcome benefit of surgical intervention. The most recent American Heart Association/American Stroke Association guidelines for ICH list early surgical intervention as a Class 1 intervention only for patients with cerebellar hemorrhage. There is equivocal evidence regarding indication and timing of surgery for ICH in other locations. Definitive treatment for an SAH due to aneurysm is surgical clipping or endovascular coiling of the aneurysm.[25] Unless otherwise contraindicated, endovascular coiling is the treatment of choice. Before repair of the aneurysm, blood pressure is maintained below 160 mm Hg to reduce the risk of rebleeding. Nimodipine administration is indicated to reduce vasospasm, which is a common cause of neurologic deterioration after aneurysmal SAH.

Surgical clipping, radiosurgical eradication, and endovascular obliteration are used to eliminate the AVM. In some cases, decompressive craniotomy may be performed at the time of rupture, but surgical control of an AVM may be delayed several weeks.[26]

Meningitis

Meningitis is an inflammation of the meningeal layers surrounding the brain and spinal cord. Causes include bacterial, viral, fungal, and parasitic factors. Viral meningitis is the most prevalent form and usually has a milder course than bacterial meningitis. Bacterial meningitis has high morbidity and mortality rates. Vaccines for *Neisseria meningitidis, Haemophilus influenzae,* and *Streptococcus pneumoniae* have reduced the incidence of bacterial meningitis. Other types of bacteria are causes of meningitis that occurs after a craniotomy or an open skull fracture. Meningitis is transmitted via the respiratory route, so patients with suspected meningitis are placed in droplet isolation.

Meningitis is frequently precipitated by flu-type symptoms such as fever, headache, and fatigue. The course of meningitis can progress very rapidly.[27] Ninety-five percent of patients with meningitis will have at least two of the three hallmark symptoms: headache, altered level of consciousness, and stiff neck. A petechial or purpuric rash is a sign of meningococcal disease. Meningococcal meningitis has a mortality rate of 15%, and another 20% of patients will have serious disability.

Diagnosis is confirmed with a lumbar puncture (LP). CSF will be cloudy, with a high white blood cell count, elevated protein, and low glucose. A Gram stain and culture are useful to identify the causative agent. Outcomes are improved when antibiotics are administered as soon as possible after the LP. Dexamethasone has been shown to improve outcomes in pneumococcal and *H. influenza* meningitis but has no benefit in meningococcal meningitis.

Purulent exudate in the subarachnoid space can lead to a communicating hydrocephalus. Hydrocephalus, abscesses, and cerebral edema can cause increased ICP. Additional care in the ED includes monitoring neurologic status and providing pain management and fever control.

Prophylactic antibiotics are indicated in meningococcal disease for family, friends, and others who have had close contact with the patient. Health care providers who have been exposed to the patient's respiratory secretions should also receive prophylactic antibiotics.

Guillain–Barré Syndrome

Guillain–Barré syndrome (GBS) is an acute immune-mediated polyneuropathy resulting in paralysis. Many distinct variants fall under the GBS umbrella. The most common types are acute inflammatory demyelinating polyneuropathy and acute motor axonal neuropathy. GBS is more common in men and in adults. The annual incidence is roughly 1 per 100,000 people in the United States.

Two-thirds of patients with GBS report a respiratory or gastrointestinal infection in the preceding weeks. *Campylobacter jejuni* is the most common identified pathogen preceding infection. Cytomegalovirus, Epstein-Barr virus, human immunodeficiency virus (HIV), influenza virus, and *H. influenza* have been associated with GBS.[28] The association between GBS and influenza vaccine has been largely disproven. The risk of GBS is higher after illness with influenza than after administration of the influenza vaccine.

The hallmark symptom of GBS is symmetric, progressive weakness along with depressed or absent deep tendon reflexes. Ninety percent of patients will have the ascending form starting in the legs. The descending form starts in the arms or face. The disease may be relatively mild or progress rapidly. Between 20% and 30% of patients will require mechanical ventilator support. Autonomic dysfunction is a common feature and manifests as cardiac dysrhythmia, postural hypotension, and ileus. Despite the motor impairment, sensory function is minimally affected. Patients will experience pain due to nerve root inflammation. Generally, GBS progresses over 2 to 4 weeks, followed by a 4-week plateau before the onset of recovery. Early intervention is imperative to slow or stop progression.

GBS is a clinical diagnosis. There are no biomarkers to confirm most variants of the disease. CSF will demonstrate elevated protein levels with normal cell counts 1 week after symptom onset. Further diagnostic testing may be necessary to rule out other causes of the patient's symptoms. ED treatment goals focus on supportive care. Patients with mild disease may be treated as outpatients, but most patients require admission to the hospital for close monitoring of respiratory function, autonomic dysfunction, and pain management. Patients should be kept NPO until a swallow evaluation is completed. Intravenous immunoglobulin (IVIG) and plasma exchange are effective in halting progression and speeding recovery. The two treatments are equally effective but have no added benefit when used together. GBS has a 3% to 7% mortality rate. At 1 year, approximately 60% of patients have full motor recovery and 84% can walk unassisted. A small percentage of patients will develop chronic demyelinating polyneuropathy.[29] Despite functional recovery fatigue, weakness and pain may continue to plague many patients for years.

Myasthenia Gravis

Myasthenia gravis (MG) is the most common neuromuscular transmission disorder. MG is an autoimmune disorder causing chronic, painless, fluctuating muscle weakness. Acetylcholine antibodies block acetylcholine receptors on the postsynaptic neuron, resulting in a failure of muscle contraction.[8] MG affects women more than men. Ptosis and diplopia are the most common presenting symptoms. MG is confined to the ocular muscles in 20% of patients. Bulbar muscle involvement causes dysphagia, speech difficulties, and flat face (inability to smile). Muscles of the trunk are the least likely to be affected. Weakness increases with repeated attempts to use the muscle.

Infection, trauma, stress, surgery, or certain medications may precipitate a myasthenic crisis. Severe muscle weakness during a crisis may lead to respiratory failure and require mechanical ventilation. In the absence of preexisting pulmonary disease, the patient will be able to maintain normal arterial blood gas levels and oxygen saturations despite poor respiratory function. Respiratory function should be monitored by trending forced vital capacity and negative inspiratory force. Plasma exchange or IVIG are useful in the treatment of an MG exacerbation.

In the ED, corticosteroids and immunosuppressants such as azathioprine or tacrolimus may be given to reduce the causative immune response. Definitive diagnosis is managed in the outpatient setting. Serum antibody testing, edrophonium testing, and electromyelography testing will confirm the diagnosis. Acetylcholinesterase inhibitors are prescribed to manage MG.

Too much acetylcholinesterase inhibitor can cause a cholinergic crisis. A cholinergic crisis presents with muscle weakness similar to that of MG. Diarrhea, increased respiratory secretions, and sweating are present in a cholinergic crisis, aiding in differentiating a myasthenic crisis from a cholinergic crisis. Treatment of a cholinergic crisis is to hold acetylcholinesterase inhibitors and the administration of pralidoxime.

Goals of ED treatment are securing ABCs, monitoring respiratory function, and providing symptom relief. Dysphagia puts the patient at risk for aspiration; keep the patient NPO if there is concern about the patient's ability to swallow. Fall precautions are initiated due to muscle weakness.

REFERENCES

1. Urden L, Stacy KM, Lough ME. *Critical Care Nursing: Diagnosis and Management.* 8th ed. Maryland Heights, MO: Elsevier; 2018.
2. Vanderah T, Gould D. *Nolte's The Human Brain.* Philadelphia, PA: Elsevier; 2016.
3. Hall J. *Guyton and Hall Textbook of Medical Physiology.* 13th ed. Philadelphia, PA: Elsevier; 2016.
4. Walls R, Hockberger R, Gausche-Hill M, eds. *Rosen's Emergency Medicine: Concepts and Clinical Practice.* Philadelphia, PA: Elsevier; 2018.
5. Headache Classification Committee of the International Headache Society. The International Classification of Headache Disorders, 3rd ed. *Cephalagia.* 2018;38(1):1–211.
6. Burch R, Loder S, Loder E, Smitherman T. The prevalence and burden of migraine and severe headache in the United States. *Headache.* 2015;55(1):21–34.
7. Orr S, Friedman B, Christie S, et al. Management of adults with acute migraine in the emergency department. *Headache.* 2016;56(6):911–940.
8. Simon R, Aminoff M, Greenberg DA. *Clinical Neurology.* 10th ed. New York, NY: McGraw-Hill Education; 2018.
9. Friedman B. Managing migraine. *Ann Emerg Med.* 2017;69(2):202–207.
10. Silberstein SD, Holland S, Freitag F, et al. Evidence-based guideline update: pharmacologic treatment for episodic migraine prevention in adults: report of the Quality Standards Subcommittee of the American Academy of Neurology and the American Headache Society. *Neurology.* 2012;78(17):1337–1345.
11. Simpson D, Hallett M, Ashman E, et al. Practice guideline summary: botulinum neurotoxin for the treatment of blepharospasm, cervical dystonia, adult spasticity, and headache. *Neurology.* 2016;86(19):1–9.
12. American Headache Society. Choosing wisely: five things physicians and patients should question. American Headache Society website. https://americanheadachesociety.org/five-things-physicians-and-patients-should-question/. Accessed May 14, 2019.
13. Koster MJ, Matteson EL, Warrington KJ. Large-vessel giant cell arteritis: diagnosis, monitoring and management. *Rheumatology.* 2018;57(suppl 2):ii32–ii42. https://doi.org/10.1093/rheumatology/kex424. Accessed May 14, 2019.
14. Docken WP. Diagnosis of giant cell arteritis. UpToDate website. https://www.uptodate.com/contents/diagnosis-of-giant-cell-arteritis?search=temporal%20arteritis&source=search_result&selectedTitle=1~125&usage_type=default&display_rank=1. Updated October 5, 2018. Accessed May 14, 2019.
15. American Epilepsy Society. FAQs. American Epilepsy Society website. https://www.aesnet.org/clinical_resources/faqs. Accessed May 14, 2019.
16. Brodie M. The 2017 ILAE classification of seizure types and the epilepsies: what do people with epilepsy and their caregivers need to know? *Epileptic Disord.* 2018;20(2):77–87.
17. Javali M, Acharya P, Shah S, Mahale R, Shetty P, Rangasetty S. Role of biomarkers in differentiating new-onset seizures from psychogenic nonepileptic seizures. *J Neurosci Rural Pract.* 2017;8(4):581–584.
18. National Stroke Association. Preventing a stroke. https://www.stroke.org/understand-stroke/preventing-a-stroke/. Accessed May 14, 2019.
19. Smith E, Kent DM, Bulsara KR, et al. Accuracy of prediction instruments for diagnosing large vessel occlusion in individuals with suspected stroke: a systematic review for the 2018 Guidelines for the Early Management of Patients With Acute Ischemic Stroke. *Stroke.* 2018;49(3):e111–e122. https://doi.org/10.1161/STR.0000000000000160.
20. Powers W, Rabinstein A, Ackerson T, et al. 2018 Guidelines for the early management of patients with acute ischemic stroke: a guideline for healthcare professionals from the American Heart Association/American Stroke Association. *Stroke.* 2018;49(3):e46–e99. https://doi.org/10.1161/STR.0000000000000158.
21. Saver J. Time is brain—quantified. *Stroke.* 2016;37(1):263–266.
22. Tsivgoulis G, Zand R, Katsanos A, et al. Safety of intravenous thrombolysis in stroke mimics: prospective 5-year study and comprehensive meta-analysis. *Stroke.* 2015;46(5):1281–1287.
23. Frontera JA, Lewin JJ, Rabinstein AA, et al. Guideline for reversal of antithrombotics in intracranial hemorrhage: a statement for healthcare professionals from the neurocritical care society and society of critical care medicine. *Neurocrit Care.* 2016;24(1):6–46.
24. Hemphill JC, Greenberg SM, Anderson CS, et al. Guidelines for the management of spontaneous intracerebral hemorrhage: a guideline for healthcare professionals from the American Heart Association/American Stroke Association. *Stroke.* 2015;46(7):2032–2060.

25. Connolly ES, Rabinstein A, Carhuapoma JR, et al. Guidelines for the management of aneurysmal subarachnoid hemorrhage: a guideline for healthcare professionals from the American Heart Association/American Stroke Association. *Stroke.* 2012;43(6):1711–1737.
26. Grotta J, Albers G, Broderick J, et al. *Stroke: Pathophysiology, Diagnosis, and Management*. 6th ed. Philadelphia, PA: Elsevier; 2016.
27. Woodward S, Mestecky A, eds. *Neuroscience Nursing*. Ames, IA: Wiley-Blackwell; 2011.
28. Willison HJ, Jacobs BC, van Doorn PA. Guillain-Barre syndrome. *Lancet.* 2016;388(10045):717–727.
29. van den Berg B, Walgaard C, Drenthen J, Fokke C, Jacobs BC, van Doorn PA. Guillain-Barre syndrome: pathogenesis, diagnosis, treatment and prognosis. *Nat Rev Neurol.* 2014;10(8):469–482.

25

Gastrointestinal Emergencies

Amy Herrington

Gastrointestinal (GI) emergencies vary from minor problems to more serious, potentially life-threatening problems. Complaints of a GI nature are a common reason for visits to the emergency department (ED). Clinical indications of a problem in the GI system include heartburn, nausea, vomiting, constipation, diarrhea, bloating, chest pain, abdominal pain, and blood in stool or vomitus. This chapter focuses on those conditions seen most often in the ED. A brief review of anatomy and physiology is followed by discussion of specific GI conditions. Trauma of the GI system is discussed in Chapter 39.

ANATOMY AND PHYSIOLOGY

Normal GI function requires ingestion of nutrients and fluids and is followed by elimination of waste products formed from metabolic actions. Major organs and structures of the GI system are the esophagus, stomach, intestines, liver, pancreas, gallbladder, and peritoneum. See Fig. 25.1.

Esophagus

The major function of the esophagus is movement of food. The esophagus, a straight, collapsible tube approximately 25 cm long and up to 3 cm in diameter, extends from the pharynx to the stomach. Distinct esophageal layers are the mucous membrane, submucosa, and muscular layer. Secretions from mucous glands spread throughout the submucosa and keep the inner lining moist and lubricated. Striated muscle in the upper esophagus is gradually replaced by smooth muscle in the lower esophagus and GI tract. The upper esophageal sphincter is at the proximal end of the esophagus, and the lower esophageal sphincter (LES; also called the cardiac sphincter) is at the distal junction of the esophagus and stomach. The LES prevents regurgitation from the stomach into the esophagus.

Stomach

The stomach is a J-shaped organ located below the diaphragm between the esophagus and small intestine. Stomach functions include food storage and combining food with gastric juices. Limited absorption occurs in the stomach before the movement of food into the small intestine. Recognized regions of the stomach are the pylorus, fundus, body, and antrum. The pyloric sphincter controls food movement from the stomach to the duodenum. Distinct layers of the stomach wall are the outer serosa, muscular layer, submucosa, and mucosa. The mucosal layer contains multiple wrinkles called rugae that straighten as the stomach fills to accommodate more volume. Completely relaxed, the stomach holds up to 1.5 L.[1] Gastric juices containing pepsin, hydrochloric acid, mucus, and intrinsic factor are secreted by glands in the submucosa. These agents begin food breakdown. Acids in the stomach maintain the pH of gastric juices at 1.0.

Intestines

The small intestine is a tubular organ extending from the pyloric sphincter to the proximal large intestine. Secretions from the pancreas and liver complete the digestion of nutrients in chyme—the semiliquid mixture of food and gastric secretions. The small intestine absorbs nutrients and other products of digestion and transports residue to the large intestine. Segments of the small intestine are the duodenum, jejunum, and ileum. The duodenum attaches to the stomach at the pyloric sphincter in the retroperitoneal space and represents the only fixed portion of the small intestine. The jejunum and ileum are mobile and lie free in the peritoneal cavity. The small intestine contains circular folds, villi, and microvilli, which leads to increased surface area for food absorption.

Segments of the large intestine are the cecum, colon, rectum, and anal canal. The large intestine is approximately 1.5 m long, beginning in the lower right side of the abdomen where the ileum joins the cecum.[1] The colon is divided into the ascending colon, transverse colon, descending colon, and sigmoid colon. Primary functions of the large intestine are absorption of water and electrolytes, formation of feces, and storage of feces. Although it is not as long as the small intestine, it is referred to as the large intestine due to the almost 3-inch diameter of the organ.

Liver

The liver, located in the right upper quadrant of the abdomen, is divided into right and left lobes. Functional units of the liver called lobules contain sinusoids and Kupffer cells. Each lobule is supplied by a hepatic artery, sublobular vein, bile duct, and lymph channel. The liver is extremely vascular; approximately 1450 mL of blood flow through the liver each minute.[1] Sinusoids in lobules act as a reservoir for overflow

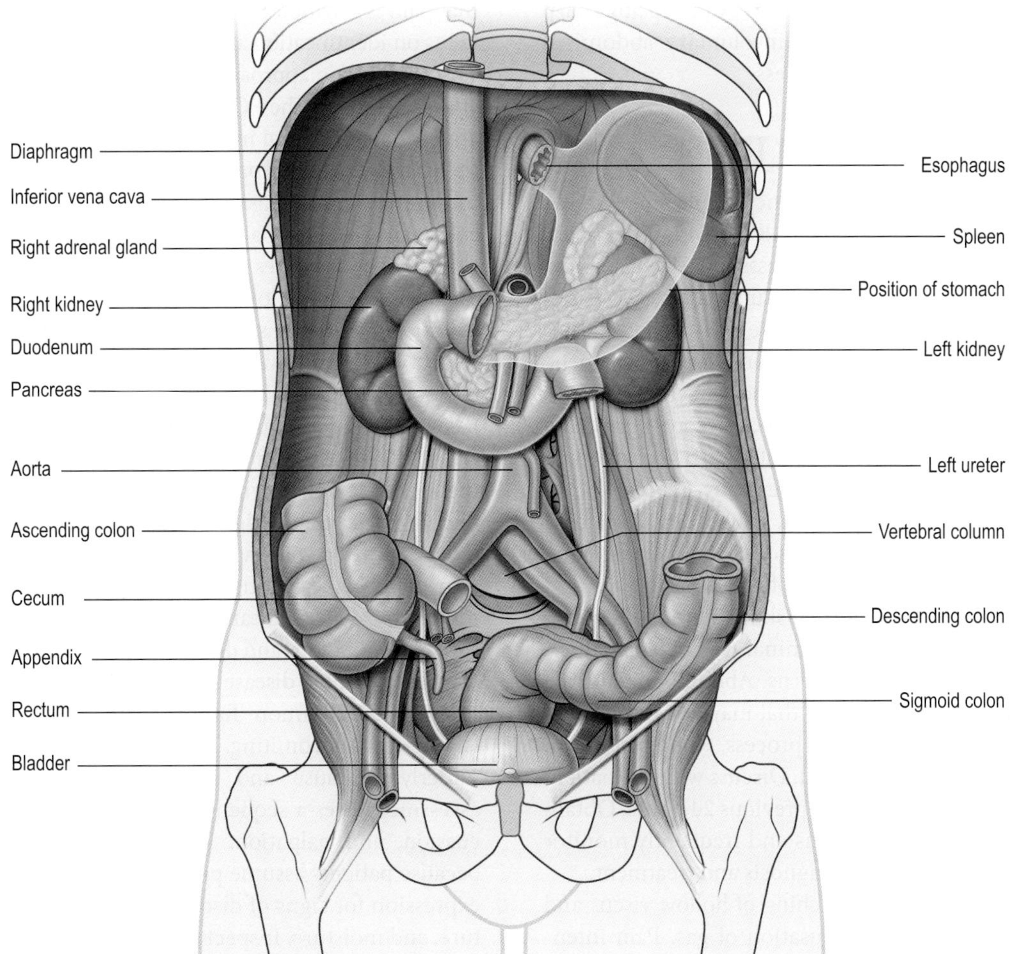

Fig. 25.1 GI Anatomy. (From Waugh A, Grant A. *Ross & Wilson Anatomy and Physiology in Health and Illness*. 13th ed. Elsevier Ltd, 2018.)

of blood and fluids from the right ventricle. A thick capsule of connective tissue known as Glisson's capsule covers the liver. The liver is involved in hundreds of metabolic functions, including metabolism of nutrients, gluconeogenesis, and drug metabolism. Production of bile is a major function of the liver; 600 to 1200 mL of bile are secreted each day.[1] Bile is essential for digestion and absorption of fats and fat-soluble vitamins and excretion of bilirubin and excess cholesterol. Bilirubin is an end product of hemoglobin destruction.

Pancreas

The pancreas is a lobulated organ behind the stomach that contains endocrine and exocrine cells. The organ is divided into the head, body, and a thin, narrow tail. Cells in the islets of Langerhans secrete insulin and regulate glucose levels. Exocrine cells called pancreatic acini secrete pancreatic juices for digestion of fats, carbohydrates, proteins, and nucleic acids. Pancreatic enzymes (i.e., lipase and amylase) enter the intestines through the pancreatic duct at the same juncture as the bile duct from the liver and gallbladder. Pancreatic and bile ducts join at a short dilated tube called the ampulla of Vater. A band of smooth muscles called the sphincter of Oddi surrounds this area and controls exit of pancreatic juices and bile.[1]

Gallbladder

The gallbladder is a pear-shaped sac located in a depression on the inferior surface of the liver. The organ's main functions are the collection, concentration, and storage of bile. Maximum volume is 30 to 60 mL; however, input from the liver can reach 450 mL over 12 hours.[1]

Peritoneum

The peritoneum is a serous membrane covering the liver, spleen, stomach, and intestines that acts as a semipermeable membrane, contains pain receptors, and provides proliferative cellular protection. Technically, all abdominal organs are behind the peritoneum and therefore are retroperitoneal; however, the liver, spleen, stomach, and intestines are suspended into the peritoneum and considered intraperitoneal organs. Omenta are folds of peritoneum surrounding the stomach and adjacent organs. The greater omentum drapes the transverse colon and loops of small intestine. It is extremely mobile and spreads easily into areas of injury to seal off potential sources of infection. The lesser omentum covers parts of the stomach and proximal intestines but is not as movable as the greater omentum.

The peritoneum is permeable to fluid, electrolytes, urea, and toxins. Somatic afferent nerves sensitize the peritoneum to all types of stimuli. In acute abdominal conditions, the peritoneum can localize an irritable focus by producing sharp pain and tenderness, voluntary or involuntary abdominal muscle rigidity, and rebound tenderness.

PATIENT ASSESSMENT AND TRIAGE

Assessment of a patient with a GI emergency should initially focus on airway, breathing, and circulation (ABCs), with the primary survey completed before the focused assessment. Determination of chief complaint; social, medical, and surgical history; reason for seeking treatment, and treatment before arrival follow the initial assessment. Information may be obtained from the patient, family members, a significant other, friends, emergency medical services personnel, or previous medical records. Historical assessment should include questions related to gynecologic and genitourinary (GU) symptoms because many gynecologic or GU conditions cause abdominal pain, nausea, and vomiting. Information related to food intake and alcohol consumption should be obtained during assessment of patient history.

Evaluate the patient for abnormal skin and mucous membrane color and temperature, abdominal wall abnormalities, pain, and alterations in bowel patterns. Abdominal pain is a common chief complaint in the ED that may be caused by an acute event or related to a chronic process. Abdominal pain may be visceral, somatic, or referred. Discuss with the patient his or her intake and output for the previous 24 hours. Obtain an initial complete set of vital signs and frequently monitor these for change affected by the diagnosis and treatment.

Visceral pain is caused by stretching of hollow viscus and is described as cramping or a sensation of gas. Pain intensifies, then decreases, and is usually centered at the umbilicus or below the midline. Diffuse pain makes localization of pain difficult. Diaphoresis, nausea, vomiting, hypotension, tachycardia, and abdominal wall spasms may be present. Conditions associated with visceral pain are appendicitis, acute pancreatitis, cholecystitis, and intestinal obstruction.

Somatic pain is produced by bacterial or chemical irritation of nerve fibers. Pain is sharp and usually localized to one area. A patient may be found lying with legs flexed and knees pulled to the chest to prevent stimulation of the peritoneum and subsequent increase in pain. Associated findings include involuntary guarding and rebound tenderness. Conditions associated with somatic pain include nerve injuries, muscle sprains/strains, and referred back pain. Somatic pain can also be chronic from previous abdominal surgery.

Referred pain occurs at a distance from the original source of the pain and is thought to be caused by the development of nerve tracts during fetal growth and development. Biliary pain can be referred to the subscapular area, whereas a peptic ulcer and pancreatic disease can cause back pain.

Individual and cultural variations in expressions of pain must be considered when assessing abdominal pain. Each person reacts differently—older adult patients may not exhibit the same level of pain as younger patients; men may hide pain because expression of pain is not considered masculine in many cultures. Conversely, dramatic expression of pain may be expected in some cultures. Emergency nurses must remember that pain is a symptom—not a diagnosis. Interventions should focus on identification and treatment of the source of pain.

A systematic approach is recommended for assessment of abdominal pain. The PQRST mnemonic can be used to obtain appropriate historical information and identification of essential characteristics of pain. *P*rovocation—Is there an action or movement that increases or changes the pain? *Q*uality or character of pain—Is the pain sharp, dull, intermittent? *R*adiation or referral of pain—Does the pain stay in the right lower quadrant or move to the left lower quadrant as well? Using an age-appropriate pain scale such as a numeric rating of 0 (no pain) to 10 (worst pain ever) can identify the intensity or *S*everity of the pain. Question the patient regarding how long the pain has lasted to determine the *T*ime of pain onset. It is important to consider the anatomy of the patient and to correlate the location of pain with the organ or system located in that region. For example, right lower quadrant pain in a female is often associated with ovarian or appendix conditions. The next step would be evaluating the descriptive information using the mnemonic discussed earlier. Final diagnosis would occur after serial examinations and diagnostics to evaluate or rule out each organ of potential disease or injury.

Another common finding with most GI emergencies is nausea and vomiting. Specific treatment varies with the underlying cause and physician preference. Abdominal assessment uses a sequence of inspection, auscultation, percussion, and palpation. Patient position should be noted because patients assume positions of comfort. Observe facial expression for signs of discomfort. Note skin color, temperature, and moisture. Inspect the abdominal wall for pulsations, movement, masses, symmetry, or surgical scars.

Auscultate bowel sounds in all four quadrants, determining frequency, quality, and pitch. Normal bowel sounds are irregular, high-pitched gurgling sounds occurring 5 to 35 times per minute. Decreased or absent bowel sounds suggest peritonitis or paralytic ileus, whereas hyperactive bowel sounds associated with nausea, vomiting, and diarrhea suggest gastroenteritis. Frequent, high-pitched bowel sounds may occur with bowel obstruction. Vascular sounds such as venous hums or bruits are abnormal findings. Auscultation should always be done before palpation because palpation may create false bowel sounds. The presence of hypoactive or hyperactive bowel sounds can be found in patients without abdominal pathologic processes. Thus bowel sounds must be evaluated in association with other abdominal findings such as guarding and tenderness with palpation. Factors such as stress and last food intake can affect bowel sounds.

Percussion is performed in all four quadrants. Dull sounds occur over solid organs or tumors, whereas tympanic sounds occur over air masses. Dull sounds may also be heard over a distended bladder or an area of bowel distended with stool. Tympany is the predominant sound heard when percussing the abdomen.

Palpation is the last step in abdominal assessment. Begin palpation away from painful sites, noting areas of tenderness, guarding, or rigidity. Assess for abnormal masses and rebound tenderness.

Concurrent findings such as fever and chills are usually found with bacterial infection, appendicitis, or cholecystitis. Other signs associated with pain are nausea, vomiting, and anorexia. Intractable vomiting or feces in emesis suggest bowel obstruction. Blood in emesis occurs with gastritis or upper GI bleeding. Assess bowel patterns for abnormalities such as diarrhea or constipation, noting stool color and consistency. Diarrhea can occur with gastroenteritis; black, tarry stools suggest upper GI bleeding; and clay-colored stools are found with biliary tract obstruction. Fatty, foul-smelling, frothy stools occur with pancreatitis.

SPECIFIC GASTROINTESTINAL EMERGENCIES

Infection, structural abnormalities, or pathologic processes may cause GI emergencies. Heredity and lifestyle also play a role. For example, excessive alcohol consumption can lead to GI bleeding, cirrhosis, or esophageal varices. Regardless of cause, nontraumatic GI emergencies are a common occurrence in any ED—ranging from minor inconvenience to life-threatening problems.

Gastrointestinal Bleeding

Bleeding can originate anywhere in the GI tract and can occur at any age. Bleeding is functionally categorized by location—upper or lower GI bleeding. Upper GI bleeding is more common in males, whereas lower GI bleeding is seen more often in females. Symptoms associated with bleeding in the GI tract include bright-red blood and/or black, "coffee grounds" material in vomitus, as well as bright-red blood from the rectum and/or black, tarry stools. Bleeding stops spontaneously in the majority of hospitalized patients.

Upper Gastrointestinal Bleeding

Upper GI bleeding refers to blood loss between the upper esophagus and duodenum at the ligament of Treitz. Bleeding is categorized as variceal or nonvariceal.[2] The risk for death is greater with variceal bleeding because of the occurrence of massive hemorrhage in these patients. Gastroesophageal varices are enlarged, venous channels that are dilated by portal hypertension. The most common cause of portal hypertension is cirrhosis. As portal hypertension increases, varices continue to enlarge and eventually rupture, causing hemorrhage. Systemic manifestations of cirrhosis vary depending on the stage of the disease. Early symptoms include generalized weakness and fatigue; intermittent low-grade fevers; ankle edema; right upper quadrant abdominal pain; and various (GI) symptoms, including anorexia, nausea and vomiting, dyspepsia, and changes in bowel pattern. As the disease progresses, jaundice, mental status changes, muscle wasting, weight loss, ascites, epistaxis, spontaneous bruising, and hypotension may occur.[3] It is during this later stage that GI bleeding becomes prevalent. Bleeding from varices requires immediate intervention and close observation after initial control of bleeding. The risk for rebleeding is high until the varices are obliterated.

Nonvariceal bleeding occurs because of the disruption of esophageal or gastroduodenal mucosa with ulceration or erosion into an underlying vein or artery. Ulcerations or erosions occur when hyperacidity, pepsin, or aspirin inhibit mucosal prostaglandins and overwhelm protective factors of the esophagus (i.e., esophageal motility, salivary secretions, and the LES) and gastric mucosa (i.e., mucus, rapid epithelial renewal, and tissue mediators). Peptic ulcer disease, an infectious process caused by *Helicobacter pylori,* renders the underlying mucosa more vulnerable to gastric acid damage by disrupting the mucosal layer and initiating an inflammatory response that perpetuates tissue damage. Peptic ulcer disease may account for more than 50% of upper GI bleeding cases.[4] Other causes of upper GI bleeding include drug-induced erosions and severe or prolonged retching and vomiting such as with bulimia.

Mallory-Weiss syndrome occurs from longitudinal tears or lacerations of the distal esophagus at the gastroesophageal junction.[5] The lacerations may result in bleeding from submucosal arteries. This syndrome is usually associated with severe retching. Mallory-Weiss syndrome has also been reported in patients with a history of straining with stools, coughing, lifting, and grand-mal seizures. Patients with a hiatal hernia are at greater risk for Mallory-Weiss syndrome.

Clinical signs and symptoms of GI bleeding are variable. Hematemesis, the vomiting of blood or coffee grounds–like material, confirms upper GI bleeding. Abdominal pain, nausea, vomiting, hematemesis, or melena (black, tarry stools) can be present. Other presenting symptoms may include pallor, dizziness, weakness, and lethargy. Signs of hypovolemia such as tachycardia, orthostatic hypotension, and syncope may also occur. Mental confusion, jaundice, or ascites are often observed in patients associated with variceal bleeding.

Management begins with maintenance of the ABCs. After ensuring the airway is patent and stable, administer oxygen via an oxygen adjunct for patients with hemodynamic compromise or indicators of hypovolemic shock to support a Spo_2 of greater than 94%. Fluid replacement begins with normal saline or lactated Ringer's solution followed by blood (packed red blood cells [PRBCs] or whole blood) replacement if the patient's condition does not improve. Using a cardiac monitor and continuous pulse oximetry is recommended for all patients with significant blood loss or bright-red bleeding. Older adult patients can experience myocardial infarction secondary to ischemia caused by hypovolemia. Monitor vital signs and level of consciousness for signs of hemodynamic compromise. A nasogastric tube is inserted for gastric lavage with saline solution to remove blood clots. Lavage also serves to clear the GI tract, which facilitates endoscopy. A urinary catheter is inserted to monitor output and fluid status.

Determine whether the patient has a history of nonsteroidal antiinflammatory drug or aspirin use and alcohol or liver disease. Baseline laboratory studies include complete blood count (CBC), type and crossmatch, electrolytes, blood urea nitrogen (BUN), creatinine, and serum glucose. Normal creatinine level with increased BUN suggests bleeding with breakdown of blood in the gut or dehydration. Liver function and coagulation studies are also recommended to rule out coagulopathies or liver disease. An upright chest radiograph can provide valuable information if perforation is suspected; however, this is not feasible if significant hemodynamic compromise is present. An electrocardiogram (ECG) should be obtained to assess for dysrhythmias or cardiac ischemic changes related to blood loss.

A variety of endoscopic methods are available to control upper GI bleeding. Endoscopic injection of sclerosing agents or cautery/thermal techniques has been used to control bleeding from peptic ulcer disease. Endoscopic band ligation and sclerotherapy are frequently used to control variceal bleeding.[6] Treatment modalities include medications and surgical interventions. Medical therapy for nonvariceal bleeding includes intravenous (IV) infusion of proton pump inhibitors such as pantoprazole. Gastroesophageal variceal bleeding is treated with IV vasopressin (20 units in 200 mL saline at 0.25–0.5 units/min) or octreotide.[3] A Sengstaken-Blakemore, Minnesota, or Linton balloon tube can be used to tamponade bleeding. Surgical intervention may be necessary in cases when the bleeding cannot be controlled via other methods. Complications related to upper GI bleeding include aspiration, pneumonia, respiratory failure, and hypovolemic shock.

Lower Gastrointestinal Bleeding

Lower GI bleeding is bleeding that occurs below the ligament of Treitz. Common causes are hemorrhoids, diverticulum, angiodysplasia, colonic polyps, colon cancer, or colitis.[7] The cardinal sign of lower GI bleeding is hematochezia, the passage of bright-red blood, maroon-colored blood, or blood clots per rectum. Diverticulum and angiodysplasia are common causes of lower GI bleeding in older adults, whereas hemorrhoids, anal fissures, and inflammatory bowel disease occur most often in younger patients. A diverticulum is a pouch or saclike protrusion of the colonic wall (Fig. 25.2). Diverticulitis represents inflammation and possible perforation of a diverticulum. Diverticular bleeding can be severe and life-threatening because diverticula often form at the site of arterial vascular penetration. Hemorrhoids are dilated submucosal veins in the anus located above (internal) or below (external) the dentate line. Serious lower GI bleeding from hemorrhoids is uncommon. The risk for

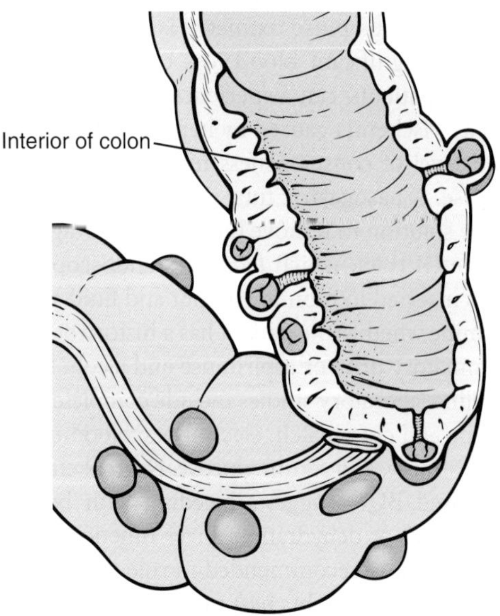

Fig. 25.2 Diverticula are outpouchings of the colon.

bleeding is increased in patients with a coagulopathy. Internal hemorrhoids are rarely associated with pain, whereas external hemorrhoids can cause significant discomfort. Angiodysplasia refers to dilated tortuous submucosal vessels. Lower GI bleeding from angiodysplasia is from a venous source and most often originates from the cecum or ascending colon.

Colitis refers to mucosal inflammation with an infectious or inflammatory cause. Inflammatory bowel disease includes both Crohn's disease and ulcerative colitis. Hematochezia is a more common initial finding in patients with ulcerative colitis. However, it is not necessary to differentiate between the two in the ED because the treatment is similar for both conditions.[7] Colon cancer is a relatively less common but serious cause of lower GI bleeding. The bleeding tends to be less severe but can occur multiple times.

Many patients with lower GI bleeding experience acute bleeds that are self-limiting and do not cause significant changes in hemodynamic status. Most patients with mild lower GI bleeding who are hemodynamically stable may be evaluated on an outpatient basis. Patients with severe symptomatic lower GI bleeding require hospital admission for resuscitation, diagnosis, and treatment. Colonoscopy should be performed to determine the source of bleeding after the patient is stabilized.

Blood originating from the left colon is typically bright red in color. Anemia may be present in patients with low-grade bleeding over time. Crampy abdominal pain may be present. Painless bleeding also occurs. Tachycardia, pallor, diaphoresis, and other indicators of hypovolemic shock indicate significant bleeding. Orthostatic changes in pulse or blood pressure occur in many patients.

Baseline laboratory studies include CBC, chemistry panels, and coagulation studies. The first priority is management of the ABCs followed by IV fluid resuscitation with normal saline or lactated Ringer's solution via large-bore catheter. Administration of PRBCs may be necessary in cases of significant blood loss. Treatment to correct coagulopathies or thrombocytopenia should be initiated. The ideal hematocrit depends on the patient's age, past medical history, and the presence of significant medical problems. For example, a young adult may tolerate a hematocrit of 25. However, the same hematocrit could be detrimental in an older adult patient with coronary artery disease.[7] Determining the source of bleeding is a priority. Colonoscopy, radionuclide imaging, or mesenteric angiography may be performed. Colonoscopy is the initial examination of choice in the majority of cases. Endoscopic therapy and interventions can be used to treat diverticula, angiodysplasia, and hemorrhoids. Surgical intervention may be required in some patients with exsanguinating lower GI bleeding.

Gastroesophageal Reflux Disease and Gastritis

Gastroesophageal reflux disease (GERD) applies to patients with symptoms or mucosal damage produced by the abnormal reflux of gastric contents into the esophagus. Most patients complain of heartburn, chest pain, regurgitation, and dysphagia. Some patients report the sensation of a lump in the throat that is not relieved with swallowing or coughing. Nausea may also be present. Bronchospasm, chronic cough, and laryngitis have also been associated with GERD. Conditions associated with GERD are decreased LES pressure, decreased esophageal motility, and increased gastric emptying time. Many foods such as fatty foods, chocolate, tea, coffee, alcohol, and foods/drinks containing caffeine can exacerbate symptoms. Some medications can also worsen or lead to GERD, and these include calcium channel blockers, theophylline, nitrates, and Valium.

The emergency nurse needs to be vigilant when reviewing home medication lists and past medical history. Look for medications or conditions that could lead to delay in gastric emptying and predispose the patient to GERD. Examples include pregnancy or the use of hormones, diabetes mellitus, scleroderma, diabetic gastroparesis, use of anticholinergics, and gastric outlet obstruction. It is of interest that acid secretion does not increase in patients with GERD. Complications associated with GERD include esophagitis and peptic stricture.

GERD-related chest pain may mimic cardiac-related chest pain and is typically described as squeezing or burning. Chest pain may be the only reported symptom. The pain may radiate to the neck, jaw, or abdomen. Similarities to the clinical presentation of ischemic heart disease require thoughtful consideration. The emergency nurse should pay close attention to patient history and to the patient for changes in condition. Other symptoms associated with GERD are nocturnal choking; sleep apnea; recurrent pneumonia; recurrent ear, nose, and throat infections; loss of dental enamel; and chronic halitosis.

Management of GERD begins with elimination of other conditions that are more lethal (e.g., ischemic heart disease and esophageal perforation). Studies such as ECG, chest radiograph, and CBC are primarily used to rule out other conditions. Additional imaging studies include endoscopy. Specific treatment in the ED includes symptomatic relief through use of antacids, H_2-blockers, and proton pump inhibitors.[8] Antacids are given with viscous lidocaine to increase effectiveness. Table 25.1 highlights specific medications and their expected outcomes.

TABLE 25.1 Drug Therapy for GERD.

Mechanism of Action	Examples
Increase Lower Esophageal Sphincter Pressure	
Cholinergic	Bethanechol (Urecholine)
Dopamine antagonist	Metoclopramide (Reglan)
Serotonin antagonist	Cisapride (Propulsid)
Acid Neutralizing	
Antacids	Gelusil, Maalox, Mylanta
Antisecretory	
Histamine H_2-receptor antagonists	Ranitidine (Zantac)
	Cimetidine (Tagamet)
	Famotidine (Pepcid)
	Nizatidine (Axid)
Proton pump inhibitors	Omeprazole (Prilosec)
	Lansoprazole (Prevacid)
	Pantoprazole (Protonix, Pantoloc)
	Rabeprazole (Aciphex)
Cytoprotective	
Alginic acid–antacid	Gaviscon
Antacids	Gelusil, Maalox, Mylanta
Acid-protective	Sucralfate (Carafate)

GERD, Gastroesophageal reflux disease.
From Lewis SM, Heitkemper MM, Dirksen SR: *Medical-Surgical Nursing: Assessment and Management of Clinical Problems.* 7th ed. St Louis, MO: Mosby; 2007.

Appendicitis

The appendix is a hollow organ. Obstruction of the appendiceal lumen appears to be the most common mechanism for the development of appendicitis. Once obstructed, the lumen becomes distended. Obstruction and distention decrease blood flow, resulting in ischemia and bacterial invasion. Untreated, inflammation progresses so that the appendix becomes nonviable and gangrenous, eventually rupturing into the peritoneal space. The incidence of appendicitis is higher in male patients than in female patients. It is also higher in the 10- to 19-year-old age-group. The diagnosis of appendicitis is challenging in young children and older adults.

Patients may have abdominal pain or abdominal cramping, nausea, vomiting, tachycardia, malaise, and anorexia. Chills and fever also occur. Abdominal pain may be initially diffuse and periumbilical in location; later the pain may become intense and localized to the lower right quadrant. Classic pain associated with appendicitis is located just inside the right iliac crest at McBurney's point. Older adult patients are often afebrile and do not exhibit this classic pain. Pressure on the lower left abdomen intensifies pain in the right lower quadrant (Rovsing's sign). Pain may not always occur in this classic location because of normal variations in the location of the appendix. The position of comfort for most patients is supine with hips and knees flexed.

If the appendix ruptures, peritoneal signs increase and involuntary guarding develops. Increased fever and rebound tenderness occur when the appendix abscesses or ruptures. Diagnosis is made by assessment of clinical signs and symptoms in concert with physical examination. Diagnostic data include elevation of white blood cell (WBC) count greater than 10,000 cells/mm^3 with increased neutrophils, specifically bands. Although leukocytosis is common, 30% of patients may have a normal WBC count. Ultrasonography point-of-care testing may demonstrate an enlarged appendix or a collection of periappendiceal fluid. Computed tomography (CT) scan is considered a more accurate diagnostic imaging test in the diagnosis of acute appendicitis. Urinalysis should be performed to rule out GU problems.

Definitive therapy for appendicitis is surgical intervention, with the laparoscopic approach as the preferred method. Obtain IV access, administer a prophylactic broad-spectrum antibiotic, and instruct the patient not to eat or drink. Complications such as perforation, peritonitis, and abscess formation can occur when treatment is delayed. Patients may develop shock as a result of these complications. Frequent reassessment of the abdomen as well as vital signs is a must.

Cholecystitis

Acute cholecystitis involves inflammation of the gallbladder and is usually associated with gallstone disease. However, approximately 10% of patients who present with acute cholecystitis will not have gallstones (acalculous cholecystitis).[9] Acalculous cholecystitis is more common in critically ill patients and is associated with a high morbidity and mortality.

Secondary infection and distention can occur if the cystic duct becomes obstructed. The most common organisms associated with the secondary infection include *Escherichia coli,* enterococcus, and *Klebsiella.* Cholecystitis can occur in both males and females. Obese, fair-skinned women of increasing age and parity may be at greater risk.

Symptoms include sudden-onset abdominal pain—usually after ingestion of fried or fatty foods. Pain is usually located in the epigastrium and/or right upper quadrant and may be referred to the right shoulder or supraclavicular area. Patients often describe the pain as steady and severe. Marked tenderness, inspiratory limitation on deep palpation under the right subcostal margin (Murphy's sign), and local and rebound tenderness may also be present. Low-grade fever (100.4°F [38°C]), tachycardia, nausea, vomiting, and flatulence are common findings. If the common bile duct is obstructed, the patient may appear slightly jaundiced. Clinical signs associated with obstructed bile flow include but are not limited to dark amber urine that foams when shaken, clay-colored stools, pruritus, and bleeding tendencies.

Diagnostic tests include urinalysis, CBC, serum electrolytes, BUN, creatinine, serum glucose, and serum bilirubin levels. A WBC count with differential often reflects leukocytosis with an increased number of band forms. The serum bilirubin level may be elevated. An elevated amylase level suggests pancreatitis rather than cholecystitis. Ultrasonography is extremely useful in the emergency setting for detection of a thickened gallbladder wall, gallstones, and pericholecystic fluid, but it may not detect smaller gallstones or sludge. A CT scan may reveal gallbladder wall edema and is useful when perforation is suspected or other diagnoses are considered. Patients with acute cholecystitis frequently require hospitalization. In these cases, a hepatobiliary iminodiacetic acid (HIDA) scan, also called cholescintigraphy, may be performed if the ultrasound scan result is negative.

Treatment of cholecystitis includes administration of IV crystalloid solution and medications for nausea and vomiting and pain. Monitor vital signs and intake and output. Broad-spectrum antibiotics are indicated for potential microbial infection. Definitive treatment for cholecystitis is surgery with traditional laparotomy or laparoscopic cholecystectomy.

Acute Pancreatitis

Acute pancreatitis is defined as an acute inflammatory process of the pancreas. The exact mechanism is not clear. Theories include bile or duodenal reflux, bacterial infection, pancreatic enzyme activation with autolysis, and ductal hypertension. Seventy to eighty percent of pancreatitis cases are due to gallstone disease or alcoholism.[10] Gallstone disease can result in ductal hypertension and pancreatic enzyme activation. Alcohol abuse causes toxic metabolites that injure the pancreas, leading to inflammation. Other causes include malignant strictures obstructing the pancreatic duct, chronic hypercalcemia, abdominal trauma, infections (e.g., mumps, cytomegalovirus infection), drugs such as antimetabolites, or toxins (e.g., organophosphate insecticides, scorpion venom). Regardless of mechanism, pancreatitis is characterized by the release of activated digestive enzymes into the pancreas and surrounding tissues. This leads to tissue damage in the pancreas, surrounding fat, and adjacent structures that results in a chemical type of burn and fluid loss, also known as third-space fluid loss. In response to the inflammation, inflammatory mediators are released into the circulation. This can also lead to systemic inflammatory response syndrome (SIRS). Complications of pancreatitis can include necrosis to segments of the pancreas, abscess formation, pseudocyst, and pulmonary capillary leak syndrome, resulting in respiratory distress syndrome.

A clinical hallmark found in 95% of patients with pancreatitis is abdominal pain, originating in the epigastric region and radiating to the back.[10] Abdominal tenderness, rebound, and guarding are common. Nausea, vomiting, and abdominal distention may be present. Patients may have a low-grade fever. Tachycardia and hypotension may be present due to the third-space fluid loss. Tachypnea is often the result of muscle splinting secondary to pain. Decreased gastric motility causes hypoactive or absent bowel sounds.

Certain laboratory values aid in the diagnosis of acute pancreatitis. Serum amylase and lipase values should be obtained in patients who are suspected of having pancreatitis. Additional serum assessments include blood glucose and triglycerides. Elevated serum amylase and lipase levels are frequently seen in pancreatitis. Amylase levels three times greater than the upper normal limit are highly suggestive of pancreatitis.[10] The amylase level may be normal in some patients with acute alcoholic pancreatitis. The lipase level is considered useful because it will stay elevated for several days after the onset of symptoms. The amylase level will lower at a faster rate compared with lipase. Leukocytosis, decreased hematocrit, hyperglycemia, and hypocalcemia may also be present. In some cases, the hematocrit may be high due to hemoconcentration from substantial third-space fluid loss.

Radiographic studies are useful in diagnosing acute pancreatitis. A chest radiograph may reveal pleural effusions or pulmonary infiltrates, and an ileus may be detected on abdominal radiographs. Abdominal ultrasonography can identify gallstones as an underlying cause. Abdominal CT scan may also contribute to the diagnosis of acute pancreatitis by identification of pancreatic edema or fluid around the pancreas.

Management includes maintaining strict NPO (nothing by mouth) status. Obtain IV access for fluid and electrolyte replacement with normal saline. Fluid resuscitation is a priority in patients with indicators of hypovolemia. Antiemetics are administered for nausea and vomiting and to minimize further fluid loss. Pain control with IV analgesics, usually narcotic, is a high priority for the patient with pancreatitis. Nasogastric suction helps alleviate nausea, vomiting, and abdominal distention. Ongoing monitoring of respiratory, cardiovascular, and renal functions is recommended. Antibiotic administration is generally limited to patients with some necrosis of the pancreas because they are at greater risk for infection.[10]

Diverticulitis

Diverticula are small pouches that develop in the large intestines secondary to aging (see Fig. 25.2). This condition, called diverticulosis, occurs in about half of all Americans aged 60 to 80 years and is found in almost all Americans older than age 80 years. Weakened areas that predispose the colon to herniation of inferior tissue layers in combination with a low-fiber diet lead to this primarily painless disorder. Less than 10% of patients with diverticulosis experience pain. However, pain is the most-reported complaint when diverticula become inflamed and diverticulitis develops. Inflammation develops when fecal material is trapped in the pouches, causing trauma to the intestinal lining, which ultimately leads to inflammation. Persistent pain associated with diverticulitis is localized in the left lower quadrant. Fever, chills, nausea, and vomiting are seen when infection is present. Other symptoms include cramping and constipation. Complications of diverticulitis include intestinal obstruction, hemorrhage, perforation, abscess, stricture, and fistula.[11]

Diagnostic evaluation includes CBC and urinalysis. Results of the CBC show a left shift resulting from infection. The presence of WBCs and red blood cells (RBCs) in urine is also a common finding. Supine and upright abdominal radiographs are obtained to rule out perforation or obstruction. Abdominal CT is the preferred diagnostic modality because it is more effective in identification of processes outside the colon's lumen (i.e., diverticulitis). Barium enema, endoscopy, and ultrasonography may also be used.

Treatment of patients with diverticulitis includes rehydration with a saline solution, resting the bowel by making the patient NPO, and inserting a gastric tube if persistent vomiting is present. Anticholinergics are used to reduce colonic spasms, with opiates reserved for more aggressive pain management. Oral or parenteral antibiotics may be given depending on clinical presentation. Emergent surgery is required when there is evidence of peritonitis.

Bowel or Esophageal Obstruction

Bowel obstruction occurs in either sex, at any age, and from a variety of causes. The most common cause is adhesions from previous abdominal surgery, followed by incarcerated inguinal hernia. Bowel obstruction can be caused by postoperative adhesions, foreign bodies, volvulus, intussusception, strictures, tumors, congenital adhesive bands, and fecal impaction.

Bowel obstructions are classified as mechanical or nonmechanical. Mechanical obstruction results from a disorder outside the intestines or blockage inside the lumen of the intestines. Intussusception, telescoping of the bowel within itself by peristalsis, is an example of a mechanical obstruction. Nonmechanical obstruction results when muscle activity of the intestine decreases and movement of contents slows (e.g., paralytic ileus).

When obstruction occurs, bowel contents accumulate above the obstruction. This leads to rapid accumulation of anaerobic and aerobic bacteria, which causes an increase in methane and hydrogen production. The more proximal the obstruction is, the quicker the onset of discomfort. Peristalsis increases, which leads to the increased release of secretions. These events worsen distention, cause bowel edema, and increase capillary permeability. Plasma leaks into the peritoneal cavity while fluid is trapped in the intestinal lumen, causing a decrease in the absorption of fluid and electrolytes.

Obstruction can be partial or complete. Strangulation with ischemia and necrosis almost always occurs in the setting of complete obstruction of the small intestines. Necrosis and perforation lead to peritonitis and sepsis.

Clinical signs vary with the location of the obstruction. With esophageal obstruction, patients may have the inability to swallow oral secretions, which may affect air patency. With intestinal obstruction, symptoms include colicky, crampy, intermittent, and wavelike abdominal pain. At times pain may be severe. Abdominal distention may also be present. Patients may have diffuse abdominal tenderness, rigidity, and constipation. Hyperactive bowel sounds or absent bowel sounds may be noted. The patient may also be febrile, tachycardic, and hypotensive with nausea and vomiting. Emesis usually has an odor of feces from proliferation of bacteria. Patients may pass some stool and flatus because the colon requires 12 to 24 hours to empty after the onset of a bowel obstruction.

Laboratory studies include CBC, BUN, serum glucose, electrolytes, serum creatinine, and arterial blood gas measurements. Leukocytosis with a left shift indicates strangulation and necrosis. The BUN may be elevated secondary to dehydration from vomiting and decreased oral intake. Metabolic acidosis can result if the bowel becomes ischemic. Metabolic alkalosis can occur in patients who have frequent emesis.[11] Upright abdominal radiographs may reveal dilated, fluid-filled loops of bowel with visible air-fluid levels. A CT scan may also be useful in determining the level and cause of obstruction. Patients with esophageal obstruction are usually able to report the cause and length of time the obstruction was present.

Treatment may include endoscopic evaluation. Similar to the treatment for other intestinal obstructions, management includes IV access for fluid and electrolyte replacement using crystalloid solution to maintain hemodynamic values and renal perfusion. Intake, output, and patient response to therapy should be monitored to prevent fluid overload. Frequently assess the abdomen for distention, tenderness, guarding to identify changes, and swallowing difficulty. A nasogastric tube may be inserted to decompress the stomach and reduce vomiting. Evaluate pain and swallowing and airway patency for worsening of the condition. Prophylactic administration of antibiotics is recommended. Surgical intervention may be required for some patients. Adults with intussusception and strangulated bowel will frequently have a laparotomy after fluid resuscitation and hemodynamic stability has been achieved. Life-threatening complications of bowel obstruction include peritonitis, bowel strangulation or perforation, renal insufficiency, aspiration, hypovolemia, intestinal ischemia or infarction, and death. Untreated obstruction that progresses to shock has a high mortality rate.[11]

Nausea, Vomiting, and Diarrhea

Nausea and vomiting with or without diarrhea is a frequent complaint of patients presenting to EDs. The etiologies for these symptoms vary from transient gastroenteritis to complications from cancer care. The ED nurse must be astute when completing the initial triage and assessment so that secondary sequelae, such as hypotension and shock, do not occur.

Cancer-Related Nausea and Vomiting

In recent years, the US Nationwide Emergency Department Sample database noted that 137.8 million ED visits occurred annually; of these, 1.6 million were due to nausea and vomiting.[12] Studies of ED use among patients with cancer are limited. The actual incidence of ED use is noted to be higher for patients with gynecologic or colon cancers, compared with those with breast, prostate, or lung cancers.[12] However, the actual number of cancer-related nausea and vomiting visits to the ED is unknown.[12] EDs affiliated with large cancer centers see many cases of cancer-associated nausea and vomiting, but presentations to EDs that are not cancer centers are becoming more prevalent due to increases in community-based cancer treatment and care.[13]

Cyclic Vomiting

Cyclic vomiting syndrome (CVS) is a chronic idiopathic functional GI disorder that is characterized by recurrent, stereotypical, disabling, discrete episodes of intense nausea and vomiting that last a few hours to days, interspersed with varying symptom-free intervals. Patients may also complain of abdominal pain and headache. This disorder is primarily recognized in children, with increasing recognition in adults. Although the exact etiology is unknown, some theorize that a dysfunctional brain-gut interaction involving corticotropin-releasing factor, dysregulation of the autonomic nervous system, and mitochondrial dysfunction may be the cause.[14,15] Additionally, this syndrome has been reported by individuals who frequently use narcotics and marijuana.[15]

Gastroenteritis

Acute gastroenteritis is one of the most common illnesses in children and adults. Gastroenteritis is an inflammation of the stomach and intestinal lining caused by viral, protozoal, bacterial, or parasitic agents. Viruses account for the majority of cases. Bacterial infection also accounts for acute diarrheal disease. Gastroenteritis may be caused by an imbalance of normal flora (*E. coli*) resulting from the ingestion of contaminated food. Patients have nausea, vomiting, diarrhea, and abdominal cramps. Hyperactive bowel sounds, fever, and headaches are also present. Anal excoriation occurs with frequent episodes of diarrhea.

For patients presenting with nausea and vomiting with or without diarrhea, triage should include assessing for signs and symptoms of dehydration, such as lethargy, decreased urinary output, dry mucous membranes, and tachycardia. Additionally, the nurse should obtain a detailed history defining signs/symptoms, length of symptoms, and medical treatment received (including the date/time of the last dose of chemotherapy and treatment provided at home or otherwise). A full set of vital signs should be obtained and frequently monitored in response to care and treatment provided in the ED. The patient should be asked about current WBC count and potential for neutropenia. All patients should be suspected to be neutropenic and isolated away from the general population.

Laboratory data include CBC, electrolytes, stool for ova and parasites, and stool culture. Obtain IV access for replacement of fluid and electrolytes. Administer antiemetics as ordered. Antibiotics are determined by patient history and presenting symptoms. Successful treatment is based on identifying the causative agent and resting the intestinal tract. Oral hydration with clear liquids is possible in most patients. Suggested fluids include cola, ginger ale, apple juice, tea, broth, and electrolyte replacement drinks such as Gatorade. Fluid replacement in children is critical to prevent dehydration. The BRAT diet (bananas, rice, applesauce, and toast) can be started as soon as diarrhea subsides. Feeding should begin as soon as possible in children and adults.

Peritonitis

Spontaneous bacterial peritonitis (SBP) is an acute bacterial infection of ascitic fluid in patients with liver disease. SBP occurs in up to a quarter of patients admitted with cirrhosis and ascites. Mortality is high in patients with cirrhosis. It is important to recognize SBP early in the course of infection because there is frequently a very short window of opportunity during which to intervene to ensure a good outcome. If the opportunity is missed, shock ensues, followed rapidly by multisystem organ failure.[16]

Peritonitis is a common and very serious problem for those individuals receiving peritoneal dialysis. Peritonitis is diagnosed when at least two of the following are present: abdominal pain; cloudy dialysis effluent; dialysis effluent WBC count above 100/µL or with over 50% of polymorphonuclear leukocytes in the differential count; and identification of infective organisms from dialysis effluent by Gram stain or culture.[16]

Assessment in the ED should include a comprehensive history because this guides the clinician to an accurate diagnosis. The nurse should obtain a medical, surgical, and social history. Patients with peritonitis may present with a constellation of symptoms including fever, abdominal tenderness, altered mental status, diarrhea, hypotension, hypothermia, and/or ileus. Abdominal assessment should be completed after the PQRST mnemonic. Frequent abdominal reassessment should occur while the patient remains in the ED. The nurse should obtain a complete set of vital signs, and these should be frequently monitored in response to treatment and to ascertain changes that may occur.

The nurse should anticipate that patients will undergo many diagnostic tests to clearly ascertain the cause of the pain. Among these tests are radiographic studies such as acute abdominal series or CT scan, CBC, comprehensive metabolic panel including amylase, lipase, alanine aminotransferase (ALT), aspartate aminotransferase (AST), and/or bilirubin. Blood and urine cultures should be collected consistent with each organization's protocols... and national sepsis guidelines. On the basis of the history, the nurse should anticipate the need to collect dialysis effluent or assist with a paracentesis for fluid analysis. Fluid resuscitation and support should be driven by the overall patient's status and the presence of any signs/symptoms of shock.

Once dialysis effluent or ascitic fluid is obtained, antibiotics should be administered. The patient receiving peritoneal dialysis should be administered intraperitoneal antibiotics, along with dialysis as the first-line treatment. However, if sepsis is present, IV antibiotics should be administered.[15] For patients diagnosed with peritonitis associated with liver failure, broad-spectrum antibiotic therapy should be administered until the results of cultures are received.

Acute Mesenteric Ischemia

Acute mesenteric ischemia (AMI) is typically defined as a group of diseases characterized by an interruption of the blood supply to varying portions of the small intestine, leading to ischemia and secondary inflammatory changes. If untreated, this process will eventuate in life-threatening intestinal necrosis.[17,18] These patients require rapid assessment and intervention to decrease mortality and morbidity.

The classic presentation for mesenteric ischemia is a sudden onset of abdominal pain, which may be associated with nausea, vomiting, and diarrhea. The abdominal pain will initially be severe and diffuse without any localization. One of the distinctive findings in mesenteric ischemia is that the abdominal pain is out of proportion to other examination findings. The patient may be screaming in pain, but the abdomen is soft, with no guarding or rebound. As the disease progresses and the bowel infarcts, the patient will develop abdominal distention with guarding, rebound, and absence of bowel sounds. Patients may develop abdominal wall rigidity. Bloody diarrhea and heme-positive stools are a late finding after the bowel has infarcted. See Table 25.2.

TABLE 25.2 Recognizing Mesenteric Ischemia.

Types	Mortality[a]	Signs/Symptoms	Risk Factors
Mesenteric artery embolus	High	• Acute onset of severe pain • Nausea/vomiting • Diarrhea with bloody stool • Abdominal distention • Peritonitis • Tachycardia, hypotension	• Arrhythmias, especially atrial fibrillation • Postmyocardial infarction with mural thrombi • Valvular heart disease • Structural heart defects • History of heart failure
Mesenteric artery thrombosis	High	• Pain progressively worsening to severe levels, especially after eating • Weight loss • Hesitation to eat/fear of eating • Nausea/vomiting • Abdominal distention • Peritonitis • Tachycardia, hypotension	• Atherosclerosis • Peripheral vascular disease • Geriatric • History of coronary artery disease • Tobacco use
Mesenteric vein thrombosis	Low	• Slow onset of vague pain • Nausea/vomiting • Peritonitis • Gastrointestinal bleeding in less than 20% of cases	• Hypercoagulable states • Recent abdominal surgery • Malignancy • Cirrhosis • History of pulmonary embolus or deep vein thrombosis (50% of cases)
Nonocclusive mesenteric ischemia	High	• Critically ill • Altered mental status • Abdominal distention and tenderness • Intolerance to eating • Peritonitis • Tachycardia, hypotension	• Cardiogenic shock • Congestive heart failure • Arrhythmias • Sepsis • Hypotensive states • Drugs causing mesenteric vasoconstriction

[a]Mortality: High = over 50%; Low = 20% to 50%.

Adapted from Bala M, Kashuk J, Moore EE, et al. Acute mesenteric ischemia: guidelines of the World Society of Emergency Surgery. *World J Emerg Surg.* 2017;12:38. https://doi.org/10.1186/s13017-017-0150-5

Long B, Koyfman A. The dangerous miss: recognizing acute mesenteric ischemia. Emergency Physicians Monthly website. http://epmonthly.com/article/the-dangerous-miss/. Published May 19, 2016. Accessed May 14, 2019.

A component of the initial evaluation for the patient with suspected mesenteric ischemia is the collection of laboratory tests, which include CBC, chemistry studies (including BUN and creatinine), coagulation panel, and type and crossmatch for blood products. The patient should be transported for radiographic studies while being hemodynamically monitored. Although CT scan of the abdomen with and without contrast media will initially be performed, it should be anticipated that this patient will require angiographic evaluation of major vessels to ascertain the location and potential treatment of occluded vessels. Frequent monitoring and assessment of vital signs and intake and output is required when caring for these patients because shock can occur abruptly. As ischemia advances and tissue necrosis occurs, rapid fluid resuscitation through a large board and the administration of broad-spectrum antibiotics will be required to stabilize the patient. If shock progresses, pressor support may be required to stabilize the patient. Invasive hemodynamic monitoring will be needed. Additionally, the nurse should have the patient ready for rapid transport to the operating room for definitive care and treatment.

SUMMARY

GI emergencies can be minor or life-threatening. Most GI emergencies present with similar clinical manifestations. Triage history and physical assessment play an important role in the management of patients with these conditions. Reassessment of signs and symptoms, such as quality and intensity of pain, vital signs, intake and output, and/or level of consciousness, should lead to rapid intervention by emergency nurses who provide care for patients with GI emergencies. The ability to differentiate GI emergency conditions requiring immediate attention is a requisite skill for the emergency nurse.

REFERENCES

1. Guyton AC, Hall GE. *Textbook of Medical Physiology*. Philadelphia, PA: Elsevier; 2006.
2. Macaluso CR, McNamara RM. Evaluation and management of acute abdominal pain in the emergency department. *Int J General Med*. 2012;5:789–797.
3. Bajaj J, Sanyal AJ. Methods to achieve hemostasis in patients with acute variceal hemorrhage. UpToDate website. https://www.uptodate.com/contents/methods-to-achieve-hemostasis-in-patients-with-acute-variceal-hemorrhage?-search=esophageal%20varices%20treatment&source=-search_result&selectedTitle=1~97&usage_type=default&display_rank=1. Updated May 5, 2017. Accessed May 14, 2019.
4. Quan S. Upper-gastrointestinal bleeding secondary to peptic ulcer disease: incidence and outcomes. *World J Gastroenterol*. 2014;20(46):17568–17577.
5. Guelrud M. Mallory-Weiss syndrome. UpToDate website. https://www.uptodate.com/contents/mallory-weiss-syndrome. Updated March 5, 2019. Accessed May 14, 2019.
6. Mugurma N, Kitamura S, Kimura T, Miyamoto H, Takayama TS. Endoscopic management of nonvariceal upper gastrointestinal bleeding: state of the art. *Clin Endosc*. 2015;48(2):96–101.
7. Strate L. Etiology of lower gastrointestinal bleeding in adults. UpToDate website. https://www.uptodate.com/contents/etiology-of-lower-gastrointestinal-bleeding-in-adults. Updated September 5, 2017. Accessed May 14, 2019.
8. Kahrilas PJ. Medical management of gastroesophageal reflux disease in adults. UpToDate website. https://www.uptodate.com/contents/medical-management-of-gastroesophageal-reflux-disease-in-adults#H671603146. Updated March 28, 2018. Accessed May 14, 2019.
9. Zakko SF. Acute cholecystitis: pathogenesis, clinical features, and diagnosis. UpToDate website. https://www.uptodate.com/contents/acute-cholecystitis-pathogenesis-clinical-features-and-diagnosis?search=algorithm%20for%20the%20diagnosis%20of%20acute%20cholecystitis&source=search_result&selectedTitle=1~150&usage_type=default&display_rank=1 updated Updated November 8, 2018. Accessed May 14, 2019.
10. Forsmark CE, Vege SS, Wilcox CM. Acute pancreatitis. *N Engl J Med*. 2016;375:1972–1981. https://doi.org/10.1056/NEJMra1505202.
11. Bordeianou L, Yeh DD. Overview of management of mechanical small bowel obstruction in adults. UpToDate website. https://www.uptodate.com/contents/overview-of-management-of-mechanical-small-bowel-obstruction-in-adults. Updated May 8, 2017. Accessed May 14, 2019.
12. Myer PA, Mannalithara A, Singh G, Singh G, Pasricha PJ, Ladabaum U. Clinical and economic burden of emergency department visits due to gastrointestinal diseases in the United States. *Am J Gastroenterol*. 2013;108(9):1496–1507.
13. Lash RS, Bell JF, Reed SC, Poghosvayn H. A systematic review of emergency department use among cancer patients. *Cancer Nurs*. 2017;40(2):135–144. https://doi.org/10.1097/NCC.0000000000000360.
14. Venkatesan T, Tarbell S, Adams K, et al. A survey of emergency department use in patients with cyclic vomiting syndrome. *BMC Emerg Med*. 2010;10:4.
15. Issenman R. A recurrent theme: a nationwide analysis of hospitalization for cyclic vomiting syndrome. *Dig Dis Sci*. 2017;62(8):1844–1846. https://doi.org/10.1007/s10620-017-4485-2.
16. Szeto CC. The new ISPD peritonitis guideline. *Renal Replacement Ther*. 2018;4:7. https://doi.org/10.1186/s41100-018-0150-2.
17. Bala M, Kashuk J, Moore EE, et al. Acute mesenteric ischemia: guidelines of the World Society of Emergency Surgery. *World J Emerg Surg*. 2017;12:38. https://doi.org/10.1186/s13017-017-0150-5.
18. Patel S. Mesenteric ischemia. *Clerkship Directors in Emergency Medicine (CDEM)*. 2018. https://www.saem.org/cdem/education/online-education/m4-curriculum/group-m4-gastrointestinal-mesenteric-ischemia. Accessed May 14, 2019.

26

Renal and Genitourinary Emergencies

Cynthia S. Baxter

Genitourinary (GU) problems are a common complaint in the emergency department (ED). In 2015 ED visits in the United States exceeded 2 million for urinary tract infections (UTIs) and 1 million for urinary calculi.[1] The incidence of end-stage renal disease (ESRD) is rising in all industrialized nations, and patients with complications of vascular or peritoneal access for life-sustaining dialysis treatments present to the ED for urgent and emergent intervention. Although they are not as common as UTIs or urinary calculi, the following GU conditions are considered emergent: testicular torsion with and without epididymitis-orchitis, priapism, rhabdomyolysis, and acute kidney injury.

ANATOMY AND PHYSIOLOGY

The GU tract consists of the kidneys, ureters, urinary bladder, urethra, and external genitalia. Urine is produced by the kidneys as a way to regulate fluid volume and acid-base and electrolyte balance. Ureters transport urine to the bladder for temporary storage. The urine is drained from the bladder to the outside by the urethra. External structures of the male GU system have reproductive functions.

The kidneys are located on the posterior abdominal wall behind the peritoneum on either side of the vertebral column inside the rib cage. The medial aspect of each kidney contains the hilum, where the renal artery and nerve enter and the renal vein and ureter exit. Blood flow to the kidney is supplied by the renal artery, which branches off the abdominal aorta and enters the kidney through the renal sinus. Blood leaves the kidney through the renal vein, which empties into the abdominal inferior vena cava.

The nephron, the functional unit of the kidney, is composed of the renal corpuscle, proximal convoluted tubule, Henle's loop, distal convoluted tubule, and collecting ducts. Each kidney contains an estimated 1 million nephrons individually capable of producing urine. These nephrons cannot be reproduced once destroyed. The renal corpuscle contains the glomerulus, a web of tightly convoluted capillaries, and Bowman's capsule, which surrounds and supports these structures. Blood flows through the afferent arteriole into the glomerulus and out the efferent arteriole. Renal blood flow accounts for 21% of cardiac output, or 1200 mL/min. Without adequate renal blood flow, the kidneys are unable to function adequately. Specialized cells called juxtaglomerular cells are located at the entrance to the glomerulus of the afferent arteriole in 15% of nephrons. These specialized cells sense changes in pressure and sodium concentration and play a role in the renin-angiotensin-aldosterone (RAA) system.

Filtration of plasma in the renal corpuscle is the first step in urine production and helps the kidneys rid the body of wastes and retain water and essential solutes. Pressure generated as blood courses through the tight web of capillaries in the glomerulus, along with oncotic pressure within the blood, is greater than pressure created by Bowman's capsule, so plasma or filtrate and small solutes cross the semipermeable epithelial capillary lining. Injury to the glomerulus, such as ischemia or inflammation, increases permeability of the capillary membrane and allows larger molecules (red blood cells [RBCs], epithelial casts, protein, or white blood cells [WBCs]) to cross. Decreased oncotic pressure, often the result of decreased serum albumin levels, or decreased pressure within the glomerulus produced by systemic hypotension decreases the glomerular filtration rate (GFR) and eventually urine output. GFR in the average adult is 125 mL/min or 180 L/day.

Tubules, Henle's loop, and collecting ducts excrete waste products (e.g., urea, nitrogen, creatinine, drug metabolites), reabsorb water and solutes (potassium, sodium, chloride, hydrogen, glucose, and amino acids) from filtrate, and secrete excess solutes the body does not need into filtrate. Osmosis, diffusion, and active transport occur between the nephron and surrounding capillaries. Hormonal control regulates reabsorption and secretion in the nephron.

The RAA system and antidiuretic hormone (ADH) are feedback-loop systems within the body that maintain homeostasis. Serum osmolarity increases and causes stimulation of the hypothalamus, which releases ADH. Nephron permeability increases, so additional water is absorbed, serum osmolarity returns to normal, and ADH release stops. Pressure changes in the glomerulus are overcome by vasodilation and constriction of the afferent arteriole by a process called autoregulation. This autoregulation keeps pressure in the glomerulus within a wide range of systolic blood pressures. When the range is exceeded, autoregulation fails and epithelial damage occurs, with eventual scarring and sclerosis followed by decreased permeability, GFR, and urine output. Inadequate nephron perfusion stimulates the juxtaglomerular apparatus to secrete renin that converts angiotensinogen to angiotensin

I, which stimulates aldosterone release from the adrenal cortex and reabsorption of sodium and water by the nephron. Conversion of angiotensin I to angiotensin II by an enzyme in the lung causes peripheral vasoconstriction. Perfusion increases to the nephron, and the cycle is altered.

Without a functioning kidney and adequate urine production, homeostasis is severely impaired. Fluid and electrolyte imbalance, accumulation of urea and creatinine, decreased excretion of drug metabolites, and inadequate reabsorption of amino acids and glucose occur. The kidneys help convert vitamin D into its active form to ensure calcium absorption from intestines and secrete erythropoietin for stimulation of RBC production in bone marrow. Consequently, altered renal function decreases bone mineralization and oxygen-carrying capacity of the blood.

The renal pelvis narrows to enter the ureter, where urine is moved to the bladder by peristaltic contractions. The muscular bladder stores urine until release to the urethra by the micturition reflex.

External genitalia are also part of the GU system. Female genitalia consist of the vestibule, the space into which the urethra and vagina open, and surrounding labia minora and majora. Anatomic position and the short length of the female urethra are responsible for the high frequency of UTIs in females.

Male external genitalia include the penis, scrotum, and scrotal contents. Scrotal contents include the testes, tubules that carry developing sperm cells and secrete testosterone, and the epididymis, which lies along the posterior testes and is the final maturation area for sperm. The prostate is glandular muscle tissue that surrounds the urethra at the base of the bladder. Enlargement of the prostate can cause outlet obstruction and urinary retention. The penis consists of three columns of erectile tissue that become engorged with blood, producing erection. Two columns of corpora cavernosa form the dorsum and sides of the penis, and the corpus spongiosum forms the base and glans. Clinical manifestations of GU disease frequently involve external genitalia.

PATIENT ASSESSMENT

Assessment of the GU system should determine history of hypertension, diabetes, previous infections, prostatitis, urethritis, bladder or urethral damage during childbirth, history of renal calculi, and recurrent UTIs. A detailed drug list, including prescription, over-the-counter (OTC), herbal preparations, and illicit drugs, should be obtained. Identification of any history of exposure to occupational chemicals or toxins may identify contact with substances that could cause nephrotoxicity. Sexual history should include discussion of risk factors that can cause GU symptoms (e.g., use of contraceptive jellies or creams, multiple partners, abnormal penile or vaginal discharges, unsafe sexual practices, history of sexually transmitted infections [STIs]). GU complaints often arise from changes in urinary patterns; for example, frequency, dysuria, urgency, dribbling, or incontinence.

Urinary disorders can be identified by the patient's own subjective interpretation (e.g., changes in output, voiding pattern, location of pain). Obtaining a urine sample for analysis can validate the nurse's suspicions. Gross visual examination for color, clarity, and amount should be done before urine is sent to the laboratory. Palpation and percussion of the kidneys may reveal costal vertebral tenderness, structural asymmetry, or the presence of masses.

Female patients, particularly those of reproductive age, warrant additional assessment for a broad spectrum of complaints. One should always consider the possibility of an unknown pregnancy and take a careful menstrual history, including use of contraceptives. If the patient is pregnant, fetal heart tones are assessed for presence, location, and rate. When a woman has a specific genital concern, a vaginal examination is indicated. Any discharge or bleeding should be noted and described by character and amount.

Males should be assessed for problems specific to their GU anatomy, including presence of a slow stream, inability to void, penile discharge, or warts.

Hematuria, the presence of blood in the urine, may be the primary complaint or may accompany other symptoms. A detailed medication and diet history may uncover other causes for discoloration of urine—foods such as beets, rhubarb, and blackberries, and medications such as phenytoin are common nonhematuric causes of red or dark urine. Hematuria can be confirmed by urinalysis (UA); however, microscopic hematuria on a single test is common. Early-stream hematuria suggests bleeding from the urethra, hematuria throughout the stream indicates upper GU tract bleeding, and bleeding at the end suggests bladder neck or urethral bleeding. Complete urinalysis and urine cytologic study may indicate the need for further diagnostic testing for urologic cancer, renal disease, infection, or renal calculi as the source of hematuria.

Pain should be assessed using the PQRST mnemonic—provocation, quality, region or radiation, severity, and time. The most severe pain associated with the GU system is renal colic caused by calculi. Increased pressure and dilation of the kidney and urinary collecting system cause sudden, unbearable pain. The patient usually presents with restlessness and pallor and complains of flank pain that often radiates to the abdomen and groin. If the stone lodges in the bladder, urinary frequency and urgency develop. Pain can cause tachypnea and tachycardia with elevated blood pressure. Oliguria, defined as urine output less than 400 mL in 24 hours, or anuria, less than 75 mL in 24 hours, may be the presenting symptom. The cause is usually obstruction; however, blood chemistry values should be evaluated for azotemia, which indicates renal failure from prolonged obstruction leading to hydronephrosis or other causes. If the patient has a urinary catheter in place, patency should be assessed. A physical examination can identify urinary retention by palpating the bladder as a firm mass above the symphysis pubis, with an urge to void on palpation; bladder scanning using ultrasonography may also be used to detect bladder distention. History should be obtained to identify drugs that contribute to retention, including OTC nasal decongestants containing anticholinergic ingredients. A neurologic examination should be performed to rule out spinal cord injury or disease that can interfere with the micturition reflex. The prostate is examined for enlargement as the cause of obstruction. After the patient has attempted to void, a urethral catheter may be inserted for residual volume. Bedside bladder ultrasonography may avoid the need for catheterization and allow assessment of prevoid and postvoid volume. If the catheter cannot be inserted without resistance, a suprapubic bladder tap or assistance from a urologist may be necessary. With a residual volume greater than 500 mL, the catheter may be left in place to allow the bladder to regain muscle tone. If residual volume is minimal, further diagnostic evaluation is aimed at identifying the cause.

SPECIFIC CONDITIONS

Acute Kidney Injury

Acute kidney injury (AKI) is an abrupt, usually reversible, decline in GFR. Classification, or more specific definitions of AKI, have been one of the focuses of the Acute Dialysis Quality Initiative (ADQI). The ADQI is an international, interdisciplinary group working to improve care in this population. In 2004 ADQI published the RIFLE criteria for classification of AKI (Table 26.1). Since then, two other scales have been developed by different groups but have not been as predictive or sensitive as the RIFLE criteria (Acute Kidney Injury Network [AKIN] and the Kidney Disease Improving Global Outcomes [KDIGO] definitions).[2] Because baseline values may not be available, the Cockcroft-Gault equation is used most often in the ED: GFR mL/min equals (140 – age in years)(weight in kg)(0.85 if female) divided by (72 × serum creatinine mol/L).[3] Azotemia, or uremia, refers to accumulation of nitrogen waste products in the blood. Acute azotemia generally refers to the patient with AKI, which usually develops over a period of days; however, patients with chronic renal failure (CRF) can experience acute episodes because of noncompliance or other medical conditions.

TABLE 26.1 RIFLE Criteria for Acute Renal Failure Classification.

Risk (R)	Increase serum creatinine level × 1.5 or decrease in GFR by 25%, or UO <0.5 mL/kg/h for 6 hours
Injury (I)	Increase serum creatinine level × 2 or decrease in GFR by 50%, or UO <0.5 mL/kg/h for 12 hours
Failure (F)	Increase serum creatinine level × 3 or decrease in GFR by 75%, or serum creatinine level ≥4 mg/dL; UO <0.3 mL/kg/h for 24 hours, or anuria for 12 hours
Loss (L)	Persistent ARF, complete loss of kidney function >4 weeks
End-stage kidney disease (E)	Loss of kidney function >3 months

ARF, Acute renal failure; *GFR,* glomerular filtration rate; *UO,* urine output.
Data from Hughes PJ. Classification systems for acute kidney injury. Medscape website. https://emedicine.medscape.com/article/1925597-overview. Updated August 7, 2018. Accessed May 14, 2019.

AKI has prerenal, intrarenal, or postrenal causes. Prerenal causes include syndromes that decrease blood flow to the kidney and therefore alter its ability to function. Those include hypovolemia, decreased cardiac output, decreased peripheral vascular resistance, or obstruction of the renal vascular system. Intrarenal complications cause damage to the kidney tubules (acute tubular necrosis) and include nephrotoxic agents (aminoglycosides, nonsteroidal antiinflammatory agents, contrast dye, crush injury, and rhabdomyolysis) or diseases damaging the vascular or interstitial tissue (hypertension, diabetes, lupus, and infectious processes). Postrenal causes result in obstruction of the urinary tract such as through calculi, prostatic hypertrophy, tumors, strictures, or neurologic causes affecting emptying of the urinary system. AKI is largely preventable. ED priorities are identification and treatment of the cause and presenting complications and removal of any active insults to the kidney. The most common cause of AKI is hypovolemia (volume depletion, third spacing, heart or liver failure, sepsis) or acute tubular necrosis (nephrotoxin exposure).

Symptoms of AKI include short-term weight gain or loss, nausea and vomiting, hematemesis, melena, dysrhythmias, dyspnea, stupor, or coma. Compromise of airway, breathing, circulation, and neurologic function requires intervention. Fever may be associated with infectious or inflammatory events. Fever reduction measures should be instituted to prevent the continued rise of nitrogenous waste products by catabolic effect of fever.

Hyperkalemia, hyponatremia, hypocalcemia, hyperphosphatemia, and volume depletion or overload (depending on cause) are the most common fluid and electrolyte imbalances resulting from loss of the kidney's ability to excrete potassium and phosphorus, conserve sodium, and eliminate excess volume. Calcium is inversely related to phosphorus. In renal failure, calcium levels decrease because of the rise in phosphorus and the inability of the kidney to convert vitamin D to its active form, which facilitates calcium absorption from the gut. The electrocardiogram (ECG) may reveal tall peaked T waves, widened QRS, and prolonged PR interval secondary to hyperkalemia.

Administration of intravenous (IV) calcium may be needed to antagonize the membrane and improve cardiac conductivity until removal of excess potassium by emergency dialysis can be initiated. IV calcium works within minutes, but duration is short, as evidenced by return of ECG changes. Administration of IV sodium bicarbonate ($NaHCO_3$), glucose, and insulin redistributes extracellular potassium into the intracellular fluid, works within 15 to 30 minutes, and lasts approximately 4 hours. Potassium can also be removed by cation exchange resin (e.g., sodium polystyrene sulfonate), but the onset of action is 60 minutes when given rectally and 120 minutes after oral administration. Urine output may be increased or decreased.

If AKI is nonoliguric, large volumes of fluid can be lost, so the patient may be dehydrated and hypotensive. Volume replacement with normal saline is recommended (1–3 L initially at 75–100 mL/h or more unless contraindicated by comorbidities) and is guided by outcome goals such as urine output and tissue oxygenation, jugular vein distention, lung auscultation, and vital signs. Invasive lines such as central venous pressure may be used for unstable patients.[4]

If AKI presents with oliguria, the patient may be volume overloaded and hypertensive, so minimal fluid is given until the volume can be removed by diuretics or through hemodialysis. Metabolic acidosis occurs because renal tubules can no longer regulate concentration of hydrogen ions. IV $NaHCO_3$ may be used unless contraindicated by volume status.

Indications for emergency dialysis include stupor or coma (caused by rising nitrogen waste products in the blood and metabolic changes), volume overload and pulmonary edema nonresponsive to diuretic therapy, and dangerous hyperkalemia and acidosis unresponsive to medical therapy. Emergency hemodialysis requires vascular access (usually a temporary femoral or subclavian dual-lumen catheter or internal shunt) and an artificial kidney (dialyzer) to act as a semipermeable membrane. The dialysate must be low in ions that the body needs to excrete and high in those to be reabsorbed. Hemodynamically unstable patients may require continuous renal replacement therapy in the intensive care unit.

After initial stabilization of the patient, history and diagnostic testing focus on identifying the cause of AKI. Tests include serial blood chemistry values, UA with sodium and potassium concentrations, chest radiograph, renal ultrasonography and Doppler studies, or computed tomography (CT) scan. Imaging procedures are usually done without contrast media because of toxic effects of the media on renal tubules. When contrast is needed, acetylcysteine or bicarbonate drip may be administered before and after the contrast study to minimize toxic renal effects.

Dialysis Access Complications

Chronic renal failure requiring dialysis is known as end-stage renal disease, or ESRD. Renal replacement therapy may be provided by peritoneal dialysis or hemodialysis. Peritoneal dialysis involves instilling 1 to 2 L of dialysate fluid containing varying amounts of glucose, magnesium, calcium, chloride, and lactate into the abdomen. The peritoneal membrane acts as a semipermeable pathway for exchange of solutes and water between the vascular peritoneal space and dialysate by osmosis and diffusion. Access to the peritoneal cavity is achieved through a plastic catheter held in place by a Dacron cuff.

Complications occurring early after surgical catheter insertion most commonly include pain, bleeding, obstruction (fluid unable to move in or out of the catheter), and infection and/or leaks.[5] Early complications are generally associated with misplacement of the catheter during insertion. Significant pain and bleeding are suspicious of perforation of an internal organ during placement. Obstruction may be related to a blockage or kink in the catheter, leaks are associated with weak abdominal wall structure or the need for placement adjustment. If early infection occurs beyond the exit site of the catheter, intraoperative contamination or perforation of the intestines may be the culprit. Late complications include pain, perforations, peritonitis, catheter obstruction, and herniation at the insertion site. Associated symptoms include abdominal pain, nausea and vomiting, fever, bleeding, distended abdomen, and cloudy dialysate fluid. Ultrasounds, or radiologic dye studies and a CT scan, may be used to further evaluate the exact cause of presenting compliant.

Depending on the infection, antibiotics may be added to the dialysate fluid or given orally or intervenously. For catheter placement complications, surgical correction may be required. For recurrent peritonitis for which antibiotic therapy is not successful, the catheter should be removed and hemodialysis initiated until peritonitis clears. Unless scarring impairs permeability of the peritoneal membrane, the catheter can be surgically replaced and peritoneal dialysis reinitiated. Care in the ED may include obtaining a sample of peritoneal fluid after installation of dialysate. During access of the peritoneal catheter, carefully adhering to aseptic technique, limiting and masking persons present in the room, and using sterile gloves to prevent contamination during access of the peritoneal catheter are extremely important to prevent infection and resultant peritonitis.

Clotted vascular access frequently brings patients with CRF to the ED. Arteriovenous fistulas are surgical connections of a native artery and vein in an extremity or insertion of Gore-Tex graft material to form the connection (Fig. 26.1). Available sites suitable for vascular access may become exhausted, so permanent subclavian dual-lumen catheters are also placed for hemodialysis. Clotted vascular access should be emergently declotted with use of locally instilled or infused fibrinolytics or surgery. Grafts, fistulas, and insertion sites also become infected and may progress to septicemia. Local symptoms include redness, drainage, or edema. Blood cultures and a complete blood count (CBC) should be obtained to rule out systemic infection. Access removal may be necessary, so temporary subclavian or femoral access (replaced every 2 or 3 days) can be used until blood is free of infection. Some type of anticoagulant will reside in the lumens of a dual-lumen dialysis catheter to prevent clotting. When accessing the catheter, failure to withdraw this anticoagulant could cause serious bleeding complications due to alteration of coagulation status.

Bleeding from vascular access sites (fistula, graph) is commonly encountered in the ED. During hemodialysis, the blood is anticoagulated with heparin to avoid clotting and blood loss during the procedure. Direct pressure that does not occlude the fistula or graph should be applied for 5 to 10 minutes. If direct pressure does not control bleeding, topical hemostatic agents may be used, such as Gelfoam pads (forms a mechanical matrix to enhance clot formation), chitosan (a fibrous complex carbohydrate that promotes adhesion), or thrombin powder. When applying a pressure dressing, avoid excess pressure and circumferential application of tape or other wrap because this may cause clotting of the vascular access. Anticoagulation studies may reveal that reversal of supratherapeutic anticoagulation is needed and protamine administration may be required.[5]

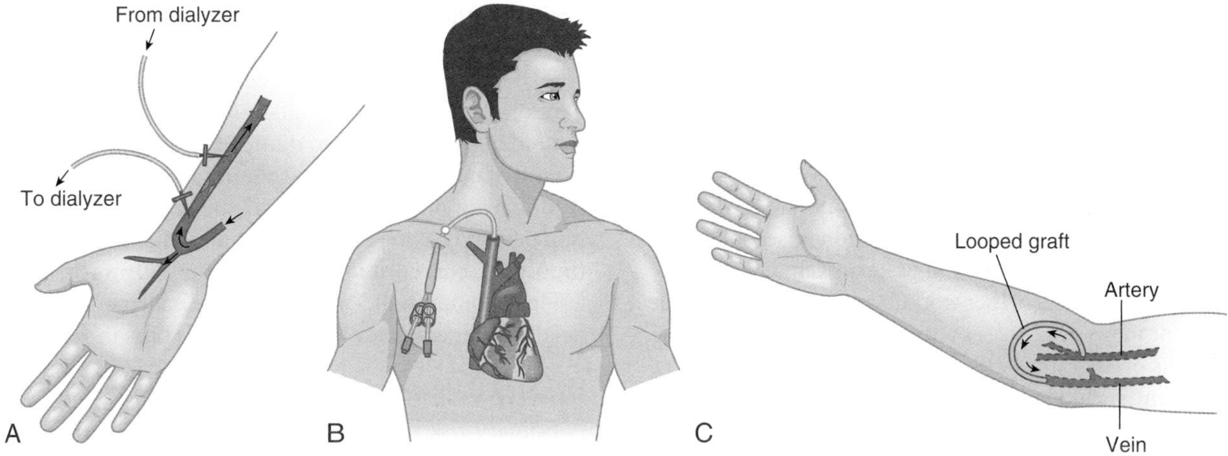

Fig. 26.1 Types of Access for Hemodialysis. (A) Forearm arteriovenous fistula. (B) Venous catheter for temporary hemodialysis access. (C) Artificial loop graft. (From National Institute of Diabetes and Digestive and Kidney Diseases. *Kidney Failure: Choosing a Treatment That's Right for You.* NIH Publication 00–2412. Bethesda, MD: National Institutes of Health; 2007.)

Rhabdomyolysis

Skeletal muscle destruction with subsequent release of myoglobin into the circulatory system causes rhabdomyolysis, which can lead to acute renal failure (ARF) from hypovolemia and obstructive tubular necrosis. There are many different causes, including crush injuries, drug or toxin ingestion (including the statin drug class for hypercholesterolemia as well as illicit drugs such as heroin, methadone, and stimulants), infection, burns, overexertion combined with use of nutritional supplements, or metabolic disturbances.[6] Crush injuries may be caused by entrapment, such as prolonged compression of the abdomen or a limb after a motor vehicle crash. Fluid shifts from the intravascular space into the interstitial space in the area of injury or systemically and can cause the patient to become profoundly hypovolemic, leading to decreased blood flow to the kidneys and resultant decrease in function. Electrolyte imbalances are also associated with the fluid shift. Hyperkalemia is predominant, but hypocalcemia and hyperuricemia are also present. There is an increase in serum creatine kinase (CK), blood urea nitrogen (BUN), creatinine, phosphate (PO_4), uric acid, aspartate aminotransferase (AST), and alanine aminotransferase (ALT). Urine will have a reddish-brown color as a result of myoglobinuria (brown urine and clear serum). Proteinuria and hematuria are noted on urinalysis; however, few or no RBCs are seen during microscopic examination.

Presenting signs and symptoms may include complaints of muscle aches or acute muscle pain but generally are nonspecific; rarely there is muscle edema unless compartment syndrome is also present. General malaise, fever, and muscle tenderness may occur, and other symptoms may be present based on the cause of rhabdomyolysis. Due to the nonspecific nature of most initial presentations, a good history is extremely helpful.

Treatment of rhabdomyolysis consists of volume replacement to prevent acute kidney injury, monitoring, and maintenance of electrolyte balance. Correcting volume depletion and using an osmotic diuretic such as mannitol, or diuretics, will increase the urine output and help flush myoglobin through the kidneys. Treatment also includes preventing myoglobin precipitation in the urine; therefore sodium bicarbonate is added to IV fluids to raise the pH of the urine and help increase excretion of myoglobin. If the patient progresses to AKI, hemodialysis may be considered.

Urinary Tract Infections

UTIs are classified as upper and lower, complicated and uncomplicated. Lower classification includes the bladder and urethra; upper includes the kidneys and ureter. Uncomplicated UTIs are those likely to improve with treatment, and complicated ones have an increased risk of failure with treatment due to comorbidities (diabetes, previous history of UTIs), pregnancy, anatomic abnormalities (including but not limited to vesicoureteral reflux, enlarged prostate, calculi), urinary tract instrumentation (i.e., catheter or stent), and infection associated with a hospital or nursing home.[7] The most common culprits for infection are the bacteria residing in the perineum and GU tract: staphylococcus, streptococcus, *Escherichia coli,* and other coliforms. UTIs of all types are more common in women and most likely associated with *E. coli.* Common symptoms of a lower UTI include signs of bladder and urethra irritability such as frequency, dysuria, urgency, microscopic hematuria, suprapubic discomfort, and cloudy urine. Upper UTI (pyelonephritis) symptoms include dull flank pain with or without costovertebral angle tenderness along with pyuria, gross hematuria, malodorous urine, chills and fever, leukocytosis, nausea, and vomiting. UTIs in children are not common but should be considered when there is irritability, decrease in appetite, and fever and should be triaged emergently because sepsis in infants may be present.

Diagnostic studies include testing a well-performed clean-catch urine specimen for uncomplicated lower UTIs. Urinalysis will be positive for leukocyte esterase and may also be positive for hematuria, WBCs, and trace protein. Other studies may also be performed in complicated lower and/or upper UTIs based on age, presenting symptom severity, and history including but not limited to urine culture and sensitivity (C&S), CBC with differential, glucose and electrolytes, BUN and creatinine, prostate studies, lumbar puncture in infants, and blood cultures. A kidneys-ureters-bladder (KUB) radiograph or ultrasound evaluation may be ordered and may show a hazy outline of the kidney secondary to edema. Ultrasound can be used in pregnant females to evaluate the GU structures. Further workup and admission may be required for more severe cases and may require cystogram or intravenous pyelogram (IVP).

Treatment includes antibiotics over a 3-day to 2-week period depending on upper or lower, complicated or uncomplicated cases. The most frequent antibiotics used, depending on local antibiogram studies for bacteria susceptibility, include ciprofloxacin, fluoroquinolones, and trimethoprim. Best practice is to administer the first dose of antibiotic in the ED before discharge or admission.

Interstitial Cystitis/Bladder Pain Syndrome

The signs and symptoms of interstitial cystitis/bladder pain (IC/BPS) vary from person to person and may vary over time but include a persistent, urgent need to void; minimal urine volumes with urination; suprapubic, perineal, or pelvic pain; and pain during intercourse. The most consistent feature of IC/BPS is increased discomfort with increased bladder filling. History may also reveal the need to void up to 60 times per day to relieve discomfort in addition to interruption of sleep to void. Women are affected five times more often than men, and IC/BPS is often associated with other chronic pain syndrome diagnoses such as irritable bowel syndrome or fibromyalgia.[8] IC/BPS is difficult to diagnose because other disorders, including UTIs, kidney stones, cancer, and STIs, are usually excluded before a diagnosis is made. Diagnosis occurs most often in women in their 30s or 40s.

Test results for UTIs will be negative; if hematuria is also present, cytology results will also be negative. Cystoscopy may be performed to observe the surface of the bladder for characteristic signs of cystitis, which include global inflammation and lesions. Although the cause is unknown, it is thought that there may be a defect in the epithelial lining of the bladder that allows irritants to penetrate the lining and activate the underlying nerve and muscle structures, causing further tissue damage. The care of the patient presenting to the ED without a current diagnosis of IC/BPS will focus on determining the differential diagnosis: infection due to urinary urgency symptoms or ruling out malignancy if hematuria is present. Postvoid bladder residual ultrasound may also be used to rule out obstruction.

Treatment focuses on symptom relief. Treatment in the ED will focus on pain management and referral to a urologist for more long-term therapy. Immediate treatment includes short-term oral analgesics and use of amitriptyline (to calm nerve irritation), pentosane polysulfate sodium (which is believed to provide a protective coating to the interior lining of the bladder), and antihistamines/leukotriene inhibitors (to reduce the inflammatory response). Application of warm or cold compresses to the perineal area may provide some relief. Long-term therapy includes keeping a dietary/voiding/pain diary to identify irritants in the diet or activity, having fluid management plans to dilute urine if concentrated urine is an irritant, using bladder training to suppress the urge to void, having physical therapy to strengthen the pelvic floor muscles, and having bladder procedures to infuse medication (lidocaine, corticosteroids, botulinum toxin) or to cauterize lesions. Common dietary irritants are caffeine, alcohol, artificial sweeteners, spicy foods, and foods high in vitamin C.[9]

Urinary Calculi

A primary risk factor for calculi is hypercalciuria; however, there is also an association with UTI, gout, excessive ingestion of certain foods, family history, dehydration, pregnancy, immobility, and warmer climates, which tend to produce more concentrated urine. Eighty percent of stones are composed of calcium combined with oxalate or phosphate; the remaining 25% are composed of struvite (associated with infection) or uric acid (associated with gout) and rarely cystine.[10] Calculi are asymptomatic until movement causes intermittent painful backache with radiation to the lower abdomen or groin, urge to void, dysuria, renal colic, and hematuria. Bacteremia and proteinuria may also be present. Diagnostic studies include CBC, BUN, creatinine, electrolytes, uric acid, UA with C&S, and helical CT scans. Helical CT has a 94% to 100% positive predictive value for urinary calculi and is currently the gold standard test for diagnosis. KUB, IVP, and ultrasound can also be used, especially in a pregnant female who cannot be scanned by CT. Fig. 26.2 shows a staghorn calculus on a KUB radiograph. Staghorn calculi can lead to decreased

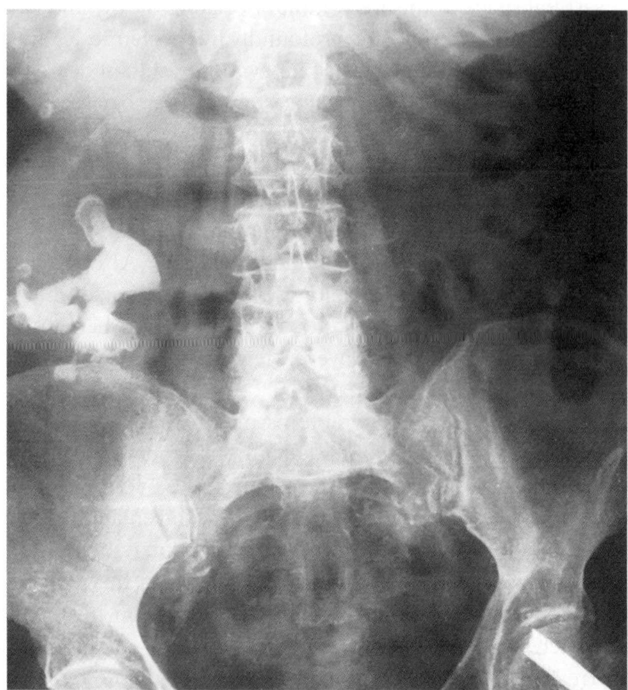

Fig. 26.2 Radiograph of a Staghorn Calculus. (Courtesy Harborview Medical Center, University of Washington, Seattle, WA.)

kidney function over time. Ninety percent of stones exit spontaneously; however, if unpassed, they may be removed by extracorporeal shock wave lithotripsy, percutaneous nephrolithotomy, or uteroscopy.

Nursing interventions include intake and output measurement, straining all urine, sending solid material for laboratory analysis, and increased fluids. Pain assessment and management are critical in these patients because of the severity of their pain. Narcotics such as morphine and hydromorphone hydrochloride may be used alone; however, combination with nonnarcotics such as ketorolac or other nonsteroidal antiinflammatory medication increases the effectiveness for most patients. Complications include ischemia at obstructive site, altered elimination, and UTI. Criteria for admission include need for frequent pain medicine, large-diameter stones, solitary kidney, ileus, bladder stones, and infection. If the patient is discharged, information should be provided about returning to the ED in case of increasing pain, vomiting, or fever and chills. Dietary restrictions should also be included for foods and drinks that contain high levels of calcium oxalate, such as beets, chocolate, coffee, cola, nuts, rhubarb, spinach, strawberries, tea, and wheat bran. Patients should be encouraged to drink large amounts of liquid, especially water, to facilitate passage of the remaining stones.

Testicular Torsion

Testicular torsion, the sudden twisting of the spermatic cord (usually internally), causes vascular compromise of the testes within 4 to 6 hours and can lead to infarction with resultant atrophy and loss of spermiogenesis.[11] Most cases occur at the beginning of adolescence; 50% occur during sleep and are associated with a congenital abnormality of the tunica vaginalis, the canal from which the testes descend. Cases can be associated with trauma to the testes, with significant swelling and sudden, rapid movement, and after heavy exercise. Clinical manifestations include upwardly retracted testes with redness and edema at the site of the torsion, abdominal pain, and nausea and vomiting. Fig. 26.3 compares normal testicular structures with testicular torsion. Manual detorsion under local anesthesia or surgery must be performed emergently to promote salvage of the involved testes. Prehn's sign may be helpful in differentiating testicular torsion from epididymitis. To assess for Prehn's sign, the scrotum is gently elevated to the level of the symphysis. In testicular torsion, pain increases; however, in epididymitis, a decrease in pain is noted. Prehn's sign is not always reliable, and definitive diagnosis is made with color Doppler ultrasonography showing decrease or absence of vascular flow. Management of the patient in the ED includes providing pain management, facilitating diagnostic and surgical interventions, and providing education about the plan of care and reassurance.

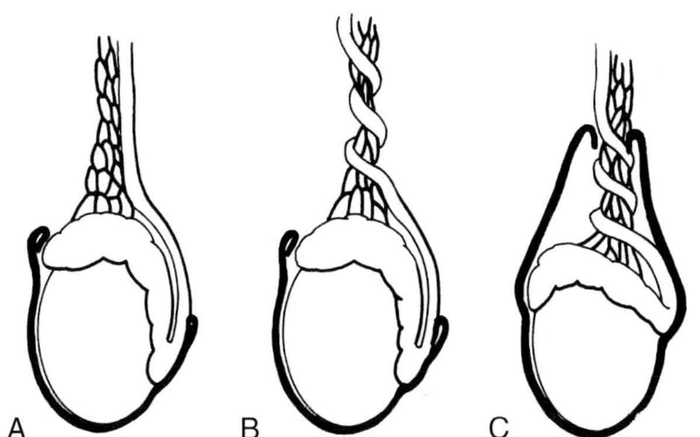

Fig. 26.3 Testicular Torsion. (A) Normal tunica vaginalis insertion. (B) Extravaginal torsion. (C) Intravaginal torsion with abnormally high vaginal insertion. (From Price SA, Wilson LM. *Pathophysiology: Clinical Concepts of Disease Processes.* 6th ed. St Louis, MO: Mosby; 2003.)

Epididymitis-Orchitis

The epididymis is a long tube located in the back of the testicle and is connected to the bladder via the vas deferens. It stores and carries sperm. Acute epididymitis results from inflammation of the epididymis predominately secondary to an STI. It is most common in sexually active males between 18 and 35 years old; the causative organism in this age-group is most often chlamydia or mycoplasma, rarely gonorrhea. It can also be caused by infection of the prostate gland or recent catheter use; this cause is more common in males aged 35 to 40 years. If the infection extends beyond the epididymis into the testes, it is termed epididymitis-orchitis. Orchitis alone is sudden swelling of the testes and is uncommon but occurs in one-third of males who contract the mump virus postpuberty; there is no spread to the epididymis. Extreme physical strain or exertion can also cause epididymitis but is not common.[12]

Signs and symptoms of epididymitis include severe scrotal pain, which can radiate into the abdomen, tenderness along the spermatic cord, edema, fever, pyuria, and possibly, urethral discharge. Orchitis will not present with urethral discharge. A positive Prehn's sign may also be observed. Diagnostic studies in the ED may include urinalysis, swab for sexually transmitted disease, and ultrasound of the testicle for differential diagnosis. Treatment depends on the cause and may include 1 to 2 weeks of antibiotic therapy, rest, medication for pain and swelling relief (most commonly nonsteroidal antiinflammatory drugs), ice used intermittently, and scrotal elevation. Rarely, hospitalization is required; it is associated with high fever and persistent nausea and vomiting and thus the need for short-term IV antibiotics.

Priapism

Priapism is a persistent, painful erection not associated with sexual desire. Engorgement is limited to the two corpora cavernosa; the corpus spongiosum and glans are not involved. Obstruction of venous drainage causes buildup of viscous deoxygenated blood, interstitial edema, and eventual fibrosis. Pain severity increases with duration. Tissue destruction begins within 4 to 6 hours of the onset of erection and leads to irreversible damage within 24 to 48 hours in ischemic priaprism.[13] With urinary obstruction and bladder distention, pain can last as long as 24 hours. Most common causes are sickle cell crisis, previous treatment of priapism (needle injury and intrapenile injection of medication), medications (antidepressants, antihypertensives), spinal cord injury, and prolonged sexual activity. Sildenafil and tadalafil are not associated with an increased incidence of priapism unless taken concomitantly with a prostaglandin inhibitor.

Ultrasound of the penis cavities will determine whether the priapism is ischemic or nonischemic. Ischemic priapism is a low–blood flow obstructive condition and can lead to compartment syndrome, tissue destruction, and loss of ability to gain an erection long term, sometimes as soon as 24 hours after erection. Nonischemic priapism is much less common and is associated with adequate blood flow, oxygenation, and usually a congenital shunt. Ischemic priapism is an emergency; pain increases with the length of time of erection. Treatment is focused on pain management and reversal of the erection. Acute detumescence is accomplished by using a large-bore needle after a regional nerve block or moderate sedation to remove blood and injection of an adrenergic agent, such as 5% phenylephrine. If acute detumescence fails, surgical stenting may be necessary to relieve obstruction. If undiagnosed sickle cell is suspected, a CBC with increased reticulocyte count may identify sickling cells as the underlying cause, so supplemental oxygen along with transfusion may be effective.

Sexually Transmitted Infections (Excluding Human Immunodeficiency Virus)

STIs spread through intimate sexual contact can present with a variety of symptoms. Risk factors include having multiple sexual partners or a new sexual partner within the last 60 days, not using condoms in nonmonogamous sexual relationships, trading sex for money or drugs, having sex with sex workers, and having anonymous sexual partners. Risk groups include men aged 15 to 24 years, men who have sex with men (MSM), and men with a history of prior STI, unmarried status, residence at a correctional facility, and illicit drug use.[14]

A careful history should be obtained in a nonjudgmental manner to gather as much information as possible to determine subsequent testing and treatment. Treatment goals are to treat the current episode, identify others at risk, and prevent further spread to other sexual partners. Left untreated, STIs can lead to further complications such as pelvic inflammatory disease, infertility, inflammatory diseases of the urinary and reproductive tracts, and endocarditis. History should include sexual practices, characteristics of any symptoms, current and past sexual partners, last menstrual cycle, and any history of previous STI. Symptoms may include discharge, pruritus, lesions, and/or burning from the vagina, penis, rectum, perineum, and oral sites.

A pelvic examination may be performed with warm water used as the only lubricant to avoid contamination of the specimen. Additional testing and general treatment[15] is listed in Table 26.2. Discharge teaching should include abstinence until treatment is completed and lesions are healed, the need for partner notification and treatment, the use of latex condoms, the importance of follow-up referral, and reporting as required by the local public health department.

PREVENTION

Disturbances involving the GU system range from life and tissue threats to communicable infections. One common denominator many of these emergencies share is that they are

TABLE 26.2 Sexually Transmitted Infections (Risk Groups, Testing, and Treatment).

Infection	Testing	Treatment
Syphilis	Serologic testing (blood)	Benzathine penicillin, doxycycline, tetracycline
Hepatitis viruses	Hepatitis B virus: antibody and antigen testing (blood) Hepatitis C virus: antibody (blood)	Postexposure prophylaxis (A & B): administer immunoglobulin and vaccine or administer booster if previously vaccinated Hepatitis C: postexposure treatment not recommended
N. gonorrhoeae *C. trachomatis*	Men (preferred): nucleic acid amplification testing (NAAT) Women (preferred): vaginal swabs May include swabs for rectal, cervical, oropharyngeal, urethral	Gonorrhea: ceftriaxone, cefixime, ciprofloxacin, ofloxacin, levofloxacin Chlamydia: azithromycin, doxycycline, erythromycin
T. vaginalis	NAAT urine testing or vaginal swabs	Antifungals: metronidazole, tinidazole
Herpes	Virologic culture swab	Acyclovir, famciclovir, valacyclovir antivirals
Human papillomavirus (HPV) infection and genital warts	Cytology swabs of cervix (Pap smear)	External warts: podofilox solution, imiquimod cream Provider administered: podophyllum resin, cryotherapy

Data from Ghanem K, Tuddenham S. Screening for sexually transmitted infections. UpToDate website. https://www.uptodate.com/contents/screening-for-sexually-transmitted-infections?search=sexually%20transmitted%20disease&source=search_result&selectedTitle=1~150&usage_type=default&display_rank=1. Updated December 7, 2017. Accessed May 14, 2019.
Workowski KA, Bolan GA. Sexually Transmitted Diseases Treatment Guidelines. 2015. *MMWR Recomm Rep.* 2015;64(RR-03):1–137.

preventable. Safe-sex practices decrease the incidence of STIs; dietary modifications may reduce the number of recurrent urinary calculi and UTIs; and changes in hygienic practices may also be helpful. Individuals who control their diabetes, hypertension, and heart failure reduce their risk for developing ESRD. ED nurses play a pivotal role in initiating strategies to protect patients from ARF: maintaining adequate intravascular volume, supporting/normalizing blood pressure, and minimizing exposure to nephrotoxic agents.

SUMMARY

GU emergencies require evaluation of renal function to rule out renal involvement. The GU system functions to maintain homeostasis, so disruption of renal function interrupts almost all organ systems. Emerging strains of resistant bacteria are challenging health care professions in treatment and prevention. Public education regarding safe sexual practice should be included in all discharge teaching for STIs. The emergency nurse has many opportunities to play an important role in the detection and prevention of GU diseases.

REFERENCES

1. Centers for Disease Control and Prevention. National Hospital Ambulatory Medical Care Survey: 2015 ED Summary Tables. https://www.cdc.gov/nchs/data/nhamcs/web_tables/2015_ed_web_tables.pdf. Published 2015. Accessed May 14, 2019.
2. Hughes PJ. Classification Systems for Acute Kidney Injury. Medscape website. https://emedicine.medscape.com/article/1925597-overview Updated August 7, 2018. Accessed May 14, 2019.
3. Okusa M, Rosher MH. Overview of the management of acute kidney injury in adults. UpToDate website. https://www.uptodate.com/contents/overview-of-the-management-of-acute-kidney-injury-in-adults?search=acute%20renal%20failure&source=search_result&selectedTitle=1~150&usage_type=default&display_rank=1. Updated November 16, 2017. Accessed May 14, 2019.
4. Simon E. The dialysis patient: managing fistula complications in the emergency department. Emdocs website. http://www.emdocs.net/dialysis-patient-managing-fistula-complications-emergency-department/. Updated September 18, 2016. Accessed May 14, 2019.
5. Fresenius Medical Care. Complications of PD catheters. https://www.advancedrenaleducation.com/content/complications-pd-catheters. Updated July 2016. Accessed May 14, 2019.
6. De Guzman MM, Jung LK, Muscal E. Rhabdomyolysis treatment and management. Medscape website. https://emedicine.medscape.com/article/1007814-treatment. Updated October 14, 2018. Accessed May 14, 2019.
7. Best J, Ou D, Kitlowski A, Bedolla J. Diagnosis and management of urinary tract infections in the emergency department. Emergency Medicine Practice (EBMedicine.net) website. https://www.ebmedicine.net/topics.php?paction=showTopic&topic_id=412. Published July 2, 2014. Accessed May 14, 2019.
8. Clemens JQ. Management of interstitial cystitis/bladder pain syndrome. UpToDate website. https://www.uptodate.com/contents/management-of-interstitial-cystitis-bladder-pain-syndrome?sectionName=THIRD-LINE%20THERAPY&topicRef=8085&anchor=H12621896&source=see_link#H12621896. Updated April 18, 2018. Accessed May 14, 2019.
9. Clemens JQ. Pathogenesis, clinical features, and diagnosis of interstitial cystitis/bladder pain syndrome. UpToDate website. https://www.uptodate.com/contents/pathogenesis-clinical-features-and-diagnosis-of-interstitial-cystitis-bladder-pain-syndrome?search=interstitial%20cystitis&source=search_result&selectedTitle=2~150&usage_type=default&display_rank=2. Updated October 17, 2017. Accessed May 14, 2019.
10. Curhan G, Aronson MD, Preminger GM. Diagnosis and acute management of suspected nephrolithiasis in adults. UpToDate website. https://www.uptodate.com/contents/diagnosis-and-acute-management-of-suspected-nephrolithiasis-in-adults?search=nephrolithiasis%20adult&source=search_result&selectedTitle=1~150&usage_type=default&display_rank=1. Updated September 21, 2018. Accessed May 14, 2019.
11. Medline Plus. Testicular torsion. Medline Plus website. https://medlineplus.gov/ency/article/000517.htm. Updated August 26, 2017. Accessed May 14, 2019.
12. Urology Care Foundation. What are epididymitis and orchitis? http://www.urologyhealth.org/urologic-conditions/epididymitis-and-orchitis. Accessed May 14, 2019.
13. Deveci S. Priapism. UpToDate website. https://www.uptodate.com/contents/priapism?search=priapism&source=search_result&selectedTitle=1~150&usage_type=default&display_rank=1. Updated November 15, 2017. May 14, 2019.
14. Ghanem K, Tuddenham S. Screening for sexually transmitted infections. UpToDate website. https://www.uptodate.com/contents/screening-for-sexually-transmitted-infections?search=sexually%20transmitted%20disease&source=search_result&selectedTitle=1~150&usage_type=default&display_rank=1. Updated December 7, 2017. Accessed May 14, 2019.
15. Workowski KA, Bolan GA. Sexually transmitted diseases treatment guidelines, 2015. *MMWR Recomm Rep*. 2015;64(RR-03):1–137.

27

Obstetric and Gynecologic Emergencies

Kathleen Sanders Jordan

Patients with obstetric and gynecologic disorders are frequently seen in the emergency department (ED). The ED nurse must have a strong knowledge base of the normal anatomy and physiology of the female reproductive system to accurately assess and provide care for this patient population. Patients with obstetric and gynecologic disorders may not disclose all of their concerns and symptoms. This could be due to a variety of reasons, including embarrassment or lack of knowledge regarding their own anatomy and physiology. Age, marital status, socioeconomic status, social support systems, and religious and cultural beliefs may also be key factors in preventing a female patient from seeking care or openly discussing problems related to the reproductive system.

ANATOMY AND PHYSIOLOGY

Obstetric and gynecologic emergencies can affect any organ in the internal or external female reproductive system. The internal reproductive organs include the vagina, cervix, uterus, fallopian tubes, and ovaries. The external genitalia include the mons pubis, labia majora and minora, clitoris, vestibular glands, hymen, vaginal orifice, urethral orifice, and the ducts of Bartholin's and Skene's glands. The perineum is the triangular area between the posterior portion of the vestibule and the anus that anatomically supports portions of the urogenital and gastrointestinal tracts.

The ovaries, fallopian tubes, and uterus are located inside the peritoneal cavity. The ovaries are bilateral oval structures, located between the uterus and lateral pelvic wall. Size of ovaries diminishes significantly after menopause. The number of ova present in the ovaries also decreases with age—from approximately 2 million at birth to 300,000 to 400,000 by puberty. During ovulation, each ovary releases a single ovum to be transported down the fallopian tubes to the uterus. The fallopian tubes (approximately 10 cm long) transport the ovum to the uterus through smooth muscle contraction. These bilateral tubes are not contiguous with the ovaries; consequently, the ovum can migrate into the peritoneal cavity. This is the basic mechanism leading to endometriosis and to ectopic pregnancy in the peritoneal space.

The uterus is a thick-walled organ shaped like an inverted pear. It is suspended in the anterior pelvis above the bladder and in front of the rectum and lengthens after pregnancy. A layer of peritoneum covers the superior portion of the uterus and forms the serous layer of the uterine wall. The middle layer of the uterine wall consists of smooth muscle with an inner mucous lining called the endometrium. The lower portion of the uterus is referred to as the cervix and provides entrance into the uterus. It is located in the vagina between the bladder on the anterior aspect and the rectum posteriorly. The top of the uterus is called the fundus.

The female reproductive cycle consists of ovulation and menstruation, with each cycle determined by the level of female hormones. Changes in hormone levels prepare the endometrium for implantation of a fertilized ovum. If the ovum is not fertilized, the endometrium sheds the inner lining as menstrual flow. A normal menstrual cycle occurs every 21 to 45 days (average of 28 days for most females), with menstruation lasting from 2 to 7 days; an average of 25 to 60 mL of blood is lost with each cycle.[1]

ASSESSMENT

An accurate history is critical to the assessment process. A patient's behavior during the assessment process may provide important clues as to the patient's feelings and attitudes regarding her illness. Pain and emotions related to one's reproductive organs and sexuality may cause a great deal of anxiety and fear for patients. The ED nurse must create an environment to establish rapport and ensure confidentiality with each individual patient to facilitate the discussion of this sensitive material. When obtaining a sexual history, a patient should be interviewed alone. All states allow minors to consent to diagnosis and treatment of sexually transmitted infections (STIs). Essential components of the history include chief complaint, pain assessment (onset, location, duration, character, aggravating factors, relieving factors, and timing), presence of vaginal bleeding, presence of vaginal discharge, menstrual history, obstetric history, sexual history, medical/surgical history, and medications and allergies. All female patients of reproductive age should be considered pregnant until pregnancy has been ruled out through a urine or serum pregnancy test. See Table 27.1 for physiologic changes related to pregnancy to consider during assessment. History of sexual activity and menstrual history should never be relied on to exclude pregnancy. Box 27.1 summarizes essential interview questions for this patient population.

TABLE 27.1 Physiologic Changes Related to Pregnancy.

Body System	Changes
Cardiovascular	Cardiac output increases 30%–40% by week 27. Placental blood flow is 625–650 mL/min. Blood volume increases by 30%.
Respiratory	Heart rate increases throughout pregnancy. Respiratory rate increases. Oxygen consumption increases by 20%. Minute volume increases by 50%. Arterial Pco_2 decreases secondary to hyperventilation.
Urinary	Rate of urine formation increases slightly. Sodium, chloride, and water reabsorption increases as much as 50%. Glomerular filtration rate increases about 50%.
Gastrointestinal	Smooth muscle relaxes, which increases gastric emptying time. Intestines are relocated to the upper abdomen.
Other	Anemia develops because of increased iron requirements by mother and fetus.

Pco_2, Pressure of carbon dioxide.

BOX 27.1 Interview Questions for Obstetric and Gynecologic Emergencies.

When was your last menstrual period? Was it normal?
How long does your period normally last?
Are you bleeding now? How much are you bleeding? How many pads or tampons have you used in the last hour? Are there any clots or tissue?
Is there a possibility you are pregnant?
If yes, when are you due and what prenatal care have you had?
How many pregnancies have you had? How many children do you have?
Do you normally have a vaginal discharge? Amount, color, odor, itching, burning? Is there anything different about your discharge today?
Are you having any bleeding, discharge, or tissue present vaginally?
Do you have any swelling, itching, redness, or pain?
Are you having other symptoms or problems, such as abdominal pain, urinary symptoms, nausea, or vomiting?
Are you sexually active?
Do you have sex with men, women, or both?
In the past 2 months, how many partners have you had sex with?
Have you ever had a sexually transmitted infection?
What type of birth control do you use? Do you consistently use it?
Do you know your blood type and Rh factor?

Patients with obstetric and gynecologic emergencies can experience significant blood loss and hypovolemia. The physical examination must include a general survey consisting of the patient's general appearance; vital signs; skin color, moisture, and temperature; and cardiovascular and respiratory status. A focused assessment should include examination of the abdominal and genitourinary systems. The abdomen should be inspected, bowel sounds auscultated, and the entire abdomen palpated for areas of tenderness, masses, and signs of peritonitis. A complete pelvic examination should be performed, including assessment of the external genitalia, vagina, and bimanual examination of the uterus and ovaries; a speculum examination is commonly performed. Specimens should be obtained for STI screening (e.g., chlamydial infection, gonorrhea, and trichomoniasis) and wet mount (i.e., normal saline and potassium hydroxide [KOH] for bacterial vaginosis and candida).

Diagnostic tests indicated for the patient with a gynecologic emergency should include a urinalysis and urine or serum tests. A catheterized urine specimen should be obtained if the patient is bleeding from the vagina. Other indicated laboratory tests include a complete blood count (CBC), prothrombin time (PT), activated partial thromboplastin time (aPTT), serum electrolyte levels, blood type and crossmatch, and C-reactive protein. Transabdominal and transvaginal ultrasonography, abdominal and pelvic computed tomography (CT), and magnetic resonance imaging (MRI) may also be useful diagnostic tests for evaluating masses and abscesses.

FIRST-TRIMESTER EMERGENCIES

Ectopic Pregnancy

Ectopic pregnancy occurs when the fertilized ovum implants anywhere other than the endometrium, such as in the fallopian tube, ovary, or abdominal cavity. Ninety-five percent of all ectopic pregnancies occur in one of the fallopian tubes, with the most common site for implantation being the ampulla, followed by the isthmus[1] (Fig. 27.1). The ovum begins to grow but may rupture, usually after the 12th week of pregnancy. Ectopic pregnancy is one of the major causes of maternal death, usually from hemorrhage.

Ectopic pregnancies often result from scarring caused by a past infection in the fallopian tubes, surgery on the fallopian tubes, or a previous ectopic pregnancy. Up to 50% of women who have ectopic pregnancies have a past history of inflammation of the fallopian tubes (salpingitis) or pelvic inflammatory disease (PID). Common presenting complaints include pelvic pain and/or vaginal bleeding. Pain may be described as mild to severe. If the ectopic pregnancy is leaking or has ruptured, the diaphragm may become irritated from blood in the peritoneum, causing referred pain to the shoulder (Kehr sign).

A pregnancy test should be obtained on all women presenting with pelvic pain and vaginal bleeding or spotting. A pelvic examination is done to evaluate the cervical os and identify the amount and source of bleeding. Bimanual pelvic examination defines uterine size and allows for identification of adnexal pain and palpation of masses outside the uterus.

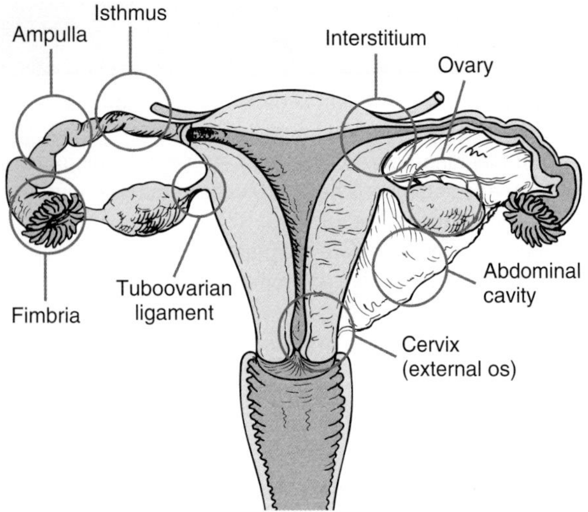

Fig. 27.1 Sites of Implantation of Ectopic Pregnancies. Order of frequency of occurrence is ampulla, isthmus, interstitium, fimbria, tuboovarian ligament, ovary, abdominal cavity, and cervix (external os). (From Lewis SL, Heitkemper MM, Dirksen SR et al: *Medical-Surgical Nursing: Assessment and Management of Clinical Problems*. 7th ed. St Louis, MO: Mosby; 2007.)

TABLE 27.2 Types of Abortion.

Type	Signs and Symptoms
Threatened	Vaginal bleeding Mild abdominal cramping Closed or slightly open os
Inevitable	Heavy vaginal bleeding Severe abdominal cramping Open os
Incomplete	Heavy vaginal bleeding Abdominal cramping Some products of conception retained
Complete	Slight vaginal bleeding No abdominal cramping All products of conception passed
Missed	Usually no maternal symptoms Discrepancy in fetal size compared with dates
Septic	Severe abdominal pain High temperature Malodorous vaginal discharge

If an ectopic pregnancy is suspected, intravenous (IV) access should be established with a large-bore IV catheter in anticipation of potential life-threatening hemorrhage. Quantitative serum β-human chorionic gonadotropin (β-hCG) level, complete blood count (CBC), and type and screen should be obtained. A transabdominal and transvaginal ultrasound is done to assist in differentiating and identifying an ectopic pregnancy.

Treatment for ectopic pregnancy includes nonoperative and operative interventions. For selected cases, ectopic pregnancy can be medically managed as an alternative to surgery. Methotrexate, a folic acid antagonist inhibiting further duplication of fetal cells, is administered intramuscularly, and the patient is followed as an outpatient with serial β-hCG levels.[2] Occasionally β-hCG levels do not fall, so additional methotrexate injections may be necessary. Operative interventions are indicated when the ectopic pregnancy has ruptured, the patient is in shock, or nonoperative interventions are unsuccessful or not appropriate.

In addition to assessment and intervention for physiologic needs, the emergency nurse must recognize the necessity of emotional support for the patient and the family. The patient may fear for her life and her future childbearing ability, feel concern because the pregnancy is not normal, or experience personal guilt related to the pregnancy.

Abortion

Abortion is defined as any interruption in pregnancy occurring before the fetus is viable. Fetal viability is usually between 20 and 24 weeks' gestation or fetal weight of 500 g. This can occur spontaneously, as a miscarriage, or be artificially induced by chemical, surgical, or other means.

Abortion is the number one cause of vaginal bleeding in women of childbearing years, with an estimated 20% to 40% of all pregnancies resulting in spontaneous abortion. This is one of the differential diagnoses for any woman of childbearing years with vaginal bleeding. Table 27.2 summarizes the types of abortion. Causes of spontaneous abortion include infection, injury, and an incompetent cervix. Many times the exact cause of a spontaneous abortion is not known.

The patient presents to the ED complaining of vaginal bleeding and pelvic pain. A missed period may or may not be reported. Gynecologic history should be elicited from the patient, including amount of bleeding.

Obtain a urine pregnancy test or serum quantitative or qualitative β-hCG level. Palpate the patient's lower abdomen for pain or tenderness, which may indicate an ectopic pregnancy. A pelvic examination should be performed to assist in determining the source of bleeding, visualize any products of conception, and assess for dilatation of the cervical os. A bimanual examination is performed to determine the size and tenderness of the uterus and tenderness of other reproductive organs. Transvaginal ultrasound is indicated to evaluate the status of the pregnancy and to exclude ectopic pregnancy.

Therapeutic interventions depend on the type of abortion. Fifty percent of threatened abortions result in complete or incomplete abortion within a few hours. A patient with a threatened abortion should be observed closely for changes in hemodynamic status. Document the amount of blood loss. If the patient exhibits signs of shock, replace blood loss with fluids or blood. Provide emotional support to the patient, significant other, and family.

If the abortion is inevitable or incomplete, obtain blood for CBC, Rh type, and type and screen. Start at least one IV line with a large-bore catheter, and administer fluids (normal saline or lactated Ringer's solution). Prepare for suction curettage, which may be performed in the operating room, labor and delivery area, or in some cases, the ED.

TABLE 27.3 **Characteristics of Mild Versus Severe Preeclampsia.**

Characteristics	Mild Preeclampsia	Severe Preeclampsia
Blood pressure	Greater than 140/90 mm Hg but less than 160/110 mm Hg 30 mm Hg systolic rise; or 15 mm Hg diastolic rise over baseline readings of early pregnancy (Readings are obtained after rest in a sitting position two times at least 6 h apart)	Blood pressure greater than 160/110 mm Hg
Proteinuria (albuminuria)	300 mg/L/24 h or two separate random daytime specimens 6 h apart (true clean-catch) of 1+, 2+	5 g or more per 24 h, 3+, 4+ in true clean-catch or catheterized specimen
Edema	Weight gain of more than 3 lbs (1.4 kg) per week or 6 lbs (2.72 kg) per month—any sudden weight gain is suspicious Minimal or marked edema 1+, 2+ of lower extremities	Weight gain advances at accelerated rate Edema more pronounced, especially of hands, face 3+, 4+ (as condition worsens, edema of lungs, brain, and other organs)
Urine output	Not below 500 mL/24 h	Oliguria less than 500 mL/24 h
Neurologic signs and symptoms	Absent or only occasional headaches, blurred vision, or spots before eyes Normal peripheral reflexes	More persistent headaches, blurred vision, and spots before eyes—retinal arteriole spasms on ophthalmic examination Hyperactive knee jerk and other tendon reflexes +3, +4 with clonus Irritability, tinnitus
Other organ involvement		Liver involvement causing epigastric or right upper quadrant abdominal pain, nausea, vomiting (often said to precede convulsion/coma or onset of eclampsia) Pulmonary edema manifested by respiratory distress, rales, cyanosis

From Novak JC, Broom BL: *Ingalls and Salerno's Maternal and Child Health Nursing*. 9th ed. St Louis, 1999, Mosby.

If the patient will be discharged, aftercare instructions should include information on pelvic rest and instructions to return to the ED or to notify the primary caregiver for increased vaginal bleeding, increasing abdominal pain, passage of tissue, fever, or chills. The patient should also be told to avoid douching and intercourse while on bed rest because these can increase vaginal bleeding, worsen cramping, or cause infection if the cervical os begins to open. The patient should be instructed to follow up with the appropriate referral caregiver. RhoGAM should be given within 72 hours if the mother is Rh negative.[2]

ANTEPARTUM EMERGENCIES

Emergencies occurring in the last months of pregnancy threaten the mother and the fetus. Neurologic sequelae such as seizures and anoxic brain damage are also possible.

Gestational Hypertension in Pregnancy: Preeclampsia/Eclampsia

Gestational hypertension in pregnancy is defined as hypertension after the 20th week of pregnancy or in the immediate postpartum period. Chronic hypertension in pregnancy is defined as hypertension existing before pregnancy, diagnosed before the 20th week of gestation, or persisting longer than 12 weeks after delivery. Gestational hypertension with proteinuria, also referred to as preeclampsia, is characterized by hypertension before 20 weeks of gestation with either a new onset of proteinuria, a sudden increase in proteinuria, or development of HELLP syndrome (hemolysis, elevated liver enzymes, and low platelets). Eclampsia is the development of new-onset seizures superimposed on preeclampsia in a woman between 20 weeks gestation and 4 weeks postpartum.[2]

Gestational hypertension with proteinuria (preeclampsia) is characterized by hypertension, proteinuria, and edema. Systolic blood pressure is greater than 140 mm Hg, or there is an increase of 30 mm Hg over the nonpregnant level. An increase of 15 mm Hg of the diastolic over baseline or diastolic blood pressure of 90 mm Hg or more is classified as hypertension. Hypertension leads to vasospasm and hemolysis and affects several organ systems.[1]

Blood pressure elevation is the paramount symptom of preeclampsia, and readings are compared with prenatal or early pregnancy blood pressure measurements. Proteinuria is a late sign and is an indicator of severity of the disease. Edema is the least reliable sign because of the normal frequency of occurrence during pregnancy. However, sudden onset of facial edema with weight gain is a significant indicator of preeclampsia (Table 27.3). Pulmonary edema may also be present. Subjective signs of worsening preeclampsia may include visual changes, headaches, epigastric pain, and decreased urination. Preeclampsia left untreated may progress to eclampsia.

BOX 27.2 Differential Diagnoses of HELLP Syndrome.

Autoimmune thrombocytopenia purpura
Chronic renal failure
Pyelonephritis
Cholecystitis
Gastroenteritis
Hepatitis
Pancreatitis
Thrombotic thrombocytopenia purpura
Hemolytic-uremic syndrome
Acute fatty liver of pregnancy

HELLP, Hemolysis, elevated liver enzymes, and low platelets.

In eclampsia the patient presents with seizures or coma. This situation is an immediate threat to the mother and the fetus.

Treatment includes oxygen, IV access, and fetal monitoring. The woman is placed in the left lateral recumbent position so the gravid uterus does not cause aortocaval compression. Pharmacologic therapy to control hypertension is usually initiated when diastolic blood pressure is higher than 90 to 100 mm Hg. Magnesium sulfate is the drug of choice to prevent seizures. Continuous monitoring, including blood pressure, pulse, and respirations every 15 to 30 minutes, is essential to identify changes in the patient's condition due to pregnancy-induced hypertension and magnesium toxicity.

Signs of magnesium toxicity include absent deep tendon reflexes, respirations less than 12 per minute, urine output less than 30 mL/h or 120 mL/4 h, and signs of fetal distress. If magnesium toxicity occurs, the patient is given calcium gluconate 1 g IV. Lorazepam can be used to control seizures, although magnesium may also be considered. Fetal monitoring is essential. Any drop in fetal heart rate or deceleration of heart rate during contractions indicates the need for immediate emergency cesarean section. Delivery does not always resolve preeclampsia. Symptoms of concern up to 6 weeks after delivery include headache, elevated blood pressure, vision changes, oliguria, and decreased platelets. These patients should receive a high priority for care.[3]

HELLP Syndrome

The HELLP syndrome is a potentially life-threatening form of preeclampsia occurring when the patient develops multiple organ damage. *H*emolysis, *E*levated *L*iver enzymes, and *L*ow *P*latelets (HELLP) affects up to 12% of women with preeclampsia-eclampsia syndrome. Unlike preeclampsia, which usually affects primigravidas,[2] HELLP syndrome is more common among the multigravida population. HELLP syndrome, characterized by complaints of epigastric or right upper quadrant pain, can imitate a variety of nonobstetric medical problems. Serious medical and surgical pathologic conditions must be ruled out (Box 27.2).

Complications associated with HELLP syndrome include disseminated intravascular coagulopathy, spontaneous hepatic and splenic hemorrhage, end organ failure, intracranial bleeding, and maternal and/or fetal death. Hypotension and tachycardia often are seen because of blood loss from significant coagulopathies. Care of the mother takes precedence, and emergent cesarean section may need to be performed, regardless of fetal viability. Intubation, ventilatory support, fluid resuscitation, and administration of blood may be required to stabilize the mother before emergent cesarean section. Delivery often reverses many of the physiologic sequelae associated with this syndrome. On rare occasions, this syndrome can occur after delivery; therefore the emergency nurse must be alert for physiologic presentation in the postpartum patient that could represent this syndrome.

THIRD-TRIMESTER EMERGENCIES

Fetal viability and the mother's survival are the primary focus for emergencies during the third trimester. Hemorrhage can be obvious or occult, so the emergency nurse must be alert to changes in the mother and fetus.

Placenta Previa

Placenta previa is a placenta extending near, over, or completely covering the cervical os. The cause of placenta previa is unknown. A low-lying or partial placenta previa is not uncommon in early pregnancy, and the placenta usually migrates to its normal position in the fundal region of the uterus as the pregnancy progresses. Three types of placenta previa are defined in relation to how much of the os is covered (Fig. 27.2)

- Complete—the placenta completely covers the os.
- Partial—the placenta partially covers the os.
- Marginal or low implantation—the placenta is adjacent to but does not extend beyond the margin of the os.[2]

Risk factors for placenta previa include previous cesarean delivery, multiple uterine surgeries, advanced maternal age, minority group status, cigarette smoking, and cocaine use. Approximately 1 in every 250 pregnancies results in placenta previa at term. Diagnostic studies include ultrasonography to determine the specific position of the placenta. A CBC, type and crossmatch for several units of blood, and clotting studies should be immediately obtained. Establish a large-bore IV line, administer a crystalloid solution for fluid resuscitation, and transfer the patient to labor and delivery for monitoring and if indicated, immediate cesarean section. Pelvic examination (speculum or digital vaginal examination) is contraindicated because of potential disruption of the cervical-placental junction that could precipitate catastrophic hemorrhage.

Assessment of vital signs should always include assessment of fetal heart rate. If fetal heart tones are not heard, this finding should be reported immediately. A normal fetal heart rate is 120 to 160 beats/min.

Abruptio Placentae

Abruptio placentae, the premature separation of a normally implanted placenta from the uterine wall, accounts for approximately 30% of episodes of bleeding in late pregnancy. The incidence of abruptio placenta is highest between the 24th and 28th weeks of pregnancy.[3] Although the majority of

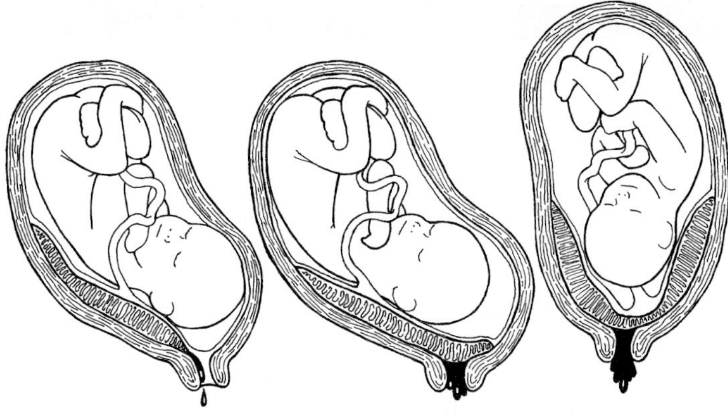

Fig. 27.2 Placenta Previa. (Modified from *AJN/Mosby Nursing Boards Review for NCLEX-RN.* 10th ed. St Louis, MO: Mosby; 1997.)

cases of abruptio placenta occur spontaneously, risk factors include abdominal trauma, cocaine use, oligohydramnios, advanced maternal age, multiparity, eclampsia, and chronic or acute hypertension. Maternal complications include coagulopathy, hemorrhagic shock, uterine rupture or multiple-organ failure. This condition can also lead to uteroplacental insufficiency causing fetal distress or demise.

Clinical features are dependent on the degree of placental abruption. A mild abruption is characterized by mild uterine tenderness, absent or minimal vaginal bleeding, normal vital signs, and variable levels of fetal distress. A severe abruption is characterized by severe uterine pain and tenderness, absent to heavy vaginal bleeding, uterine contractions, maternal hypotension, shock, and fetal distress. Abruptio placentae should be considered in any woman in the third trimester who presents to the ED with vaginal bleeding and abdominal pain or contractions. This is an emergency requiring immediate intervention.

Maternal assessment with vital signs and fetal heart rate is essential. At least one IV line should be started with a large-bore IV catheter and crystalloid solution. A CBC and type and crossmatch should be sent to the laboratory immediately. Fetal monitoring is essential. The patient should be sent to labor and delivery for monitoring and if indicated, immediate cesarean section.

DELIVERY

With decreasing access to prenatal care, the probability of deliveries occurring in prehospital care settings and the ED is high. If a patient in labor arrives in the ED and time permits, rapid obstetric examination should be performed and a brief obstetric history obtained. An in-depth, rapid maternal assessment should be completed.

The first stage of labor is the time from onset of regular contractions until complete cervical dilation. This is generally the longest of the three stages of labor. The second stage of labor is the time from full cervical dilation until delivery of the baby. The mother may have the urge to push in this stage. The average time for stage two is 20 minutes to 1 hour. The third stage of labor is from delivery of the baby until delivery of the placenta. This stage usually lasts from 5 to 15 minutes. In cases where the placenta fails to detach from the uterine wall, it may be necessary to manually remove the placenta.

When a woman in labor arrives at the ED, if time permits, a brief physical examination should be performed. Fetal heart tones should be assessed; normal fetal heart tones between 120 and 160 beats/min. Prolonged fetal bradycardia or tachycardia may indicate fetal distress. If this occurs, place the mother on her left side and give supplemental high-flow oxygen. Arrange for immediate obstetric consultation for possible emergency delivery by cesarean section.

After the fetus is determined to be in no distress, examine the mother's abdomen and measure uterine height. A full-term fetus elevates the uterus to the level of the xiphoid. Palpate contractions as they occur. Help the mother relax between contractions. The emergency nurse involved in a delivery should remember the mother does most of the work. Some of the roles of the nurse are to provide psychological support, "coach" the mother, and ensure the infant, once delivered, is breathing adequately, has a good pulse, and is kept warm.

If crowning is not present, a manual vaginal examination using sterile technique is performed to determine dilation, effacement, and station of the fetus. If fluid is present, identify if it is amniotic fluid by determining acidity of the fluid. Amniotic fluid is neutral, whereas normal vaginal secretions are acidic. If the test is equivocal because of the presence of blood, assume the membranes have ruptured and amniotic fluid is present.

A rapid decision should be made as to whether delivery is imminent and the baby will be delivered in the ED or, if time permits, transport of the mother to labor and delivery. If there is any indication the mother will deliver imminently (i.e., crowning), keep her in the ED for delivery.

If an emergent delivery is imminent, place the mother on a stretcher and obtain equipment necessary for delivery of the fetus. Sterile disposable delivery kits usually have most

TABLE 27.4 Apgar Score.

	SCORE		
Assessment	**0**	**1**	**2**
A Appearance (color)	Blue	Blue limbs, pink body	Pink
P Pulse (heart rate)	Absent	<100 beats/min	>100 beats/min
G Grimace (muscle tone)	Limp	Some flexion	Good flexion
A Activity (reflexes irritable)	Absent	Some motion	Good motion
R Respiratory effort	Absent	Weak cry	Strong cry

equipment necessary for an emergent delivery. Do not place equipment between the mother's legs; place it on a surface beside the stretcher. Minimum essential equipment includes cord clamps, scissors, towels, and bulb syringe.

Support the mother through delivery of the infant's head. Suction, first the mouth, then the nose, gently with a bulb syringe. Support the head through the delivery of the shoulders. After the shoulders are delivered, the delivery of the rest of the infant's body occurs rapidly. If needed, suction the nose and mouth again. If spontaneous breathing or crying does not occur, gently rub the infant's back with a towel to stimulate breathing.

If not already done, clamp the umbilical cord in two places at least 6 inches from the umbilicus. The cord can be cut as soon as it is convenient, usually when it has stopped pulsating.

Place the infant in a warmed environment. Assess airway, breathing, and circulation (ABCs). If necessary, open the infant's airway with a slight chin lift, being careful not to overextend the neck. If breathing is absent or the heart rate is less than 60 beats/min despite 30 seconds of assisted ventilation, begin resuscitation measures following current American Heart Association guidelines for neonatal resuscitation.[1]

Determine the infant's Apgar score at delivery, and repeat 5 minutes after delivery (Table 27.4). The Apgar score is a system used to predict health outcomes by scoring and totaling five key factors. Each factor is scored from 0 to 2. Zero is a poor response or absence of the factor being measured, 1 indicates some response, and 2 indicates a normal finding. A total score of 10 is possible, with 7 to 10 considered very good. A score of 4 to 6 indicates a moderately depressed infant, whereas a score of 0 to 3 indicates a severely depressed infant.

After ensuring the health of the infant and its continued warmth, place the infant skin-to-skin on the mother's abdomen and encourage the mother to breastfeed the infant if appropriate. Be sure to cover the mother and baby to keep the baby warm. Sucking stimulates the uterus to contract, reassures the mother the infant is fine, and helps keep the infant warm. Put an identification band on the infant's wrist and ankle.

After delivery of the infant, the third stage of labor begins. Palpate the uterus through the abdominal wall. Prepare for delivery of the placenta; this usually occurs 5 to 10 minutes after the infant is born. A sudden gush of blood occurs when the placenta separates from the uterine wall; the uterus rises into the abdomen and the umbilical cord protruding from the vagina lengthens. Do not pull on the umbilical cord; this could cause uterine inversion.

When the placenta has separated, apply slight traction to the umbilical cord and place your hand on the dome of the uterus, pressing downward slightly toward the suprapubic area. As the placenta enters the vaginal area, continue applying gentle traction to the umbilical cord and carefully remove the placenta.

Complicated Deliveries

Prolapsed Cord

A prolapsed umbilicus occurs when the umbilical cord precedes the fetus through the birth canal, becomes entrapped when the fetus passes through the birth canal, and obstructs fetal circulation. A prolapsed cord constitutes an obstetric emergency.

There are three variations of this condition. The first is a situation in which uterine membranes are intact; the cord is compressed by fetal parts but is not visible externally. This variation should be suspected when there are signs of fetal distress, most prominently bradycardia. This variation is actually called "cord presentation" rather than true prolapse.

In the second variation the cord may not be visible but can be felt in the vagina or cervix. In the third and most extreme variation, the umbilical cord actually protrudes from the vagina.

Cord compression can be determined in two ways. First, on examination the cord is felt as the presenting part. However, cord compression is usually identified when the fetus suddenly develops distress, which is noted on the fetal monitor as a decreasing fetal heart rate or decelerations.

Therapeutic intervention is aimed at relieving pressure on the cord and minimizing fetal anoxia. Either elevate the mother's hips, or place the mother in the knee-chest position with the bed in Trendelenburg's position. Instruct her to not push because this may cause further compression of the cord. Administer oxygen via nonrebreather mask at 100%. An exposed cord dries out, so cover it with saline-moistened sterile gauze. If the cervix is completely dilated, forceps may be used to rapidly deliver the baby. If the cervix is not fully dilated, emergency cesarean section is performed.

Shoulder Dystocia

Risk factors associated with shoulder dystocia include large infants, prolonged second stage of labor, and use of high forceps during delivery. Whatever the cause, the infant's shoulder has difficulty passing through the pelvis. Shoulder dystocia is an emergency presenting in fewer than 2% of deliveries. After the head is delivered, the shoulders cannot pass through the pelvis. Compression of the shoulders can lead to cord compression and subsequent fetal distress. Rapid delivery is critical. Call for obstetric support if possible. Positioning the mother with legs hyperflexed over the abdomen (McRoberts' maneuver)[4] may disengage the anterior shoulder and make delivery possible. If this maneuver does not work, application of suprapubic pressure will be attempted to try to facilitate delivery. Infant complications of shoulder dystocia include asphyxia, traumatic brachial plexus injuries, fractured clavicle or humerus, and Erb palsy. Maternal complications include tears to the cervix, vagina, perineum, or rectum.

Breech Delivery

With breech delivery, the head—the largest fetal body part—is delivered last. A woman whose fetus is a breech presentation is often scheduled for cesarean section. Unfortunately, in the emergency setting, when a woman arrives in labor with delivery imminent and the fetus is in a breech position, there may not be time to arrange for cesarean section. Delivery must be completed in the ED, especially if the fetus has been delivered to the level of the umbilicus.

Categories of breech presentation are frank breech, full or complete breech, and footling breech. Frank breech is the most common variation, occurring when fetal legs are extended across the abdomen toward the shoulders and the buttocks are presenting. Full (or complete) breech is reversal of the usual cephalic presentation. The head, knees, and hips are flexed, but the buttocks are presenting. Footling breech is when one or both feet present. With any breech presentation, call for obstetric support if possible.

Meconium Aspiration Syndrome

Meconium aspiration syndrome occurs when meconium enters fetal lungs during delivery. Relaxation of the anal sphincter in utero caused by fetal hypoxia leads to meconium staining of amniotic fluid. Staining is seen most often in postterm deliveries. Meconium staining of amniotic fluid can be an emergency for the fetus, but delivery must be adapted to address potential fetal respiratory distress. The 2005 American Heart Association recommendations no longer advise routine intrapartum oropharyngeal and nasopharyngeal suctioning for infants born to mothers with meconium-stained amniotic fluid. For meconium-stained infants who are not born vigorous (strong respiratory effort, good muscle tone, and heart rate greater than 100 beats/min), endotracheal suctioning with a meconium aspirator should be performed immediately after birth.[1]

Multiple Fetuses

With delivery of twins or other multiple births, there are additional concerns. Often multiple-birth neonates are premature or have multiple other medical problems. The initial and most important objective is to ensure safe delivery of all fetuses. The best advice is to take one fetus at a time, as they come. Both neonates should be suctioned as they are delivered. Both cords should be clamped and both neonates should receive identification bands. Multiples increase the risk for complications; if at all possible, there should be two teams available in the event neonatal resuscitation is required.

Amniotic Fluid Embolism

Amniotic fluid embolism is a catastrophic event with high maternal mortality because amniotic fluid leaks into the mother's venous circulation during labor or delivery. This embolus of squamous epithelial cells, lanugo, and vasoactive chemicals travels to the pulmonary circulation, causing sudden, severe obstruction and respiratory arrest, which is usually followed quickly by cardiac arrest.

Amniotic fluid emboli are seen most commonly with placenta previa, abruptio placentae, precipitate labor in the multiparous woman, and intrauterine fetal death. Amniotic fluid emboli occur in about 1 of every 100,000 deliveries. The mother may initially demonstrate profound hypotension, tachycardia, tachypnea, cyanosis, and hypoxia followed by cardiopulmonary arrest. Coagulopathies can also occur.

Therapeutic interventions must be rapid and aggressive. Administer oxygen at high-flow via a nonrebreather mask. Rapid endotracheal intubation and mechanical ventilation with positive end-expiratory pressure is required for many patients. Crystalloid solutions and blood products should be administered. Fresh frozen plasma may be infused for identified coagulopathies.

POSTPARTUM EMERGENCIES

Postpartum Hemorrhage

Postpartum hemorrhage, defined as 500 mL or more of blood, is the most common complication of labor and delivery.[1] Bleeding can occur immediately (within 24 hours) after delivery or be delayed (24 hours to 6 weeks). The main causes of postpartum bleeding are uterine atony, which can cause subinvolution; a decreased or absent decrease in size of the uterus; retained products of conception, such as pieces of the placenta or membranes; and vaginal or cervical tears incurred during delivery. Subinvolution usually occurs 7 to 14 days after delivery when thrombi detach from placental-attachment sites and those sites begin to bleed. If involution does not occur, the gravid uterus will not return to the nonpregnant state and life-threatening hemorrhage can occur. Retention of membranes or placental fragments can also cause sudden hemorrhage because they interfere with the involutional process. The emergency nurse should also be aware of a condition known as placenta accreta. When the placenta fails to separate from the uterine wall after delivery because it has grown into the uterine muscle itself, postpartum bleeding results and immediate surgery is indicated. Cervical tears and vaginal lacerations can also cause postpartum hemorrhage.

When assessing the patient with postpartum bleeding, assess the patient's general condition. Note the presence or absence of pain, skin color, posture, gait, motor activity, and facial expression. The following information should be elicited when obtaining history of the problem:

- Quantity, character, and duration of bleeding. How does it compare with the patient's normal menstrual period? How many pads has she used in the past hour? During the past 24 hours? How does it compare with the number she normally requires during a period?
- Menstrual history. When was the date of her last period?
- Does she have pain? What is the nature of the pain—dull, achy, cramping, constant, or radiating? Where is the pain? How long has she had it? Was onset gradual or sudden?
- Is there any history of trauma?
- When did she deliver? Has she ever had any infections of the reproductive system? Has she had previous episodes of bleeding?

Continued assessment should include vital signs, palpation of the uterine fundus for firmness, and evaluation of vaginal bleeding. If the fundus is boggy and relaxed, gently massage it until firm. Check the pad the patient is wearing to objectively evaluate the amount of bleeding. Note presence or absence of clots or odor. Examine and save any clots or tissue the patient may have brought with her for laboratory examination. If bleeding is profuse, establish two IV lines with large-bore catheters for administration of warmed crystalloids and blood. If respirations are labored, administer oxygen. Obtain a CBC, sedimentation rate, and type and crossmatch.[1]

Postpartum bleeding generally responds to administration of IV oxytocin, bed rest, and fundal massage. If bleeding continues, prepare the patient for operative evaluation of bleeding. Treatment of retained products of conception includes removal of the offending piece by dilation and curettage and a thorough exploration of the uterus after the patient is under general anesthesia. Suturing of vaginal lacerations can be performed in the ED. However, with the possibility of damage at the cervix, suturing is best performed after general anesthesia. A complete pelvic examination can also be performed after anesthesia.[5]

Disseminated Intravascular Coagulation

Disseminated intravascular coagulation is characterized by acceleration and hyperactivity of clotting mechanisms in pregnancy. This condition of simultaneous bleeding and clotting is seen most often in severe cases of abruptio placentae in the form of hypofibrinogenemia but can also occur after excessive blood loss, amniotic fluid embolus, or fetal death in utero. In this hypercoagulable state, clotting factors are consumed before the liver has time to replace them. See Chapter 29 for additional discussion of disseminated intravascular coagulation.

Postpartum Infection

Vaginal lacerations, cervical tears, episiotomy sites, placental implant sites, and retained tissue can become host sites for infection. Patients develop fever and abdominal or pelvic pain and occasionally have foul-smelling lochia. Therapeutic interventions include culture of drainage and administration of antibiotics as indicated. In rare cases the postpartum patient may become septic and require fluid resuscitation and stabilization.

OTHER OBSTETRIC EMERGENCIES

Molar Pregnancy (Hydatidiform Mole)

Molar pregnancy occurs when trophoblast villi grow very rapidly and then die. If an embryo is formed, it dies very early. As trophoblast cells degenerate, they fill with a jellylike fluid. The cells become vesicles resembling grapes filled with fluid. Bleeding occurs early in the second trimester as these vesicles enlarge and rupture. There is a definite association between hydatidiform mole and choriocarcinoma, which is a rapidly growing carcinoma, so early diagnosis is critical.

Because the trophoblast secretes hCG and grows very rapidly, the uterus grows larger than expected for the due date. At about 16 weeks' gestation, the woman develops vaginal bleeding. Bleeding may be mixed with clear fluid as the vesicles begin to rupture. The patient will have a positive pregnancy test with enlarging uterus; however, fetal heart tones cannot be auscultated. A viable fetus is not evident on pelvic ultrasonography.[3]

Intervention for molar pregnancy is removal of the mole. The patient should be prepared for suction dilation and curettage. The patient and family require emotional support. They now know this is an abnormal pregnancy (without a fetus) and must also worry about the possibility of a tumor.

SPECIFIC GYNECOLOGIC EMERGENCIES

Vaginal Bleeding/Dysfunctional Uterine Bleeding

Vaginal bleeding in the nonpregnant patient can be due to a variety of causes, including hormonal imbalance; vaginal, cervical, or uterine disorders; trauma; infection; malignancies; systemic disease; medications; or blood dyscrasias. Up to 20% of women with heavy uterine bleeding have an underlying coagulation disorder. Eating disorders, excessive weight loss, stress, and exercise can also cause abnormal vaginal bleeding or amenorrhea. More than 8 saturated pads per day or 12 tampons per day is considered excessive bleeding, although blood loss is difficult to estimate depending on the frequency of pad or tampon changes. Vaginal bleeding is abnormal in prepubertal females and necessitates a full diagnostic workup. Terms used to define abnormal uterine bleeding[1] are listed in Box 27.3.

Dysfunctional uterine bleeding (DUB) is the most common cause of vaginal bleeding during a woman's reproductive years. The diagnosis of DUB is a diagnosis of exclusion and should only be made when other organic and structural causes for the abnormal bleeding have been ruled out.

BOX 27.3 Terms Used to Define Abnormal Uterine Bleeding.

Amenorrhea—no menstruation
Oligomenorrhea—too few episodes of bleeding
Menorrhagia—too much blood loss
Metrorrhagia—too many episodes of bleeding
Menometrorrhagia—too much and too many episodes of bleeding

DUB may occur at any age; however, because most cases are due to anovulation, it is most common at the extremes of the reproductive years. Most cases in adolescent girls occur during the first 18 months after the onset of menstruation because of immaturity of their hypothalamic-pituitary axis. In the perimenopausal period, DUB may be an early manifestation of ovarian failure. Vaginal bleeding in the postmenopausal patient should be considered a malignancy until this is ruled out.

Assessment of the nonpregnant patient with vaginal bleeding includes a detailed history followed by an abdominal and pelvic examination. The history should include the amount and duration of bleeding the patient has experienced. The patient with an established menstrual history should be asked to compare the number of pads used per day in a normal menstrual cycle with the number used at this time. The average tampon holds 5 mL of blood, and the average pad 5 to 15 mL of blood. Additional information should be obtained regarding the presence or absence of pain; date of last normal menstrual period (LNMP), including duration and flow; menstrual regularity; obstetric history; contraceptive use; and sexual history. Additional information should be obtained regarding comorbidities and medications taken.

A physical examination should be conducted to assess volume status, hemodynamic stability, and extent of bleeding. Laboratory specimens should be obtained for urinalysis, urine or serum pregnancy test, and CBC. Other indicated laboratory tests include PT, aPTT, liver function tests (in the presence of liver disease), and type and crossmatch. A pelvic or intravaginal ultrasound examination may be obtained to evaluate for structural abnormalities.

In the presence of hemodynamic instability, nursing interventions should be directed at immediate resuscitation and stabilization. An emergent gynecologic consultation should be obtained. If bleeding is severe and the patient is not responsive to initial fluid resuscitation, a 25-mg dose of IV conjugated estrogen should be administered. Repeat doses every 2 to 4 hours may be administered as needed. A course of oral estrogen therapy may also be prescribed for cessation of bleeding. Perimenopausal women may be treated with cyclic oral contraceptives three times per day for a period of 7 days to control and regulate bleeding.[1,3] Patients who are discharged should be given a referral to a gynecologist for further workup. All patients with anemia should be advised to take an iron supplement.

Pelvic Pain

Pelvic pain is a common presenting chief complaint in patients seeking care in the ED. Pain in the lower abdomen or pelvis may be due to a variety of causes. The uterus, cervix, and adnexa share the same visceral innervation as the lower ileum, sigmoid colon, and rectum. It may be difficult to distinguish pain originating in the gynecologic organs from pain originating in the gastrointestinal organs. Poorly localized visceral pain originates in organs and viscera innervated by autonomic nerves. This may be caused by distention of a hollow viscus (e.g., fallopian tube or bowel), distention of the capsule of a solid organ, or stretching of pelvic ligaments or adhesions. In contrast, well-localized pain originates from somatic nerve irritation, such as irritation of the peritoneum caused by an inflamed organ (e.g., endometritis, appendicitis) or the presence of blood or purulent fluid (e.g., ruptured ectopic pregnancy or ovarian cyst).[4] Pelvic pain is classified as acute, chronic, or cyclic. Box 27.4 outlines the causes of pelvic pain originating from the reproductive organs. An accurate history and physical examination are crucial in this patient population because the condition causing the pain may be life-threatening.[4]

BOX 27.4 Causes of Pelvic Pain of Gynecologic Origin.

Acute Pelvic Pain
- Abortion (threatened or incomplete)
- Ectopic pregnancy
- Ovarian cyst
- Ovarian torsion
- Acute pelvic inflammatory disease
- Tuboovarian abscess
- Endometritis
- Degenerating fibroid

Cyclic Pelvic Pain
- Mittelschmerz
- Endometriosis
- Dysmenorrhea
- Adenomyosis

Chronic Pelvic Pain
- Adhesions
- Chronic pelvic inflammatory disease

Dysmenorrhea

Pain with menstruation is a common gynecologic complaint, particularly in adolescents and young women. Primary dysmenorrhea is defined as pelvic pain during menstruation in the absence of other pelvic pathologic conditions. It typically develops 1 to 3 years after menarche with an increasing incidence through the early to mid-twenties as ovulatory cycles are established. Primary dysmenorrhea is the most common form of pain during menstruation. This problem may be significant, causing up to 10% of women to miss days of school or work.[6] It is most severe in young, nulliparous women. Primary dysmenorrhea is characterized by crampy, low midline pain, which occurs secondary to progesterone-mediated uterine contractions and arteriolar vasospasm. The pain typically precedes menstrual flow by up to 24 hours and subsides after menses begins. There may be associated nausea, vomiting, back pain, headache, and irritability.

Secondary dysmenorrhea is cyclic menstrual pain associated with a pelvic pathologic condition. This is most frequently caused by endometriosis or pelvic inflammatory disease (PID). Other causes include intrauterine devices, adhesions, and benign tumors of the uterus.

Management of primary dysmenorrhea includes the use of nonsteroidal antiinflammatory drugs (NSAIDs) to inhibit the synthesis of prostaglandins; narcotics should be avoided. To maximize pain relief, NSAIDs should be administered before the onset of menses. If NSAIDs fail to provide relief, cyclic oral contraceptives (COCs) should be started to inhibit ovulation, which will decrease the amount of menstrual pain and bleeding. If dysmenorrhea persists despite the use of COCs, a secondary cause of dysmenorrhea should be considered and an appropriate diagnostic workup should be pursued. Sympathetic reassurance is helpful after other causes of acute pelvic pain have been ruled out. Gynecologic follow-up is indicated.[6]

Endometriosis

Endometriosis is a common cause of cyclic pain in menstruating women. Endometrial tissue develops outside of the uterus, causing pain with menses. Organs involved may include the ovaries, posterior cul de sac, fallopian tubes, and uterosacral ligaments. Despite the abnormal location of endometrial tissue growth, the tissue sloughs and bleeds just as the uterine tissue does. As the disease progresses, pelvic adhesions may develop. Pain is cyclic or constant and may vary in character and intensity. It is generally worse just before or during menses. The character of the pain may range from midline pelvic cramping to severe diffuse pain.

Endometriosis may be strongly suspected, but it is not a diagnosis made in the ED. Laparoscopy is the standard modality used to definitively diagnose endometriosis. ED management focuses on pain control through the use of NSAIDs. Further therapy depends on the severity of symptoms, stage of the disease, and desire for future fertility. Hormonal therapy may be used to mimic pseudopregnancy, chronic anovulation, and pseudomenopause.

Mittelschmerz

Pain with ovulation, referred to as mittelschmerz, is a transient, midcycle pelvic pain occurring during or just after ovulation. Pain is usually mild and lasts from a few hours to a few days. The cause is increasing ovarian capsular pressure before the follicle erupts and leakage of prostaglandin-containing follicular fluid associated with ovulation. Mittelschmerz is characterized by sudden, sharp, and unilateral pelvic pain. Treatment includes antiprostaglandin therapy with NSAIDs for pain relief. Sympathetic reassurance is helpful after other causes of acute pelvic pain have been ruled out.[6]

Ovarian Cyst

An ovarian cyst is a fluid-filled or semi–fluid-filled sac in an ovary developing at any time from the neonatal period to postmenopause. For most patients, ovarian cysts cause no symptoms and are an incidental finding during ultrasonography performed for another reason. Follicular cysts of the ovary are the most common cystic structure found in healthy ovaries, and they develop during the first 2 weeks of the menstrual cycle; most rupture at ovulation.[7] This type of cyst results from either failure of the mature follicle to rupture or failure of an immature follicle to undergo the normal maturation process. A follicular cyst may grow to a size of 8 to 10 cm, and stretching of the capsule is the cause of pelvic discomfort. Most of these cysts regress spontaneously over 1 to 3 months. Follicular cysts are thin walled and may rupture during sexual intercourse or strenuous exercise. The symptoms of a ruptured follicular cyst include sharp pelvic pain of sudden onset that resolves over a few days.

Corpus luteal cysts develop during the latter half of the menstrual cycle during the luteal phase, and most regress at the end of the menstrual cycle. However, persistent corpus luteal cysts are blood filled and may rupture, producing sharp pelvic pain, intraperitoneal irritation, and bleeding, which may progress to anemia and hypovolemia. Bleeding from a ruptured corpus luteal cyst is usually self-limited but in rare cases may progress to hemorrhage and hypovolemic shock.[7] Hemorrhagic cysts occur when a blood vessel in the cyst wall ruptures. A dermoid cyst is a germ cell neoplasm containing tissue including fat, skin, hair, and teeth. Most are benign, and usually occur in individuals between the ages of 10 and 30.

Diagnostic studies include a pregnancy test, urinalysis, and CBC. Definitive diagnosis is made through pelvic ultrasonography and/or laparoscopy. Ovarian cysts that are < 8 cm, unilateral, and unilocular are generally managed through observation because they typically resolve. Treatment of ruptured ovarian cysts is directed at pain control with NSAIDs and/or narcotics and treatment of complications, including hypovolemia and hemorrhage. Patients may need admission for observation and serial hematocrit determinations to monitor bleeding. Surgical intervention is usually not required except for the rare case of continued intraperitoneal hemorrhage.[7]

Ovarian Torsion

Twisting of the ovary or fallopian tube is referred to as torsion and represents a surgical emergency. Most ovarian torsions result secondary to an ovarian cyst (most commonly dermoid cysts) or mass. The enlargement of the ovary causes it to twist, leading to ischemia and necrosis of the ovary. The pain is due to ischemia and is usually described as acute, severe, and unilateral. Pain may be intermittent or constant. Associated symptoms commonly include nausea and vomiting, low-grade fever, and leukocytosis. Diagnostic studies include a pregnancy test, CBC, and transvaginal ultrasound with Doppler. Patients with torsion require hospital admission for surgical intervention. If untreated, an ovarian torsion can lead to infertility, infection, and eventual necrosis of the affected ovary or fallopian tube.

Vaginal Discharge and Vaginitis

Discharge from the vagina that is odorless and clear to milky in color is normal and the body's physiologic way of keeping the vagina healthy. A complex and intricate balance of microorganisms maintain the normal vaginal flora. Factors influencing and altering the composition of the vaginal flora include age, stress, hormonal balance, sexual activity, contraceptives, hygiene products, antibiotics, and general health status. Any change in the amount, color, odor, and/or associated symptoms of itching, burning, or irritation may indicate a change in this chemical balance in the vagina and lead to an infection. Vaginitis is common in postpubertal adolescents and adult women but relatively uncommon in prepubertal females. The most common cause of vaginitis is bacterial vaginosis (40%–50%), followed by *Candida albicans* (20%–25%), and *Trichomonas vaginalis* (15%–20%).[1]

Bacterial Vaginosis

Bacterial vaginosis (BV) occurs when the normal bacterial flora in the vagina is replaced with *Gardnerella vaginalis* and *Mycoplasma hominis.* BV is characterized by a vaginal discharge that is thin, homogeneous, malodorous, and white to gray in color. Up to 50% of women with BV are asymptomatic. The Centers for Disease Control and Prevention (CDC) state that three of the following signs and symptoms must be present for this condition to be diagnosed: (1) a homogeneous, white, noninflammatory discharge that coats the vaginal walls; (2) the presence of clue cells on microscopic examination; (3) pH greater than 4.5; and (4) a fishy odor to the discharge after the addition of KOH (positive whiff test).[8] BV has also been associated with PID, endometritis, and vaginal cuff cellulitis after surgical procedures. Complications of BV in pregnancy include preterm labor, premature rupture of membranes and low infant birth weight. Metronidazole and clindamycin are both effective for the treatment of BV. Both of these pharmacologic agents may be administered orally or intravaginally.[8]

Candidiasis

Vaginal candidiasis is caused by vaginal colonization of the airborne fungi of the *Candida* species. Most commonly, the organisms gain access to the vaginal lumen from the adjacent perianal area. Risk factors for the development of vaginal candidiasis include oral contraceptive use, intrauterine device (IUD) use, young age at first intercourse, increased frequency of intercourse, diabetes, human immunodeficiency virus (HIV) or other immunocompromised states, chronic antibiotic use, and pregnancy. Symptoms include pruritus (the most common symptom); thick, odorless, white vaginal discharge (with an appearance similar to cottage cheese; Fig. 27.3); vulvar burning; dyspareunia; and vulvar dysuria. Erythema and swelling of the labia may be present, with the vaginal discharge adhering to the walls of the vagina. Diagnosis is made microscopically by examining a wet mount sample of vaginal secretions for yeast buds and pseudohyphae. Treatment options include a 1-day treatment with oral fluconazole or the use of intravaginal azole preparations (fungistatic agents) with regimens ranging from 1 to 7 days.[1]

Trichomoniasis

Trichomoniasis infection is caused by the protozoan *Trichomonas vaginalis.* Trichomoniasis is almost always an STI and is the most common nonviral STI in the world. It is estimated that 3.7 million American women contract the disease annually.[8] There is a high incidence of coinfection with gonorrhea in women with *T. vaginalis* infection. Risk factors include multiple sexual partners, early initiation of sexual activity, increased frequency of sexual activity, poverty, and lower educational level. Infection can range from an asymptomatic carrier state to severe, acute inflammatory disease. Symptoms commonly include a malodorous, copious, frothy discharge that is white to greenish-yellow; vulvovaginal soreness, fullness, and irritation; pruritus; dysuria; and dyspareunia. Gynecologic examination may reveal erythema of the cervix and upper portion of the vagina (strawberry cervix). Diagnosis is made microscopically through the examination of a wet mount sample for the presence of trichomonads. Diagnostic accuracy may be improved with a culture. The most effective treatment is metronidazole either in a single dose or a 7-day course. The single-dose treatment is preferable because of the lower cost, fewer side effects, and greater patient compliance[1]

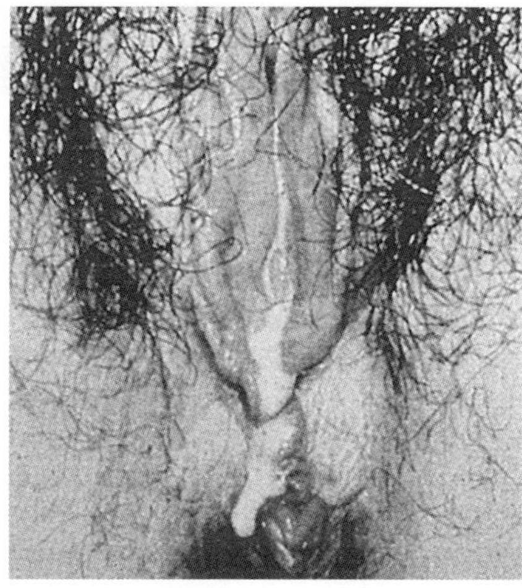

Fig. 27.3 *Candida albicans.* (From Zitelli BJ, Davis HW. *Atlas of Pediatric Physical Diagnosis.* 4th ed. St Louis, MO: Mosby; 2002.)

Pelvic Inflammatory Disease

Pelvic inflammatory disease is a term used to describe infection of the upper reproductive tract, including the endometrium, fallopian tubes, ovaries, pelvic peritoneum, and/or the pelvic connective tissue. PID may be acute, subacute, or chronic. The two most common organisms causing PID are *Neisseria gonorrheae* and *Chlamydia trachomatis,* which frequently coexist. Other aerobic and anaerobic organisms may also cause PID. Most cases of PID originate from STIs of the lower genital tract followed by an ascending infection to the upper tract. Another cause of PID is the introduction of microorganisms through instrumentation such as endometrial biopsy, curettage, and hysteroscopy. Factors facilitating the ascending migration of microorganisms include menses-related loss of the cervical barrier and hormonal changes reducing the bacteriostatic properties of the cervical mucus.[9] Risk factors for PID include multiple sexual partners, increased frequency of sexual activity, IUD use, history of other STIs, substance abuse, and frequent vaginal douching.

The most common symptom of PID is lower abdominal or pelvic pain increasing with movement—to limit this pain with walking, patients with PID characteristically shuffle (the

BOX 27.5 CDC Criteria for Identification of Pelvic Inflammatory Disease.

Cervical motion tenderness OR uterine tenderness OR adnexal tenderness
Oral temperature >101°F (>38.3°C)
Abnormal cervical or vaginal mucopurulent discharge
Presence of abundant numbers of WBC on saline microscopy of vaginal secretions
Elevated erythrocyte sedimentation rate
Elevated C-reactive protein
Laboratory documentation of cervical infection with *Neisseria gonorrheae* or *Chlamydia trachomatis*

CDC, Centers for Disease Control and Prevention; *WBC*, white blood cell.

"PID shuffle"). Other symptoms include abnormal vaginal discharge, vaginal bleeding, postcoital bleeding, dyspareunia, fever, malaise, nausea, and vomiting. Gynecologic examination usually reveals lower abdominal tenderness, mucopurulent cervicitis, cervical motion tenderness, and bilateral adnexal tenderness. Laboratory evaluation should include a pregnancy test, urinalysis, CBC, C-reactive protein and/or sedimentation rate, wet mount sample, and cervical culture and Gram stain. DNA probes for gonorrhea and chlamydial infection should also be included. An elevated white blood cell count and sedimentation rate and/or C-reactive protein support the diagnosis of PID. Imaging studies may include a pelvic sonogram, abdominal/pelvic CT scan, and/or MRI. Laparoscopy may also be performed for definitive diagnosis. Box 27.5 outlines the CDC diagnostic criteria for PID.[9]

Complications of PID can include tubo-ovarian abscess, chronic pelvic pain, dyspareunia, infertility, and tubal adhesions and scarring, which increase the risk for ectopic pregnancy. The patient may also develop perihepatic inflammation, including right upper quadrant or pleuritic pain (Fitz-Hugh-Curtis syndrome). The goals of treatment are to control pain, eliminate the acute infection, and prevent complications. Effective analgesia should be provided. Early initiation of empiric, broad-spectrum antibiotic therapy either on an outpatient or inpatient basis is critical to cover likely pathogens. Parenteral and oral therapy appear to have similar efficacy in achieving successful clinical outcomes in patients with mild to moderate PID. Hospital admission is suggested for patients who meet any of the following criteria: (1) surgical emergencies (appendicitis) cannot be excluded; (2) the patient is pregnant; (3) the patient does not respond clinically to oral antimicrobial therapy; (4) the patient is unable to follow or tolerate an outpatient oral regimen; (5) the patient has severe illness, nausea and vomiting, or high fever; or (6) the patient has a tubo-ovarian abscess.[1]

Tuboovarian Abscess

A tuboovarian abscess (TOA) is a complication of PID and salpingitis with bacterial invasion into the disrupted capsule of the ovary. If the TOA ruptures, bacteria spill into the peritoneal space, which may lead to bacteremia and septic shock. The patient with a TOA is ill appearing and presents with acute, severe pelvic pain. Associated symptoms include fever (which may be as high as 104°F [40°C]), nausea, vomiting, purulent vaginal discharge, and vaginal bleeding. Diagnostic studies include a pregnancy test, CBC, urinalysis, C-reactive protein, cervical culture, and Gram stain. DNA probes for gonorrhea and chlamydial infection should also be included. Imaging studies include pelvic ultrasonography, CT scan, or MRI. Treatment includes hospital admission, pain control, IV antibiotics, and surgical intervention for incision and drainage. Complications from TOA include chronic pelvic pain, pelvic adhesions, tubal factor infertility, and ectopic pregnancy.[1]

Bartholin Gland Abscess

The Bartholin glands are located within the vestibule at the 5 and 7 o'clock positions. The glands secrete a clear viscous fluid that lubricates the vaginal vestibule. Under normal circumstances the glands cannot be palpated or visualized. Occasionally a Bartholin gland forms a cyst or an abscess (see Fig. 27.3). A cyst develops when the duct of the gland becomes distended and gets occluded. A cyst is characterized by a small, painless lump. In the absence of infection, warm sitz baths are usually the only treatment required. An abscess is a primary infection of the gland with bacteria. Infection is generally the result of vaginal and fecal organisms (*Escherichia coli, G. vaginalis,* and other anaerobic bacteria); however, STIs such as *N. gonorrheae* and *C. trachomatis* have also been cultured. The patient with an abscess complains of a progressive increase in unilateral pain, swelling, and redness of the labia. On physical examination there will be a labial mass that is erythematous, tender, and fluctuant on palpation. Treatment of a Bartholin gland abscess is incision and drainage with possible placement of a Word catheter; a wound culture should be obtained. If used, the Word catheter should remain in place for several weeks to prevent abscess recurrence. The patient should be advised to avoid sexual intercourse until the catheter has been removed. Other discharge instructions include sitz baths, pain control with NSAIDs or short-term narcotics, and gynecologic follow-up.

Sexually Transmitted Infections

STIs are frequently encountered in the ED because the ED is used as initial entry into the health care system. The primary STIs include gonorrhea, chlamydial infection, trichomoniasis, syphilis, bacterial vaginosis, genital warts, genital herpes, hepatitis, and HIV infection. (See Chapter 19 for discussion of hepatitis and HIV.) The CDC estimates that 19 million new infections occur each year, almost half of them among young people[8] aged 15 to 24. STIs are associated with significant physiologic and psychological morbidity. Complications associated with STIs include vaginitis, cervicitis, PID, infertility, urethritis, epididymitis, pharyngitis, proctitis, skin and mucous membrane lesions, and acquired immunodeficiency syndrome (AIDS) associated with the HIV virus (Table 27.5). Early diagnosis and treatment are critical in the prevention of the sequelae associated with STIs. Overall, prevention of

STIs is possible; therefore primary prevention through health counseling should be a goal for all emergency care providers.

Genital Herpes

Genital herpes is most often caused by herpes simplex virus type 2 (HSV-2). However, 10% to 50% of infections are due to herpes simplex virus type 1 (HSV-1). The virus is transmitted through microabrasions on mucosal surfaces during oral, vaginal, or rectal intercourse with an infected person. There may also be perinatal transmission of the herpes virus. Once the virus initially infects the mucosal surface, it enters the neurons, where it migrates to the ganglia. Viral replication occurs in the ganglia. Virus latency may be maintained in the ganglia, where it can undergo periods of reactivation and replication.

Up to 1 million new cases occur each year, with up to 50% of cases being asymptomatic.[8] The incubation period for a primary infection is 2 to 12 days (average, 4 days). If symptoms of the primary infection do develop, they are manifested by multiple, painful grouped vesicles or ulcerative and crusted external lesions on an erythematous base on the genitalia, buttocks, and/or thighs. The most common sites in females include the vulva and cervix and in males, the prepuce and glans penis (Fig. 27.4). Systemic symptoms are common in primary infection and include fever, malaise, headache, myalgias, regional lymphadenopathy, and dysuria. Females may also develop urinary retention secondary to severe dysuria. The primary illness lasts 10 to 20 days. An estimated 50% to 80% of patients will experience recurrent or reactivation eruptions 5 to 8 times per year because the virus remains latent. These recurrent eruptions are not as severe as the primary infection, and systemic symptoms usually do not develop.

Definitive diagnosis of genital herpes is through viral culture. Treatment of this chronic illness is palliative and includes the use of antiviral therapy such as acyclovir, famciclovir, or valacyclovir. These drugs are reported to reduce both the severity and duration of symptoms in primary cases and may reduce recurrence. Once-daily suppressive therapy reduces the frequency of genital herpes recurrences in up to 80% of patients who have frequent recurrence (up to six per year). Analgesics and sitz baths may also be used to reduce pain. Recurrences often occur during times of stress; therefore rest, a balanced diet, and stress reduction are part of the treatment regimen. All patients should be counseled regarding the transmission of the virus. Sexual activity should be avoided during the 24-hour prodromal period and for the duration of the outbreak until the time at which all lesions are dry.

Genital Warts

Human papillomavirus (HPV) is the etiologic agent responsible for the development of genital warts (condylomata acuminata). Genital warts are considered to be the most common cause of STIs in the world. More than 24 million Americans are infected with HPV, and 50% of sexually active men and women will acquire HPV at some point in their lives. More than 100 strains of HPV have been isolated thus far, and more than 30 of the viruses are transmitted sexually. Many of these viruses have been

TABLE 27.5 Complications Caused by Sexually Transmitted Organisms.

Complication	Causative Organisms
Salpingitis, infertility, and ectopic pregnancy	*Neisseria gonorrhoeae* *Chlamydia trachomatis* *Mycoplasma hominis* *Ureaplasma urealyticum*
Reproductive loss (abortion/miscarriage)	*Neisseria gonorrhoeae* *Chlamydia trachomatis* *Herpes simplex virus* *Mycoplasma hominis* *Ureaplasma urealyticum* *Treponema pallidum*
Puerperal infection	*Neisseria gonorrhoeae* *Chlamydia trachomatis*
Perinatal infection	Hepatitis B virus Human immunodeficiency virus Human papillomavirus *Neisseria gonorrhoeae* *Chlamydia trachomatis* *Herpes simplex virus* *Treponema pallidum* Cytomegalovirus Group B streptococcus
Cancer of genital area	*Chlamydia trachomatis* Herpes simplex virus Human papillomavirus
Male urethritis	*Mycoplasma hominis* Herpes simplex virus *Neisseria gonorrhoeae* *Chlamydia trachomatis* *Ureaplasma urealyticum*
Vulvovaginitis	Herpes simplex virus *Trichomonas vaginalis* Bacteria causing vaginosis *Candida albicans*
Cervicitis	*Neisseria gonorrhoeae* *Chlamydia trachomatis* Herpes simplex virus
Proctitis	*Neisseria gonorrhoeae* *Chlamydia trachomatis* Herpes simplex virus *Campylobacter jejuni* *Shigella species* *Entamoeba histolytica*
Hepatitis	*Treponema pallidum* Hepatitis A, B, and C virus
Dermatitis	*Sarcoptes scabiei* *Phthirus pubis*
Genital ulceration or warts	*Chlamydia trachomatis* Herpes simplex virus Human papillomavirus *Treponema pallidum* *Haemophilus ducreyi* *Calymmatobacterium granulomatis*

From Ignatavicius DD, Workman ML. *Medical-Surgical Nursing: Critical Thinking for Collaborative Care*. 5th ed. Philadelphia, PA: Saunders; 2006.

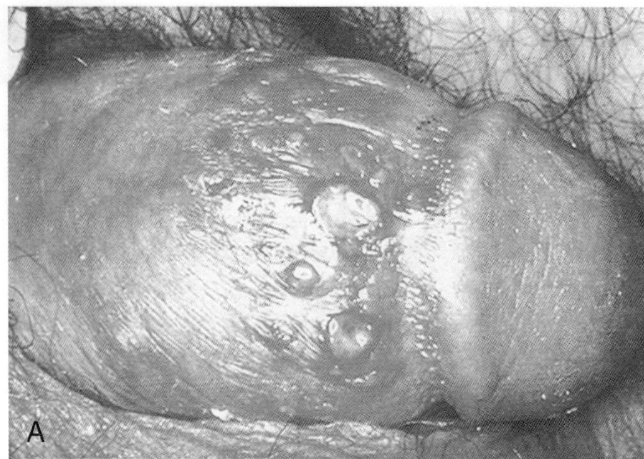

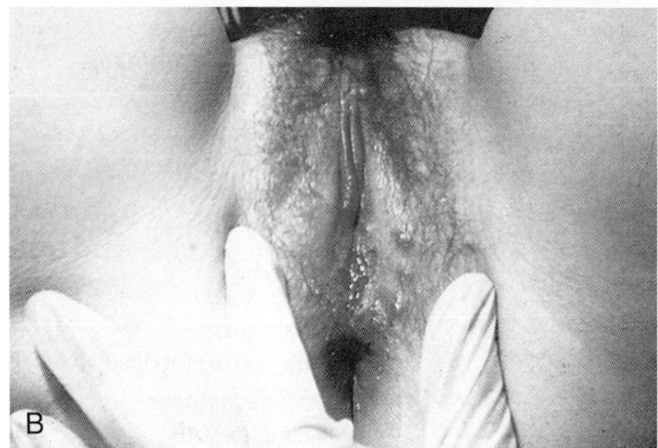

Fig. 27.4 Genital herpes in a male (A) and in a female (B). (From Lewis SM, Collier IC, Heitkemper MM: *Medical-Surgical Nursing: Assessment and Management of Clinical Problems.* 4th ed. St Louis, MO: Mosby; 1996.)

associated with an increased neoplastic risk in both men and women; squamous cell cervical cancer is firmly linked to HPV.

The virus invades the epidermal layer, penetrating skin and mucosal microabrasions in the genital and perineal area of males and females. A latency period of months to years may follow the initial virus transmission. After the latency period, host cells become infected and genital warts develop. Warts are typically single or multiple papular eruptions of varying shapes, such as cauliflower or plaquelike. The color may vary from that of the skin to erythema or hyperpigmentation. The sites where warts are most commonly found include the vulva, perineum, cervix, penis, and perianal areas (Fig. 27.5). Lesions may also be found in the mouth, pharynx, and larynx. The diagnosis of genital warts is established by appearance of the lesions without biopsy. The patient should be tested for other STIs.[8]

There is no evidence that treatment of genital warts will eradicate the virus or reduce the risk for neoplasm. If left untreated, visible genital warts can undergo spontaneous resolution, increase in size and number, or remain unchanged. The goal of treatment is removal of symptomatic warts to induce wart-free periods. Treatment can be accomplished through cryotherapy, electrodessication, curettage, surgical excision, or carbon dioxide laser therapy. The patient may also use home medications such as imiquimod cream, podofilox gel or solution, or antiproliferative compounds. In June 2006, Gardasil, a vaccine licensed by the US Food and Drug Administration (FDA) to prevent cervical cancer and other diseases caused by HPV in females, was released. This vaccine is recommended to be administered to 11- to 12-year-old girls; it may be given in patients as young as 9 years. The vaccine is also recommended for 13- to 26-year-old females who have not yet received or completed the vaccine series. Gardasil is administered in three separate doses; the initial dose is followed by a second and third dose at 2 and 6 months after the first dose, respectively.[9] Emergency care providers are in an excellent position to educate patients regarding the importance of this vaccine.

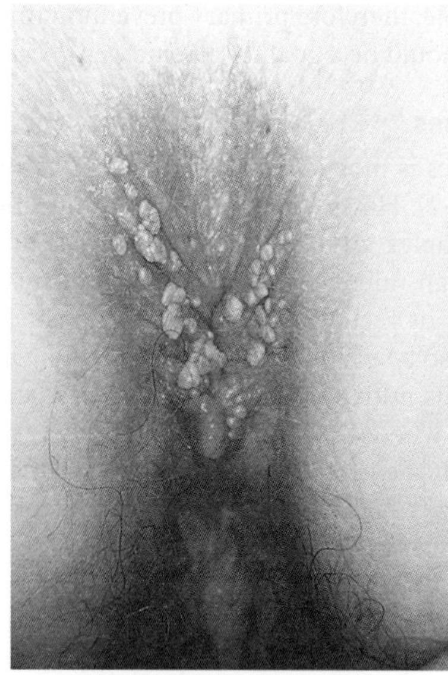

Fig. 27.5 Genital Warts (Condylomata Acuminata). (From Black JM, Hawks JH. *Medical-Surgical Nursing: Clinical Management for Positive Outcomes.* 8th ed. Philadelphia, PA: Saunders; 2009.)

Chancroid

The causative agent for chancroid is *Haemophilus ducreyi,* a gram-negative rod. It is a highly contagious disease most commonly found in third-world and developing countries. However, the incidence and prevalence in the United States is increasing. Coinfection with herpes or syphilis is found in 10% of patients with chancroid. An incubation period of 2 to 10 days is followed by the development of a papule or pustule developing into a painful, shallow ulcer surrounded by an erythematous ring. The borders of the lesions are irregular, with a purulent exudate covering the base. Multiple lesions are common and may coalesce into a large ulceration. The lesions are most commonly found on the fourchette, the vestibule, the clitoris, and the labia. There may be associated dyspareunia, vaginal discharge, fever, or weakness. Painful inguinal lymphadenopathy, referred to as buboes, is found in up to 50% of patients.[1] Lymphadenopathy occurs within 1 to 2 weeks after the ulcer formation.

Cultures are insensitive and unreliable to confirm the diagnosis of chancroid. The World Health Organization (WHO) and the CDC suggest a positive diagnosis be made if the patient has one or more painful ulcers without evidence of syphilis or HSV.[8] Serologic testing for syphilis, HIV, and other STIs should be performed, with a retest in 3 months if the initial test results are negative. Chancroid is one of the STIs associated with an increased risk for transmission of HIV. Treatment is with oral antibiotics. All patients should be counseled regarding safe-sex practices and cautioned not to engage in sexual activity until the ulcers are healed.[8]

Syphilis

Syphilis is caused by the spirochete *Treponema pallidum*. The disease is almost always transmitted through direct contact with an infected lesion; however, perinatal and transfusion-related transmissions have occurred. The incidence of syphilis in the United States has increased, particularly among men who have sex with men. The spirochete penetrates abraded skin or intact mucous membranes easily and disseminates rapidly. There are numerous presentations of syphilis mimicking several other infections; thus it is referred to as "the great imposter."

Syphilis is characterized by episodes of active disease and periods of latent infection. The disease occurs in three distinct phases: primary, secondary, and tertiary (latent). Primary syphilis is manifested by a single, painless genital ulcer, referred to as a chancre, which develops approximately 10 to 90 days after exposure. There is associated nontender inguinal adenopathy. The secondary phase of syphilis occurs 6 to 20 weeks after exposure. Secondary syphilis is manifested by a dull symmetric rash involving the palms and soles of the feet, fever and chills, lethargy, lymphadenopathy, patchy alopecia, loss of the lateral third of the eyebrow, and other nonspecific findings such as malaise, sore throat, and headache. The tertiary (latent) phase of syphilis develops years after the initial exposure and is manifested by neurologic findings, including meningitis, general paresis, progressive dementia, neuropathy, and tremulous extremities. Urinary incontinence may also occur. Cardiovascular complications of tertiary syphilis include aortic insufficiency and thoracic aneurysm. Figs. 27.6 and 27.7 depict the clinical appearance of primary and secondary syphilis, respectively.

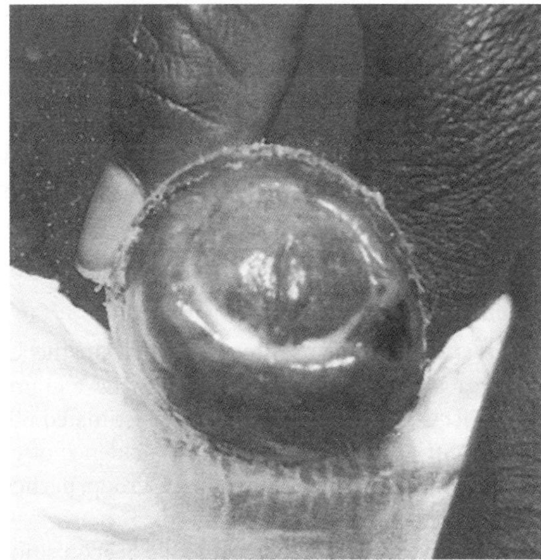

Fig. 27.6 Primary Syphilis in the Male. (From Greenberger NJ, Hinthorn DR. *History Taking and Physical Examination: Essentials and Clinical Correlates.* St Louis, MO: Mosby; 1993.)

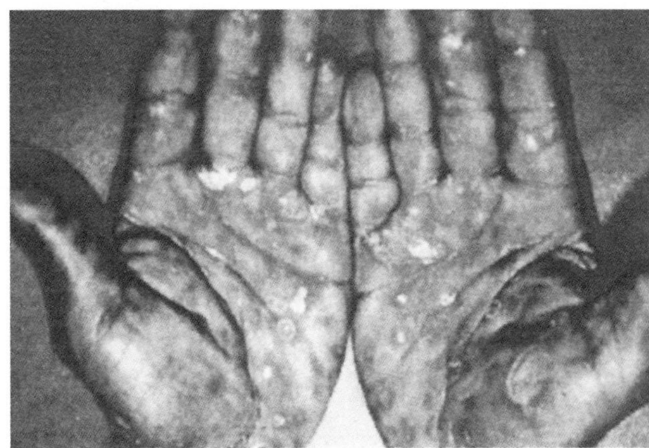

Fig. 27.7 Secondary Syphilis. (From Goldstein BG, Goldstein AO. *Practical Dermatology.* 2nd ed. St Louis, MO: Mosby; 1997.)

Early identification and antibiotic therapy are the keys to eradicating syphilis and the devastating complications associated with advanced disease. *T. pallidum* is too small to be visualized under a light microscope and cannot be cultivated in vivo; therefore diagnosis is made through serologic testing. The Venereal Disease Research Laboratories (VDRL) test and the rapid plasma reagent (RPR) test are the screening tests most commonly used. Confirmatory tests include the specific treponemal antibody tests, which are more specific.

Chlamydia

Chlamydial genital infection is the most frequently reported STI in the United States. The causative organism is *C. trachomatis*. The prevalence is highest among persons 25 years of age or younger, and within this young adult population 15- to 19-year-old adolescents are most frequently affected. An estimated 2.8 million Americans are infected with chlamydial infection each year.[8] Asymptomatic infection is common in both men and women, and therefore underreporting of this STI is substantial. Annual screening of all sexually active women age 25 years or younger is recommended, as is screening of older women who are at risk for contracting chlamydial infection. Risk factors include those who have a new sex partner or multiple sexual partners.

Chlamydial infection can be transmitted during vaginal, oral, or anal sexual contact with an infected person. In females the sequelae associated with chlamydial infection include cervicitis (most common), urethritis, bartholinitis, PID, and infertility. In males the resulting complications can include epididymitis, prostatitis, and Reiter syndrome (arthritis, urethritis, and conjunctivitis). Chlamydial infection can also cause lymphogranuloma venereum, an uncommon STI characterized by unilateral, painful lymphadenitis. Chlamydial infection can also be transmitted to neonates passing through an infected birth canal, with resulting conjunctivitis and/or neonatal pneumonia. Approximately 70% of women will be asymptomatic or have minimal symptoms such as dysuria, mild abdominal pain, or a vaginal discharge. Infected males may experience dysuria, urethral itching, and a thin, mucopurulent discharge, although 50% of men are asymptomatic.[1]

Diagnosis of chlamydial infection can be done through urine tests or vaginal/urethral swabs. Urine polymerase chain reaction (PCR), direct fluorescent antibody (DFA), nucleic acid amplification, and enzyme-linked immunoassay may all be used depending on the clinical site and test availability. Selected oral antibiotic treatment regimens should be effective against both *C. trachomatis* and *N. gonorrheae* because of the high frequency of concomitant infection.[1]

Gonorrhea

Gonorrhea is the second most common STI in the United States. The causative organism is *N. gonorrheae,* a gram-negative diplococcus. In the United States an estimated 600,000 new cases occur each year. The greatest incidence of gonorrhea is found in the 15- to 19-year-old age-group, particularly among females.[8]

The organism causes infection at the site of acquisition and commonly results in mucopurulent cervicitis and urethritis. Three patterns of disease have been identified in females with gonorrhea: (1) asymptomatic carrier, (2) cervicitis, and (3) PID. Between 30% and 40% of females are asymptomatic. Gonococcal infection may involve the periurethral Skene's glands, labial Bartholin glands, rectum, pharynx, and conjunctiva. Men are almost always symptomatic. In males the infection may involve the urethra, epididymis, and prostate gland. The infection may disseminate via the hematogenous route and lead to involvement of the joints, skin, meninges, and endocardium. Fever, chills, and a rash characterize disseminated gonococcal infections. Perinatal transmission may result in neonatal meningitis, sepsis, and ophthalmia neonatorum.

Diagnostic testing for *N. gonorrhea* can be done using endocervical, vaginal, male urethral, or urine specimens. Culture, nucleic acid hybridization tests, and nucleic acid amplification are available for the diagnosis of gonorrhea. Patients infected with gonorrhea are frequently coinfected with *C. trachomatis;* therefore it is recommended that patients should be treated concurrently for chlamydial infection.

In many geographic areas and populations there has been an increasing resistance to quinolones for the treatment of gonorrhea. Quinolone resistance has developed in parts of Europe, the Middle East, Asia, and the Pacific. In the United States, quinolone resistance is becoming increasingly common. This has led to changes in the recommended treatment regimens. The current CDC recommendation for treatment of uncomplicated gonococcal infections of the cervix, urethra, and rectum is to administer single-dose oral or intramuscular antibiotics.[8]

SUMMARY

The patient with an obstetric or gynecologic emergency presents challenging opportunities to the ED nurse. This patient population may have complex physiologic and psychosocial needs, particularly because a large proportion of this population is made up of adolescents and young adults. In addition to meeting the physical needs of a patient, the ED nurse is afforded a great opportunity for patient teaching and counseling.

REFERENCES

1. Tintinalli J, Stapczynski JS, Ma OJ, Yealy D, Meckler G, Cline D. *Tintinalli's Emergency Medicine: A Comprehensive Study Guide.* 8th ed. New York, NY: McGraw-Hill; 2016.
2. Emergency Nurses Association. *Emergency Nursing Core Curriculum.* 7th ed. St Louis, MO: Elsevier; 2018.
3. Angelini DJ, LaFontaine DF. *Obstetric, Triage, and Emergency Care Protocols.* 2nd ed. New York, NY: Springer; 2017.
4. Stratton P. Evaluation of acute pelvic pain in non-pregnant women. UpToDate. https://www.uptodate.com/contents/pelvic-inflammatory-disease-treatment-in-adults-and-adolescents. Updated May 09, 2019. Accessed May 14, 2019.
5. Barbieri R. *Emergency Department Management of Obstetric Complications.* New York, NY: Springer; 2017.
6. Marcdante KJ, Kliegman RM. *Nelson Essentials of Pediatrics.* Philadelphia, PA: Elsevier Saunders; 2018.
7. Sharp HT. Evaluation and management of ruptured ovarian cyst. UpToDate. https://www.uptodate.com/contents/evaluation-and-management-of-ruptured-ovarian-cyst?search=sharp%20ruptured%20ovarian%20cyst&source=search_result&selectedTitle=1~150&usage_type=default&display_rank=1. Updated Oct 09, 2018. Accessed May 14, 2019.
8. Centers for Disease Control and Prevention. *Sexually Transmitted Diseases Treatment Guidelines. Centers for Disease Control and Prevention Website*; 2015. https://www.cdc.gov/std/tg2015/default.htm. Published June 4, 2015. August May 14, 2019.
9. Wiesenfeld HC. Pelvic inflammatory disease: treatment in adults and adolescents. UpToDate. https://www.uptodate.com/contents/pelvic-inflammatory-disease-treatment-in-adults-and-adolescents. Updated Jan 2, 2019. Accessed May 14, 2019.

Endocrine Emergencies

Catherine T. Recznik

The endocrine system is an integrated complex of hormone-secreting glands. This system is instrumental in regulating metabolism, tissue function, growth and development, and emotions. The endocrine system works constantly to maintain homeostasis in response to physiologic stress, and dysfunction of one endocrine gland can affect the physiology of the entire body. Without prompt assessment, identification, and management, endocrine disturbances may result in life-threatening emergencies. The majority of endocrine emergencies encountered in the emergency department (ED) are related to diabetes mellitus. This chapter addresses selected endocrine disorders, including those related to diabetes, as well as pituitary, thyroid, and adrenal pathology. This chapter also addresses alcoholic ketoacidosis, a metabolic emergency.

ENDOCRINE SYSTEM PHYSIOLOGY

The endocrine system consists of the hypothalamus, pituitary, thyroid, parathyroids, adrenals, pancreas, testes, and ovaries (Fig. 28.1). Each gland produces and stores one or more hormones that have specific, unique functions. Table 28.1 identifies the hormones produced by the major endocrine glands, their target tissue, and their functions. Activities of the testes and ovaries are discussed in Chapters 26 and 27.

Hormone activity is the result of feedback loops, nerve stimulation, and intrinsic rhythms. Internal factors, such as renal and liver function, and external factors, such as pain, stress, or fear, all affect hormone release. Excessive amounts of circulating hormones inhibit additional hormone release, whereas low levels lead to increased hormone release. Neural stimulation triggers increased glandular activity and the release of hormones. Intrinsic rhythms vary from hours to weeks and provide another method of hormone control.

Hypothalamus

The hypothalamus creates part of the walls and floor of the third ventricle of the brain. Various centers in the anterior and posterior hypothalamus control most endocrine functions and influence many emotional behaviors. Nerve tracts from the hypothalamus join the posterior pituitary, which lies just below it. Posterior pituitary hormones are synthesized in the hypothalamus and then transferred along axons for storage in the posterior pituitary. The hypothalamus regulates anterior pituitary action by inhibiting or releasing additional hormones.

Pituitary

The pituitary gland, approximately 1 cm in all directions, lies within the sella turcica of the middle cranial fossa. Two physiologically distinct areas are found in the pituitary. The anterior pituitary contains secretory cells, whereas the posterior pituitary consists of neural cells that serve as a supporting structure for nerve fibers and nerve endings. Hormones secreted by the anterior pituitary include growth hormone, adrenocorticotropic hormone (ACTH), thyroid-stimulating hormone (TSH), prolactin, follicle-stimulating hormone,

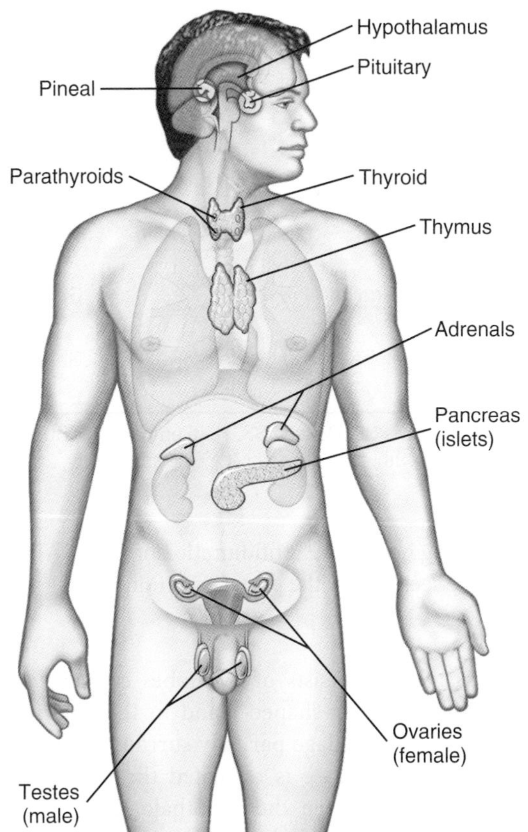

Fig. 28.1 Location of the Major Endocrine Glands. The parathyroid glands lie on the posterior surface of the thyroid gland. (From Lewis SL, Dirksen SR, Heitkemper MM, Bucher L, Harding MM. *Medical-Surgical Nursing: Assessment and Management of Clinical Problems.* 9th ed. St Louis, MO: Elsevier-Mosby; 2014.)

TABLE 28.1 Major Endocrine Glands and Hormones.

Hormones	Target Tissue	Functions
Anterior Pituitary (Adenohypophysis)		
Thyroid-stimulating hormone (TSH) or thyrotropin	Thyroid gland	Stimulates synthesis and release of thyroid hormones, growth and function of thyroid.
Adrenocorticotropic hormone (ACTH) or corticotrophin	Adrenal cortex	Fosters growth of adrenal cortex; stimulates secretion of glucocorticoids.
Posterior Pituitary (Neurohypophysis)		
Antidiuretic hormone (ADH) or vasopressin	Renal tubules, vascular smooth muscle	Promotes reabsorption of water. Raises blood pressure by inducing moderate vasoconstriction.
Thyroid		
Thyroxine (T_4)	All body tissues	Precursor to T_3.
Triiodothyronine (T_3)	All body tissues	Regulates metabolic rate of all cells and processes of cell growth and tissue differentiation.
Adrenal Medulla		
Epinephrine (adrenalin)	α- and β-adrenergic receptors	Increases heart rate and stroke volume, dilates pupils, constricts arterioles in the skin and digestive system, dilates arterioles in skeletal muscles. Relaxes bronchial smooth muscles. Triggers the release of glucose from energy stores.
Norepinephrine	α- and β-adrenergic receptors	Effects similar to epinephrine although longer acting. Also increased alertness and arousal.
Adrenal Cortex		
Corticosteroids (e.g., cortisol, hydrocortisone)	All body tissues	Maintains blood glucose, suppresses the immune response, and is released as part of the body's response to stress.
Mineralocorticoids (e.g., aldosterone)	Kidney	Regulates sodium and potassium balance and thus water balance.
Pancreas		
Insulin (from beta cells)	General	Promotes movement of glucose out of blood and into cells.
Glucagon (from alpha cells)	General	Promotes movement of glucose from storage and into blood.

Modified from Lewis SL, Dirksen SR, Heitkemper MM, Bucher L, Harding MM. *Medical-Surgical Nursing: Assessment and Management of Clinical Problems*. 9th ed. St Louis, MO: Elsevier-Mosby; 2014.

and luteinizing hormone.[1] Antidiuretic hormone (ADH) and oxytocin are secreted by the posterior pituitary.[1]

Thyroid

The thyroid gland consists of two lobes connected by an isthmus. This butterfly-shaped gland in the anterior neck below the cricoid cartilage partially surrounds the trachea. Thyroid hormone release is regulated through a complex feedback system between the hypothalamus and anterior pituitary. This main metabolic regulator contains follicular cells that secrete thyroxine (T_4) and triiodothyronine (T_3) in response to stimulation by the pituitary. Calcitonin originating in parafollicular cells in the thyroid affects calcium metabolism.

Parathyroids

The parathyroid glands are four small glands located on the posterior surface of the thyroid gland. The purpose of these glands is to maintain the body's calcium level within a very narrow range so that the nervous and muscular systems can function normally.

Adrenals

The adrenal glands, located in the retroperitoneal area above the upper pole of each kidney, consist of an outer cortical layer and inner medullary layer. The adrenal cortex produces mineralocorticoids (e.g., aldosterone), glucocorticoids (e.g., cortisol), and androgens. Aldosterone is critical for maintaining internal fluid balance, whereas glucocorticoids are major

BOX 28.1 Nursing Interventions for Suspected Endocrine Emergencies.

- Assess ABCs
- Intravenous access
- Laboratory testing:
  - Bedside glucose
  - Venous or arterial blood gases (POCT if possible)
  - Serum electrolytes
- Cardiac monitoring
- Strict intake and output
- Careful fluid replacement
- Focused history and physical
- Thorough cardiovascular, pulmonary, and neurologic assessments

POCT Point of care testing.

contributors to the body's ability to resist stress. The adrenal medulla releases the catecholamines epinephrine and norepinephrine in response to sympathetic stimulation.

Pancreas

The pancreas is situated behind the stomach in the retroperitoneal space. The body of the pancreas extends horizontally across the abdominal wall, with the head in the curve of the abdomen and the tail touching the spleen. Exocrine and endocrine cells are found in the pancreas. Acini are exocrine cells that release digestive enzymes, including amylase and lipase. Within the islet of Langerhans, two major types of cells are alpha cells, which secrete glucagon, and beta cells, which produce insulin.[1]

PATIENT ASSESSMENT

The endocrine system affects most, if not all, body systems. Complaints most commonly associated with endocrine disorders include fatigue, weakness, polyuria, polydipsia, weight changes, and mental status changes. The focused assessment should target the specific presenting complaint. When a critically ill patient presents to the ED, an endocrine etiology should be considered as part of the differential diagnosis. Care of the patient begins with assessment and stabilization of the airway, breathing, and circulation (ABCs) as well as a neurologic assessment. The neurologic assessment includes evaluation of possible causes of altered consciousness such as trauma, blood glucose abnormalities, stroke, or toxins. Identification of a stressor or precipitating event may be elicited through patient history, family interviews, laboratory findings, radiographic analysis, or other diagnostic procedures. The emergency nurse should expect to perform a standard set of interventions for any patient with a suspected endocrine emergency, as seen in Box 28.1.

SELECTED ENDOCRINE EMERGENCIES

The emergency nurse will encounter patients with varied severity of endocrine dysfunction. Selected conditions covered in this chapter include those situations that may lead to hemodynamic instability or altered neurologic function. Awareness of the potential for endocrine system abnormalities in every critical patient is extremely important for the ED nurse.

Diabetic Emergencies

Diabetes mellitus (DM) is a chronic condition characterized by hyperglycemia and disturbances of carbohydrate, fat, and protein metabolism. Two major types of DM exist: type 1, in which there is a failure of the beta cells to produce insulin, producing an absolute insulin deficiency, and type 2, which is characterized by impaired insulin secretion, peripheral insulin resistance, and inappropriate hepatic glucose production.[1] Type 2 accounts for at least 90% of all diabetes in the United States, with obesity as a major risk factor for the development of this disorder.[2]

Hypoglycemia

Hypoglycemia is a potentially life-threatening emergency commonly affecting patients with diabetes, as well as those without diabetes who are very young, very old, or critically ill. Hypoglycemia is defined as a pathologic state characterized by a low serum glucose level. The precise level of glucose that is low enough to be considered hypoglycemia depends on the measurement method, the age of the patient, the presence or absence of symptoms, and the purpose of the definition. For adults, children, and infants older than 24 hours of age, glucose levels under 70 mg/dL are indicative of hypoglycemia,[2] although this value may vary based on an individual's normal levels and institutional policy. The rapidity at which the serum glucose decreases can influence the patient's symptoms; if glucose levels drop too quickly in relation to the body's compensatory ability, the patient may become symptomatic at higher serum glucose levels.[1] Hospital policies should reflect the need for the nurse to assess for signs and symptoms, which may also influence treatment options. The American Diabetes Association (ADA) advocates for the adoption of nurse-initiated treatment protocols for patients experience symptomatic and laboratory-defined hypoglycemia. Low serum glucose level is a common cause of ED presentations.[3] The most dramatic effects of hypoglycemia are neurologic because glucose is the most important source of energy for the brain. The brain requires continuous delivery of glucose to function adequately[1]; all unresponsive or neurologically altered patients should be promptly evaluated for hypoglycemia.

Medications, infections, liver disease, and congenital metabolic abnormalities are all possible causes for symptomatic hypoglycemia.[2–4] In addition to insulin, oral antidiabetics, such as sulfonylureas and meglitinides, are associated with hypoglycemia, whereas α-glucosidase inhibitors, biguanides, and thiazolidinediones alone do not normally cause hypoglycemia.[5] Factors that contribute to hypoglycemia include lack of dietary intake, increased physical stress, changes in type of insulin or oral agents, pregnancy, alcohol ingestion, and certain drugs.

Normally the body senses declining serum glucose levels and releases glucagon and epinephrine to stimulate release

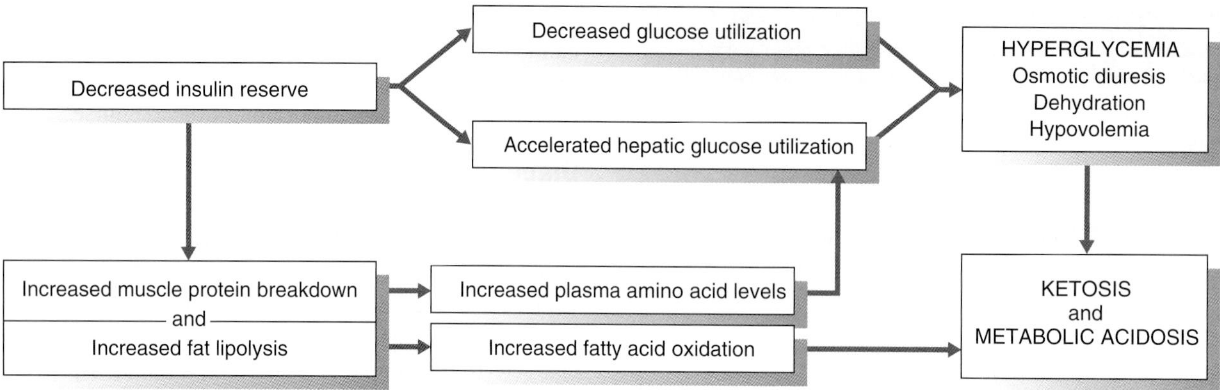

Fig. 28.2 Pathophysiology of Diabetic Ketoacidosis.

of glycogen by the liver. Glycogen functions as an alternate energy source; however, in acute hypoglycemia, glycogen stores cannot be broken down quickly enough to overcome the effects of insulin. Epinephrine release decreases utilization of existing glucose. Common symptoms of hypoglycemia, including shakiness, anxiety, palpitations, sweating, dry mouth, pallor, pupil dilation, and hunger, are attributed to epinephrine release.[1] The known patient with diabetes can usually recognize these symptoms and self-treat. β-Blocker therapy masks this sympathetic response; it is important to provide appropriate education to patients prescribed these medications who are already at risk for low blood glucose.[6]

As the brain becomes deprived of glucose, symptoms including abnormal mentation, irritability, confusion, difficulty speaking, ataxia, headaches, and stupor occur.[1] The patient may or may not be able to self-treat or seek treatment at this point. Without treatment, neuroglycopenia can lead to seizures, coma, and even death. Patient and family education is essential, as often the family must initiate treatment if severe hypoglycemia occurs.

In the hospital setting, priorities include supporting the ABCs, ensuring patient safety, and initiating treatment. Treatment of the conscious patient consists of oral intake of 10 to 15 g of simple carbohydrates, usually in the form of glucose gel, juice, or hard candy, followed by a more complex carbohydrate snack or small meal. In the lethargic or unconscious patient, rapid administration of intravenous (IV) dextrose remains the treatment of choice (20–50 g of 50% dextrose for an adult).[1] If IV access cannot be obtained, intramuscular glucagon 1 mg (adult dose) should be administered.[6] Glucagon stimulates the liver to release glycogen, which is converted to glucose; patients must have adequate glycogen stores for this therapy to be effective. Because vomiting is common after the administration of glucagon, the patient should be positioned to minimize the risk for aspiration. Unresponsive patients receiving insulin via an insulin pump should have the pump disconnected or delayed until the patient has regained their faculties.

Laboratory study results obtained before glucose administration may provide helpful information, but administration of glucose should not be delayed to obtain laboratory samples. Severe neurologic deficits can result if the central nervous system (CNS) is left without glucose. Once alert, the patient should be given additional food, including complex carbohydrates, to maintain an adequate glucose level.[2] If the cause of the episode is identified and resolved, the patient may be discharged after a meal, observation, and confirmation that the glucose level has stabilized. Patients for whom a clear cause is not identified should have further evaluation and testing.

With the current focus on tight glycemic control and intensive insulin therapy, the risk for hypoglycemia is increased.[3] Maintaining euglycemia decreases many of the microvascular complications associated with DM.[1] Patients receiving intensive insulin therapy have a greater incidence of severe, disabling hypoglycemia than those receiving conventional insulin therapy. Intensive insulin therapy is not recommended as a therapy in older adults or for critically ill patients receiving intensive care.[2] After treatment of the acute event, it is important to obtain a careful history, including medication use, current illness, and activity level. This can be a key opportunity for patient teaching for prevention and management of future episodes.

Diabetic Ketoacidosis

Diabetic ketoacidosis (DKA) develops when a patient experiences relative or absolute depletion of circulating insulin. This potentially life-threatening condition may occur in up to two-thirds of previously undiagnosed pediatric patients, leading to the initial diagnosis of diabetes (particularly type 1).[7] For patients with previously diagnosed diabetes, infection, illness, pregnancy, or situational stressors can create a relative insulin deficiency. In other patients, excess circulating glucose secondary to poor dietary management can overwhelm an already stressed system. Absolute deficiency can occur in patients who fail to follow their prescribed insulin regimen, experience insulin delivery failure, or are unable or unwilling to take adequate insulin. The latter example demonstrates why diabetic education is critical.

After prolonged insulin deficiency, the patient can present with four acute problems: hyperglycemia, dehydration, electrolyte depletion, and metabolic acidosis (Fig. 28.2). Stress causes release of counterregulatory hormones, which leads to gluconeogenesis. Severe hyperglycemia increases serum osmolality and leads to osmotic diuresis, resulting in significant dehydration. Osmotic diuresis leads to urinary losses of water, sodium, potassium, magnesium, calcium, and phosphorus. The typical total body water loss in DKA is 6 to 9 L in adult patients.[8]

Despite gluconeogenesis, without insulin, the newly liberated glucose cannot be used, further increasing serum blood glucose levels, urine glucose concentrations, and osmotic diuresis.[1] Fats and muscle proteins are metabolized for energy. This lipolysis causes a buildup of fatty acids, which overcomes the body's natural buffering system, resulting in acidosis. As this acidosis worsens, it is sometimes detected by noting the presence of a fruity odor on the patient's breath.

DKA develops over a relatively short time, even just hours after a triggering event.[9] The patient describes a steady progression of symptoms, including polydipsia, polyuria, polyphagia, fatigue, and weakness. Patients with new-onset diabetes may report recent weight loss. As ketoacidosis worsens, nausea, vomiting, decreased appetite, and abdominal cramping occur. The patient appears in moderate to severe distress with possible alteration in level of consciousness, confusion about recent events, or slow response to questions. Lethargy can progress to coma, and hyperthermia may be present.

In response to the acidosis, the body compensates by triggering rapid, deep breathing called Kussmaul respirations. This respiratory compensation serves to improve the pH by "blowing off" CO_2. The skin is usually hot and dry, skin turgor is diminished, and mucous membranes are dry. Hypotension can result from severe dehydration. The most frequently seen cardiac rhythm is sinus tachycardia, but dysrhythmias related to electrolyte disturbances also occur. In pregnancy this can have deleterious effects on the fetus, and early identification and aggressive interventions are critical to minimize the effects of DKA on the fetus and the mother.

Initial laboratory studies should be obtained early and fluid therapy started on arrival to the ED. A serum glucose level higher than 250 mg/dL, a pH under 7.3, and the presence of serum or urine ketones are expected findings.[9] In addition, potassium levels may be normal or elevated, and creatinine and blood urea nitrogen (BUN) levels may be elevated as a result of dehydration. Serum ketone testing based on the measurement of β-hydroxybutyrate (β-OHB, the main ketoacid causing acidosis) is recommended for diagnosis and monitoring,[10] with a β-OHB level of >3.8 mmol/L being considered "positive."[9] Blood gas values from a patient with DKA demonstrate decreased pH, decreased HCO_3, decreased PCO_2, and normal arterial oxygen pressure (PaO_2); although traditionally arterial blood gases (ABGs) were used to establish the presence of acidosis, some guidelines now recognize the utility of venous blood gases (VBGs),[10] and recent studies have found that VBGs can be used in place of ABGs for the treatment of DKA.[11] Because infection can precipitate DKA, blood and urine cultures should be obtained when infection is suspected. After cultures are obtained, antibiotic therapy should begin; as in all critically ill patients, antibiotic administration should not be delayed to obtain cultures. Radiology studies may also be useful in determining the primary site of infection.

Management in the ED should be aggressive. Treatment focuses on correction of hyperglycemia, dehydration, electrolyte imbalances, and metabolic acidosis. Close monitoring with frequent reassessment is essential to prevent complications. Serum glucose and potassium levels should be monitored every 1 to 2 hours, and pH should be monitored every 2 to 4 hours.[9]

IV fluid replacement should start immediately with 15 to 20 mL/kg of normal saline over the first 1 to 2 hours of treatment for adults.[9] As mentioned earlier, the adult patient may require up to 9 L of fluid.[8] In children the initial fluid bolus is typically 10 mL/kg of either 0.9% or 0.45% saline solution[12]; volume replacement is carefully titrated because of the high risk for cerebral edema in the pediatric population. At the time of this writing, a recently published study refutes the previously proposed theory that the rate and sodium content of fluid replacement has a relationship with cerebral edema and neurologic outcomes in pediatric patients.[13] In fact, Kuppermann et al., in a large, randomized trial, demonstrated no statistically significant neurologic difference among groups that received 0.9% sodium chloride versus 0.45% sodium chloride and fast versus slow rehydration.[13] The authors suggest cerebral edema may be a symptom, rather than the cause, of cerebral edema, and suggest that cerebral hypoperfusion during DKA may actually be the cause of the brain injuries incurred during DKA.[13] Another recent paper proposes benefits by use solutions that are not sodium-chloride based.[14] Close observation of intake and output is essential; placement of a urinary catheter ensures accurate output assessment, but the risk of catheter-associated complications should be carefully weighed against the benefit of more accurate measurement of urinary output. After fluid resuscitation has begun, current guidelines recommend the initiation of a continuous IV infusion of regular insulin at 0.1 units/kg per hour[10] with the goal to stop ketogenesis and achieve a steady decrease in serum glucose level of no greater than 90 mg/dL per hour[10]; in adult patients, an initial IV bolus of 0.1 units/kg of regular insulin may also be used.[8] Regular insulin is the only insulin that can be administered IV, and in DKA IV administration is the standard of care. It is also important to note that the IV tubing should be "primed" with 20 mL of the insulin-containing solution, as the insulin itself is known to adhere to the tubing. This ensures the patient receives the ordered rate of insulin infusion.[15]

After serum glucose level reaches 200 to 250mg/dL,[8] fluids should be converted to dextrose-containing solutions to prevent hypoglycemia. In pediatric populations, this is often achieved through the use of a "two bag" system.[12] Resolution of the hyperglycemic emergency occurs when the serum glucose level is less than 200 mg/dL, serum bicarbonate level is greater than or equal to 18 mEq/L, and in DKA, the venous pH is greater than 7.3.[10]

Fluid replacement dilutes serum potassium and promotes diuresis, so potassium replacement should begin after the first IV fluid bolus, even when initial values are normal.[9] Potassium levels frequently drop precipitously in the first few hours after treatment has been initiated as potassium moves back to the intracellular space along with the insulin and existing glucose. Serum potassium levels must be repeated

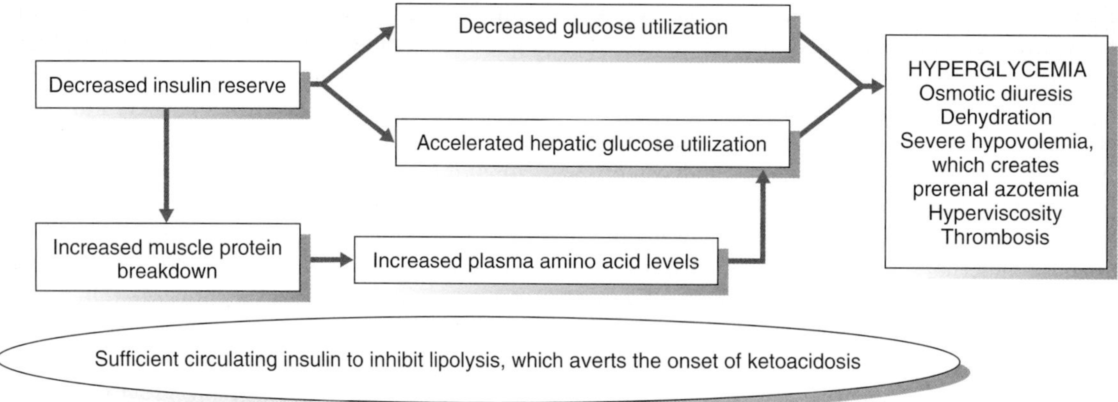

Fig. 28.3 Pathophysiology of Hyperosmolar Hyperglycemic State.

every 1 to 2 hours during initial management. Cardiac monitoring is essential because dysrhythmias can develop with significant hypokalemia. If the serum potassium is less than 3.3 mEq/L, insulin replacement should be delayed until the serum potassium level is in normal range.[9]

Additional considerations are resolution of acidosis and treatment of presenting signs and symptoms. Acidosis generally corrects with fluid and insulin therapy. Insulin allows the cells to use available glucose for energy, leading to decreased proteolysis and lipolysis, and the ketoacidosis resolves. Insulin infusion should be continued until the pH or serum bicarbonate level has normalized; acidosis in DKA is not routinely treated with sodium bicarbonate because sodium bicarbonate does not appear to confer benefit.[9] Treatment of signs and symptoms, such as nausea, vomiting, and pain, should also be prioritized, as this will not only improve patient comfort but also prevent worsening dehydration. Providing a quiet, calm environment can improve patient comfort. Thorough explanation of treatment, medications, and plan of care can alleviate stress related to hospitalization. Potential complications include hypoglycemia, hypokalemia, dysrhythmias, and cerebral edema. Monitor serum glucose levels, electrocardiogram (ECG) tracings, laboratory values, vital signs, intake and output, and neurologic status carefully. Care should be taken to carefully transition the patient's glucose and pH levels back to normal, as rapid shifting has been associated with complications.[10]

Hyperosmolar Hyperglycemic State

Hyperosmolar hyperglycemic state (HHS), also known as hyperosmolar hyperglycemic nonketotic coma, is a life-threatening emergency characterized by marked elevation of blood glucose level, hyperosmolarity, and little or no ketosis.[10] HHS threatens patients with type 2 diabetes with mortality rates as high as 20%.[16] With the increase in the prevalence of type 2 DM, this condition is likely to be encountered more frequently in the future.[17] The precipitating causes are numerous, with infections being the most common.[17] Other causes include medication and treatment noncompliance, undiagnosed diabetes, substance abuse, and coexisting disease.[9] Physical findings include those associated with profound dehydration and various neurologic symptoms such as coma. Typically, patients presenting with HHS are older than 50 years of age, but the incidence in pediatric patients is increasing.[17] Patients with a diagnosis of HHS are frequently on medications that aggravate the problem, such as diuretics that cause mild dehydration.[17] When a diagnosis is established, identifying contributing or additional diagnoses is warranted.[1]

When stressed with illness, surgery, or injury, the body responds by increasing serum glucose levels. Patients with type 2 DM produce enough insulin to avoid ketoacidosis but not enough to prevent profound hyperglycemia. This increased serum glucose level acts as an osmotic diuretic, leading to severe dehydration with serum hyperosmolarity. Patients are unable to replace lost fluids, so their condition progressively worsens. Because insulin is present, the metabolizing of fats is minimal, and serum ketones are usually absent or only present in trace amounts.[16,17] The persistently inadequate level of insulin is insufficient to ensure cellular access to glucose, additional hepatic gluconeogenesis occurs, compounding existing hyperglycemia. Underlying renal disease or decreased intravascular volume may also decrease the glomerular filtration rate and cause an even more rapid rise in serum glucose. Fig. 28.3 explains HHS pathophysiology.

Onset of symptoms in HHS is much more insidious than with DKA, developing over days or even weeks. Subtlety of symptoms may account for delay in seeking treatment. The patient may notice decreased appetite, polydipsia, and polyuria. As the disease progresses, neurologic symptoms such as headaches, blurred vision, confusion, decreasing level of consciousness, seizure, or even coma may develop.[17] At the time of presentation, tachycardia, hypotension, and decreased urinary output may be present.[17] Respirations may be increased but do not have the fruity smell associated with DKA. The decrease in mental status often prompts the ED visit, especially as the neurologic signs and symptoms may mimic a stroke.[1]

Laboratory studies should include complete blood count (CBC), electrolytes, urinalysis, and venous or ABGs. Typical laboratory findings in HHS include blood glucose levels greater than 600 mg/dL, serum osmolality greater than 320 mOsm/kg, pH levels greater than 7.30, and mild or absent ketonemia.[17] Serum potassium levels may be high, low, or normal depending on the level of dehydration, whereas serum sodium is typically falsely low.[17]

TABLE 28.2 **Comparison of Classic Presentations of Diabetic Ketoacidosis (DKA) and Hyperglycemic Hyperosmolar State (HHS).**

Clinical Picture	DKA	HHS
Patient's age	Usually younger	Usually older adults
Type of diabetes mellitus	Type 1	Type 2
Duration of symptoms	Hours to days	Several days
Neurologic symptoms and signs	Rare except as complication	Very common
Glucose level	≥250 mg/dL	>600 mg/dL
Ketones	Moderate or large	Small or absent
Serum sodium	Likely to be low or normal	Low or normal
Serum potassium	High, normal, or low	High, normal, or low
Serum bicarbonate	Low	Normal
Blood pH	Low	Normal
Serum osmolality	Typically normal	>320 mOsm/L
Thrombosis	Rare	Frequent

Although acidosis is not present, the initial treatment for HHS is the same as that for DKA, although the fluid deficit is often more extreme.[9] Careful assessment of laboratory findings, IV fluid replacement, potassium administration, and IV insulin are cornerstones of therapy. Admission and treatment for underlying conditions should also be prioritized, and education and follow-up should focus on prevention of future episodes and treatment of underlying disease. Due to the average older age of patients with HHS, volume overload is more likely, despite the severe dehydration; in addition, the incidence of cerebral edema is also higher in patients of all ages with HHS.[16,17] Otherwise, the same careful monitoring and interventions as for DKA apply.

In HHS, resolution of disease is defined as normalization of mental status and return to a serum osmolarity under 320 mOsm/kg.[9] Adequate fluids must be given before initiating insulin therapy because hypotension may worsen if insulin is administered before fluids.[9] In addition, interventions aimed at stabilizing glucose levels begin when the serum glucose level reaches a slightly higher target of 250 to 300 mg/dL; when this occurs, it is recommended that dextrose replacement be initiated and that the insulin infusion be decreased to 0.02 to 0.05 U/kg per hour.[10] Finally, because patients with HHS are at increased risk for thrombus formation, the prevention and management of this condition should be included in the treatment plan.[16]

Differentiation between HHS and DKA may be initially difficult; however, this should not alter the basic course of treatment. Management of ABCs remains the top priority of emergency care, and IV fluid therapy should begin immediately in both cases. Nursing actions are similar in both instances and include close observation of vital signs and laboratory values to prevent complications of therapy. Table 28.2 compares the clinical features of DKA and HHS.

Alcoholic Ketoacidosis

Alcoholic ketoacidosis (AKA) is an acute metabolic emergency that generally occurs 24 hours or more after a patient who has been ingesting large amounts of alcohol abruptly stops drinking.[18] AKA is most common in adults with chronic alcohol abuse and a recent history of binge drinking, persistent vomiting, and decreased food intake.[18] It is thought that alcoholic ketoacidosis is underdiagnosed in some countries.[19] AKA is characterized by elevated serum ketone levels, decreased bicarbonate level, and theoretically, a glucose level that is only mildly elevated.[20] Unfortunately, complicating the diagnosis of AKA is the fact that patients can present with higher glucose levels, leading to an incorrect diagnosis of DKA.[19] Once placed on an insulin drop per DKA treatment protocols, these patients can develop life-threatening hypoglycemia that must be promptly treated[19]; the consideration of alternative diagnoses, including AKA and starvation ketosis, must be considered for these patients.[20]

Patients with alcoholism often do not maintain adequate nutritional intake. During periods of starvation, insulin levels are decreased, making glucose utilization difficult.[18] When these patients drink a substantial amount of alcohol and then suddenly stop, the body breaks down fats and lipids, producing ketones as a byproduct.[20] Dehydration, a common finding in patients who abuse alcohol, can produce a state of lactic acidosis, and the byproducts of alcohol are themselves acidic.[21] The presentation of AKA is thought to be a culmination of these factors.[21]

Patients present with abdominal pain, nausea, vomiting, and signs of alcohol withdrawal.[21] Physical findings include tachypnea, tachycardia, and alteration in mental status; AKA should be included in the differential diagnosis when acute alcohol intoxication is suspected.[18] Initial laboratory studies may show decreased pH, although serum pH levels can be misleading because patients with AKA may have a mixed acid-base disorder due to vomiting, dehydration, or compensatory hyperventilation.[20]

Management in the ED is focused on ABCs and correction of volume loss, glycogen stores, and electrolyte imbalance. Once the diagnosis of AKA is established, the treatment is hydration with dextrose-containing IV fluids, which leads to an increase in serum insulin levels and suppression of the release of glucagon and other counterregulatory hormones.[20]

Electrolyte levels should be carefully evaluated and deficiencies treated promptly.[21] Because patients with alcoholism often have underlying nutritional deficiencies, consideration should be given to the administration of thiamine before or together with dextrose-containing fluids, although the quality of evidence to support this recommendation is low.[22] Ongoing thiamine deficiency may result in Wernicke's encephalopathy, a syndrome characterized by ataxia, confusion, and vision changes.[18,22] Throughout treatment, the patient with AKA requires close monitoring, seizure precautions, and supportive care. Frequent assessment of vital signs, intake and output, neurologic status, and electrolyte values is necessary to monitor effectiveness of therapy and to ensure an uncomplicated return to the patient's normal metabolic state.

Pituitary Disorders

Diabetes Insipidus

Diabetes insipidus (DI) is characterized by excretion of large volumes of dilute urine and can be life-threatening if not properly diagnosed and managed. The two main types of DI can be described as one of two different disturbances, inadequate or impaired secretion of ADH (central) or inadequate renal response to ADH (nephrogenic).[23] Determining the type of disturbance is essential for effective treatment. In addition to passing large amounts of dilute urine, patients typically present with extraordinary thirst despite copious water intake, dry skin, tachycardia, and progressive hemodynamic instability.[1]

Central DI results from any condition that impairs the secretion and release of ADH. Central DI can be idiopathic, genetic, or acquired, such as from head injury or brain surgery.[1] In nephrogenic DI there is sufficient ADH, but the kidneys do not properly concentrate the urine. Nephrogenic DI may be genetic or acquired, with children typically presenting with a genetic cause and adults typically presenting with an acquired one.[23] Acquired nephrogenic DI can be permanent or transient, and can be caused by drugs, particularly lithium; vascular damage, such as in sickle cell anemia; or profound electrolyte imbalance, including hypokalemia and hypercalcemia.[23]

Diagnosis is made by measurement of urine osmolality, which helps in determining whether polyuria is due to DI. A urine osmolality less than 300 mOsm/kg in the presence of polyuria is makes DI extremely likely.[24] Determination of the type of DI is essential, as replacement of ADH is the treatment for central DI but would be ineffective in the setting of nephrogenic DI.

ED testing includes measurement of urine osmolality, serum electrolytes, and serum osmolality, but after patient stabilization, further diagnostic testing for identification of the type of DI includes the water deprivation test. This test consists of withholding all fluids for a period lasting up to 7 hours, with frequent measurements of body weight, urine osmolality, and serum osmolality until the patient experiences a 5% decrease in body weight or variability in urine samples ceases.[4,24,25] At the conclusion of the water deprivation test, exogenous ADH (vasopressin) is provided and a final measurement of serum and urine osmolality is conducted.[25] Patients with central DI will increase their urine osmolality; patients with nephrogenic DI will not.[24]

For central DI, therapy focuses on administration of ADH as well as fluid volume replacement. Fluid administration that is too rapid can lead to volume overload or a rapid change in serum sodium levels, and the patient should be monitored carefully.[26] ADH replacement is achieved primarily with the use of desmopressin,[26] although additional drugs such as carbamazepine can be used to decrease the necessary dose.[23] Nephrogenic DI does not respond to ADH; therefore treatment includes adequate oral intake, electrolyte management, dietary salt restrictions, and identification and removal of possible causes.[24] In addition, thiazide diuretics can be used in the treatment of both central and nephrogenic DI.[24,25] Although the administration of a diuretic is counterintuitive, the use of a thiazide diuretic leads to activation of the renin-angiotensin system, which in turn increases the amount of sodium and water that is reabsorbed.[27]

Emergency management of the patient with DI includes close monitoring of fluid status, neurologic status, electrolyte levels, and resulting ECG rhythm or other systemic disturbances. Close monitoring of fluid intake, output, and urine osmolality, in addition to prompt distinction between central and nephrogenic DI, will determine the course of treatment.

Syndrome of Inappropriate Antidiuretic Hormone

Syndrome of inappropriate antidiuretic hormone (SIADH) occurs when the feedback system that regulates the ADH level fails, causing the pituitary gland to release excessive amounts of ADH. A patient with SIADH may present to the ED with dilutional hyponatremia, which can lead to seizures and death if left untreated.[28] Because ADH is generated in the hypothalamus and stored in the pituitary gland, any disease process or pharmacotherapy that alters the function or pathways of these endocrine systems can precipitate SIADH.[1,28] Thyroid and pituitary lesions, drugs, including diuretics and carbamazepine, and head trauma or stroke can precipitate SIADH.[1,28] Other associated disorders include pain, emotional stress, positive pressure ventilation, pneumonia, and tuberculosis.[1,28]

In SIADH, excess ADH causes increased distal renal tubular permeability to water, causing the kidneys to retain fluid and produce decreased urine volumes. Serum osmolality and circulating blood volume typically influence ADH release; however, in patients with SIADH vasopressin (ADH) continues to be released into circulation despite the decreasing serum osmolarity (typically under 275 mOsmol/kg[4]). Signs and symptoms of SIADH are caused by the resulting fluid overload and associated hyponatremia.[28]

Subjective complaints include weakness, nausea, vomiting, abdominal and muscle cramps, sudden weight gain without edema, headache, and fatigue.[1,4] The patient or caregiver may note decreased urinary output despite regular oral intake; the greatest changes, however, may be in neurologic and cardiac function. The patient appears confused and disoriented with possible seizure activity as the hyponatremia worsens. Severe hyponatremia leads to fluid shifts, which can cause cerebral edema, pulmonary edema, hypertension, and jugular vein distention.[7] Laboratory tests may reveal marked hyponatremia (<125 mEq/L[4]), low serum osmolality (<280 mOsm/kg[1]), and decreased creatinine.[7] Urine osmolality, sodium, and specific gravity are increased; urine is hyperosmolar compared with the plasma.[4,7]

Management of SIADH is related to the severity of hyponatremia. Free water restriction is sufficient in mild cases. For adults, fluid restrictions often start at 800 to 1000 mL/day; however, restrictions as severe as 500 mL/day may be required.[1,28] Acute, severe hyponatremia (<121 mmol/L) is often associated with neurologic symptoms such as seizures and should be treated urgently because of the high risk for cerebral edema.[28] The initial correction rate with hypertonic saline should not exceed 1 to 2 mEq/L per hour unless severe neurologic symptoms are present.[28] The importance of accurate intake and output monitoring cannot be overemphasized, with especially careful attention to any signs or symptoms of fluid overload. Once the serum sodium is at least 125 mEq/L, small amounts of loop diuretics may be administered to increase urinary output and improve hypervolemia.[1,28] Demeclocycline can be given to interfere with ADH action; however, this simply augments fluid restriction therapy.[1]

Ultimately, serum sodium and osmolality should improve. Serial electrolyte evaluations help avoid complications in therapy and assist in monitoring therapy progress. After the patient stabilizes, identification and treatment of the precipitating event is prioritized. Close observation, timely management, and adequate education ensure patient safety and prevent complications.

Thyroid Emergencies

True thyroid emergencies are rare, but can be life-threatening. The thyroid gland regulates the body's metabolic rate through the hypothalamic-pituitary-thyroid counterregulatory system. Thyroid gland activity depends on the hypothalamus secreting thyrotropin-releasing hormone (TRH), which is responsible for release of TSH by the anterior pituitary, which causes the release of T_4. Circulating T_4 is converted to T_3 in the peripheral system. The amount of TSH depends on the amount of TRH, which can be influenced by physical stressors such as surgery, infection, and extreme temperatures. Circulating levels of T_3 and T_4 also affect the amount of TRH released through negative feedback. If any part of this system malfunctions, the resulting hyperactivity or hypoactivity of the thyroid gland can lead to multisystem symptoms.

Hyperthyroidism

Hyperthyroidism can be caused by multiple disturbances. True hyperthyroidism is characterized by an overactive thyroid gland and excessive production of thyroid hormones. Graves' disease, an autoimmune disorder in which thyroid-stimulating immunoglobulins increase thyroid activity,[29] is responsible for as much as 80% of all cases of hyperthyroidism.[1] Other possible causes include tumors, thyroiditis, and ingestion of thyroid hormones (intentionally or unintentionally).[29,30] Certain drugs, such as amiodarone, can also induce hyperthyroidism.[31]

Thyroid Storm

Thyroid storm is an acute, life-threatening complication of poorly managed hyperthyroidism or thyrotoxicosis (symptomatic hyperthyroidism).[29] One study found an inpatient mortality rate of 10.1% but described rates as high as 25% in previous studies.[32] Rapid elevation in thyroid hormone levels results in a decompensated state of severe hypermetabolism, characterized by hyperthermia, agitation, tachydysrhythmias, and tremors.[1] Elevated hormone levels can occur in response to hospitalization, surgery, infection, trauma, or overmanipulation of the thyroid.[29]

Gathering a concise history regarding illnesses, current medications, and family history of any autoimmune diseases is important. The patient may have recently discontinued a medication or experienced a recent change in therapy. The patient commonly has a history of Graves' disease. Patients often report recent weight loss despite increased appetite and increased caloric intake. The patient may be restless with a shortened attention span; children may have a recent decline in school performance.[7] Tremors and manic behaviors are also common. In late stages the patient may have altered mental status progressing to coma.[1] Hyperthermia may be extreme with temperatures as high as 105.3°F (40.7°C).[1] Cardiac complications, including atrial fibrillation and heart failure, are common comorbidities at the time of diagnosis.[32] As the condition persists, signs and symptoms of dehydration become more evident, particularly as a result of gastrointestinal losses related to nausea, vomiting, and diarrhea.[33] Goiter, an enlarged thyroid gland, develops as the condition progresses.[7] Eyes become protuberant (exophthalmus) and the patient may have a staring gaze with heavy eyelids.[1,7] Laboratory testing typically demonstrates decreased TSH with increased T_3 and T_4 levels.[7] If thyroid storm is suspected, rapid, aggressive therapy is essential to reduce hormone levels and preserve hemodynamic integrity.

Immediate goals for management of thyroid storm include inhibiting thyroid hormone synthesis and release, blocking peripheral thyroid hormone effects, and supportive care such as management of ABCs and control of hyperthermia and sympathomimetic symptoms. β-Blockers are given to inhibit adrenergic effects but should be used with caution in older patients, and those with preexisting heart or lung disease, including asthma.[6] Antithyroid drugs, including propylthiouracil (PTU) and methimazole (MMI), are used to block further synthesis of thyroid hormone, with MMI as the first-line agent given the significant side effects that can occur with PTU.[34] Both medications are given orally, with their peak effect at 4 to 10 weeks.[6] Iodides can be given to block the conversion of T_4 to T_3 and to inhibit hormone release, but must be given at least 1 hour after antithyroid medication is initiated; if given sooner, the iodine may be used to create new hormone.[33] Patients in thyroid storm may also require stress-dose corticosteroids, if there is potential adrenal insufficiency.[33] In addition to preventing adrenal compromise and inhibiting production of additional hormone, large doses of steroids[33] also inhibit T_4 conversion to T_3.

Treatment of elevated body temperature is also important and can be accomplished with antipyretic medications and with cooling measures such as cooling blankets. Aspirin must be avoided because it can displace thyroid hormones from binding sites and worsen the patient's condition.[33] IV fluid therapy and electrolyte replacement should also be implemented.[29] Provision of supplemental oxygen assists with increased multisystem oxygen demands.

After the patient stabilizes, close evaluation and assessment are necessary to identify the aggravating agent or illness. Laboratory analysis may include cultures, toxicology screens, thyroid function studies, electrolyte levels, and CBC. Radiology studies should be utilized to rule out potential infectious, oncologic, or traumatic causes. Antibiotic therapy should be initiated if infection is suspected as a causal agent.

Myxedema Coma

Myxedema coma is an extreme complication of hypothyroidism in which patients exhibit multiple-organ dysfunction and progressive mental deterioration; although the term "coma" is used, patients may not be comatose but rather have some level of altered mental status.[35] Myxedema coma usually occurs in older patients, with more cases associated with colder weather and poorly heated homes.[35] Older adult women with a known diagnosis of hypothyroidism appear to be at highest risk for the development of myxedema coma[29]; with women in general being diagnosed with hypothyroidism more often compared with men.[1] Mortality rates for myxedema coma may be as high as 60% even with treatment.[29]

The initial thyroid dysfunction is most often "primary" and may be related to autoimmune thyroiditis (e.g., Hashimoto's disease), ablation therapy (treatment for hyperthyroidism), iodine deficiency, tumor activity, or drug therapy.[1] Secondary hypothyroidism stems from pituitary dysfunction and is much less common.[36] Medications, including lithium, amiodarone, and interferon-alpha, can precipitate myxedema coma.[36] Additionally, significant stressors such as infections or heart failure can precipitate myxedema coma.[29]

In patients with a hypoactive thyroid, the entire metabolic system slows down. Symptom onset may occur over long periods, making it difficult to recognize, particularly in the older adult patient.[1,36] Nonspecific symptoms include complaints of pronounced fatigue, decreased appetite, dyspnea, arthralgia, and weight gain.[1] Tongue swelling (macroglossia) may also occur.[36] Patients may exhibit significant confusion. Altered mental status can progress to coma. "Myxedema madness" refers to acute-onset psychosis in the setting of severe hypothyroidism.[36]

Support of the ABCs is essential in patients with myxedema coma. The thick tongue can obstruct the airway in a semiconscious or unconscious patient. Weak respiratory effort with decreased respiratory drive leads to alveolar hypoventilation, predisposing the patient to pulmonary infection and increasing the chances that the patient will need ventilator support. Alveolar hypoventilation also leads to hypercarbia, which can further confound an altered mental status. Supportive care and careful monitoring are essential, with the recognition that the need for mechanical ventilation can occur at any time.

Patients with hypothyroidism have an increased risk for cardiac complications such as coronary artery disease.[37] Patients presenting with ongoing hypothyroidism may exhibit decreased heart rate, decreased stroke volume, decreased cardiac output, and prolonged QT intervals.[37] Patients with untreated hypothyroidism can also have elevated serum creatinine kinase (CK) levels, which may or may not be related to an actual myocardial infarction.[37] Inability to maintain body temperature is common, and patients frequently present with low body temperature, under 95°F (35°C)[38]; at times hypothermia may be so profound it can go unrecognized if only a conventional thermometer is used.[35] In addition, renal impairment, pulmonary edema, low serum sodium, decreased gastrointestinal motility, and hypoglycemia are common manifestations.[38]

Diagnostic tests reveal decreased free T_4 and free T_3 levels, and with elevated TSH if primary hypothyroidism is the cause.[35] In addition, anemia is common,[37] although the overall white blood cell count may not be elevated even in the presence of infection.[35] Care focuses on thyroid hormone replacement along with stabilization and support of ABCs. As mentioned previously, the patient may require mechanical ventilation to maintain adequate oxygenation and ventilation.[35] A chest radiograph can quickly shed light on potential cardiac and pulmonary complications.[35]

Treatment with the necessary thyroid hormone should be initiated rapidly, as myxedema coma has a high mortality even with treatment.[29] The most current guidelines from the American Thyroid Association Task Force on Thyroid Hormone Replacement (2014) recommend initial hormone replacement in the form of IV T_4, levothyroxine (strong recommendation), with an additional weak recommendation to add liothyronine, IV T_3, in small doses. Monotherapy with liothyronine is not recommended given the known increased mortality related to adverse cardiac effects.[39] It is important to note that IV levothyroxine should be administered via syringe, instead of using infusion tubing, as this hormone adheres easily to available IV tubing and the patient would not be receiving the ordered dose.[29] In addition to the replacement of thyroid hormone, glucocorticoid administration is recommended to mitigate actual or potential adrenal crisis.[39] After the patient can tolerate PO intake, oral T_4 therapy may begin.[35] Additional scans, radiographs, and further diagnostic tests are performed after the patient stabilizes. Slow, careful rewarming measures should be employed, with careful attention to the patient's cardiovascular, respiratory, and neurologic status. Passive, slow warming with blankets and a warm room is recommended because rapid rewarming increases oxygen demands and adds stress to an already overstressed system.[29,35] Ongoing intensive care management is expected until the patient is awake, alert, and has no need for further respiratory assistance.[35]

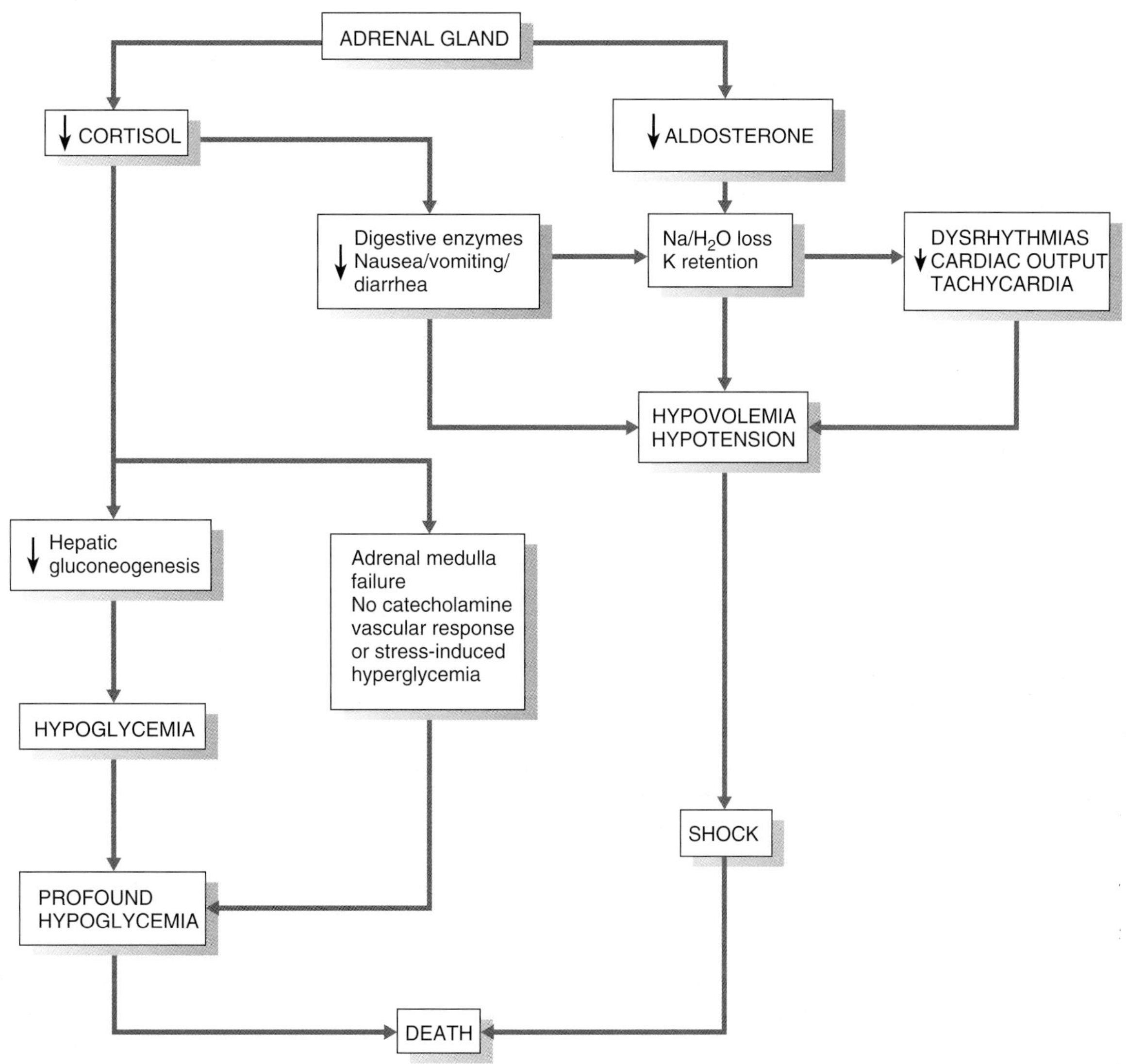

Fig. 28.4 Pathophysiology of Acute Adrenal Crisis.

Adrenal Disorders

Acute Adrenal Insufficiency

Acute adrenal insufficiency, also known as adrenal crisis or Addisonian crisis, is a rare occurrence with life-threatening potential characterized by depletion of adrenal glucocorticoids and mineralocorticoids. The crisis can occur in a person with Addison's disease or may be caused by sudden withdrawal of long-term steroid therapy, removal or injury of the adrenal glands, or destruction of the pituitary gland.[1] Other risk factors include stress, trauma, surgery, or infection in a patient with Addison's disease.[1,40] Massive bilateral adrenal hemorrhage can occur after major surgery, and is associated with severe physiologic stress such as myocardial infarction, septic shock, or complicated pregnancy.[41]

Normally stress increases cortisol output from the adrenal system; therefore inability to meet these increased demands begins the sequence of events that leads to a crisis,[1] as seen in Fig. 28.4. When the adrenal system fails, the resulting decrease in cortisol and aldosterone levels leads to sodium and water loss, primarily from the kidneys, but also from the integumentary and gastrointestinal systems.[42] Water loss results in hypotension and hypovolemia, which can progress to cardiovascular collapse, coma, and death.[43] As sodium decreases and kidney function declines, hyperkalemia results, which can lead to potentially fatal dysrhythmias. Gluconeogenesis, the normal hepatic response to stress, fails without sufficient levels of cortisol; therefore hypoglycemia can also occur.[42] Decreased cortisol levels also alter activities of the adrenal medulla, which normally responds to stress through the release of catecholamines to increase heart rate and serum glucose.[1] Without a catecholamine response, the severity of hypoglycemia and hypotension is magnified, and may be unresponsive to standard therapies.[43]

Diagnosing adrenal insufficiency can be difficult because symptoms often are insidious and nonspecific. An accurate history of prior illnesses, recent medication changes, recent surgery, or injury helps determine precipitating factors. The patient may complain of fatigue, weakness, and weight loss, as well as gastrointestinal symptoms such as nausea, anorexia, and chronic diarrhea.[42] Reported symptoms of adrenal crisis can include sudden pain in the abdomen, lower back, or legs[42]; severe vomiting and diarrhea[1]; and profound weakness.[42]

Physical findings are nonspecific and may include resting tachycardia, orthostatic hypotension, and signs of dehydration such as dry mucous membranes, delayed capillary refill, and poor skin turgor. If infection is a precipitating cause, fever may be present.[42] If there is chronic primary adrenal insufficiency, diffuse hyperpigmentation of the buccal mucosa and skin, especially over the elbows, knuckles, and axillary folds may be present.[43]

Laboratory studies typically demonstrate hyponatremia, hyperkalemia, hypoglycemia, and hypercalcemia, as well as elevated BUN and hematocrit relative to dehydration.[42,43] The effects of the hyperkalemia may be seen in the ECG, with findings such as peaked T waves and a widening QRS.[44] After the patient has been stabilized, an ACTH stimulation test can be conducted for patients without a history of adrenal insufficiency, but this is not a useful test in the emergency setting given the length of time that it takes to perform.[1,44]

Maintenance of ABCs, replacement of glucocorticoids, and correction of fluid and electrolyte disturbances are cornerstones of care for the patient with adrenal crisis. Although shock and dehydration should be treated with appropriate fluid resuscitation and vasopressors, it is important to note that these may be minimally effective without the administration of exogenous steroids.[43] Hydrocortisone is the primary synthetic glucocorticoid used to treat acute adrenal crisis,[6,43] although any glucocorticoid can be utilized.[44] If it is possible to obtain blood specimens for ACTH and cortisol before administration of the steroid, these levels can be used to assist with the diagnosis of adrenal insufficiency.[44]

Rapid IV fluid replacement assists in correcting volume deficit, which can be significant.[44] A bedside glucose level should be obtained and hypoglycemia corrected with dextrose-containing IV fluids if needed.[44] The hyperkalemia associated with adrenal crisis is usually mild and will resolve with IV fluids and glucocorticoids, even to the point of hypokalemia necessitating replacement.[42] Clinical judgment should be applied, however, and patients with clinical signs of hyperkalemia (muscle paralysis) or ECG changes (peaked T waves, widening QRS) should be treated appropriately.[45] Continuous cardiac monitoring, careful neurologic assessment, strict measurement of intake and output, and accurate measurement of vital signs are all essential components of care. Frequent reassessment of glucose and electrolyte levels is necessary for ongoing management and prevention of complications. Once the patient has stabilized, additional testing can seek the cause for the acute presentation.[44]

Cushing's Syndrome

Cushing's syndrome is caused by prolonged exposure to elevated levels of either endogenous or exogenous glucocorticoids; the majority of cases result from the administration of exogenous steroids, especially glucocorticoids.[46] Patients affected with this disorder develop a characteristic appearance due to increased adipose tissue in the face (moon face), upper back at the base of the neck (buffalo hump), and above the clavicles.[1]

Although Cushing's syndrome is not a medical emergency, exposure to excess glucocorticoids results in multiple medical problems, including hypertension, obesity, glucose intolerance, osteoporosis and fractures, impaired immune function, and impaired wound healing.[1] In addition, these patients are at risk for developing adrenal crisis if steroids are abruptly stopped or dosage is not increased during an acute illness.[1] The emergency nurse needs to be alert to the multisystem consequences of Cushing's syndrome when providing care for these patients in the ED, and maintain awareness of the potential need to increase or continue steroid dosing during treatment for other acute illnesses. Finally, the emergency nurse must recognize that patients who have had surgery to address Cushing's disease will have permanent, acquired adrenal insufficiency.[46]

Pheochromocytoma

A pheochromocytoma is a rare catecholamine-producing tumor, most commonly found in the adrenal medulla.[47] This tumor secretes catecholamines, including norepinephrine and epinephrine, and the clinical manifestations result from excessive (intermittent or continuous) catecholamine secretion.[47] Patients characteristically present with severe hypertension accompanied by a triad of headache, palpitations, and diaphoresis.[1] A sense of impending doom, fatigue, anxiety, pallor, tremors, chest pain, abdominal pain, and palpitations may also be noted.[47] Intermittent episodes may be triggered by medications, abdominal palpation, position change, or emotional trauma.[47] Pheochromocytoma has been associated with life-threatening events such as myocardial infarction and cardiomyopathy.[48] The diagnosis of pheochromocytoma should be suspected based on history and clinical findings and should be considered in patients with sudden or severe unexplained hypertension.[47] An abdominal computed tomography scan or magnetic resonance imaging may detect an adrenal mass. A 24-hour urine collection for catecholamines and metanephrines may be obtained.[47]

Emergent care of the patient with pheochromocytoma entails controlling the effects of excessive catecholamine secretion while preparing the patient for surgery.[47] Intravenous α-blocking agents (e.g., phentolamine) and nitroprusside are commonly used to manage hypertensive crisis.[49] β-blockers, particularly the nonselective beta-adrenergic receptor blocker, propranolol, can be used as an adjunct therapy if needed.[49] Unopposed beta blockade should be avoided, because this may paradoxically increase blood pressure.[47] The patient requires continuous cardiac monitoring to allow rapid detection and treatment of dysrhythmias. IV fluids are administered to maintain a normal circulating volume. Surgical resection of the tumor is the primary treatment for pheochromocytoma and should result in resolution of the hypertension.[49]

SUMMARY

Endocrine emergencies affect all body systems because of the diversity of hormones and their effects. Rapid assessment and initiation of treatment is often needed. Support of hemodynamic functions, identification of precipitating events, and detection of potential complications through careful monitoring and reassessment are essential for the survival of these patients.

REFERENCES

1. Lewis SL, Dirksen SR, Heitkemper MM, Bucher L, Harding MM. *Medical-Surgical Nursing: Assessment and Management of Clinical Problems.* 9th ed. St Louis, MO: Elsevier-Mosby; 2014.
2. American Diabetes Association. Standards of medical care in diabetes—2018. *Diabetes Care J Clin Appl Res Ed.* 2018;41(S1).
3. Kumar JG, Abhilash KP, Saya RP, Tadipaneni N, Bose JM. A retrospective study on epidemiology of hypoglycemia in emergency department. *Indian J Endocrinol Metab.* 2017;21(1):119–124.
4. Rudd K, Kocisko DM. *Pediatric Nursing: The Critical Components of Nursing Care.* Philadelphia, PA: FA Davis; 2014.
5. Joslin Diabetes Center. Oral Diabetes Medications Summary Chart. http://www.joslin.org/info/oral_diabetes_medications_summary_chart.html. Accessed May 20, 2019.
6. Vallerand AH, Sanoski CA. *Davis's Drug Guide for Nurses.* 15th ed. Philadelphia, PA: FA Davis; 2017.
7. Ball J, Bindler RM, Cowen KJ, Shaw MR. *Principles of Pediatric Nursing: Caring for Children.* 7th ed. Hoboken, NJ: Pearson Education; 2017.
8. Gosmanov AR, Gosmanova EO, Dillard-Cannon E. Management of adult diabetic ketoacidosis. *Diabetes Metab Syndr Obes.* 2014;7:255–264.
9. Gosmanov A, Gosmanova E, Kitabchi A. Hyperglycemic crises: diabetic ketoacidosis (DKA), and hyperglycemic hyperosmolar state (HHS). In: Feingold KR, Anawalt B, Boyce A, et al., eds, *Endotext [Internet].* South Dartmouth, MA: MDText.com, Inc.; original publication; 2000. https://www.ncbi.nlm.nih.gov/books/NBK279052/. Updated May 17, 2018. Accessed May 20, 2019.
10. Dhatariya KK, Vellanki P. Treatment of diabetic ketoacidosis (DKA)/Hyperglycemic Hyperosmolar State (HHS): novel advances in the management of hyperglycemic crises (UK Versus USA). *Curr Diab Rep.* 2017;17(5):33.
11. Mohan N, Kumar KPG, Sreekrishnan TP, et al. Can venous blood gases replace arterial blood gases in diabetic ketoacidosis/renal failure induced metabolic acidosis? *Uni J Med Sci.* 2015;3(3):65–69.
12. Hsia DS, Tarai SG, Alimi A, Coss-Bu JA, Haymond MW. Fluid management in pediatric patients with DKA and rates of suspected clinical cerebral edema. *Pediatr Diabetes.* 2015;16(5):338–344.
13. Kuppermann N, Ghetti S, Schunk JE, et al. Clinical trial of fluid infusion rates for pediatric diabetic ketoacidosis. *N Engl J Med.* 2018;378(24):2275–2287.
14. Oliver WD, Willis GC, Hines MC, Hayes BD. Comparison of Plasma-Lyte A and sodium chloride 0.9% for fluid resuscitation of patients with diabetic ketoacidosis. *Hospital Pharm.* 2018. 0018578718757517.
15. Thompson CD, Vital-Carona J, Faustino EV. The effect of tubing dwell time on insulin adsorption during intravenous insulin infusions. *Diabetes Technol Ther.* 2012;14(10): 912–916.
16. Pasquel FJ, Umpierrez GE. Hyperosmolar hyperglycemic state: a historic review of the clinical presentation, diagnosis, and treatment. *Diabetes Care.* 2014;37(11):3124–3131. http://care.diabetesjournals.org/content/37/11/3124.short. Accessed May 20, 2019.
17. Adeyinka A, Kondamudi NP. *Hyperosmolar Hyperglycemic Nonketotic Coma (HHNC, Hyperosmolar Hyperglycemic Nonketotic Syndrome). StatPearls.* Treasure Island FL: StatPearls Publishing. https://www.ncbi.nlm.nih.gov/books/NBK482142/. Updated March, 2019. Accessed May 20, 2019.
18. Brutsaert EF. *Alcoholic ketoacidosis. Merck Manuals Professional Edition [Online Version].* Kenilworth, NJ: Merck & Co. https://www.merckmanuals.com/professional/endocrine-and-metabolic-disorders/diabetes-mellitus-and-disorders-of-carbohydrate-metabolism/alcoholic-ketoacidosis. Updated Jan, 2019. Accessed May 20, 2019.
19. Chandrasekara H, Fernando P, Danjuma M, Jayawarna C. Ketoacidosis is not always due to diabetes. *BMJ Case Rep.* 2014;2014. https://doi.org/10.1136/bcr-2013-203263.
20. Howard RD, Bokhari SRA. *Alcoholic Ketoacidosis (AKA). StatPearls.* Treasure Island FL: StatPearls. https://www.ncbi.nlm.nih.gov/books/NBK430922/. Updated April 1, 2019. Accessed May 20, 2019.
21. Noor NM, Basavaraju K, Sharpstone D. Alcoholic ketoacidosis: a case report and review of the literature. *Oxf Med Case Rep.* 2016;2016(3):31–33.
22. Schabelman E, Kuo D. Glucose before thiamine for Wernicke encephalopathy: a literature review. *J Emerg Med.* 2012;42(4):488–494.
23. Kalra S, Zargar AH, Jain SM, et al. Diabetes insipidus: the other diabetes. *Indian J Endocrinol Metab.* 2016;20(1):9–21.
24. Hechanova LA. *Nephrogenic Diabetes Insipidus. Merck Manuals Professional Edition [Online Version].* Kenilworth, NJ: Merck & Co. https://www.merckmanuals.com/professional/genitourinary-disorders/renal-transport-abnormalities/nephrogenic-diabetes-insipidus. Updated Jan, 2019. Accessed May 20, 2019.
25. Chapman IM. *Central Diabetes Insipidus. Merck Manuals Professional Edition [Online Version].* Kenilworth, NJ: Merck & Co. https://www.merckmanuals.com/home/hormonal-and-metabolic-disorders/pituitary-gland-disorders/central-diabetes-insipidus. Updated Nov, 2018. Accessed May 20, 2019.
26. Khardori R, Ullal J, Cooperman M. Diabetes Insipidus Treatment and Management. Medscape Website. https://emedicine.medscape.com/article/117648-treatment. Updated February 21, 2018 Accessed May 20, 2019.
27. Sands JM, Klein JD. Physiological insights into novel therapies for nephrogenic diabetes insipidus. *Am J Physiol Renal Physiol.* 2016;311(6):F1149–F1152.
28. Lewis JL. *Hyponatremia. Merck Manuals Professional Edition.* Kenilworth, NJ: Merck & Co. https://www.merckmanuals.com/professional/endocrine-and-metabolic-disorders/electrolyte-disorders/hyponatremia. Updated March, 2018. Accessed May 20, 2019.

29. Leung AM. Thyroid emergencies. *J Infus Nurs*. 2016;39(5):281–286.
30. Xue J, Zhang L, Qin Z, et al. No obvious sympathetic excitation after massive levothyroxine overdose: a case report. *Med (Baltimore)*. 2018;97(23):e10909.
31. Amor MMI, Adedayo AM, Singh S, Grayver E. Refractory atrial fibrillation secondary to contrast-induced thyroid storm in a patient with amiodarone-induced hyperthyroidism. *J Am Coll Cardiol*. 2016;67(13):1230.
32. Ono Y, Ono S, Yasunaga H, Matsui H, Fushimi K, Tanaka Y. Factors associated with mortality of thyroid storm: analysis using a national inpatient database in Japan. *Med (Baltimore)*. 2016;95(7):e2848.
33. Schraga ED. Hyperthyroidism, Thyroid Storm, and Graves Disease (Clinical Presentation). Medscape Website. https://emedicine.medscape.com/article/767130-overview. Updated April 3, 2018. Accessed May 20, 2019.
34. Hershman JM. *Hyperthyroidism (Thyrotoxicosis). Merck Manuals Professional Edition [Online Version]*. Kenilworth, NJ: Merck & Co. https://www.merckmanuals.com/professional/endocrine-and-metabolic-disorders/thyroid-disorders/hyperthyroidism. Updated April, 2018. Accessed May 20, 2019.
35. Eledrisi MS. Myxedema Coma or Crisis. Medscape Website. https://emedicine.medscape.com/article/123577-overview#a5. Updated October 10, 2018. Accessed May 20, 2019.
36. Hershman JM. *Hypothyroidism (Myxedema). Merck Manuals Professional Edition [Online Version]*. Kenilworth, NJ: Merck & Co. https://www.merckmanuals.com/professional/endocrine-and-metabolic-disorders/thyroid-disorders/hypothyroidism. Updated April, 2018. Accessed May 20, 2019.
37. Klein I, Danzi S. Thyroid disease and the heart. *Curr Probl Cardiol*. 2016;41(2):65–92.
38. Popoveniuc G, Chandra T, Sud A, et al. A diagnostic scoring system for myxedema coma. *Endocr Pract*. 2014;20(8):808–817.
39. Jonklaas J, Bianco AC, Bauer AJ, et al. Guidelines for the treatment of hypothyroidism: prepared by the American Thyroid Association Task Force on thyroid hormone replacement. *Thyroid*. 2014;24(12):1670–1751.
40. Johannsson G, Falorni A, Skrtic S, et al. Adrenal insufficiency: review of clinical outcomes with current glucocorticoid replacement therapy. *Clin Endocrinol (Oxf)*. 2015;82(1):2–11.
41. Logaraj A, Tsang VH, Kabir S, Ip JC. Adrenal crisis secondary to bilateral adrenal haemorrhage after hemicolectomy. *Endocrinol Diabetes Metab Case Rep*. 2016;2016:16–0048.
42. Grossmann AB. *Addison Disease. Merck Manuals Professional Edition [Online Version]*. Kenilworth, NJ: Merck & Co. https://www.merckmanuals.com/professional/endocrine-and-metabolic-disorders/adrenal-disorders/addison-disease. Updated Jan, 2018. Accessed May 20, 2019.
43. Puar TH, Stikkelbroeck NM, Smans LC, Zelissen PM, Hermus AR. Adrenal crisis: still a deadly event in the 21st century. *Am J Med*. 2016;129(3):339.e331–e339.
44. Rathbun KM, Singhal M. *Addisonian Crisis. StatPearls*. Treasure Island FL: StatPearls Publishing. https://www.ncbi.nlm.nih.gov/books/NBK441933/. Updated March, 2019. Accessed May 20, 2019.
45. Mishra A, Pandya HV, Dave N, Sapre CM, Chaudhary S. Hyperkalemic paralysis in primary adrenal insufficiency. *Indian J Crit Care Med*. 2014;18(8):527–529.
46. Raff H, Carroll T. Cushing's syndrome: from physiological principles to diagnosis and clinical care. *J Physiol*. 2015;593(3):493–506.
47. Grossmann AB. *Pheochromocytoma. Merck Manuals Professional Edition [Online Version]*. Kenilworth, NJ: Merck & Co. https://www.merckmanuals.com/professional/endocrine-and-metabolic-disorders/adrenal-disorders/pheochromocytoma. Updated January 2018. Accessed May 20, 2019.
48. Riester A, Weismann D, Quinkler M, et al. Life-threatening events in patients with pheochromocytoma. *Eur J Endocrinol*. 2015;173(6):757–764.
49. Blake MB. Pheochromocytoma. Medscape Website. https://emedicine.medscape.com/article/124059-overview. Updated August 10, 2018. Accessed June 25, 2018.

29

Hematologic and Oncologic Emergencies

Wanda S. Pritts

The hematologic system (blood components and the organs that form them) plays a vital role in maintaining homeostasis of the whole body, affecting multiple cellular activities, including oxygen transport and delivery, hemostasis, and immune response. In turn, oncologic conditions and their treatments may have detrimental effects on the hematologic system. Patients with hematologic and oncologic disorders may present for emergency department (ED) care for an acute onset of a new condition, a sudden exacerbation of an existing disease, or a therapy-related complication of their underlying disease. This chapter provides an overview of blood physiology, discusses general assessment of individuals with hematologic and oncologic emergencies, and describes specific hematologic and oncologic emergencies, including anemia, sickle cell disease (SCD), leukemia, thrombocytopenia, hemophilia, disseminated intravascular coagulation (DIC), fever and neutropenia, tumor lysis syndrome (TLS), syndrome of inappropriate antidiuretic hormone secretion (SIADH), superior vena cava syndrome, and spinal cord compression.

ANATOMY AND PHYSIOLOGY

Blood is a collection of erythrocytes, leukocytes, platelets, and other particulate material in an aqueous colloid solution. This suspension provides a medium for exchange between fixed cells in the body and the external environment. Nutrients such as oxygen and glucose are carried to each cell, whereas cellular wastes such as carbon dioxide and nitrogen are removed. Other essential functions include regulation of pH, temperature, and cellular water; prevention of fluid loss through coagulation; and protection against toxins and foreign microbes.

Plasma

Plasma is the clear aqueous part of blood containing blood cells, electrolytes, gases, amino acids, sugars, lipids, and nonprotein nitrogens such as urea, creatine, and uric acid.[1] These and other substances may be dissolved in the plasma or may bind with various plasma proteins for transport. Albumin, the primary plasma protein, maintains blood volume by providing colloid osmotic pressure, buffering capacity to regulate pH and electrolyte balance, and transporting substances, including drugs.

Erythrocytes

Adults have approximately 5 million erythrocytes, or red blood cells (RBCs), per microliter of blood. The number of RBCs is slightly higher in men. Natives living at altitudes greater than 14,000 feet may have as many as 7 million/μL. The primary role of RBCs is transport of oxygen and carbon dioxide. Erythrocytes' average life span is 120 days, so new cells must be constantly produced.[2] Production of erythrocytes occurs in the bone marrow but is regulated by the kidneys. When oxygen levels drop, the kidneys release erythropoietin, which stimulates RBC production by the bone marrow. Reticulocytes are erythrocyte precursors that mature within 24 to 48 hours of release into the circulation. Increased reticulocytes indicate increased bone marrow activity.

Erythrocytes are soft, pliable cells that change shape easily, thereby increasing the cell's oxygen-carrying capability by increasing surface area. The outer stroma, or support, of the cell contains antigens A and B and Rh factor, whereas the inner stroma contains hemoglobin, the primary vehicle for oxygen transport. Hemoglobin molecules are so small they would leak across the blood vessel's endothelial membrane if left floating free in plasma. There are 300 different types of genetically determined hemoglobin (Hb). With the exception of normal fetal hemoglobin (Hb F), normal adult hemoglobin (Hb A), and sickle cell hemoglobin (Hb S), hemoglobins are identified by sequential letters of the alphabet. Abnormal hemoglobin molecules are produced in response to molecular abnormalities within blood. Tests such as hemoglobin electrophoresis are used to differentiate normal and abnormal hemoglobin. The most common hemoglobins are described in Table 29.1.

Red cell indices provide information about the size and weight of average red cells and are used to differentiate acute and chronic anemias. Mean corpuscular volume, mean corpuscular hemoglobin content, and mean corpuscular hemoglobin concentration values provide information on how well red cells function. Table 29.2 includes normal values for these indices as well as the other components of a complete blood count (CBC).

Erythrocyte sedimentation rate (ESR) measures the time required for erythrocytes in a whole blood specimen to settle to the bottom of a vertical tube. ESR is a product of red cell volume, surface area, density, aggregation, and surface charge.[2] Increased ESR occurs with widespread inflammation, red cell aggregation, pregnancy, and some malignancies, whereas polycythemia, SCD, and decreased plasma proteins are associated with decreased ESR.

Leukocytes

The body's primary defense against infection is leukocytes, or white blood cells (WBCs). Six types of leukocytes normally occur in the blood: neutrophils, eosinophils, basophils, monocytes, lymphocytes, and occasionally, plasma cells (Table 29.3). The WBC count quantifies the total number of leukocytes in the circulation, whereas the differential count quantifies the percentage of each type.

Neutrophils

Neutrophils are the primary defense against bacterial infection. Bone marrow contains a reserve approximately 10 times greater than daily neutrophil production. About one-half of all mature neutrophils adhere to vessel walls and are not measured by the traditional WBC count. The bone marrow reserve and the number of neutrophils on vessel walls allows for a sudden increase in the circulating WBC count in response to stress or infection. After being released into the circulation, neutrophils live 4 to 8 hours. Immature neutrophils are called bands (also called stabs); mature neutrophils are called polymorphonuclear neutrophil leukocytes (PMNs, or segs). An increased number of bands, sometimes called a "left shift," indicates acute infection.[2]

Eosinophils

Eosinophils accumulate at the site of allergic reactions. Increases also occur during asthma attacks, drug reactions, and parasitic infections. Eosinophils decrease in response to stressors such as trauma, shock, or burns. The cell half-life is approximately 4 to 5 hours after release into the circulation.

Basophils

Basophils contain histamine, heparin, bradykinin, serotonin, and lysosomal enzymes. During allergic reactions, basophils rupture and release these substances. This accounts for many of the clinical manifestations of an allergic reaction. High counts of basophils are associated with allergies, parasitic infections, and hypothyroidism. Low counts are associated with pregnancy, stress, and hyperthyroidism.[2]

Monocytes

Monocytes remain in the circulation less than 20 hours before moving into surrounding tissue to become macrophages. A macrophage acts as a "garbage collector," consuming bacteria, foreign pathogens, worn-out erythrocytes, and other debris. Macrophages can live for months or even years. Monocytes are the body's second line of defense and are usually associated with chronic infection.

Lymphocytes

Lymphocytes play a major role in immunity against acquired infections. Their life span may be weeks, months, or years, depending on the body's needs. The three major groups include natural killer cells, B cells, and T cells.[2] Natural killer

TABLE 29.1 Types of Hemoglobin.

Type	Significance
Hb A	Normal adult hemoglobin
Hb A_{1c}	Glycosylated hemoglobin
Hb A_2	β-Thalassemia, makes up 2% of hemoglobin in normal adults
Hb F	Fetal hemoglobin, thalassemia after 6 months
Hb C	Hemolytic anemia
Hb S	Sickle cell anemia
Hb M	Methemoglobinemia

Hb, Hemoglobin.

TABLE 29.2 Components of Complete Blood Cell Count.

Component	Normal Values	Comments
White blood cell count	5000–10,000/mm³	
Red blood cell count	Male: 4.6–6.2 million/mm³ Female: 4.2–5.4 million/mm³	
Hemoglobin level	Male: 14–18 g/dL Female: 12–16 g/dL	A conjugated protein responsible for oxygen and carbon dioxide transport in the blood
Hematocrit	Male: 40%–54% Female: 37%–47%	Proportion of blood that consists of packed red blood cells; expressed as a percentage by volume
Mean corpuscular volume	82–92 μm³	Average volume of red blood cells in a sample
Mean corpuscular hemoglobin content	27–37 mcg	Average hemoglobin content of red blood cells in a sample
Mean corpuscular hemoglobin concentration	32%–36%	Average hemoglobin content in 100 mL of blood
Platelets	150,000–400,000/μL	Aid in hemostasis and maintenance of vascular integrity

TABLE 29.3 Leukocytes: Functions and Characteristics.

Name	Percentage of Total WBCs	Function	Circulatory Life Span
Neutrophils	62.0	Attack and destroy bacteria and viruses through phagocytosis	4–8 h
Eosinophils	2.3	Attach to surface of parasites, then release substances that kill the organism; detoxify inflammatory substances that occur in allergic reactions	4–8 h
Basophils	0.4	Prevent coagulation and speed fat removal from blood after a fatty meal	4–8 h
Monocytes	5.3	Consume bacteria, viruses, necrotic tissue, and other foreign material	10–20 h
Lymphocytes	30.0	Provide immunity against acquired infections; basis for antibody formation	2–3 h
Plasma cells	—	Produce γ-globulin antibodies in response to specific antigens	Varies with need for antibodies

WBCs, White blood cells.

cells recognize "nonself" cells (e.g., cancer cells or infected cells) and provide generalized, nonspecific immunity. B-cell lymphocytes become antibodies and are responsible for humoral immunity. T-cell lymphocytes are responsible for cell-mediated immunity. At least three major types of T-cell lymphocytes have been identified: helper T cells, cytotoxic T cells, and suppressor T cells (Table 29.4). Lymphocyte increases are associated with viral infection.

TABLE 29.4 Types of T-Cell Lymphocytes.

Name	Function
Helper T cells	Regulate immune functions by forming lymphokines or protein mediators such as interleukin and interferon; inactivated or destroyed by AIDS virus
Cytotoxic T cells	Also called killer T cells; capable of direct attack on microorganisms and on the body's own cells; role in destroying cancer cells and heart transplant cells
Suppressor T cells	Protect from attack by the person's own immune system; suppress helper and cytotoxic T-cell functions

AIDS, Acquired immunodeficiency syndrome.

Plasma Cells

Plasma cells produce γ-globulin (gamma globulin) antibodies in response to a specific antigen. Production continues until plasma cells die of exhaustion days to weeks later.

Platelets

Platelets, or thrombocytes, provide hemostasis at the site of injury. These granular, disk-shaped fragments form when a megakaryocyte cell breaks into cell fragments.[2] Platelet life span is 9 to 12 days. Approximately one-third of the body's platelets are stored in the spleen as a reserve. Clotting factors V, VIII, and IX are found on the platelet's surface. Platelets provide hemostasis by clumping at the site of injury to form a platelet plug and seal bleeding capillaries. Substances such as ethanol and salicylates interfere with platelet aggregation by impairing their ability to clump. Decreased platelet aggregation leads to increased bleeding.[2]

Hemostasis

Hemostasis refers to processes that prevent blood loss after vascular damage (i.e., vascular spasm, platelet aggregation, coagulation, and fibrinolysis). When vessel injury occurs, the initial response is reflex vasoconstriction. Arterioles contract, decreasing blood flow by decreasing vessel size and pressing endothelial surfaces together. Next, serotonin and histamine release cause immediate vasoconstriction and decrease blood flow to the injured area. Vasoconstriction is followed by platelet aggregation at the injury site. This temporary measure prevents bleeding by sealing capillaries.

Platelet aggregation is followed by clot formation, which requires activation of the coagulation cascade. The coagulation cascade is a complex network of 12 different clotting factors (Table 29.5). A defect of any clotting factor or an injury that overwhelms the entire system can cause failure of the coagulation cascade and lead to life- or limb-threatening hemorrhage. The cascade may be activated by intrinsic factors, such as damage to a vessel wall, or extrinsic factors, such as damage to surrounding tissue. Regardless of the method of activation, the end result of the coagulation cascade is formation of a clot (a protein mesh made of fibrin strands).

The final step in hemostasis is clot resolution via the fibrinolytic system. Clot resolution maintains blood in a fluid state by removing clots that are no longer needed. Without this system, circulation to affected areas may be permanently lost because of obstructed blood vessels.

TABLE 29.5 **Coagulation Factors.**

Factor	Synonyms	Pathway	Description/Function
I	Fibrinogen	Common	Fibrin precursor
II	Prothrombin	Common	Thrombin precursor
III	Tissue thromboplastin or tissue factor	Extrinsic	Activates prothrombin
IV	Calcium	Both	Essential for prothrombin activation and fibrin formation
V	Labile factor, proaccelerin	Both	Accelerates conversion of prothrombin to thrombin
VII	Prothrombin conversion accelerator	Extrinsic	Accelerates conversion of prothrombin to thrombin
VIII	Antihemophilic factor A	Intrinsic	Associated with factors IX, XI, and XII; essential for thromboplastin formation (deficiency results in hemophilia A)
IX	Christmas factor, antihemophilic factor B	Intrinsic	Associated with factors VIII, XI, and XII; essential for thromboplastin formation (deficiency results in hemophilia B)
X	Thrombokinase factor, Stuart-Prower factor	Both	Triggers prothrombin conversion; requires vitamin K
XI	Plasma thromboplastin antecedent, antihemophilic factor C	Intrinsic	Formation of thromboplastin in association with factors VIII, IX, and XII (deficiency results in hemophilia C)
XII	Contact factor, Hageman factor	Intrinsic	Activates factor XI in thromboplastin formation
XIII	Fibrin-stabilizing factor	—	Strengthens fibrin clot, slows fibrinolysis

PATIENT ASSESSMENT

The type and severity of hematologic or oncologic emergency depend on the individual's condition. Assessment is often complicated by vague complaints, and it is therefore important to assess the patient specifically for hematologic/oncologic problems, such as pale, jaundiced, or cyanotic skin. Ecchymosis, purpura, petechiae, and ulcerations may be present. Evaluate skin for temperature, diaphoresis, texture, and turgor. Observe for joint deformity, edema, redness, limitation of movement, and difficulty with ambulation or inability to ambulate. Obtain vital signs, noting pulse pressure; orthostatic blood pressure, pulse rate, and capillary refill.

Of concern are new onset of fever, weakness, cough, rash, dyspnea, and increased or unusual bruising. Does the patient complain of spontaneous bleeding, such as epistaxis or menorrhagia? Are bleeding gums, hematemesis, melena, dark urine, or hemoptysis present? These symptoms suggest a hematologic/oncologic problem and indicate the need for more detailed evaluation. Identify existing hematologic/oncologic diseases and family history of such disorders. Obtain medication history, including use of prescription and over-the-counter medications. It is also important to ask the patient about herbals that may affect clotting. For example, evening primrose, garlic, and skullcap increase clotting time, whereas ginseng, cinnamon, and parsley decrease clotting time. Document allergies, exposure to toxic substances, and dietary history.

Complete Blood Cell Count

The CBC is used to determine the patient's hematologic status. A CBC is reported in two parts: the cell count and the differential count. The cell count is done by machine; if the differential count is abnormal, a manual count will be done. The cell count of the CBC provides normal values for leukocytes, erythrocytes, hemoglobin, and hematocrit (see Table 29.2). Normal CBC values vary with the age and sex of the patient. The differential count provides information on red cell morphology and the percentage distribution of leukocytes.[1]

SPECIFIC HEMATOLOGIC EMERGENCIES

Anemia

Anemia is a reduction in the total number of RBCs or a deficiency in the cells' ability to transport oxygen. Anemia may be acute or chronic. Severity depends on the patient's ability to compensate for RBC loss and provide essential oxygen to the cells. Oxygenation depends on blood flow and on hemoglobin's oxygen-carrying capacity and affinity for oxygen. A defect in any of these factors affects cellular oxygen.

Acute Anemia

Acute anemia is usually the result of blood loss. Causes include trauma, gastrointestinal hemorrhage, vaginal bleeding, and uterine rupture. Response to blood loss depends on the patient's age, physical condition, and rate of blood loss. Signs and symptoms may include tachycardia; cool, clammy skin with prolonged capillary refill; decreased blood pressure; narrowing pulse pressure; tachypnea; postural hypotension; and decreased urinary output. Thirst and complaints of "feeling cold" are early clues to acute blood loss. A decreased level of consciousness may also occur.

Treatment begins with stabilization of the patient's airway, breathing, and circulation. Large-bore intravenous (IV) catheters and fluid resuscitation with normal saline or lactated Ringer's solution are used for volume replacement. Initial laboratory studies include CBC, type and crossmatch, prothrombin time (PT), partial thromboplastin time (PTT), international normalized ratio (INR), and serum electrolytes. Supplemental oxygen is indicated because these patients have lost a major source of oxygen delivery to the cells. Blood replacement therapy may be necessary in severe anemia. Care should be taken to maintain normothermia during fluid and blood replacement therapy. Hypothermia alters the coagulation cascade, increasing stimulation of the fibrinolytic system and resulting in increased bleeding.[2] Other causes of anemia may include SCD, massive burns, DIC, toxins, infections, ABO incompatibility, transfusion reactions, carbon monoxide poisoning, and medications. Most chemotherapy agents adversely affect RBC production in some manner.[3]

Chronic Anemia

Chronic anemia is not considered life-threatening, has an insidious onset, and is often diagnosed before an ED visit. Patients may complain of fatigue, headache, irritability, dizziness, and shortness of breath. Diagnosis is made by clinical assessment, history, and laboratory analysis, including a CBC with leukocyte differential, RBC indices, peripheral smear, and reticulocyte count. Patients are usually treated as outpatients unless they have acute shortness of breath, chest pain, severe dizziness, or altered level of consciousness.

Diminished RBC production occurs in iron deficiency anemia, vitamin B_{12} deficiency, thalassemia, lead poisoning, chronic liver and renal disease, hypothyroidism, some forms of cancer, lupus, and rheumatoid arthritis.[2] Decreased bone marrow production causes aplastic anemia. Other causes of anemia include increased destruction of RBCs resulting from enzyme defects (e.g., glucose-6-phosphate dehydrogenase deficiency), cell membrane abnormalities, or abnormalities of the hemoglobin molecule, such as SCD).[1]

Sickle Cell Disease

SCD is a genetically determined, inherited disorder primarily characterized by pain. Chronic pain with acute exacerbation is the most common reason for the nearly 200,000 annual ED visits, with 29% of those visits resulting in hospital admission.[4] Individuals of African, Caribbean, Central and South American, Saudi Arabian, Indian, and Mediterranean descent experience the highest rates of SCD, with most being African American. Incidence occurs in approximately 1 in 500 African Americans.[4] The disease is usually diagnosed in the first few years of life secondary to presentation of initial symptoms. In SCD, erythrocytes or RBCs contain Hb S, an abnormal hemoglobin that may precipitate into long crystals when exposed to low oxygen concentrations, dehydration, infection, high altitudes, intense stress, or strenuous exercise. The resulting sickle shape of the cell gives the disorder its name. Organ damage occurs from the repeated vasoocclusion, infarction, and chronic anemia. This contributes to high use of health care facilities, poor quality of life, and shortened survival.[5] Sickle cell anemia is an autosomal recessive disorder. An individual who inherits one abnormal gene for sickle hemoglobin (Hb S) has sickle cell trait and may pass this gene on to their offspring. An individual with both genes for Hb S will have sickle cell disease.[5]

In SCD, as cells become hypoxic and sickling occurs, the cells are no longer flexible enough to pass through the smaller vessels and begin to clump in various parts of the body. The life span of RBCs that sickle is approximately 10 to 20 days compared with the 120-day life span of normal RBCs, leading to chronic anemia and a chronically elevated reticulocyte count. These sickle-shaped cells adhere to each other and to blood vessel walls, blocking blood flow and decreasing circulation to tissues and causing organ damage, inflammation, and pain. This ischemic event is known as a vasoocclusive crisis.[5] Pain occurs most often in long bones, large joints, and the spine, but every organ is affected by the ischemia.

Early and aggressive management includes effective pain control, adequate fluid infusion, adequate oxygen therapy, correction of metabolic acidosis, and transfusion of RBCs.[3] Sickle cell crisis or vasoocclusive crisis is the most common painful complication of SCD and a primary reason for seeking medical care. Acute episodes cause severe pain; however, research demonstrates that for many complex factors, providers are often reluctant to administer patients adequate doses of narcotics.[4] Pain management in SCD should be individualized, and treatment should be driven by pain assessment, associated symptoms, outpatient analgesic use, and the patient's past experience with side effects.[4] Drug therapy should be adjusted for drug tolerance and follow an analgesic ladder, using appropriate nonsteroidal antiinflammatory drugs and opioids such as codeine or hydrocodone for mild to moderate pain. Moderate to severe pain should be treated with an opioid such as morphine or hydromorphone. Meperidine is not recommended for pain control because the metabolite normeperidine may cause seizures with long-term use. Ineffective pain management has the potential to increase prolonged admissions and/or readmissions for this patient population.[4]

Acute chest syndrome (ACS) is the second most common cause of hospitalization and the leading cause of mortality and morbidity in SCD.[6] Symptoms of ACS include chest pain, dyspnea, cough, fever, wheezing, and hypoxemia, with pulmonary infiltrates that show up as a total white-out on chest x-ray film. ACS may rapidly progress to pulmonary failure, so immediate aggressive intervention is needed. This treatment includes broad-spectrum antibiotics, aggressive oxygen delivery therapies, analgesics, and careful acid/base and volume management.[6]

Over the past few decades, early detection and early intervention have increased the life expectancy of the individual with SCD, but still many patients die[5] before age 50. Ongoing research into the disease may change this dismal outlook through stem cell and bone marrow transplants. Currently, management is primarily aimed at symptoms and complications including effective pain management, transfusion of packed RBCs, chelation of iron, infection prevention, and administration of hydroxyurea.[5] Hydroxyurea is thought to work by increasing the level of fetal hemoglobin in RBCs, reducing the concentration of sickle hemoglobin and sickling itself. In general, effective management requires vigilant surveillance for complications associated with SCD: septicemia, acute myocardial infarction, priapism, stroke, acute kidney injury, acute limb ischemia, anemia, hepatomegaly, jaundice, pneumonia, meningitis, and shock.[6]

Leukemia

Leukemia is a malignant disorder of blood and blood-forming organs characterized by excessive, abnormal growth of leukocyte precursors in the bone marrow. An uncontrolled increase in immature leukocytes decreases production and function of normal leukocytes. Leukemia is classified as lymphogenous or myelogenous. Lymphogenous leukemias are caused by cancerous production of lymphoid cells, whereas myelogenous leukemias begin as the cancerous growth of myelogenous cells in bone marrow. Both types may be acute or chronic.[7]

Acute lymphocytic leukemia (ALL) is most common in children younger than 10 years of age but also has another peak incidence after the age of 50 years.[7] Newer therapies have increased the life expectancy for the childhood form. Presenting signs and symptoms are usually nonspecific and include fatigue, easy bruising, infections, and dyspnea. Diagnosis is made by the WBC count and confirmed by bone marrow examination. When the WBC counts rise above 50,000, the potential for leukostasis (a clumping or aggregation of WBCs) occurs. The organs most affected by leukostasis are the brain and lungs, potentially precipitating stroke or pulmonary infarcts. Chronic lymphocytic leukemia (CLL) is the most common leukemia seen in patients older than age 50 years. Signs and symptoms include spleen and liver enlargement, fatigue, easy bruising, infections, and weight loss. Leukostasis is rarely seen in CLL.[7]

Acute myelogenous leukemia (AML) is the most common type of acute leukemia and has its highest incidence in the population older than 60 years of age. It has an association with some genetic disorders, such as Down syndrome, Klinefelter's syndrome, and Fanconi's anemia and has also been associated with radiation exposure and specific medications. Presentation includes fever, dyspnea, pulmonary infiltrates that resemble pneumonia, fatigue, bruising, and volume overload.[8] Chronic myelogenous leukemia (CML) is the least common form but does occur most commonly in individuals older than 40 years of age. Manifestations include weight loss, sweating, fatigue, headache, vertigo, dyspnea, and enlarged spleen.[8] These patients are at risk for TLS and leukostasis.

Regardless of type, leukemic cells invade the spleen, lymph nodes, liver, and other vascular regions. Clinical manifestations of leukostasis by system may include (1) central nervous system symptoms of headache, dizziness, confusion, seizures, neurologic deficits, or intracranial hemorrhage; (2) ophthalmologic symptoms of blurred or loss of vision, papilledema, or retinal hemorrhage; (3) pulmonary symptoms of tachypnea, hypoxia, pulmonary infiltrates, or respiratory failure; (4) cardiovascular symptoms of chest pain or myocardial ischemia; and (5) general symptoms, such as fever, renal failure, priapism, elevated uric acid levels, lymph node enlargement, hepatomegaly, splenomegaly, disseminated intravascular coagulation, or TLS.[8]

Treatment includes adequate hydration, uric acid–lowering agents, hydroxyurea, chemotherapy, immunotherapy, and leukocytapheresis. Blood transfusions, antibiotics, antifungal agents, and antiviral agents may also be used. These patients are at significant risk for infection from their disease and their treatment; therefore it is critical that the patient be protected against exposure to potential infectious agents.[3]

Thrombocytopenia

Normal platelet count is 150,000 to 450,000/μL. Thrombocytopenia is an abnormal decrease in circulating platelets: a platelet count less than 150,000/μL. Effect on the platelet count is multifactorial and is seen primarily either as decreased platelet production or increased platelet destruction. Reduced platelet formation occurs with deficiencies in iron, folic acid, or vitamin B_{12}; certain chemotherapeutic agents; leukemia and lymphoma; or congenital or acquired disorders such as decreased bone marrow production, alcohol abuse, and liver disease. Autoantibody-mediated platelet destruction may be induced by drugs, infections, DIC, drug-induced thrombocytopenia, heparin-induced thrombocytopenia, preeclampsia, and HELLP syndrome (hemolysis, elevated liver enzymes, and low platelets), or autoimmune disorders.[9]

Immune thrombocytopenic purpura (ITP), also known as idiopathic thrombocytopenic purpura, the most common form of thrombocytopenia, is an acquired disease in which increased platelet destruction is caused by immune autoreactive antibodies.[10] Acute ITP usually is usually noted in children 1 to 3 weeks after a viral infection or a live virus vaccination. Acute ITP is self-limiting and typically resolves spontaneously within 6 months. Peak incidence is between 2 to 4 years of age. Bruising and petechiae are considered universal presenting symptoms for acute ITP. Three to four percent of patients may also present with purpura, epistaxis, mucous membrane bleeding, gastrointestinal bleeding, hematuria, and retinal bleeding. The diagnosis of ITP is based on patient history and confirmed with a platelet count. Treatment is generally unnecessary, but fresh frozen plasma (FFP), IV immunoglobulin, and splenectomy may be instituted for severe cases of spontaneous bleeding.[10]

Chronic ITP most commonly affects individuals 20 to 50 years of age, with a higher incidence in women. Chronic ITP is an autoimmune disorder; platelet life span is shortened to a few hours. Early symptoms are vague and include ecchymoses, menorrhagia, mucous membrane bleeding, and epistaxis. The decision to treat is based on the platelet count and on risk factors for bleeding (e.g., recent surgery or trauma) or prophylaxis to prevent hemorrhage, particularly spontaneous intracranial hemorrhage.[10] A patient with a platelet count above 30,000/μL usually requires no treatment. For patients with platelet counts below 30,000/μL and/or with additional risk factors, the first line of treatment is usually corticosteroids, followed by cyclosporine, administration of FFP, therapeutic plasma exchange, or potentially, splenectomy.[3] Confirming the cause of the thrombocytopenia, decreased platelet production, increased platelet destruction, or increased sequestration in the spleen directs the specific therapies.

Hemophilia

Hemophilia refers to several clotting disorders, including hemophilia A, hemophilia B, and von Willebrand's disease.[2] Hemophilia is an inherited, sex-linked disorder that occurs almost always in males. Females carry the disease and pass it on to their children. Severity ranges from mild to severe. The primary defect in hemophilia is absence or dysfunction of a specific clotting factor. Hemophilia A, or classic hemophilia, is due to a factor VIII disorder and affects approximately 1 in 10,000 people, primarily males. In most patients with hemophilia A, factor VIII is not missing. It may even be present in excess quantities; however, available factor VIII does not function adequately. Disease severity is directly related to the functional activity of factor VIII.[11] Hemophilia B, or Christmas disease, occurs less often than hemophilia A and is reported in 1 in 50,000 people. It is caused by the absence or functional deficiency of factor IX.[11]

Von Willebrand's disease is usually less acute than hemophilia A or B and occurs in both sexes. It is estimated that 1% of the population manifests the disease. Women experience bleeding challenges of menstruation and childbirth and hence are disproportionately affected by von Willebrand's disease. The specific coagulation defect in this type of hemophilia results from a deficiency of normal von Willebrand factor; hence, those affected have decreased platelet adherence and decreased levels of factor VIII.[12]

Hemophilia A and hemophilia B have similar clinical presentations. Patients with von Willebrand's disease exhibit less severe symptoms, with a lower incidence of bleeding into joints and deeper tissues. When a patient has hemophilia, even minor trauma can cause major bruises, visceral bleeding, and subdural hematomas. With the exception of lacerations or major trauma, one of the worst features of hemophilia is hemarthrosis—bleeding into a joint. Hemarthrosis usually begins in adolescence and involves primarily the knees, ankles, and elbows. Patients usually present to the ED with severe pain associated with hemarthrosis rather than actual bleeding.[11] Improperly managed hemarthrosis can lead to arthritis and ultimately joint destruction. Platelet-mediated hemostasis does not depend on factor VIII or factor IX; therefore the affected extremity should be elevated whenever possible. Identification of the specific type of hemophilia is crucial because hemophilia A and hemophilia B present the same clinical picture but require treatment with different clotting factors. A bleeding history should be obtained from all patients with abnormal bleeding. A screening coagulation panel should also be considered.

FFP has been used to treat hemophilia A and von Willebrand's disease. Unfortunately, FFP contains relatively small amounts of factor VIII per unit of volume, so large quantities are required for successful treatment.[10] Cryoprecipitate is rich in factor VIII per unit of volume. Fortunately, recent product modifications have reduced the risk of disease transmission and reduced the cost of production. Most individuals with hemophilia A are treated with replacement of factor VIII, either from pooled plasma or from a genetically engineered source. Antibody-purified factor IX is the treatment for patients with hemophilia B with limited prior exposure to cryoprecipitate who are negative for human immunodeficiency virus. Mild to-moderate bleeding may be treated with FFP.[11]

Disseminated Intravascular Coagulation

DIC is an acquired dysfunction of the clotting system due to excessive stimulation of the coagulation cascade from both the intrinsic and extrinsic pathways. Activation of the coagulation cascade leads to accelerated clotting. This in turn triggers thrombosis as excessive fibrin is released into the circulation, causing microclots and obstructing blood flow in the small vessels. As coagulation continues at this accelerated rate, it exceeds the capacity of the fibrinolytic system. Consequently, platelets, clotting factors, and fibrinogen are consumed faster than the body can replace them and, as the system becomes overwhelmed, simultaneous bleeding and clotting occur.[3,13]

Conditions that may trigger DIC include (1) infections, especially gram-negative sepsis; (2) obstetric issues (50% of cases are related to obstetrics, particularly amniotic fluid embolism, incomplete abortion, placental abruption, HELLP syndrome, retained placenta, and fetal demise); (3) toxins, allergic reactions, or overdoses such as those involving amphetamines; (4) inflammatory states (e.g., acute pancreatitis); (5) vascular stimulation from crush injuries and severe trauma; and (6) malignancy or liver disease.[3,9,13] In most cases DIC presents with bleeding, although some patients present with organ ischemia related to microthrombi and impaired blood flow. This is the result of two mechanisms: thromboses that occur in the microcirculation from the overfunction of the coagulation process and bleeding resulting from the consumption of platelets, fibrin, and clotting factors. Thrombosis-related signs include cyanosis; gangrene of fingers, toes, nose, and ears; bowel infarction; and renal failure.[10] Hemorrhagic signs include petechiae, purpura, bleeding from IV sites and surgical sites, epistaxis, altered level of consciousness, menorrhagia, hemoptysis, gastrointestinal bleeding, and hematuria. Other systemic signs may include cough, dyspnea, confusion, fever, and tachypnea. Diagnostic laboratory studies include PT, PTT, fibrinogen levels, platelet levels, fibrin split products, and fibrin degradation products (D-dimer).[9]

DIC is frequently a life-threatening condition frequently progressing to multiple-organ failure and death. There are three components of treatment for DIC, and they should be accomplished simultaneously: (1) identify and treat or remove the trigger; (2) maintain or restore tissue perfusion; and (3) balance clot formation, clot breakdown, and clot prevention.[10] Identifying DIC may be difficult, and the diagnosis is made by exclusion of other conditions such as hemodilution by bleeding/massive transfusion, heparin-induced thrombocytopenia, vitamin K deficiency, and liver failure.[3]

DIC both causes and is exacerbated by ischemia and necrosis; therefore adequate oxygenation and perfusion are essential in its treatment. Supplemental oxygen should be given to maintain oxygen saturation.[10] Volume replacement with IV fluids and packed RBCs may help restore intravascular volume. Vasopressors, such as dopamine, may be prescribed to maintain blood pressure and tissue perfusion. Achieving a balance in the coagulation process among clot formation, breakdown, and prevention may be a difficult process. Replacement of the depleted clotting factors is one of the first orders of treatment and includes transfusions of FFP, packed RBCs, cryoprecipitate, and platelets. Packed RBCs will help restore the oxygen-carrying capacity of the blood. FFP replaces clotting factors, and cryoprecipitate replaces fibrin.

Heparin has been used to prevent the formation of new clots, but its use is controversial. It is contraindicated in some instances such as recent surgery, gastrointestinal bleeding, or central nervous system bleeding.[3] It has been used when there is evidence of organ damage or when loss of life or limb is imminent. Heparin has also been used with success in some obstetric-related cases of DIC, such as retained placenta and incomplete abortion.[13] Each case of DIC is unique, and therapy should be tailored to the underlying condition, with supportive therapy.

SPECIFIC ONCOLOGIC EMERGENCIES

Oncology-related emergencies are structural or metabolic problems that fall into three categories: cytopenias related to bone marrow suppression caused by disease process or treatment (anemia, neutropenia, and thrombocytopenia), electrolyte and fluid imbalances (hyperuricemia, TLS, and SIADH), and tumor-mediated compression of surrounding structures (superior vena cava syndrome and spinal cord compression). Structural emergencies are most often recognized by physical assessment, clinical findings, and imaging studies, whereas metabolic emergencies are confirmed by physical assessment, clinical findings, and laboratory values.

Fever and Neutropenia

Infections are common in patients with cancer and are a major contributor to morbidity and mortality. Neutropenia is a condition in which the absolute neutrophil count is less than 1000 cells/mm³ and indicates a moderate risk for infection.[8] Neutropenia can be the result of a neoplastic process, medication/drug effects, or infection and is commonly associated with chemotherapy, radiation therapy, and bone marrow transplant.[8] The nadir (the period when neutrophil levels are at their lowest point) differs with each chemotherapeutic agent but usually occurs 10 to 14 days after the administration of chemotherapy. Many patients receive growth factors (e.g., filgrastim and pegfilgrastim) as a preventative measure to decrease the severity of neutropenia, although some patients may still continue to progress to a severe state of neutropenia. The ED nursing assessment should include asking the patient if he or she is taking any of these growth factors.

Infection in patients with neutropenia often presents only as fever (febrile neutropenia). Sepsis is the leading cause of death in patients with cancer, and in immunosuppressed patients, there may be few signs of infection/sepsis (fever, hypotension, site for infection focus). Development of an infection while the patient is neutropenic may result in death within hours.[13] Febrile neutropenia is defined as either a single temperature greater than or equal to 101°F (38.3°C) or a temperature of 100.4°F (38°C) sustained for more than 1 hour.[8,14] Initial workup for febrile neutropenia should include two or more blood cultures from separate sites, one being from the patient's central venous access device; CBC; electrolyte levels; kidney and liver function tests; chest x-ray examination; urinalysis; urine culture and sensitivity; and cultures of throat, stool, and any skin lesions.[8,13] Examination of cerebrospinal, pleural, or peritoneal fluids may also be indicated. Initial antibiotic therapy recommendations are for empirical broad-spectrum antibiotic therapy initiated within 1 hour after fever or blood cultures.[13] Admission should be to a private room, preferably with a positive-pressure airflow, and the patient should wear a mask when being transported throughout the hospital. Patients at higher risk for complications from febrile neutropenia are those who are older than 65 years of age, have comorbid chronic disease, have impaired renal or liver function, have been neutropenic for more than 1 week, or are status-post stem cell or bone marrow transplantation.[13,14]

Tumor Lysis Syndrome

TLS is a constellation of metabolic derangements resulting from the death of neoplastic cells, which then release their intracellular contents into the circulation. Although it may occur spontaneously, TLS is usually a direct result of treatment (chemotherapy or radiation therapy).[8] The destroyed cells release their intracellular contents into the bloodstream, with hyperkalemia and resulting life-threatening cardiac arrhythmias frequently the first presentation. The catabolism of nucleic acids results in hyperuricemia. The high concentrations of uric acid will lead to crystallization within the renal tubules and result in acute kidney injury. The release of phosphates from the neoplastic cells leads to hyperphosphatemia, which in turn binds calcium and leads to hypocalcemia.[8,15]

The diagnosis of TLS is based on laboratory tests, patient history, and clinical manifestations.[8,15] Symptoms depend on the extent of the electrolyte imbalance and include fatigue, nausea, anorexia, muscle cramps, paresthesias, widened QRS, dysrhythmias, abdominal cramps, diarrhea, flank pain, and renal failure.[3,8] Hydration is the single most important intervention for TLS because it facilitates excretion of the excessive electrolytes. IV administration of sodium bicarbonate alkalinizes the urine to prevent renal failure from uric acid deposits in the kidneys. Diuretics may be given to increase the excretion of uric acid and electrolytes. Allopurinol prevents the formation of uric acid. Hyperkalemia is managed by the administration of sodium polystyrene sulfonate to pull potassium into the gastrointestinal tract for excretion and by the IV administration of calcium chloride/calcium gluconate, sodium bicarbonate, hypertonic glucose, and insulin to move potassium from the serum into the intracellular spaces and/or nebulized administration of albuterol. Emergency dialysis may be required. Phosphate-binding agents, such as aluminum hydroxide gel, help eliminate the hyperphosphatemia.[3,8]

Syndrome of Inappropriate Antidiuretic Hormone

Under usual circumstances, the pituitary gland produces and releases vasopressin (antidiuretic hormone, ADH) to manage increased serum osmolarity by reducing urine output. In certain types of cancers, especially small cell lung cancer, the tumors themselves release ADH, leading to an increase in fluid retention by the kidneys. This water intoxication results in a dilutional hyponatremia (serum sodium level less than 129 mEq/L). The excess fluid moves by osmosis into the cells, causing cellular swelling. Cerebral edema may be the most life-threatening sequela.[16,17]

Symptoms of SIADH include headache, personality changes, mental status changes, irritability, lethargy, confusion, nausea, vomiting, anorexia, diarrhea, and muscle cramps.[17] As the hyponatremia becomes more severe, symptoms progress to seizure activity, papilledema, coma, and death. Diagnosis is confirmed by laboratory tests: serum sodium levels, blood urea nitrogen, creatinine, and urine osmolality. Treatment is dictated by the degree of hyponatremia and includes fluid restrictions, cautious administration of hypertonic sodium chloride infusions, diuretics, and a vasopressin receptor antagonist, tolvaptan (Samsca).[18] Care must be taken to correct sodium slowly, keep appropriate seizure precautions in place, and monitor carefully.[18]

Superior Vena Cava Syndrome

Superior vena cava syndrome results from obstruction of the major blood vessels draining the head, neck, and upper torso.[19] This obstruction may arise from outside the vena cava as compression by a tumor or an enlarged lymph node, or the obstruction may arise from within the superior vena cava by the formation of a thrombus caused by position of a venous access device. Advanced lung cancer accounts for approximately 75% of cases.[19] Much of the time, superior vena cava syndrome develops slowly, allowing collateral circulation to develop. Symptoms may be grouped: (1) respiratory: stridor, dysphagia, dyspnea, orthopnea, laryngeal edema, chest pain, cough, or pleurisy; (2) neurologic: malaise, visual disorders, headache, vertigo, or coma; and (3) facial: swelling, lip edema, nasal obstruction or epistaxis, and vessel dilation of the neck, face, or arms.[3] Symptoms accompanying a rapid onset of superior vena cava syndrome may include life-threatening manifestations such as cerebral edema (mental status changes, dizziness, visual changes) and airway obstruction from laryngeal swelling.[19]

A definitive diagnosis of the cause and the type of tumor will direct the treatment regimen; therefore referral to an oncologist is of prime importance. Drug-sensitive tumors will be treated with chemotherapy; others will be treated with radiation therapy. Potentially emergency surgery or stent placement may be required. If the obstruction was caused by a thrombosis arising from a vascular access device, treatment modalities will include vascular catheter removal, fibrinolytic therapy, or anticoagulation. Other supportive measures might include corticosteroids, oxygen therapy, and diuretics.[3,8] The patient should be placed in the semi-Fowler's position to facilitate breathing and to decrease facial and upper body swelling.

Spinal Cord Compression

Spinal cord compression is a common oncologic emergency.[20] The most frequent oncologic cause of spinal cord compression is vertebral body erosion from tumors, usually arising from breast, lung, and prostate cancer, and melanomas and lymphomas. It is estimated that 40% of patients with cancer will develop metastatic spinal disease, with 10% to 20% of these patients developing symptoms of spinal cord compression.[20] Symptomatic compression of the cord is an oncologic emergency because irreversible neurologic damage may occur in hours.[3]

The most frequently reported symptom is back pain worsened by movement, coughing, sneezing, or by supine positioning. Many patients with cancer have chronic back pain; therefore any new pain or a worsening or change in existing pain (such as sensory and/or motor deficits) necessitates further assessment.[20] More specific symptoms depend on the location of the compression (most often thoracic) and may include lower extremity weakness progressing to paralysis, paresthesias, sensory losses, and loss of deep tendon reflexes, along with bowel and bladder dysfunction.

Evidence of loss of neurologic function is an indication for emergent treatment to prevent further loss of function. Lost function is rarely regained. Diagnostic evaluation includes magnetic resonance imaging to rule out other causes of cord compression. Emergent treatment includes IV dexamethasone and radiation therapy with potential preparation for decompressive surgery.[3] Less emergent symptoms (pain without loss of neurologic function) may respond well to other treatment modalities such as chemotherapy or percutaneous vertebroplasty.[20] These patients need to be referred to their oncologist for timely intervention.

SUMMARY

Hematologic and oncologic emergencies cover an array of clinical conditions and represent a broad spectrum of patient acuity. Knowledge of the common disease processes and astute assessment skills enhance the ability of the emergency nurse to appropriately prioritize care to ensure optimal patient outcome.

REFERENCES

1. Ostrowski SR. Blood components—so much more than clots and oxygen delivery! *ISBT Sci Ser*. 2017;12(4):463–470. https://doi.org/10.1111/voxs.12352.
2. Betts JG, DeSaix P, Johnson E, Johnson JE, Korol O, Kruse D, et al. *Anatomy and Physiology*. Houston, TX: OpenStax; 2017.
3. Nifosi G. Hematologic emergencies. *Open J Int Med*. 2016;6(3):83–92. https://doi.org/10.4236/ojim.2016.63014.
4. Matthie N, Jenerette C. Sickle cell disease in adults: developing an appropriate care plan. *Clin J Oncol Nurs*. 2015;19(5):562–567.
5. Ware RE, de Montalembert M, Tshilolo L, Abboud MR. Sickle cell disease. *Lancet*. 2017;390(10091):311–323. https://doi.org/10.1016/S0140-6736(17)30193-9.

6. Mekontso Dessap AM, Fartoukh M, Machado RF. Ten tips for managing critically ill patients with sickle cell disease. *Intensive Care Med.* 2017;43(1):80–82. https://doi.org/10.1007/s00134-016-4472-7.
7. Terwillinger T, Abdul-Hay M. Acute lymphoblastic leukemia: a comprehensive review and 2017 update. *Blood Cancer J.* 2017;7(6):e577. https://doi.org/10.1038/bcj.2017.53.
8. Halfdanarson TR, Hogan WJ, Madsen BE. Emergencies in hematology and oncology. *Mayo Clin Proc.* 2017;92(4):609–641. https://doi.org/10.1016yj.mayocp.2017.02.008.
9. Ali N, Auerbach HE. New-onset acute thrombocytopenia in hospitalized patients: pathophysiology and diagnostic approach. *J Community Hosp Intern Med Perspect.* 2017;7(3):157–167. https://doi.org/10.1080/20009666.2017.1335156.
10. Retter A, Barrett NA. The management of abnormal haemostasis in the ICU. *Anaesthesia.* 2015;70(suppl 1):121–127. https://doi.org/10.1111/anae.12908.
11. Rosen M, Quint E. Bleeding disorders: when to worry, how to help. *Contemporary OB/GYN.* 2017;62(7):15–23.
12. James A. Von Willebrand: an underdiagnosed disorder. *Contemporary OB/GYN.* 2017;62(5):20–43.
13. Toepke McLean M. Marion's message: disseminated intravascular coagulation. *Midwifery Today Int Midwife.* 2015 Summer;114:7.
14. Bryant AL, Walton A, Albrecht TA. Management of febrile neutropenia in a patient with acute leukemia. *J Emerg Nurs.* 2014;40(4):377–381. https://doi.org/10.1016/j.jen.2013.07.021.
15. Smith LT, Venella K. Cytokine release syndrome. *Clin J Oncol Nurs.* 2017;21(2):29–34. https://doi.org/10.1188/17.CJON.S2.29-34.
16. Goldvaser H, Rozen-Zvi B, Yerushalmi R, Gafter-Gvili A, Lahav M, Shepshelovich D. Malignancy associated SIADH: characterization and clinical implications. *Acta Oncologica.* 2016;55(9/10):1190–1195. https://doi.org/10.3109/0284186X.2016.1170198.
17. Frazer C. Syndrome of inappropriate antidiuresis. *MEDSURG Nursing.* 2017;26(5):346–348.
18. Peñas R, Ponce S, Henao F, et al. SIADH-related hyponatremia in hospital day care units: clinical experience and management with tolvaptan. *Support Care Cancer.* 2016;24(1):499–507. https://doi.org/10.1007/s00520-015-2948-6.
19. Koetters KT. Superior vena cava syndrome. *J Emerg Nurs.* 2012;38(2):135–138. https://doi.org/10.1016/j.jen.2010.08.019.
20. Bowers B. Recognizing metastatic spinal cord compression. *Br J Commun Nurs.* 2015;20(4):162–165.

Environmental Emergencies

Gordon H. Worley

Humans may be exposed to environmental hazards and extremes under a wide variety of circumstances. These include voluntary participation in activities such as outdoor recreation, military service, work, or travel; or involuntary exposure caused by accidents, lack of experience, disaster events, lack of shelter (homelessness), confusion, inattention, mental illness, alcohol, or drugs.

THERMAL EMERGENCIES

Normothermia is the maintenance of a normal body core temperature of 37°C (98.6°F) ± 1.0°C. Body heat is generated by metabolism, and body temperature is regulated by dissipating or retaining heat. Heat may be dissipated from the body by radiation into the environment, convection from air movement over the body surface, evaporation of sweat or other liquids, or conduction into a solid object. When the body is exposed to extremes of temperature without appropriate thermal protection, heat can be gained or lost beyond the body's ability to thermoregulate.[1,2]

Heat Illness

Heat illness is a significant cause of morbidity and mortality. The estimated annual death rate from heat-related illness in the United States is 600 deaths per year.[3] Heat illnesses represent a spectrum ranging from mild (heat exhaustion) to severe and life-threatening (heat stroke and exercise-associated hyponatremia). See Table 30.1. Young children and infants are at increased risk of heat illness due to their higher body surface area to weight ratio, which accelerates heat gain or loss. A particular risk for young children is being left alone in a hot car. Older adults and the chronically ill may have comorbidities or may use medications predisposing them to heat illnesses.[4,5]

Heat Exhaustion

Heat exhaustion is a mild-moderate heat illness resulting from exposure to high environmental temperatures or strenuous exercise in warm or hot environments. Elevated body temperature and fluid loss due to heavy perspiration and inadequate fluid replacement lead to volume depletion.[4] Heat exhaustion occurs most often in individuals working or exercising in hot environments, such as laborers, athletes, firefighters, and military personnel, and among older adults and children.[4,5]

Heat exhaustion is characterized by a body core temperature of 38.5ºC to 40.0º C (101.3ºF to 104.0ºF) accompanied by tachycardia and orthostatic hypotension. Patients may demonstrate nausea, vomiting, thirst, fatigue, headache, anxiety, dizziness, syncope, and collapse. Diaphoresis may or may not be present. Mental status will be normal or mildly altered. Unrecognized or untreated heat exhaustion can progress to heat stroke.[4,5]

Initial treatment includes moving the patient to a cool environment and initiating cooling measures. Wetting the patient's clothing and fanning the patient can help dissipate heat by evaporation and convection. If the patient can tolerate oral fluids, fluid and electrolyte replacement should be provided using cool isotonic drinks. Body core temperature should be monitored. Laboratory studies should include electrolytes, glucose, renal and liver function tests, complete blood count (CBC), and urinalysis.[4,5] Serum sodium should be checked rapidly to differentiate exercise-associated hyponatremia (EAH) from other forms of heat illness.[6] EAH is discussed later in this chapter.

If the patient is hypotensive, or is nauseated or vomiting, intravenous access and fluid resuscitation using 0.9% normal saline solution should be initiated. Patients with hypotension or a history of cardiac disease should be placed on a cardiac monitor.[4,5,7,8]

Heat Stroke

Heat stroke is a severe, life-threatening illness resulting from the body's loss of its intrinsic thermoregulatory mechanisms. It is characterized by a body core temperature ≥40ºC (104ºF) accompanied by central nervous system (CNS) dysfunction.[7] Classic heat stroke occurs from passive exposure to high environmental temperatures. It may progress gradually or occur suddenly. Older adults, the chronically ill, and young children and infants are at highest risk. Mortality from classic heat stroke can be as high as 65%.[4]

Exertional heat stroke (EHS) is most common among young, physically fit individuals such as athletes, laborers, members of the military, and firefighters. Heat production from vigorous exercise exceeds the body's ability to dissipate heat into the environment, leading to increasing core temperature. EHS can occur in hot environments or when there are barriers to heat dissipation, such as heavy protective clothing (a firefighter's turnout gear, etc.).[4]

TABLE 30.1 Heat Illness.

Condition	Core Temperature	Mental Status	Vital Signs	Other Findings
Heat exhaustion	38.5°C (101.3°F) to 40.0°C (104.0°F)	• Normal or only mildly altered	• Tachycardia • Orthostatic hypotension	• Nausea and vomiting • Diaphoresis • Extreme thirst • Fatigue • Headache • Anxiety • Dizziness • Syncope • Collapse
Heat stroke	≥ 40°C (104°F)	• Anxiety • Ataxia • Poor coordination • Slurred speech • Agitation • Delirium • Seizures • Coma	• Tachycardia • Hypotension	• Diarrhea • Vomiting • Hyperventilation • Decreased urine output • Sweating may or may not be present
Exercise-associated hyponatremia	Normal or mildly elevated	• Dizziness • Headache • Confusion • Agitation • Delirium • Ataxia • Seizures • Coma	• Tachycardia • Orthostatic hypotension	• Serum sodium below 130 mmol/L • Nausea and vomiting • Puffiness/peripheral edema • Body weight gain from baseline

From Leon LR, Kenefick RW. Pathophysiology of heat-related illness. In: Auerbach PS, Cushing TA, Harris NS, eds. *Auerbach's Wilderness Medicine.* 7th ed. Philadelphia, PA: Elsevier; 2017:259–274; Platt M, Vicario S. Heat illness. In: Marx JA, ed. *Rosen's Emergency Medicine: Concepts and Clinical Practice.* 8th ed. Philadelphia, PA: Elsevier; 2014:1896–1904.
Bennett BL, Hew-Butler T, Hoffman MD, Rogers IR, Rosner MH, Wilderness Medical Society. Wilderness Medical Society practice guidelines for treatment of exercise-associated hyponatremia: 2014 update. *Wilderness Environ Med.* 2014;25(suppl 4):S30–S42.
Lipman GS, Eifling KP, Ellis MA, et al. Wilderness Medical Society practice guidelines for the prevention and treatment of heat-related illness: 2014 update. *Wilderness Environ Med.* 2014;25(suppl 4):S55–S65.
Hew-Butler T, Loi V, Pani A, Rosner MH. Exercise-associated hyponatremia: 2017 update. *Front Med.* 2017;4(3):370–310.

The cardinal sign of heat stroke is altered mental status or other CNS dysfunction in the setting of elevated body temperature. Early neurologic signs can include anxiety, ataxia, poor coordination, and slurred speech. Later signs include agitation, delirium, seizures, and coma. Symptoms related to multisystem involvement can include diarrhea, vomiting, hyperventilation, and decreased urine output.[4,7,8,9] Sweating may or may not be present. The absence of sweating is not a diagnostic sign for heat stroke,[4] but the loss of this cooling mechanism can accelerate the rise in body temperature. Other possible causes of elevated body temperature should be considered, including infection, thyroid storm, and drug-induced hyperthermia.

Anyone who develops mental status changes during or after exercise in warm weather and has no evidence of trauma, and all older adult or chronically ill patients with mental status changes associated with heat exposure should be treated as having heat stroke. Heat stroke can be fatal despite rapid and appropriate treatment.[4,5]

Treatment of Heat Stroke. As soon as safety allows, the patient should be moved to a cooler area and the patient's clothing wetted with tepid water and fanned. Cold packs may be applied to the axillae and groin. Large-bore intravenous (IV) access should be obtained and fluid resuscitation initiated with cool fluids (4ºC/39ºF). Fluid resuscitation recommendations vary, but the most common recommendation is administering 1 to 2 L of 0.9% saline solution over the first 4 hours. Rapid fluid resuscitation is not usually indicated, unless the patient is hypotensive.[8]

Ice-water or cold-water immersion is an effective method of rapidly lowering core body temperature and has been shown to be safe in patients with EHS.[7,9] Spraying the patient with tepid (40ºC/104ºF) water and using fans to continuously blow air over the patient is the recommended treatment for patients with classic heat stroke. This is an effective cooling method and requires little specialized equipment.[8,10] Cooling should be continued until mental status returns to baseline and the rectal temperature is ≤102.0°F (38.8°C).[8] Core temperature should be monitored using a rectal probe for all patients with suspected heat stroke, particularly during the cooling phase, to prevent inadvertent hypothermia.

Prompt measurement of serum sodium is important to differentiate EAH from other forms of heat illness, as described in the next section.[6] Additional laboratory studies include electrolytes, glucose, renal and liver function tests, creatinine kinase, CBC, prothrombin time/partial thromboplastin time (PT/PTT), and urinalysis. Antipyretics (aspirin, ibuprofen, acetaminophen) and dantrolene sodium have not been shown to be useful in heat stroke and are not recommended.[5,7] Benzodiazepines may be useful to control shivering from rapid cooling and to manage seizures.[5] A urinary catheter should be inserted and urine output maintained at ≥1 to 2 mL/kg per hour. Urine color and urine myoglobin should be monitored for signs of rhabdomyolysis. Coagulopathies including disseminated intravascular coagulation (DIC) can occur, most commonly on the second or third day of the illness.[5]

Exercise-Associated Hyponatremia

EAH is a life-threatening condition most common among endurance athletes and others who exert themselves in high-temperature conditions. Hyponatremia is defined as a serum sodium level below 135 mmol/L (or the low-normal for the specific laboratory). Severe hyponatremia is usually defined as a serum sodium level ≤125 mmol/L, although some patients may be symptomatic with levels between 125 and 130 mmol/L.[6,11]

The pathophysiologic mechanism of EAH is the excess consumption of water or other hypotonic fluids beyond what is necessary to replace fluid loss from sweating. All documented fatalities from EAH have been associated with excessive water consumption. The resulting dilutional hyponatremia causes osmotic fluid shifts from the extracellular to the intracellular space. These fluid shifts can result in cerebral edema and neurologic symptoms. Severe cases can cause significant brain swelling with brain stem herniation.[6,11,12]

Symptoms of mild EAH include dizziness, nausea, puffiness/peripheral edema, and body weight gain from baseline. Signs and symptoms of severe EAH include headache, vomiting, confusion, ataxia, delirium, agitation, seizures, and coma. The most severe cases may show signs of noncardiac pulmonary edema or decorticate posturing and other signs of impending brain stem herniation.[6,11]

Patients may be significantly hyponatremic without overt symptoms. Unrecognized EAH that is treated as other heat illness can worsen the hyponatremia and may cause asymptomatic EAH to progress to symptomatic EAH. Endurance athletes with nonspecific symptoms and any patient who has been exercising in the heat and demonstrates altered mental status without elevated body temperature should raise suspicion for EAH.[6,11,12]

Rapid measurement of the serum sodium level is key to the diagnosis of EAH. Treatment of confirmed or suspected EAH is aimed at rapid correction of the hyponatremia with hypertonic saline (HTS) solution, such as 3% sodium chloride. If EAH is suspected but serum sodium measurement is not rapidly available, the recommended treatment is to administer HTS. If HTS is unavailable, it is generally the best approach to avoid the use of large volumes of isotonic or hypotonic fluids such 0.9% saline until the serum sodium level is known.[6,11,12]

Cold-Related Emergencies

Accidental Hypothermia

Accidental hypothermia is the most dangerous cold-related emergency condition. Although cold weather, wet weather, and immersion in cold water pose the highest risk of hypothermia, this condition can occur in temperate and even tropical climates when heat loss exceeds body heat production. Accidental hypothermia may result from outdoor occupational or recreational activities, disasters, homelessness, or substance abuse, or secondary to trauma, sepsis, hypoglycemia, and other medical conditions. Intentional targeted temperature management is discussed in Chapter 23.

There are 1300 to 1500 reported deaths due to hypothermia in the United States each year.[3,13,14] Most reported hypothermia fatalities (67%) occur in males, and death rates are highest for patients aged 65 years or older. About 10% are related to drug or alcohol use.[13] Iatrogenic hypothermia occurs when ill or injured patients are not adequately protected from heat loss during resuscitation and can contribute to mortality from other conditions, such as trauma.[1,14]

Accidental hypothermia is defined as an unintentional decrease in body core temperature below 35°C (95°F). This decrease in core temperature results in neurologic impairment, depressed cardiac output, dysrhythmias, metabolic derangement, coagulopathy and, eventually, death if not reversed.[1]

In mild hypothermia (32°C–35°C/90°F–95°F), thermoregulatory mechanisms remain intact but are under stress. The patient will generally be awake, alert, and vigorously shivering. Skin cooling induces shivering, which increases metabolism and heat production by muscular activity. Tachycardia and rapid respirations may be present, progressing to bradycardia and respiratory depression as the core temperature drops. Glucose stores may become depleted with prolonged shivering. Patients may show progressive neurologic impairment, demonstrating poor judgment, lack of coordination, slurred speech, amnesia, apathy, and ataxia.[15]

Moderate hypothermia (28°C–32°C/82°F–90°F) represents the progressive failure of the patient's thermoregulatory mechanisms. As the core temperature drops, shivering becomes more intense, then begins to decrease below 31°C (88°F), ultimately ceasing at about 30°C (86°F). There is a progressive decrease in level of consciousness and in cardiopulmonary function. Patients will demonstrate bradycardia, bradypnea, dysrhythmias, and electrocardiogram (ECG) changes including development of a J wave, a positive deflection at the beginning of the ST segment, as illustrated in Fig. 30.1. A rare and puzzling response to worsening hypothermia is paradoxical disrobing, where the hypothermic individual undresses despite the cold.[15]

In severe hypothermia (less than 28°C/82°F), thermoregulatory mechanisms have failed and shivering is absent. The patient may be unresponsive and have absent reflexes. There is usually profound bradycardia and respiratory depression, and vital signs may be undetectable. The ventricular fibrillation (VF) threshold is decreased and the heart muscle is very irritable. Rough handling or sudden position changes can induce

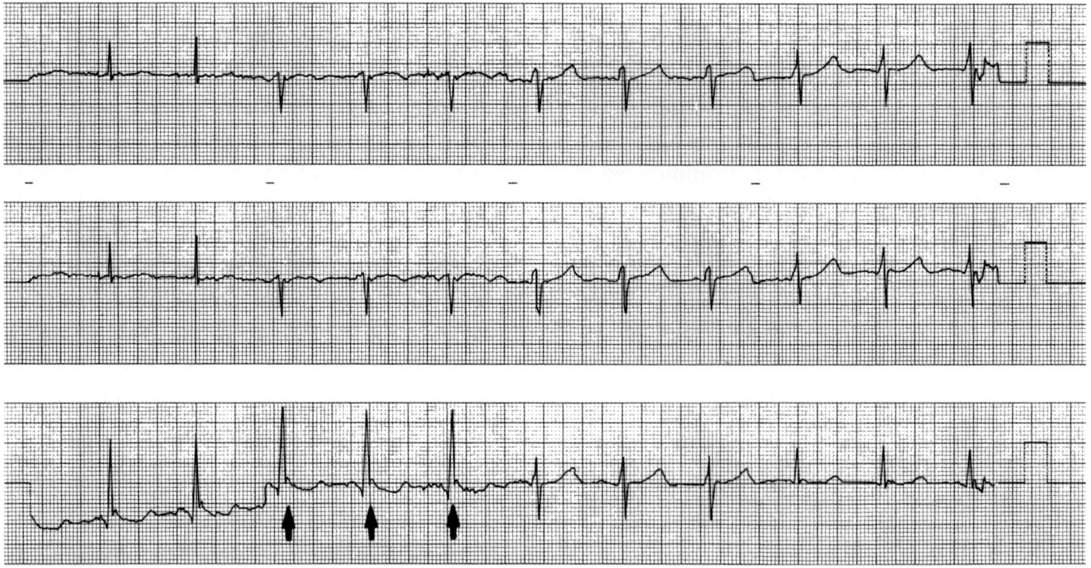

Fig. 30.1 Hypothermic J Waves. (From Rosen P, Barkin RM, Hockberger RS, eds. *Emergency Medicine: Concepts and Clinical Practice*. 3rd ed. St Louis, MO: Mosby: 1999.)

VF. Laboratory tests will demonstrate elevated potassium, acid-base disturbances, and coagulation abnormalities.[15]

Afterdrop should be anticipated in all patients with hypothermia. This phenomenon occurs after removal from the cold environment and initiation of rewarming. Core temperature continues to decrease due to conduction of heat from the core into colder peripheral tissues and the circulation of colder blood from the periphery back to the core. Afterdrop may result in an additional decrease in core temperature of as much as 5°C to 6°C before the body temperature begins to rise again.[2]

Treatment of Hypothermia. The first step in the management of all patients with hypothermia is to safely remove them from the cold environment to a warmer, sheltered location. Gentle handling is very important to protect the irritable heart muscle from sudden shocks.[1] The mildly hypothermic patient who is alert and shivering is usually able to self-rewarm. Treatment involves preventing further heat loss and providing passive external rewarming by removing wet clothing and providing insulation and a vapor barrier.[1,14,16] External sources of heat can assist in rewarming and improve patient comfort but are not usually required. Giving the patient warm oral fluids containing carbohydrates can provide additional calories to support heat production.[1] See Table 30.2.

Moderately hypothermic patients have a diminished or absent ability to rewarm themselves and will require active external rewarming. Core temperature should be continuously monitored using an esophageal probe in the distal esophagus, and afterdrop should be anticipated. Rectal probes, oral thermometers, and temperature-sensing urinary catheters are not recommended. They lag behind actual core temperature by as much as an hour in the patient with hypothermia.[1,2]

The most effective and practical method of active external rewarming in the emergency department (ED) is a commercial forced-air warming blanket. Radiant heat lamps, hot water bottles placed in the axillae and groin, and large, chemical heat pads are also effective. Heat should be concentrated on the chest, axillae, and back. Gastric lavage with warmed fluids, warmed oxygen, and warm water mattresses may be useful as adjuncts but are usually not adequate to achieve effective rewarming on their own.[2,15] IV fluids should be warmed to 40°C to 42°C (104°F–108°F).[2,17] Immersion in warm water or warm showers should not be used for rewarming in hypothermia; this technique has been associated with cardiovascular collapse and death.[1,17]

Severely hypothermic patients may be divided into two groups: those who have detectable vital signs and those who do not. The latter group may appear to be dead, with no discernible respirations or pulse, fixed and dilated pupils, and the appearance of rigor mortis. Assessment for breathing and circulation should be performed for at least 1 minute. Respirations may be easier to detect than a carotid pulse; if respirations are present, assume there is cardiac output. Ultrasound and ECG monitoring can be helpful in detecting cardiac activity.[1,17]

For patients with detectable signs of life, including organized electrical activity on the cardiac monitor or heart wall motion on ultrasound, aggressive external rewarming is the primary treatment. Some patients may require endotracheal intubation or placement of supraglottic airway to support ventilation or prevent aspiration. All patients should have continuous ECG, end-tidal CO_2 ($EtCO_2$), and temperature monitoring.[2,17]

Cardiopulmonary resuscitation (CPR) should be initiated on patients with no detectable cardiac or respiratory activity. IV access should be obtained and warmed dextrose-containing fluids such as D_5/0.9 % normal saline administered. Aggressive rewarming should continue. If the cardiac monitor shows pulseless ventricular tachycardia (pVT) or VF, defibrillate with a single shock at the maximum power setting. If this is unsuccessful, wait to repeat the shock until the patient has been rewarmed at least 1°C to 2°C. Once the core

TABLE 30.2 Management of Hypothermia.

Classification	Core Temperature	Signs and Symptoms	Treatment
Mild hypothermia	32°C–35°C (90°F–95°F)	• Awake and alert • May have mildly altered mentation • Poor judgment • Slurred speech • Amnesia • Apathy • Lack of coordination • Ataxia • Vigorously shivering	• Able to self-rewarm • Protect from environment • Insulate • Encourage shivering • Warm sweetened beverages • External heat helpful, but required
Moderate hypothermia	28°C–32°C (82°F–90°F)	• Shivering above 30°C (86°F) • Loss of shivering below 30°C • Decreasing loss of consciousness • Bradycardia • Bradypnea • Dysrhythmias • J-wave on ECG (Fig. 30.1)	• Not able to effectively self-rewarm • Active external rewarming indicated • Keep NPO • Handle gently
Severe hypothermia	<28°C (82°F)	• Shivering absent • Profound bradycardia • May appear dead, vital signs may be undetectable • Heart muscle very irritable, high risk of ventricular fibrillation	• Handle very gently • Active external or internal rewarming required for survival

ECG, Electrocardiogram; *NPO*, nil by mouth.
From Zafren K, Giesbrecht GG, Danzl DF, et al. Wilderness Medical Society practice guidelines for the out-of-hospital evaluation and treatment of accidental hypothermia: 2014 update. *Wilderness Environ Med.* 2014;25(suppl 4):S66–S85; Haverkamp FJC, Giesbrecht GG, Tan ECTH. The prehospital management of hypothermia—an up-to-date overview. *Injury.* 2018;49(2):149–164; Danzl DF, Huecker MR. Accidental hypothermia. In: Auerbach PS, Cushing TA, Harris NS, eds. *Auerbach's Wilderness Medicine.* 7th ed. Philadelphia, PA: Elsevier; 2017:135–162.
Zafren K, Giesbrecht G. State of Alaska: Cold injuries guidelines. http://dhss.alaska.gov/dph/Emergency/Documents/ems/documents/Alaska%20DHSS%20EMS%20Cold%20Injuries%20Guidelines%20June%202014.pdf. Published July 2014. Accessed May 30, 2018.

temperature reaches 30°C, follow standard advanced cardiac life support (ACLS) guidelines.[2,18]

Drug metabolism will be significantly reduced below 30°C, and unmetabolized medications can build up with repeated doses, resulting in toxic levels once the patient is rewarmed. Withhold resuscitation medications below 30°C, double the interval between doses above 30°C, and use normal ACLS dosing and intervals above 35°C.[17,18]

Severely hypothermic patients may require internal or extracorporeal rewarming. Peritoneal, mediastinal, and thoracic lavage with warmed saline will serve to directly warm the core organs and the blood as it passes through these areas. Endovascular devices in large veins can warm the blood as it passes by the device. Extracorporeal warming may be performed using hemodialysis machines, continuous arteriovenous rewarming (CAVR) using catheters in the contralateral femoral artery and vein, and cardiopulmonary bypass (CPB) or extracorporeal membrane oxygenation (ECMO) systems.[15]

Frostbite

Frostbite is a freezing injury of the skin and deeper tissues. It can occur as the result of exposure to cold weather, contact with cold objects or snow, evaporative cooling (particularly from volatile liquids like gasoline or propane), or convective cooling from windchill. Other factors that can predispose or worsen frostbite include inadequate insulation from the cold or wind, constrictive clothing or footwear, circulatory disease, fatigue, alcohol or drug use, smoking, injuries, dehydration, and hypothermia.[2] Urban frostbite is often associated with homelessness and alcohol intoxication.[19]

Initial skin cooling causes vasoconstriction and ischemia, with further cooling resulting in the formation of ice crystals in the tissue. Ice formation causes electrolyte and fluid shifts within the cells and fluid shift out of the cells, resulting in cellular dehydration, cell membrane injury, and cell death. Thawing of the frozen tissue results in reperfusion injury and an inflammatory response. Later stages involve formation of intravascular thrombi and a worsening inflammatory cascade, leading to progressive tissue ischemia and infarction.[19,20]

Superficial frostbite involves freezing injury of the upper skin layers with little or no anticipated tissue loss. It commonly involves the fingertips, ears, nose, toes, and cheeks. Initial symptoms include numbness and a pale, waxy appearance to the skin. Affected skin feels cold and firm, but not hard. In more involved cases, superficial blisters filled with milky fluid may appear.[17,19,20] Deep frostbite involves freezing

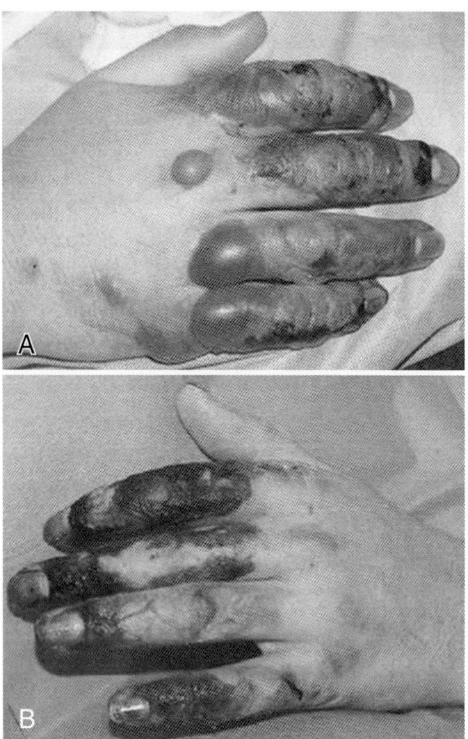

Fig. 30.2 Early (A) and later (B) appearance of deep frostbite of the hand. (From Freer L, Handford C, Imray CHE. Frostbite. In: Auerbach PS, Cushing TA, Harris NS, eds. *Auerbach's Wilderness Medicine.* 7th ed. Philadelphia, PA: Elsevier; 2017.)

of the dermis and subdermal layers and may extend into the underlying muscles, tendons, and bones. Deep frostbite appears white or yellow-white and is hard, cool, and insensitive to touch. The formation of blisters is an indication the area has partially or totally thawed. Deeply injured tissue will eventually become necrotic and will require amputation.[17] See Fig. 30.2.

Treatment of Frostbite. Prehospital treatment should focus on identifying and treating hypothermia and other life-threatening conditions, protecting the frostbitten tissues from further injury, and providing prompt transport to a facility capable of performing appropriate rewarming. The injured tissue should not be rubbed with snow. Field rewarming of frostbite is not recommended in most circumstances. Refreezing of frostbitten and subsequently thawed tissue will result in devastating tissue loss and must be prevented at all costs.[17]

Rewarming in the ED setting should be accomplished immediately after stabilization of life-threatening conditions. Rapid thawing is accomplished by immersion of the frostbitten tissue in a gently circulating warm-water bath at 37°C to 39°C (99°F–102°F). It is important to maintain the water temperature within this range until the tissue is thawed. Rewarm until the tissue becomes erythematous and pliable to the distal part of the frozen area; this will generally take 20 to 45 minutes.[17,19,20]

Rewarming frozen tissue is very painful. IV access should be obtained early and parenteral opioids should be administered as needed. Once the tissue has thawed, it should be evaluated for the severity (depth) of injury. Superficially damaged tissue will be erythematous but have minimal other changes. Deep frostbite will result in fluid-filled blebs or blisters. Clear fluid-filled blisters with swelling suggest shallower damage, whereas blood-filled blisters without swelling indicate deeper tissue injury. Large blisters containing clear or cloudy fluid may be drained by needle aspiration; blood-filled blisters should be left intact.[17,20]

The damaged tissue should be protected from further injury. Cotton padding should be placed between frostbitten digits, bed cradles should be used to prevent sheets and blankets from pressing into injured tissues, and the injured extremities should be elevated at or above heart level to reduce swelling. Topical aloe vera gel should be applied to the thawed tissue. Whirlpool baths and topical antiseptics should be used to keep the injured areas clean.[17,19,20]

Nonsteroidal antiinflammatory drugs (NSAIDs) such as aspirin or ibuprofen are often used to block the production of thromboxanes and prostaglandins and reduce tissue damage. Regional nerve blocks and epidural anesthesia can be used to control pain and promote vasodilation.[17,20] Ultrasound, magnetic resonance imaging (MRI), and nuclear medicine scans are often used to assess the extent of tissue damage.[19] IV and intraarterial tissue plasminogen activator (tPA) have been shown to improve limb salvage and reduce amputations.[21,22] Most patients with frostbite will need to be admitted to the hospital, ideally under the care of a specialist with experience in the care of frostbite.[19]

DROWNING

Drowning is a significant public health problem across the globe, with an estimated 372,000 fatal drownings every year worldwide.[23] In the United States, there are almost 4000 deaths from drowning each year,[24] with an estimated 15,000+ persons treated in EDs annually for nonfatal drowning.[25,26] Drowning is the leading cause of injury death in the United States for children 1 to 4 years of age and is one of the top five causes of death for all ages.[24,27] Alcohol is implicated in a significant percentage of adult and adolescent drownings.[25,28] Ethnic minorities demonstrate a significantly higher rate than Caucasians of fatal and nonfatal drowning.[26,29]

The World Health Organization (WHO) defined drowning in 2002 as "the process of experiencing respiratory impairment from submersion/immersion in liquid."[23,30] Terms such as *near-drowning, secondary drowning, wet drowning, dry drowning, active drowning,* and *passive drowning* have historically been used to classify drownings. These terms should be avoided; the preferred terminology is *drowning death* for fatal drownings, and *drowning with morbidity* and *drowning without morbidity* for nonfatal events.[25,27,28,30]

Unexpected submersion in water will cause the victim to reflexively hold their breath, panic, and struggle to reach the surface. The victim will rapidly become hypoxic and hypercapnic, develop profound air hunger, and may swallow some water. As hypoxia worsens, the breath-holding reflex is overcome and the patient begins to gasp and aspirate water. Some victims may experience laryngospasm, which can prevent or reduce immediate aspiration. Worsening hypoxia, hypercapnia, and respiratory acidosis lead to loss of consciousness and cardiac arrest. The drowning process usually occurs in a few seconds to a few minutes, but in cases of cold-water submersion and hypothermia, the process may take up to an hour.[25,27,28]

For drowning victims who are rescued alive, their clinical condition will be related to the amount of water aspirated and the duration of the hypoxic state. Water in the alveoli interferes with surfactant and creates an osmotic gradient that damages the alveolar-capillary membrane. This results in reduced lung compliance, impaired gas exchange, bronchospasm, pulmonary edema, and a progressively worsening VQ mismatch. Aspiration of salt water and aspiration of fresh water cause similar degrees of pulmonary injury, and their management is the same. CNS injury is the result of hypoxemia.

Presenting symptoms can range from mild lethargy to coma with fixed and dilated pupils. The extent of neurologic injury is the major determining factor in survival and long-term recovery.[25,28,31] Multisystem involvement can include hypothermia, lactic acidosis, cardiac dysrhythmias, rhabdomyolysis, acute kidney injury, and coagulopathies. Other reasons for the patient's condition should be considered for all patients found unresponsive in the water. The patient's condition, or the drowning event itself, could be the result of trauma, hypoglycemia, seizure, alcohol or drug intoxication, child abuse or neglect, or attempted suicide or homicide.[28]

Care of patients with drowning with morbidity includes safely removing them from the water; attention to their airway, breathing, and circulation (ABCs); and assessment for other conditions such as trauma and hypothermia. For victims who are rescued without vital signs, CPR should be initiated promptly, before removal from the water if this can be performed safely. All patients who have suffered a drowning event should be evaluated at a medical facility.[27,28,31]

On ED arrival, resuscitative measures including CPR should be continued as warranted. The patient's core temperature should be measured and continuous cardiac and pulse oximetry monitoring initiated. Hypothermic patients should be rewarmed as described in the previous section. IV access should be established and a CBC, electrolytes, glucose, and renal and liver function studies obtained. Arterial blood gases, coagulation studies, and toxicology screening should be performed as indicated. An ECG and a chest x-ray (CXR) should be obtained. The initial CXR may not demonstrate the full extent of the pulmonary injury. Patients in severe respiratory distress or those who are deteriorating may require endotracheal intubation and mechanical ventilation.[25,28,31]

All symptomatic drowning patients and those with abnormal laboratory results or x-ray findings should be admitted. Patients who are asymptomatic on ED arrival, have a normal CXR, and remain stable with normal pulse oximetry may often be safely discharged home after 6 to 8 hours of observation, with explicit instructions to return for any worsening of their condition.[25,28,31]

The number of drowning deaths has been decreasing since the 1990s in the United States, likely due to drowning prevention efforts.[28] There is still room for improvement and for ongoing public education on drowning prevention, including close supervision of children around water, use of personal flotation devices by children and while boating, the risks of drinking alcohol around water, and the instillation of pool and spa fences.[23,28,32]

DIVING EMERGENCIES

Diving with self-contained underwater breathing apparatus (scuba) has been a popular recreational pastime for more than 60 years. Diving also has many scientific, public safety, military, and commercial applications. There are an estimated 2.3 to 3.1 million active recreational divers in the United States.[33] Recreational diving requires that the diver complete a basic level of training and be certified. Many levels of advanced and specialty training are also available.[34]

When proper safety rules and practices are followed, diving can be a safe sport, but the ocean is an unforgiving environment. In 2015 there were 43 reported diving-related deaths in the United States and Canada, and more than 3500 injuries reported to the Divers Alert Network (DAN) emergency hotline.[35] Recreational and other types of diving occur across the country, and the ability of divers to easily travel to and from dive destinations means that diving-related emergencies have the potential to present to EDs virtually anywhere.[36]

Diving Physics and Physiology

Scuba diving involves breathing compressed air at the ambient pressure of the water surrounding the diver. Pressure is a factor of depth; at sea level the ambient pressure is one atmosphere (1 atm/760 mm Hg/14.7 psi). As the diver descends, the ambient pressure increases by one atm for every 10 m (33 feet) of seawater.[37] The scuba regulator delivers gas at the ambient pressure of the surrounding water, so as the diver descends the pressure of the inspired gas increases.[34]

Boyle's law states that at a constant temperature the volume of a gas is inversely proportional to its absolute pressure. As pressure increases, volume decreases. The gas in any air-filled structures (lungs, sinuses, ears, bowel, etc.), or any gas bubbles in the diver's tissues, will shrink as depth increases and expand as depth decreases.[36,37]

Henry's law states that at a constant temperature, the amount of a gas dissolved in a liquid is directly proportional to the partial pressure of the gas in equilibrium with the liquid. The gas that is of primary concern in diving emergencies is nitrogen, which makes up roughly 78% of room air. As a diver descends, the amount of dissolved nitrogen in the tissues increases as a factor of depth and time—the longer and deeper the dive, the more nitrogen is dissolved in the body tissues. Nitrogen can also have a narcoticlike effect on the neurologic system at depths of 30 m (100 feet) or greater, a condition called nitrogen narcosis. This effect can impair cognitive function and coordination and may lead to unconsciousness.[36,37]

Barotrauma

Barotrauma is tissue injury caused by changes in pressure. In divers it can occur during descent or ascent. Gas-filled spaces such as the sinuses, middle ears, and the diver's facemask will be compressed as ambient pressure increases on descent, resulting in a relatively lower pressure inside these spaces. This pressure differential can cause injury to the sinuses, the eardrums, or the facial structures under the mask. These effects can be painful and carry the risk of permanent injury. Divers are taught techniques to equalize these pressures while descending or ascending.[36,38,39]

The most dangerous type of barotrauma is to the lungs. It is the result of not equalizing pressures on ascent, when the volume of gas in the lungs is expanding due to decreasing ambient pressure. The depth change need not be large; pulmonary barotrauma has been reported with ascent from depths as little as 1.3 M (4 feet).[37,38] If divers hold their breath during ascent or do not exhale adequately, or if there is air-trapping from mucous plugging or bronchospasm, intrapulmonary pressures increase, resulting in alveolar distention and rupture. This allows gas bubbles to enter the mediastinum (pneumomediastinum), the pleural space (pneumothorax), the soft tissues, the chest wall and neck (subcutaneous emphysema), or the pulmonary capillary circulation (arterial gas embolism).[36,38,39]

Decompression Illness

Decompression illness (DCI) is the term used to describe both arterial gas embolism resulting from barotrauma and decompression sickness resulting from nitrogen bubble formation in the tissues. There can be considerable similarity in patient presentation, and it may be difficult to discriminate between these two disorders in the field or on initial presentation to the ED.[36]

Arterial Gas Embolism

The most common cause of death in diving accidents is drowning, as noted earlier; the second most common cause is arterial gas embolism (AGE).[35] An AGE occurs when pulmonary barotrauma injects gas bubbles into the pulmonary circulation. These bubbles are then distributed throughout the body via the arterial circulation. They can cause direct vascular occlusion, resulting in immediate ischemia of the brain, spinal cord, heart, or other tissues, and a variety of vascular injuries and inflammatory changes.[36,38,39]

Patients who have AGE will generally demonstrate signs and symptoms within 10 minutes of surfacing. Signs and symptoms are widely variable, with neurologic symptoms being the most common. Findings are often suggestive of an acute stroke, including loss of consciousness, widespread or focal paralysis, paresthesia, seizures, aphasia, confusion, blindness, and visual field deficits. Bubbles in the vascular system can lead to a variety of hematologic and biochemical abnormalities, organ injury, damage to the vascular endothelium, and an inflammatory cascade.[36,38,39] About 4% of divers who have an AGE will have immediate collapse and cardiopulmonary arrest on surfacing.[39] All patients with signs of AGE, or a history worrisome for AGE or other pulmonary barotrauma (rapid uncontrolled ascent or loss of consciousness after surfacing), should be placed on high-flow oxygen and transported to an appropriate medical facility for evaluation.[36,38,39]

Decompression Sickness

As a diver descends to and remains at depth, the increased partial pressure of nitrogen in the inspired air results in increased gas absorption by body tissues. The longer the diver stays at depth, the more nitrogen is absorbed by the tissues. As the diver ascends, these tissues become supersaturated with nitrogen. A gradual, controlled ascent permits this excess nitrogen to diffuse from the tissues and be exhaled by the lungs (off-gassing). If the diver remains at depth too long and develops too great a tissue nitrogen load or ascends too rapidly, the level of nitrogen dissolved in the tissues can exceed the solubility threshold. When this occurs, the excess nitrogen comes out of solution and forms bubbles in the tissues and venous circulation. This condition is known as decompression sickness (DCS).[36,38,39]

Certified divers are trained to plan their dives to reduce the risk of DCS. Dive tables or dive computers are used to calculate the safe "no decompression" depth and time limits for each dive. Dive computers and tables are based on mathematical models of nitrogen absorption and release; they do not directly monitor the individual diver's tissue nitrogen load. These methods are generally very safe, but even if the diver strictly follows the dive plan indicated by the computer or tables, there is still a risk of developing DCS.[34,38]

Symptoms of DCS will generally appear within 3 hours of surfacing. Severe cases may be symptomatic within 10 minutes, and some cases may take up to 24 hours to develop symptoms.[38,39] Type 1 DCS, also called pain-only DCS or "the Bends," typically involves musculoskeletal pain, itching, and mild rashes. Pain in type 1 DCS is gradual in onset and involves the joints; it is typically described as dull, deep, and aching or "boring" in character, but may also be sharp and stabbing or tearing. Movement of the joint may worsen the pain. These symptoms can easily be mistaken for pain from an injury. One way of differentiating the two is to wrap a blood pressure cuff around the painful joint and inflate it to 150 to 250 mm Hg. If this relieves the pain, it is suggestive of gas bubbles in the tendons and ligaments of the joint. Mild pruritic rashes may be present in type 1 DCS, but the presence of skin mottling suggests the development of type 2 DCS.[36,38]

Type 2 DCS is more serious, with patients having symptoms resulting from bubble formation in the brain and the spinal cord, heart, pulmonary circulation, or inner ear. Neurologic symptoms can include numbness, tingling, weakness, ataxia, loss of coordination, urinary incontinence, paralysis, and altered mental status. Patients may also report headache, nausea, vomiting, and fatigue. Cardiopulmonary symptoms, also known as "the Chokes," result from air emboli in the pulmonary vascular bed and include a dry cough, substernal pain, dyspnea, and pink-stained, frothy sputum. Inner ear symptoms include hearing loss, tinnitus, vertigo, nausea, and loss of balance.[38,39]

Symptoms of DCS can develop slowly or rapidly, and patients may deny the seriousness of their symptoms. Any patient who has been breathing air under pressure and develops symptoms should be considered to have DCS until proven otherwise. Laboratory tests should be obtained but may not reveal any acute abnormalities. A chest x-ray should be obtained for all patients with any cardiopulmonary findings to rule out pneumothorax, pulmonary edema, or other abnormalities. Computed tomography or MRI scans can be useful for patients with neurologic symptoms.[38,39]

Treatment of Decompression Illness

The initial treatment of DCI in the field or on a dive boat is administration of high-flow oxygen (10 LPM by nonrebreather face mask or via demand valve), which creates a higher partial-pressure gradient to encourage off-gassing of nitrogen and provides additional oxygen to ischemic tissues. The definitive treatment for both DCS and AGE is recompression in a hyperbaric chamber. Patients may be in remote locations, so initiation of rapid transport to a recompression facility should not be delayed. Life-threatening conditions, such as pneumothorax, should be addressed as indicated.[38,39] IV access should be obtained and isotonic fluids administered to maintain hydration.[38] If air transport is required, pressurized aircraft should maintain a sea-level cabin pressure, and helicopters should ideally stay below an altitude of 1000 feet, but always below 3000 feet.[40]

Recompression treatment reduces bubble size, restores circulation, drives nitrogen back into solution, and reverses some of the secondary inflammation and endothelial damage. Treatment should be initiated as rapidly as possible, but treatment even several days after the initial injury has been found to be of benefit.[38] There are roughly 1375 hyperbaric chambers in the United States, with about 130 able to accept patients on an emergency basis.[41] It is recommended for EDs to contact the 24-hour Divers Alert Network (DAN) emergency hotline at +1-919-684-9111 for consultation on the management of diving emergencies and for assistance in locating available hyperbaric chambers. See Fig. 30.3. DAN also maintains a Medical Information line[35] at 919-684-2948.

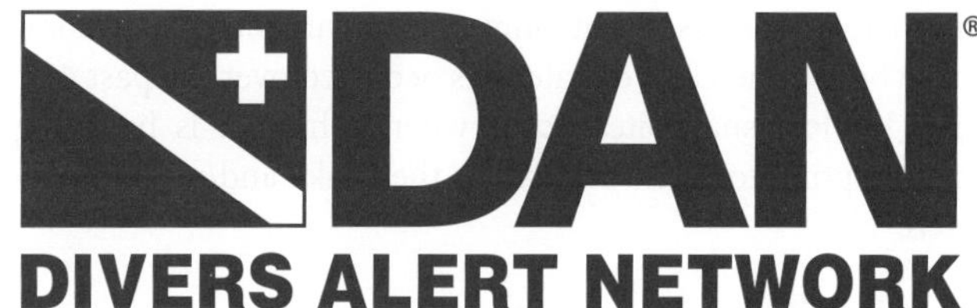

24-Hour Emergency Hotline
+1-919-684-9111

DAN Medical Information Line
919-684-2948
www.DAN.org/Health

Fig. 30.3 The Divers Alert Network. (Used with permission of the Divers Alert Network.)

VENOMOUS BITES AND STINGS

Venomous reptiles, fish, insects, arachnids, and other animals can be found throughout the world. Morbidity and mortality from envenomation may be the result of the direct toxic effects of the venom, from allergic or anaphylactic reactions to the venom or to the antivenom used as a treatment, or due to sequalae such as organ failure. Treatment of anaphylaxis is discussed in Chapter 21.

Snakebite

Two families of venomous snakes are native to North America. The Crotalids, or pit vipers (Family *Viperidae,* subfamily *Crotalinae*), which includes rattlesnakes, copperheads, and cottonmouths, are found throughout North and Central America. Coral snakes (family *Elapidae*) are found in the southern and southwestern United States and Mexico.

Pit vipers can be identified by their characteristic broad, triangular head, narrow neck, and thick body. Other identifying features include vertical elliptical pupils ("cat's eyes"), heavy brow ridges, and heat-sensing pits between the eye and nostril, from which they get their common name. Rattlesnakes (genera *Crotalus* and *Sistrurus*) have a row of rattles at the

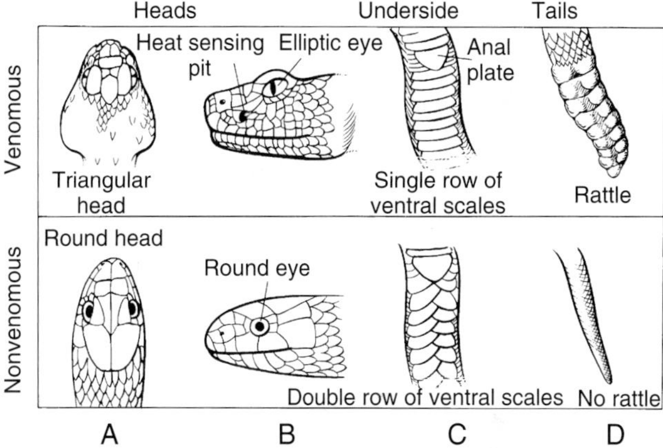

Fig. 30.4 Identification of Venomous Pit-Vipers. (A) Triangular head, (B) elliptic pupil of eye; heat-sensing facial pits on sides of head near nostrils, (C) single row of ventral scales leading up to the anal plate, (D) rattles on tail (baby rattlesnakes have only "buttons" but are still quite venomous), copperheads and cottonmouths have a pointed tail. (From Auerbach PS, Constance BB, Freer L, et al. *Field Guide to Wilderness Medicine.* 4th ed. St Louis, MO: Elsevier; 2013.)

tail, formed when the snake sheds its skin. Cottonmouths and copperheads (genus *Agkistrodon*) have tapered, pointed tails without rattles. All North American pit vipers have a single row of ventral scales at the base of the tail, behind the anal plate.[42] See Fig. 30.4.

Coral snakes (genera *Micrurus* and *Micruroides),* and all nonvenomous North American snakes, have slender bodies, round pupils, and split ventral scales. The eastern coral snake is found in Florida and surrounding states, the Texas coral snake in Texas and western Louisiana, and the Sonoran coral snake in southern Arizona, New Mexico, and northern Mexico.[42,43]

Annual rates of snakebite in the United States have been reported at between 4700 to 7000 per year, almost all from crotalids, but there are likely many unreported bites.[42-46] An average of 2 to 3 deaths occur per year in the United States from crotalid bites,[42,44] with occasional fatalities from exotic (nonnative) species,[42] but only one documented fatal coral snake bite in the United States has occurred over the past 40+ years.[47] Most snakebites occur when a human is handling or attempting to catch or pick up the snake and/or is intoxicated.[42,44,46]

Crotalid (Pit Viper) Envenomation

Pit vipers have long, folding fangs that are used to inject venom into their prey. When stalking prey or when threatened, they coil themselves and strike out very quickly, opening their mouths and extending their fangs. The venom is expelled from glands near the base of the jaw through the fangs. Pit vipers can strike and bite from any position, so a snake uncoiled is still a hazard.[48] Bites without envenomation are referred to as "dry bites." The reasons for dry bites have been hypothesized to be poor timing by the snake, intentional restriction of venom release, or if the snake has used up its venom while hunting. It is estimated that 20% to 25% of pit viper bites with visible fang marks are dry bites.[42,46]

Crotalid venom is a complex combination of as many as 100 enzymes, glycoproteins, peptides, and other substances with hemotoxic, cardiotoxic, myotoxic, and neurotoxic effects. It serves to immobilize or kill the prey and begin the digestive process. Pit viper venom is primarily hemotoxic and myotoxic, but some species such as the Mohave (or Mojave) rattlesnake have a neurotoxic venom. Clinical presentations associated with envenomation are the result of the effects of the various venom components, which break down muscle tissue, damage cell membranes, initiate an inflammatory cascade, inhibit neurotransmitters, and induce coagulopathies.[42,44,46]

Presenting signs and symptoms will depend on the location and depth of the bite, species and size of the snake, amount of venom injected, age and health of the patient, number of bites, and time elapsed since the envenomation. Upper extremity bites are most often the result of the patient interacting with the snake (picking it up, tormenting it, trying to catch it, etc.), whereas lower extremity bites are more often accidental. Bites to the head, face, or neck are less common but can cause rapid, severe swelling, resulting in airway compromise that requires endotracheal intubation or surgical cricothyrotomy.[42,46]

One to four fang marks are the universal indicator of a crotalid bite. Fang marks in the absence of any local, systemic, or coagulopathic findings generally represent a dry bite. Patients with a presumed dry bite should be observed for 8 hours or longer for signs of a delayed reaction or neurotoxic effects.[42,49]

Most pit viper envenomations result in severe, burning pain and swelling at the site of the bite within a few minutes. The swelling will then progress proximally from the bite. The extent of the swelling and the speed of its advance vary depending on the severity of the envenomation. There is typically bruising around the fang marks and oozing of bloody fluid from the punctures. Localized blebs may be present around the bite.[49] Over the hours to days after the bite, blood or serum-filled vesicles and bullae can appear around and proximal to the bite site. This is more likely if there is a delay in obtaining treatment.[42]

Bites from the Mohave rattlesnake with its neurotoxic venom may not present with the common findings of pain, ecchymosis, and swelling.[42] The Mohave rattlesnake is found in Arizona, New Mexico, Nevada, Utah, Texas, and southern California.[50] Neurotoxic venom has also been isolated from the Southern Pacific rattlesnake in southern California.[51] In these areas, identification of the snake species involved can be particularly valuable. It is never advisable to attempt to capture or kill the snake, as this creates the risk of a second bite victim. Taking a digital photograph for later expert evaluation is the recommended approach to species identification. Prehospital and ED personnel should be familiar with the snake species found in their area.[42,46]

Common systemic symptoms include nausea (with or without vomiting), numbness and tingling to the mouth or tongue, and an odd taste in the mouth variously described as metallic, rubbery, or minty. More severe systemic symptoms include respiratory distress due to neurotoxic venom components, myocardial depression, hypotension and shock, and allergic or anaphylactic reactions to the venom. Myotoxic effects can cause muscle fasciculations or twitching, which in severe cases can result in respiratory compromise. Other neurotoxic effects can include paresthesia, motor weakness, numbness, altered mental status, cranial nerve dysfunction, and diplopia. Hemotoxic venom factors can lead to coagulopathies. Significant bleeding is a rare but can be life-threatening. Rhabdomyolysis and kidney injury can occur. Patients with significant comorbidities such as cardiovascular or respiratory disease are at higher risk for life-threatening complications.[42,46]

Initial evaluation and treatment focus on getting the patient to a safe location and ensuring a patent airway and adequate breathing and circulation. The patient should be kept calm and any constrictive jewelry or clothing near the bite should be removed. The involved extremity should be immobilized and kept at a level near the heart.[49] As much information about the snake as possible should be obtained (species, size, etc.). As noted earlier, there should not be attempts to catch or kill the snake or to bring it to the hospital. The patient should be transported to a hospital using whatever method of transportation is available. To minimize the risk of systemic spread of the venom, patients should not walk or exert themselves unless there is no alternative.[42,46]

Over the years, many treatments for pit viper bites have been used, including tourniquets, constricting bands, incision and suction, suction alone, ice, alcohol, and electric shock. None of these has been found to be effective, and in fact most have been proved to be harmful; therefore none are recommended.[42,52] The Australian pressure wrap is not recommended for North American crotaline envenomation. It has not been shown to be helpful and has been found to worsen local tissue damage.[53] Appropriate prehospital treatment is rapid transport to a hospital for evaluation and antivenom therapy. If a tourniquet, pressure wrap, or other venom sequestration technique has been applied, it is recommended to leave it in place until antivenom therapy has been initiated to prevent the release of a venom bolus into the systemic circulation.[42,46]

On arrival to the ED, the patient should be evaluated for signs of potentially life-threatening reactions such as facial or airway swelling, angioedema, or shock. The basic steps discussed earlier should be performed, followed by an assessment of the severity of swelling and pain. The margin of the swelling should be marked on the skin and the circumference of the involved extremity measured at the level of the bite, as well as proximal to and distal to the bite. These measurements should be recorded and repeated every 15 to 30 minutes to track the rate of progression of the swelling and the response to antivenom therapy.[49] IV access should be obtained (two sites are recommended) and baseline laboratory tests obtained, including a CBC, coagulation studies (PT, PTT, fibrinogen, D-dimer), electrolytes, glucose, liver and kidney function studies, creatinine kinase, urinalysis, and type and screen.[42] In patients with preexisting cardiac disease or who have chest pain, an ECG and troponin-I measurement are recommended.[46]

IV fluid resuscitation using 0.9% saline or lactated Ringer's solution should be initiated, and hypotension or tachycardia treated with fluid boluses. If the patient continues to have inadequate organ perfusion after aggressive fluid boluses (2000 mL in adults or 20–40 mL/kg in children), 5% human albumin should be administered (250–500 mL for adults or 15–20 mL/kg for children). Vasopressors should not be used to treat venom-induced shock until after adequate volume replacement has been completed and antivenom therapy has been started.[42]

Pain control using opioid analgesics and antiemetics should be provided. NSAIDs are not recommended for crotalid bites, due to their potential to worsen coagulopathies. The wound should be washed with soap and water. Prophylactic antibiotics are not generally recommended. Tetanus status should be determined and a booster immunization administered if indicated.

There are two crotaline Fab-fragment antivenoms (FabAV) available in the United States: Crotaline polyvalent immune fab, ovine (CroFab, BTG International, West Conshohocken, PA) approved by the US Food and Drug Administration (FDA) in 2000 and Antivipmyn, equine (Anavip, Instituto Bioclon S.A. de C.V., Mexico City, Mexico), which became available in the United States in late 2018.[54] FabAV therapy is indicated for any clinically significant signs of envenomation. These include any swelling beyond minimal local swelling, progressive swelling, elevated PT, decreased fibrinogen or platelets, or any systemic symptoms. Most guidelines advocate early contact with a Poison Center to help guide treatment.[49] A nursing consideration with FabAV treatment is to know that FabAV can take up 20 to 25 minutes to reconstitute each vial. Larger volumes of diluent can decrease the reconstitution time.

Control of envenomation is demonstrated when the progression of swelling and tenderness stops or begins to reverse, when laboratory values (PT, fibrinogen, and platelets) are normal or improving, the patient is hemodynamically stable, and there are no signs of neurotoxicity. All patients who have received antivenom should be observed in the hospital for at least 18 to 24 hours. Serial laboratory tests and physical examination, including measurement of swelling, are indicated for all patients who have received antivenom therapy. Local and systemic recurrence of symptoms can occur between 6 and 36 hours after the time of initial control, with delayed symptoms reported up to 10 days after initial treatment. Repeat dosing with antivenom may be required as often as every 6 hours.[46,49] Patients who develop severe systemic symptoms or fail to respond to FabAV treatment need to be admitted and followed by a specialist with experience in managing envenomated patients.

Compartment syndrome is a rare complication of crotalid snakebite. If the involved extremity becomes increasingly swollen and tense despite appropriate antivenom treatment, compartment pressures should be measured and an orthopedic consult obtained. Fasciotomy is usually only indicated if compartment pressures remain persistently elevated despite appropriate treatment with antivenom.[46]

Coral Snake Envenomation

Coral snakes have slender bodies and round pupils, the same as their nonvenomous relatives. The distinctive feature of coral snakes is their color pattern of alternating bands of red, yellow, and black, with the red bands adjoining the yellow bands. Other nonvenomous species such as king snakes have similar color patterns, but with the red and black bands together. The common rhyme to help remember this is, "Red on yellow, kill a fellow; Red on black, venom lack."

Elapids have small, fixed fangs located in the front of the mouth. They are shy and inoffensive creatures but can bite very quickly. Coral snakes account for about 2% of reported snakebites in the United States, with only about 40% of these bites resulting in envenomation. Coral snake venom is less complex than crotalid venom. The potentially lethal component is a potent neurotoxin, but their venom also has myotoxic components. Eastern coral snake bites tend to be the most severe, and those of the Texas coral snake are typically less severe. Bites by the Sonoran coral snake are usually of minimal severity.[42]

Early symptoms of coral snake envenomation include transient pain and fang marks (which may be difficult to see) with minimal or no swelling. More severe symptoms may occur up to 13 hours after the bite and include abdominal pain, headache, diaphoresis, pallor, paresthesia, and altered mental status. In very severe cases, myocardial depression with hypotension and respiratory failure requiring endotracheal intubation and mechanical ventilation can occur. Laboratory results may show elevated creatine kinase (CK) and myoglobinuria but generally do not show other significant abnormalities.[42]

Venom sequestration techniques such as pressure immobilization have been used effectively in Australia for field management of elapid snake bites. This technique has been advocated as effective for coral snake envenomation but has not been specifically studied. It should only be performed by individuals familiar with the technique.[55] There is no FDA-approved coral snake antivenom available in the United States.[56]

Arthropod Envenomation

Arthropods (insects and arachnids) are the most common animals on planet Earth. Some species of arthropods are venomous, and several present significant health risks to humans.[57]

Hymenoptera

Bees, wasps, hornets, yellow jackets, and fire ants are all members of the order *Hymenoptera.* This group is the most medically significant of the venomous insects. Hymenoptera stings cause an average of 60 reported deaths annually in the United States, accounting for more deaths than any other type of envenomation.[58] Venom glands are located at the posterior aspect of the insect's abdomen and are connected to a stinging apparatus that can pierce the skin and inject the venom. Venom composition varies among species and consists of a mix of antigenic, cytotoxic, hemolytic, and vasoactive compounds.[57,59] Honeybees will sting once, whereas most other species may sting repeatedly. Africanized hybrid honeybees are found in south and central America and have migrated into some southern states. Their venom is not significantly more toxic than that of native bees, but they are much more aggressive and victims often have more severe reactions from multiple stings after being swarmed by a colony.[57,59,60]

Local reactions consist of mild to moderate stinging or burning, swelling, and itching. Systemic toxic reactions, often associated with multiple stings, include nausea and vomiting, headache, fever, edema, and liver enzyme and coagulation abnormalities. Toxic reactions may also induce bronchospasm mimicking an anaphylactic reaction.[57]

Most fatalities from Hymenoptera stings are due to anaphylactic reactions, which usually occur within 10 to 15 minutes of the sting. Patients exhibit urticaria, pruritus, flushing, edema, nausea, vomiting, bronchospasm, laryngeal edema, stridor, and hypotension. The severity of the reaction is not related to the number of stings; a single sting can elicit a life-threatening reaction.[60] Treatment of anaphylaxis is discussed in Chapter 21.

Treatment begins with removal of the stinger as quickly as possible to prevent injection of additional venom. Scrape the stinger away by using a dull object such as the side of a credit card, knife blade, or needle. The classic advice has been to not grasp or squeeze the stinger with forceps or tweezers because this may squeeze out more venom; however, current recommendations are to remove the stinger as soon as possible using whatever method is most readily available.[57] Application of ice packs to the site will reduce pain and may be the only treatment required. Oral antihistamines will block some effects of the venom and of endogenously released histamine. Most stings resolve with no residual effects.[57,59]

Patients may become sensitized to Hymenoptera venom and develop more severe reactions, including anaphylaxis, to subsequent stings. Patients with a known or suspected severe allergic or anaphylactic reaction should be prescribed an epinephrine autoinjector and instructed in its use. They should also be encouraged to wear a medical identification bracelet or tag.[57]

Spider (Arachnid) Bites

There are roughly 40,000 species of spiders worldwide, and virtually all are venomous; however, most species do not have fangs long enough to penetrate the skin and are consequently not harmful to humans. Only a few species of spiders in North America cause significant risk to humans.[59-61]

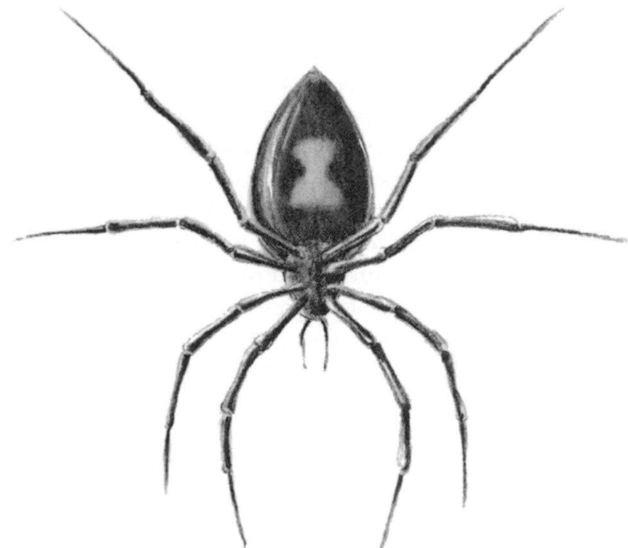

Fig. 30.5 Female black widow spider (*Latrodectus mactans*) with typical hourglass marking on the abdomen. (From Davis JH, Sheldon GF, Druckec WR, et al. *Surgery: A Problem Solving Approach.* 2nd ed. St Louis, MO: Mosby; 1995.)

Many patients will blame a spider bite for any localized necrotic skin lesion, even if they did not see a spider. It is important to consider other possible causes for the chief complaint of "spider bite." These include skin cancer, bites or stings by other creatures, viral infections such as herpes zoster, and bacterial infections including methicillin-resistant *Staphylococcus aureus* (MRSA) and cutaneous anthrax.[59,61,62]

Black Widow Spider. The black widow spider (genus *Latrodectus*) is found in temperate zones across the world. In the United States they are found in every state except Alaska. They are nocturnal and live in secluded, dimly lit locations such as outhouses, woodpiles, barns, stables, and under stones or logs. They are not aggressive, biting only when disturbed. Black widow spiders spin webs and await their prey. These webs may be found around outdoor toilet seats, resulting in bites on or near the genitalia.[59]

The adult female is considered venomous and is of most concern; males have smaller jaws and minimal venom production. The adult female is recognizable by her large, shiny black body with a bright red or orange hourglass marking on the abdomen (Fig. 30.5). The black widow's venom is neurotoxic.[60] An average of 2600 black widow bites are reported to US Poison Centers annually, with one-third reported as moderate and only 1.4% reported as severe.[61] Deaths are rare worldwide, with no recent reported deaths in the United States.[60]

The bite will produce localized pain ranging from a pinprick sensation that often goes unnoticed to more severe, sharp pain, which may be out of proportion to the apparent injury. Two small fang marks may be visible. Local irritation with erythema, induration, a small papule, urticaria, or a halo-shaped lesion may develop over the next few hours. The majority of bites will only produce local symptoms.[60,61]

More severe cases will progress to muscle pain and spasms of the abdomen, lower back, and chest. Bites of the upper extremities typically result in pain concentrated in the chest, whereas lower extremity bites cause pain in the lower back and abdomen. Abdominal pain and rigidity can be mistaken for an acute abdomen. Systemic symptoms occur in about one-third of patients and can include nausea, vomiting, diaphoresis, hypertension, and elevated temperature. Patients may also develop respiratory difficulty, headache, syncope, weakness, priapism, and seizures.[60] Children are at higher risk for severe or fatal reactions to black widow envenomation.[60,61]

Initial treatment of a black widow spider bite includes stabilization of the ABCs and application of ice to the bite area to slow the action of the neurotoxin and relieve pain. IV access should be established and a CBC, electrolytes, blood glucose, liver and kidney function studies, and urinalysis obtained. IV opioids and large doses of benzodiazepines may be required to control pain and muscle spasms. In these cases, monitor the patient's airway and ventilatory status closely because both the spider venom and these medications may lead to respiratory depression. Tetanus immunization should be updated as needed. A Poison Center should be contacted for consultation and advice.[60,61]

A *Latrodectus* antivenom (Black Widow Spider Antivenin [equine]; Merck & Co., Kenilworth, NJ) is available, but its use is limited to severe cases and for those patients who are at high risk for severe complications. In most cases, pain and other symptoms will resolve over several hours, but some patients may have symptoms for 2 to 3 days. Patients who received antivenom may develop serum sickness symptoms up to 1 to 3 weeks after treatment. Any patient who has cardiovascular or respiratory compromise, seizures, or is pregnant, and all pediatric patients, should be admitted for observation.[60]

Brown Recluse Spider. The brown recluse spider (*Loxosceles reclusa*), also known as the fiddleback spider, is the most prevalent and medically significant of the six *Loxosceles* species native to the United States. Brown recluse spiders are light-brown in color with a dark-brown fiddle-shaped mark extending down their back (Fig. 30.6). They are most active at night from April through October.[60,63] The brown recluse spider is native to an area from southeastern Nebraska and southern Ohio south into western North Carolina, northern Georgia, and Texas. Brown recluse spiders are seldom identified outside their native range, and spiders found elsewhere or outside the spring and summer months and presumed to be brown recluse spiders are most likely other species.[64]

Recluse spiders are reclusive, as their name suggests. They prefer dark, dry, and undisturbed locations, such as the undersides of logs, boards, and rocks, and inside barns and garages. Within homes they are found in attics, closets, and storage areas for bedding, clothing, and furniture. Both the male and female spiders are venomous. Bites are rare, even in houses heavily infested with brown recluse spiders.[60]

The venom of the brown recluse spider is cytotoxic and hemolytic. Bites of the recluse spider can cause a condition termed necrotic arachnidism or loxocolism. The bite is initially painless, with subsequent itching, tenderness, swelling, and erythema at the bite site. Over the next few hours the bite may progress to a central blue-gray macule with a halo of pallor, surrounded by erythema—sometimes called the "red, white, and blue sign." Over the next 48 to 72 hours

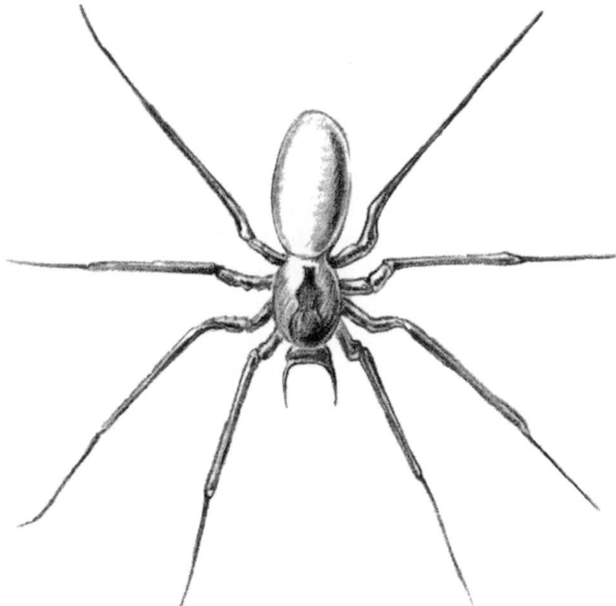

Fig. 30.6 Brown recluse spider (*Loxosceles reclusa*) with typical dark violin-shaped marking on the cephalothorax. (From Davis JH, Sheldon GF, Druckec WR, et al. *Surgery: A Problem Solving Approach.* 2nd ed. St Louis, MO: Mosby; 1995.)

a necrotic base with a central black eschar forms, which then develops into a necrotic ulceration over the subsequent 7 to 14 days. Although most recluse bites heal uneventfully, 10% have a protracted course, with the wound taking months to resolve completely. Bites in areas with increased adipose tissue such as the thighs, buttocks, and abdomen are at higher risk for severe necrosis than bites occurring at other sites.[60,61]

Systemic reactions are rare but can be life-threatening. They do not typically correlate with the severity or size of the skin lesion. Onset is within 24 to 72 hours of envenomation, with the patient experiencing fever, chills, myalgias, and arthralgias. Severe systemic reactions may present with hemolytic anemia, hematuria, coagulopathies, DIC, jaundice, hypotension, kidney failure, and seizures.[60,61]

Treatment for the bite of the brown recluse is dependent on its severity. General care includes cleaning the wound and immobilizing and elevating the injured extremity to help reduce pain and swelling. Ice will help reduce the extent of the local wound reaction and reduce pain. Analgesics should be provided, and severe pain may require opioid medications. Tetanus immunization should be administered as needed. Antibiotics are usually not indicated unless there is suspicion of a secondary infection.[60,61] Some authorities recommend steroids to help stabilize red blood cell membranes and reduce hemolysis.[60] An *L. reclusa* antivenom is not commercially available in the United States.[61]

Predicting whether a necrotic lesion will occur is difficult during the initial stages. If a necrotic lesion appears, it is difficult to predict whether it will progress to a severe, disfiguring lesion. Debridement of necrotic ulcers is usually indicated, but early excision of the ulcer is not recommended.[60] Patients should be referred to follow-up with a plastic surgeon familiar with the care of brown recluse bites.[60,61]

Scorpion Stings

Scorpions are the oldest living terrestrial animals and cause significant morbidity and mortality in tropical and subtropical areas worldwide. In the United States they are primarily found in the warm southern and southwestern states. The long, mobile tail of the scorpion ends in a telson containing two venom glands and a stinger. A unique characteristic of scorpions is that they fluoresce under ultraviolet light.[59,60,65]

There are more than 40 native species of scorpions in North America, and all are capable of inflicting painful stings, but only the bark scorpion (*Centruroides sculpturatus*) is considered to be potentially lethal. The bark scorpion is yellow-brown in color, varying in length from 1.3 to 7.6 cm. It is found throughout Arizona and in parts of California, Nevada, Texas, New Mexico, and northern Mexico.[66] Deaths from *Centruroides* envenomation were common in the early 20th century, but only two deaths have been reported[65,67] since 1970.

Scorpions are not aggressive creatures; stings typically occur when the human steps on or crushes the scorpion. When hunting or when threatened, the scorpion rapidly swings its tail forward and injects its venom. Scorpion venom is a complex mixture of enzymes, histamines, and toxins, with neurotoxins being the most important component in human envenomation. Envenomation by most scorpions produces immediate local pain and tenderness aggravated by tapping over the sting site (tap test). Most scorpion stings will result in mild, localized symptoms that only require symptomatic treatment. Children are at higher risk of death or severe complications due to their smaller body mass. Roughly 25% of children envenomated by the bark scorpion have severe systemic reactions, compared with 6% of adults.[65,67]

Treatment of most milder scorpion stings consists of ice and analgesics to reduce pain. Local infiltration anesthesia or digital blocks can be helpful for more severe pain. Patients with these symptoms should be observed for several hours for progression of the envenomation and worsening symptoms. The wound should be thoroughly washed and tetanus immunization updated as needed.[65] As with other envenomations, consultation with a Poison Center should be obtained early in the course of treatment.

For more severe cases, IV access and appropriate fluid resuscitation is indicated. These patients usually require admission to an intensive care unit for supportive therapy tailored to their condition. Opioid analgesics should be used with caution because there may be an additive respiratory depressant effect when combined with the scorpion venom.[68] A bark scorpion antivenom (Centruroides [Scorpion] Immune F[ab']2, equine [Anascorp]; Rare Disease Therapeutics, Franklin, TN) has been approved by the FDA as an "orphan drug" and is available in Arizona and surrounding areas.[65]

TICK-BORNE ILLNESS

Tick Removal

The first step in the management of all tick-borne illnesses is the removal of the tick. Tick removal is performed using fine-point forceps or a specialized tick removal tool. Gently grasp the tick as close to the skin as possible and pull at a 90-degree angle to the skin surface in a steady motion, tenting the skin. It may require several minutes of steady, gentle pulling before the tick disengages from the skin. Do not jerk or apply heavy pressure; this will most likely break off the tick's head, leaving the head or mandibles imbedded in the skin. See Fig. 30.7. After the tick is removed, cleanse the skin with soap and warm water or a topical antiseptic.[68]

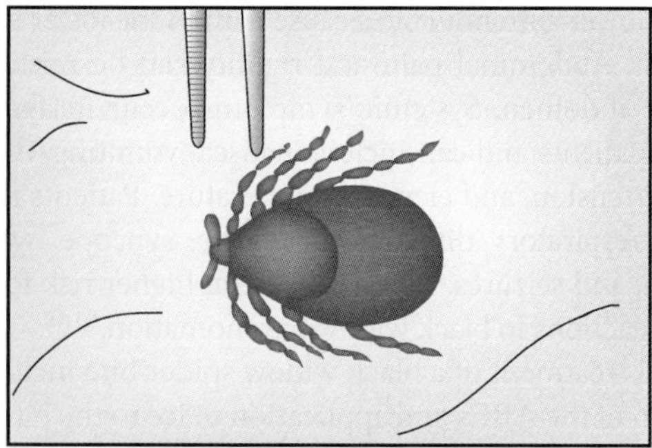

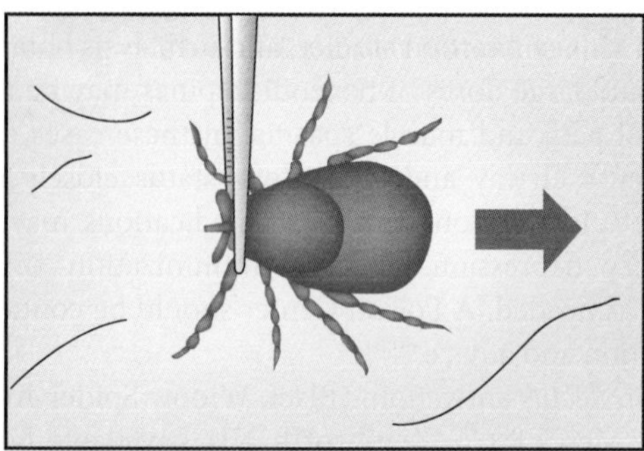

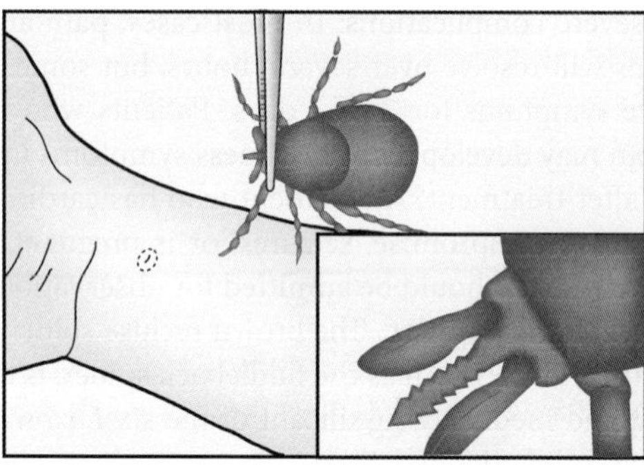

Fig. 30.7 Tick Removal. Grasp the tick near the skin surface and withdraw from the skin in a steady, constant motion. Do not turn, jerk, or twist. (From Auerbach PS, Constance BB, Freer L, et al. *Field Guide to Wilderness Medicine.* 4th ed. St Louis, MO: Elsevier; 2013.)

Lyme Disease

Lyme disease is caused by the spirochete *Borrelia burgdorferi,* which is transmitted via the bite of the *Ixodes* tick and accounts for more than 90% of the reported cases of vector-borne illness in the United States. Lyme disease has been found in all 50 states, with the northeastern states accounting for the vast majority of cases. Tick attachment for less than 24 hours carries a low risk of transmission. Attachment for more than 48 to 72 hours is more likely to transmit the disease.[69]

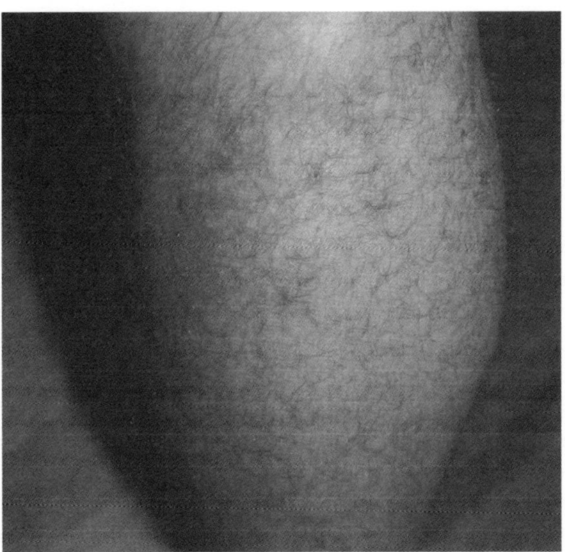

Fig. 30.8 Classic *erythema migrans* rash seen in Stage 1 Lyme disease. (From Cummins GA, Traub SJ. Tick-borne diseases. In: Auerbach PS, Cushing TA, Harris NS, eds. *Auerbach's Wilderness Medicine.* 7th ed. Philadelphia, PA: Elsevier; 2017.)

Lyme disease is classified into three stages. Stage I (early localized disease) usually begins 5 to 7 days after the tick bite, with flulike symptoms and an expanding, red "bulls-eye" rash (erythema migrans), as shown in Fig. 30.8. The rash generally disappears with or without antibiotic treatment, but untreated patients are at risk for developing disseminated disease. Stage II (early disseminated disease) occurs days to weeks after the tick bite. Patients may exhibit neurologic, cardiac, and musculoskeletal complications such as meningitis, hepatitis, cranial neuropathies, atrioventricular blocks, cardiomyopathies, and arthralgias. Stage III (late disease) is characterized by chronic arthritis and less commonly neurologic symptoms including encephalopathy, peripheral nervous system abnormalities, and psychiatric disturbances.[69,70]

Antibiotics are the treatment for Lyme disease, started as early in the course of the disease as possible. The choice of antibiotic depends on the stage of the disease and the patient's symptoms. Prophylactic antibiotic treatment of asymptomatic tick bites is controversial, especially when the attachment time is less than 24 to 36 hours. Some references recommend not treating these patients, whereas others recommend a single dose of doxycycline 200 mg within 72 hours of tick removal for tick bites in endemic areas if the tick was attached, or is suspected to have been attached, for more than 36 hours.[69,70]

Rocky Mountain Spotted Fever

Rocky Mountain spotted fever (RMSF) is caused by the bacterium *Rickettsia rickettsii,* which is transmitted via the bite of an *Ixodes* tick. *R. rickettsii* is endemic across North America, but despite its name it is most prevalent in the south Atlantic and south-central states. Most cases are reported between April and September, when ticks are most active. The incubation period for RMSF is 2 to 14 days. Major symptoms include fever, chills, malaise, myalgias, and headache. During the first 10 days 85% to 90% of patients develop a pink, macular rash over the palms, wrists, hands, feet, ankles, and other parts of the body.[69]

Patients may go on to develop neurologic symptoms, including encephalopathy, ataxia, delirium, and seizures. Severe cases may develop myocarditis, ECG changes, noncardiac pulmonary edema, gastrointestinal hemorrhage, vasculitis, and coagulation abnormalities. Treatment involves antibiotic therapy and supportive care.[69]

Tick Paralysis

Tick paralysis is an ascending paralysis caused by a neurotoxic venom transmitted by the bite of a female *Dermacentor andersoni* (wood tick) or *Dermacentor variabilis* (dog tick). Other tick species have also been implicated. Most cases occur in the southeastern, northwestern, and Rocky Mountain states during the months of April through June.[69,70]

Symptoms typically begin after the tick has been attached for 5 to 6 days. Early symptoms include irritability and paresthesia of the hands and feet. Over the following 1 to 2 days, patients develop a progressive ascending, symmetric, flaccid paralysis with loss of deep tendon reflexes. Some cases may progress to respiratory paralysis requiring endotracheal intubation and mechanical ventilation. Treatment involves tick removal and supportive care, including ventilatory support, until the symptoms resolve. No antivenom is available.[69]

MAMMAL BITES

More than 5 million mammal bites are reported in the United States each year. Dogs and cats are by far the most common animals involved, followed by humans.[71] Other animals involved include rodents, ferrets, and rabbits. Large carnivore (bear, cougar, etc.) bites are rare. Animal bite injuries account for roughly 1% of annual US ED visits.[72]

There are common features in the management of most mammalian bites. All patients who experienced a bite should be quickly assessed for life-threatening injuries, particularly if the injury involves the head or neck, or if there is significant bleeding. Once this has been addressed and stabilized, assessment should focus on the type and extent of the bite injuries. The size and depth of the wounds should be documented, using photographs when possible. Range of motion of any involved joints should be assessed and x-rays performed for any concern of fracture, foreign body, or deep puncture wounds potentially extending to the bone. Ultrasound may be used to evaluate for possible vascular injuries. The wound should be evaluated for signs of infection.[71,72]

Pain control should be provided using oral or parenteral medications. Local infiltration anesthesia or regional nerve blocks should be performed after a careful neurologic examination. The wounds should then be thoroughly irrigated, cleaned, and explored for foreign bodies. Tetanus immunization should be administered if indicated.

The risk of rabies exposure should be explored, and the animal's immunization status documented (if known). Rabies prophylaxis should be considered in cases of raccoon, skunk, fox, or bat bites, unimmunized pets, or unprovoked attack by an unknown animal. Local public health officials should be contacted for guidance about postexposure prophylaxis. Animal bites must be reported to health authorities according to local and state regulations.[72,73]

Suturing of animal bite wounds is controversial.[74–76] It is typically only indicated for facial wounds or for large and potentially disfiguring wounds. Other wounds should be evaluated on an individual basis for risk of infection. Puncture wounds, crush injuries, extremity wounds more than 12 hours old, facial wounds more than 24 hours old, human bites to the metacarpophalangeal joints, or bite wounds in immunocompromised patients or patients with diabetes carry a high risk of infection and should not be sutured.[71,74–76]

Prophylactic antibiotics are indicated for high-risk animal bite injuries such as bites to the hands, face, or genital area, puncture wounds, most cat bites, crushing injuries, wounds near joints, all wounds considered moderate or severe, and wounds more than 6 to 12 hours old (12–24 hours for facial wounds). Amoxicillin/clavulanate is the most commonly prescribed antibiotic for animal and human bites. In patients allergic to β-lactam, clindamycin plus ciprofloxacin or clindamycin plus sulfamethoxazole/trimethoprim are recommended.[72,74,75] Clear aftercare instructions for follow-up and wound care should be given to the patient and family with an explicit explanation of the signs and symptoms of infection and instructions to have the wound reevaluated if any signs of infection develop.

Dog Bites

Dog bites account for 80% to 90% of all bites treated in EDs and for roughly 34 fatalities annually in the United States.[58,74] Most victims know the dogs that bite them, with children being the population at greatest risk. The most common sites of injury in children younger than 10 years of age are the head and neck, with the extremities being the most common site in older children and adults.[74] Dogs have powerful jaws, which can cause puncture wounds, deep open lacerations, crush injuries, and the tearing away of tissue. Wounds should be thoroughly cleansed and irrigated as previously described and may require surgical debridement.[71,72,74,76] The infection rate for dog bite injuries is ~15% to 25%.[76]

Cat Bites and Scratches

Cat bites are far less common than dog bites, accounting for 5% to 10% of all reported bites in the United States each year.[72] A cat's teeth are long, slender, and sharp. They can cause lacerations and deep puncture wounds that may involve the tendons and joint capsules.[71] The hands and arms are the most common sites for cat bite injuries.[74]

The infection rate for cat bites is more than double that for dogs, ranging from 30% to 80%.[71,76] Cats are hunters and often come in contact with bacteria-infected rodents, which contaminate their mouths with *Pasteurella multocida.* This bacterium is also found in the mouths of dogs, but *P. multocida* is present in the mouths of 90% of cats.[76] Cat scratches can also transmit *P. multocida.* Signs of *Pasteurella* infection such as pain, swelling, and erythema will typically appear rapidly, usually within 12 to 24 hours of the bite.[74]

Human Bites

Human bites are the third most common cause of bite wounds, accounting for 2% to 3% of bite wounds seen in US EDs, although the actual incidence is likely higher because many bites are probably not reported. Human bites may occur as the result of altercations, physical or sexual assault, domestic violence, self-defense, child abuse, or sexual activities. The most common site of injury is the metacarpophalangeal (MCP) joint of the hand in males, caused by the impact of a clenched fist against the teeth of another individual, often referred to as a "fight-bite." Occlusive bites are caused by the teeth closing directly on tissue and may occur on the arms, legs, breasts, genitals, and in other locations.[74,77]

Bite wounds to the hand may be deceiving, appearing to be small but causing significant injury to the underlying tendons, bones, blood vessels, and joint structures, and having a high risk of bacterial contamination. Patients may deny or not recognize the severity of these wounds and not seek care until the wound has become infected. These wounds need to be carefully examined for possible injury to underlying structures. X-rays can help identify fractures, impaction injuries, foreign bodies such as tooth fragments in the wound, and air in the joint or soft tissue. Referral to a hand specialist for surgical exploration and debridement may be necessary. Suturing of human bites to the hand is generally not recommended.[74,77]

The human mouth harbors a wide range of bacteria, and human bites to the hand and elsewhere carry a high risk of infection. Thorough wound care and antibiotic prophylaxis as described earlier are indicated. If blood is present in the mouth of the individual whose teeth caused the injury, there is a risk of transmission of human immunodeficiency virus and hepatitis B and C. In significant infections, hospital admission for IV antibiotics may be necessary.[74,77]

WILDERNESS MEDICINE

The study of environmental illnesses and injuries and their treatment is a part of the growing specialty of wilderness medicine, which also includes caring for patients under austere or remote conditions. This chapter has highlighted several common environmental illnesses and injuries, but there is not space to go into great detail on any of them. A wilderness medicine textbook that explores the topics covered in this chapter in more detail can be a worthwhile addition to the professional library of any emergency nurse or ED. The Wilderness Medical Society publishes regularly updated, evidence-based practice guidelines on a wide range of conditions in the WMS journal *Wilderness and Environmental Medicine* which are available online at https://wms.org/research/guidelines.

REFERENCES

1. Zafren K, Giesbrecht GG, Danzl DF, et al. Wilderness Medical Society practice guidelines for the out-of-hospital evaluation and treatment of accidental hypothermia: 2014 update. *Wilderness Environ Med.* 2014;25(suppl 4):S66–S85.
2. Zafren K. Out-of-hospital evaluation and treatment of accidental hypothermia. *Emerg Med Clin North Am.* 2017;35(2):261–279.
3. Berko J, Ingram DD, Saha S, Parker JD. Deaths attributed to heat, cold, and other weather events in the United States, 2006-2010. *Natl Health Stat Report.* 2014;(76):1–15.
4. Leon LR, Kenefick RW. Pathophysiology of heat-related illness. In: Auerbach PS, Cushing TA, Harris NS, eds. *Auerbach's Wilderness Medicine.* 7th ed. Philadelphia, PA: Elsevier; 2017:259–274.
5. Platt M, Vicario S. Heat illness. In: Marx JA, ed. *Rosen's Emergency Medicine: Concepts and Clinical Practice.* 8th ed. Philadelphia, PA: Elsevier; 2014:1896–1904.
6. Bennett BL, Hew-Butler T, Hoffman MD, Rogers IR, Rosner MH, Wilderness Medical Society. Wilderness Medical Society practice guidelines for treatment of exercise-associated hyponatremia: 2014 update. *Wilderness Environ Med.* 2014;25(suppl 4):S30–S42.
7. Lipman GS, Eifling KP, Ellis MA, et al. Wilderness Medical Society practice guidelines for the prevention and treatment of heat-related illness: 2014 update. *Wilderness Environ Med.* 2014;25(suppl 4):S55–S65.
8. O'Brien KK, Leon LR, Kenefik RW, O'Connor FG. Clinical management of heat-related illnesses. In: Auerbach PS, Cushing TA, Harris NS, eds. *Auerbach's Wilderness Medicine.* 7th ed. Philadelphia, PA: Elsevier; 2017:259–274.
9. Walter E, Steel K. Management of exertional heat stroke: a practical update for primary care physicians. *Br J Gen Pract.* 2018;68(668):153–154.
10. Gaudio FG, Grissom CK. Cooling methods in heat stroke. *J Emerg Med.* 2016;50(4):607–616.
11. Hew-Butler T, Loi V, Pani A, Rosner MH. Exercise-associated hyponatremia: 2017 update. *Front Med.* 2017;4(3):370–310.
12. Hew-Butler T, Rosner MH, Fowkes-Godek S, et al. Statement of the 3rd international exercise-associated hyponatremia consensus development conference, Carlsbad, California, 2015. *Br J Sports Med.* 2015;49(22):1432–1446.
13. Meiman J, Anderson H, Tomasallo C. Hypothermia-related deaths—Wisconsin, 2014; and United States, 2003-2013. *MMWR.* 2015;64(6):141–143.
14. Haverkamp FJC, Giesbrecht GG, Tan ECTH. The prehospital management of hypothermia—An up-to-date overview. *Injury.* 2018;49(2):149–164.
15. Danzl DF, Huecker MR. Accidental hypothermia. In: Auerbach PS, Cushing TA, Harris NS, eds. *Auerbach's Wilderness Medicine.* 7th ed. Philadelphia, PA: Elsevier; 2017:135–162.
16. Henriksson O, Lundgren PJ, Kuklane K, et al. Protection against cold in prehospital care—wet clothing removal or addition of a vapor barrier. *Wilderness Environ Med.* 2015;26(1): 11–20.
17. Zafren K, Giesbrecht G. *State of Alaska: Cold injuries guidelines*; 2014. http://dhss.alaska.gov/dph/Emergency/Documents/ems/documents/Alaska%20DHSS%20EMS%20Cold%20Injuries%20Guidelines%20June%202014.pdf. Published July 2014. Accessed May 28, 2019.
18. American Heart Association. *Advanced Cardiovascular Life Support Provider Manual.* Dallas, TX: American Heart Association; 2016:92–109.
19. Freer L, Handford C, Imray CHE. Frostbite. In: Auerbach PS, Cushing TA, Harris NS, eds. *Auerbach's Wilderness Medicine.* 7th ed. Philadelphia, PA: Elsevier; 2017:197–222.
20. McIntosh SE, Opacic M, Freer L, et al. Wilderness Medical Society practice guidelines for the prevention and treatment of frostbite: 2014 update. *Wilderness Environ Med.* 2014;25(suppl 4):S43–S54.
21. Jones LM, Coffey RA, Natwa MP, Bailey JK. The use of intravenous tPA for the treatment of severe frostbite. *Burns.* 2017;43(5):1088–1096.
22. Wexler A, Zavala S. The use of thrombolytic therapy in the treatment of frostbite injury. *J Burn Care Res.* 2017;38(5): e877–e881.
23. World Health Organization. *Global report on drowning: Preventing a leading killer.* 2014. http://www.who.int/violence_injury_prevention/global_report_drowning/en/. Published 2014. Accessed May 28, 2019.
24. Centers for Disease Control and Prevention. Drowning—United States, 2005-2009. *MMWR Morb Mortal Wkly Rep.* 2012;61(19):344–347.
25. Szpilman D, Bierens JJLM, Handley AJ, Orlowski JP. *Drowning. N Engl J Med.* 2012;366(22):2102–2110.
26. Felton H, Myers J, Liu G, Davis DW. Unintentional, non-fatal drowning of children: US trends and racial/ethnic disparities. *BMJ Open.* 2015;5(12):e008444–e008448.
27. Sempsrott J, Schmidt AC, Hawkins S, Cushing T. Drowning and submersion injuries. In: Auerbach PS, Cushing TA, Harris NS, eds. *Auerbach's Wilderness Medicine.* 7th ed. Philadelphia, PA: Elsevier; 2017:1530–1549.
28. Richards DB, Jacquet GA. Drowning. In: Marx JA, ed. *Rosen's Emergency Medicine: Concepts and Clinical Practice.* 8th ed. Philadelphia, PA: Elsevier; 2014:1941–1945.
29. Gilchrist J, Parker EM. Racial/ethnic disparities in fatal unintentional drowning among persons aged <= 29 years United States, 1999-2010. *MMWR.* 2014;63(19):421–426.
30. Van Beeck EF, Branche CM, Szpilman D, Modell JH, Bierens JJLM. A new definition of drowning: towards documentation and prevention of a global public health problem. *Bull World Health Organ.* 83(11):853–856.
31. Cico SJ, Quan L. Drowning. In: Tintinalli JE, ed. *Tintinalli's Emergency Medicine: A Comprehensive Study Guide.* 8th ed. New York, NY: McGraw-Hill; 2016:1395–1397.
32. Szpilman D, Webber J, Quan L, et al. Creating a drowning chain of survival. *Resuscitation.* 2014;85(9):1149–1152.
33. SCUBA diving participation in 2014. *Divers Alert Network. The Dive Lab Website.* 2014. https://thedivelab.dan.org/2014/12/17/scuba-diving-participation-in-2014/Posted Dec 17, 2017. Accessed May 28, 2019.
34. Professional Association of Dive Instructors. *PADI open water diver manual.* Rancho Santa Margarita, CA: Professional Association of Dive Instructors; 2016.
35. Buzzacott PL. *Divers Alert Network Annual Diving Report 2017 Edition—A Report on 2015 Diving Fatalities, Injuries, and Incidents.* 2017. https://www.diversalertnetwork.org/medical/report/AnnualDivingReport-2017Edition.pdf, Accessed date: May 28, 2019. Published.
36. Bove AA. Diving medicine. *Am J Respir Crit Care Med.* 2014;189(12):1479–1486.

37. National Oceanic and Atmospheric Administration. *NOAA Diving Manual.* 6th ed. Washington, DC: National Oceanic and Atmospheric Administration; 2017. 2-1 to 2-17.
38. Pollock NW, Buteau D. Updates in decompression illness. *Emerg Med Clin North Am.* 2017;35(2):301–319.
39. Van Hoesen KB, Lang MA. Diving medicine. In: Auerbach PS, Cushing TA, Harris NS, eds. *Auerbach's Wilderness Medicine.* 7th ed. Philadelphia, PA: Elsevier; 2017:1583–1618.
40. Swearingen C. Transport physiology. In: Holleran RS, Wolfe AC, Frakes MA, eds. *Patient Transport: Principles & Practice.* St Louis, MO: Elsevier; 2018:27–42.
41. McCafferty M. Why are fewer chambers available for emergencies? *Alert Diver.* 2016;32(4):54–55.
42. Norris RL, Bush SP, Cardwell MD. Bites by venomous reptiles in Canada, the United States, and Mexico. In: Auerbach PS, Cushing TA, Harris NS, eds. *Auerbach's Wilderness Medicine.* 7th ed. Philadelphia, PA: Elsevier; 2017:729–760.
43. Corbett B, Clark RF. North American snake envenomation. *Emerg Med Clin North Am.* 2017;35(2):339–354.
44. Seifert SA, Boyer LV, Benson BE, Rogers JJ. AAPCC database characterization of native U.S. venomous snake exposures, 2001-2005. *Clin Toxicol.* 2009;47(4):327–335.
45. Ruha A-M, Kleinschmidt KC, Greene S, et al. The epidemiology, clinical course, and management of snakebites in the North American Snakebite Registry. *J Med Toxicol.* 2017;13(4):309–320.
46. Kanaan NC, Ray J, Stewart M, et al. Wilderness Medical Society practice guidelines for the treatment of pitviper envenomations in the United States and Canada. *Wilderness Environ Med.* 2015;26(4):472–487.
47. Norris RL, Pfalzgraf RR, Laing G. Death following coral snake bite in the United States: first documented case (with ELISA confirmation of envenomation) in over 40 years. *Toxicon.* 2009;53(6):693–697.
48. Higham TE, Clark RW, Collins CE, Whitford MD, Freymiller GA. Rattlesnakes are extremely fast and variable when striking at kangaroo rats in nature: three-dimensional high-speed kinematics at night. *Sci Rep.* 2017;7:40412.
49. Lavonas EJ, Ruha AM, Banner W, et al. Unified treatment algorithm for the management of crotaline snakebite in the United States: results of an evidence-informed consensus workshop. *BMC Emerg Med.* 2011;11:2.
50. Bush SP, Cardwell MD. Mojave rattlesnake (Crotalus scutulatus scutulatus) identification. *Wilderness Environ Med.* 1999;10(1):6–9.
51. French WJ, Hayes WK, Bush SP, Cardwell MD, Bader JO, Rael ED. Mojave toxin in venom of Crotalus helleri (Southern Pacific Rattlesnake): molecular and geographic characterization. *Toxicon.* 2004;44(7):781–791.
52. Bush SP. Snakebite suction devices don't remove venom: they just suck. *Ann Emerg Med.* 2004;43(2):187–188.
53. American College of Medical Toxicology, American Academy of Clinical Toxicology, American Association of Poison Control Centers. European Association of Poison Control Centres, International Society of Toxinology, Asia Pacific Association of Medical Toxicology. Pressure immobilization after North American Crotalinae snake envenomation. *J Med Toxicol.* 2011;7(4):322–323.
54. Arizona poison centers welcome approval of new snake antivenom, plan research. University of Arizona website; 2015. http://opa.uahs.arizona.edu/newsroom/news/2015/arizona-poison-centers-welcome-approval-new-snake-antivenom-plan-research. Published 2015. Accessed May 28, 2019.
55. Norris RL, Ngo J, Nolan K, Hooker G. Physicians and lay people are unable to apply pressure immobilization properly in a simulated snakebite scenario. *Wilderness Environ Med.* 2005;16(1):16–21.
56. Expiration date extension for North American coral snake antivenin (Micrurus fulvius) (Equine origin) Lot L67530 through January 31, 2020. US Food and Drug Administration website; 2018. https://www.fda.gov/vaccines-blood-biologics/safety-availability-biologics/expiration-date-extension-north-american-coral-snake-antivenin-micrurus-fulvius-equine-origin-lot-1, Accessed May 28, 2019.
57. Erickson TB, Marquez A. Arthropod envenomation and parasitism. In: Auerbach PS, Cushing TA, Harris NS, eds. *Auerbach's Wilderness Medicine.* 7th ed. Philadelphia, PA: Elsevier; 2017:936–968.
58. Forrester JA, Weiser TG, Forrester JD. An update on fatalities due to venomous and nonvenomous animals in the United States (2008-2015). *Wilderness Environ Med.* 2018;29(1):36–44.
59. Otten EJ. Venomous animal injuries. In: Marx JA, ed. *Rosen's Emergency Medicine: Concepts and Clinical Practice.* 8th ed. Philadelphia, PA: Elsevier; 2014:794–807.
60. Erickson TB, Cheema N. Arthropod envenomation in North America. *Emerg Med Clin North Am.* 2017;35(2):355–375.
61. Boyer LV, Binford GJ, Degan JA. Spider bites. In: Auerbach PS, Cushing TA, Harris NS, eds. *Auerbach's Wilderness Medicine.* 7th ed. Philadelphia, PA: Elsevier; 2017:993–1016.
62. Vetter RS, Pagac BB, Reiland RW, Bolesh DT, Swanson DL. Skin lesions in barracks: consider community-acquired methicillin-resistant *Staphylococcus aureus* infection instead of spider bites. *Mil Med.* 2006;171(9):830–832.
63. Delasotta LA, Orozco F, Ong A, Sheikh E. Surgical treatment of a brown recluse spider bite: a case study and literature review. *J Foot Ankle Surg.* 2014;53(3):320–323.
64. Vetter RS. Arachnids submitted as suspected brown recluse spiders: Loxosceles spiders are virtually restricted to their known distributions but are perceived to exist throughout the United States. *J Med Entomol.* 2005;42(4):512–521.
65. Suchard JR. Scorpion envenomation. In: Auerbach PS, Cushing TA, Harris NS, eds. *Auerbach's Wilderness Medicine.* 7th ed. Philadelphia, PA: Elsevier; 2017:1017–1032.
66. Kang AM, Brooks DE. Geographic distribution of scorpion exposures in the United States, 2010-2015. *Am J Public Health.* 2017;107(12):1958–1963.
67. Skolnik AB, Ewald MB. Pediatric scorpion envenomation in the United States: morbidity, mortality, and therapeutic innovations. *Pediatr Emerg Care.* 2013;29(1):98–106.
68. Auerbach PS, Constance BB, Freer L, et al. *Field Guide to Wilderness Medicine.* 4th ed. St Louis, MO: Elsevier; 2013:472.
69. Cummins GA, Traub SJ. Tick-borne diseases. In: Auerbach PS, Cushing TA, Harris NS, eds. *Auerbach's Wilderness Medicine.* 7th ed. Philadelphia, PA: Elsevier; 2017:968–993.
70. Bolgiano EB, Sexton J. Tick-borne illnesses. In: Marx JA, ed. *Rosen's Emergency Medicine: Concepts and Clinical Practice.* 8th ed. Philadelphia, PA: Elsevier; 2014:1785–1808.
71. Phillips LL, Semple J. Bites and injuries inflicted by wild and domestic animals. In: Auerbach PS, Cushing TA, Harris NS, eds. *Auerbach's Wilderness Medicine.* 7th ed. Philadelphia, PA: Elsevier; 2017:618–645.

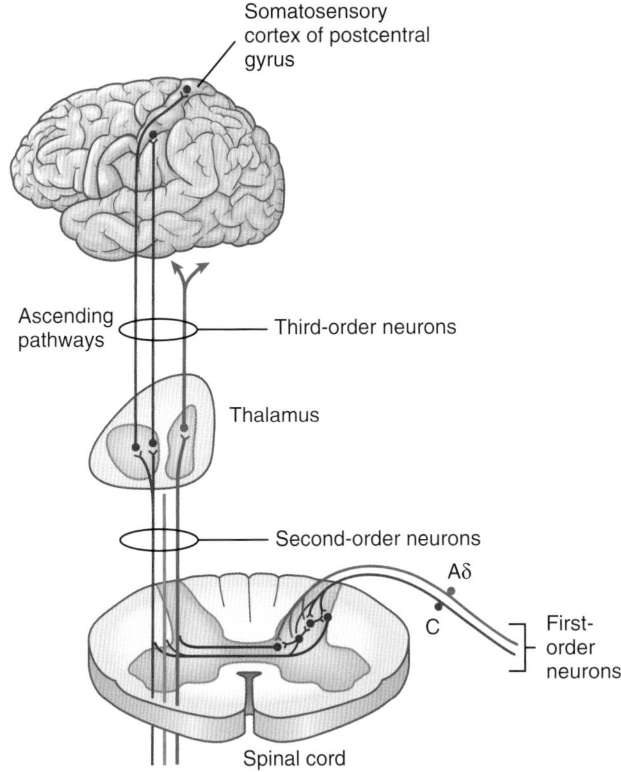

Fig. 10.1 Nociception Pathways. A-delta and C fibers constitute the primary, first-order sensory afferents coming into the gate at the posterior part of the spinal cord. Here we see second-order neurons crossing the cord (decussating) and ascending to the thalamus as part of the spinothalamic tract. Third-order afferents project to higher brain centers of the limbic system, the frontal cortex, and the primary sensory cortex of the postcentral gyrus of the parietal lobe. (From McCance KL, Huether SE: *Pathophysiology: The Biologic Basis for Disease in Adults and Children*. 8th ed. St Louis, MO: Mosby; 2019.)

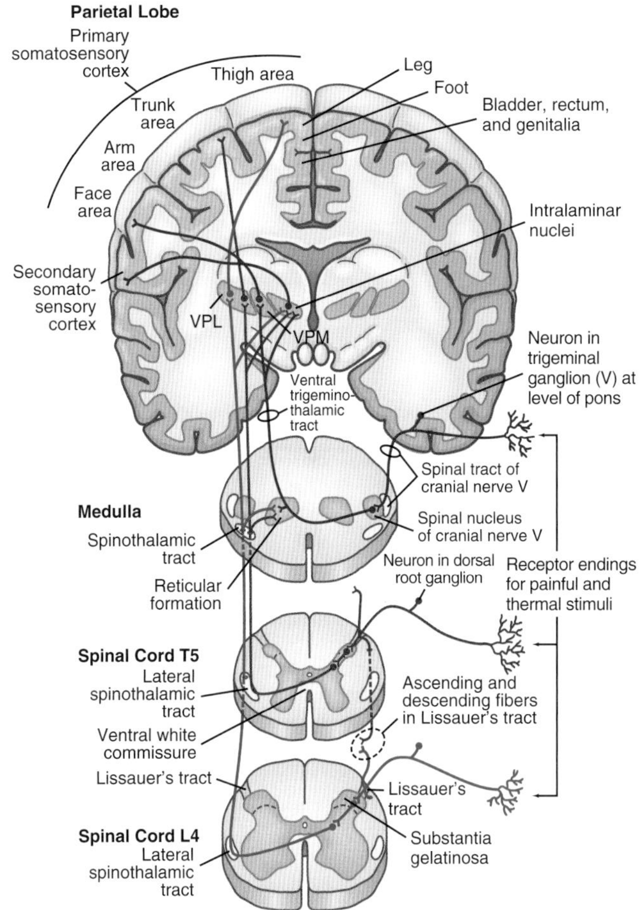

Fig. 10.2 Central Nervous System Pathways Mediating the Sensations of Pain and Temperature. VPL, Ventral posterior lateral thalamic nuclei; VPM, ventral posterior medial thalamic nuclei. (From McCance KL, Huether SE: *Pathophysiology: The Biologic Basis for Disease in Adults and Children*. 8th ed. St Louis, MO: 2019, Mosby.)

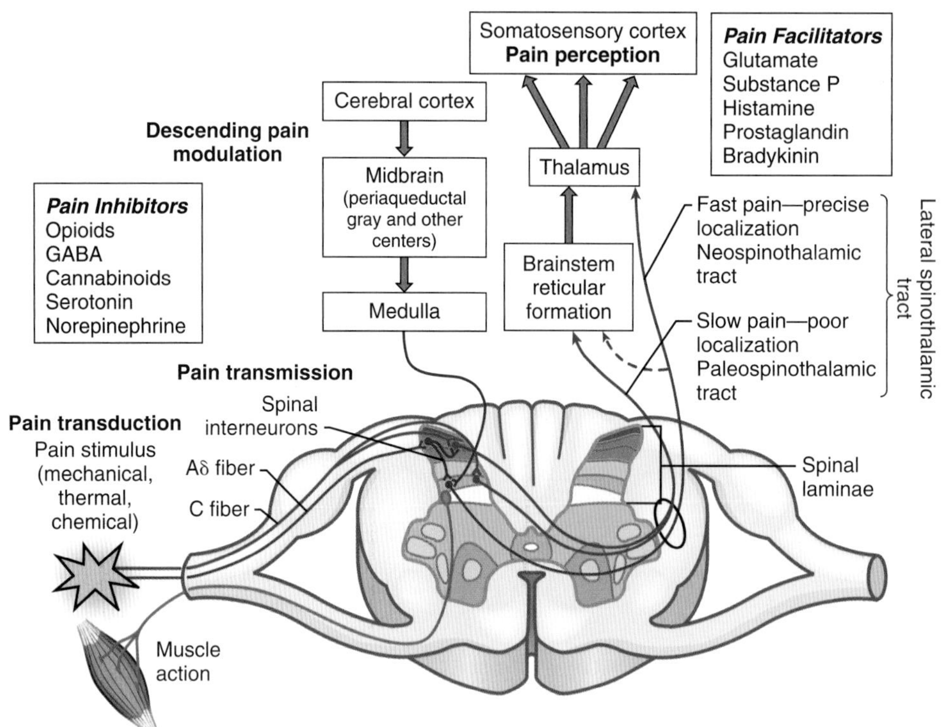

Fig. 10.3 Pain Fibers That Terminate Primarily in Laminae II and V of the Dorsal Horn. The myelinated Aδ fibers (fast localized pain) synapse on a second set of neurons that carry the signal to the thalamus via the neospinothalamic tracts. The C fibers (slow pain) synapse on laminae II and V interneurons that connect with neurons in laminae II, IV, and V and carry the pain signal to the reticular formation and midbrain via the paleospinothalamic tract. The axons of the spinothalamic tracts cross over the spinal cord to ascend in the anterior and lateral spinal cord white matter. (From McCance KL, Huether SE: *Pathophysiology: The Biologic Basis for Disease in Adults and Children*. 8th ed. St Louis, MO: 2019, Mosby.)

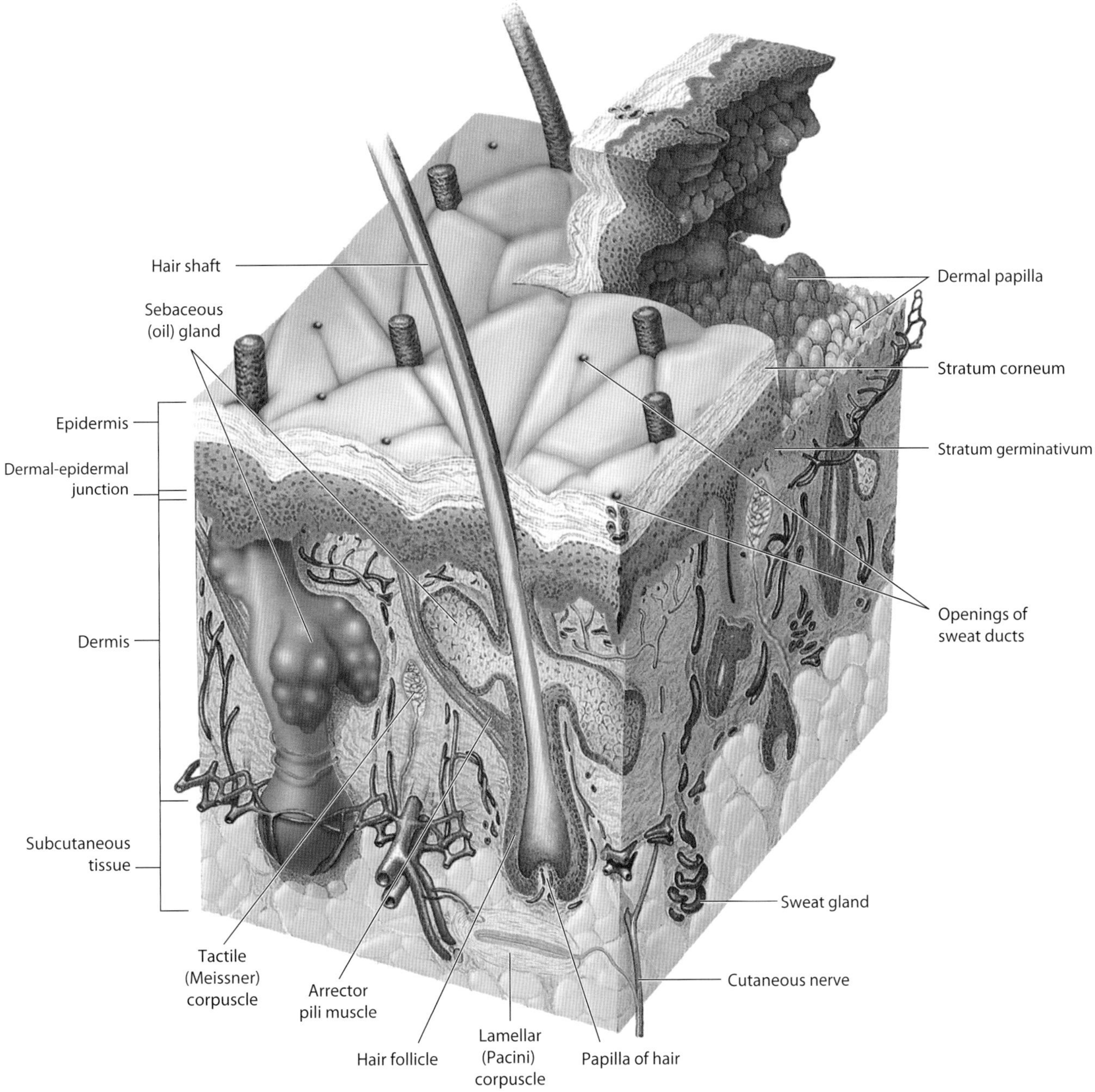

Hair shaft
Sebaceous (oil) gland
Epidermis
Dermal-epidermal junction
Dermis
Subcutaneous tissue
Tactile (Meissner) corpuscle
Arrector pili muscle
Hair follicle
Lamellar (Pacini) corpuscle
Papilla of hair
Cutaneous nerve
Sweat gland
Openings of sweat ducts
Stratum germinativum
Stratum corneum
Dermal papilla

Fig. 11.1 Anatomy of the Skin. (From Patton KT, Thibodeau GA. *Structure and Function of the Body.* 15th ed. St Louis, MO: Mosby; 2016.)

Coagulation
Inflammation
Polymorphonuclear neutrophils predominant
Macrophages predominant
Fibroplasia and granulation tissue formation
50% of normal tissue strength
Vasoconstriction
Maturation and remodeling
Vasodilation
Angiogenesis
Epithelialization
- incomplete basement membrane
- complete basement membrane
Contraction
1 2 3 4 5 10 20 30 minutes
1 60 2 3 4 5 6 12 hours
1 24 2 48 3 4 5 6 days 7
1 2 14 3 weeks
1 2 3 4 5 6 7 10 months
1 12 2 years

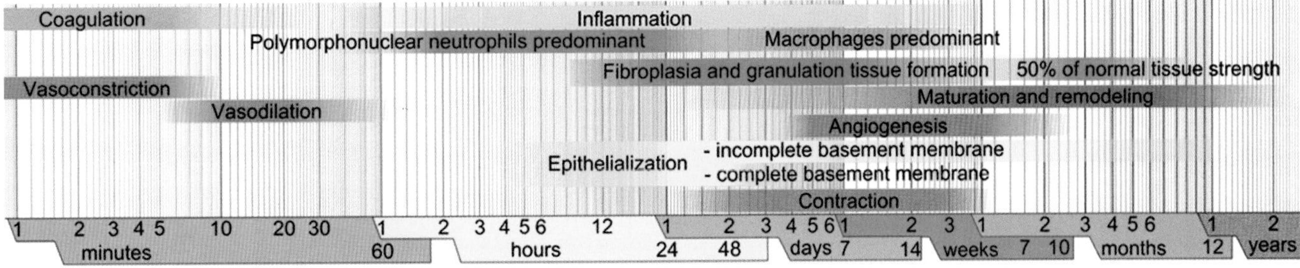

Fig. 11.2 Wound Healing Timeline. (By Mikael Häggström, used with permission.)

Wound Tape Application

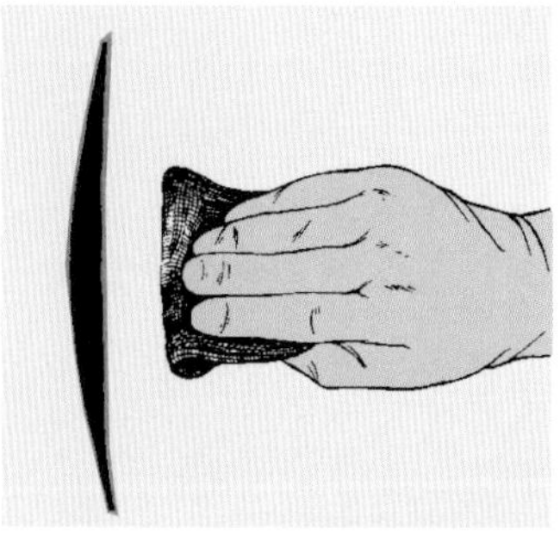

1. After wound preparation (and placement of deep closures, if needed), dry the skin thoroughly at least 2 inches around the wound. Failure to dry the skin and failure to obtain perfect hemostasis are common causes of failure of tape to stick to the skin.

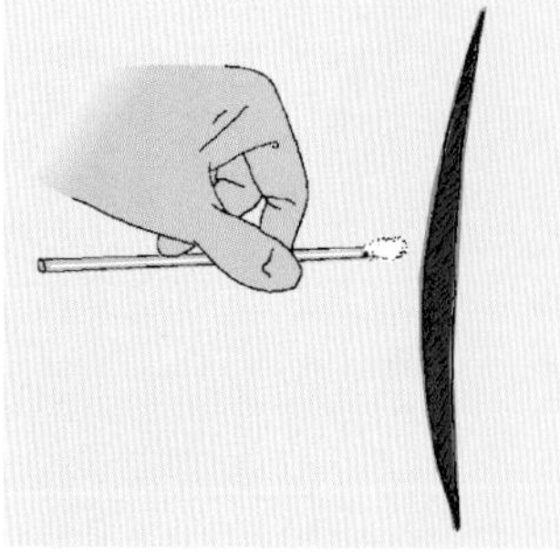

2. Apply a thin coating of tincture of benzoin around the wound to enhance tape adhesiveness. Benzoin should not enter the wound because it increases the risk of infection. Do not allow benzoin to enter the eye.

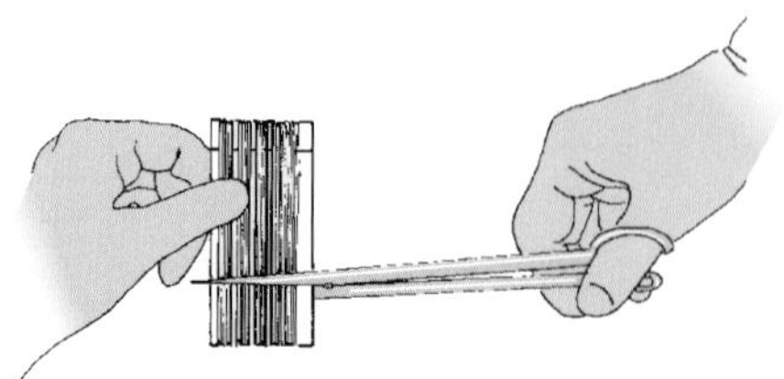

3. Cut the tape to the desired length before removing the backing.

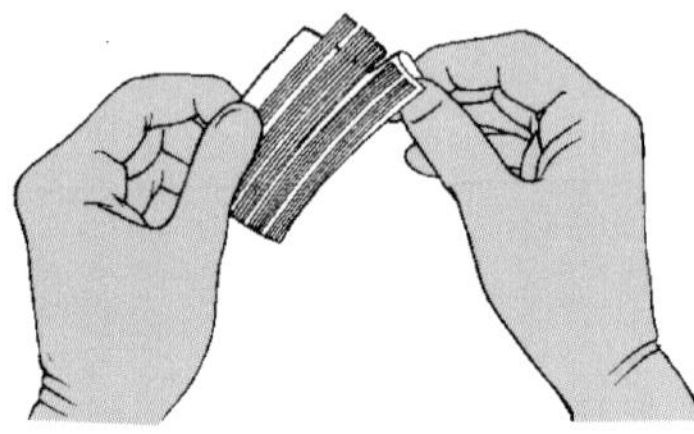

4. The tape is attached to a card with perforated tabs on both ends. Gently peel the end tab from the tape.

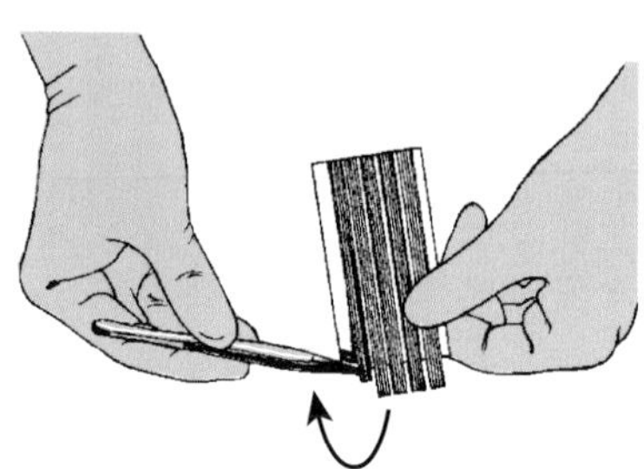

5. Use forceps to peel the tape off the card backing. Pull directly backward, not to the side.

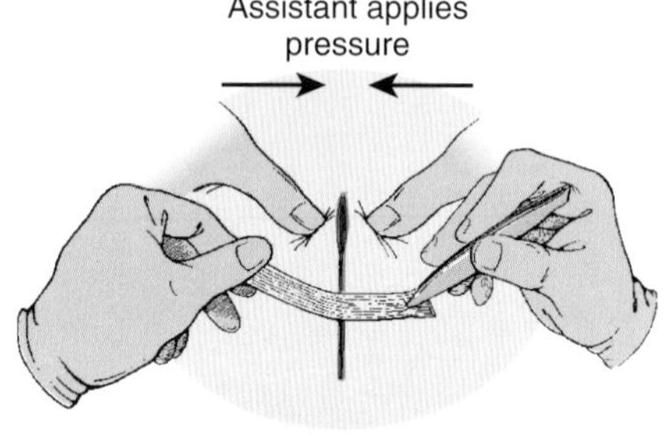

6. Place half of the first tape at the midportion of the wound; secure firmly in place.

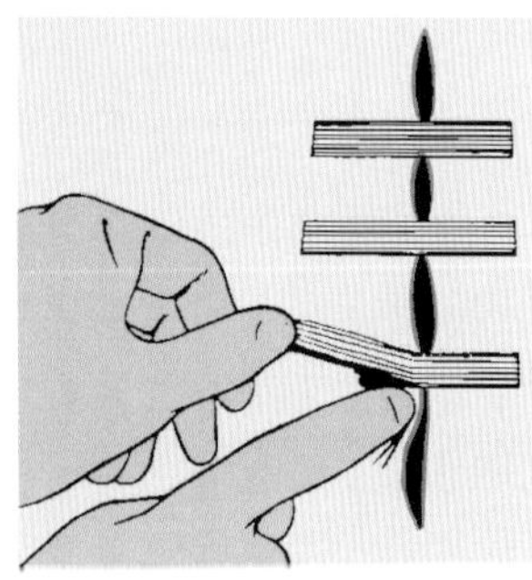

7. Gently but firmly appose the opposite side of the wound with the free hand or forceps. If an assistant is not available, the operator can approximate the wound edges. The tape should be applied by bisecting the wound until the wound is closed satisfactorily.

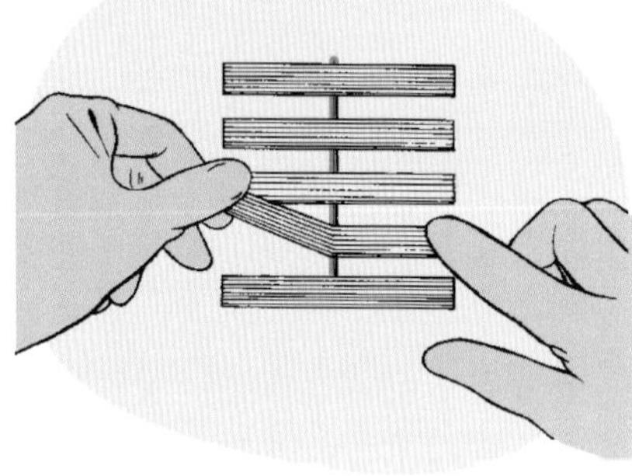

8. Wound margins are completely apposed without totally occluding the wound.

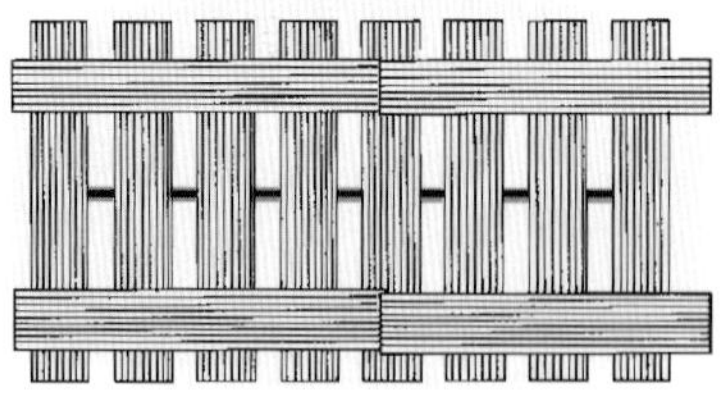

9. Only if using woven tape strips, additional supporting strips of tape are placed approximately 2.5 cm from the wound and parallel to the direction of the wound. Taping in this manner prevents the skin blistering that may occur at the ends of the tape.

Fig. 11.4 Wound Tape. (From Roberts JR, Custalow CB, Thomsen T, eds. *Robert's and Hedge's Clinical Procedures in Emergency Medicine and Acute Care*. 7th ed. Philadelphia, PA: Elsevier; 2018.)

Wound Staples

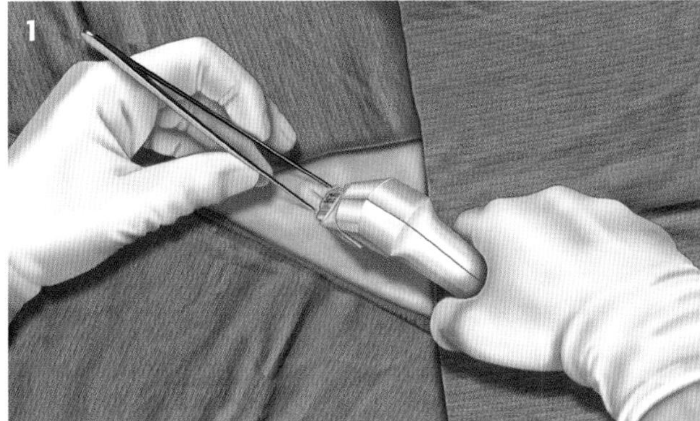

Approximate and evert the skin edges by hand or with forceps before they are secured with staples. If possible, have an assistant perform this duty. Failure to evert the wound edges is a common error that may cause an unacceptable result.

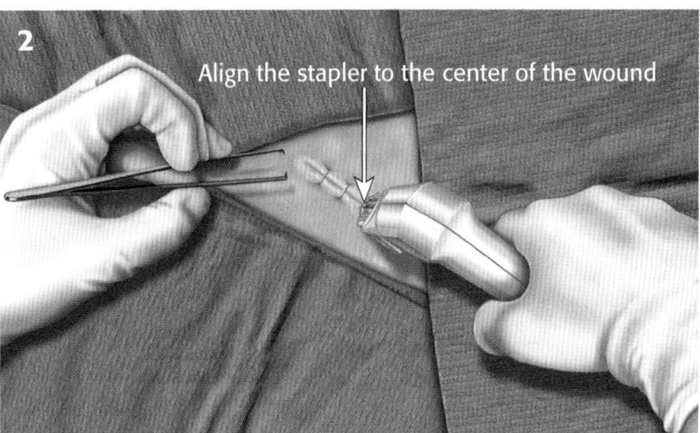

Align the center of the stapler over the center of the wound. Squeeze the stapler handle to advance one staple into the wound margins. Do not press too hard on the skin to prevent placing the staple too deeply.

3

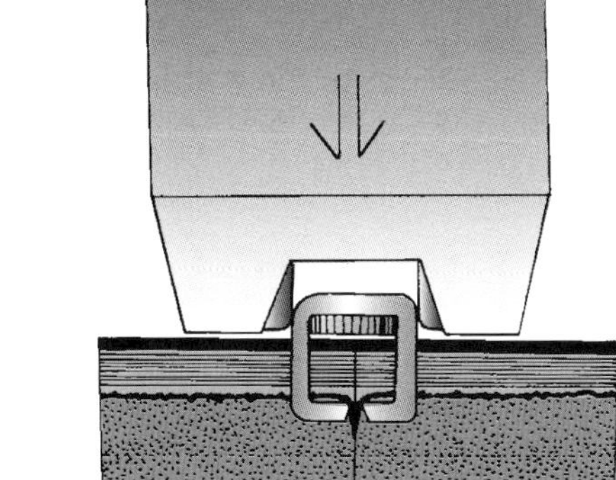

As the handle is squeezed, an anvil automatically bends the staple to the proper configuration.

4

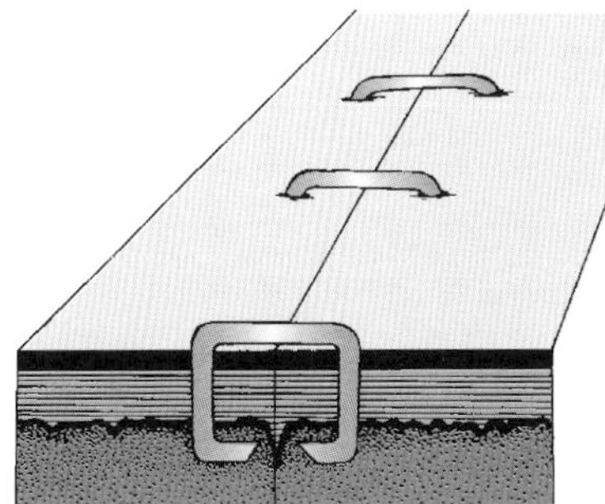

Allow a small space to remain between the skin and the crossbar of the staple. Excessive pressure created by placing the staple too deep causes wound edge ischemia, as well as pain on removal. Note that the staple bar is 2 to 3 mm above the skin line.

5

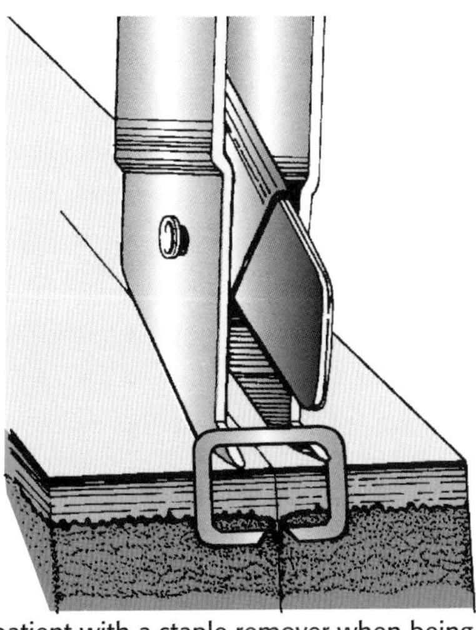

Supply the patient with a staple remover when being referred to an office for removal or for self-removal. To remove the staple, place the lower jaw of the remover under the crossbar of the staple.

6

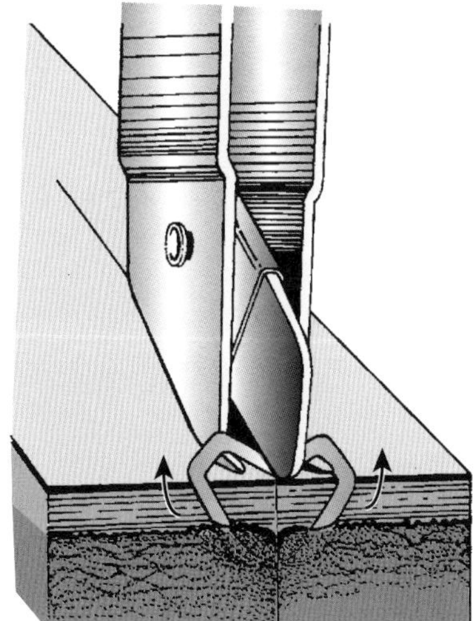

Squeeze the handle gently, and the upper jaw will compress the staple and allow it to exit the skin.

Fig. 11.5 Application of Skin Staples. (From Roberts JR, Custalow CB, Thomsen T, eds. *Robert's and Hedge's Clinical Procedures in Emergency Medicine and Acute Care*. 7th ed. Philadelphia, PA: Elsevier; 2018.)

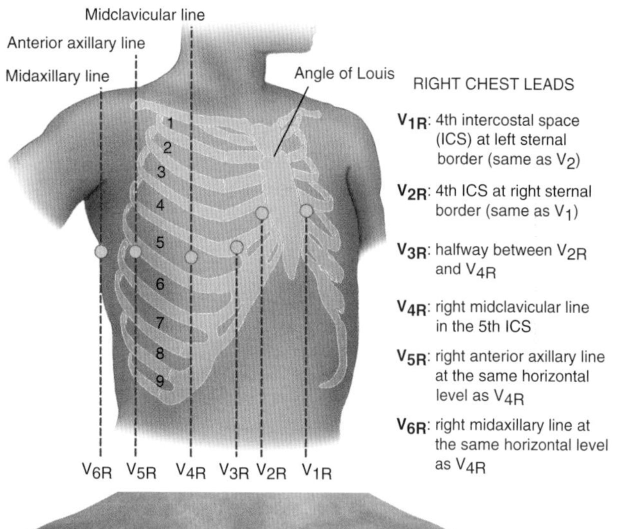

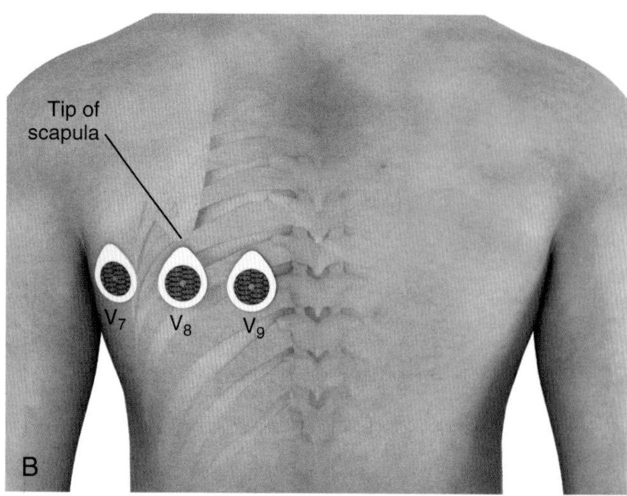

Fig. 23.15B Right ventricular (b) electrocardiogram lead placement.

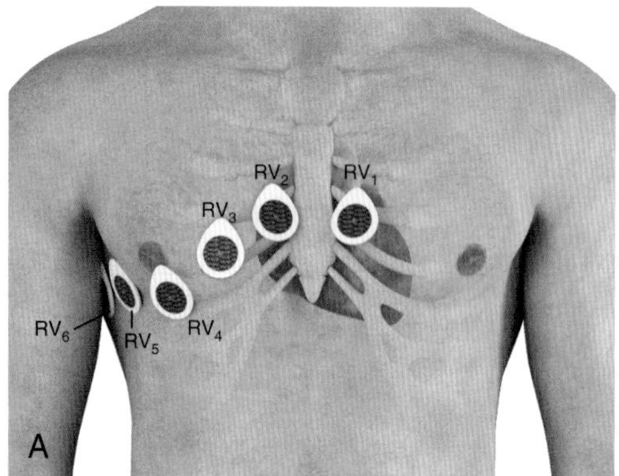

Fig. 23.15A Right ventricular (a) and posterior wall

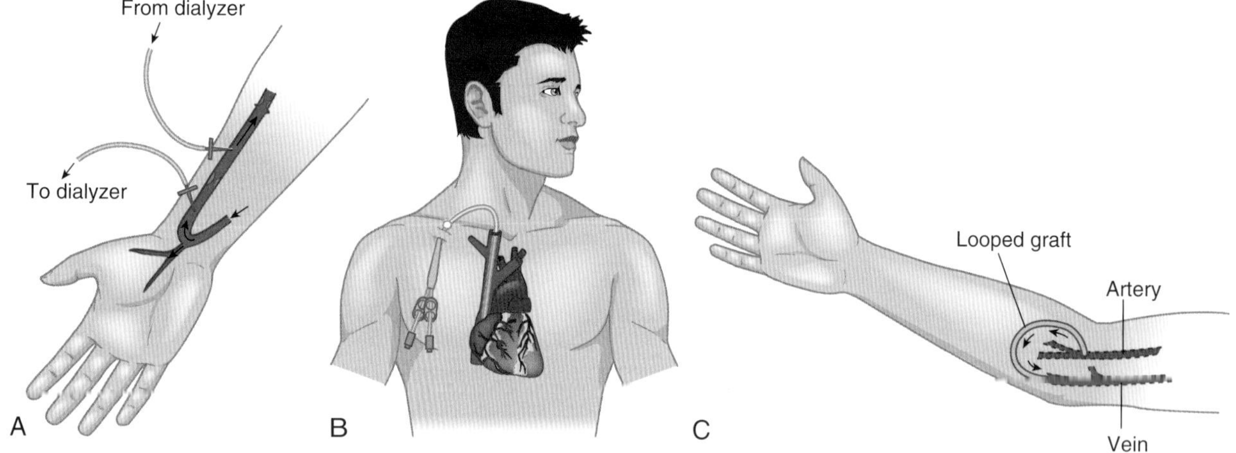

Fig. 26.1 Types of Access for Hemodialysis. (A) Forearm arteriovenous fistula. (B) Venous catheter for temporary hemodialysis access. (C) Artificial loop graft. (From National Institute of Diabetes and Digestive and Kidney Diseases. *Kidney Failure: Choosing a Treatment That's Right for You*. Bethesda, MD: National Institutes of Health; 2007. NIH publication 00–2412.)

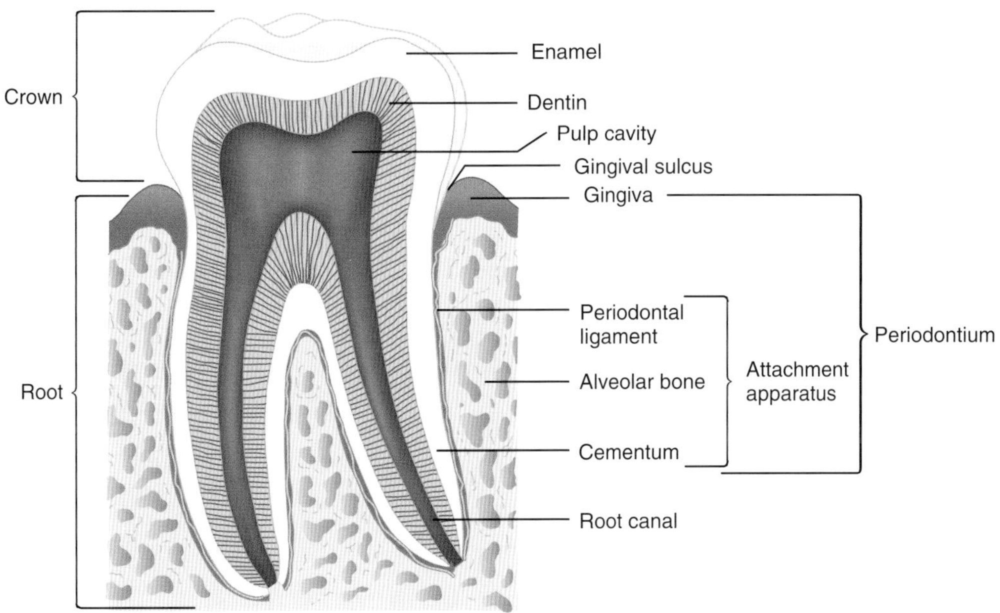

Fig. 32.1 Dental Anatomic Unit and Attachment Apparatus. (From Walls RM, Hockberger RS, Gausche-Hill M, ed. *Rosen's Emergency Medicine: Concepts and Clinical Practice*. Philadelphia, PA: Elsevier; 2018:771-790.)

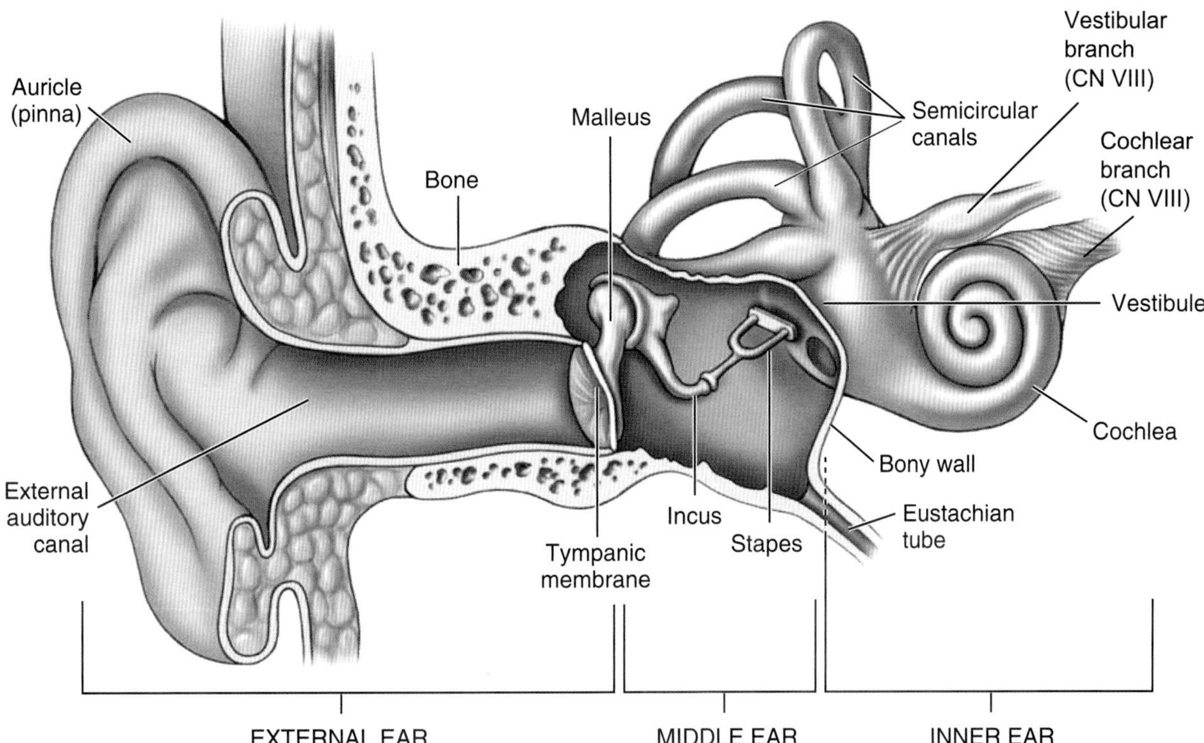

Fig. 32.2 Cross-Sectional View of the External, Middle, and Inner Ear. (From Herlihy B. *The Human Body in Health and Illness*. 6th ed. St Louis, MO: Elsevier, 2017.)

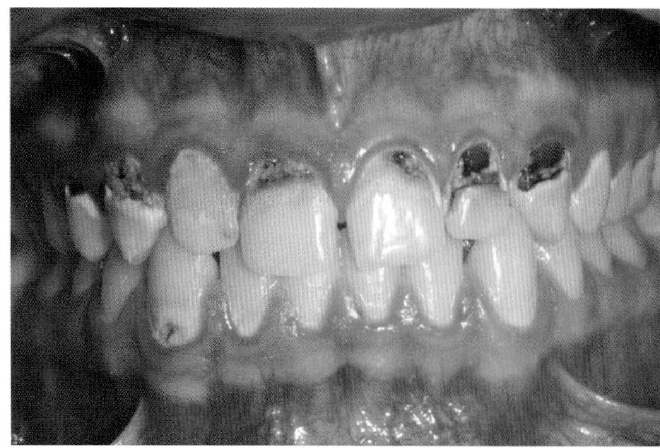

Fig. 32.3 Dental Caries. (From Neville BW, Damm DD, Allen CM. Physical and chemical injuries. In: *Oral and Maxillofacial Pathology*. 4th ed. Elsevier; 2016:259-302.)

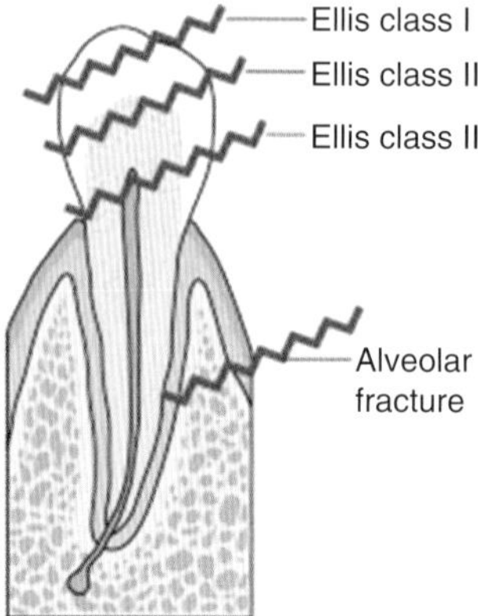

Fig. 32.4 Dental Fractures With Ellis Fracture Classification. (From Pfenninger JL, Fowler GC: *Pfenninger and Fowler's Procedures for Primary Care*. Philadelphia, PA: Elsevier/Mosby: 2011.)

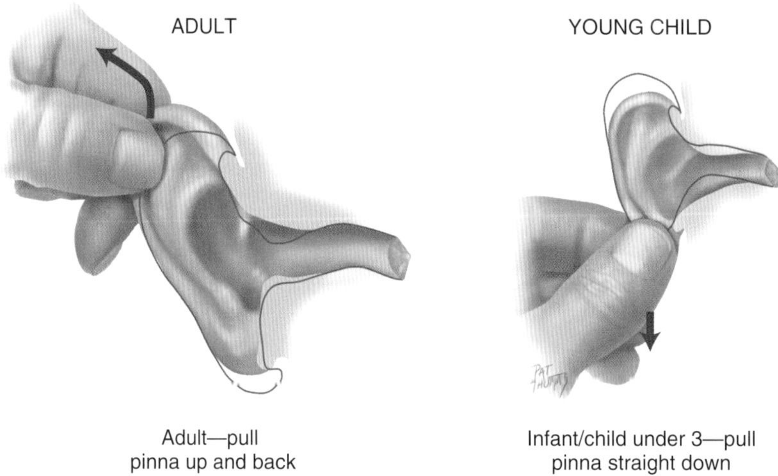

Fig. 32.5 Ear Positioning for Assessment and Drop Instillation. (From: Jarvis C. Ears. In: *Physical Examination and Health Assessment*. 7th ed. St Louis, MO: Elsevier, 2016:325-351.)

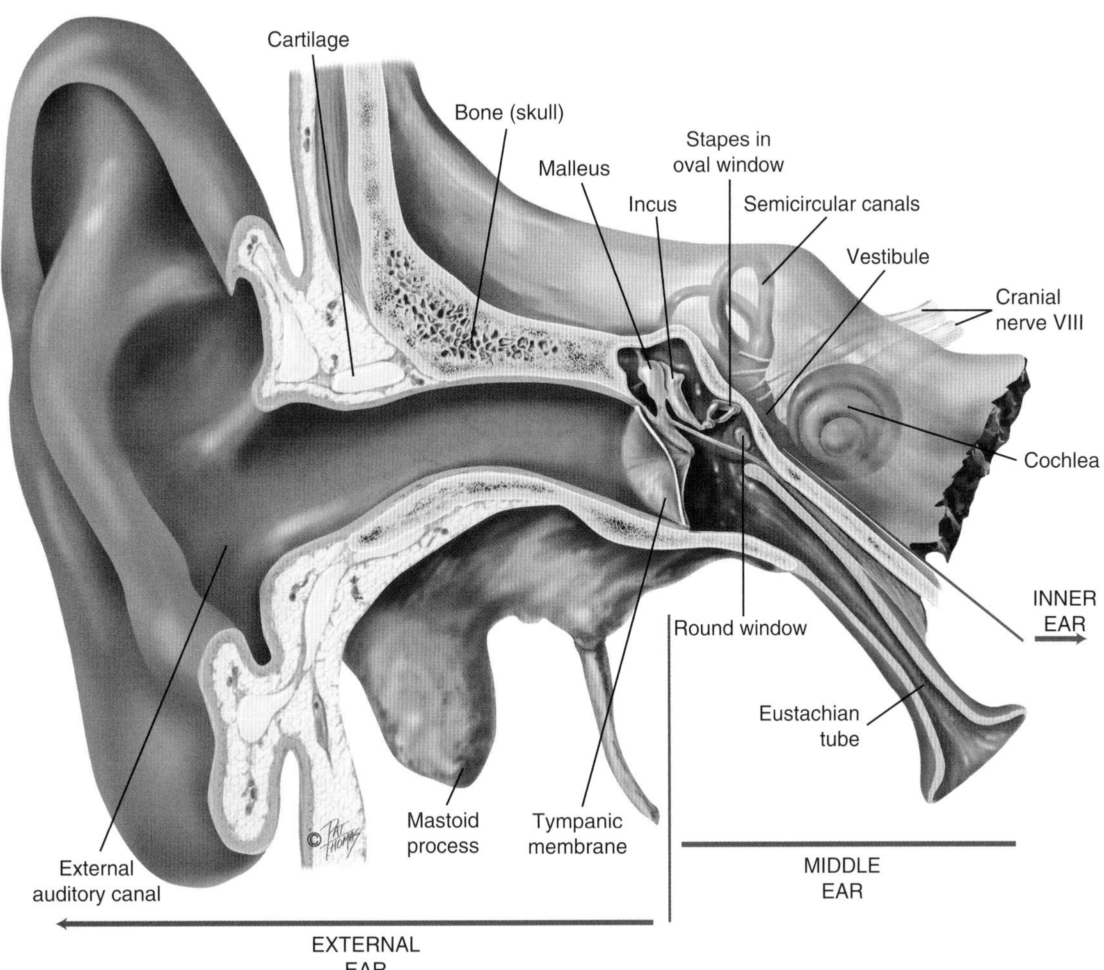

Fig. 32.6 Otitis Externa (Swimmer's Ear). (From: Jarvis C. Ears. In: *Physical Examination and Health Assessment*. 7th ed. St Louis, MO: Elsevier, 2016:325-351.)

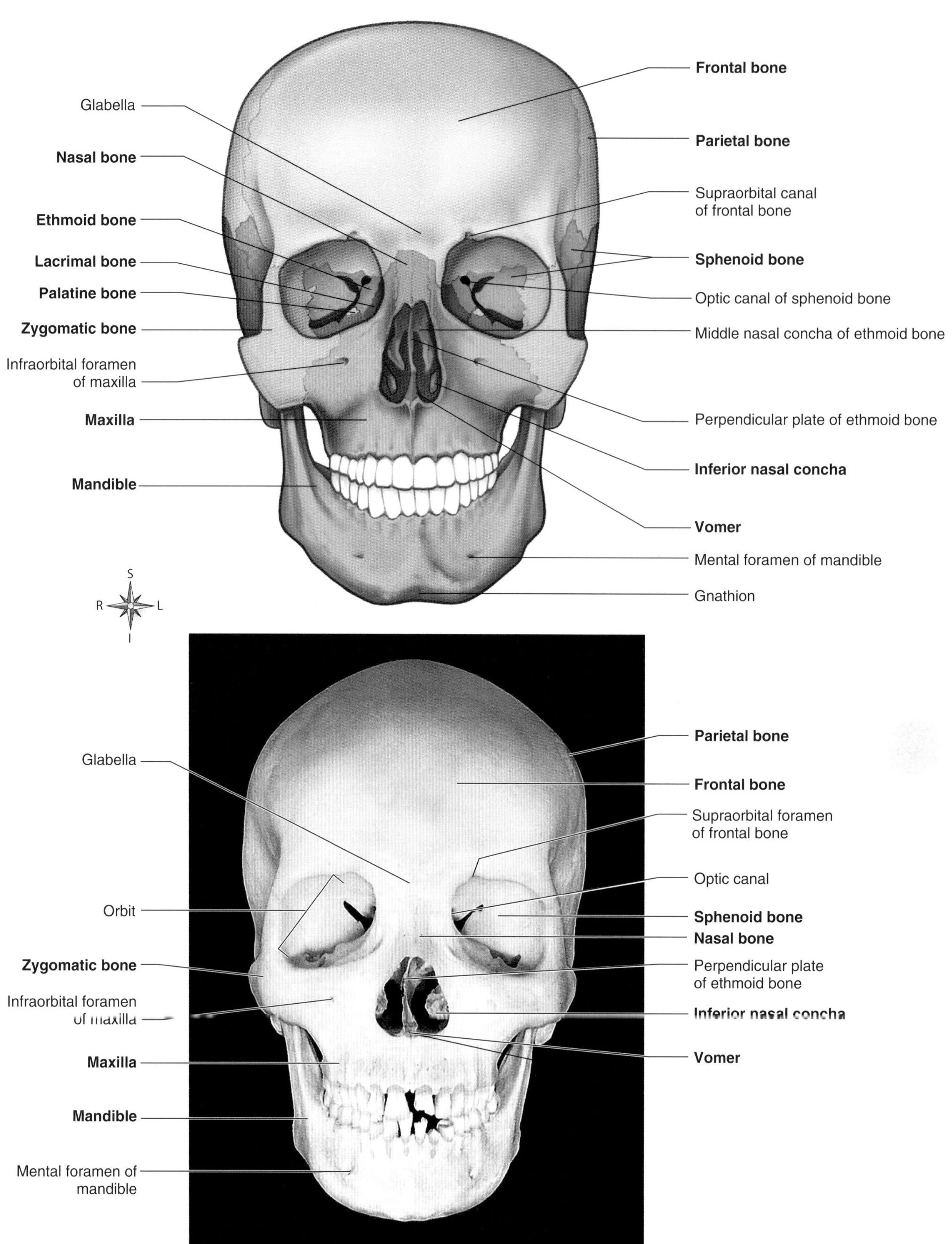

Fig. 36.1 Facial Bones. (From Patton KT. *Anatomy & Physiology*, 7th ed. St Louis, MO: Elsevier; 2010.)

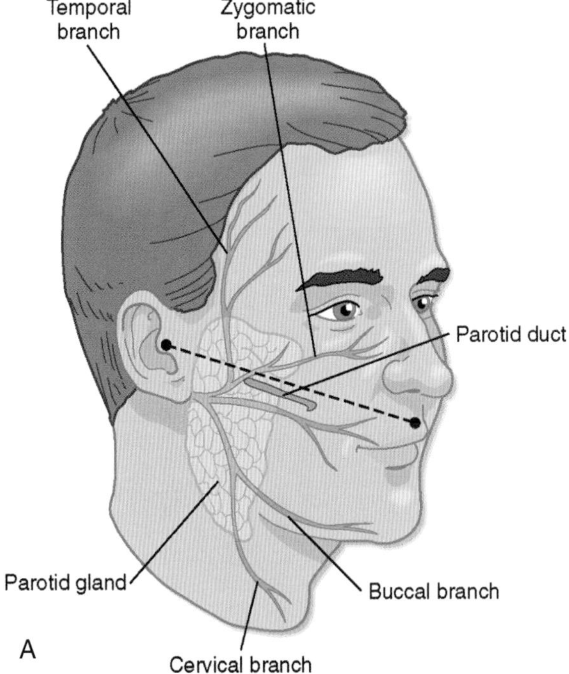

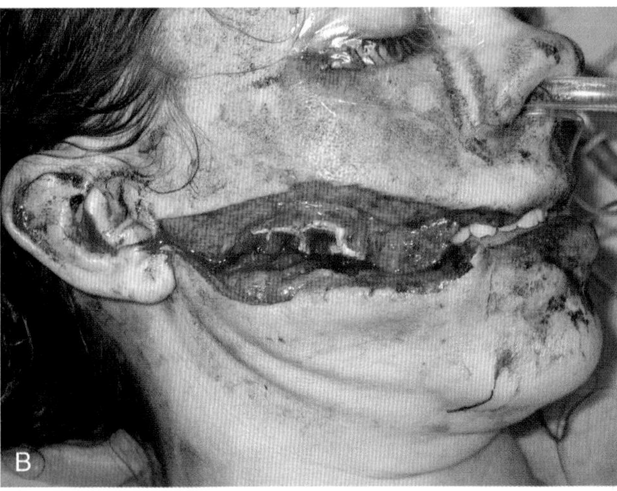

Fig. 36.2 (A) A line drawn from the tragus of the ear to the middle of the upper lip approximates the course of the parotid duct. Injury to the parotid gland duct is usually located at or distal to the anterior border of the masseter muscle along this line. (B) Facial laceration with high risk of injury to parotid gland and duct. (A from Adams J, Barton E, Collings J, et al. *Emergency Medicine*. St Louis, MO: Saunders; 2008. B from Fonesca RJ, Walker RV, Barber HD, et al. *Oral & Maxillofacial Trauma*. 4th ed. St Louis, MO: Elsevier Saunders, 2013.)

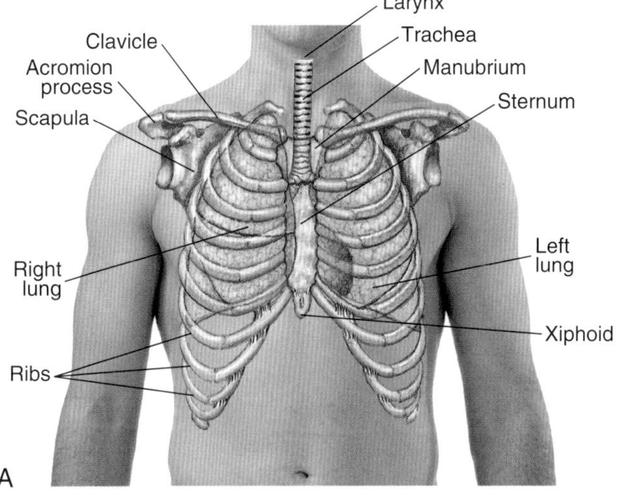

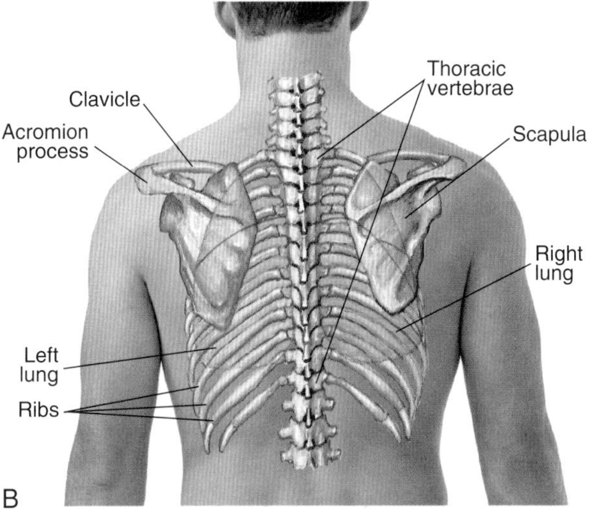

Fig. 38.1 Chest and Anatomic Landmarks. (From Thompson JM, Wilson SF. Health assessment for nursing practice. St Louis, MO: Mosby; 1996. In: Ball JE, Dains JW, Flynn JA, Solomon B, Stewart RW. *Seidel's Guide to Physical Examination: An Interventional Approach*. 9th ed. St Louis, MO: Elsevier; 2017.)

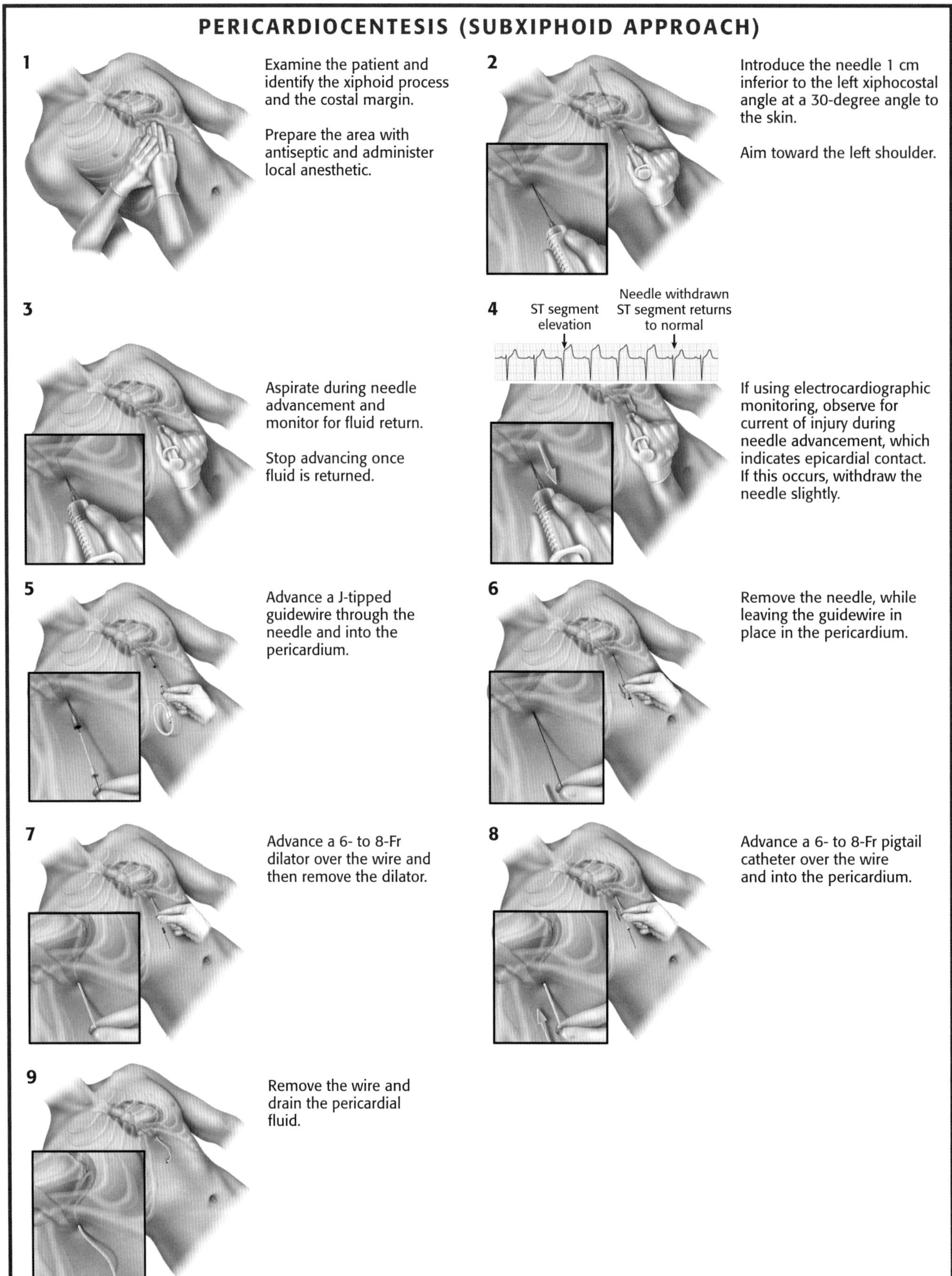

Fig. 38.14 Pericardiocentesis. (From Custalow CB: *Color Atlas of Emergency Department Procedures*. Philadelphia, PA: Saunders: 2005. In: Roberts JR, Custalow CB, Thomsen TW, eds. *Roberts and Hedges' Clinical Procedures in Emergency Medicine and Acute Care*. 7th ed. Philadelphia, PA: Elsevier; 2019.)

72. Rasmussen D, Landon A, Powell J, Brown GR. Evaluating and treating mammalian bites. *JAAPA*. 2017;30(3):32–36.
73. Lanteri CA, Nguyen K, Gibbons RV. Rabies. In: Auerbach PS, Cushing TA, Harris NS, eds. *Auerbach's Wilderness Medicine*. 7th ed. Philadelphia, PA: Elsevier; 2017:645–673.
74. Aziz H, Rhee P, Pandit V, Tang A, Gries L, Joseph B. The current concepts in management of animal and human bite wounds. *J Trauma Acute Care Surg*. 2015;78(3):641–648.
75. Ellis R, Ellis C. Dog and cat bites. *Am Fam Physician*. 2014;90(4):239–243.
76. Esposito S, Picciolli I, Semino M, Principi N. Dog and cat bite-associated infections in children. *Eur J Clin Microbiol Infect Dis*. 2013;32(8):971–976.
77. Kennedy SA, Stoll LE, Lauder AS. Human and other mammalian bite injuries of the hand: evaluation and management. *J Am Acad Orthop Surg*. 2015;23(1):47–57.

31

Toxicologic Emergencies

Michael De Laby

Toxicologic emergencies include acute poisonings and intake of substances of abuse. These situations pose a unique challenge to the emergency department (ED) nurse. The American Association of Poison Control Centers' annual report for 2016 stated that 93% of cases occurred in the home, with 46% occurring in children younger than 6 years old and the highest incidence occurring in 1- and 2-year-olds. In addition, 87.9% of toxic exposures were acute and 70% were unintentional. Therapeutic medication errors, such as double dosing or taking the wrong medicine, accounted for more than 12.5% of all poisonings.[1] Ingestion or co-ingestion of over-the-counter (OTC) drugs such as antihistamines, antidiarrheals, or indigestion remedies in potential poisonings may cloud or mask true symptoms of acute poisoning. In 2011 more than 5 million ED visits were associated with drugs of abuse or misuse, including prescription and OTC drugs, inhalants, and illicit drugs.[2] Patients may also use more than one drug in combination with alcohol, leading to fatalities.

PATIENT MANAGEMENT

Determining the precise agent or agents involved in a toxicologic emergency can be challenging due to the vast number of potentially toxic substances. Consideration must be given to the causes such as thyroid disease, hypoglycemia, hypoxia, or the purposeful or accidental exposure to a toxin or chemical when dealing with patients with an altered level of consciousness. Poison control centers act as a resource for information on various drugs, potential toxicity, and patient management. Poison control centers, available nationwide through the telephone number 1-800-222-1222 and staffed by nurses and/or pharmacists, provide professionals and the public with 24-hour telephone access to evidence-based treatment regimens.

Symptoms of toxic exposures range from minor to severe and vary widely with the causative agent, dose, and extent of exposure. Toxins are capable of affecting every body system, and certain toxins produce predictable clinical signs and symptoms. Patient assessments should include a detailed history from the patient, family, or prehospital care providers to assist in identifying information related to exposure to substances or toxins, such as the dosage, duration, and form of exposure. Consider the possibility of ingestion of or exposure to a toxic agent if the patient presents with a decreased level of consciousness without an identifiable cause. Table 31.1 describes essential assessment information related to toxic exposure.

Provision of supportive care, identification of patients requiring treatment with an antidote, and appropriate use of methods limiting poison absorption or increasing elimination remain priorities of management[3] for patients presenting with toxicologic emergencies.

General Interventions

Stabilization of airway, breathing, and circulation are priorities when caring for an individual with a toxicologic emergency. Protect the airway, ensure adequate oxygenation and ventilation, and support the cardiovascular system while attempting to identify specific toxins involved. Significant exposures may require endotracheal intubation, mechanical ventilation, and medications providing hemodynamic support.

Substance-to-substance variations in toxicologic management exist; however, ensuring patient safety and providing emotional support are common to all poisonings. Knowledge of common toxidromes and interventions associated with each will assist the emergency nurse in the management of the patient with a toxicologic emergency. Treatment is directed at preventing or decreasing absorption of the toxic substance (Table 31.2). This can be accomplished using measures to enhance elimination of the substance (Table 31.3) or by administering specific antidotes to counteract the toxic substance (Table 31.4).

SPECIFIC TOXICOLOGIC EMERGENCIES

Patients may present with toxicity from a single agent or from ingestion of multiple agents. Caregivers should never assume the patient with a toxicologic emergency ingested only one pill or one type of pill. Specific toxicologic emergencies are reviewed in the following section.

Salicylates

Salicylates have analgesic, antiinflammatory, and antipyretic properties, making them frequent components of both prescription and nonprescription drugs. More than 200 products contain aspirin or salicylates. Toxicity may result from either short-term or long-term exposure, particularly in children and older adults. Aspirin (acetylsalicylic acid) is the most

TABLE 31.1 Essential Assessment Information for Toxic Exposure.

Item	Description
Substance	If possible, visually confirm substance(s) involved. Ask what medications the patient takes at home.
Time of exposure	Time since exposure influences both symptoms and treatment.
Acute or chronic	Acute exposures have different presenting symptoms and are managed differently than chronic exposures.
Amount of toxin	Determine the maximum quantity possible. Count pills in the bottle; confirm when the prescription was filled.
Signs and symptoms	Assess for symptoms in all systems. Toxins can affect every tissue in the body.
Prior treatment	Clarify any interventions provided by lay and prehospital personnel. Some home remedies can be detrimental.
Intentional or accidental	Poisoning is a popular form of suicide and suicidal gesture. Have there been previous suicide attempts? Does the patient have a history of depression or preexisting mental health problems? Was the poisoning recreational? Is this a possible homicide attempt?

readily available salicylate. Oil of wintergreen (methyl salicylate) is a highly toxic, liquid form of salicylate used in products such as BENGAY. Bismuth subsalicylate is an ingredient in Pepto-Bismol. The incidence of acute salicylate ingestion has dropped in the United States over the past two decades because of increased use of acetaminophen and ibuprofen. However, acute and chronic overdoses of salicylates continue to occur.

Clinical findings vary significantly with patient age, amount of salicylate consumed, and whether ingestion was chronic or acute. Acute salicylate ingestions can be divided into mild, moderate, and severe based on the dose ingested and the symptoms. Mild toxicity occurs with an ingested dose of more than 150 mg/kg. Symptoms of mild toxicity include nausea, vomiting, dizziness, and tinnitus. Moderate toxicity occurs with an ingested dose of more than 250 mg/kg, and symptoms include tachypnea, hyperpyrexia, sweating, dehydration, agitation, and ataxia. Severe toxicity is associated with an ingested dose of more than 500 mg/kg. Patients with severe toxicity (more than 700 mg/dL) may exhibit hypotension, metabolic acidosis, renal failure, coma, and convulsion. Acidosis can lead to cardiac dysrhythmias and cardiac failure.

Chronic toxicity may occur with ingestion of more than 100 mg/kg per day for 2 or more days. Symptoms include lethargy, confusion, dehydration, hallucinations, pulmonary edema, elevated liver enzymes, and prolonged prothrombin time (PT). Direct gastrointestinal (GI) irritation causes nausea, vomiting, and hematemesis. Patients may also exhibit hyperthermia, renal failure, tinnitus, and hypoglycemia.

Salicylates stimulate the respiratory center of the brain stem, resulting in hyperventilation and respiratory alkalosis. They also decrease adenosine triphosphate (ATP) production, which leads to metabolic acidosis. Metabolic acidosis decreases the renal elimination of salicylates and increases central nervous system (CNS) toxicity. Children tend to present to the ED with metabolic acidosis, whereas adults often present with respiratory alkalosis. Decreased platelet function can lead to petechiae. Hypoglycemia is more common in children.

Diagnostic studies include serial measurements of salicylate levels, arterial blood gases, electrolytes (particularly potassium), glucose, blood urea nitrogen (BUN), creatinine, platelets, PT, and urine pH. Obtain a serum salicylate level initially or at least within 4 hours after ingestion and then approximately every 4 hours until the concentration has peaked. Peak serum levels usually occur 6 hours after short-term ingestion, but levels may not peak for 12 to 18 hours after ingestion of enteric-coated tablets.

Initial treatment consists of administration of activated charcoal. Repeat doses of activated charcoal should be administered at 2-hour intervals until serum levels start decreasing. Gastric lavage may be considered if patients present within 1 hour of ingestion of more than 500 mg/kg. Urinary alkalinization is an effective method of increasing renal excretion of salicylates in patients who exhibit moderate toxicity.[4] This can be accomplished by adding 100 mEq of sodium bicarbonate to each liter of intravenous (IV) fluid and infusing at 200 to 300 mL/h. Potassium may be added to the IV fluid to avoid potassium loss associated with alkaline diuresis. Hemodialysis is very effective for poisonings not responding to simpler measures and should be considered in patients with a salicylate level of more than 700 mg/dL who exhibit symptoms of severe toxicity not improving with treatment. Patients in significant metabolic acidosis may require 50 mL of 8.4% sodium bicarbonate IV push. Short-acting benzodiazepines should be used for emergency treatment of salicylate-induced seizures.

Acetaminophen

As with salicylates, acetaminophen is a common ingredient in many OTC analgesics, antipyretics, and cold remedies. Acetaminophen is also used in combination with narcotics, and assessment of possible acetaminophen overdose should be considered in patients who present with narcotic overdose. Acetaminophen overdoses are usually unintentional in the pediatric patient and intentional in adults. Although initial symptoms are mild, severe acetaminophen poisoning causes life-threatening hepatotoxicity. Hepatotoxicity may occur through therapeutic medication errors, in patients concurrently using acetaminophen and abusing alcohol, or in patients taking other medications metabolized by the liver.[5]

Acetaminophen is rapidly absorbed from the gut and broken down by the liver, forming a toxic metabolite. In therapeutic doses, endogenous hepatic enzymes rapidly detoxify this intermediary product. However, toxic doses deplete these essential enzymes, damaging both the liver and kidneys as

TABLE 31.2 Measures to Prevent or Decrease Absorption of Drugs or Chemicals.

Procedure	Indications	Contraindications	Comments
Ocular Decontamination			
Irrigation with water or saline, use Morgan lens as indicated		Alkali solution requires longer periods of irrigation Ensure pH is neutral before discontinuing	Refer to ophthalmology for alkali or continued irrigation
Dermal Decontamination			
Remove all contaminated clothing Flush surfaces with water or saline, including hair and under nails	Organophosphate insecticides Gasoline, hydrocarbons Acids, alkali Any chemical that may burn skin	Ensure chemical is not combustible with use of water	Ensure protective gear is used
Gastrointestinal Decontamination in Oral Ingestions			
Gastric: Emptying with syrup of ipecac		Contraindicated use in drugs causing central nervous system depression, inducing seizures (e.g., tricyclic antidepressants), caustic or corrosives, or having a potential for aspiration	Use is controversial American Academy of Pediatrics Policy Statement (2003) and American Association of Poison Control Center Guideline (2005) issued recommendations limiting or discouraging use in out-of-hospital situations No recommendations regarding emergency department use have been made
Gastric: Lavage Use large-lumen (36–40 F) orogastric tube Best initiated within 60 min of ingestion		Potential for aspiration Caution in ingestion of caustic corrosives Contraindicated in coingestion of sharp objects and nontoxic ingestions	Benefit is controversial
Cathartic Administration: Use magnesium sulfate, magnesium citrate, sorbitol Mix and administer with activated charcoal orally or via lavage/nasogastric tube Use single doses; do not repeat	May be used to enhance elimination of activated charcoal	Contraindicated with absent bowel sounds and preexisting renal and cardiac failure	May cause vomiting or severe diarrhea
Whole Bowel Irrigation (controversial): Use nonabsorbable evacuant solution via nasogastric tube/lavage (GoLYTELY, CoLyte)	Used in enteric-coated or sustained-released products, drugs that may form concentrations (e.g., aspirin), body packers, drugs not absorbed by activated charcoal (e.g., iron, lithium)	Contraindicated in preexisting gastrointestinal disease, presence or risk of ileus, perforation, obstruction Precaution in pediatric patients	May cause nausea, vomiting, abdominal cramping, risk of electrolyte imbalance
Prevent or Limit Absorption/Adsorption of Drugs or Chemicals in Oral Ingestions			
Activated charcoal Adults: 1g/kg body weight Pediatrics: 0.5 g/kg	Used to adsorb most chemicals ingested	Contraindicated in corrosive or caustic ingestions, decreased or absent bowel sounds, toxins not bound by activated charcoal (iron, lead, lithium)	Specific substances may require multiple doses (e.g., aspirin)

TABLE 31.3 **Measures to Enhance Elimination of Drugs or Chemicals.**

Measure	Procedure	Indications	Contraindications/ Precautions	Comments
Urinary alkalization using sodium bicarbonate	Use of intravenous sodium bicarbonate	Used with chemicals altering pH (e.g., aspirin)	Contraindicated in presence of pulmonary edema or renal failure; fluid overload possible	Frequent pH and electrolyte levels indicated, particularly potassium
Hemodialysis	Venous blood sent across membrane and treated with dialysate, toxins removed	Salicylates/aspirin, valproic acid, methanol, ethylene glycol, others Renal dysfunction with long-term drug use (e.g., lithium)	Caution in patients with bleeding disorders	Drugs with large volumes of distribution not always dialyzable
Hemoperfusion	Similar to hemodialysis, charcoal filter often used	Phenobarbital, theophylline, others	May cause thrombocytopenia	Although clearance rates are frequently higher, it is not the treatment of choice

TABLE 31.4 **Specific Antidotes.**

Antidote	Poisoning	Antidote	Poisoning
N-acetylcysteine Mucomyst (oral formations) Acetadote (intravenous formulation)	Acetaminophen (Tylenol)	Ethanol intravenously 10%	Ethylene glycol, methanol
Atropine	Organophosphate, carbamate, insecticide Bradycardia caused by toxins	Flumazenil (Romazicon)	Benzodiazepine
Antivenins Polyvalent equine Polyvalent immune Fab-Ovine/Cro-Fab Black widow spider	Rattlesnake, copperhead envenomation Rattlesnake, copperhead envenomation Black widow spider bite	Folic acid	Methanol
Dimercaprol (BAL in oil)	Heavy metal	Fomepizole (4 MP) (Antizol)	Ethylene glycol, methanol
Botulinum antitoxin	Botulism	Glucagon	β-blocker, calcium channel blocker
Calcium chloride or gluconate	Calcium channel blocker, hydrofluoric acid: skin exposure or poisoning, hypocalcemia	Methylene blue	Methemoglobinemia
Cyanide antidote kit	Cyanide	Naloxone (Narcan)	Narcotic overdose
Deferoxamine	Iron	Oxygen, hyperbaric oxygen	Carbon monoxide
Dextrose	Hypoglycemia caused by toxin	Octreotide (Sandostatin)	Oral sulfonylurea Hypoglycemia
Digoxin Fab	Digoxin, oleander	Physostigmine/Antilirium	Anticholinergic
DMSA (Succimer) (Chemet)	Heavy metal (especially lead, mercury)	Pralidoxime (2-PAM) (Protopam)	Organophosphate
Edetate disodium, d-Penicillamine	Heavy metal	Protamine	Heparin
		Pyridoxine	Isonicotinic acid hydrazide (INH), ethylene glycol
		Prussian blue	Thallium, radioactive cesium
		Sodium bicarbonate	Sodium channel blockers, alkalinization of urine or serum
		Sodium thiosulfate	Cyanide
		Thiamine	Ethylene glycol, Wernicke's syndrome, *Gyromitra* mushrooms, hydrazine
		Vitamin K	Warfarin (Coumadin), warfarin-based rodenticides

TABLE 31.5 Acetaminophen Toxicity.

Stage	Time Frame	Symptoms
I	0–24 hours	May be asymptomatic or experience lethargy, diaphoresis, mild gastric upset, including nausea, vomiting, and anorexia
II	24–48 hours	May have no complaints or develop liver failure, abnormal liver function tests, prolonged partial thromboplastin time, increasing bilirubin levels, right upper quadrant pain, hepatomegaly, oliguria
III	72–96 hours	Massive hepatic dysfunction, liver enzymes >100 times normal, hypoglycemia, jaundice; patient appears acutely ill; can progress to hepatic failure, encephalopathy, and death
IV	4 days to 2 weeks	If patient survives Stage III, enters recovery phase characterized by slow resolution of hepatic dysfunction

metabolites accumulate. An acute toxic dose of acetaminophen for children older than 6 years is 10 g or 200 mg/kg, and 7.5 g is considered an acute toxic dose in adults.[6] Higher levels are tolerated in pediatric patients without toxicity because of their ability to better metabolize the drug.

Serum acetaminophen levels of 200 mcg/mL or greater 4 hours after ingestion are considered toxic, and treatment should be initiated. Levels may continue to rise up to 4 hours after ingestion of a toxic amount. Individuals at risk for acetaminophen toxicity at lower doses include those with malnutrition or preexisting hepatic dysfunction and those taking anticonvulsant medications such as phenytoin or carbamazepine.

Signs and symptoms of acetaminophen toxicity develop slowly and can be overlooked until significant damage has occurred. The clinical course of acetaminophen toxicity occurs in 4 phases. Table 31.5 describes the time frame and symptoms for each stage. Initial acetaminophen levels should be drawn 4 hours after ingestion. Plotting the 4-hour acetaminophen value on published, evidence-based resources, such as the Rumack-Matthew nomogram, determines whether the patient is at risk for potential hepatotoxicity. This nomogram is useful only for acute, single-dose poisonings not combined with other agents (such as opioids or anticholinergics), which delay absorption. Obtain liver function studies, PT, complete blood count, BUN, and creatinine levels for patients who present with clinical symptoms and those whose levels fall within the "possible hepatic toxicity" range on the nomogram.

If a patient's 4-hour serum acetaminophen level remains below the identified level on the nomogram, no further treatment is required and serial acetaminophen levels are not indicated.[7] If the patient's serum acetaminophen level is above the potential risk line on the nomogram, antidotal treatment is indicated. *N*-Acetylcysteine is the antidote for acetaminophen and the preferred treatment for patients who have a hepatotoxic level. *N*-Acetylcysteine is available in an oral form (NAC, Mucomyst) and in an IV form (Acetadote). The oral and IV forms appear to be equally effective when administered within 8 to 10 hours of acetaminophen ingestion. *N*-Acetylcysteine is most useful when administered within 8 to 10 hours of ingestion but may be administered up to 24 hours after ingestion. *N*-Acetylcysteine works by replenishing the liver's supply of essential enzymes, allowing removal of acetaminophen metabolites.

Activated charcoal reduces acetaminophen absorption from the GI tract if administered within 2 hours of ingestion. Do not administer activated charcoal if more than 2 hours have elapsed since the time of ingestion unless delayed absorption is suspected. Repeat doses or multiple doses of charcoal do not decrease serum acetaminophen concentration. Activated charcoal does not reduce the effectiveness of *N*-acetylcysteine. However, oral *N*-acetylcysteine has been shown in vitro to diminish the efficacy of activated charcoal in binding to acetaminophen.[8]

Because effective therapy depends on early initiation of oral *N*-acetylcysteine, it is important to treat nausea and vomiting with antiemetics. All patients with a serum acetaminophen level falling into the "possible hepatic toxicity" range should receive *N*-acetylcysteine. Patients with significant poisoning suspected should begin *N*-acetylcysteine therapy on arrival without waiting for results of the serum acetaminophen level.[9]

The standard initial dose of oral *N*-acetylcysteine is 140 mg/kg, followed by half the calculated amount every 4 hours for 17 additional doses. Continue to treat if the patient remains symptomatic. Because of the foul taste and odor, *N*-acetylcysteine is usually given through a gastric tube or diluted in fruit juice or soft drinks. If the patient vomits within 1 hour of ingestion, the dose should be repeated.

Anaphylactic reactions with *N*-acetylcysteine are rare but have been reported to occur more frequently in patients receiving the IV form. Thus the oral form should be considered for patients with hypersensitivity reactions.[10] Administration of *N*-acetylcysteine in the United States generally occurs via the oral route unless the patient has refractory vomiting. Because acetaminophen crosses the placenta and can cause fetal liver toxicity, *N*-acetylcysteine should not be used in pregnant patients.

Nonsteroidal Antiinflammatory Drugs

Nonsteroidal antiinflammatory drugs (NSAIDs) are a class of drugs aimed at decreasing inflammation mediated by prostaglandins. Ibuprofen is the most common NSAID. Toxic ingestions of NSAIDs typically present with GI upset, with hemorrhage and renal damage with larger doses. Ibuprofen ingestion of more than 100 mg/kg is associated with GI symptoms, including abdominal pain, vomiting, and diarrhea. Very large ingestions may cause drowsiness, coma, acidosis, apnea, bradycardia, and renal failure. Management of patients primarily consists of detoxification measures and supportive and symptomatic care. Patients presenting within 1 to 2 hours of an ingestion of more than 100 mg/kg of ibuprofen or 10 tablets of any other NSAID should receive activated charcoal. Symptoms of gastric irritation can be treated with antacids, a mucosal protective agent, or a proton pump inhibitor.

Central Nervous System Stimulants

CNS stimulants are a loosely related group of legal and illegal drugs simulating or mimicking the sympathetic branch of the autonomic nervous system. Illicit CNS stimulants include cocaine and methamphetamines. Street names for cocaine include crack, rock, coke, snow, and blow. Street names for methamphetamines include speed, meth, chalk, ice, crystal, crank, glass, and grit. Some CNS stimulants are available by prescription for the treatment of narcolepsy, obesity, and attention-deficit/hyperactivity disorder in children. Other CNS stimulants such as caffeine, phenylpropanolamine, and pseudoephedrine are common ingredients in OTC diet pills, cold remedies, and alertness aids. Legitimate CNS stimulants are less potent and produce fewer euphoric or psychotic effects than their illegal counterparts; however, sufficient doses produce similar physiologic responses. CNS stimulants can be ingested, injected, inhaled, snorted, and absorbed rectally or vaginally.

Although CNS stimulants are not all the same, their actions, side effects, and hazards are similar. Table 31.6 lists the effects of a stimulant based on the degree of intoxication. Street drugs, such as cocaine and amphetamines, are often diluted or "cut" with other CNS stimulants (e.g., caffeine, phenylpropanolamine, or phencyclidine hydrochloride [PCP]), making precise identification of specific agents difficult. CNS stimulants are rapidly absorbed from the gut, with onset of action minutes after injection or inhalation. These stimulants have relatively short half-lives and produce varying degrees of α-, β_1-, and β_2-adrenergic receptor innervation.

Patients present with a wide range of responses and symptoms related to the drug and quantity consumed (see Table 31.6). The patient may experience a sense of omnipotence, excitement, hyperalertness, hyperactivity, hypersexuality, anxiety, agitation, aggression, hallucinations, mania, or paranoia. Tachycardia, hypertension, cardiac dysrhythmias, hemorrhagic stroke, coronary artery spasms, and myocardial infarction can also occur. Neurologic effects include pupil dilation, tremors, restlessness, delirium, seizures, and coma. Stimulation of the GI tract produces nausea, vomiting, and diarrhea. Other effects include hyperthermia, rhabdomyolysis, piloerection (goose bumps), and coagulopathies.

The toxic dose is highly variable and depends on the agent or agents involved, route of entry, individual tolerance, and drug amount. Toxicologic screening of urine or blood provides a rapid qualitative test for common CNS stimulants; quantitative measures do not correlate well with clinical status. Initial care addresses airway, breathing, and circulatory issues; ongoing care is performed based on specific symptoms exhibited by the patient. Because of an increased metabolic

TABLE 31.6 Clinical Effects of Central Nervous System Stimulants.

Degree of Intoxication	Effects
Mild	Insomnia, talkativeness, restlessness, garrulousness, agitation, aggression, tremor, hyperactivity
Moderate	Mydriasis, headache, nystagmus, hypertension, tachycardia, chest pain, dysrhythmias, hallucinations
Severe	Paranoia, shock, hyperthermia, rhabdomyolysis, acute tubular necrosis, acidosis, hyperkalemia, seizures, coma, myocardial infarction
Late	Chronic abusers may be exhausted after bingeing due to intense exertion and dopamine depletion; may sleep for hours; can be difficult to awaken, but when aroused, the patient is oriented

rate, diaphoresis, and drug-induced diuresis, this population is frequently dehydrated. Adequate fluid volume is essential to minimize complications such as tachycardia, hyperthermia, and myoglobinuric renal failure.

Gastric lavage may be performed if oral ingestion was within an hour of arrival to the ED, there is no potential of airway compromise, and the risk for seizure is low. The treatment of choice is activated charcoal. Administer a single dose of activated charcoal as soon as possible. Gastric decontamination has no benefit when these drugs are inhaled, snorted, or injected. "Body packers" who have ingested cocaine-filled balloons or condoms may receive activated charcoal to absorb cocaine from the GI tract in case the containers rupture.

No specific measures are used to promote CNS stimulant elimination. Urinary acidification enhances excretion of some CNS agents but places patients at risk for rhabdomyolysis. Whole bowel irrigation has been used successfully to remove swallowed body-packed or body-stuffed drugs. Endoscopic or surgical removal may be necessary if packets rupture.

Treatment of CNS stimulant toxicosis is largely symptomatic. Symptoms can progress rapidly, mandating diligent observation. Continuous cardiac and blood pressure monitoring detects tachycardia, dysrhythmias, and hypertension. A 12-lead ECG is indicated for patients with chest pain or shock. The risk for acute coronary syndrome is highest in the first hour, but the syndrome may occur 4 to 6 hours after cocaine use.[11] Cocaine-induced coronary artery vasospasm reduces myocardial oxygen supply when there is a greater myocardial oxygen demand. Cocaine-induced coronary artery vasospasm is more pronounced in smokers. Cocaine increases platelet activation and aggregation and produces vascular endothelial damage, which can lead to greater coronary artery damage in long-term users. Due to the potential for rapid onset of severe hyperthermia, check body temperature frequently until symptoms subside.

The patient with a significant CNS stimulant overdose can be paranoid, incredibly strong, and anesthetized to pain. Prevent injury to the patient and others by sedating psychotic patients with benzodiazepines. Exclusive use of physical restraints can cause extreme agitation and intense muscle activity, contributing to hyperthermia and rhabdomyolysis. After the patient is under control, provide a minimal-stimulation environment.

CNS stimulants affect the sympathetic nervous system, so a β-blocker (e.g., propranolol, esmolol) may be used for treatment of significant overdoses, sometimes given in combination with a vasodilator. Intense muscle activity and increased metabolic rate can rapidly produce core temperatures greater than 104°F (40°C). Cool patients aggressively.

IV benzodiazepines are the agents of choice for treatment of actual or impending seizures. Adequate seizure control is essential because strenuous muscle use contributes significantly to hyperthermia.

Opiates

Originally derived from the opium poppy, opiates are among the oldest known analgesic agents, having been used for thousands of years. Today opium is refined into many different drugs. Numerous synthetic opioids are also available. In the United States, single-agent and multidrug formula opiates can be legally obtained only by prescription. Narcotic toxicosis is often associated with IV abuse. Overdoses result from both pharmacologically prepared and "street drug" versions. Illicitly obtained opiates may be cut with caffeine, amphetamines, PCP, strychnine, lactose, or powdered sugar. Cointoxicants may be responsible for many of the patient's symptoms.

Although there are significant differences among opiate agents, all act on the CNS, producing variable degrees of sedation, euphoria, analgesia, and amnesia. Their psychic effects make opiates popular drugs of abuse. CNS depression sufficient to induce coma can occur with large drug doses or with relatively small amounts in novice users. Death occurs from the side effects of the drug, most notably respiratory arrest and pulmonary edema. Tolerance and dependence are common phenomena; addiction may follow chronic use. Table 31.7 lists potential effects of narcotic abuse and toxicity.

Opiates also act on the respiratory center in the brain stem, producing depression and apnea. These agents slow the GI system, making constipation a common side effect. Opiates such as paregoric and diphenoxylate hydrochloride with atropine (Lomotil) are prescribed specifically for this action. Signs and symptoms of opiate toxicity and abuse can be related to specific effects of the agent, substance abuse, lifestyle, or acute drug withdrawal.[12]

A qualitative toxicologic screen documents recent opiate use, but levels do not correlate with clinical presentation because of the number of substances available and the wide range of individual tolerance. Oral ingestions of opiates should be treated as soon as possible with activated charcoal, which effectively binds and reduces absorption into the circulation. Gastric emptying is not necessary if activated charcoal can be given promptly. Cathartic agents, in conjunction with charcoal, may be useful for enhancing drug elimination in opiate toxicity because of drug-induced intestinal hypomotility. However, they should be implemented only in patients with a secure airway.

TABLE 31.7 Effects of Narcotic Abuse and Toxicity.

Etiology	Potential Effects
Narcotic	Pinpoint pupils, respiratory depression, mental changes, hypotension, visual hallucinations, analgesia, amnesia, sleep, coma
Lifestyle	Skin abscesses, cellulitis, endocarditis, septicemia, track marks, malnutrition, dental disease, hepatitis, human immunodeficiency virus infection, tuberculosis, pulmonary edema, fecal impaction, septic arthritis, frequent trauma
Withdrawal	Rhinorrhea, tearing, yawning, dilated pupils, abdominal pain, diarrhea, diaphoresis, nasal congestion, vomiting, headache, piloerection, chills, fever, joint pain, agitation, confusion, hyperactivity

Naloxone is the antidote for opiate poisoning or toxicity. Administer naloxone at 0.2-mg increments until the patient's respiratory status and level of consciousness improve. Naloxone may require redosing every 20 to 60 minutes in some patients. Naloxone can be administered intravenously, intramuscularly, subcutaneously, or intranasally. It antagonizes opiate receptor sites in the CNS, reversing opioid effects of respiratory depression and decreased level of consciousness. Doses of 4 mg or higher may be used in cases of severe opiate toxicity. Full and sudden awakening is rarely desirable. Naloxone has a ½- to 2-hour duration of action, which may be less than that of the particular narcotic involved. Repeat doses or continuous IV naloxone infusions may be indicated and should be titrated to clinical response.

Sedative-Hypnotics and Barbiturates

Sedative-hypnotics are CNS depressants. Their chief effect is respiratory depression, which can be increased by the coingestion of alcohol or other depressant medications. These medications are commonly prescribed to induce sleep and allay anxiety. Sedative-hypnotics include the following: barbiturates such as phenobarbital; nonbarbiturates such as the benzodiazepines diazepam (Valium), alprazolam (Xanax), flurazepam (Dalmane), and chlordiazepoxide (Librium); and antihistamines such as hydroxyzine (Atarax, Vistaril).[5] This class contains a large number of substances with broad variation in their indications, potency, and duration of effect.

Benzodiazepines potentiate effects of the inhibitory neurotransmitter γ-aminobutyric acid (GABA), producing CNS depression. The toxic effects of benzodiazepines are an extension of their therapeutic effects, and a milligram-per-kilogram toxic dose has not been established.

Qualitative serum benzodiazepine levels confirm the presence of these agents. Quantitative levels are not particularly useful because of significant individual variability. Therefore interventions are dictated by the patient's clinical status rather than by serum drug levels.

The clinical features of benzodiazepine intoxication include slurred speech, incoordination, unsteady gait, drowsiness, lethargy, hypothermia, confusion, and coma. Profound coma suggests involvement of other CNS depressants. Significant circulatory compromise after isolated benzodiazepine ingestion is rare, so other causes should be considered.

Benzodiazepines have a low order of toxicity when ingested alone and rarely cause death, whereas the others may cause hypotension and deep coma. Barbiturates are highly toxic, have a high abuse potential because of their euphoric effects, and are classified according to their duration of action.

Gastric emptying is of no additional value if activated charcoal can be given promptly. Administer a cathartic agent along with the charcoal to counteract GI hypomotility and enhance fecal drug elimination. Hemodialysis and charcoal hemoperfusion have little benefit in benzodiazepine overdose. Flumazenil (Romazicon) is the antidote for benzodiazepines. Flumazenil competes directly with benzodiazepines at their receptor sites. However, flumazenil administration can induce seizures in those with benzodiazepine addiction and in those with concomitant tricyclic antidepressant (TCA) overdose. Therefore, because benzodiazepine toxicosis is associated with low morbidity and mortality, the decision to administer flumazenil must be considered carefully. The starting dose is 0.2 mg IV over 30 seconds. An interval of at least 30 seconds should pass before administering the next dose of 0.3 mg. Further doses of 0.5 mg may be administered every 60 seconds up to a total dose of 3 mg.

Tricyclic Antidepressants

There are a variety of TCA drugs available, including amitriptyline (Elavil), trazodone (Desyrel), nortriptyline, imipramine (Tofranil), desipramine (Norpramin), and doxepin (Sinequan). The use of TCAs has decreased during the past decade because of the increase of selective serotonin reuptake inhibitors (SSRIs) for the management of depression. Along with depression, TCAs are used for patients with chronic pain, panic disorder, and obsessive-compulsive disorder. TCA overdoses are usually associated with suicidal intent.

TCAs inhibit the cardiac fast-sodium channels, α-adrenergic receptors, and histamine receptors. They are well absorbed from the GI tract and are difficult to remove from the body once absorbed. Toxicity may not be closely associated with a milligram-per-kilogram ingested dose. The lethality of these drugs is related to their very narrow therapeutic index. Generally, an ingestion of greater than 10 mg/kg is likely to produce significant toxicity. Serum levels do not correlate well with clinical effects. A qualitative urine study is sufficient to confirm ingestion.

Because TCAs produce neurotoxicity, cardiotoxicity, and anticholinergic effects, signs and symptoms of TCA poisoning fall into three general categories. Neurotoxicity is characterized by lethargy, confusion, delirium, and hallucinations. CNS depression, coma, and seizures can occur. Profound CNS depression can lead to apnea and respiratory failure. Cardiac manifestations include hypotension and numerous ECG changes such as prolonged PR intervals, prolonged QRS intervals, prolonged QT intervals, ST- and T-wave abnormalities, conduction blocks, and tachycardia. Sinus tachycardia is a common rhythm seen in the early presentation of the patient. Ventricular tachycardia and fibrillation are more frequent in severe poisonings complicated by acidosis, hypotension, and extreme QRS prolongation. Polymorphic tachycardia (e.g., torsades de pointes) is not commonly associated with TCA overdose. TCA poisoning should be suspected in any patient with lethargy, coma, or seizures accompanied by QRS prolongation. A major cause of death from TCA poisoning is refractory hypotension due to decreased contractility and peripheral vasodilation.

Anticholinergic effects include mydriasis, flushed skin, dry mucous membranes, anxiety or psychosis, tachycardia, elevated body temperature, and urinary retention.

Respiratory arrest can occur quickly, and death from TCA toxicity may happen within a few hours of admission. Do not attempt to induce vomiting because CNS depression can develop rapidly. For large overdoses, protect the patient's airway with endotracheal intubation, then administer activated charcoal. Activated charcoal effectively binds TCAs, dramatically reducing their half-life. Gastric emptying is not recommended in the routine management of patients with TCA poisoning.[13] Because of TCA's anticholinergic effects, intestinal transit time is significantly lengthened; administering activated charcoal with sorbitol can increase drug elimination and prevent GI obstruction. TCAs are highly tissue-bound, so hemodialysis is not effective.

Continuous cardiac monitoring is imperative for all significant TCA ingestions. Treat ventricular dysrhythmias with amiodarone or lidocaine. Do not administer procainamide (Pronestyl) or other type 1A antidysrhythmic agents. This class of antidysrhythmic has been associated with the development of QRS widening progressing to asystole. Serious conduction blocks may occur with acute TCA overdose; pharmacologic therapy is rarely helpful, and external pacing is usually the only effective intervention.

Systemic alkalinization with sodium bicarbonate is indicated in patients with QRS widening, ventricular dysrhythmias, and/or hypotension.[14] Sodium bicarbonate can narrow the QRS, improve systolic pressure, and control ventricular dysrhythmias. The increase in pH lowers free drug concentrations, making it less available to bind to sodium channels. Sodium bicarbonate is administered initially as a 1- to 2-mEq/kg bolus. Further doses are titrated to maintain a systemic pH of 7.5 to 7.55. This can be accomplished by the addition of sodium bicarbonate to IV fluids, guided by arterial blood gas values. Potassium chloride 10 to 20 mEq may be added to IV fluids to prevent hypokalemia secondary to sodium bicarbonate administration. Hypotension is initially managed with normal saline boluses; however, catecholamine vasopressors (e.g., norepinephrine, phenylephrine) are necessary for refractory hypotension. Treat seizures acutely with a short-acting benzodiazepine such as diazepam or lorazepam. Phenytoin is a sodium channel–blocking drug and should not be used to treat TCA-induced seizures.

Toxic Alcohols

In addition to ethanol, three other alcohols can cause severe poisoning. Toxic alcohols exist in many common household products not generally considered dangerous. Methanol, also known as "wood alcohol," is found in windshield wiper fluid, canned fuel (Sterno), and solvents such as paint removers. Isopropanol is a major component of rubbing alcohol, disinfectants, cleansers, and nail polish removers. Ethylene glycol is an odorless substance contained in antifreeze, detergents, paints, polishes, and coolants. Its sweet taste and fluorescent color are particularly appealing to children and pets. Toxic alcohol ingestions can be accidental, recreational, or suicidal or may occur in desperate alcohol abusers unable to obtain ethanol. In addition to oral ingestion, toxic alcohols may be inhaled or topically absorbed.

These alcohols are relatively nonpoisonous before hepatic conversion, by the enzyme alcohol dehydrogenase, to their toxic metabolites. The toxins—glycolaldehyde (ethylene glycol), formaldehyde and formic acid (methanol), and acetone (isopropanol)—produce widespread damage and metabolic dysfunction.

Clinical findings of alcohol intoxication include CNS and respiratory depression. Methanol toxicity causes nausea, vomiting, abdominal pain, blindness, and coma. The patient with isopropanol ingestion presents with acetone breath odor, vomiting, and possibly significant hypotension. Ethylene glycol causes seizures, ataxia, coma, nystagmus, cardiac conduction disturbances, and dysrhythmias. Profound acidosis, renal failure, and pulmonary edema may also occur. If untreated in a timely manner, overdose will lead to death.

Appropriate laboratory studies should be performed to detect the following predicted abnormalities. In methanol intoxication, pronounced metabolic acidosis results from accumulation of formic acid. Isopropanol poisoning causes elevated serum acetone levels with ketones present in blood and urine. Hyperglycemia may also occur. With significant ethylene glycol toxicity, both anion gap metabolic acidosis and a large osmolar gap are evident.

Gastric lavage may be used in severe cases to remove any alcohol remaining in the stomach. Because of the rapid absorption of alcohols, the effectiveness of gastric lavage and activated charcoal is limited. The lungs are responsible for eliminating a significant amount of toxic alcohols; therefore intubation and mechanical ventilation can be used to maximize respiratory excretion in severe poisoning. Hemodialysis both effectively removes toxic metabolites and reverses acidosis.[15]

Ethanol and each of the toxic alcohols rely on the enzyme alcohol dehydrogenase for metabolism; however, the liver preferentially metabolizes ethyl alcohol. Administration of IV ethanol (100 mg/kg per hour) saturates available alcohol dehydrogenase molecules and slows methanol and ethylene glycol degradation, preventing accumulation of toxic metabolites. Ethanol infusions must be continued during dialysis with the rate increased to maintain a serum ethanol level of 100 mg/dL. The antidote, fomepizole (Antizol), can be substituted for ethanol in the treatment of ethylene glycol and methanol poisoning.[16] Fomepizole is a competitive inhibitor of alcohol dehydrogenase and inhibits the metabolism of ethylene glycol and methanol to their respective toxic metabolites. Neither fomepizole nor ethanol is indicated for isopropanol toxicity.

Other treatable causes of altered level of consciousness such as hypoglycemia and opiate ingestion cannot be overlooked. Fifty percent dextrose in water ($D_{50}W$) is given to reverse hypoglycemia; however, thiamine should be given concurrently because it allows the brain to metabolize the glucose. Naloxone is used to reverse opiate toxicity.

Organophosphates

Organophosphates are major active ingredients in insecticides such as ant sprays, flea sprays, and insect sprays, powders, and liquids. Toxicity varies significantly among chemical formulations. Organophosphates can be ingested, inhaled, or absorbed topically. Mass poisoning occasionally occurs from ingestion of unwashed produce or airborne contamination during crop spraying. Tabun (GA), sarin (GB), and soman (GD) are three examples of such agents falling into the organophosphate category.

The neurotransmitter acetylcholine is released into synaptic junctions in response to parasympathetic and sympathetic impulses. Acetylcholine plays a role in activation of specific smooth and skeletal muscles. Normally, cholinesterase enzymes rapidly break down acetylcholine, halting its action until another stimulus is received. Organophosphates aggressively bind to cholinesterase molecules, inhibiting their effect and allowing acetylcholine to remain unopposed in the neural synapse. This leads to "overactivity" and specific signs and symptoms. Organophosphate-cholinesterase bonds do not spontaneously reverse. After 24 to 48 hours of continuous binding, cholinesterase molecules are destroyed. Complete regeneration of cholinesterase can take weeks or even months.

Clinical findings depend on the specific organophosphate and amount of poison involved. Most oral or respiratory exposures will produce signs and symptoms within 3 hours. Symptoms from toxic dermal exposures may be delayed up to 12 hours. A few lipophilic organophosphates such as dichlofenthion, fenthion, and malathion may not produce significant distress for 1 to 5 days. Acute toxicity from organophosphates presents with manifestations of cholinergic excess. Primary toxic effects involve the autonomic nervous system, neuromuscular junctions, and CNS. The dominant clinical features of cholinergic toxicity include bradycardia, miosis, lacrimation, salivation, increased respiratory secretions, bronchospasm, urination, emesis, and diarrhea. Other symptoms are based on the nicotinic effects and include fasciculations, muscle weakness, and paralysis. Delirium, coma, and seizures may occur. Respiratory arrest may occur because of paralysis of the respiratory muscles.

Dermal exposures necessitate removal of all clothing and jewelry, followed by copious soap and water skin cleansing. Contaminated irrigation fluid should be considered hazardous waste.[17]

Interventions are largely supportive. Severely poisoned patients with a markedly depressed mental status should receive 100% oxygen and intubation. Effective antidote therapy counteracts organophosphate effects, although recovery requires synthesis of new cholinesterase. Because organophosphates produce a cholinergic syndrome, anticholinergics are the treatment of choice. Immediate therapy includes administration of IV atropine titrated to the therapeutic end point of clearing of respiratory secretions and cessation of bronchospasms and bronchoconstriction. Atropine should be administered beginning at 2 to 5 mg IV for adults and 0.05 mg/kg IV for children. Cases of severe poisoning may necessitate up to 5 mg of atropine every 3 to 5 minutes. The presence of tachycardia is not a contraindication to atropine administration in the organophosphate-poisoned patient. Atropine does not treat neuromuscular dysfunctions such as muscle fasciculations and weakness. Pralidoxime (2-PAM) may decrease or inhibit the effects of organophosphates on nicotinic receptors. It should be administered once atropine therapy is initiated. The initial IV dose is 30 mg/kg (adults) and 25 to 50 mg/kg (children) administered slowly over 20 to 30 minutes and based on severity of symptoms.[18] An initial bolus is followed by additional boluses every 1 to 2 hours or by a continuous infusion of at least 8 mg/kg per hour in adults and 10 to 20 mg/kg per hour for children.[19] Seizures should be treated with diazepam. Phenytoin is not recommended for seizures induced by organophosphates.

The organophosphate-intoxicated individual is at significant risk for contaminating others. Perform resuscitation and decontamination in a well-ventilated, isolated area. All people coming into contact with the poisoned individual require full personal protective equipment, including gloves and goggles. The patient's clothing is considered contaminated. Vomitus, gastric lavage material, and stool must be handled with caution, followed by careful disposal, to avoid secondary contamination.

Carbon Monoxide Poisoning

Carbon monoxide (CO) is a colorless odorless, and tasteless gas that binds to hemoglobin. Once combined with hemoglobin, it forms COHb, limiting the ability of hemoglobin to carry oxygen. This leads to severe hypoxia in patients with CO exposure. Length of exposure to the gas contributes to the extent of the poisoning, and symptoms rarely correlate with the serum level of COHb. Pregnant patients pose additional challenges because the exposure to CO lends itself to great risk to the fetus. CO is produced from multiple sources, including auto exhaust systems, smoke from wood fires, propane heaters, hibachi grills, and barbecues, Sterno (canned heat) stoves, and faulty furnaces. Patients can present with confusion, altered level of consciousness, hypotension, and seizures and appear in moderate to severe distress. A classic sign of CO poisoning is cherry-red skin and mucous membranes on physical examination. Death is usually the result of dysrhythmias. The half-life of COHb is 4 to 5 hours, and treatment with high-flow 100% oxygen will decrease the half-life. Patients with severe CO poisoning may require transfer to a facility with hyperbaric oxygen (HBO) therapy.[5]

Heavy Metals

Heavy metals involved in poisoning include lead, mercury, zinc, arsenic, and cadmium. Because heavy metals are a byproduct of the industrial age, all inhabitants of developed countries have measurable serum heavy metal levels. Intoxication by these agents is often chronic and subtle, making diagnosis difficult. For example, lead exposure may be related to daily use of glazed ceramic dinnerware or occasional ingestion of paint chips by a small child. Industrial exposure to button batteries, dental cement, marine paints, solder, and countless other products and manufacturing processes puts individuals at risk for heavy metal poisoning. Water pollution can cause mercury toxicity from seafood ingestion.

Absorption of these metals can occur through inhalation and ingestion. Chronic toxicities have a different presentation than acute poisonings. Exposure to an inorganic metal versus an organic metal salt also causes different effects. Heavy metal toxicosis is frequently associated with other poisons such as hydrocarbons (leaded gasoline), organophosphates (arsenic-containing pesticides), and carbon monoxide (mercury released in fuel burning). Without careful assessment and diagnostic evaluation, such polytoxicities can easily be missed.

Heavy metals have no known beneficial physiologic activity in humans and are not metabolized, so they accumulate in the tissues. The metals bind with reactive protein groups and enzymes, disrupting enzymatic function. Excretion from the body is slow, making the effects long term. Although symptoms vary with type of metal and extent of exposure, GI disturbances—ranging from nausea, vomiting, and diarrhea to GI hemorrhage—are frequently found. Central and peripheral nervous system effects include tremors, peripheral neuropathies, neuropsychiatric disturbances, and seizures. Acute inhalation produces chemical pneumonitis, pulmonary edema, and lung cancer.

Serum levels generally provide the best evaluation of heavy metal exposure, although urine and hair samples are sometimes tested. A plain film of the abdomen may show recently ingested metals in the GI tract. Therapeutic intervention is determined by extent of exposure and patient symptomatology. With certain chronic exposures, terminating contact with the offending agent or environment is all that is required. For very recent ingestions, standard gastric-emptying techniques can be employed; however, this is of no benefit for chronic ingestion or inhalation. Activated charcoal does not absorb metals.

Because heavy metals accumulate in tissues and are not metabolized, chelation therapy is the best means of eliminating these substances from the body. Chelating agents—administered orally, intramuscularly, or intravenously—bind to metals and facilitate excretion. Three chelating drugs are commonly used: dimercaprol, penicillamine, and ethylene-diaminetetraacetic acid (EDTA). The particular agent selected and route of administration vary with the toxin involved. Dosage is dependent on patient size and symptom severity. Because of the highly individualized circumstances surrounding each exposure, consultation with poison control center personnel should be undertaken before administering any chelating drug. Other supportive measures are largely determined on a patient-by-patient basis as symptoms dictate. Fluid volume deficits, anemia, cardiopulmonary dysfunction, and renal failure require intervention as appropriate.

Iron

Iron overdose is one of the most common and severe poisonings in children younger than 6 years. Unlike heavy metals, iron plays an important physiologic role. Its therapeutic usefulness has made iron widely available in many OTC formulations containing varying amounts of elemental iron. Iron toxicity begins with a direct corrosive effect on GI mucosa, leading to perforation, hemorrhage, and necrosis. After it is absorbed, iron initiates cellular toxicity by interfering with aerobic metabolism, causing lactic acidosis and producing free radical injury.

Doses less than 20 mg/kg of elemental iron are generally asymptomatic. Ingestions between 20 and 40 mg/kg may produce self-limited vomiting, abdominal pain, and diarrhea. Doses higher than 40 mg/kg are considered serious, and doses greater than 60 mg/kg may be lethal.[20]

Classically, the iron-poisoned patient passes through four clinical stages. In stage I, iron can produce GI corrosion. Symptoms of stage II range from nausea to massive hemorrhage. Patients who survive stage II may experience a latent period of apparent improvement over the next 12 hours. Stage III is signaled by abrupt onset of coma, shock, seizures, metabolic acidosis, coagulopathies, and hepatic failure. Survivors eventually enter stage IV, the recovery phase.

Diagnosis of iron ingestion is based on a history of exposure. Suggestive laboratory tests include elevated white blood cell count (greater than or equal to 15,000/mm^2 and hyperglycemia (greater than 150 mg/dL). Mild to moderate toxicity generally manifests with serum iron levels of 350 to 500 mcg/dL. Hepatotoxicity is observed at levels greater than 500 mcg/dL. Iron tablets may also be visible on abdominal radiographs.

If the acutely iron-toxic patient presents in hemorrhagic shock, early management focuses on basic stabilization. Gastric lavage may be considered if exposure was recent, tablets were chewed, or a liquid iron preparation was ingested. However, intact tablets are large and are unlikely to pass through a lavage tube. Activated charcoal does not absorb iron and is not recommended unless other drugs were ingested. Whole bowel irrigation is effective and can be considered. Massive ingestions may result in bezoar formation (i.e., a hard ball developing in the stomach), requiring endoscopic or surgical removal.

Deferoxamine, the specific antidote for iron poisoning, is indicated in cases of serious intoxication.[5] This chelating agent is generally given intravenously by constant infusion at a rate of 15 mg/kg per hour. The chelated deferoxamine-iron complex is excreted in urine, usually producing a characteristic orange or pink-red color. Therapy may be stopped when urine color or serum iron levels return to normal or the patient's symptoms have resolved.

Calcium Channel and β-Blockers

Calcium channel blockers are used for the management of angina, hypertension, dysrhythmias, and migraine prophylaxis. Some of the common calcium channel blocker agents include verapamil, nifedipine, diltiazem, bepridil, and mibefradil. Calcium channel blockers are rapidly emerging as one of the most lethal prescription drug ingestions. Children can become symptomatic with as little as one tablet. Overdose by short-acting agents is characterized by rapid progression to cardiac arrest. Overdose from extended-release agents results in delayed onset of dysrhythmias, shock, cardiac collapse, and bowel ischemia. Calcium channel blockers result in peripheral vasodilation, decreased heart rate, decreased contractility, and decreased conduction. Significant bradycardia, hypotension, and heart blocks are classic symptoms of calcium channel blocker poisoning. Hyperglycemia may occur because calcium channel blockade inhibits insulin release. Serum drug levels may be obtained but often take hours to perform. Treatment must be instituted based on symptoms and history. A 12-lead ECG should be obtained and continuous cardiac monitoring implemented. Cardiac markers may help differentiate drug-induced bradycardia from ischemic causes. Atropine may be tried if the patient has a hemodynamically unstable bradycardic rhythm; however, atropine is often not effective in calcium channel blocker toxicity. Transcutaneous pacing may be required for a hemodynamically unstable heart block. Dopamine at 5 to 10 mcg/kg per minute may improve heart rate and contractility. Administer a fluid bolus of normal saline for hypotension if there is no evidence of decompensated heart failure. Administer 5 to 15 mg of glucagon IV if hypotension persists; glucagon is the accepted antidote for β-blockers. Glucagon competes for receptor sites and neutralizes the effects of β-blockers. Either calcium chloride or calcium gluconate (up to 4 g) may be administered for hypotension or heart block associated with acute or chronic calcium channel blocker toxicity. Calcium is essential for contractility; calcium channel blockers stop the movement of calcium, resulting in diminished perfusion. If performed within 1 to 2 hours of ingestion, gastric lavage may be helpful for ingestion of extended-release formulas. Activated charcoal is recommended for calcium channel poisoning.

β-Adrenergic antagonists (β-blockers) are used in the treatment of hypertension, glaucoma, and various other disorders. They decrease cardiac rate and contractility. Recent data from the American Association of Poison Control Centers reported 2467 significant toxic ingestions.[21] Propranolol is considered the most toxic β-blocker. Immediate-release β-blockers are rapidly absorbed from the GI tract. The first critical signs of overdose may appear within 20 minutes but are more commonly observed within 1 to 2 hours. Bradycardia with hemodynamic compromise from hypotension is considered severe β-blocker toxicity and can lead to rapid clinical deterioration. Hypotension usually does not occur before the onset of bradycardia. β-Blockers may be associated with hypoglycemia, especially in patients with diabetes and in children. A 12-lead ECG and continuous cardiac monitoring are essential. Consider cardiac markers to rule out cardiac reasons for bradycardia and hemodynamic compromise. Glucagon may enhance cardiac contractility and conduction; the initial IV bolus is 3 to 10 mg. Transcutaneous pacing may be indicated in hemodynamically unstable bradycardic rhythms. Activated charcoal is indicated for the treatment of β-blocker poisoning.

Digitalis Glycosides

Digitalis glycosides are available in pharmaceutical preparations such as digoxin and digitoxin and can also be found in homes and yards in oleander, lily of the valley, rhododendron, and foxglove plants. At therapeutic and toxic doses, digitalis glycosides block the sodium-potassium-adenosine triphosphatase pump. With high serum concentrations, both vagal and sympathetic tone increase.

Clinical symptoms can be vague and difficult to diagnose, particularly with chronic overdoses in older adult patients. Findings include drowsiness, lethargy, and coma. Cardiac conduction disturbances (first-, second-, and third-degree heart block), ventricular dysrhythmias (premature ventricular contractions, ventricular tachycardia, and ventricular fibrillation), asystole, and profound hypotension also occur. (See Chapter 23 for discussion of management of various dysrhythmias.) Visual changes include the appearance of yellow or green halos around objects. The patient may experience anorexia, nausea, and vomiting, especially in cases of chronic poisoning. Elevated potassium levels are a prominent feature of cardiac glycoside poisoning, and hyperkalemia (greater than 5.5 mEq/L) must be treated aggressively.

Quantitative serum levels of digoxin or digitoxin can be useful for assessing an individual's degree of toxicity. Complete tissue distribution of cardiac glycosides requires at least 12 hours. Although serum levels are routinely drawn when toxicity is first suspected, samples collected before that time may not reflect a state of blood-tissue equilibrium. Because toxicosis can occur at various serum concentrations, symptomatology must guide therapy. Activated charcoal absorbs digitalis glycosides from the GI tract, decreasing systemic absorption. Multiple doses of activated charcoal have been suggested for the treatment of digoxin and digitoxin overdose, although limited clinical experience with this treatment has been reported.

High serum digitalis concentrations are an indication for antidote treatment. Digoxin immune Fab (Digibind), an ovine-derived antibody, attaches to digitalis glycosides and renders them inactive. Indications for Digibind are the presence of two or more of the following: life-threatening dysrhythmias, serum potassium levels higher than 5 mEq/L, and serum digoxin concentration greater than 10 ng/mL. The Digibind manufacturer also suggests administration if a single digitalis dose of more than 4 mg has been ingested by a child or more than 10 mg by an adult. An appropriate Digibind dosage is calculated based on a pharmacokinetic determination of total digoxin/digitoxin body load.[22]

Hydrocarbons

Hydrocarbons are found in petroleum, natural gas, coal, and bitumen. Exposure may be caused by inhalation, dermal contact, or ingestion. Accidental exposures are common in children younger than 5 years of age with access to kerosene, gasoline, or lighter fluid. Adults are usually poisoned as a result of occupational contact.

The effects of hydrocarbon toxicity can be divided into pulmonary aspiration and systemic absorption. The potential for pulmonary aspiration is inversely related to the substances' viscosity—the more viscous the hydrocarbon, the less toxic the substance. Aspiration of tiny amounts of low-viscosity hydrocarbons (gasoline, turpentine, lighter fluid, kerosene, petroleum, and ether) causes coughing and wheezing and can progress to a life-threatening chemical pneumonitis within hours. Systemic absorption occurs from ingestion, inhalation of hydrocarbon vapors, or dermal contact. Systemic manifestations of hydrocarbon toxicity vary widely by substance and time since exposure. Neurologic symptoms include confusion, headache, lethargy, ataxia, and coma. Hydrocarbons affect the heart's conduction system, causing complete heart block, asystole, and ventricular fibrillation. Nausea, vomiting, and GI bleeding have also been reported. Hepatic failure, renal failure, or hemolysis can occur days or even weeks after exposure. Dermal contact causes local irritation and chemical burns.

Exposure to high-viscosity substances (lubricating oil, petroleum jelly, grease, diesel oil, tar, and paraffin) with a low systemic toxicity potential requires no treatment. Chemicals with a low potential for systemic problems, but with high risk for aspiration pneumonitis, only require observation for pulmonary embarrassment, with appropriate respiratory support, should complications occur. Gastric suctioning and activated charcoal administration are indicated for recent ingestion of substances with low viscosity and high potential for systemic toxicity. A cuffed endotracheal tube must be inserted before gastric lavage to protect the patient from aspiration. Continuous cardiac and oxygen saturation monitoring is recommended. Remove clothing, and wash contaminated skin with copious amounts of soap and water. IV access should be established for emergency medications; however, fluids should be administered judiciously because of the potential for pulmonary edema development. Position the patient carefully to minimize risk for aspiration. Obtain a chest radiograph to rule out early pulmonary alterations. All symptomatic patients should be observed for 24 hours for pulmonary and cardiac problems. Patients who remain asymptomatic can be discharged after 4 to 6 hours.

Toxic Plants

Many plants found in the home and surrounding environment contain toxic substances. In fact, there are more than 100 species of toxic mushrooms alone. Some plants contain hallucinogenic, narcotic, or anticholinergic toxins, making them popular substances of abuse; others have neurotoxic or cardiotoxic effects. Many are simply GI irritants. Plants frequently associated with intentional or unintentional poisoning include poinsettia, jimsonweed, lily of the valley, and oleander. Cardiac glycoside plants such as oleander, foxglove, and lily of the valley cause a loss of cardiac excitability and hyperkalemia. Plants with anticholinergic properties (jimsonweed, deadly nightshade, and potato leaves) antagonize acetylcholine at the neuroreceptor site and cause a typical anticholinergic presentation of tachycardia, mydriasis, and fever.[5] Consult poison control to determine interventions for toxic plant exposures.

SUMMARY

Toxicologic emergencies are a routine cause of ED visits. The initial focus of care in any intoxicated patient is always stabilization of cardiopulmonary or hemodynamic issues. Treatment priorities include limiting poison absorption, enhancing substance elimination, and providing toxin- and patient-specific supportive interventions. The reader is referred to a detailed toxicology text or the experts at a poison control center for further information on any of the toxicities discussed in this chapter.

REFERENCES

1. Emergency Nurses Association. *Emergency Nursing Core Curriculum*. 7th ed. St Louis, MO: Elsevier; 2018.
2. Gummin DD, Mowry JB, Spyker DA, et al. 2016 Annual Report of the American Association of Poison Control Centers' National Poison Data System (NPDS): 34th annual report. *Clin Toxicol (Phila)*. 2017; 55(10):1072–1252. https://www.aapcc.org/annual-reports/. Accessed May 23, 2019.
3. Greene SL, Dargan PI, Jones AL. Acute poisoning: understanding 90% of cases in a nutshell. *Postgrad Med J*. 2005;81(954):204–216.
4. Proudfoot AT, Krenzelok EP, Vale JA. Position paper on urine alkalinization. *J Toxicol Clin Toxicol*. 2004;42(1):19.
5. Alymara V, Bourantas D, Chaidos A. Effectiveness and safety of combined iron chelation therapy with deferoxamine and deferiprone. *Hematol J*. 2004;5(6):477.
6. Farrell SE, Defendi GL. Acetaminophen toxicity. https://emedicine.medscape.com/article/820200-overview. Published January 22, 2018. Accessed May 23, 2019.
7. Olson K. Acetaminophen. In: Olsen K, ed. *Poisoning and Drug Overdose*. 3rd ed. Stamford, CT: Appleton & Lange; 1999.
8. Tenebein PK, Sitar DS, Tenebein M. Interaction between N-acetylcysteine and activated charcoal: implications for the treatment of acetaminophen poisoning. *Pharmacotherapy*. 2001;21(11):1333.
9. Hendrickson RG, Traub SJ, Grayzel J. Gastrointestinal decontamination of the poisoned patient. UpToDate. http://www.uptodate.com/online/content/topic.do?topicKey=ad_tox-/2200&selectedTitle=1~133&source=search_result. Published 2018. Updated March 15, 2019. Accessed May 23, 2019.
10. Kanter MZ. Comparison of oral and IV acetylcysteine in the treatment of acetaminophen poisoning. *Am J Health Syst Pharm*. 2006;63(19):1825.
11. Mittleman MA, Mintzer D, Maclure M, Tofler GH, Sherwood JB, Muller JE. Triggering of myocardial infarction by cocaine. *Circulation*. 1999;99(21):2739–2741.
12. Karch S, Stephens MG. Toxicology and pathology of deaths related to methadone: a retrospective review. *West J Med*. 2000;172(1):11–14.
13. Dargan PI, Coldbridge MG, Jones AL. The management of tricyclic antidepressant poisoning. *Toxicol Rev*. 2005;24(3):193.
14. Salhanick SD, Traub SJ, Grayzel J. Tricyclic antidepressant poisoning. UpToDate. http://www.uptodate.com/online/content/topic.do?topicKey=ad_tox/10025&selectedTitle=6~133&-source=search_result. Published July 2018. Updated March 1, 2018. Accessed May 23, 2019.
15. Unsal A, Basurk T, Sakac T, Ahbap E, Koc Y, Yilmaz M. Epidemic acute methanol intoxication as a result of illicit alcohol ingestion. *Nephro-Urol Mon*. 2012;4(1):366–371.
16. Lai MW, Klein-Schwartz W, Rodgers GC, et al. 2005 Annual Report of the American Association of Poison Control Centers' national poisoning and exposure database. *Clin Toxicol*. 2006;44(6-7):803–932.
17. Stacey R, Mofrey D, Payne S. Secondary contamination in organophosphate poisoning: analysis of an incident. *QJM*. 2004;97(2):75–80.
18. Eddleston M, Szinicz L, Eyer P, Buckley N. Oximes in acute organophosphorous pesticide poisoning: a systematic review of clinical trials. *Q J Med*. 2002;95(5):275–283.
19. Pawar KS, Bhoite RR, Pillay CP, Chavan SC, Malshikare DS, Garad SG. Continuous pralidoxime infusion versus repeated bolus injection to treat organophosphorus pesticide poisoning: a randomized control trial. *Lancet*. 2006;368(9553):2136–2141.
20. Morris C. Pediatric iron poisonings in the United States. *South Med J*. 2000;93(4):352–358.
21. Watson WA, Litovitz TL, Rodgers GC Jr , et al. 2004 Annual report of the American Association of Poison Control Centers Toxic Exposure Surveillance System. *Am J Emerg Med*. 2005;23(5):600.
22. Kawasaki C, Nishi R, Uekihara S, Hayano S, Otagiri M. Charcoal hemoperfusion in the treatment of phenytoin overdose. *Am J Kidney Dis*. 2000;35(2):323–326.

32

Dental, Ear, Nose, Throat, and Facial Emergencies

Joni Lee Winter

Emergencies involving the mouth, ears, nose, throat, and face are often associated with discomfort and pain. Some conditions can become life-threatening if associated edema compromises the airway. Infectious processes in the mouth and face can spread to the brain with potentially fatal systemic effects. Other concerns include functional, cosmetic, and psychological effects. This chapter describes conditions of the mouth, ears, nose, throat, and face that are commonly seen in the emergency department (ED). A brief review of anatomy is provided. Refer to the chapter on patient assessment for assessment parameters for head, ears, nose, and throat.[1]

ANATOMY

Structures of the mouth, ears, nose, throat, and face are intimately connected and encompass vital sensory organs. Injury or infection to one area may involve or affect adjacent areas.[1]

Mouth

Dentition consists of two main structures: the teeth and periodontium. Teeth encompass pulp, dentin, enamel, and root (Fig. 32.1). The pulp, located at the center of the tooth, provides neurovascular supply and produces dentin. Dentin is a microtubular structure that overlays the pulp, provides hydration, and cushions teeth during mastication. Enamel, which covers the crown, is the visible part of the tooth and the hardest substance in the body. The root anchors the tooth into alveolar tissue and bone. The periodontium is made up of gingiva and the attachment apparatus. Gingiva, or gums, is a mucous membrane with supporting fibrous tissue encircling the teeth and covering teeth not yet erupted. The attachment apparatus consists of the cementum, periodontal ligament, and alveolar bone.[2] In children, onset of primary and permanent teeth is important in determining management of injuries. Normal primary dentition begins erupting at 6 months, with 20 teeth by age 3 years. Permanent dentition begins at 5 to 6 years with eruption of the first molar and is usually completed by age 16 to 18, for a total of 32 teeth.[2,3]

Ears

The ear is divided into three sections: external, middle, and inner ear (Fig. 32.2). The external ear consists of the auricle (pinna), ear canal, and tympanic membrane (TM). The auricle is a cartilaginous skin appendage, which collects and directs sound to sensory organs within the ear. The S-shaped ear canal is approximately 2.5 to 3.0 cm long in adults, terminating at the TM. Glands lining the canal secrete cerumen, a yellow, waxy substance that lubricates and protects the ear.[4]

The TM, or eardrum, is a thin, translucent, pearly gray oval disk separating the external ear from the middle ear. It protects the middle ear and conducts sound vibrations to the ossicles.[3] On inspection with an otoscopic light, a cone of light at the anteroinferior aspect of the TM should normally be visible. Another landmark is the handle of the malleus (manubrium), which divides the TM anteriorly and posteriorly.[4,5]

The middle ear, an air-filled cavity inside the temporal bone, consists of the ossicles, windows, and eustachian tube. Three tiny ear bones, or ossicles, that conduct sound from the TM are the malleus, incus, and stapes. Round and oval windows open into the inner ear, where sound vibrations enter. The eustachian tubes connect the middle ear with the nasopharynx, allowing passage of air to equalize pressure on either side of the TM. They also provide drainage for middle ear and inner ear secretions into the nasopharynx. The inner ear houses the bony labyrinth, which provides the sensory organs for equilibrium and hearing.[4,5]

Nose

Externally the nose is a triangular, mostly cartilaginous structure that warms, filters, and moistens inhaled air, provides a sense of smell, and is the primary passageway for inhaled air to the lungs. The upper third of the nose, where the frontal and maxillary bones form the bridge, is bony. Two nares at the base of the triangle allow air to enter and pass into the nasopharynx. The internal nose is structured by hard and soft palatine (floor), frontal and sphenoid bones (roof), and inferiorly and superiorly by the cribriform plate of the ethmoid bone. Branches of the olfactory nerve pass through the cribriform plate. The nasal cavity is separated by the septum, which forms two anterior vestibules. The septum is usually deviated slightly to one side. Lateral walls are formed by three parallel bony projections—the superior, middle, and inferior turbinates—that help increase surface area to warm inhaled air.[1,5,6]

Blood supply to the nose originates from the internal and external carotid arteries. The internal maxillary artery branch of the external carotid artery supplies the posterior nasal septum and lateral wall of the nose. As a branch of the internal carotid artery, the anterior ethmoidal artery supplies blood

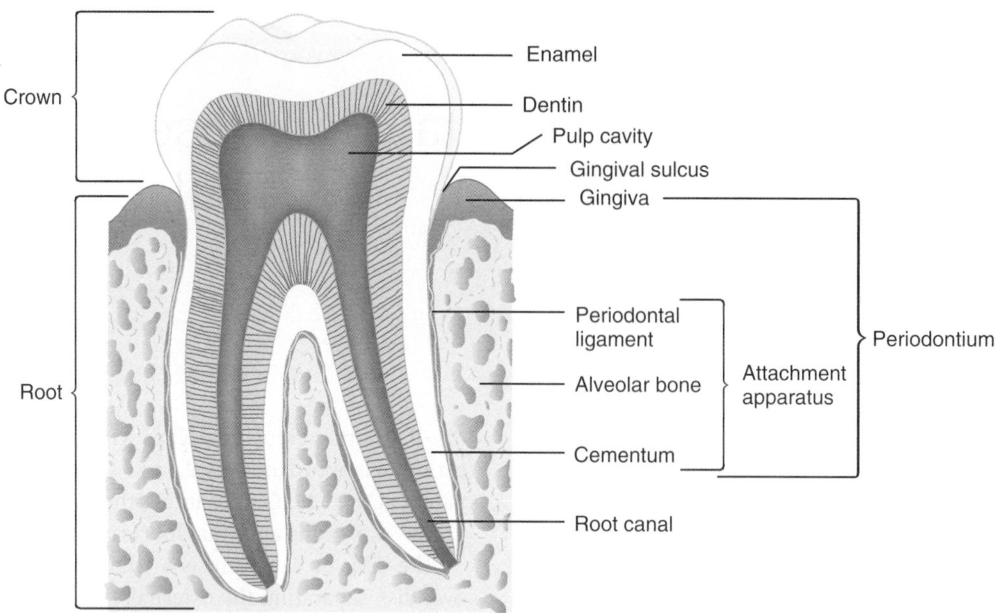

Fig. 32.1 Dental Anatomic Unit and Attachment Apparatus. (From Walls RM, Hockberger RS, Gausche-Hill M, ed. *Rosen's Emergency Medicine: Concepts and Clinical Practice*. Philadelphia, PA: Elsevier; 2018:771–790.)

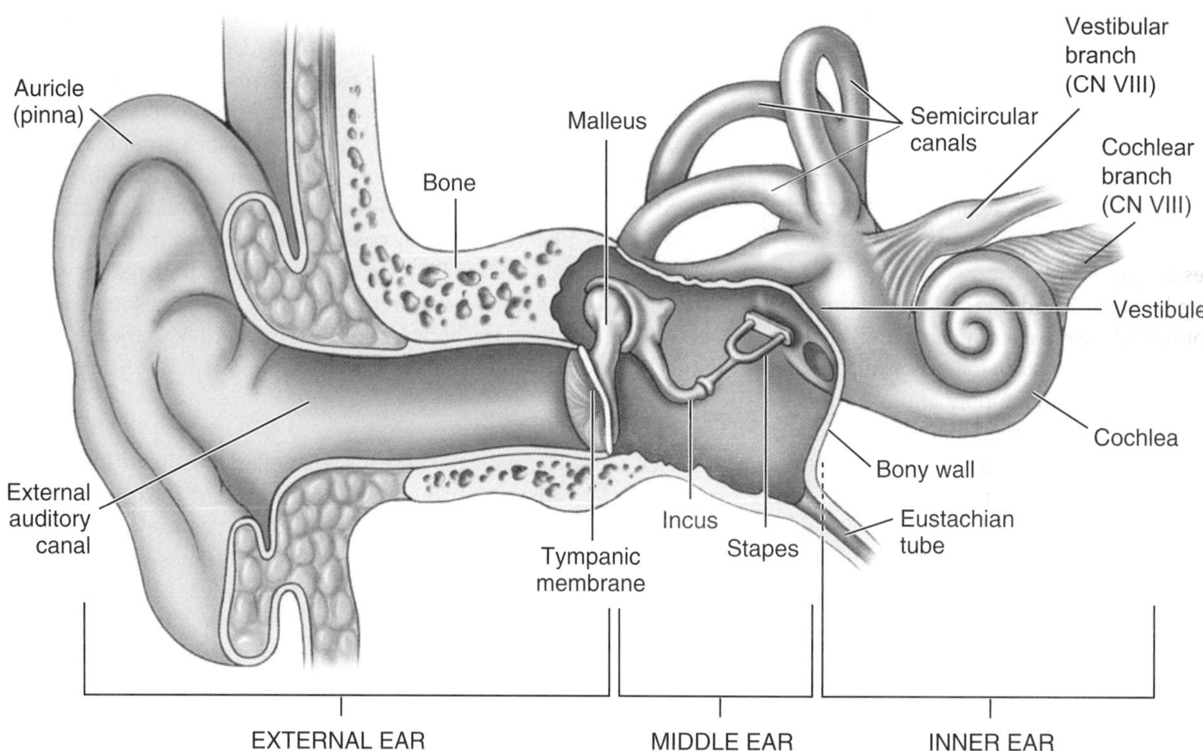

Fig. 32.2 Cross-Sectional View of the External, Middle, and Inner Ear. (From Herlihy B. *The Human Body in Health and Illness*. 6th ed. St Louis, MO: Elsevier; 2017.)

to the anterior septum at Kiesselbach's plexus in Little's area. This area is also supplied by the septal branches on the sphenopalatine and superior labial arteries.[5,6,7]

Throat

The throat, or pharynx, comprises the nasopharynx, oropharynx, and laryngopharynx (hypopharynx). The nasopharynx is positioned behind the nasal cavities and extends to the plane of the soft palate. The pharyngeal tonsils, or adenoids, and eustachian tube openings are located in this area. The oropharynx, a common passageway for both air and food, extends downward from the inferior soft palate to the level of the hyoid bone. The palatine tonsils, lymphoid tissue that filters microorganisms to protect the respiratory and gastrointestinal tracts, are found here. The laryngopharynx extends from the hyoid bone to the opening of the larynx anteriorly and the esophagus posteriorly. The pharynx allows passage of air into the larynx and enables speech and swallowing.[8,9] Pharyngeal constrictor muscles propel food or liquid into the esophagus. These muscles are also responsible for the cough and gag reflexes, which are controlled by the cranial nerves.[9,10] The larynx, or voice box, is a tubular, mostly cartilaginous structure that connects the trachea and pharynx; its main purpose is to allow air into the trachea. The epiglottis, a large, leaf-shaped piece of cartilage, lies on top of the larynx. This structure prevents aspiration by forming a lid over the glottis (the space between the vocal cords) so that liquids and food are routed into the esophagus and away from the trachea. The larynx is also responsible for voice production via the vocal cords.[8 10]

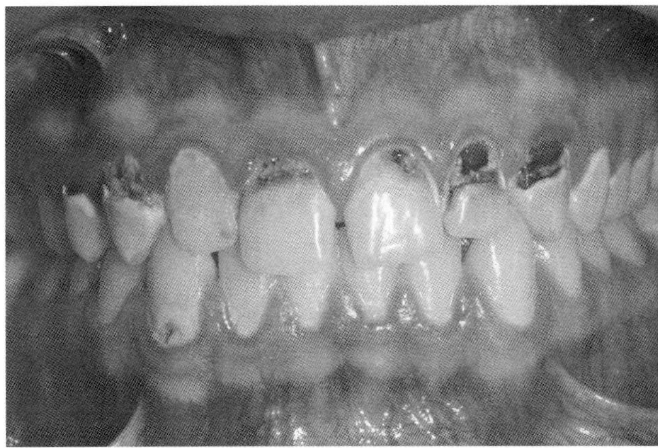

Fig. 32.3 Dental Caries. (From Neville BW, Damm DD, Allen CM. Physical and chemical injuries. In: *Oral and Maxillofacial Pathology*. 4th ed. Elsevier; 2016:259–302.)

Face

The bony structures of the face are symmetric and consist of a single vomer and mandible and the following pairs of bones: maxillae, palatine, zygomatic, lacrimal, nasal, and inferior nasal conchae. The 14 bones shape the facial skeleton and provide attachment for muscles that move the jaw and control facial expressions.[11] Cranial nerves V (trigeminal) and VII (facial) are responsible for facial innervation and movement, respectively.[1] The paranasal sinuses are sterile, air-filled pockets situated around the nose, eyes, and cheeks. The sinuses provide resonance for speech, shock absorption, and warm, humidify, and move secretions into the nasopharynx via ciliated mucous membranes. Four pairs of sinuses are named for their craniofacial location.[1,12] The ethmoidal and maxillary sinuses are present at birth, whereas the sphenoid and frontal develop between 5 and 8 years of age. However, most sinuses are not fully developed until adolescence.[13]

The temporomandibular joint (TMJ) is the point where the mandible connects to the temporal bone of the skull; it can be palpated bilaterally just anterior to the tragus of the ear. The TMJ is a synovial joint that allows hinge action to open and close the jaws, gliding action for protrusion and retraction, and gliding for side-to-side movement of the lower jaw.[14]

DENTAL EMERGENCIES

Dental emergencies affect the teeth and gums. Specific emergencies involve infection, eruption of new teeth, or trauma. The most common emergencies seen in the ED are related to pain. Common causes of dental pain include dry socket, fractured teeth, periodontal disease, dental abscess, erupting teeth, maxillary sinusitis, and post root canal surgery.[2,15]

Odontalgia

Dental caries is the most frequent cause of dental pain, or odontalgia (Fig. 32.3).[2] Too much sugar in the diet is largely responsible for decay. Dental caries is also caused by poor oral hygiene, which allows bacterial plaque to develop, which in turn form acids that break down and decalcify tooth enamel. Sodium fluoride, found in toothpaste, oral rinses, and public drinking water, helps stabilize the integrity of tooth enamel to prevent this breakdown. Affected teeth are usually tender to percussion and sensitive to heat, cold, or air.[16] If left untreated, decay progresses and invades dentin and pulp, eventually producing a hyperemic response. The pulp becomes inflamed, leading to pulpitis and finally pulpal necrosis. Occasionally pus leaks from the apex of the affected tooth as a periapical abscess forms.[15,17] Toothaches accompanied by facial or neck swelling should be assessed and promptly treated to prevent spread of infection. Clinical management includes antibiotics, topical anesthetics, nerve blocks, and analgesics, including parenteral narcotics, as palliative treatment until the patient receives definitive care from the dentist.[2,15–17]

Tooth Eruption

Between 6 months and 3 years of age, children's primary teeth erupt, causing a variety of symptoms including pain, irritability, disrupted sleep, nasal discharge and crying. Increased salivary gland production causes diarrhea as well as significant drooling. Decreased fluid intake related to dental pain may cause dehydration and low-grade fever. Care must be taken not to attribute significant fevers to this relatively benign process. Tonsillar or throat infections, thrush, other oral lesions, and respiratory emergencies such as epiglottitis (especially with excessive drooling) should be considered. In the second decade of life, third molars, or wisdom teeth, begin erupting, causing pain in adolescents and adults. Gingival inflammation secondary to wisdom tooth eruption may cause pericoronitis.

Topical anesthetics such as benzocaine are used sparingly to prevent sterile abscess formation. Acetaminophen is useful for analgesia in young children. To maintain hydration, popsicles are usually well received and also provide pain relief. When there is minimal oral intake, rehydration therapy may be necessary. In adults, frequent saline irrigation may be used to remove debris from the affected tooth. Nonnarcotic analgesia is effective for pain relief in adult patients. Any consistent swelling or drainage from the eruption site requires referral to a dentist or oral surgeon.[2,15–19]

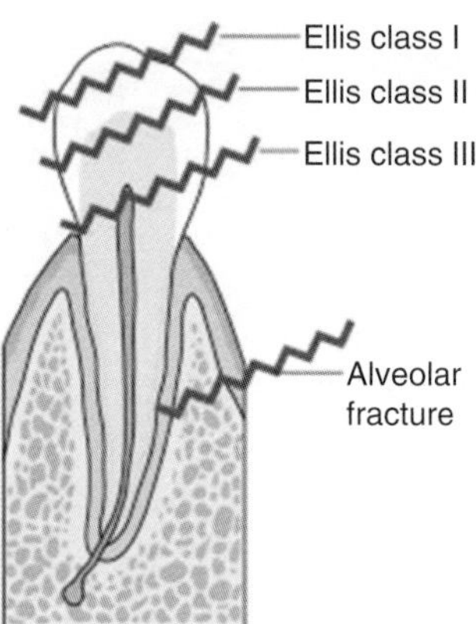

Fig. 32.4 Dental Fractures With Ellis Fracture Classification. (From Pfenninger JL, Fowler GC. *Pfenninger and Fowler's Procedures for Primary Care.* Philadelphia, PA: Elsevier/Mosby; 2011.)

Pericoronitis

If erupting molars become impacted or crowded, food and debris lodge under the pericoronal flap, causing gingival inflammation or pericoronitis. Pericoronitis is extremely painful, especially with opening and closing of the mouth. Earache on the affected side, sore throat, and fever may also occur. Surrounding tissues appear red and inflamed, with submandibular lymphadenopathy and trismus noted in some patients.

Warm saline or peroxide irrigation and mouth rinses are helpful in early stages of pericoronitis. When pus is present, incision and drainage may be necessary. However, antibiotic therapy is indicated. Follow-up with an oral-maxillofacial surgeon within 24 to 48 hours for removal of the affected third molar is highly recommended.[2,15–19]

Fractured Tooth

The most frequently seen dental emergency in the ED is a chipped or broken tooth, usually anterior maxillary teeth. Trauma to dentition occurs as a result of sports activity, motor vehicle collisions, propulsive objects, falls, convulsive seizures, and physical assaults or abuse. Child abuse should be considered in children sustaining physical trauma in the head and neck region.[20] The emergency nurse should assess for concurrent head injury or maxillofacial trauma. Aspiration of a tooth or fragment or an embedded tooth should also be considered.

Management of fractures of the anterior teeth is determined by the relationship of the fracture to the pulp as well as patient age. The Ellis classification system is used to describe location of tooth fractures (Fig. 32.4). Class I fractures are the most common, involving only enamel. Injured areas appear chalky white. Cosmetic restoration is possible with dental referral within 24 to 48 hours. Class II fractures pass through the enamel and expose dentin. The fracture area appears ivory-yellow. Fractures are urgent for children because there is little dentin to protect pulp. Bacteria pass easily into pulp, causing an infection or abscess if exposed for longer than 6 hours. Adults may be treated up to 24 hours later because the pulp is protected by a thicker layer of dentin, which reduces potential for infection. Class III fractures are a dental emergency. Injury to the enamel, dentin, and pulp cause a pink or bloody tinge to the fractured area. Exposure of pulp also exposes the nerve, causing significant discomfort. Apply calcium hydroxide paste to minimize discomfort from thermal sensitivity and to decrease infection risk. The patient should be referred to a dentist with follow-up within 24 hours. Oral analgesics or a nerve block is usually effective for pain control. Tetanus immunizations should be administered as appropriate. Patients will be placed on a liquid diet with ability to advance to soft foods after 1 week. Reassure the patient that cosmetic restoration is possible with enamel-bonding plastic materials.[2]

With facial trauma, assess the airway, breathing, and circulation (ABCs) before assessing the dental problem. History should include mechanism of injury, concomitant injuries, and tissue loss. Consider abuse in children, older adults, or disabled adults when the history does not correlate to the injury. Assess for tooth pain, thermal sensitivity, stability of the tooth in the socket, and malocclusion. Complications of tooth fractures include infection (pulpitis), malocclusion, embedded tooth fragments, aspiration of tooth fragments, color change, and loss of affected teeth.[1,2]

Tooth Avulsion

Tooth avulsion is a dental emergency. When a tooth has been torn from the socket, tissue hypoxia develops, followed by eventual necrosis of the pulp. Reimplantation within 30 minutes greatly increases chances for successful reimplantation and healing. The periodontal ligament cells die if the tooth is out of the socket for more than 60 minutes. Determine the mechanism and time of injury immediately on arrival. Handle the avulsed tooth by the crown to avoid damage to attached periodontal ligament fragments. These fragments aid in healing of the reimplanted tooth. Ideally the tooth should be rinsed and placed back in the socket as soon as possible. Immediate reimplantation is not always possible because of lack of patient cooperation, life-threatening injuries, or other factors at the scene of injury. In these cases, the tooth should be transported in Hank's solution (pH-preserving fluid), milk, saline, oral rehydration solution, or under the tongue of an alert patient. Use discretion with children, who may swallow or aspirate the tooth. Primary teeth (6 months to 6 years) are not reimplanted because fusion with the bone interferes with permanent tooth eruption and can cause cosmetic deformities. If the tooth cannot be found, examine the oral cavity and face to ensure the tooth is not embedded in soft tissue. A chest x-ray examination is recommended to rule out tooth aspiration.[1,2]

Symptoms include pain and bleeding at the site of the avulsion. Assess for concomitant head, neck, or maxillofacial injuries. Moist saline gauze may be applied to exposed oral tissues for comfort and to control bleeding. Administer analgesics and tetanus prophylaxis as indicated. Instruct the patient not to bite into anything with the affected tooth and to avoid hot or cold substances. Antibiotics and a referral to a dentist or oral surgeon for definitive care is recommended.

Patients should be advised to use a soft toothbrush and rinse with chlorhexidine.[2]

Dental Abscess

Primary dental abscesses are periapical and periodontal. Periapical abscesses occur as an extension of pulpal necrosis from a decayed tooth or traumatic injury. A pocket of plaque and food debris between the tooth and the gingiva causes localized swelling at the apex of the tooth, which leads to periodontal abscess formation. Normally abscesses are confined; however, certain infectious processes can spread to facial planes of the head and neck. The upper half of the face is affected with extension of infection from the maxillary teeth. Cellulitis in the lower half of the face and neck extends from the infection of the mandibular teeth. With localized abscesses the patient may have severe pain unrelieved by analgesics, fever, malaise, foul breath odor, and slight facial swelling near the affected tooth. An extensive abscess causes facial and neck edema, trismus, dysphagia, difficulty handling secretions, and potential airway obstruction.[2,21]

The typical therapy includes oral or parenteral narcotics, antipyretics, and antibiotics. If abscess fluctuance is present, incision and drainage with culture and sensitivity of the exudate are required. The patient should be instructed to take medications as directed, use warm saline rinses, and follow up with an oral surgeon, dentist, or ear, nose, and throat (ENT) specialist within 24 to 48 hours for definitive care. Admission for further diagnostic studies and intravenous (IV) antibiotics may be necessary if the patient has abnormal vital signs or is unable to take oral medications.[2,21]

Gingivitis

Gingivitis, or inflammation of the gums, is usually caused by poor dental hygiene, allowing for the accumulation of food debris and plaque in crevices between the gums and teeth. This periodontal disease, along with periodontitis (loss of supporting bony structure of the teeth), affects many adults. It is the most common cause of tooth loss today. Gingivitis may also occur with vitamin C deficiency or in pregnancy and puberty because of changing hormone levels.[2,4,21] If inflammation continues, alveolar bone is lost, leading to periodontitis and eventual loss of teeth. Visual evidence of gingivitis includes red, swollen gum margins and possible bleeding. Pain unrelieved by over-the-counter analgesics, difficulty chewing, and low-grade fever also occur. Topical anesthetics, analgesics, and oral antibiotic therapy/rinses are indicated. Patient teaching regarding good oral hygiene, including brushing and flossing three to four times a day with peroxide and warm water rinses twice daily, is extremely important to prevent extension of gingivitis.[2,21]

Ludwig's Angina

Ludwig's angina is the spread of an existing, untreated dental infection or cellulitis into three mandibular spaces: submandibular, sublingual, and submental. Infection spreads downward from the jaw to the mediastinum and is characterized by bilateral, boardlike, brawny induration of involved tissues and elevation of the tongue. The inherent danger with Ludwig's angina is respiratory distress and airway obstruction.[2,21]

The patient develops significant swelling of the anterior and lateral neck. Swelling of the submandibular tissue displaces the tongue superiorly. Other symptoms include pain and tenderness, trismus, muffled voice, dysphagia, drooling, and fever or chills. Dyspnea and decreased oxygen pressure occur secondary to edematous tissues. The patient may be anxious or restless. Offer reassurance, check the patient frequently, and explain all procedures to ease fears.

Priorities in the ED include maintaining ABCs, pain relief, and IV antibiotics. Elevate the head of the bed to prevent aspiration of secretions. Administer supplemental oxygen in concert with continuous pulse oximetry monitoring. Respiratory and mental status should be continuously monitored. Provide prescribed analgesics appropriate for the patient's degree of pain. Insert an IV catheter for IV fluids to prevent dehydration, to administer broad-spectrum antibiotics, and as an access for emergency medications. Diagnostic procedures such as determination of arterial blood gas levels, complete blood count (CBC) with differential, culture and sensitivity of exudate, and soft tissue x-ray films, or computed tomography (CT) scan of the neck, may be ordered. Definitive care by an oral-maxillofacial surgeon includes determining site of the initial infection, surgical drainage of pus with removal of necrotic tissue, and continued antibiotic therapy.[2,21]

EAR EMERGENCIES

Ear emergencies commonly seen in the ED involve infection, pain, foreign body in the ear canal, and injury of the TM. Most ear emergencies require instillation of some type of otic drops and otoscopic examination. To visualize for assessment and/or instill drops, one must pull the pinna up and back on the adult and straight down for pediatrics (Fig. 32.5).

Otitis

Otitis, or inflammation of the ear, may occur in any section of the ear. Symptoms vary with location; however, almost all cases of acute otitis cause significant discomfort.

Otitis externa is inflammation of the external ear canal and auricle. Also known as swimmer's ear, this condition is seen most often during the summer. Factors that predispose the patient to otitis externa include soaking or swimming in contaminated water, exposure to chemical irritants, cleaning the ear canal with a foreign object, regular use of ear devices, and a perforated TM. The most common infectious agents are usually bacteria, such as *Pseudomonas aeruginosa* or *Staphylococcus aureus* species. However, dermatologic and fungal conditions could be the source. Symptoms include pain, swelling, redness, and purulent drainage of the auricle and ear canal (Fig. 32.6). Pain is usually worsened by chewing or movement of the tragus or pinna. Regional cellulitis, partial hearing loss, and lymphadenopathy may also be present. Basic treatment measures cure >90% of patients without complications. Treatment includes keeping the ear dry, cleansing the external canal, ear wicks, and providing analgesics and

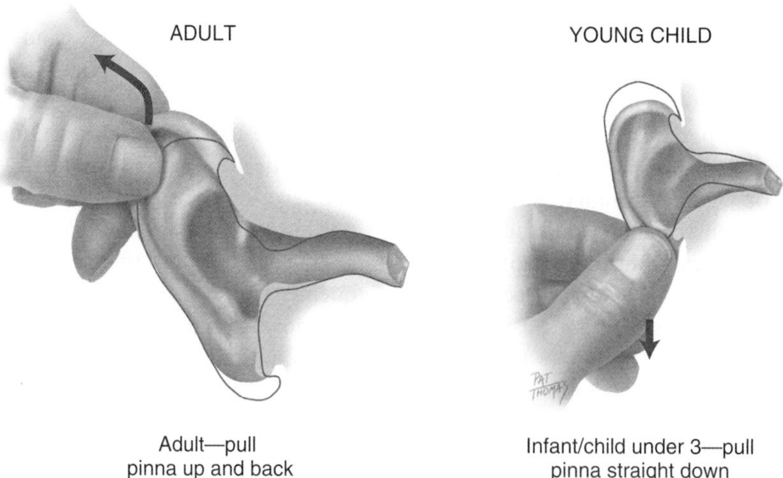

Fig. 32.5 **Ear Positioning for Assessment and Drop Instillation.** (From Jarvis C. Ears. In: *Physical Examination and Health Assessment.* 7th ed. St Louis, MO: Elsevier; 2016:325–351.)

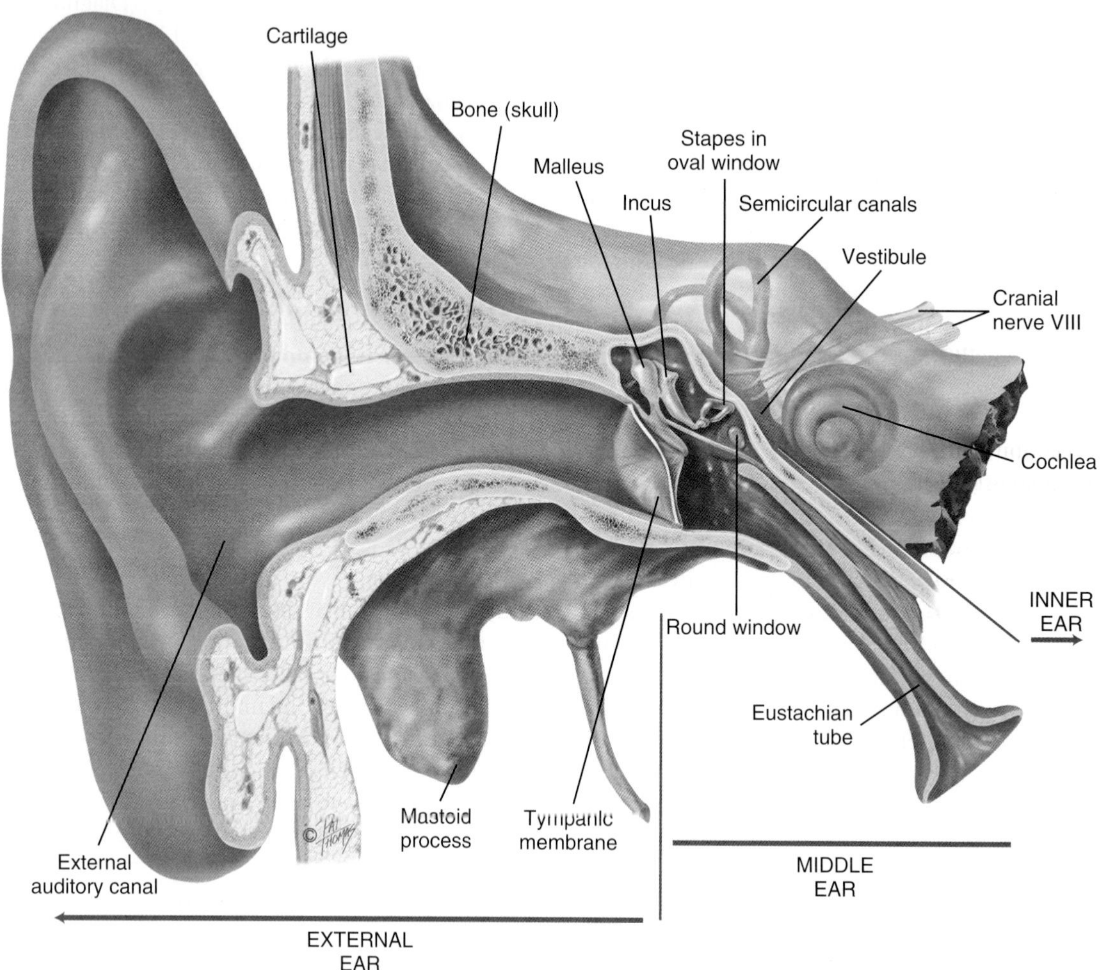

Fig. 32.6 **Otitis Externa (Swimmer's Ear).** (From: Jarvis C. Ears. In: *Physical Examination and Health Assessment.* 7th ed. St Louis, MO: Elsevier; 2016:325–351.)

antibiotics without or without topical steroids. Topical or otic antibiotics are used unless the patient has a persistent fever or regional cellulitis, in which case hospitalization and high-dose antibiotic therapy is needed. Otitis externa usually resolves in 7 days but frequently recurs. Patients should be instructed to use earplugs lightly coated with petroleum jelly for 2 to 4 weeks to protect the ear canal from water.[22–24]

Otitis media (OM), or infection of the middle ear, occurs most often in children under the age of 5. *Streptococcus pneumoniae, Haemophilus influenza,* and *Moraxella catarrhalis* are the most common causative bacterial organisms. However, bacterial OM may follow a viral infection and/or present as a coinfection. Acute OM is characterized by rapid onset of ear pain, headache, tinnitus, hearing loss, and nausea or vomiting. Infants and young children may present with irritability, crying, rubbing or pulling the ears, restless sleep, and lethargy. Other symptoms such as fever, rhinitis, cough, otorrhea secondary to rupture of the TM, and conjunctivitis occur at any age. Visualization of the TM, necessary for diagnosis, usually reveals a dull light reflex and whitish-yellow opacity. Bulging may also occur as the infection progresses. Redness of the TM is an inconsistent finding because it may be caused by crying or fever. Sinusitis and purulent rhinitis may frequently accompany otitis, especially in pediatrics.

Acute OM is treated with antibiotics, antipyretics, and analgesics such as acetaminophen or ibuprofen. Topical anesthetic otic solutions (e.g., Auralgan) for pain relief should be warmed before instilling. Treatment recommendations include immediate antibiotics for special populations or observation for 48 to 72 hours in those not meeting criteria, with initiation of antibiotic therapy if there is no resolution of symptoms. If not treated, acute OM can cause serious complications such as ruptured TM, meningitis, acute mastoiditis, intracranial abscess, neck abscess, facial nerve damage, or permanent hearing loss. First-line treatment is amoxicillin. Patients should complete the full course of antibiotic therapy and be reevaluated if there is no improvement in 48 to 72 hours. Encourage parents to ensure children finish prescribed medications and to keep follow-up appointments. For cases of OM with an effusion, patients should be reevaluated at 3-month intervals to determine whether the middle ear effusion persists. Chronic or persistent pediatric OM requires further intervention with quinolone antibiotics and referral to an otolaryngologist for myringotomy tube placement due to risk of hearing loss.[22–25]

Labyrinthitis, or inflammation of the inner ear, is rare. Causes include acute febrile illnesses, such as viral, bacterial, and autoimmune etiologies. The inner ear is the body's center of balance. The patient usually develops severe vertigo with nausea, vomiting, and gait disturbance. Vertigo usually lasts 3 to 5 days but may persist for weeks. Treatment includes bed rest, meclizine (Antivert) to control vertigo, antiemetics, and fluids for dehydration secondary to vomiting. Antibiotics are indicated for suppurative labyrinthitis.[26]

Ruptured Tympanic Membrane

A ruptured TM is most often the painful result of a bacterial infection—acute or chronic OM. Trauma such as skull fracture, foreign body insertion (e.g., cotton swabs, hairpins), explosions, or blows to the ear also rupture the TM. Children, especially those with chronic ear infections, are most often victims of this disorder. Symptoms include pain, bloody or purulent discharge, hearing loss, vertigo, and fever or the patient may be pain-free because pain and pressure are relieved with rupture. In trauma-related TM rupture, ear drainage should be checked for the presence of cerebrospinal fluid, which is indicative of basilar skull fracture. Otoscopic examination reveals the TM as slit-shaped or irregular. X-ray and/or CT examination of the skull, temporal bone, and cervical spine may be indicated with trauma. Hearing loss may be present in the affected ear, so speak slowly and clearly toward the unaffected ear while facing the patient. Large perforations require myringoplasty. If the middle ear is also involved, a tympanoplasty is performed. Perforations with 25% or less TM involvement heal spontaneously within a month.[27,28]

Management includes antibiotics, analgesics, and antipyretics. Carefully clean the ear canal of blood or debris with gentle suction, and obtain a culture and sensitivity of drainage. Irrigation is contraindicated with TM rupture. Instillation of quinolone otic drops is often done. The patient should be instructed to keep water out of the ears because this provides an environment conducive to bacterial or fungal growth. A piece of cotton lightly coated with petroleum jelly and placed in the affected ear helps repel water. The patient should follow up with an otolaryngologist for definitive care.[27,28]

Foreign Body

Cerumen is a common obstructive material in adults and pediatrics, often caused by cotton swabs pushing wax and cotton fibers deeper into the ear canal. Therefore education surrounding avoiding routine use of cotton swabs for ear cleaning is imperative. Cerumen color varies from yellow-brown to gray-black, with textures ranging from moist to dry waxy material. The wax can obstruct the view of the TM and impede hearing, so it must be removed. Approximately 57% of aging adults are prone to impacted cerumen. Use of hearing aids is a contributing factor because of increased cerumen production and obstruction of natural outflow from the ear.[4]

The patient who presents with a foreign body in the ear is most often a child younger than 8 years of age. Beads, small stones, toys, food, and insects are common culprits. Parents, often unaware of the foreign body, bring the child to the ED with an earache or purulent, foul-smelling ear discharge. Older children and adults may complain of decreased hearing and fullness in the affected ear. Insects, including roaches, can fly or crawl into the ear and become trapped, moving and buzzing in the ear, causing great discomfort and anxiety for the patient. Children with insects in the ear may be extremely frightened.[29,30]

Before attempting removal of impacted cerumen or a foreign body, evaluate for a history of ruptured TM or current infection. Explain the procedure to the patient in terms that are appropriate for his or her age. Cooperation is elicited from a child whose trust is not violated. Conscious sedation or restraints may be required in difficult situations. Methods for foreign body removal include suctioning, irrigation, and use of special tools under direct visualization. A good light source such as an operating otoscope or head lamp is imperative for these procedures. To best expose the ear canal, pull the auricle up and back for adults, down and back for children. Vegetables or other soft materials that may absorb water should not be irrigated. Subsequent swelling caused by water absorption makes removal more difficult. Live insects can be

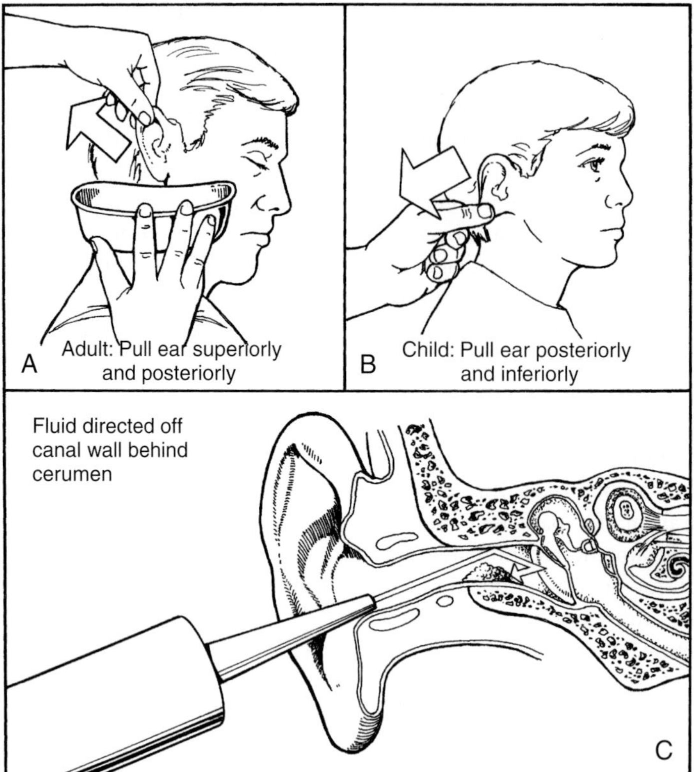

Fig. 32.7 Ear Irrigation. (A) The external auditory canal in the adult can best be exposed by pulling the earlobe upward and backward. (B) The same exposure can be achieved in the child by gently pulling the auricle of the ear downward and backward. (C) An enlarged diagram showing the direction of irrigating fluid against the side of the canal. Note: This is more effective in dislodging cerumen than if the flow of solution were directed straight into the canal.

killed by placing a few drops of mineral oil in the ear or by filling the ear canal with 2% lidocaine. The dead insect can then be removed with direct instrumentation. If removal is difficult or involves a button battery or a penetrating object, urgent referral to an ENT specialist is recommended.[4,29,30]

Irrigation, often the safest and most effective method for removal of impacted cerumen, is contraindicated with a history of TM rupture, infection, a soft or vegetable-like foreign body, or in children younger than age 5. Any solutions for the ear should be lukewarm or room temperature before instillation to prevent inner ear stimulation. Suggested guidelines for ear irrigation are illustrated in Fig. 32.7.[4,29,30]

Other methods of foreign body removal include use of an ear curette, right-angle hook, small suction catheter, alligator forceps, and cyanoacrylate glue. Warmed mineral oil and hydrogen peroxide may soften cerumen for ease of removal. If an impacted foreign body cannot be removed, urgently refer the patient to an ENT specialist. Emergent referral is necessary with severe pain or presence of a caustic foreign body substance. Antibiotics may be prescribed to prevent or treat an existing infection. Complications include hearing loss, TM rupture, and acute OM or otitis externa from injury during attempted foreign body removal or from retained foreign

NASAL EMERGENCIES

Nasal emergencies involve infection, hemorrhage, or a foreign body. Most problems are minor such as infection or nasal fracture. However, life-threatening hemorrhage can also occur.

Rhinitis

Rhinitis is inflammation of the nasal mucosa, which usually accompanies a viral upper respiratory infection (URI) such as the common cold. Acute rhinitis, the most prevalent disease among all age-groups, is spread by droplet contact. Upper respiratory viruses are the most common causative organisms. Symptoms include copious, mucopurulent nasal secretions; red and swollen nasal mucosa; mild fever; and decreased sense of smell. Allergic rhinitis may be perennial or seasonal—caused by pollens, grasses, trees, or flowers. Perennial allergic rhinitis is a chronic condition caused by environmental factors such as dust, animal dander, mold, and foods. Perennial rhinitis is characterized by nasal mucosa that appears pale to bluish and swollen, tearing, periorbital edema, and thin, watery nasal discharge.[22,31,32]

The single most effective treatment for all forms of rhinitis is warm saline irrigation; however, not all patients are willing to continue this treatment on their own. Systemic or topical antihistamines are used to shrink swollen nasal tissues. Systemic or topical decongestants and steroids are other modalities. Instruct the patient on appropriate use of nasal sprays. Analgesics and antipyretics are administered as necessary. The patient should be instructed to drink plenty of clear fluids, humidify the home environment, avoid allergens, and rest. Complications associated with rhinitis include fatigue, headaches, sleep disturbance, serous OM, sinusitis, and exacerbation of asthma.[22,31,32]

Epistaxis

Epistaxis, or nosebleed, is seen frequently in the ED. Causes include infection, trauma, local irritants, foreign bodies, anticoagulant drug therapy, congenital or disease-induced coagulation disorders, and tumors. However, the most common causes are URIs and nose picking. Bleeding may occur anteriorly or posteriorly. Anterior bleeding is usually acute and almost always originates at Kiesselbach's plexus, a highly vascularized area in the anteroinferior nasal septum. Posterior epistaxis is usually chronic and common in older adults. Bleeding is more profuse, involving posterior branches of the sphenopalatine artery. Hypertension can worsen the bleed but has not been shown to cause epistaxis. In mild cases bleeding may stop spontaneously within minutes or by simply pinching the nares. Bleeding may be profuse and continuous with potential for hypovolemia, requiring aggressive management and ENT consult for embolization.[22,33]

The patient usually presents clutching bloody tissues or towels to the nose and can be extremely anxious. A calm, reassuring systematic approach by the emergency nurse helps ease anxiety and allows efficient management. Obtain a quick history, including duration, frequency, and amount of bleeding; recent trauma or surgery; nausea or vomiting; recreational drug use; and pertinent medical history. All staff caring for this patient should observe universal precautions including gloves, goggles, mask, and gown because potential for blood splashing is high.

Maintain the patient in an upright seated position with the head tilted downward and nostrils pinched. Assess ABCs, and initiate appropriate interventions such as suction, IV access, cardiac monitor, and oxygen saturation monitor. Obtain CBC, prothrombin time, partial thromboplastin time, and type and crossmatch as ordered. The bleeding site is determined after clearing the nose of clots by having the patient blow the nose or with suction using a small Frazier catheter. A nasal speculum and appropriate lighting are required to visualize the posterior nasal cavity. Treatment of anterior epistaxis begins with identification of the bleeding site followed by application of topical Afrin, direct pressure for 5 to 10 minutes, chemical (silver nitrate) or electrical cautery, and packing if necessary. Some patients may require anxiolytics to help with anxiety. Nasal packing may be done with standard petrolatum-iodoform gauze or newer commercial products such as the Merocel nasal sponge or Gelfoam, which eventually dissolve and do not require removal. Coat packing material with antibiotic ointment before insertion to help prevent sinusitis and toxic shock. Anterior nasal packing is left in place for 48 hours. The patient should follow up with ENT or return to the ED immediately for persistent bleeding or dislodged nasal packing.[22,33]

Bleeding with posterior epistaxis is more difficult to manage and requires insertion of posterior nasal packing or a balloon catheter.[33] Devices used in posterior epistaxis include Merocel nasal sponges, nasal balloon catheters, 10 Fr to 14 Fr urinary catheters, and thrombogenic foams/gels. These devices should be removed within 48 hours. Posterior nasal packing predisposes the patient to hypoxia, so admission is necessary for monitoring of airway, sedation, and cardiac effects. Surgical ligation of vessels may be required for control of severe posterior epistaxis.[22,33] Antihypertensive agents may be needed for patients whose blood pressure remains elevated.

Complications of anterior and posterior epistaxis include hypoxia, dislodged nasal packing, airway occlusion, hypovolemia, severe discomfort, sinusitis, toxic shock, cardiac dysrhythmias, and respiratory or cardiac arrest. With severe blood loss, blood transfusion may be necessary. Posterior epistaxis is often associated with significant atherosclerosis and can precipitate myocardial or cerebral infarction.[22,33]

Foreign Body

Nasal foreign bodies usually occur in children and are often discovered when a purulent nasal discharge is noticed. Usually self-inserted, foreign bodies in the nose may also occur with trauma and involve various shapes and sizes. Presentation may include pain and fullness from a recently placed foreign body or with purulent, foul-smelling nasal discharge, recurrent epistaxis, sinus pain, fever, and edematous nasal mucosa. Care should be taken to prevent damage to the highly vascular nasal septum and mucosa during removal. Children may require conscious sedation, restraint, topical anesthetic agents, and nebulized vasoconstrictive agents. Ask the patient to occlude the unobstructed nostril and apply positive pressure insufflation via parent mouth to mouth, manual ventilation, or patient induced from blowing. If unsuccessful, other methods include utilizing a blunt right-angle probe, forceps, balloon catheters, suction, and magnets for metal objects. Take care not to dislodge the foreign body deeper because this poses a risk for aspiration. Referral to an otolaryngologist is indicated with traumatic or complicated removals, suspected necrosis, batteries, or inability to remove the foreign body.[29]

THROAT EMERGENCIES

Throat emergencies represent a threat to the patient's airway. The emergency nurse should evaluate the patient's ABCs carefully and monitor for significant changes in breathing and mentation.

Pharyngitis

Pharyngitis is an inflammation of the pharynx and may include the following symptoms: red throat, swollen tonsils, white or yellow exudate on tonsils and pharynx, swollen uvula, and enlarged, tender cervical and tonsillar nodes. The patient may complain of sore throat, fever, dysphagia, and halitosis. Treatment for pharyngitis depends on the underlying pathologic condition. A throat culture and sensitivity should be obtained to distinguish bacterial or viral causes. Many EDs use a rapid strep test to screen for streptococcal infections. Most sore throats in adults are viral and do not warrant antibiotics. For bacterial pharyngitis (i.e., streptococcal pharyngitis), treatment consists of antibiotics, antipyretics, steroids, and analgesics. Stress the importance of bed rest, increased fluid intake, and completing the full course of antibiotics. A tonsillectomy may be necessary in severe or recurrent cases. Complications include retropharyngeal abscess, mastoiditis, cervical lymphadenitis, and acute rheumatic fever.[10]

Laryngitis

Acute laryngitis, inflammation of the vocal cords, is caused by the following etiologies: overuse, trauma, allergies, irritants, acid reflux, and viral or bacterial infections. The patient presents with partial or complete voice loss, with or without URI symptoms. Dyspnea or stridor should be evaluated and treated immediately as potential airway obstruction. Throat culture, CBC, and direct laryngoscopy can be useful diagnostic procedures. Treatment includes voice rest, steam inhalations, increased fluid intake, and topical anesthetic throat lozenges. Patient teaching should emphasize preventive therapy, avoiding airway irritants such as cigarette smoke and loud or excessive use of the voice. In the presence of infection, administer antibiotics and instruct the patient to complete the entire course. Complications of laryngitis are aspiration with decreased cough reflex and airway compromise or obstruction.[34]

Tonsillitis

Tonsillitis refers to inflammation of the palatine tonsils. Tonsils are lymphatic tissue that filters microorganisms to prevent infection in the body. Culture for streptococcus bacteria may be taken because it is the most common and complicated form. Viruses are also a leading cause of tonsillitis. Symptoms resemble pharyngitis and include the following: red, swollen tonsils; a feeling of fullness/pain in the throat; malaise; fever; otalgia; difficulty speaking or swallowing; white or yellow exudate on tonsils; and halitosis. Rapid strep test, throat culture and sensitivity, CBC, and monospot test may be ordered. As with pharyngitis, treatment is geared toward the cause. Topical anesthetics, analgesics, antipyretics, steroids, and antibiotics (usually penicillin unless allergic) may be utilized. Surgery may be recommended for recurrent streptococcal infections or complicated courses predisposing patients to airway obstruction.[10]

Peritonsillar Abscess

Untreated acute or chronic suppurative tonsillitis may evolve into a peritonsillar abscess caused by extension of the infection into deep soft tissue. The abscesses are often polymicrobial; however *Fusobacterium necrophorum* and β-lactamase organisms are the most common. The abscess is usually unilateral with dysphagia, drooling, hot potato/muffled voice, dysphagia, trismus, and anxiety present. Fever, malaise, and dehydration are usually seen. Abscess treatment includes fluid resuscitation, antipyretics and analgesics as needed, antibiotics, possible steroids, and needle aspiration and/or surgical incision and drainage. Patients can be managed on an outpatient basis unless they show signs of sepsis, airway compromise, or complications.[10,34]

In more severe cases with airway compromise, stability of ABCs takes priority, with upright positioning until airway is secured. These patients require IV fluids and medications, oxygen therapy, cardiac monitoring, and advanced airway management followed by IV antibiotic therapy and surgical incision and drainage. Dangerous sequelae associated with a peritonsillar abscess include aspiration, airway obstruction, parapharyngeal abscess, sepsis, septic embolization, and possible spread to cerebral or cardiac structures.[10,34]

FACIAL EMERGENCIES

Facial emergencies affect structures of the face such as the nerves, bones, and sinuses. These emergencies may be secondary to infection or other disease processes.

Sinusitis

Acute sinusitis, inflammation of mucous membranes in any of the paranasal sinuses, generally occurs because of blockage and backup of secretions. The causes are usually attributed to URI or allergic rhinitis with symptom duration less than 1 month. Other causes include foreign bodies, trauma, inhalation of irritants such as cocaine or cigarette smoke, deviated nasal septum, polyps, and tumors. Secretions are retained in the sinus cavity as a result of altered ciliary activity and obstruction of the sinus ostia. Negative pressure and air-fluid levels result from fluid accumulation and reabsorption of air in the sinus. Fluid accumulation forms a medium for bacteria to grow and multiply, resulting in bacterial sinusitis. *H. influenzae, S. pneumoniae,* and *M. catarrhalis* are common causative organisms.[12,13,34] Subacute sinusitis is defined as symptom duration lasting 1 to 3 months.[13]

Chronic sinusitis is a result of unresolved acute sinusitis for more than 12 weeks. In chronic sinusitis, the mucous membrane becomes permanently thickened from prolonged or repeated inflammation or infection. The patient with sinusitis complains of dull, achy pain over the affected sinus. In adults, frontal sinusitis with periorbital and forehead pain that worsens when bending over is common.[12,13,34] Ethmoidal sinusitis, common in children, causes pain at the bridge of the nose and behind the eyes. Fever, decreased appetite, and nausea may also be present. Ethmoidal sinusitis is especially serious in children because of the tendency for the infection to extend toward the retroorbital area and central nervous system.[13] The patient has tenderness to palpation over the involved sinus; swollen, erythematous mucosa with purulent nasal discharge; and diminished transillumination. Radiographic studies are not always conclusive or reliable in the diagnosis of sinusitis. Some reliable findings include sinus opacity, air-fluid level, displacement of sinus wall, or increased mucosal thickening. Absence of radiographic evidence does not exclude the diagnosis of sinusitis. Other diagnostic methods include CT scan, magnetic resonance imaging, sinus endoscopy, and sinus culture and biopsy.[12,13,34]

In most patients, treatment is targeted at symptom management because acute sinusitis can resolve spontaneously. Over-the-counter nasal decongestant sprays (e.g., Afrin or Neo-Synephrine) may provide immediate relief; however, topical decongestants should not be used for more than 3 to 5 days because of a dangerous rebound effect. Isotonic saline nose drops may also help. Encourage increased fluid intake and use of a humidifier in the home. Warm, moist compresses to the sinus areas promote drainage and comfort. Administer antibiotics and analgesics as prescribed. Instruct the patient to avoid environmental irritants and avoid bending over because this increases sinus pressure and pain. If the condition worsens despite antibiotic therapy for 3 to 5 days, the patient should return to the ED immediately or see an ENT specialist. Complications of undertreated acute sinusitis are chronic sinusitis, orbital or periorbital cellulitis or abscess, cavernous sinus thrombosis, sepsis, brain abscess, meningitis, and osteomyelitis of the frontal bone.[12,13,34]

Temporomandibular Joint Dislocation

TMJ dislocation refers to anterior and superior bilateral displacement of the jaw. Unilateral dislocation rarely occurs but will deviate to the opposite side. Jaw muscles attempt to close the mandible, but the resulting spasm prevents condyles from returning to normal position in the mandibular fossae. TMJ dislocation usually occurs when opening the mouth too wide or too long, as in yawning, laughing, or dental procedures. Trauma or dystonic reaction to drugs may also be responsible. The patient usually presents with the chin protruding from anterior displacement, the mouth open, drooling, and pain related to muscle spasms. The patient cannot close the mouth, talk, or swallow and may be extremely anxious. Diagnostics include Panorex or CT scan of facial bones with pre- and post-reduction films. Muscle relaxants may be administered to reduce muscle spasm and relax the patient.[2]

To reduce the dislocation, provide procedural sedation and analgesia and position the patient facing or in front of the physician. The physician places the thumbs intraorally onto the lower molar ridge and applies a downward and backward pressure to return the condyle to the normal position. The physician should pad the thumbs with a thick layer of gauze around a tongue blade because the strong masseter muscles of the jaw contract with great force with reduction of the TMJ. Postreduction pain is typically minimal and can be treated with warm compresses, nonsteroidal antiinflammatory drugs, and muscle relaxants. Instruct the patient to avoid stress on the TMJ by consuming a soft diet for 1 week and avoid extreme mouth opening. Referral to an otolaryngologist is recommended if dislocation was concurrent with a fracture. Referral is also indicated for any TMJ dislocation because it predisposes the patient to further dislocations.[2]

SUMMARY

Emergencies of the mouth, face, nose, and ears are a routine part of emergency nursing. Most are not life-threatening. However, the ability to discern problems that represent a potential threat to the patient's life is a requisite skill for the emergency nurse.

REFERENCES

1. Mayersak RJ. Facial trauma. In: Walls RM, Hockberger RS, Gausche-Hill M, eds. *Rosen's Emergency Medicine: Concepts and Clinical Practice*. 9th ed. Philadelphia, PA: Elsevier; 2018:330–348.
2. Pedigo RA, Amsterdam JT. Oral medicine. In: Walls RM, Hockberger RS, Gausche-Hill M, eds. *Rosen's Emergency Medicine: Concepts and Clinical Practice*. 9th ed. Philadelphia, PA: Elsevier; 2018:771–790.
3. American Academy of Pediatric Dentistry Reference Manual. Guidelines on management of acute dental trauma. *Am Acad Pediatr Dent*. 2011;34(6):230–238.
4. Jarvis C. Ears. In: *Physical Examination and Health Assessment*. 7th ed. Philadelphia, PA: Elsevier; 2016:325–352.
5. Swartz MH. The ear and nose. In: *Textbook of Physical Diagnosis*. 7th ed. Philadelphia, PA: Elsevier; 2014:249–277.
6. Ball JW, Dains JE, Flynn JA, Solomon BS, Stewart RW. Ears, nose, and throat. In: *Seidel's Guide to Physical Examination*. 8th ed. St Louis, MO: Elsevier; 2015:231–259.
7. MacArthur FJD, McGarry GW. The arterial supply of the nasal cavity. *Eur Arch Otorhinolaryngol*. 2016;274(2):809–815. https://doi.org/10.1007/s00405-016-4281-1.
8. Swartz MH. The oral cavity and pharynx. In: *Textbook of Physical Diagnosis*. 7th ed. Philadelphia, PA: Elsevier; 2014:278–314.
9. Pandolfino JE, Kahrilas PJ. Esophageal neuromuscular function and motility disorders. In: Feldman M, Friedman LS, Brandt L, eds. *Sleisenger and Fordtran's Gastrointestinal and Liver Disease*. 10th ed. Philadelphia, PA: Elsevier; 2016:701–732.
10. Kaji AH. Sore throat. In: Walls RM, Hockberger RS, Gausche-Hill M, eds. *Rosen's Emergency Medicine: Concepts and Clinical Practice*. 9th ed. Philadelphia, PA: Elsevier; 2018:184–189.
11. Swartz MH. The head and neck. In: *Textbook of Physical Diagnosis*. 7th ed. Philadelphia, PA: Elsevier; 2014:145–160.
12. Demuri GP, Wald ER. Sinusitis. In: Bennett JE, Dolin R, Blaser MJ, eds. *Mandell, Douglas, and Bennett's Principles and Practice of Infectious Diseases, Updated Eighth Edition*. 8th ed. Philadelphia, PA: Elsevier; 2015:774–784.
13. Pappas DE, Hendley JO. Sinusitis. In: Kliegman RM, Stanton BF, St Geme JW, Schor NF, eds. *Nelson Textbook of Pediatrics*. 20th ed. Philadelphia, PA: Elsevier; 2016:2014–2017.
14. Drake RL, Vogl AW, Mitchell AWM. Head and neck. In: *Gray's Anatomy for Students*. 3rd ed. Philadelphia, PA: Elsevier; 2015:835–1135.
15. Cameron P. Dental emergencies. In: Cameron P, Jelinek G, Kelly AM, Brown A, Little M, eds. *Textbook of Adult Emergency Medicine*. 4th ed. Philadelphia, PA: Elsevier; 2015:616–619.
16. Karami S, Ghobadi N, Karami H. Diagnostic and preventive approaches for dental caries in children: a review. *J Pediatr Review*. 2017;5(2):1–7. https://doi.org/10.5812/jpr.10222.
17. Benko K. Dental emergencies. In: Adams JG, ed. *Emergency Medicine*. 2nd ed. Philadelphia, PA: Elsevier; 2013:236–248.
18. Beale T, Brown J, Rout J. ENT, neck and dental radiology. In: Adams A, Dixon AK, Gillard JH, Schaefer-Prokop CM, eds. *Grainger & Allison's Diagnostic Radiology*. 6th ed. Philadelphia, PA: Elsevier; 2015:1590–1647.
19. Un Lam C, Hsu CS, Yee R, et al. Early-life factors affect risk of pain and fever in infants during teething periods. *Clin Oral Investig*. 2016;20(8):1861–1870. https://doi.org/10.1007/s00784-015-1658-2.

20. Tinanoff N. Dental trauma. In: Kliegman RM, Stanton BF, St Geme JW, Schor NF, eds. *Nelson Textbook of Pediatrics*. 20th ed. Philadelphia, PA: Elsevier; 2016:1776–1778.
21. Stallard TC. Emergency disorders of the ear, nose sinuses, oropharynx, & mouth. In: Stone CK, Humphries RL, eds. *Current Diagnosis & Treatment Emergency Medicine*. 7th ed. New York, NY: McGraw-Hill; 2011:513–536.
22. Pfaff JA, Moore GP. Otolaryngology. In: Walls RM, Hockberger RS, Gausche-Hill M, eds. *Rosen's Emergency Medicine: Concepts and Clinical Practice*. 9th ed. Philadelphia, PA: Elsevier; 2018:820–846.
23. Heward E, Cullen M, Hobson J. Microbiology and antimicrobial susceptibility of otitis externa: a changing pattern of antimicrobial resistance. *J Laryngol Otol*. 2018;132(4):314–317. https://doi.org/10.1017/S0022215118000191.
24. Waitzman AA, Elluru RG. Otitis externa treatment & management. Medscape website. https://emedicine.medscape.com/article/994550-overview. Published March 30, 2018. Accessed May 23, 2019.
25. Dye LD. Acute otitis media. https://www-clinicalkey-com.libproxy.usouthal.edu/#!/content/clinical_overview/67-s2.0-45be9d84-7a11-4658-931b-3f8ca04dec19?scrollTo=%23toc-9. Published March 14, 2018. Accessed May 23, 2019.
26. Boston ME, Strasnick B. Labyrinthitis. https://emedicine.medscape.com/article/856215-overview. Published January 23, 2017. Accessed May 23, 2019.
27. Pelton S. Acute Otitis Media in Children: Treatment. https://www.uptodate.com/contents/acute-otitis-media-in-children-treatment. Published February 15, 2018. Accessed May 23, 2019.
28. Evans AK, Handler SD. Evaluation and management of middle ear trauma. https://www.uptodate.com/contents/evaluation-and-management-of-middle-ear-trauma?search=tympanic%20membrane%20perforation&source=search_result&selectedTitle=1~71&usage_type=default&display_rank=1. Published March 19, 2018. Accessed May 23, 2019.
29. Thomas SH, Goodloe JM. Foreign bodies. In: Walls RM, Hockberger RS, Gausche-Hill M, eds. *Rosen's Emergency Medicine: Concepts and Clinical Practice*. 9th ed. Philadelphia, PA: Elsevier; 2018:674–689.
30. Isaacson GC, Aderonke O. Diagnosis and management of foreign bodies of the outer ear. https://www.uptodate.com/contents/diagnosis-and-management-of-foreign-bodies-of-the-outer-ear?search=cerumen%20impaction&source=search_result&selectedTitle=8~13&usage_type=default&display_rank=8#H19482771. Published January 13, 2017. Updated January 8, 2019. Accessed May 23, 2019.
31. Beard S. Rhinitis. In: Kellerman RD, Bope ET, eds. *Conn's Current Therapy 2018*. 10th ed. Philadelphia, PA: Elsevier; 2018:54–57.
32. Peden D. An overview of rhinitis. https://www.uptodate.com/contents/an-overview-of-rhinitis?search=rhinitis&source=search_result&selectedTitle=1~150&usage_type=default&display_rank=1. Published July 23, 2018. Accessed May 23, 2019.
33. Alter H. Approach to the adult with epistaxis. https://www.uptodate.com/contents/approach-to-the-adult-with-epistaxis?search=epistaxis&source=search_result&selectedTitle=1~150&usage_type=default&display_rank=1. Published May15, 2018. Accessed May 23, 2019.
34. Melio FR. Upper respiratory tract infections. In: Walls RM, Hockberger RS, Gausche-Hill M, eds. *Rosen's Emergency Medicine: Concepts and Clinical Practice*. 9th ed. Philadelphia, PA: Elsevier; 2018:857–870.

33

Ocular Emergencies

Laurie Nolan-Kelley

The human eye transmits messages of light, color, movement, and spatial relations and can display changes in brain function, body chemistry, and emotion. Its ability to track, focus, and adapt to changes in the environment were critical to human survival throughout evolution. Although the human eye does not have the precision possessed by the eyes of many other species, most humans have natural or corrected visual acuity that permits us to safely conduct activities of daily living. Eye injury or disease, or the threat of lost or impaired vision, brings patients to emergency departments (EDs) every day. The emergency nurse must be prepared to assess the patient who has an ocular complaint and recognize the signs and symptoms of the uncommon presentations that are true ocular emergencies. This chapter will review ocular anatomy and physiology and assessment of the eye and of visual acuity, and it will describe the conditions that can cause vision loss or permanent impairment.

EPIDEMIOLOGY

According to the US Nationwide Emergency Department Sample (NEDS), from 2006 to 2011, about 2 million ED visits per year were for ocular or ophthalmic complaints. Most patients, more than 90%, are discharged. The most common diagnosis is conjunctivitis (28%). The most common eye injuries are corneal abrasion (13.7%) and a foreign body on the external eye (7.5%).[1]

The typical ocular emergencies treated in the ED include corneal or conjunctival foreign body, conjunctivitis, and corneal abrasion. These conditions do not cause significant morbidity; however, the patient does experience discomfort, and this may interfere with daily life.[1] Burns, penetrating trauma, angle-closure glaucoma, globe rupture, and retinal artery occlusion can result in permanent visual impairment or vision loss and are true ocular emergencies.

ANATOMY AND PHYSIOLOGY

To conduct a thorough assessment of the eye, the emergency nurse must understand its anatomy. Fig. 33.1 illustrates the structures of the eye. The bony structures surrounding the eye, the eyelids, and the sclera protect it. Lacrimal glands secrete tears, which continuously bathe the eye to decrease friction and remove minor irritants. Zeis and Meibomian glands are sebaceous glands that service the eyelashes and prevent the tear film from evaporating, respectively.

Light enters the eye through the cornea, passes through the lens, and is reflected off the retina. The amount of light entering the posterior chamber is controlled by the iris as it expands and contracts to open and close the pupil. Six oculomotor muscles control movement of the eye itself. The external muscles are innervated by cranial nerves III, IV, and VI, the oculomotor, trochlear, and abducens nerves, respectively. The intrinsic muscles are innervated by the parasympathetic component of cranial nerve III and the ascending cervical sympathetic system.

PATIENT ASSESSMENT

Triage of the patient who presents with an ocular complaint includes assessment of the risk of loss of vision. Symptoms posing a threat to vision are triaged as emergent. A patient with a reddened eye, controlled eye pain, or irritation with no potential for loss of vision and without other problems may be triaged as nonurgent.

After a brief assessment to ensure that airway, breathing, and circulation (ABCs) are stable and there is no obvious, life-threatening bleeding, the patient is evaluated to identify potential threats to vision. Focused assessment includes determination of precipitating events, duration of symptoms, and identification of anything that worsens or improves symptoms. When the patient verbalizes discomfort, a description of the discomfort helps clarify the patient's problem. Does the patient describe itching, burning, or the sensation of something in the eye? Determine the degree of pain and where the pain occurs. Clarify reported visual changes to determine whether the impairment is partial or complete and in one or both eyes. The sensation of a something in the eye or sudden pain with a known or suspected foreign body suggests a corneal abrasion or retained foreign material. Biocular changes (vision changes in both eyes) suggest a neurologic condition rather than an ocular condition, whereas the presence of "floaters" suggests a retinal tear.

If there is a report of eye injury, as with any trauma, determine the mechanism of injury and when it occurred. If the injury occurred as a result of a motor vehicle crash, determine if the patient was restrained, if the eyes were exposed to flying debris or chemicals, and if the air bag

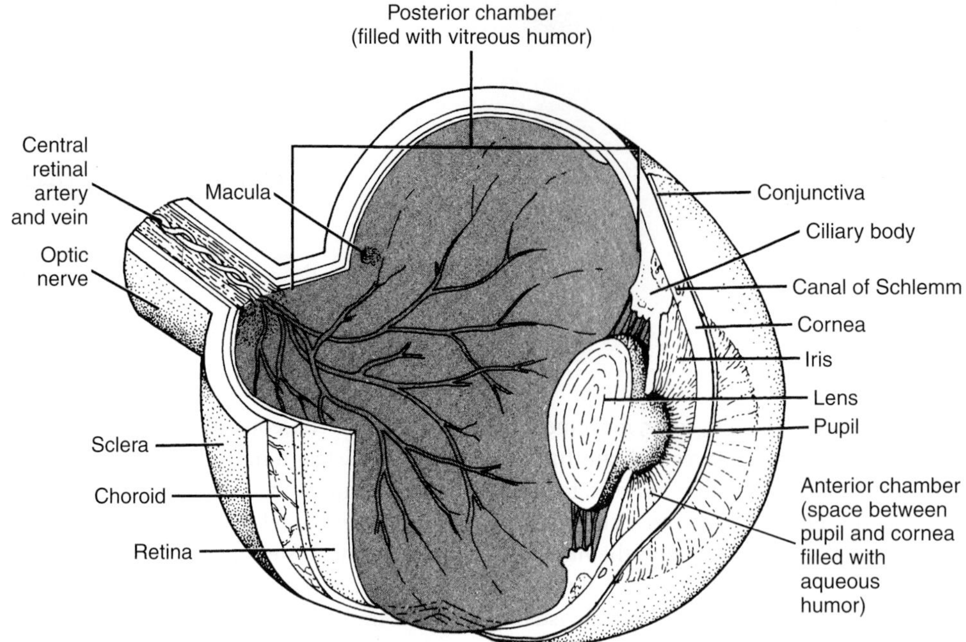

Fig. 33.1 Anatomy of the Eye. (From Rumack BH, Matthew H. Acetaminophen poisoning and toxicity. *Pediatrics.* 1975;55:871.)

was deployed. Injuries associated with air-bag deployment include orbital fractures, retinal detachment, hyphema, and globe rupture. The emergency nurse should be aware that alkaline powder in air bags can cause significant eye irritation.[2] Determine whether the patient was wearing protective eyewear, glasses, or contact lenses. Evaluate medical history, including ocular history, use of corrective lenses, medications, past ocular surgery, and disease such as diabetes and cardiovascular disease. Tetanus status should be determined if signs of ocular trauma are noted. Some medications and many recreational drugs will influence the ocular assessment, so query the patient regarding current prescribed and over-the-counter medications, as well as alcohol and other substance use.

The primary elements of the ocular examination for all patients are visual acuity and evaluation of external features, pupils, anterior segment, and extraocular movement (EOM).[1,2] A systematic process of assessing visual acuity and inspecting for injury is recommended.[3]

Visual Acuity

When there is no other serious complaint or life threat, visual acuity testing should occur at triage. Visual acuity is a vital sign for patients with an ocular concern and is part of the focused assessment. This simple test is done on all patients presenting with any type of ocular or vision complaint.[3,4] Physical examination begins with visual acuity unless the patient has sustained ocular exposure to a chemical. In these situations, irrigation takes priority over determination of visual acuity.[5] Measure visual acuity both with and without the patient's corrective lenses. When corrective lenses are not available, the pinhole test can be used for measurement of visual acuity. This is accomplished by punching a hole in a note card with an 18-gauge needle. Looking through a pinhole usually corrects any refractory error[5] to at least 20/30. Test the affected eye first, then the unaffected eye, and finally both eyes.

The Snellen chart is the standard method for determination of visual acuity. For the examination, have the patient stand 20 feet from the chart and cover the eye without applying pressure to the orbit. Alternative techniques for visual acuity when a Snellen chart is not available are using a pocket Rosenbaum vision screener held 14 inches from the nose or having the patient read a newspaper and record the distance at which the paper must be held for the patient to read. If the patient is unable to read, hold fingers up, record the distance at which the patient can see your fingers, and then ask the patient how many fingers you are holding up. If the patient cannot see fingers moving, record the distance at which the patient perceives hand motion. If the patient is unable to see hand motion, determine whether the patient is able to perceive light. Table 33.1 describes documentation of visual acuity for the Snellen chart and alternative techniques for reporting visual acuity.

For people who are illiterate or do not speak English, there is an E chart where the patient indicates the direction of the letter *E*. The Allen card of objects is used for children. Be sure to name the objects before the test so that they are identified correctly. The patient with a corneal abrasion or foreign body may have difficulty with photophobia (painful sensitivity to light), pain, and tearing. Placing a drop of topical anesthetic in the affected eye can provide temporary relief and may assist in accomplishing an accurate visual acuity evaluation in these patients.[3,5]

TABLE 33.1 Examples of Visual Acuity Examination.	
20/20	Standing at 20 feet, patient can read what the normal eye can read at 20 feet.
20/20 2	Standing at 20 feet, patient can read what the normal eye can read at 20 feet; however, missed two letters.
20/200	At 20 feet, patient can read what the normal eye can read at 200 feet. Patient is considered legally blind if reading is obtained while wearing glasses or contact lenses.
10/200	When patient cannot read letters on the Snellen chart, have patient stand half the distance to the chart. Record findings at the distance the patient is standing from the chart over the smallest line he or she can read.
CF/3 ft	Patient can count fingers at a maximum distance of 3 feet.
HM/4	Patient can see hand motion at a maximum distance of 4 feet.
LP/position	Patient can perceive light and determine the direction from which it is coming.
LP/no position	Patient can perceive light but is unable to tell the direction from which it is coming.
NLP	Patient is unable to perceive light.

External Features

External examination of ocular complaints begins by inspecting the patient.[6] Observe for bruising, lacerations, lesions, and other differences between the eyes. Assess eyelids, lashes, and how the eyes rest in the sockets. Examine the conjunctiva and sclera for abnormal color.

Pupil Examination

Pupil examination includes assessment of shape, size, and reactivity. Testing should be performed in a dimly lit examination room. Pupils are normally round, black, and equal in size. Variations may indicate a potentially serious problem or may reflect a normal physiologic variation. For some people, unequal pupils (physiologic anisocoria) is a normal finding.[7] Physiologic anisocoria is a normal finding when the difference in pupils is 1 mm or less and both pupils react briskly to light.[3] An oval pupil may be caused by a tumor or retinal detachment. A pupil that is the shape of a teardrop suggests a ruptured globe, with the teardrop pointing to the rupture site.[4,7] Pupil size is measured in millimeters. Assess and document the change in size that occurs in each pupil in response to direct and consensual light stimulation. Normally, both pupils constrict equally when a strong light is directed at one eye (a direct response occurs in the eye to which light is directed, and a consensual response occurs in the other eye).[7] This is noted in the medical record as: "Pupils equal and reactive to light and accommodation," or "PEARLA."

Anterior Segment

The anterior segment is composed of the sclera, conjunctiva, cornea, anterior chamber, iris, lens, and ciliary body.[6] The conjunctiva, or the white of the eye, should be inspected for changes in color, swelling (chemosis), discharge, foreign bodies, and laceration. The cornea should be clear. The cornea is stained with fluorescein to inspect for the presence of any abrasions. The anterior chamber is inspected for hyphema (blood in the anterior chamber) or hypopyon (pus in the anterior chamber). To inspect the anterior chamber, hold a light tangential or at a 90-degree angle to the eye. A slit lamp is used to perform an adequate assessment of the anterior chamber.[6]

Ocular Motility

Evaluate the patient's ability to move the eyes through six cardinal positions of gaze by asking the patient to follow your finger as you move it through these positions. Ocular movement is controlled by the cranial nerves that regulate the oculomotor muscles. Fig. 33.2 shows these positions of gaze and identifies the specific oculomotor muscles and cranial nerves involved. Impaired ocular movement may occur with an entrapped muscle secondary to a blowout fracture, muscular injury, orbital cellulitis, or underlying central nervous system problem. Evaluation of ocular motility in children requires patience and creativity. Hold toys, keys, or lights in different areas so that the child glances in that direction. Children become easily bored with the same object, so a general rule of thumb is to use a different toy for each position.[7]

Other Examinations

Other techniques used to evaluate ocular function include fluorescein staining, measurement of intraocular pressure (IOP), and funduscopic examination. Fluorescein is used to determine whether the corneal epithelium is intact. Before staining is done, the patient should remove his or her contact lenses. Explain the procedure to the patient. Moisten end of a sterile fluorescein strip with normal saline solution. Pull down on the lower lid and touch the moistened fluorescein strip to the inner canthus of the lower lid. Ask the patient to blink several times before examining the patient with a cobalt blue light; disruptions of the corneal epithelium appear as a bright yellow spot. After fluorescein application, flush the eye with normal saline and instruct the patient not to insert contact lenses for at least 3 to 5 hours.[8]

IOP is measured with a Schiøtz tonometer (Fig. 33.3) or a Tono-Pen. This procedure is contraindicated in patients with possible globe rupture. The Tono-Pen is a handheld instrument that has gained popularity because of its ease of use and decreased incidence of contamination; the sterile, disposable cover over the tip is for a single use and is discarded after each patient contact. Regardless of technique, the cornea

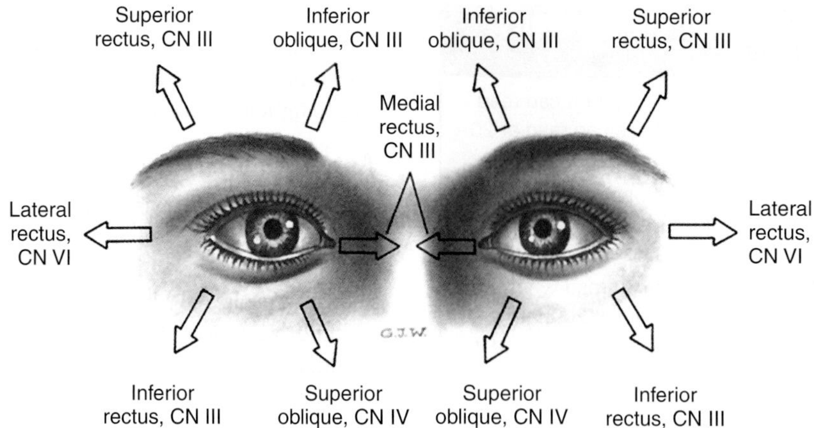

Fig. 33.2 Innervation and Movement of Extraocular Muscles. *CN,* Cranial nerve. (From Thompson JM, McFarland GK, Hirsch JE, et al. *Mosby's Clinical Nursing.* 5th ed. St Louis, MO: Mosby; 2002.)

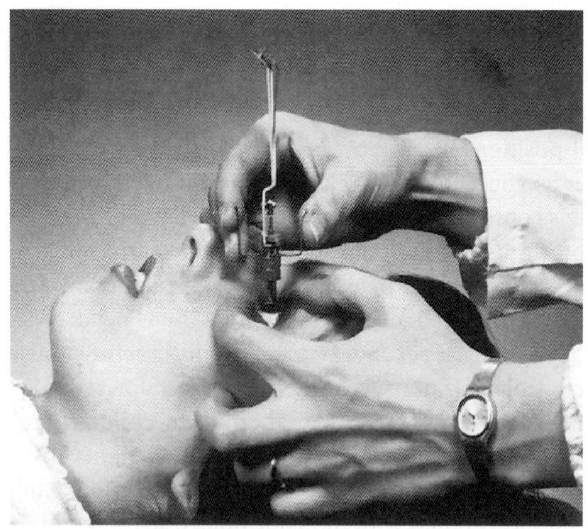

Fig. 33.3 Measurement of Ocular Tension With Schiøtz Tonometer. (From Newell FW. *Ophthalmology: Principles and Concepts,* 8th ed. St Louis, MO: Mosby; 1996.)

must be anesthetized before measurement. Normal IOP is 10 to 21 mm Hg. A low reading indicates decreased IOP, whereas a high reading indicates increased IOP. Any obstruction to aqueous outflow, such as glaucoma, can result in an elevated IOP.[4,5]

Direct ophthalmoscopy, or funduscopic evaluation, is used to evaluate the posterior chamber of the eye using a light beam directed through the pupil.[6] Mydriatic drops may be administered to dilate the pupil and make visualization of the disc, retinal artery, and macula easier; however, they are contraindicated in patients who have sustained a head injury.[5] Ophthalmoscopes provide different shapes and colors of light beams to assist in detecting various abnormalities.

PATIENT MANAGEMENT

General management of ocular emergencies includes removal of contact lens, instillation of ocular medication, and irrigation. Recommendations surrounding eye patching vary and are evolving.[5,7,8]

Eye drops and ophthalmic ointments are used to decrease pain, provide antibiotic therapy, change pupil size, reduce allergic reactions in the eye, and cleanse the eye. Topical ophthalmic medications are prepared under sterile conditions and distributed in single-dose containers. Container caps are color coded by the medication's effect on the pupil. For example, a red cap indicates a mydriatic (pupil-dilating) medication; a green cap, a pupil constrictor (miotic); a white cap, a topical anesthetic; a blue cap, an irrigating or lubricating agent; and a yellow cap, medication that decreases aqueous humor production.

Instilling eye drops or ointments requires attention to detail to prevent contamination and minimize systemic effects of the medication. Topical anesthetics may be used to facilitate the examination but should not be prescribed for continuous use because these agents retard epithelial healing. During instillation of eye drops and ointments, have the patient gaze upward because this will help to ensure the patient does not blink at an inopportune time. Monitor patients carefully after instillation of eye drops; systemic effects secondary to eye drops may occur. These systemic effects can be minimized by instructing patients to apply pressure to the medial canthus for several minutes after medication instillation to close the nasolacrimal duct. If more than one type of drop is ordered, wait several minutes between applications to allow maximal exposure for each drop.

Irrigation is used to remove chemicals, small foreign bodies, and other substances. Isotonic saline or lactated Ringer's solution are the fluids of choice for ocular irrigation.[5,9] Dextrose solutions should not be used because they are sticky and irritate the eye. Irrigation is contraindicated in the patient with a possible ruptured globe. There is no documented literature on the correct length of tubing to be used; however, the shorter the tubing, the faster the flow. Before irrigating the eye, make sure the outer aspects of the eye are cleansed so that additional debris does not inadvertently contaminate the eye and cause further problems.

In the case of a chemical exposure, a baseline pH measurement of the eye should be obtained by placing pH paper in the conjunctival sac before irrigation is initiated. Irrigation is continued until the pH of the tear film is neutral (normal conjunctival pH is 7.1). This may require several liters of fluid with intermittent checks of pH. The eyes can be irrigated simultaneously by connecting a nasal cannula to the hanging fluid and positioning the cannula over the bridge of the nose. This method is better tolerated and does not carry the risk of injury of more invasive irrigation tools.[9]

Eye patching is performed to minimize ocular stimulation by reducing movement and limiting light exposure. Current evidence does not support use of eye patching.[5] Eye patches should not be used when there is an increased risk for a *Pseudomonas* organism infection, for example, in the contact lens wearer. Although not widely available in the ED, a collagen shield that is similar to a contact lens is being used by ophthalmologists for corneal erosions.[5] Studies indicate that patients may be safely discharged with a prescribed ocular anesthetic to use for 24 hours, allowing improved pain management after corneal abrasion.[10]

SPECIFIC OCULAR EMERGENCIES

Injury or disease may cause ocular emergencies. Comprehensive discussion of every disease process is beyond the scope of this text; however, situations encountered most often by the emergency nurse are discussed.

Trauma

General principles pertaining to ocular examination are essentially the same as for the patient with an eye injury; however, the patient's ABCs should be evaluated, bleeding controlled, and the patient stabilized before interventions for the ocular problem. Ocular injury often occurs in conjunction with head and facial trauma; therefore these patients should be carefully evaluated for an associated eye injury. Check for contact lenses in the unconscious patient, and remove them as soon as possible. Do not instill eye drops before evaluation of ocular injury. Severe pain associated with ocular trauma can be minimized without medication by patching both eyes to reduce consensual eye movement. When the patient cannot blink, protect the cornea from drying with ophthalmic ointment or artificial tears. The eyes may be taped shut when ointment is used.

Obtain pertinent details of the traumatic event, including mechanism of injury, time of injury, energy source, material involved when there is ocular penetration, and use of protective eyewear. If the foreign material is organic, there is increased risk for infection, whereas metallic materials cause vitreous and ocular reactions.

Blunt Trauma

Blunt trauma to the eye may be caused by a motor vehicle collision, assault with various weapons, or a fall. The most commonly seen ocular injury is periorbital contusion, or a black eye. This injury is usually benign, but the patient should be assessed for more serious injury, such as a hyphema, blood in the anterior chamber of the eye, or basilar skull fracture. Symptoms usually include ecchymosis of the lids, which can make it very difficult to visualize the globe. If the globe appears intact, rule out orbital fracture and hyphema. If no obvious associated problems are identified, therapeutic interventions such as ice, head elevation, and reassurance are initiated. Resolution of uncomplicated periorbital ecchymosis usually occurs within 2 to 3 weeks.[4]

Orbital fractures. Orbital fractures involve the bones of the orbital floor and the orbital rim. A fracture of the orbital floor, sometimes called a blowout fracture, is serious and usually results from direct blunt trauma to the eye. A blowout fracture occurs when direct trauma increases IOP to the point where the orbital floor fractures. Orbital contents may herniate into the maxillary or ethmoid sinuses and trap the inferior rectus muscle in the defect. A blowout fracture is diagnosed by history and observation of periorbital ecchymosis, subconjunctival hemorrhage, periorbital edema, enophthalmos (sunken eye), an upward gaze, and a complaint of diplopia.[7] The latter three conditions occur when the inferior rectus and oblique muscles are trapped in the fracture defect. Computed tomography (CT) scan is most often used for the diagnosis of orbital fractures; facial radiographs are rarely used. CT scan or magnetic resonance imaging is more helpful in identification of muscle entrapment than plain radiographs are.[4,7]

Orbital fractures are not considered an ocular emergency unless visual impairment or globe injury is present. Surgical intervention is usually delayed until swelling resolves in 7 to 10 days. Patients without eye injury or entrapment may be referred to an ophthalmologist and treated conservatively. Patients who have fractures involving the sinuses should receive a prescription of antibiotics. At discharge, instruct the patient on application of ice packs and caution against Valsalva maneuvers, sneezing, and nose blowing (activities that increase IOP).[4,7]

Hyphema. Hyphema refers to blood accumulation in the anterior chamber of the eye, usually secondary to blunt trauma (Fig. 33.4). It occurs when blood vessels of the iris rupture and leak into the clear aqueous fluid of the anterior chamber and is usually painful. Hyphema size varies from microscopic to total involvement of the anterior chamber. A large clot can obstruct aqueous outflow and lead to secondary glaucoma. A patient with a hyphema requires evaluation by an ophthalmologist.[11]

Symptoms of hyphema include pain, photophobia, and blurred vision. Blood in the anterior chamber may be easily seen in patients with lighter-colored eyes but may be extremely difficult to see in dark-eyed patients. Suspect concurrent head injury if the patient has an altered level of consciousness. Patients with bleeding disorders, diabetes, anticoagulant therapy, kidney disease, liver disease, or sickle cell disease have an increased risk for complications; therefore these patients should be monitored carefully for increased bleeding. The most common complication of hyphema is rebleeding, which occurs in 30% of patients, usually within 2 to 5 days, but it can occur up to 14 days after the initial injury.[12] Other complications include corneal blood staining, secondary acute glaucoma, loss of vision, and loss of the eye.

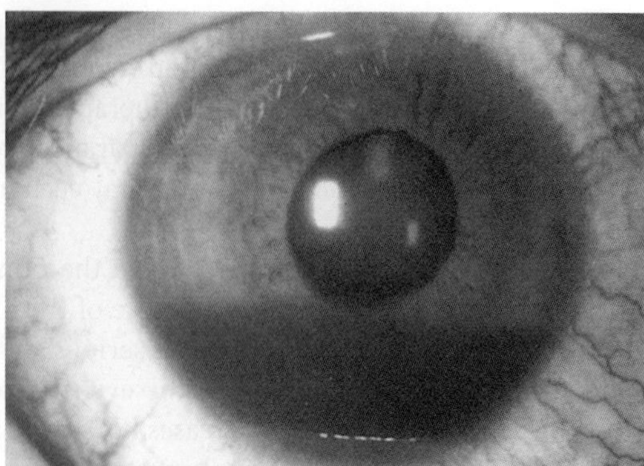

Fig. 33.4 **Traumatic Hyphema.** (From Abrams D. *Ophthalmology in Medicine: An Illustrated Clinical Guide.* St Louis, MO: Mosby; 1990.)

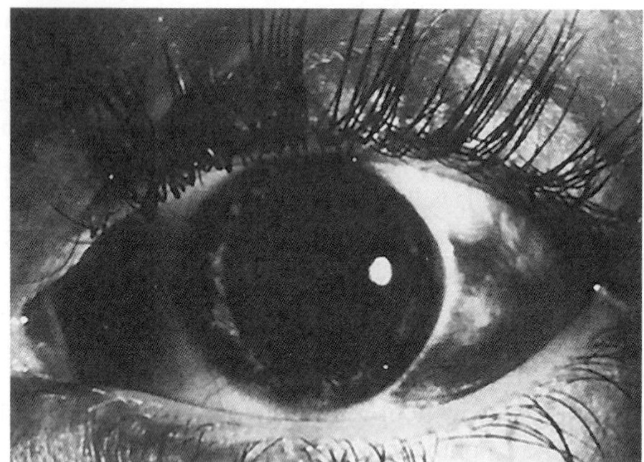

Fig. 33.5 **Subconjunctival Hemorrhage.** (From Stein HA, Slatt BJ, Stein RM. *The Ophthalmic Assistant.* 7th ed. St Louis, MO: Mosby; 2000.)

Management of hyphema includes bed rest with the head of the bed elevated 30 to 45 degrees or very limited activity, with monitoring for spontaneous rebleeding. The eye may be patched. Conservative therapy is considered for patients at low risk for complications, children, and older adults. Hospitalization should be considered for patients with higher risk profiles.[13] Pharmacologic management varies and often includes cycloplegics, steroids, and antiglaucoma medications to control swelling and rising IOP and reduce the risk of rebleeding. There is controversy surrounding treatment of hyphema because no strong evidence indicates that current treatment medications provide benefit. Topical nonsteroidal antiinflammatory drugs (NSAIDs) have been demonstrated to reduce pain and inflammation and reduce the need for oral pain medications. It is imperative that all patients with a hyphema are referred to an ophthalmologist for follow-up.[14,15]

Subconjunctival hemorrhage. Subconjunctival hemorrhage is a harmless ocular condition that startles and frightens patients by its appearance. It is usually caused by trivial trauma such as a cough, sneeze, or the Valsalva maneuver. This condition is caused when a small blood vessel underneath the conjunctiva ruptures and bleeds (Fig. 33.5). The symptoms include a painless, bright red flat patch on the sclera. Most patients usually discover a subconjunctival hemorrhage as a surprise when looking in the mirror. Although a subconjunctival hemorrhage is benign, if there has been facial trauma and the bleeding tracks posteriorly, it may indicate presence of an orbital fracture. No treatment is required for an atraumatic subconjunctival hemorrhage; blood will usually reabsorb in 2 to 3 weeks.[15]

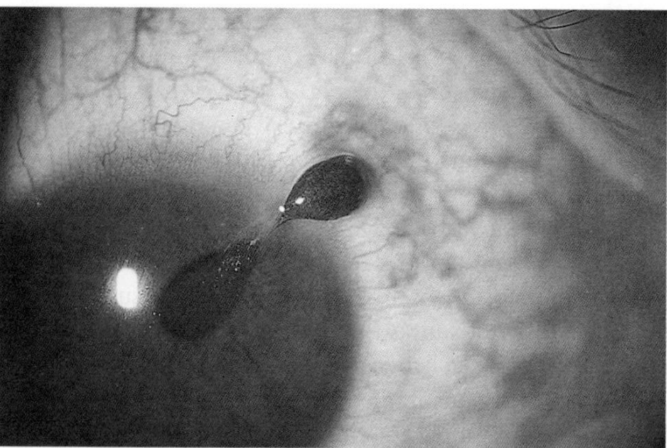

Fig. 33.6 **Ruptured Globe.** (From Auerbach PS. *Wilderness Medicine.* 5th ed. St Louis, MO: Mosby; 2007. Courtesy Steve Chaflin, MD, University of Texas Health Science Center, San Antonio, TX.)

Penetrating Trauma

A penetrating injury to the eye may occur during work or play and is often associated with lack of protective eyewear. Injury may affect surface structures, such as the cornea, or involve damage to the globe.

Periorbital wounds. Periorbital wounds involve injury to the eyelids and surrounding tissue. Tissues lie in close proximity to the globe, so wounds should be examined carefully for globe penetration. Depending on the mechanism of injury, careful examination for foreign bodies should be part of the examination. Therapeutic interventions for lacerations include wound care and early closure, with careful approximation of wound edges before edema develops. For major lacerations or injuries with missing tissue, a plastic surgeon is recommended.[4] Bedside ultrasound can aid in identifying foreign bodies and diagnosing injury to the structures of the eye when edema and ecchymosis make examination challenging.[15]

Globe rupture. Globe rupture is an ocular emergency resulting from blunt or penetrating trauma. Rupture occurs at a point of weakness in the ocular structures, usually at the insertion of the extraocular muscles or the corneoscleral junction (limbus). Penetrating injuries to the globe are caused by perforation with a sharp object such as a knife, stick, or projectile object. Blunt forces cause globe rupture secondary to an abrupt rise in IOP.

Signs and symptoms of globe rupture include an unusually deep or shallow anterior chamber, altered light perception, hyphema, and occasionally vitreous hemorrhage (Fig. 33.6). The pupil assumes a teardrop shape with the tip pointing to the perforation. A Seidel test is conducted by instilling a large amount of fluorescein. A globe rupture is diagnosed when a dark streak interrupts the flow of fluorescein. Pain and nausea should be treated aggressively. Severe pain or vomiting will increase IOP and the risk of expulsion of intraocular contents.

When globe rupture is suspected, further eye manipulation should be avoided. If an impaled object is present, do not remove it. Secure the object, if possible. Detailed examination is not performed until the ophthalmologist arrives; during this time a CT scan may be ordered. General anesthesia may be necessary to perform an adequate examination. Eye drops should not be used when globe rupture is suspected. Tetanus immunization should be updated. While the patient is waiting for the ophthalmologist, a shield or other protective device can be placed over the affected eye. The unaffected eye should also be patched to minimize consensual eye movement. Keep the patient NPO (nothing by mouth), and prepare for surgery.[4,7,15]

Superficial Trauma

Corneal abrasion. Corneal abrasions are a common injury seen in the ED. The cornea is damaged when dirt, a contact lens, or another foreign body scratches, abrades, or denudes the epithelium. Damage to the cornea exposes superficial corneal nerves, causing tearing, eyelid spasms, and pain. The patient will usually complain of a foreign body sensation, photophobia, and acute onset of pain.

Instillation of a drop of topical anesthesia will assist in obtaining a visual acuity. It will also alleviate the sensation of a foreign body and decrease pain. The upper eyelid should be inverted to ensure that no foreign body is found. Diagnosis is made with fluorescein staining and examination with a cobalt light and a slit-lamp examination. If the abrasion is large, cycloplegics may be prescribed to decrease ciliary spasms; however, there is no supporting evidence for this treatment. Good evidence shows that application of topical NSAIDs is effective in relieving pain in the first 24 to 48 hours without interfering with healing. Topical antibiotics are usually prescribed to prevent secondary infection. Patching is not recommended. The injury should be reevaluated in 24 hours.[15]

Corneal lacerations. Corneal lacerations present similarly to corneal abrasions; they may be small or large. Small lacerations are treated as corneal abrasions, or a corneal band aid may be applied. Larger corneal lacerations may require surgery to preserve the integrity of the intraocular contents. Corneal lacerations are identified by the Seidel test described earlier. An ophthalmology consult is indicated for these patients.[15]

Foreign Body

Conjunctival/corneal foreign body. A patient with a retained foreign body presents with complaints similar to those for a corneal abrasion. The foreign body is most often a speck of dirt or dust. It may be flushed out with normal saline irrigation. Using a topical anesthetic will aid the nurse in examination of the eye, including folding back the upper lid. When visualized, the foreign body can often be removed with a cotton swab moistened with sterile saline.[8]

With a suspected foreign body in the conjunctiva and cornea, determine the identity of the foreign body (what the patient believes is in the eye). A history of high-speed projectiles should increase the index of suspicion for an intraocular foreign body. Organic foreign bodies have a higher incidence of infection, whereas metallic objects leave a rust ring unless the object is removed within 12 hours. Inert foreign bodies do not cause infection but have a greater risk for penetration.

Never use a dry cotton-tipped swab on the cornea because it may create a large corneal defect. If the foreign body adheres to the cornea, a topical anesthetic is applied, and then a 25- to 27-gauge needle is used at a tangential angle to remove the object. Larger embedded objects are referred to the ophthalmologist for removal or follow-up. After the foreign body is removed, the cornea should be carefully examined for other objects, a rust ring, or corneal abrasion. Ocular burr drills are also used to remove rust rings and may be used to free foreign bodies stuck to the cornea. Treat subsequent corneal abrasions. If the patient has a rust ring, an ophthalmologic referral should be arranged so that the patient is seen within the next 24 hours.[15]

Intraocular foreign body. Intraocular foreign bodies are usually small and easily overlooked. The entry site may be small and difficult to locate. A high index of suspicion is required to prompt a vigorous evaluation for this type of injury. Many patients experience only slight discomfort. Visual acuity may be significantly decreased or may be normal. The pupil may assume the shape of a cat's eye, which may indicate a ruptured globe. Ocular ultrasound or CT scan can aid in diagnosing and locating the foreign body. More than 90% of patients with an intraocular foreign body require surgery. Prompt surgical intervention to remove the object is necessary to preserve vision and prevent further injury or infection.[16]

Ocular Burns

Ocular burns pose an immediate threat to the patient's vision. Burns to the eye may result from a chemical, a heat source such as a fire or household appliance, or radiation. Regardless of cause, these injuries cause significant discomfort and can lead to vision impairment or loss. The limbic cells repair and maintain the corneal epithelium. A burn leading to limbic ischemia causes permanent damage to vision and disfigures the eye.[15]

Chemical trauma. A chemical burn is the most urgent of all ocular emergencies. Chemical burns from acids, alkalis, or petroleum-based products occur at home and work. These substances, particularly alkalis, have a devastating effect on the eye. Acid burns cause immediate damage to the cornea by denaturing the tissue, so the cornea appears white and opaque. No further damage occurs after the initial impact because the acid is neutralized on contact. Conversely, alkalis such as concrete, lye, and drain cleaners also cause opacification of the cornea; however, alkalis continue to penetrate and damage the cornea until the substance is removed. Urgent and copious irrigation is indicated. Irrigation with normal saline, or lactated Ringer's solution is preferred, but tap water can be used if these are not readily available.[15]

With alkaline burns, irrigation should continue until ocular pH reaches approximately 7.5 to 8. Irrigation for a minimum of 30 minutes with 2 L of fluid is the norm, and the nurse should measure pH periodically during and after the initial irrigation. Patients should receive topical antibiotics. Parenteral or oral narcotic analgesia is also recommended. Administer a tetanus immunization as appropriate. Obtain an ophthalmologic consult for all ocular burns and guidance on medical management.[15]

Thermal burns. Thermal burns affect the eyelids but rarely involve the globe because of reflex lid closure. Thermal burns are treated similarly to other burns that occur on the body. If the lids are damaged so they do not close adequately, special attention must be given to ensure that the globe is not injured. Burns to the eyelids may cause lid contracture, which is disfiguring and affects vision. Data comparing the efficacy of therapeutic interventions are lacking. Treatment often includes topical antibiotics, artificial tears, and topical steroids.[15]

Radiation burns. Radiation burns may be ultraviolet or infrared. Severity of the burn depends on wavelength and degree of exposure. Ultraviolet burns occur in welders, snow skiers, ice climbers, people who read on the beach, and those who use sun lamps. Ultraviolet radiation is absorbed by the cornea and produces keratitis, conjunctivitis, or both. Pain, tearing, photophobia, and a foreign body sensation usually begin 8 to 12 hours after exposure. Ultraviolet burns are considered the most painful of all ocular burns. Visual acuity is usually decreased. Therapeutic interventions include topical NSAIDs and antibiotics, cycloplegics to reduce ciliary spasm, and light avoidance (e.g., sunglasses). The cornea usually heals within 24 hours without residual scarring. Slit-lamp examination with fluorescein staining reveals superficial punctate keratitis that looks like small microdots on the corneal surface.[7,9,15]

Infrared burns are more serious than radiation burns, but they are uncommon primarily because of the use of protective eyewear. In the past, infrared injuries were associated with eclipses and atomic bomb detonation. In recent years, however, the laser has been implicated in causing infrared burns. A laser pointer shone into the eye creates a hole in the macula and causes retinal damage. Vision deteriorates over days to weeks. Surgery is required to close the hole and restore vision.[17]

Medical Problems Involving the Eye

Many ocular problems that present to the ED are not related to trauma. Problems may be a minor annoyance or represent a significant threat to the patient's vision. The most common medical conditions seen in the ED are described in the following section.

Infections

Lid infections

Hordeolum. Hordeolum, commonly called a stye, is an infection of an eyelash oil gland of Zeis or Moll. The patient develops a small external abscess, pain, redness, and swelling (Fig. 33.7). Therapeutic intervention includes application of warm compresses four times per day until the abscess erupts, which may occur spontaneously. Massage after warm compresses will encourage drainage of the clogged duct. Massage

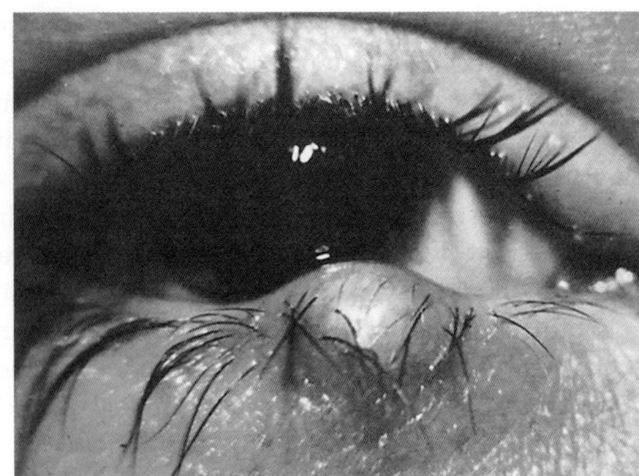

Fig. 33.7 Acute Hordeolum of the Lower Eyelid. (From Newell FW. *Ophthalmology: Principles and Concepts.* 8th ed. St Louis, MO: Mosby; 1996.)

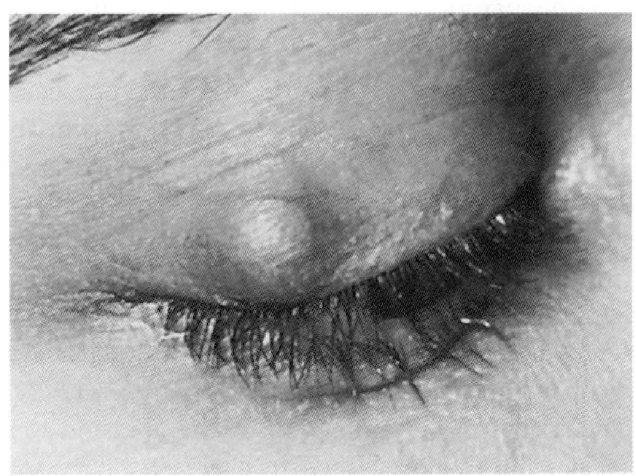

Fig. 33.8 Chronic Chalazion of Meibomian Gland of the Upper Eyelid. (From Newell FW. *Ophthalmology: Principles and Concepts.* 8th ed. St Louis, MO: Mosby; 1996.)

should be gentle, without squeezing the abscess, because squeezing can spread infection and worsen the condition.[18] If the condition is unresponsive to conservative therapy, including antibiotic administration, the patient should be referred to an ophthalmologist for consideration of incision and drainage.

Chalazion. A chalazion is an internal hordeolum caused by chronic granulomatous inflammation of the Meibomian gland (Fig. 33.8). The patient usually presents with several weeks of painless, localized swelling. A chalazion is differentiated from a hordeolum by the absence of acute inflammation. Treatment options include steroid injection or surgical incision and curettage.[19]

Corneal infections

Keratitis. Keratitis is a generic term for inflammation of the cornea. The inflammation may be caused by a bacterial, fungal, or protozoan infection or a corneal ulcer. It is often associated with contact lens use. The cornea becomes light sensitive, red, and painful, with profuse tearing. The typical presentation is conjunctivitis, pain, photophobia, mucopurulent discharge, and decreased vision. Pus in the anterior chamber (hypopyon) may also be present. Culture and sensitivity should be obtained to determine the specific cause of the infection.

Therapeutic interventions include warm compresses, broad-spectrum antibiotics, and topical antimicrobials. In the most severe cases, steroids are an effective treatment. The eye should not be patched. Referral to an ophthalmologist within 24 hours is required to confirm microbe susceptibility and to prevent further complications.[20]

Viral keratoconjunctivitis. Viral keratoconjunctivitis is an acute conjunctivitis and keratitis most commonly caused by an adenovirus. The patient complains of redness to the eye, tearing, and pain. Photophobia may occur several days later. Eyelids and conjunctiva become swollen. In adults, this condition is confined to the eye; however, children may have fever, pharyngitis, and diarrhea. Therapeutic intervention is usually supportive; including fluids and management of discomfort and fever with over-the-counter remedies. Antibiotics will be ineffective against viral infection. Testing with point-of-care pathogen screening assists with diagnosis and guides treatment.

Investigation into the effectiveness of topical antivirals is ongoing. Viral conjunctivitis and keratoconjunctivitis infections spread easily. To prevent further transmission of the disease, it is critical that the patient, family members, coworkers, and health care providers avoid touching the infected eye and perform scrupulous hand washing. All instruments used on the patient should be sterilized.[21]

Herpes simplex. Herpes simplex infection can affect the eyelids, conjunctiva, and cornea. Symptoms include watery discharge, burning, and a foreign body sensation. Skin involvement includes vesicular lesions. The conjunctiva appear inflamed. Fluorescein staining reveals a corneal dendrite. Outbreaks on the lids and conjunctiva can be treated with oral and topical antiviral agents. Steroids are contraindicated.[21]

Herpes zoster ophthalmicus. Herpes zoster ophthalmicus represents shingles in the ophthalmic division of the trigeminal nerve. Patients will often have prodromal signs of fever, fatigue, and malaise before the eruption of vesicles along the affected dermatome. They often have significant pain and scalp tenderness on half of the forehead. If the tip of the nose is involved, ocular involvement is more likely (Hutchinson's sign). Standard management includes local wound care, analgesics, and antiviral therapy. Topical steroids may be indicated for ocular involvement, and antibiotics may be required for secondary bacterial infection of the lesions. Administration of antivirals is recommended, ideally within 72 hours of vesicular eruption. Complications, including postherpetic neuralgia or vision loss, can occur. Zoster infections can be avoided with vaccination. The nurse should educate patients on the vaccines recommended by the National Center for Immunization and Respiratory Diseases.[22]

Conjunctivitis. Conjunctivitis, often called pink eye, is the most frequently seen ophthalmic problem in the ED and has multiple etiologic origins: bacterial, viral, chemical, and allergic. Viral and bacterial conjunctivitis are highly contagious, and patients often report that close contacts are also affected.

Viral conjunctivitis is most common, implicated in up to 80% of cases. Eye discharge with viral infection is clear or watery. Infection spreads easily, transmitted on contaminated hands or personal items or in the water in swimming pools and hot tubs. With viral infection, the patient is more likely to present with lymphadenopathy, bilateral eye infection, fever, or sore throat. Antiviral medications are not shown to be effective, but antihistamine eye drops and artificial tears may provide symptom relief. Often misdiagnosed as bacterial and treated inappropriately with antibiotics, viral conjunctivitis may be exacerbated by antibiotic treatment when patients spread the virus from one eye to the other on the medication dropper.[23,24]

Bacterial conjunctivitis usually presents with a yellow-green purulent discharge. Drainage from the eye is reported. Often the drainage will dry during sleep, making it difficult to open the eyes upon waking. The drainage can assist in differentiating among viral, bacterial, and allergic conjunctivitis. Purulent or mucopurulent drainage suggests a bacterial infection. Bacterial conjunctivitis infection may be caused by *Streptococcus pneumoniae, Staphylococcus aureus,* and *Moraxella* and *Haemophilus* organisms. Symptoms are most often unilateral. Discharge teaching includes instruction to use warm compresses for comfort and to observe strict hand hygiene.[8]

Conjunctivitis secondary to *Neisseria gonorrheae* is rare but is seen in patients with systemic gonorrhea and neonates exposed to untreated gonorrheal infection in the mother.[25] The patient presents with red, swollen conjunctiva and copious purulent drainage. Microbiology determines the presence of *N. gonorrheae.* Treatment follows guidelines for systemic sexually transmitted disease, including intramuscular ceftriaxone and oral azithromycin therapy for the patient and his or her sexual contacts. Because gonorrheal conjunctivitis can cause ocular injury leading to vision loss, patients must be referred for close ophthalmology follow-up.[25] The neonate should be admitted for parenteral antibiotic therapy and close monitoring. The mother should also be treated.

Allergic conjunctivitis is usually caused by an allergen that makes the eyes tear and the lids itch. Treatment is supportive and may consist of eye drops containing antihistamines, decongestants, and/or nonsteroidal agents; cool compresses; and systemic antihistamines.[23]

Uveitis/iritis. Uveitis/iritis is an inflammation of the uveal tract, including the iris, ciliary body, and choroid. Uveal inflammation usually affects the anterior portion of the uveal tract and is categorized as iritis. It can be caused by inflammation, infection, or trauma. The patient presents with complaints of decreased vision, photophobia, and pain with direct and consensual light reflex, reddened eye, and excessive tearing. Initial treatments include cycloplegics and topical steroids for relief of photophobia and inflammation; however, anterior uveitis and iritis must be evaluated by an ophthalmologist. Viral uveitis may be caused by herpes zoster or varicella zoster. Syphilis serology is useful to rule out syphilis infection in bacterial uveitis.[21,26,27]

Orbital cellulitis. Orbital cellulitis (Fig. 33.9), an infection deep into the orbital septum, can be life-threatening. The usual causes are *S. pneumoniae, S. aureus,* and *Haemophilus influenzae.* Frequently, the orbital infection is secondary to a sinus infection. Symptoms include pain, fever, and impaired EOM.

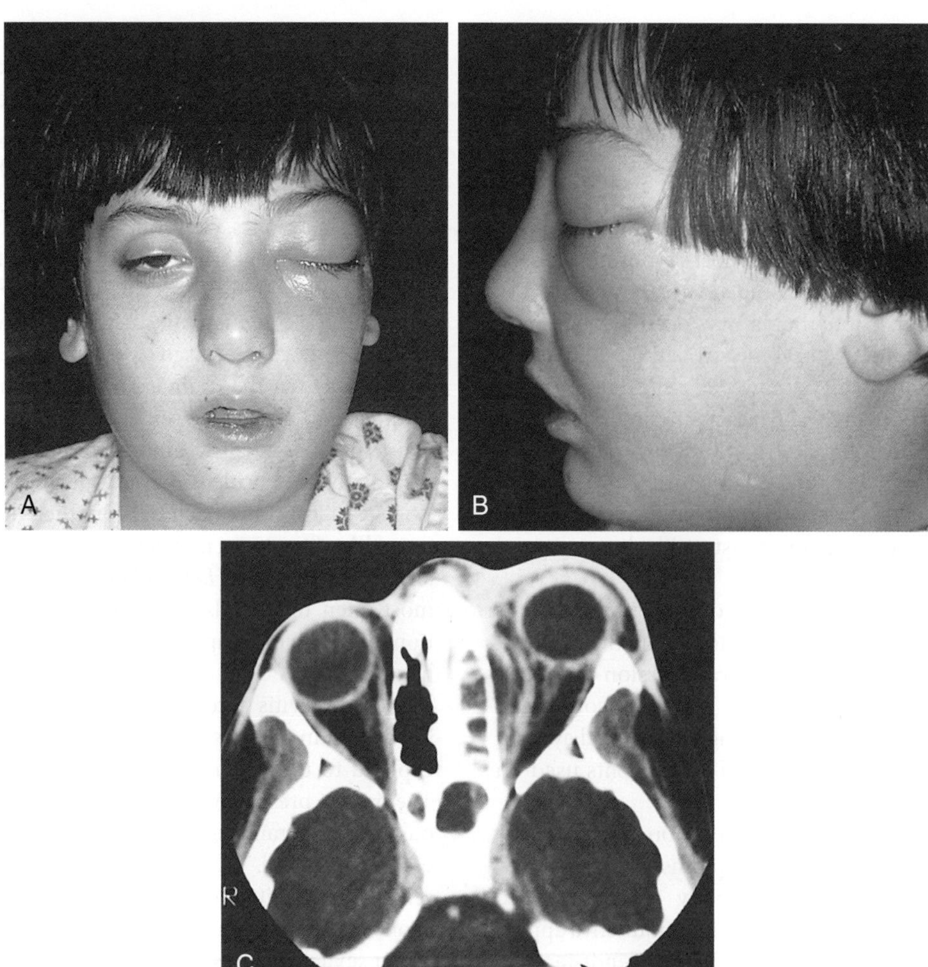

Fig. 33.9 Orbital Cellulitis. (A and B) This child had a fever, severe toxicity, and marked lethargy. He experienced intense orbital and retroorbital pain and showed a limited range of ocular motion. (C) This computed tomography scan shows preseptal swelling, proptosis, and lateral displacement of the globe and orbital contents by a subperiosteal abscess. (From Zitelli B, Davis H. *Atlas of Pediatric Physical Diagnosis*. 4th ed. St Louis, MO: Mosby; 2002.)

Impaired EOM is a crucial clue in differentiating between periorbital cellulitis and orbital cellulitis. With periorbital cellulitis, there is no impairment of the extraocular muscles.

Bacterial infection of the orbit endangers vision and can be life-threatening. Studies indicate a trend toward mixed aerobic and anaerobic pathogens in orbital cellulitis. In addition, with the emergence of virulent antibiotic-resistant bacteria, including methicillin-resistant *Staphylococcus aureus* (MRSA), treatment with broad-spectrum antibiotics is recommended. Nasal spray to encourage drainage of the infected sinus is also advised. The patient must be assessed for signs and symptoms of systemic infection such as fever, chills, lethargy, and headache. In rare cases, the infection spreads to the cavernous sinus and can pose a threat to life or vision. Patients with suspected or confirmed diagnosis of orbital cellulitis require a prompt ophthalmology consultation.[28]

Retinal Emergencies

Central retinal artery occlusion. Central retinal artery occlusion (CRAO) is sometimes called an eye stroke. It is a true medical emergency. Occlusion of the artery, most often by a thrombus, leads to retinal ischemia. Patients with a history of cardiac disease, hypertension, or stroke are at increased risk.[8,29] Conservative treatment, such as medication to reduce intraocular pressure, vasodilation techniques (such as blowing into a paper bag), and ocular massage are not shown to be reliable for restoring or recovering sight. Early studies of the use of systemic fibrinolytic therapy are promising. Reestablishing circulation is time sensitive, and prompt intervention is imperative.[29,30]

Retinal detachment. Retinal detachment occurs when the retina tears and allows vitreous humor to seep between the retina and the choroid. The normal function of the retina is to perceive light and send an impulse to the optic nerve. When the retina is torn, impaired circulation of blood, oxygen, and nutrients renders the retina unable to perceive light. The patient may complain of "flashing lights," "floaters," or a "veil" or "curtain effect" in the visual field. Diagnosis is made by patient history and symptoms, along with diagnostic imaging. Early studies show bedside ocular ultrasound is highly accurate in diagnosing retinal detachment.[15,20,30]

Glaucoma

Glaucoma is a leading cause of blindness worldwide and is characterized as open-angle glaucoma or angle-closure glaucoma. In the United States, more than 80% of patients diagnosed with glaucoma have open-angle disease. However, angle-closure glaucoma is more likely to cause severe vision impairment or vision loss. Risk increases with age and a family history of the disease. Elevated intraocular pressure leading to glaucoma may also occur with poorly controlled diabetes and cardiovascular disease. Glaucoma is a degenerative, neuropathic disease affecting neurons whose cell bodies are in the retina with axons in the optic nerve. Glaucoma occurs when aqueous humor cannot escape from the anterior chamber, causing volume to increase and IOP to rise. In normal, healthy eyes, aqueous humor leaves the anterior chamber and enters the vascular system via Schlemm's canal. With glaucoma, increased anterior chamber pressure decreases circulation to the retina and increases pressure on the optic nerve.

Early diagnosis and treatment are most effective in preventing progression of the disease. The resultant increased pressure eventually leads to blindness. Examination of the optic nerve head with direct ophthalmoscopy may reveal structural changes suspicious of disease. Patients must be referred for an ophthalmology consult. Emerging technologies, including optical coherence tomography and confocal scanning laser ophthalmoscopy, have been shown to be effective and reliable in detecting increased IOP, facilitating early diagnosis and sight-saving intervention.[31-33]

Acute angle-closure glaucoma. Contrary to the far more common open-angle glaucoma, which often progresses slowly and without symptoms, primary acute angle-closure glaucoma (PACG) occurs suddenly and is characterized by severe, sudden eye pain, often accompanied by headache, nausea, and vomiting. PACG is a true ocular emergency. It occurs when aqueous humor is unable to flow from the posterior to the anterior chambers of the pupil, resulting in a rapid and dramatic increase in IOP. PACG is more common in women, and risk increases with age. Acute angle-closure glaucoma occurs with blockage of the anterior chamber angle near the root of the iris (Fig. 33.10). IOP greater than 60 to 70 mm Hg damages the corneal endothelium, lens, iris, optical nerve, and retina. Antiemetics and narcotics may be useful for symptom management. PACG is treated with laser iridotomy. The laser relieves the pressure by creating a hole in the iris, thus eliminating the pupillary block.[31,32]

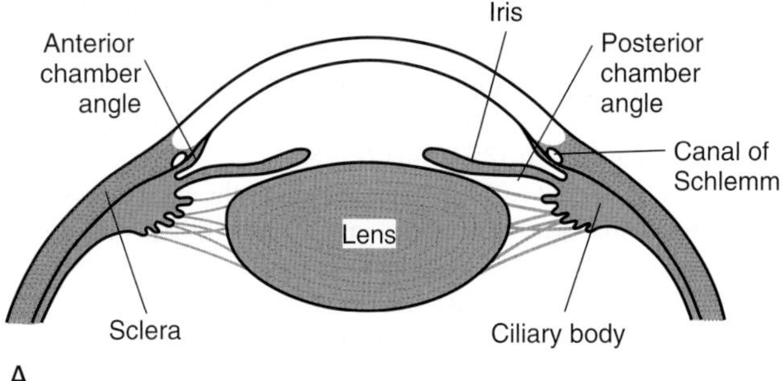

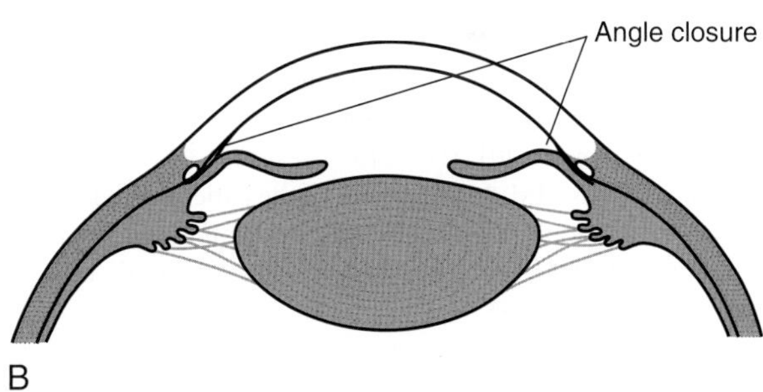

Fig. 33.10 Comparison of normal angle of eye (A) with closed angle in angle-closure glaucoma (B).

SUMMARY

Although ED visits by patients with eye complaints are not uncommon, true ocular emergencies, those posing a threat to the patient's vision, are rare. Injury to the eye and orbit are evaluated as part of a trauma examination. Illnesses causing pain or irritation of the eye have many causes, and preferred treatment is often supportive care. The emergency nurse assesses and evaluates the patient and can aid in identifying symptoms of illness or injury that suggest actual or potential risk of vision loss, responding with actions to best protect and preserve the patient's ocular health.

REFERENCES

1. Channa R, Zafar SN, Canner JK, Haring RS, Schneider EB, Friedman DS. Epidemiology of eye-related emergency department visits. *JAMA Ophthalmol.* 2016;134(3):312–319.
2. Yan H, Wang J, Li Y, Meng X, Yao X. Patient care process of ocular emergency. In: Yan H, ed. *Ocular Emergency*. Singapore, Singapore: Springer; 2018:19–28.
3. Emergency Nurses Association. *Emergency Nursing Core Curriculum*. 7th ed. St Louis, MO: Elsevier; 2018.
4. Mitchell JD. Ocular emergencies. In: Tintinalli JE, Kelen GD, Stapczynski JS, eds. *Emergency Medicine: A Comprehensive Study Guide*. 6th ed. New York, NY: McGraw-Hill; 2004.
5. Knoop KJ, Dennis WR, Hedges JR. Ophthalmologic procedures. In: Roberts JR, Hedges JR, eds. *Clinical Procedures in Emergency Medicine*. 4th ed. Philadelphia, PA: Saunders; 2004.
6. Guluma K. An evidence-based approach to abnormal vision. *Emerg Med Pract.* 2007;9(9):1.
7. Kim G, Witt M. Ocular trauma: an evidence-based approach to evaluation and management in the ED. *Pediatr Emerg Med Pract.* 2006;3(11):1.
8. Quigley MT. Tonometry. In: Proehl JA, ed. *Emergency Nursing Procedures*. 3rd ed. St Louis, MO: Saunders; 2004.
9. Wade RG, Peacock D. Bilateral eye irrigation: a simple and effective hands-free technique. *Eur J Emerg Med.* 2014;21(4):305–307.

10. Waldman N, Winrow B, Densie I, et al. An observational study to determine whether routinely sending patients home with a 24-hour supply of topical tetracaine from the emergency department for simple corneal abrasion pain is potentially safe. *Ann Emerg Med*. 2018;71(6):767–778.
11. Sowka JW, Kabat AG. A pop fly straight to the eye: a refresher on hyphema management, just in time for wiffleball season. *Review of Optometry*. 2017;154(6):98–101. https://www.reviewofoptometry.com/article/ro0617-a-pop-fly-straight-to-the-eye. Accessed May 28, 2019.
12. Shaik N, Arora J, Liao J, Rizzuti AE. Trauma to the anterior chamber and lens. In: Kaufman SC, Lazzaro DR, eds. *Textbook of Ocular Trauma: Evaluation and Treatment*. Cham, Switzerland: Springer; 2017:17–31.
13. American College of Surgeons Committee on Trauma. *Ocular trauma. Advanced Trauma Life Support*. Chicago, IL: American College of Surgeons; 2012:311–315.
14. Wierda SB, Ariss MM. Management of the patient with hyphema. In: Traboulsi EI, Utz MV, eds. *Practical Management of Pediatric Ocular Disorders and Strabismus*. New York, NY: Springer; 2016:149–153.
15. Hooker EA. Ocular injuries: new strategies in emergency department management. *Emerg Med Pract*. 2015;17(11):1–21.
16. Feldman M, Shigyo K, Kaji A. Intraocular foreign body: ultrasound and CT findings. *JETem (Journal of Education & Teaching in Emergency Medicine)*. 2017;2(1). https://doi.org/10.21980/J8JS3M.
17. Dhoot DS, Xu D, Srivastava S. High-powered laser pointer injury resulting in macular hole formation. *J Pediatr*. 2014;164(3):668.
18. Bragg KJ, Le JK. *Hordeolum. StatPearls [Internet]*. Treasure Island, FL: StatPearls Publishing. https://www.ncbi.nlm.nih.gov/books/NBK441985/, Updated May 4, 2019. Accessed May 28, 2019.
19. Aycinena ARP, Achiron A, Paul M, Burgansky-Eliash Z. Incision and curettage versus steroid injection for the treatment of chalazia: a meta-analysis. *Ophthalmic Plast Reconstr Surg*. 2016;32(3):220–224.
20. Zimmerman AB, Nixon AD, Rueff EM. Contact lens associated microbial keratitis: practical considerations for the optometrist. *Clin Optometr. (Auckl.)*. 2016;8:1–12.
21. Sendrowski DP, Maher J. Claim victory over viral conjunctivitis: adenovirus and herpes virus are highly contagious pathogens, but you can put a stop to them if you diagnose them quickly and manage them appropriately. *Rev Optometr*. 2016;153(6):78–84.
22. Lu P, O'Halloran A, Williams WW, Harpaz R. National and state-specific shingles vaccination among adults aged ≥60 years. *Am J Prev Med*. 2017;52(3):362–372.
23. Azari AA, Barney NP. Conjunctivitis: a systematic review of diagnosis and treatment. *JAMA*. 2013;310(16):1721–1730. https://doi.org/10.1001/jama.2013.280318.
24. Keen M, Thompson M. Treatment of acute conjunctivitis in the United States and evidence of antibiotic overuse: isolated issue or a systematic problem? *Ophthalmology*. 2017;124(8):1096–1098.
25. Costumbrado J, Ghassemzadeh S. *Gonococcal conjunctivitis. StatPearls [Internet]*. Treasure Island, FL: StatPearls Publishing; 2018. Published January 2018. https://www.ncbi.nlm.nih.gov/books/NBK459289, Updated February 15, 2019. Accessed May 28, 2019.
26. Tugal-Tutkun Ilknur, Cimino L, Akova YA. Review for disease of the year: varicella zoster virus-induced anterior uveitis. *Ocul Immunol Inflamm*. 2018;26(2):171–177.
27. Seve P, Cacoub P, Bodaghi B, et al. Uveitis: diagnostic work-up. A literature review and recommendations from an expert committee. *Autoimmun Rev*. 2017;16(12):1254–1264.
28. Liao JC, Harris GJ. Current guidelines for the management of orbital cellulitis. In: Yen MT, Johnson TE, eds. *Orbital Cellulitis and Periorbital Infections*. Cham, Switzerland: Springer; 2018:55–63.
29. Callizo J, Feltgen N, Pantenburg S, et al. Cardiovascular risk factors in central retinal artery occlusion: results of a prospective and standardized medical examination. *Ophthalmology*. 2015;122(9):1881–1888.
30. Vrablik ME, Snead GR, Minnigan HJ, Kirschner JM, Emmett TW, Seupaul RA. The diagnostic accuracy of bedside ocular ultrasonography for the diagnosis of retinal detachment: a systematic review and meta-analysis. *Ann Emerg Med*. 2015;65(2):199–203.
31. Weinreb RN, Aung T, Medeiros FA. The pathophysiology and treatment of glaucoma: a review. *JAMA*. 2014;311(18):1901–1911.
32. Kansal V, Armstrong JJ, Pintwala R, Hutnik C. Optical coherence tomography for glaucoma diagnosis: an evidence based meta-analysis. *PloS One*. 2018;13(1):e0190621.
33. Chan TCW, Bala C, Siu A, Wan F, White A. Risk factors for rapid glaucoma disease progression. *Am J Ophthalmol*. 2017;180:151–157.

UNIT V

Trauma Emergencies

34

Epidemiology and Mechanisms of Injury

Cynthia Blank-Reid
Paul C. Reid

Epidemiology and mechanism of injury (MOI) are separate and distinct disciplines, yet they are closely intertwined in the trauma literature. Epidemiology is the branch of medicine studying the causes, distribution, and control of disease in populations.[1] It defines the scope of injuries in terms of their incidence and identifies associated factors and determinants of specific types of injury. Mechanism of injury is the study of how energy is transferred from the environment to the individual. An understanding of MOI equips health care providers with the knowledge to anticipate injuries, diagnosis, treatments, and complications of traumatic injury. Common patterns of injury are observed with specific mechanisms, and this knowledge can assist with the rapid detection of suspected injuries. Unless death occurs immediately, the outcome of an injured person depends not only on injury severity but also on the speed and appropriateness of treatment.

Knowledge of both epidemiology and MOI helps shape health care by allowing providers to deliver evidence-based care and understand what populations are at risk for particular injuries and those who need to be targeted for specific prevention programs. It also provides the ability to evaluate the effectiveness of these programs over time. Nurses who care for trauma patients clearly recognize the need for prevention and control strategies to curb mortality and morbidity. The perception of trauma as preventable events rather than acts of random unexpectedness ("accidents") is essential for the success of prevention programs. Throughout this chapter, the terms *trauma* and *injury* are used interchangeably.

EPIDEMIOLOGY

The epidemiology of trauma is particularly important because of the implications for social and public policy, legislation, and injury-prevention programs.[1] Understanding the scope of any problem is central to successful planning and implementation of legal, environmental, and educational remedies. Data elements such as incidence, prevalence, age, sex, race or ethnicity, geographic distribution; and morbidity or mortality are the sources of epidemiologic surveillance and serve to quantify aggregates.

Trauma is a disease that remains a leading cause of death for Americans of all ages regardless of gender, race, or economic status. Millions of Americans are injured each year and survive.[2] Whether the injury is fatal or not, the patient and his or her family, friends, and employers will all have to face adjustments in their lives. Refer to Table 34.1, the Centers for Disease Control and Prevention's (CDC's) 10 leading causes of death by age-group.

Trauma is the leading cause of death for children older than 1 year and adults younger than 45 years of age. Trauma is also the primary cause for loss of work years because it predominately affects a younger population who are in their prime working years. (Refer to Table 34.2). The great social, personal, and economic costs associated with traumatic injuries makes trauma a major public health problem in the United States.

Trauma in the United States

Age

For children younger than 1 year of age, the leading cause of a fatal injury is unintentional suffocation due to choking or strangulation. For those aged 1 to 4 years, drowning is the leading cause of death, followed by motor vehicle crashes (MVCs). MVCs are a leading cause of death from ages 2 to 24 years. Young children are frequently unrestrained passengers and innocent participants in the MVC.[3]

The high rate of injury for older individuals (15–24 years of age) involved in MVCs is multifactorial and frequently the result of high-speed driving, distracted driving, inexperience with poor weather or other road hazards, experimentation with drugs and alcohol in combination with poor judgment, and risk taking behaviors. Statistics for teenagers, though, are changing. A total of 2820 teenagers aged 13 to 19 died in MVCs in 2016. This is 68% fewer than in 1975 and 3% more[4] than in 2015. The risk for MVC is higher among 16- to 19-year-olds than in any other age-group. Drivers in this age-group are four times more likely than older drivers to crash, based on number of miles driven.[4] Teenage drivers, though, continue to be at high risk because of the following:

- *Inexperience:* They often fail to recognize or underestimate the dangers in hazardous situations. They are more likely to be distracted by technology, speed, run red lights, make illegal turns, ride with an intoxicated driver, and drive after using alcohol or drugs.[5]

TABLE 34.1 Ten Leading Causes of Death by Age-Group in the United States for 2016, All Races, Both Sexes

	AGE-GROUPS										
Rank	<1	1–4	5–9	10–14	15–24	25–34	35–44	45–54	55–64	65 +	Total
1	Congenital Anomalies 4816	Uninten-tional Injury 1261	Unintentional Injury 787	Unintentional Injury 847	Uninten-tional Injury 13,895	Uninten-tional Injury 23,984	Unintentional Injury 20,975	Malignant Neoplasms 41,291	Malignant Neoplasms 116,364	Heart Disease 507,118	Heart Disease 635,260
2	Short Gestation 3927	Congenital Anomalies 433	Malignant Neoplasms 449	Suicide 436	Suicide 5723	Suicide 7366	Malignant Neoplasms 10,903	Heart Disease 34,027	Heart Disease 78,610	Malignant Neoplasms 422,927	Malignant Neoplasms 598,038
3	Sudden Infant Death Syndrome 1500	Malignant Neoplasms 377	Congenital Anomalies 203	Malignant Neoplasms 431	Homicide 5172	Homicide 5376	Heart Disease 10,477	Unintentional Injury 23,377	Unintentional Injury 21,860	Chronic Low. Respiratory Disease 131,002	Unintentional Injury 161,374
4	Maternal Pregnancy Complica-tions 1402	Homicide 339	Homicide 139	Homicide 147	Malignant Neoplasms 1431	Malignant Neoplasms 3791	Suicide 7030	Suicide 8437	Chronic Low Respiratory Disease 17,810	Cerebro vascular 121,630	Chronic Low Respiratory Disease 154,596
5	Unintentional Injury 1219	Heart Disease 118	Heart Disease 77	Congenital Anomalies 146	Heart Disease 949	Heart Disease 3445	Hormade 3369	Liver Disease 8364	Diabetes Mellitus 14,251	Alzheimer's Disease 114,883	Cerebro vascular 142,142
6	Placenta Cord. Mem-branes 841	Influenza & Pneumonia 103	Chronic Low. Respiratory Disease 68	Heart Disease 111	Congenital Anomalies 388	Liver Disease 925	Liver Disease 2851	Diabetes Mellitus 6267	Liver Disease 13,448	Diabetes Mellitus 56,452	Alzheimer Disease 116,103
7	Bacterial Sepsis 583	Septicemia 70	Influenza & Pneumonia 48	Chronic Low/ Respiratory Disease 75	Diabetes Mellitus 211	Diabetes Mellitus 792	Diabetes Mellitus 2049	Cerebro vascular 5353	Cerebro vas-cular 12,310	Unintentional Injury 53,141	Diabetes Mellitus 80,058
8	Respiratory Distress 488	Perinatal Period 60	Septicemia 40	Cerebrovas-cular 50	Chronic Low Respiratory Disease 206	Cerebrovas-cular 575	Cerebrovas-cular 1851	Chronic Low. Respiratory Disease 4307	Suicide 7759	Influenza & Pneumonia 42,479	Influenza & Pneumonia 51,537
9	Circulatory System Disease 460	Cerebrovas-cular 55	Cerebrovas-cular 38	Influenza & Pneumonia 39	Influenza & Pneumonia 189	Human Immuno-deficiency Virus 546	Human Immuno-deficiency Virus 971	Septicemia 2472	Septicemia 5941	Nephritis 41,095	Nephritis 50,046
10	Neonatal Hemor-rhage 398	Chronic Low Respiratory Disease 51	Benign Neo-plasms 31	Septicemia 31	Complicated Pregnancy 184	Complicated Pregnancy 472	Septicemia 897	Homicide 2152	Nephritis 5650	Septicemia 30,405	Suicide 44,965

CDC Produced by: National Center for Injury Prevention and Control, CDC using WISQARS™.
Data source: National Vital Statistics System. National Center for Health Statistics. From Centers for Disease Control and Prevention, National Center for Injury Prevention and Control: Web-based Injury Statistics Query and Reporting System (WISQARS). 2016. http://www.cdc.gov/ncipc/wisqars.

TABLE 34.2 **Ten Leading Causes of Nonfatal Injury, United States 2016, All Races, Both Sexes, Disposition: All Cases**

	AGE-GROUPS										
Rank	**<1**	**1–4**	**5–9**	**10–14**	**15–24**	**25–34**	**35–44**	**45–54**	**55–64**	**65+**	**All Ages**
1	Unintentional Fall 122,266	Unintentional Fall 750,052	Unintentional Fall 588,689	Unintentional Fall 490,255	Unintentional Struck by/ Against 843,602	Unintentional Fall 718,186	Unintentional Fall 661,809	Unintentional Fall 872,377	Unintentional Fall 1,072,216	Unintentional Fall 3,175,414	Unintentional Fall 9,194,403
2	Unintentional Struck by/ Against 28,224	Unintentional Struck by/ Against 282,087	Unintentional Struck by/ Against 348,333	Unintentional Struck by/ Against 482,632	Unintentional Fall 742,092	Unintentional MV-Occupant 592,609	Unintentional Overexer-tion 477,104	Unintentional Other Specified 439,928	Unintentional Other Specified 309,663	Unintentional Struck by/ Against 344,769	Unintentional Struck by/ Against 4,043,802
3	Unintentional Other Bite/ Sting 10,649	Unintentional Other Bite/ Sting 137,409	Unintentional Other Bite/ Sting 98,268	Unintentional Overexer-tion 250,247	Unintentional MV-Occupant 665,419	Unintentional Struck by/ Against 590,710	Unintentional Struck by/ Against 427,935	Unintentional Struck by/ Against 405,938	Unintentional Struck by/ Against 289,371	Unintentional Overexer-tion 257,602	Unintentional Overexer-tion 2,968,273
4	Unintentional Foreign Body 10,046	Unintentional Foreign Body 117,387	Unintentional Cut/Pierce 88,241	Unintentional Cut/Pierce 112,638	Unintentional Overexertion 580,343	Unintentional Overexertion 562,016	Unintentional MV-Occu-pant 417,169	Unintentional Overexertion 405,475	Unintentional Overexer-tion 283,343	Unintentional MV-Occu-pant 241,134	Unintentional MV-Occu-pant 2,723,012
5	Unintentional Other Specified 8857	Unintentional Cut/Pierce 70,899	Unintentional Overexer-tion 80,651	Unintentional MV-Occu-pant 71,252	Unintentional Cut/Pierce 387,016	Unintentional Other Spec-ified 454,527	Unintentional Other Specified 375,750	Unintentional MV-Occupant 372,488	Unintentional MV-Occu-pant 270,408	Unintentional Cut/Pierce 177,209	Unintentional Other Spec-ified 2,182,292
6	Unintentional Fire/Burn 7081	Unintentional Overexertion 67,790	Unintentional MV-Occu-pant 60,722	Unintentional Unknown/ Unspecified 66,312	Unintentional Other Specified 348,726	Unintentional Cut/Pierce 408,160	Unintentional Poisoning 312,902	Unintentional Poisoning 360,752	Unintentional Poisoning 245,288	Unintentional Poisoning 141,837	Unintentional Cut/Pierce 1,994,265
7	Unintentional Inhalation/ Suffocation 5111	Unintentional Other Spec-ified 59,638	Unintentional Foreign Body 54,978	Unintentional Other Bite/ Sting 60,262	Other Assault[a]- Struck by/ Again 333,051	Unintentional Poisoning 358,454	Unintentional Cut/Pierce 285,165	Unintentional Cut/Pierce 254,245	Unintentional Cut/Pierce 206,002	Unintentional Other Specified 137,863	Unintentional Poisoning 1,711,836

TABLE 34.2 Ten Leading Causes of Nonfatal Injury, United States 2016, All Races, Both Sexes, Disposition: All Cases—cont'd

	AGE-GROUPS										
Rank	**<1**	**1–4**	**5–9**	**10–14**	**15–24**	**25–34**	**35–44**	**45–54**	**55–64**	**65+**	**All Ages**
8	Unintentional Unknown/ Unspecified 5002	Unintentional Unknown/ Unspecified 39,644	Unintentional Pedal Cyclist 48,196	Unintentional Pedal Cyclist 59,702	Unintentional Poisoning 237,982	Other Assault[a] Struck by/ Again 343,026	Other Assault[a] Struck by/ Again 218,273	Other Assault[a] Struck by/ Again 167,942	Unintentional Other Bite/ Sting 117,195	Unintentional Other Bite/ Sting 107,023	Other Assault[a] Struck by/ Again 1,250,382
9	Unintentional Cut/Pierce 4463	Unintentional Fire/Burn 39,079	Unintentional Dog Bite 36,934	Unintentional Other Transport 48,951	Unintentional Other Bite/ Sting 161,344	Unintentional Other Bite/ Sting 176,116	Unintentional Other Bite/ Sting 143,424	Unintentional Other Bite/ Sting 142,524	Other Assault[a] Struck by/ Again 81,739	Unintentional Unknown/ Unspecified 99,146	Unintentional Other Bite/ Sting 1,154,289
10	Unintentional MV-Occu- pant 3879	Unintentional Poisoning 30,671	Unintentional Other Transport 31,934	Other Assault[a] Struck by/ Again 48,914	Unintentional Unknown/ Unspecified 132,613	Unintentiona Unknown/ Unspecified 131,119	Unintentional Unknown/ Unspeci- fied 106,005	Unintentional Unknown/ Unspecified 109,922	Unintentional Unknown/ Unspecified 81,296	Unintentional Other Transport 95,027	Unintentional Unknown/ Unspecified 800,719

[a]The 'Other Assault' category includes all assaults that are **not** classified as sexual assault. It represents the majority of assaults.
MV, Motor vehicle.
Produced by: Office of Statistics and Programming, National Center for Injury Prevention and Control, CDC.
Data source: NEISS All Injury Program operated by the Consumer Product Safety Commission (CPSC).

- *Alcohol and driving:* Studies show 25% of teenage drivers who died in an MVC had a blood alcohol concentration (BAC) of 0.08% or higher, which is above the legal BAC limit for adult drivers.[6,7]
- *Texting:* The prevalence of texting while driving among US high school students was higher in states with lower minimum learner's permit ages and in states where a larger percentage of students drove.[8]

The 65 years and older age-group is the fastest-growing segment of the US population. As the US population grows older, more and more people become vulnerable and are dependent on others to meet their most basic needs. Individuals older than 75 years of age have the highest death rate from injuries, which is attributed to multiple factors, including their frailer state of health and preexisting medical conditions. Older drivers drive less, but they are more likely to crash and die in the collision.[9,10] Estimates indicate more than 40 million older adults will be licensed drivers in 2020.[2,10] In addition, age is a major factor in determining the risk for a cervical spine injury in injuries from collisions between autos and pedestrians. Those older than 65 years are 12 to 14 times more likely to sustain a cervical spine injury than pediatric patients.[11]

Of the 11 million people aged 65 years and older who are hospitalized annually, a significant percentage (52%) of people admitted for injury-related conditions have fractures.[2,10] Falls continue to be the most common cause of nonfatal and fatal injuries in adults ages 65 and older.[3] They also continue to be the primary cause of hip fractures. Although hip fractures are still highest among older adult females, they also affect males. Studies have shown that rates of hip fractures sustained by men are highest among white males and lowest for Asian men. One-year mortality was similar for white, black, and Hispanic men but significantly lower for Asians.[12] Interestingly, medical costs for the geriatric population are 2.5 times greater than for younger patients with similar injuries; this is due to longer lengths of stay, a higher incidence of complications, and more intensive care unit days.[13,14]

Gender

Gender, along with age variances, is related to the incidence and type of injury incurred. A total of 2820 teenagers aged 13 to 19 years died in MVCs in 2016. About two of every three teenagers killed in crashes in 2016 were males. Since 1975, teenage crash deaths have decreased more among males (72%) than among females (57%).[4] Males are 2.5 times more likely to be injured than females. This statistic is significant because of their participation in more hazardous activities and greater risk taking. This fact continues throughout the life span, as rates for motor vehicle (MV)–related injuries are twice as high for older men than women.[3] The pedestrian fatality rate is also more than twice as high for men as for women.[3]

Race/Ethnicity

Injury and death rates vary with race and income. The reasons for these variations are multifactorial and not completely understood. However, knowledge of the differences observed has been used to target prevention programs toward specific populations or geographic areas. For African Americans and whites, no matter what the MOI, the higher the income, the lower the death rate. The number of MVCs decreases in a depressed economy, whereas homicides and suicides increase. The highest homicide rate occurs in the African American population, the highest suicide rate is seen in whites and Native Americans, and the lowest death rate occurs in Asian Americans.[15]

African Americans have a pedestrian death rate 1.7 times that of whites.[3] African American men age 65 and older have one of the highest MV-related death rates when sorted by age, sex, and race.[3] Homicide is the leading cause of death for African Americans aged 10 to 24 years.[3] The drowning rate for 5- to 14-year-old African Americans is 3.2 times higher than that of whites.[16,17]

Asian-Pacific and Native American women age 65 years and older have the highest death rates when sorted by age, sex, and race.[3] Homicide is the second leading cause of death for Asian-Pacific Islanders aged 10 to 24 years.[3]

Hispanics have a mortality rate 1.8 times higher than non-Hispanics if they are a pedestrian who has been injured.[3] Homicide is the second leading cause of death for Hispanics among people aged 10 to 24 years.[3]

Native Americans 19 years of age and younger are at greater risk for preventable injury-related deaths than are all other children and youth in the United States. They have twice the average rate of traumatic deaths than their counterparts in any other racial group. Injuries and violence account for 75% of all deaths among Native Americans in this age-group. MVCs are the leading cause of fatality, followed by homicide, drowning, and fires.[2] The rates for pedestrian deaths in auto-pedestrian injuries are three times higher for Native Americans and Alaska Natives than whites.[3] The drowning rate overall for Native Americans and Alaska Natives is 1.8 times higher than that for whites; in children aged 5 to 14 years, the drowning rate is 2.6 times higher.[17,18] Native American men aged 20 years and older are (1) twice as likely to die in an MVC, (2) nearly twice as likely to die of fire and burn injuries, and (3) five times more likely to drown than their counterparts in other races. They are also four times more likely to commit suicide and three times more likely to be murdered.[19-21]

Firearm-Related Injuries

The CDC began tracking firearm injuries in the early 1960s. Firearm violence and firearm-related deaths have been increasing at a steady rate for decades.[3] Firearm injury disproportionately affects young people, resulting in lives cut short or forever affected as a result of their use. Firearms (especially handguns) are effective lethal weapons with the capability to escalate often-impulsive acts of interpersonal violence or suicidal thoughts into death. The United States has wrestled with firearms and the consequences of their use and misuse for more than half a century. Compared with other industrialized countries, the firearm death rate in the United States is eight times the average rate of its economic counterparts.[22] Among all industrialized countries, more men are killed by firearms than women; however, women in the United States die at a much higher rate from firearm injuries than their counterparts in other high-income countries.[22] Research has shown that restrictive firearm legislation is associated with decreased pediatric, unintentional, suicide, and overall firearm-related fatality rates. Unfortunately, homicide and the firearm-related fatality rate among African Americans appears unaffected by restrictive firearm legislation.[22,23]

Alcohol and Drugs

Alcohol plays a significant role in all types of trauma, including MVCs, family violence, suicides, homicides, and altercations. Alcohol alters judgment and coordination, so it frequently contributes to injury-producing events.

An alcohol-related MVC kills someone every 31 minutes and nonfatally injures someone every 2 minutes.[6,24] The CDC's research has found that about 68% of the children killed in alcohol-related crashes were riding in cars driven by drivers who had been drinking.[4] One study demonstrated that child passenger restraint use decreased as the BAC of the child's driver increased.[25]

Although the overall use of drugs is less common among fatally injured older adult drivers, compared with younger drivers, driving under the influence of prescription medication may be a relevant traffic safety concern for the older adult population. With the increase in life expectancy of senior citizens, there is an increase in the number of older adults driving. Although many factors influence how many decades an individual may drive, the issues of increased frailty of health, increased use of prescription drugs, and the significance of medical conditions cannot be overlooked.[10]

Insurance Status

The role insurance plays in patient care and outcomes has been studied much more frequently during the past 25 years. Insurance has become as significant part of the discussion in health care disparities and race/ethnicity. Research has shown that insurance status can significantly affect patient outcomes. Frequently, this is related to better and earlier access to health care to treat preexisting conditions and the ability to transfer patients and have health care providers provide treatment, rehabilitation, medication, diagnostic studies, equipment, and so on.

MECHANISM OF INJURY

Trauma is now recognized as a disease process, with MOI as part of its etiology. Strong assessment skills are essential for health care providers because treatment of trauma patients is contingent on identifying all injuries. Unfortunately, even when the clinician has strong assessment skills, some injuries go undetected if the "index of suspicion" is not sufficient. Understanding MOI and maintaining a high index of suspicion enable caregivers to predict and locate occult injuries more quickly and save time initiating essential treatment. Injury should be considered present until definitively ruled out in the hospital setting.

Human beings are exposed to potential injury in multiple forms during the course of a normal day. Injury, defined as trauma or damage to a part of the body, occurs when an uncontrolled or acute source of energy makes contact with the body and the body cannot tolerate exposure to it. Energy originates from numerous sources, including kinetic (motion or mechanical), chemical, electrical, thermal, and radiation. The absence of heat and oxygen causes injuries such as frostbite, drowning, or suffocation. Kinetic energy is defined as energy resulting from motion.[13,26,27] Most traumatic injuries are caused by absorption of kinetic energy. Box 34.1 defines essential concepts for understanding mechanisms of injury.

Severity of trauma depends on the wounding agent. The three major classifications of traumatic disease are blunt injury, penetrating injury, and thermal injury. Energy transfer can result in any one of these individual categories or in any combination of these wounding forces.

Kinematics

Kinematics is the process of looking at an event and determining what injuries are likely to occur given the forces and motion involved. Physics is the foundation on which kinematics is based. Understanding essential laws of physics is the first step toward understanding kinematics.

Newton's First Law of Motion

Newton's first law of motion states that a body at rest remains at rest and a body in motion remains in motion unless acted on by an outside force. Pedestrians struck by a vehicle, patients who have a blast injury, and people with gunshot wounds (GSW) reflect examples of when stationary objects are set in motion by energy forces. Moving objects interrupted or acted on to stop their motion are illustrated by people falling from a height, vehicles hitting a tree, or vehicles braking to a sudden stop.[26,27]

Law of Conservation of Energy

The law of conservation of energy states that energy is neither created nor destroyed but changes form. As a car decelerates slowly, the energy of motion (acceleration) is converted to friction heat in braking (thermal energy).[26,27]

Newton's Second Law

Newton's second law states that force equals mass multiplied by acceleration or deceleration.[28]

Kinetic Energy

Kinetic energy (KE) equals one-half the mass (M) multiplied by the velocity squared (V^2).[26] This law is evidenced in firearm injuries—the mass (the bullet) is small, but because of the velocity (speed) with which the bullet is propelled, substantial energy is transferred to the body.

Patient Assessment

Initially, trauma patients may not appear seriously injured because of strong compensatory mechanisms that maintain adequate vital signs. All members of a trauma team

BOX 34.1 Essential Concepts for Mechanisms of Injury

Acceleration	Increase in Velocity or Speed of a Moving Object
Acceleration-deceleration	Increase in velocity or speed of object followed by decrease in velocity or speed.
Axial loading	Injury occurs when force is applied upward and downward with no posterior or lateral bending of the neck.
Cavitation	Creation of temporary cavity as tissues are stretched and compressed.
Compression	Squeezing inward pressure.
Compressive strength	Ability to resist squeezing forces or inward pressure.
Deceleration	Decrease in velocity or speed of a moving object.
Distraction	Separation of spinal column with resulting cord transection, seen in legal hangings.
Elasticity	Ability to resume original shape and size after being stretched.
Force	Physical factor changing the motion of body at rest or already in motion.
High velocity	Missiles compressing and accelerating tissue away from the bullet, causing a cavity around the bullet and the entire tract.
Inertial resistance	Ability of body to resist movement.
Injury	Trauma or damage to some part of the body.
Kinematics	Process of looking at an accident and determining what injuries might result.
Kinetic energy	Energy resulting from motion.
Low velocity	Missiles localizing injury to a small radius from center of the tract with little disruptive effect.
Muzzle blast	Cloud of hot gas and burning powder at the muzzle of a gun.
Shearing	Two oppositely directed parallel forces. It is the tissue's ability to resist a force parallel to the tissue. An example is the coup/contrecoup head injury.
Stress	Internal resistance to deformation, or internal force generated from application load.
Tensile strength	Amount of tension tissue can withstand and ability to resist stretching forces. Tendons, ligaments, and muscles most commonly become overstretched.
Tumbling	Forward rotation around the center; somersault action of the missile can create massive injury.
Yaw	Deviation of bullet nose in longitudinal axis from straight line of flight.

must anticipate injuries by recognizing potential patterns of injury related to the energy and force of the trauma. Assessment, resuscitation, and stabilization efforts based on this knowledge enable health care providers to evaluate hidden or internal injuries according to these predicted patterns. Health care providers should correlate reported mechanisms to actual or potential injuries. Patients, family, and friends may have reasons to fabricate, falsify, or deny the actual event. Consequently, injuries identified in the examination may not correspond to the reported mechanism. Eliciting a careful history of the injury during initial assessment is vital. Accurate information, especially about MOI, can reduce morbidity and mortality in many circumstances.

When assessing a trauma patient, the emergency nurse should identify mechanisms associated with major force or energy transfer (e.g., a pedestrian hit by a vehicle traveling faster than 20 mph, falls from more than 20 feet, MVCs with major vehicular damage, a speed change of more than 20 mph, vehicle rollover, ejected occupant, or death of occupant). Some injuries are significant because of potential complications, such as two or more long-bone fractures; flail chest; penetrating trauma to the head, neck, chest, abdomen, or groin; and any combination of these patterns with burns over the head, face, or airway.[26,13] Patients with significant injuries require close monitoring for complications or changes in hemodynamic stability.

Certain questions elicit valuable information regarding the MOI and are helpful in assessing potential injuries. When an MV is involved, asking the following questions is important:

- What type of vehicle was the patient driving (large or small)?
- What was the estimated speed at the time of the crash?
- Were seat belts or restraint devices used? Were the devices applied appropriately? Did the air bags deploy?
- Where was the patient in the vehicle (driver, front-seat passenger, or rear-seat passenger)? If ejected, how far was the patient thrown or found from the vehicle?
- How much damage was done to the vehicle? Where was the majority of the damage? Was there intrusion into the passenger space? How much?
- Was there any steering wheel deformity?

If the patient was involved in a fall, the following questions should be asked:

- What was the approximate height of the fall?
- Were any objects struck during the fall?
- What was the surface where the patient landed?
- In what position was the patient found after the fall?

With penetrating injury, the following questions should be asked:

- What was the wounding agent (e.g., knife, gun, arrow, ice pick)?
- What was the size and length of the agent?
- If a firearm was used, what was the caliber? What was the distance between the fired weapon and the patient?

Patients with penetrating trauma must be assessed for other types of trauma, such as falls or assaults. Patients may be exposed to more than one wounding force.

Obtaining a detailed history is not always possible and often impractical. Valuable information can be obtained from family members, prehospital personnel, police, firefighters, bystanders, or eyewitnesses, but these resources are often overlooked or are unavailable in a hectic emergency department (ED). Management of life-threatening injuries must take priority over obtaining a detailed history; however, every effort should be made to obtain as much historical data as possible.

After airway/cervical spine protection, breathing, circulation, and neurologic function have been assessed and supported, a rapid head-to-toe assessment should be performed. Patients with penetrating trauma are generally easier to assess than those with blunt trauma because injuries are usually focused in one area. Surface trauma may or may not be present with blunt injuries; therefore assessment tends to be more difficult. During the secondary survey, injuries can be found by systematically examining the patient when the patient is completely undressed. Maintaining a high index of suspicion for probable injuries based on certain MOIs and performing a detailed physical assessment will minimize the risk for missed injuries.

Blunt Injury

Blunt trauma is characterized as an injury with no opening in the skin or communication to the outside environment. Definitive diagnosis of blunt trauma is challenging. The extent of injuries is not always obvious; however, these injuries may indeed be life-threatening. Depending on the tissue injured and properties associated with this tissue, certain diagnostic studies are more helpful than others. Air-filled organs, such as the lungs and bowel, are subject to blast and compressive injuries. Crush injuries to solid organs (e.g., liver and spleen) may present with minimal external signs of injury, but because energy associated with blunt trauma is transmitted in all directions, organs and tissues can rupture or break if pressure is not released.[13,26]

Examples of blunt force events include MVCs, falls, contact sports (see Table 34.3), and assaults. Direct impact causes the greatest injury. Injuries result when energy is released on impact with the body. Various body tissues respond differently; tissue may move and displace with impact or rupture from the force.

Forces commonly associated with blunt trauma include acceleration, deceleration, shearing, and compression forces. Acceleration injuries occur when velocity (speed) is transferred to a stationary or slower-moving object; deceleration injuries occur when velocity or forward momentum is abruptly stopped. Shearing injuries occur when two oppositely directed parallel forces are applied to tissue. Compression injuries occur with a squeezing inward pressure applied to tissues. An example of these forces is seen with blunt injury to the thoracic aorta. Rapid deceleration causes the aorta to bend and stretch. Shearing damage occurs when stretching forces exceed vessel elasticity. Shearing damage causes the aorta to dissect, rupture, tear, or form an aneurysm.[29]

TABLE 34.3 Sports-Related Injuries

Sport	Potential Injuries
Boxing	Cumulative brain damage, ocular injuries, lacerations, nasal fractures, hand fractures
Gymnastics	Spinal cord injuries, extremity fractures, sprains, strains
Football	Spinal cord injuries, head injuries, knee strains, fractures, lacerations
Skiing	Head injuries, lower extremity fractures, and exposure to elements
Ice hockey	Facial fractures, soft-tissue injuries, lacerations
Running	Lower extremity injuries, strains, sprains
Baseball	Head injuries, ocular injuries, fractures, lacerations, sprains, strains
Basketball	Lower extremity sprains, strains, fractures, lacerations, contusions
Horseback riding	Head injuries, bite wounds, crush wounds
Inline skates	Wrist fractures, head injuries, lower extremity fractures
Bungee jumping	Major impact-related injuries, intraocular hemorrhages, spinal cord injuries, peroneal nerve injuries, soft-tissue injuries

Data from Centers for Disease Control and Prevention: Preventing injuries in America: public health in action, 2004. Centers for Disease Control and Prevention website. http://www.cdc.gov; Published July 17, 2007.

Motor Vehicle Collisions

Before a collision, the occupant and the vehicle are moving at the same speed. At the time of collision, the vehicle and the occupant decelerate to a speed of zero, but at different rates. Deceleration forces are transferred to the body in three points of collision (Fig. 34.1).[13,26] The first collision occurs when the vehicle strikes another object. As the vehicle stops, the driver or occupant continues to move forward. The second collision occurs when the driver or occupant strikes the steering column, windshield, restraint system, or another structure in the car. The body stops; however, internal organs continue to move until they collide with another organ, cavity wall, or structure or they are restrained suddenly by vasculature, muscles, ligaments, or fascia—the third collision point. A fourth collision may occur when unsecured objects in the vehicle collide with the occupant (e.g., unrestrained passengers, bottled drinks, sports equipment). Different damage occurs with each collision; therefore each collision point must be considered separately to avoid missed injuries.

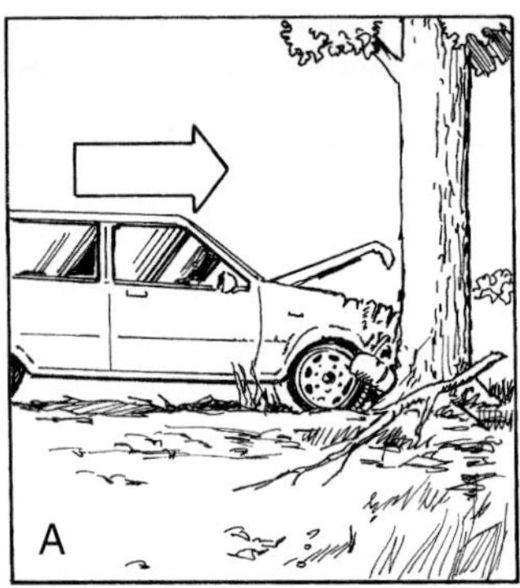

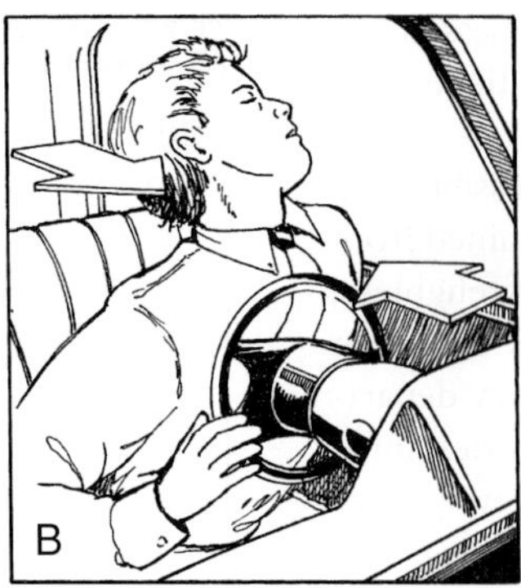

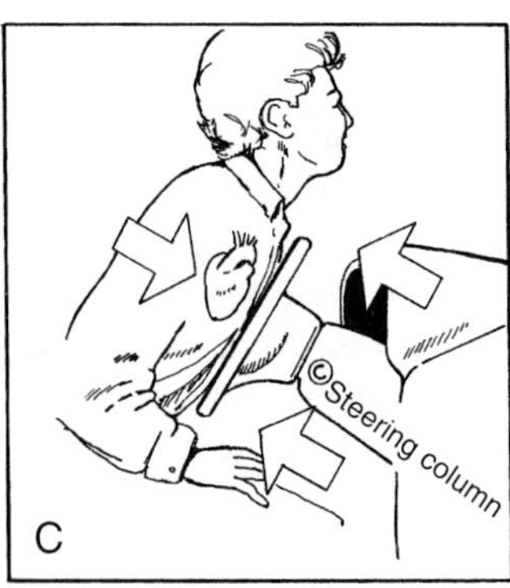

Fig. 34.1 The Three Collisions of a Motor Vehicle Collision. (A) Auto hits tree. (B) Body hits steering wheel, causing broken ribs. (C) Heart strikes chest wall, causing blunt cardiac injury.

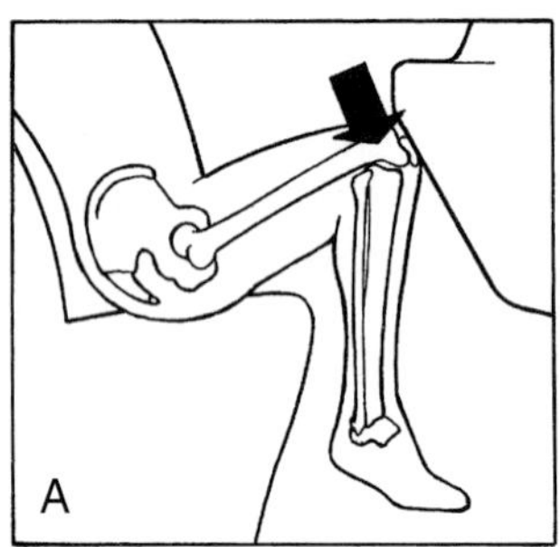

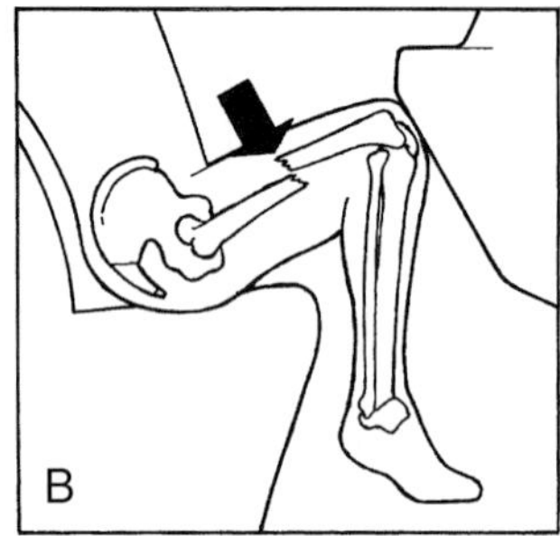

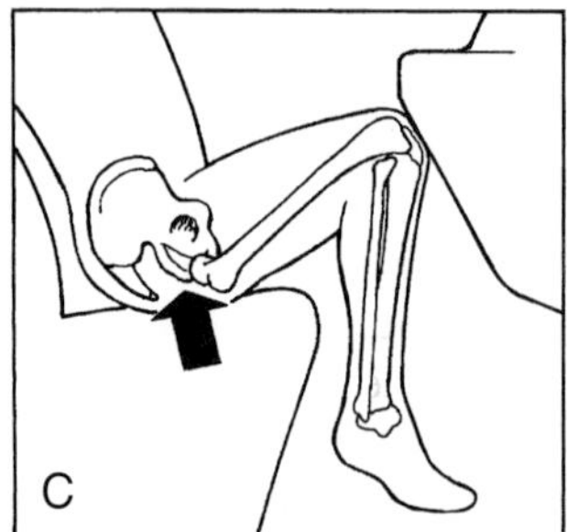

Fig. 34.2 Down and Under Pathway. (A) Dislocation of the knee. (B) Fracture of the femur. (C) Dislocation from the acetabulum.

One way to estimate injuries in an MVC is for members of the trauma team to be able to look at the vehicle. Because this is not possible in the ED, the emergency nurse should ask prehospital providers about vehicular damage—interior and exterior. Some prehospital personnel take instant photographs (i.e., digital), allowing hospital providers to see vehicular damage firsthand. The picture can then either be downloaded or printed out and become a permanent part of the medical record.

Frontal impact. Frontal impact occurs when the front of a vehicle impacts another object (e.g., another vehicle, tree, bridge abutment). The first collision results in damage to the front end. The more severe the damage and the faster the vehicle was traveling, the greater the probability for severe injury due to the amount of energy transferred.

Multiple injuries may occur when a person comes to a sudden stop. The use of restraints does reduce the energy absorbed by the body, minimize direct contact with nonyielding interior structures, and prevent ejection from the vehicle. Interior structures, such as the windshield, steering wheel, dashboard, or instrument panel, injure the occupants when direct contact is made. After the vehicle stops, occupants in the front seat continue to move down and under, or up and over, the dashboard.

Down and under. One path an occupant may travel after a frontal impact is down and under. The occupant continues forward movement downward into the steering column or dashboard. The person's knees impact the dashboard; however, the upper legs absorb most of the energy. This mechanism may cause patellar dislocations, midshaft femur fractures, and posterior dislocations or fractures of the acetabulum or femoral head (Fig. 34.2). When one of these injuries is identified, the patient should be carefully evaluated for the other associated injuries.

Up and over. Continued forward motion from a frontal collision can carry the body up and over, so the head, chest, and/or abdomen strike the steering column, dashboard, or windshield. Head injuries, such as contusions and scalp lacerations, skull fractures, facial fractures, cerebral hemorrhage, or cerebral contusions can occur.

The brain does not stretch easily, so if one part of the brain moves in one direction, the rest follows. The skull stops suddenly after striking the steering wheel, windshield, or another stationary object, but the brain continues to move forward and strikes the inside of the skull.[13,26] This area of the brain is compressed and may sustain ecchymosis, edema, or contusion. This type of injury is called a "coup injury," and it occurs when the damaged area forms directly at the site of contact. As this injury is occurring, the other side of the brain continues to move forward and may be disrupted and shear away from tissue and vascular attachments (Fig. 34.3). A contrecoup injury occurs on the side opposite the direct contact because of the movement of the brain within the skull (recoil or "bounce-back"). This impact can cause two separate injuries, shear injury and compression injury, to the same organ, the brain.

When the head collides with an object, injury to the cervical spine can also occur. The spiderweb effect of a broken windshield suggests the possibility for cervical spine injury. If prehospital providers report a spiderweb effect,

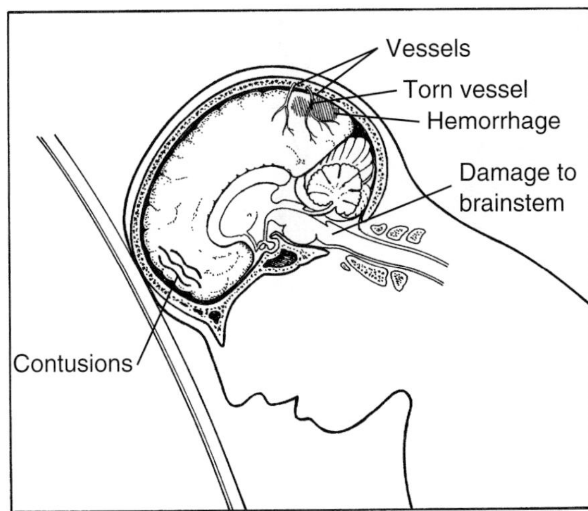

Fig. 34.3 Brain Injury.

caregivers must maintain a high index of suspicion for a spinal injury.

Chest injuries occur when the thorax is compressed against the steering column. Injuries include fractured ribs and sternum, anterior flail chest, blunt cardiac injury, and pulmonary contusion. Thoracic vertebral injuries occur as energy travels up or down the thoracic spine; however, these injuries are less common because the thoracic vertebrae are so well protected.

Compression injuries to the abdomen may result in ruptured hollow organs (e.g., the stomach or intestines), which spill their contents into the abdominal cavity, whereas fractured or lacerated solid organs (e.g., the liver and spleen) are associated with significant blood loss. Organs in the abdominal cavity are attached to the abdominal wall by the mesentery, ligaments, and vasculature. As organs continue their forward motion, attachments can be torn or lacerated.

The steering column is often referred to as a modern-day battering ram and can be the most lethal part of a vehicle.[13,26] When a steering wheel deformity is reported, the index of suspicion for neck, face, thoracic, or abdominal injuries should increase significantly. Injuries caused by this collision may or may not be readily visible. Lacerations of the chin and mouth, contusion and ecchymosis of the neck, traumatic tattooing of the chest and abdomen, and bruising of the chest and abdomen may be obvious or subtle. Internal occult injuries may be secondary to compression forces, shearing forces, and displacement of kinetic energy.[13,26]

Certain organs are more susceptible to shear injuries because of ligamentous attachments (e.g., liver, spleen, bowel, kidneys, and aortic arch). Compression forces commonly injure the lungs, diaphragm, heart, and bladder. Respiratory distress in trauma patients may be caused by injuries such as a pneumothorax, flail chest, and pulmonary contusion. A diaphragmatic hernia or a ruptured diaphragm can also cause respiratory distress and is characterized by bowel sounds in the chest. If a trauma patient has a contused chest wall, a blunt cardiac injury should be considered.

In frontal and lateral impacts, a mechanism sometimes called the "paper bag effect" leads to pneumothorax. The driver or occupant sees the collision about to happen, inhales deeply, and holds his or her breath. The glottis closes and seals the lungs. As the chest impacts, the lungs burst like paper bags (Fig. 34.4).

Frontal impacts are also characterized by extremity injuries. Fractures of the lower extremities, ankles, and feet occur when the occupant extends the feet or are secondary to vehicle intrusion into the passenger compartment. An unrestrained back-seat passenger doubles the risk for injury to front-seat occupants during frontal impact.

Rear impact. Rear-impact collisions occur when a stationary object or a slower-moving object is struck from behind. Initial impact accelerates the slower-moving or stationary object and may force the vehicle into a frontal collision. When the vehicle suddenly decelerates, hyperextension of the neck may occur, especially when headrests are not properly positioned. Neck ligaments may be strained or torn. If the vehicle strikes another object or is slowed by the driver applying the brake, rapid forward deceleration occurs. The crash then involves two points of impact, rear and frontal, which increases the chance for occupant injuries. Injuries common to each mechanism must be assessed.

Lateral or side impact. When a vehicle is struck on either side ("T-boned"), most injuries are dependent on vehicle deformity because the vehicle either remains in place or moves away from the point of impact. If the vehicle remains in place, energy is transferred or changed to vehicle damage rather than the energy of motion. Trauma to the occupants can be more severe because of intrusion into the interior compartment. The greater the intrusion, the more significant the injury can be. More than 10 to 12 inches of intrusion is considered significant.

With side-impact or lateral collisions, occupants generally receive most injuries on the same side of their body as the vehicle impact. A second collision may occur between occupants if another passenger is in the vehicle. The head and shoulder of one occupant may impact the other occupant's head and shoulder. When a patient has an injury on the side opposite impact, caregivers should assess both occupants for associated injuries.

Fig. 34.5 illustrates injuries from a side-impact collision. Flail chest, pulmonary contusion, and rib fractures are possible chest injuries. Numerous musculoskeletal injuries can occur. Energy from an impact can pin the occupant's arm against the car, causing injury to the chest wall and clavicle or force the femoral head through the pelvis, causing a pelvic or acetabulum fracture.[13,26] Strain on the lateral neck can cause spinal fractures or ligament tears. Side impacts can cause spine fractures, with associated neurologic deficit, more often than rear collisions. Other injuries may include a splenic injury when impact is on the driver's side and liver injury when the impact is on the passenger side.

Rotational impact. Rotational impact occurs when the corner of one vehicle strikes another stationary vehicle, a vehicle traveling in the opposite direction, or a slower vehicle. The point of impact on the second car stops forward motion, and then the rest of the vehicle rotates until

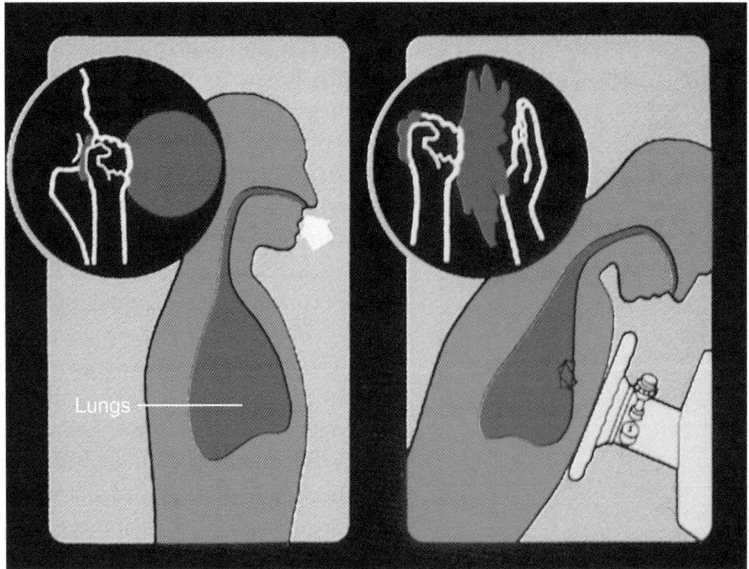

Fig. 34.4 Compression of the lung against the closed glottis by impact on anterior or lateral chest wall produces effect like that of compressing a paper bag when the opening is closed tightly by hands: the paper bag ruptures, and so does the lung. (From National Association of Emergency Medical Technicians. *PHTLS: Prehospital Trauma Life Support.* 8th ed. St Louis, MO: Jones and Bartlett Learning; 2014.)

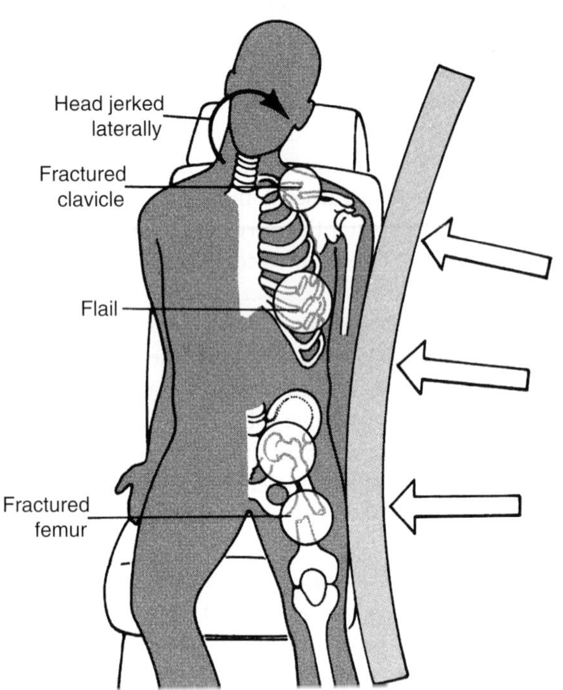

Fig. 34.5 Potential Injury Sites in Lateral-Impact Collision. Injury is still possible in lateral crash with air bag inflation; however, injuries are usually fewer with air bag inflation than without. (From Neff JA, Kidd PS: *Trauma Nursing: The Art and Science.* St Louis, MO: Mosby; 1993.)

all energy is transformed. As the car is hit, the occupant's forward motion continues until it impacts with the side of the car as the vehicle begins rotating. Injuries occurring in rotational impacts are a combination of those seen in frontal and lateral impacts.

Vehicle rollover. Vehicular rollover is when a vehicle flips over, regardless of whether the motion is end over end, or side over side. In rollovers, injuries are sometimes difficult to predict. Occupants frequently have injuries in the same body areas where damage occurs to the vehicle. Just as the vehicle impacts at different angles, several times, so does the occupant's body and internal organs. In the rollover mechanism, the chance for axial loading injuries is increased.

Ejection. Ejection is when an occupant is thrown from the vehicle. Occupants who are ejected sustain injuries at the point of impact and when energy is transferred to the entire body; spinal fractures and severe traumatic brain injuries occur at a higher rate in ejections. Occupants who are ejected have a much greater chance of dying than occupants who remain in the vehicle, and those at greatest risk are unrestrained occupants.[2]

Restraint systems. The first mandatory child restraint use law was enacted in Tennessee in 1978, and now all 50 states and the District of Columbia have child restraint laws. The first mandatory seat belt law was enacted in New York state in 1984, and every state and the District of Columbia have since enacted seat belt laws. Restraint systems are designed to prevent injuries and decrease their severity by allowing occupants to decelerate at the same rate as the vehicle rather than being thrown against interior structures or being ejected from the vehicle. Restraints also keep occupants from striking each other within the compartment. Worn properly, safety restraints reduce fatalities and the severity of injuries.

The most effective restraint system is the three-point restraint, which is a shoulder harness and lap belt. Three-point restraints decrease severity of the "second" collision, reducing facial, head, and abdominal injuries and long-bone fractures.[13,26] The National Highway Traffic Safety Agency (NHTSA) has reported lap and shoulder safety belts "reduce the risk of fatal injury to front-seat passenger car occupants by 45% and the risk of moderate-to-critical injury by 50%." More people are now using occupant protection.[24,30]

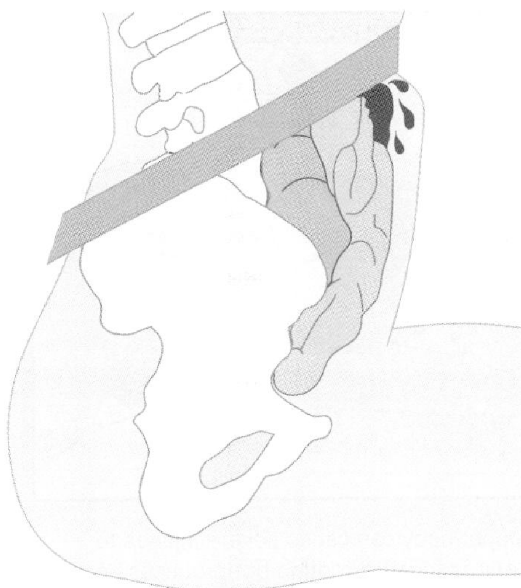

Fig. 34.6 A seat belt that is positioned above the rim of the pelvis allows the abdominal organs to be trapped between the moving posterior wall and the belt. Injuries to the pancreas and other retroperitoneal organs, as well as blowout ruptures of the small intestine and colon, result. (From McSwain N, Paturas J: *The Basic EMT: Comprehensive Prehospital Patient Care.* 2nd ed. St Louis, MO: Mosby; 2003.)

Injuries caused by a shoulder-lap belt fastened loosely or worn above the anterior iliac crest (Fig. 34.6) include compression to abdominal organs such as the pancreas, liver, and spleen; possible rupture of the diaphragm with herniation of abdominal organs; and anterior compression fractures of the lumbar spine. Diaphragmatic rupture occurs from increased intraabdominal pressure from the misplaced lap belt. Fig. 34.7 illustrates the consequences of incorrect use of lap belts and shoulder straps. Lap belts worn alone allow injuries to the face, head, neck, and chest, whereas shoulder belts worn without a lap belt can cause severe neck injuries.

Properly used restraints transfer energy from the impact to the restraint system instead of to the occupant. Injuries received when seat belts are used properly are generally not life-threatening, or the chance of sustaining a life-threatening injury is greatly reduced. Box 34.2 describes injuries occurring even with proper seat belt use.

Air bags. Air bags were designed to protect front-seat occupants in frontal deceleration collisions by inflating from the center of the steering column or the dashboard or both at impact (Fig. 34.8), cushioning the head and chest, and then rapidly deflating. Since 1998, all new passenger cars have been equipped with driver and front-seat passenger air bags. Some newer vehicles also have side-impact air bags. Injuries reported from air bag deployment include facial trauma, such as tattooing, ecchymosis, and corneal abrasions. Abrasions and ecchymosis from air bag deployment are seen on forearms. Air bags, however, are not considered primary restraint systems but are "supplemental" to lap and shoulder belts. An ongoing Special Crash Investigation Program sponsored by NHTSA provides data associated with adult passengers, drivers, and children who sustain fatal or serious injuries in "minor or moderate severity air bag deployment crashes."[30]

Drivers and passengers should sit at least 10 inches away from the steering column/dashboard and tilt the seat rearward for vehicles with air bags. Serious injuries have been reported in small drivers who adjust the seat closer to the steering wheel. Infants and children placed in the front seat have been seriously injured or killed by inflating air bags. The NHTSA website (https://www.nhtsa.dot.gov) has a section discussing the most updated information on the rules and regulations governing on and off switches for air bags. The following points regarding driving in a car equipped with air bags are recommended by the NHTSA[30]:

- Children 12 years and younger should ride in the back seat of cars.
- Never use a rear-facing child-restraint seat in a seat with an air bag.
- Always wear a lap and shoulder belt even in vehicles equipped with air bags.
- When driving a car equipped with an air bag, sit at least 10 inches away from the steering wheel and tilt the seat rearward.
- There are some situations authorized by the NHTSA permitting air bag deactivation if the vehicle is not equipped with an air bag off switch.

MVC preventive measures. Because MVCs account for more than half the injuries associated with blunt trauma, preventive measures are an ongoing concern. Research has shown the number of MVCs can be reduced by highway design changes, enforcement of speed limits, and improvements in vehicle design. Safety changes made in highway design include separating opposing streams of traffic, installing breakaway barriers and nonskid road surfaces, and removing obstacles from the roadside. Enforcing the speed limit also reduces injuries from MVCs because speed is a determining factor in the severity of injuries. The greater the speed or velocity, the more energy dissipated and the more severe the injury. The size and design of vehicles also affect injury. Small cars are associated with more injuries and deaths than larger cars. Changes in interior design can decrease injuries seen in occupants. Examples of this include incorporation of side air bags and additional padding on dashboards.

Farm Equipment

Most fatalities associated with tractors are crushing injuries when the tractor overturns.[31] When tractors turn over, it is generally to the side; however, they can overturn to the rear. Rear overturns do not allow the driver to jump free or be thrown clear. Other mechanisms of injury include thermal burns from ignited fuel or hot engine parts and chemical burns from diesel fuel, hydraulic fluid, gasoline, or battery acid.[31]

Pedestrian Injuries

When a vehicle strikes a pedestrian, injuries can be predicted based on the person's age or size. Children and adults have different patterns of injuries because of their size differences and orientation to the vehicle.

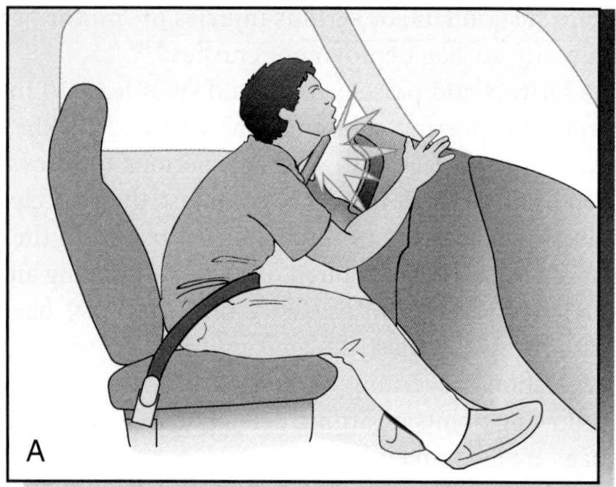

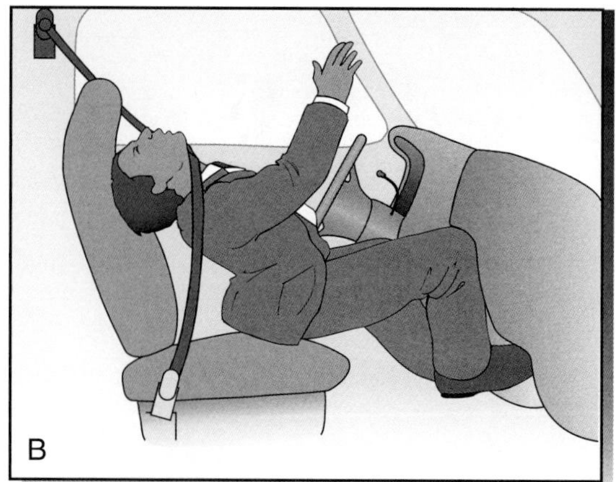

Fig. 34.7 (A) Without the diagonal strap, the forward motion of the upper body can cause severe injuries to the face, head, and neck. (B) When worn alone, the diagonal strap retards forward motion but produces an excessive force on the neck. Neck injuries as severe as decapitation have been reported. (From McSwain N, Paturas J: *The Basic EMT: Comprehensive Prehospital Patient Care.* 2nd ed. St Louis, MO: Mosby; 2003.)

BOX 34.2 Injuries With Appropriate Restraint Systems

Spinal

- Cervical vertebral fractures from flexion forces
- Neck sprains secondary to hyperextension
- Lumbar vertebral fractures secondary to flexion-distraction forces

Thoracic

- Soft-tissue injuries of the chest wall associated with belt placement
- Sternal fractures with or without blunt cardiac injury
- Fewer than three rib fractures if restrained; more than four if unrestrained
- Trauma to breast in females

Abdominal

- Soft-tissue injuries (contusions, abrasions, ecchymosis)
- Seat belt friction burns or abrasion where seat belt rests
- Injuries to small bowel secondary to crushing and deceleration
- Ruptured aorta secondary to longitudinal stretching of the vessel
- Injuries to the liver, pancreas, gallbladder, and duodenum secondary to crushing forces

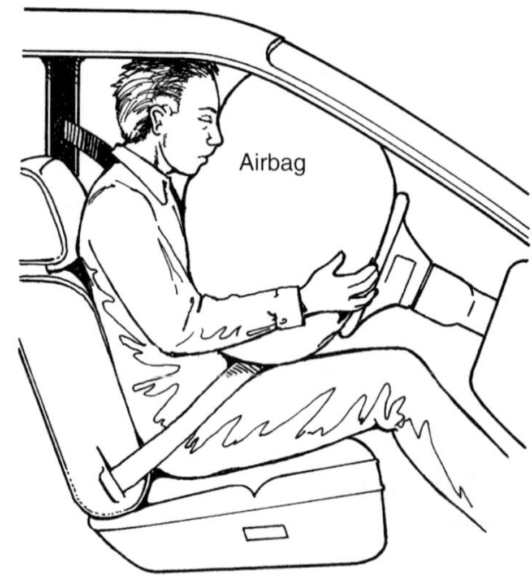

Fig. 34.8 Inflated Air Bag.

In children, frontal impacts usually occur because children tend to freeze and face the approaching vehicle. The femur or chest of the child impacts the bumper or hood depending on the child's height. The child is then thrown backward with his or her upper back or head impacting the ground or pavement, where contralateral skull injuries occur. Very small children are rarely thrown clear of the vehicle because of their low center of gravity, size, and weight. A child may be knocked down and under the vehicle, then run over or dragged. Multisystem trauma should be suspected in any child hit by a car. A combination of injuries referred to as Waddell's triad often occurs when a child is struck by a car (Fig. 34.9). Waddell's triad is characterized by injuries to the chest, head, and femurs.

Adults struck by a vehicle sustain injuries to the lower extremities along with head, chest, and abdominal injuries. Adults try to protect themselves by turning sideways, so the impact is usually lateral. Upper and lower leg impact with the bumper and hood of the car causes bowing of both legs with fractures above and below the joint of impact. This may also cause ligament damage to the opposite knee from associated strain. Fig. 34.10 shows points of impact when an adult is struck by a vehicle.

Another common injury in an adult pedestrian is a fractured pelvis. As the patient folds over, the upper femur and pelvis strike the front of the hood while the abdomen and chest strike the top of the hood. The head may also strike the hood of the car or the angle where the hood meets the windshield. The patient then rolls off the hood and onto the pavement or into the windshield. The victim may be able to protect the face and head with the arms during this forward

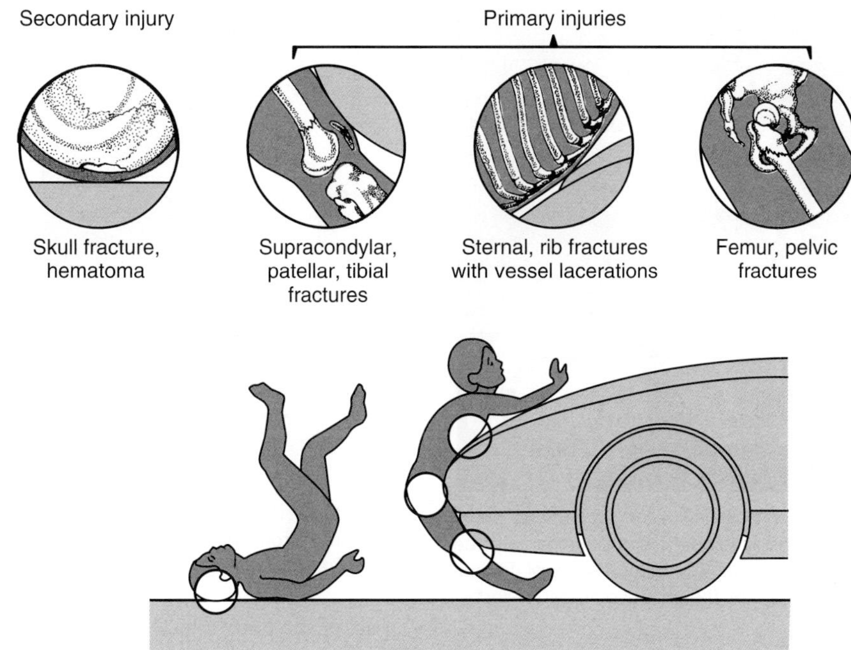

Fig. 34.9 Potential Primary Injury Sites of Child Pedestrian. (Modified from Neff JA, Kidd PS: *Trauma Nursing: The Art and Science.* St Louis, MO: Mosby; 1993.)

motion. If the victim is thrown any distance, he or she can be run over by a second vehicle. Tire mark impressions may be found on the clothing or skin of victims who are run over.

School Buses

Although the incidence of crashes involving school buses is low, the general public is concerned that safety restraints are not standard equipment. Understanding the epidemiology associated with school bus injuries and deaths is an example of how a problem must be identified before implementing those strategies that will have the most effect on prevention of such injuries. Most deaths involving school buses are not to bus occupants. Data indicate that promoting safety around school buses being used for transport of children is one of the necessary prevention strategies.[14] NHTSA has a free school bus safety program for teaching children how to be cautious and vigilant around school buses.

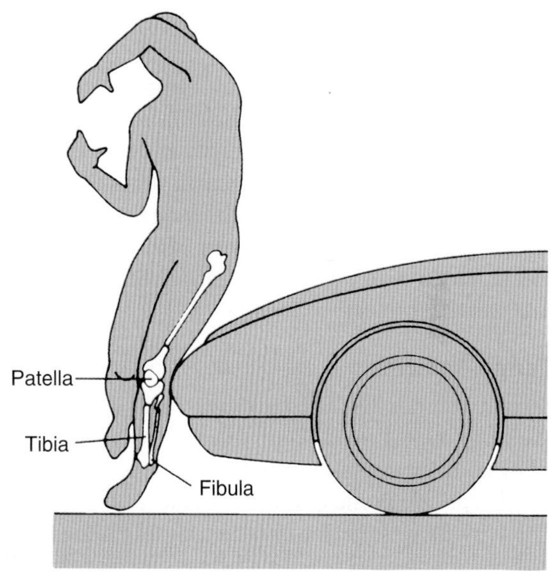

Fig. 34.10. Potential Primary Injury Sites of Adult Pedestrian. (From Neff JA, Kidd PS: *Trauma Nursing: The Art and Science.* St Louis, MO: Mosby; 1993.)

Motorcycle Crashes

Injuries occurring from motorcycle crashes (MCCs) depend on the amount and type of kinetic energy and part of the body impacted. Head, neck, and extremity injuries occur more frequently with MCCs because of the lack of protection afforded the riders. Clues to the amount of force sustained during a collision include the length of skid marks, deformity of the motorcycle, and stationary objects impacted. The condition of an MCC rider is often similar to that of an occupant ejected from a vehicle (Fig. 34.11). The next four sections describe four types of motorcycle impacts with predictable injuries.

Head-on impact. The motorcycle impacts an object head-on, and the cycle flips forward, so the rider strikes or travels over the handlebars. As the rider strikes the handlebars, abdominal and chest injuries and shearing fractures of the tibia can occur. Bilateral femur fractures occur if the rider's feet are trapped by the foot pegs at the time of impact. A helmet will provide limited protection to the rider's head, but it will not protect the neck.

Angular impact. The cycle is struck at an angle and falls on the rider so one side of the rider's body is crushed between the motorcycle and the ground or the object struck. Injuries tend to occur to the lower extremities, such as open fractures of the tibia or fibula, crushed legs, ankle dislocation, and soft tissue injuries.

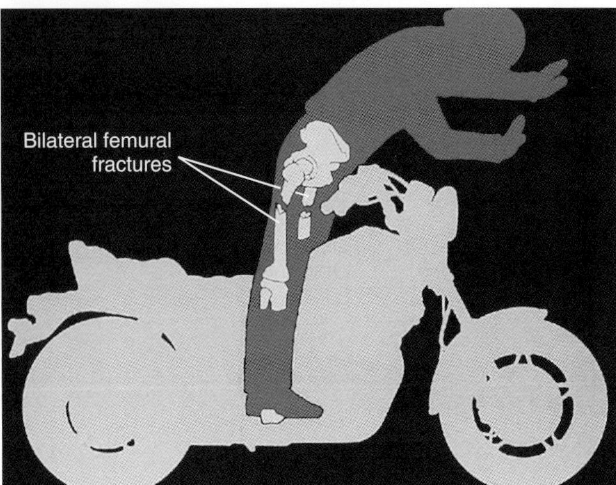

Fig. 34.11 The body travels forward and over the motorcycle, pushing the thighs and femurs into the handlebars. The driver can also be ejected. (From National Association of Emergency Medical Technicians. *Prehospital Trauma Life Support.* 6th ed. St Louis, MO: Mosby; 2007.)

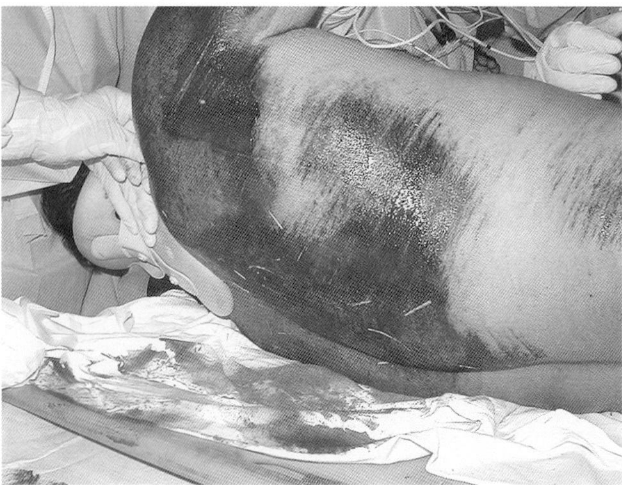

Fig. 34.12 Road burns after a motorcycle crash without protective clothing. (From McSwain N, Paturas J: *The Basic EMT: Comprehensive Prehospital Patient Care.* 2nd ed. St Louis, MO: Mosby; 2003.)

Ejection. When a rider is ejected from the motorcycle, injuries occur to the body part that is hit at the time of impact and the point of impact when the body lands. Energy from the impact is absorbed by the rest of the body. Ejection from a motorcycle has a high potential for severe injuries.

Laying the bike down. This maneuver is used by professional riders to separate themselves from their bikes when they see an impending collision. This maneuver slows down the rider as the bike is turned sideways, and the rider drags the inner leg. The most common injuries seen with laying the bike down are minor fractures, abrasions, and crush injuries to lower legs. Fig. 34.12 shows road burns which occurred in a rider who was not wearing protective clothing.

All-Terrain Vehicles

All-terrain vehicles (ATVs) have two basic designs: three-wheeled or four-wheeled. Four-wheeled ATVs offer easier handling and more stability than three-wheeled, which when turned sharply are prone to rollover because of a higher center of gravity. Some states have enacted laws defining the minimum operator age and requiring helmets for all riders.

The most common MOIs associated with ATVs are rollovers, the rider falling off, and the vehicle hitting a stationary object and causing forward deceleration of the rider. Injuries depend on which part of the rider's anatomy is struck and the mechanism involved. Head, spine, and chest injuries involving the ribs, sternum, and clavicles have been reported.

Snowmobiles

Snowmobiles are used for work and play. Injuries commonly seen are similar to those associated with ATVs. The snowmobile has a low center of gravity and low clearance. Crush injuries are frequently seen because snowmobiles turn over more easily and are heavier than most ATVs. Significant neck injuries can occur if the rider runs into an unseen wire fence or rope. Patterns of injury depend on the mechanism and the part of the body affected. Hypothermia is a significant risk if the rider is not adequately clothed for the weather or is not found immediately after the injuring event.

Watercraft

Watercraft or boating injuries can occur from colliding with another boat or an obstruction in the water. Occupants of boats are not provided with restraint systems, and, unlike cars, boats are not built to absorb the energy associated with impacts. There is also the potential for drowning or hypothermia when occupants are ejected into the water. Other injuries may be similar to those seen in people ejected from a vehicle. It is always advisable for watercraft users of all ages and even the most experienced of swimmers to use Coast Guard–approved personal floatation devices.[32]

Personal watercraft (PWC), such as wave runners and jet skis, are popular recreational vehicles. The injury rate is approximately eight times higher with PWCs than with motorboats. Different styles allow the driver to sit or stand while operating the watercraft, with some PWCs large enough to carry two to three passengers. A high speed can be obtained quickly with most PWCs, so collisions can occur with other watercraft or objects in the water. The potential for injury is very similar to the injury patterns seen with ATVs. Rectal, vaginal, and perineal trauma may occur when passengers or drivers hit the water (buttocks first) or seat at high speeds. Drowning and hypothermia are additional complications associated with PWC accidents. Alcohol use is the leading known contributing factor in fatal boating incidents.[32]

Bicycle Crashes

Several mechanisms for bicycle collisions exist; the most common are collisions with a MV or pedestrian and falling off the bicycle. Most deaths related to bicycles are the result of a collision with a MV. A rider usually loses control and falls off because of hazardous ground surfaces, performing stunts, speeding, or generalized lack of skill.

Bicycle crashes have common patterns of injuries. The spokes of a bicycle wheel can fracture the feet when feet are caught in the wheel. These injuries may cause the person to be thrown and sustain other injuries. Properly installed wheel guards decrease spoke-related injuries.

When a rider is thrown over the handlebars as a bike impacts an object and tips forward, the rider without a helmet may suffer injuries similar to someone ejected from a MV (e.g., head, neck, abdomen, and chest injuries). If the rider impacts the middle bar or seat, straddle injuries such as vaginal tears, scrotal injuries, and perineal contusions occur. Riders can also sustain serious abdominal injuries from coming into contact with the bicycle handlebars. These injuries can range from pancreatic, liver, and spleen tears to stomach injuries to bowel perforations.

Bicycle-mounted child seats are another cause of injuries with bicycle use. The child may fall from the seat, the seat can detach from the bicycle, the bike can tip over, or the child's extremity may be caught in wheel spokes. Head and facial injuries are common and often severe. Child seats mounted on bicycles do not provide protection to the child's head and face, and the child is not developmentally ready for self-protection; therefore helmets should be worn by all children in bicycle-mounted seats.

Injuries can occur to bicycle riders from rear-view mirrors extending from trucks or vans. Significant head, neck, and facial injuries and severe deep lacerations to the head and neck can occur and can be fatal.

Falls

Vertical deceleration is the wounding force associated with falls. Severity and types of injuries seen depend on the height of the fall, area of the body impacted, and the landing surface. Falls are more likely to result in severe injury when the distance is three times greater than the victim's height; however, any fall greater than the person's standing height has the potential for significant injury. Different patterns of injuries are seen with different types of falls. Small children tend to land on the head because it is the largest/heaviest part of their body. Certain injuries occur when a person falls from a height and lands feet first. A trio of injuries, called the Don Juan syndrome, includes bilateral calcaneus fractures, compression fractures of the vertebrae (usually thoracolumbar), and bilateral Colles fractures. Energy transfer initially causes bilateral calcaneus fractures, then displaces upward and causes other injuries, including femur fractures, hip dislocations or fractures, vertebral compression fractures, and basilar skull fractures. Wrist fractures occur from acute flexion as the person falls forward onto his or her outstretched arms. Deceleration forces of this nature can also cause secondary renal injuries.

If a person lands on other areas of the body, injuries occur at those impact points and to the rest of the body. If impact is on the wrist, energy is transferred upward through the elbow and shoulder, whereas impact on the knee transfers energy upward to the hip. Another point of impact may be the head, as seen in diving injuries. With this impact, injuries occur because the weight and force of the torso, pelvis, and legs bear down on the head and cervical spine. This type of injury is known as a compression injury or axial loading injury. Vertebral bodies are compressed and wedged, producing vertebral fragments that can penetrate the spinal cord.[33]

Falls affect older adults in a significant way. It is estimated that one in three adults aged 65 and older falls per year, and 50% of those hospitalized are at risk for death within a year's time of the fall.[3,13,26,33] Falls resulting in fractures of the hip in adults aged 65 and older have some particular characteristics: (1) 84% of them occur at home, (2) 76% occur indoors, (3) 76% occur while the victim is standing, (4) 72% fall in a sideways direction, (5) 47% occur when the victim is moving forward, (6) very few falls (10%) are related to wet or slippery surfaces, and (7) 13% of falls occur as a result of some manifestation of another medical condition, such as dizziness, seizures, or sudden paralysis. Research has been replicated that demonstrates extrinsic factors, such as objects in the environment (e.g., furniture, cords, loose mats), are associated with only 25% of falls and that intrinsic factors, such as balance and gait, are more frequently associated with falls that result in fractures.[26,27,32] Factors increasing the probability of falls in older adults include deterioration in health, physical changes associated with aging (i.e., loss of visual acuity), use of prosthetic devices (e.g., canes, walkers), and environmental hazards (e.g., slippery surfaces, stairs, poor lighting, unexpected objects in walkways).

To lessen the chances of falls, floor surfaces should be covered with nonslip materials and handgrips provided on both sides of walkways. Handgrips are especially helpful in bathrooms. Floors and stairs can be covered with resilient materials that lessen the chance of injury if a fall occurs. Improved lighting in hallways and on stairs helps older adults avoid tripping. Lighting should be concentrated on landings, where falls are most likely to occur. The strength of lighting should be uniform so older adults do not have to make rapid visual adjustments to variable light intensity.

Sports- and Recreation-Related Injuries

Injuries associated with sports are generally caused by compressive forces or sudden deceleration as well as by twisting, hyperflexion, and hyperextension. Factors contributing to injuring events include a lack of protective equipment, a lack of conditioning, and inadequate training of the participant. Mechanisms associated with recreational sports and sports-like activities are similar to those involved in MVCs, motorcycle collisions, and bicycle crashes. Potential mechanisms associated with individual sports are numerous; however, the general principles are the same as with falls and MVCs.[34–36]

- What energy or forces impacted the individual?
- What parts of the body are affected by the energy or force?
- What are the obvious injuries?
- What injuries are associated with the involved energy or force?

Damaged equipment, such as broken snow skis or football, lacrosse, or bicycle helmets, can help establish impact sites. See Table 34.3 for descriptions of injuries associated with various sports.

Adolescents 10 to 14 years of age have the highest rates of sports- and recreation-related injury.[28] An estimated 1.6 to 3.8 million sports- and recreation-related traumatic brain injuries occur in the United States every year.[13,27] Collegiate and high school football players who have at least one concussion are at an increased risk for another concussion.[34,36]

Scooters

For this discussion, scooters will be divided into two types. The first is a powered stand-up scooter using a small gas engine or an electric motor that is used primarily by younger individuals. The second type is a mobility aide, equivalent to a wheelchair, but it has an electric motor. Mobility scooters are primarily used by disabled individuals and older adults. Most of those injured on mobility scooters tend to have injuries occur when the scooter is involved in a collision with a car. Most of those injured from stand-up scooters are children younger than 15 years of age and male. Injuries from using scooters include fractures or dislocations, lacerations, contusions and abrasions, and strains and sprains. Injuries are predominately to the arms and hands, the head and face, and the leg and foot. The National Highway Traffic Safety Administration has made the following recommendations for stand-up scooter use[30]:

- Scooter riders should wear helmets meeting Consumer Product Safety Commission standards.
- Scooter riders should wear knee and elbow pads.
- Scooters should be used on "smooth, paved surfaces without traffic."
- Scooters should not be used on "water, sand, gravel, or dirt."
- Scooter riding should be avoided at night.
- Supervision should be provided for young children using scooters.

Penetrating trauma

Penetrating injuries are caused by foreign objects in motion that penetrate the body. Energy created by the foreign object dissipates into the surrounding tissues. Evaluation and assessment of penetrating trauma depends on the wounding agent, how the energy dissipates, the distance from the patient to the weapon, and the characteristics of the tissues struck. Examples of penetrating trauma include GSWs, stab wounds, and impalements. The tissue penetrated and underlying structures damaged determine the severity of the injury. Patients sustaining penetrating trauma may also suffer blunt injuries; for instance, falling down a flight of stairs after being shot.[28,37]

Ultimately, the extent of damage will be governed by an interaction of three factors: (1) the character of the wounding instrument (e.g., knife, gun, bomb fragment), (2) its velocity at the time of impact, and (3) the characteristics of the tissue through which it passes.

STAB Wounds

Stab wounds are considered low-velocity injuries and therefore low energy transfer. Damage is the result of the sharp cutting edge of the wounding agent; minimal secondary trauma occurs. A narrow, pointed object (e.g., an ice pick) will cause a microscopic crush injury, which will be confined to the path of the instrument's apex. If the instrument is tapered and flat (e.g., a dagger), there will also be fraying and crushing in the tissues as they are stretched to accommodate the wide edge of the blade close to the shaft. If a blunter instrument is used (e.g., an axe), there will be a greater area of crushed tissue and the force applied to achieve the same degree of penetration will also include blunt injury.

For patients with penetrating trauma from a stab wound, knowing the position of the attacker and the patient, the type of weapon used, and the gender of the attacker can identify the projected path of the weapon. Women tend to stab downward, whereas men tend to stab upward.

Damage from a stab wound depends on the location of the penetrating object. Tissue damage is generally isolated to the area of penetration (Fig. 34.13); however, a single wound can penetrate several body cavities, causing lethal injuries. For example, the weapon can enter the thoracic and abdominal cavities with just one penetration. Chest wounds at the level of the nipple or below can involve the abdominal cavity and underlying organs.

More than one wound may exist. It is also important to remember that small wounds can hide extensive internal damage caused by weapon movement. Internal damage is directly proportional to the length of the wounding object and to the density of tissue affected.

Impalements

Impalements are generally low-velocity injuries occurring from falls or MVCs or secondary to a flying or falling object. Impaled objects should be stabilized and removed only when the patient is in a controlled environment, such as an operating room, where surgical support and intervention are immediately available.

Gunshot Wounds

Handguns, shotguns, and rifles are responsible for most firearm injuries. Ballistics is the science of the study of the motion of projectiles. A penetrating wound occurs when the missile remains in the body and there is only an entrance wound; a perforating wound occurs when the missile passes out of the body and thus creates an entrance and an exit wound (Fig. 34.14). The size of the entrance wound will vary directly with the size (caliber) of the missile. The size and shape of the wound are also subject to the missile's flight pattern at the time of impact (yaw). (Fig. 34.15 demonstrates these movements.) Also affecting the size and shape of the wound is the shape of the projectile (i.e., a smooth bullet or a jagged shell fragment). Once the missile is inside the body, the degree of damage is a result of the interaction between the body itself and the projectile and depends on the consistency of the tissues being traversed by the missile and the characteristics of the weapon that launched it.

Missile velocity determines tissue deformation and extent of cavitation.[26] Velocity is generally described as low or high.

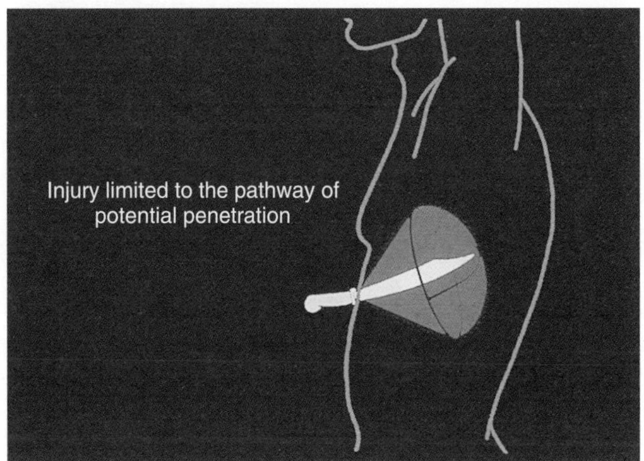

Fig. 34.13 Movement of a knife blade inside a victim produces damage, limited to path of penetration. (Modified from Prehospital Trauma Life Support Committee of the National Association of Emergency Medical Technicians in cooperation with the Committee on Trauma of the American College of Surgeons. *PHTLS: Basic and Advanced Prehospital Life Support.* 4th ed. St Louis, MO: Mosby; 1999.)

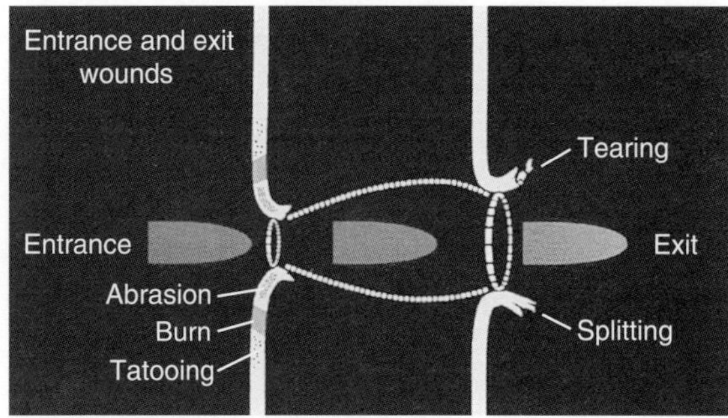

Fig. 34.14 A spinning missile produces a 1- to 2-mm abraded edge along the wound if it enters straight. If it enters at an angle, the abraded side is on the bottom of the missile, with more skin contact, and covers a much wider area. Difference in entrance and exit wounds is also depicted. Exit wounds are generally longer and more explosive. (Modified from Prehospital Trauma Life Support Committee of the National Association of Emergency Medical Technicians in cooperation with the Committee on Trauma of the American College of Surgeons. *PHTLS: Basic and Advanced Prehospital Life Support.* 4th ed. St Louis, MO: Mosby; 1999.)

Low-velocity missiles travel at speeds below 2500 ft/sec and have little disruptive effect on tissues. Injuries are localized at the center of the tract with a small radius of distribution. The temporary cavity is two to three times the diameter of the missile.[13,26] Low-velocity missiles push tissues aside along the path. Side arms such as pistols and submachine guns fall into this type of category.

High-velocity missiles (HVMs) travel at speeds above 2500 ft/sec and cause more serious injuries because of high cavitation and energy transfer.[26] High-velocity missiles create a cavity around the bullet and the bullet tract by compressing and displacing tissue. As kinetic energy is transferred from the bullet to the tissue, the cavity enlarges. A tract temporarily displaces tissue laterally and forward as the missile moves forward. Behind or following the missile, negative pressure contaminates the wound by pulling in foreign material. These cavities can be 30 to 40 times the diameter of the bullet. Fig. 34.16 describes the cavitational differences between low-velocity and high-velocity bullets. High-velocity wounds often require debridement because of extensive tissue disruption. An example of this type of missile would be one fired from a modern-day rifle.

Entrance and exit wounds with HVMs differ with types of tissues and body areas hit.[13] Exit wounds may be larger when the missile travels through smaller structures such as an extremity because all the energy has not dissipated by the time the bullet exits; cavitation and missile movement is still occurring. Exit wounds tend to be small in dense tissue because cavitation is complete and most energy is dissipated. If the bullet fragments while traveling through the tissues, no exit wound is found. Because entrance and exit wounds may have differing characteristics in differing circumstances, documentation should include only a description of the wound and not identification as either an entrance or exit wound.

Deformation of the bullet is another important factor when assessing GSWs. Energy production increases when missiles change shape on impact. Types of bullets that

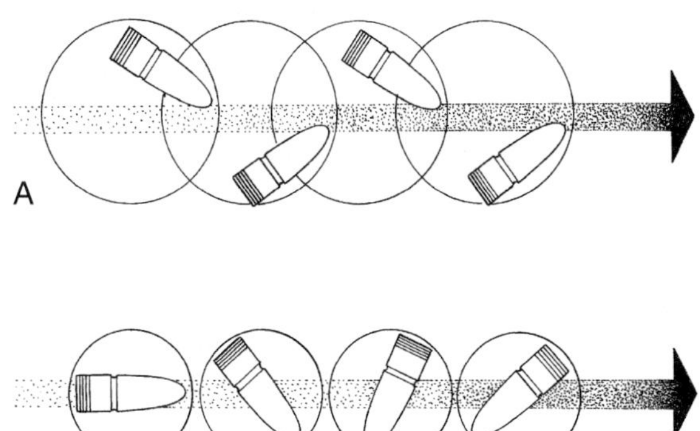

Fig. 34.15 Effect of Bullet Movement on Wounding Potential. (A) Yawing. (B) Tumbling.

produce greater kinetic energy include soft-nosed, flat-nosed, and hollow-point bullets that mushroom on impact. Refer to Table 34.4 for the characteristics of bullets by shape.

Another feature of GSWs is the muzzle blast seen with close-range wounds or when the gun is pressed against the skin. Immediately on firing, a cloud of burning powder and hot gas is released from the muzzle. If a muzzle blast is evident, tattooing from burning particles, abrasions, and burn marks at the entrance wound are seen.

Blast injuries

Blasts are not as common in the United States as in some other countries; however, the potential for hazardous explosions at chemical plants, oil refineries, shipyards, and other industrial settings does exist. Terrorist activity has increased the concern for explosions in urban areas. Explosions can occur anywhere because of the large amount of volatile materials carried by rail or truck. Blasts occur when explosives are detonated and changed to gases. As the gas expands, an equal volume of air is displaced and travels after the blast wave. Disruption of tissue, evisceration, and traumatic amputation

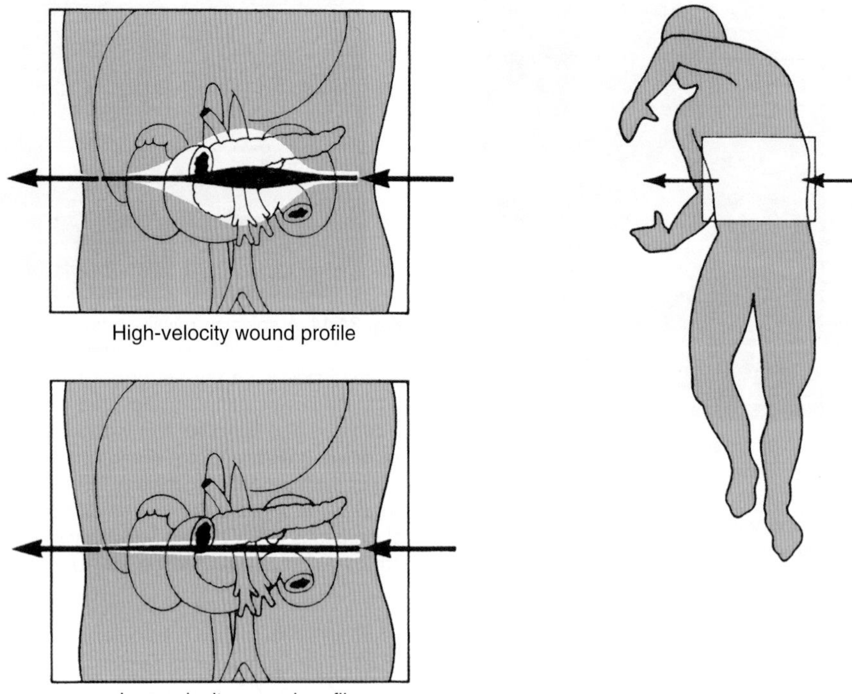

Fig. 34.16 Potential Injury Path of High- and Low-Velocity Bullets. (From Neff JA, Kidd PS: *Trauma Nursing: The Art and Science.* St Louis, MO: Mosby; 1993.)

can occur from this mass movement of air. When the explosive casing ruptures, the casing fragments become high-velocity projectiles.[26,27]

The greater density of water allows a blast wave to travel more rapidly and farther in water than air. Consequently, injuries associated with underwater blasts are usually more severe. Closed-area explosions cause more damage than open-area ones because of the potential inhalation of smoke and toxic gases.

Blast injuries occur in three phases or impact points. Fig. 34.17 diagrams how injuries occur from an explosive blast, and Table 34.5 describes common injuries. As explosives change to an expanding mass of heated gas, primary injuries occur because of the concussive effects of the pressure wave. Concussion injuries are frequently overlooked because they are not obvious and may occur without external signs of trauma; however, these injuries are usually the most severe. Injuries associated with this mechanism include brain and spinal cord injuries, rupture of air-containing organs, and tearing of membranes and small vessels. The associated heat wave can also cause burns on areas of the body facing the explosion.

Fragments of glass, rocks, or metal debris become high-velocity projectiles and can cause secondary injuries, including impalements, fractures, traumatic amputations, burns, and soft-tissue injuries such as contusions, abrasions, and lacerations.

The third point of impact occurs when the victim is thrown through the air and becomes a missile. Tertiary injuries associated with this mechanism are similar to those seen when people are ejected from vehicles or fall from heights, and these injuries generally occur at the point of impact. Structural collapse during the blast can lead to crush injuries.

TABLE 34.4 Classification of Bullets by Shape

Shape	Composition
Pointed nose Round nose	Certain kinds are called "soft points" and on impact will flatten and "mushroom" back on themselves, increasing the amount of damage.
Hollow-Pointed nose	Made with a depression at the tip of their noses and deform on impact. It is thought that by becoming deformed, these bullets will increase the amount of damage.
Flat nose	One type is "Dum-Dum" bullets, which were developed by the British in 1897 at their garrison in Dum Dum, India. The Hague Convention outlawed them for military use.

Reprinted from Emergency Nurses Association: *Trauma Nursing Core course: Provider Manual.* 7th ed. Des Plaines, IL: Emergency Nurses Association; 2014.

Specific mechanisms of injury

Burns

Data reveal that, on average, in the United States, someone dies in a fire approximately every 2.5 hours. Most fires (73%) take place in the home. Cooking and barbequing are the primary causes of residential fires. Smoking is also a significant

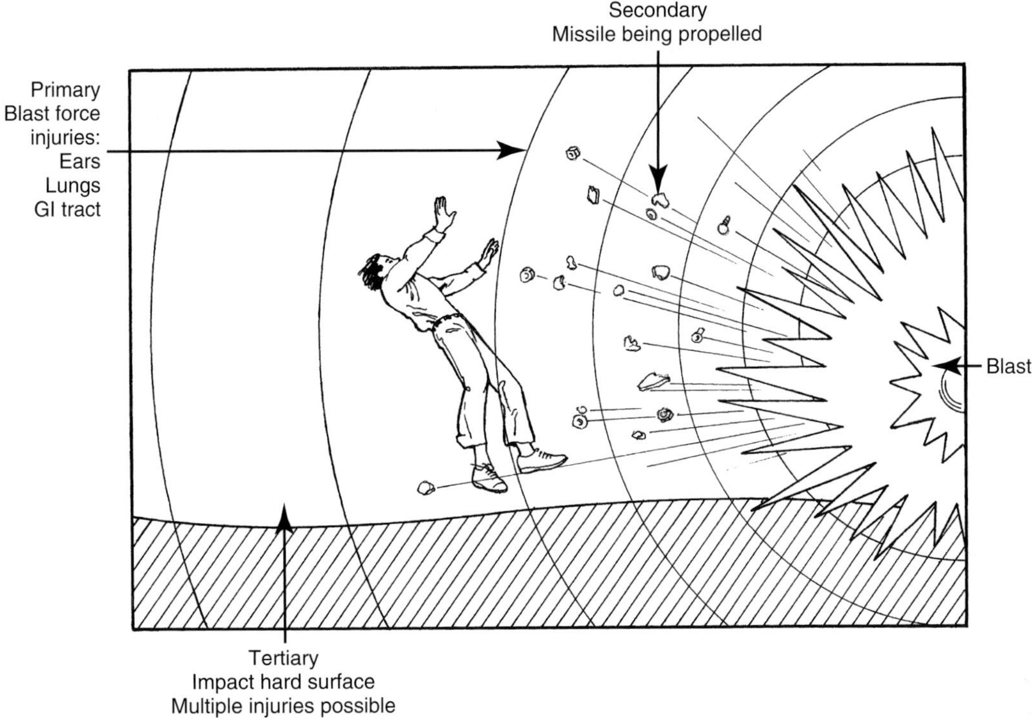

Fig. 34.17 Effects of an Explosive Blast.

TABLE 34.5 Mechanisms of Blast Injuries

Mechanism	Causation	Primary Organs Affected
Primary	Initial blast or air wave. It is important to try and determine what type of blast occurred (steam, chemical, gas, electrical, etc.) so prehospital providers can be safe and secondary complications can be avoided with the patients.	Affects primarily air-filled organs: Tympanic membranes—rupture and permanent deafness can occur Lungs—pneumothorax, alveolar rupture, air embolus GI—intestinal and stomach contusions and rupture CNS—concussion syndrome, various types of focal and diffuse cerebral hemorrhage, cerebral air embolism
Secondary	Flying debris, which act as projectiles	Injuries will vary depending on the size of the projectiles and what and where they hit
Tertiary	The distance an individual's body travels from the blast and where it has impacted	Injuries are similar to those in an individual who has been ejected from an MVC or fallen from a great height. Miscellaneous: Lungs, skin, eyes. Inhalation of dust or toxic gases, thermal burns, radiation, etc.

CNS, Central nervous system; *GI,* gastrointestinal; *MVC,* motor vehicle crash.
Reprinted from Emergency Nurses Association: Trauma nursing core course: provider manual, ed 7, Des Plaines, IL, 2014, The Association.

cause of fire-related deaths. Alcohol contributes to about 40% of residential fire deaths.[38] Those at greatest risk for fire-related deaths and sustaining burns are the following:

- children aged 4 years and younger
- adults aged 65 and older
- those living in poverty
- African Americans and Native Americans
- those living in rural areas
- those living in manufactured homes or substandard housing

Although the number of fatalities and injuries caused by residential fires has declined gradually over the past several decades, many residential fire–related deaths remain preventable and continue to pose a significant public health problem. Those younger than age 5 and older than age 65 are the most susceptible to scald burns from hot liquids. Those older than age 65 sustain the majority (75%) of burns from clothing ignition resulting from cigarette smoking or the use of stoves and space heaters.

Submersion Injuries

Submersion (drowning and near-drowning) results in injury secondary to oxygen deprivation. Blunt trauma is frequently associated with these events due to the increased use of watercraft and the reality that the individuals involved were not able to be rescued or able to rescue themselves. Males account for 80% of drownings in the United States.[3,32] Alcohol is involved in about 25% to 50% of adolescent and adult deaths associated with water recreation.[35] Alcohol influences balance, coordination, and judgment, and its effects are heightened by sun exposure and heat.[30] Up to 70% of boating-related deaths were the result of drowning; 86% of the people who drowned were not wearing personal flotation devices.[3,32] Most drownings occur at sites without lifeguards.[3,32]

For every child 14 years of age or younger who drowns, three will receive ED care for nonfatal submersion injuries. Nonfatal incidents can cause brain damage, resulting in long-term disability ranging from memory problems and learning disabilities to a persistent vegetative state. Children younger than the age of 1 year most often drown in bathtubs or toilets.[3] The overall age-adjusted drowning rate for African Americans is 1.4 times higher than for whites.[17]

Violence-Related Injuries

Violence-related injuries are defined as those resulting from the intentional use of physical force or power against oneself, another person, or a group or community. This definition encompasses violence, intimate partner violence, and other types of assaults. It also includes acts of self-directed violence such as suicide, suicide attempts, and self-mutilation. Violence adversely affects the health and welfare of all Americans through premature death, disability, medical costs, and lost productivity. Medical costs and productivity losses due to interpersonal and self-directed violence in the United States are significant and difficult to quantify.[22,28,37] See Chapters 48 to 51 for further discussion of abuse and neglect, intimate partner violence, and sexual assault.

School Violence

The number of incidents involving firearms on school properties has been increasing over the past decade, along with the number of multiple-victim incidents. More than 50% of school-associated violent deaths occurred at the beginning or end of the school day or during lunch. School-associated homicide rates are highest near the start of each school semester; suicide rates are generally higher in the spring semester.[3]

Suicide/Self-Inflicted Violence

Suicide rates have increased in nearly every state over the past two decades, and half of the 50 states have seen suicide rates rise more than 30%. CDC suicide data indicate that although females attempt suicide more often than males, males are four times more likely to die of suicide. Suicide is the third leading cause of death among young people aged 15 to 24 years.[39] Suicide rates are highest among those aged 65 and older. Data indicate that Americans older than age 65 average one suicide every 90 minutes, with men constituting 85% of these suicides.[3] Standard definitions for suicide do not exist, and the definitions used in federal and state legislation vary drastically. These inconsistencies contribute to confusion and a lack of consensus about the magnitude of the problem. Although there are numerous methods for suicide (e.g., toxicologic overdose, hanging, asphyxiation), 56% of suicides are committed with a firearm.[15,39]

Overall, poisoning (66%) and cuttings/piercings (18%) are the most common forms of self-inflicted injuries. Males are six times more likely to sustain a firearm injury, whereas self-inflicted poisonings were 60% higher for females than males.[2,15]

PREVENTION

Traumatic injuries have physical, emotional, and financial consequences that can affect the lives of individuals, families, and society. Some injuries can result in temporary or permanent disability or death. Because of this, injury-prevention programs have been developed in the hopes of stopping the injury from ever occurring.[40]

The Haddon Injury Matrix is the most widely used epidemiologic model of injury prevention.[3] This model describes a two-dimensional approach to injury and its causes. The first dimension encompasses the three factors of injury: host or human factors, the agent or vector of energy transfer, and the physical and social environment. The second dimension in this model is the phase of injury. The prevent phase is amenable to primary prevention strategies designed to stop the injuring event from occurring by acting on its cause (e.g., installing pool fences or divided highways). The injury event phase is amenable to secondary prevention strategies attempting to prevent an injury or reduce the seriousness of an injury when an event actually occurs (e.g., wearing safety restraints or bicycle helmets). The postinjury event phase is amenable to tertiary prevention strategies that attempt to reduce the seriousness of an injury after the event has occurred by providing adequate care (e.g., trained prehospital and ED staff). Injury-prevention programs can be constructed to target specific factors or phases of injury or both. Table 34.6 describes possible injury-prevention strategies to reduce falls in older adults using the Haddon matrix. In general, most injury-control strategies can be classified according to three E's: engineering and technologic interventions, enforcement and legislative interventions, and education and behavioral interventions. For example, a program designed to prevent falls in older adults may include engineering/technologic innovations such as specially designed padded underwear, enforcement/legislation interventions such as regulations related to restraint use, and education/behavioral interventions such as the CDC's Check for Safety: A Home Fall Prevention Checklist for Older Adults.

The Emergency Nurses Association (ENA) offers a wide variety of injury-prevention programs and materials through the Injury Prevention Institute; programs include alcohol prevention education, bike and helmet safety, child passenger safety, gun safety, and healthy aging. An example of an injury-prevention strategy adopted at the state level is the gradual

TABLE 34.6 The Haddon Injury Matrix to Plan Prevention Strategies

Phases	Human Factors	Vehicle or Vector Factors	Environmental Factors
Prevent	Reduce use of sedatives	Correct defects in safety equipment (e.g., walkers, wheelchairs)	Use of safety bars, handrails, side rails on beds
Event	Consider reduction in severity of preexisting medical conditions (e.g., vertigo, imbalance)	Cover exposed skin areas with protective barriers to reduce severity of injury (e.g., elbow and knee pads)	Reduction of clutter in the patient's environment
Post event	Consider if patient is on anticoagulants or other medications and their effects on subsequent bleeding or physiologic response to shock and trauma	Have patients avoid areas where they could become trapped after a fall and where access to help is minimal	Implementation of comprehensive emergency response protocols and systems

phasing in of licensing of young drivers so they drive mainly in the daylight, have no other teenagers in the car, and need to be with an experienced driver. Additional examples of injury programs are the ThinkFirst diving program and the National Rifle Association's Eddie the Eagle gun safety program for children.

Not all injury-prevention programs are successful. The key is to implement an evaluation system measuring the impact of the program. Some may view the prevention of one death or one injury as a success, but when scarce resources are available in public health, the impact of expense must be justified.

It is difficult to determine the effect of some programs; for example, those that encourage people to tie a red ribbon around one's side-mounted mirror or educational programs for teens and drunk-driving prevention.

Access to the Internet provides innumerable resources for prevention programs through federal, state, and local nonprofit and private organizations, companies, and foundations. The key to preventing many unintentional injury deaths and disabling injuries among children is effective supervision, yet this behavioral component of injury prevention lacks conceptual and methodological clarity.[3]

SUMMARY

Treatment of trauma patients depends on identifying all injuries and rapidly intervening to correct those which are life-threatening. Consideration of mechanisms of injury is essential to identifying patients with possible underlying injuries who require further evaluation and treatment.

REFERENCES

1. *Epidemiology. American Heritage Dictionary*. 3rd ed. Boston, MA: Houghton Mifflin; 1992.
2. Centers for Disease Control and Prevention. 10 leading causes of death by age group, United States—2016. https://www.cdc.gov/injury/wisqars/pdf/leading_causes_of_death_by_age_group_2016-508.pdf, 2016. Accessed June 1, 2018.
3. Centers for Disease Control and Prevention. 10 leading causes of nonfatal injury, United States—2016. https://www.cdc.gov/injury/wisqars/pdf/leading_cause_of_nonfatal_injury_2016-508.pdf, 2016. Accessed June 1, 2018.
4. Insurance Institute for Highway Safety. Highway Loss Data Institute. Teenagers. Arlington, VA: Insurance Institute for Highway Safety. https://www.iihs.org/topics/teenagers. Accessed May 27, 2019.
5. Jonah BA, Dawson NE. Youth and risk: age differences in risky driving, risk perception, and risk utility. *Alcohol Drugs Driving*. 1987;3(3-4):13–29.
6. Centers for Disease Control and Prevention. Impaired driving: fact sheet. Centers for Disease Control and Prevention website. 2007. https://www.cdc.gov/motorvehiclesafety/impaired_driving/. Accessed May 27, 2019.
7. National Highway Traffic Safety Administration, US Department of Transportation. *Traffic Safety Facts 2003. Data: Young Drivers*. Washington, DC: National Highway Traffic Safety Administration; 2004.
8. Li L, Shults RA, Andridge RR, Yellman MA, Xiang H, Zhu M. Texting/emailing while driving among high school students in 35 states, United States, 2015. *J Adolesc Health*. 2018; pii.
9. Chang YS, Lee WJ, Lee JH. Are there higher pedestrian fatalities in larger cities? a scaling analysis of 115 to 161 largest cities in the United States. *Traffic Inj Prev*. 2016;17(7):720–728.
10. Rudisill TM, Zhu M, Abate M, et al. Characterization of drug and alcohol use among senior drivers fatally injured in U.S. motor vehicle collisions, 2008-2012. *Traffic Inj Prev*. 2016;17(8):788–795.
11. Yanar H, Demetriades D, Hatzizacharia P, et al. Pedestrians injured by automobiles: risk factors for cervical spine injuries. *J Am Coll Surg*. 2007;205(6):794–799.
12. Liu LH, Chandra M, Gonzalez JR, Lo JC. Racial and ethnic differences in hip fracture outcomes in men. *Am J Manag Care*. 2017;23(9):560–564.
13. Moore EE, Feliciano DV, Mattox KL, eds. *Trauma*. 8th ed. New York, NY: McGraw-Hill; 2017.
14. McQuillan K, Whalen E, Makic MBF, eds. *Trauma Nursing: From Resuscitation Through Rehabilitation*. 4th ed. Philadelphia, PA: Elsevier; 2008.
15. Greenfield N. CDC: US suicide rates have climbed dramatically. National Public Radio website. https://www.npr.org/sections/health-shots/2018/06/07/617897261/cdc-u-s-suicide-rates-have-climbed-dramatically, Published June 7, 2018. Accessed July 1, 2018.

16. Brenner RA, Trumble AC, Smith GS, Kessler EP, Overpeck MD. Where children drown, United States, 1995. *Pediatrics*. 2001;108(1):85–89.
17. El Sibi R, Bachir R, El Sayed M. Submersion injuries in the United States: patients' characteristics and predictors of mortality and morbidity. *Injury*. 2018;49(3):543–548.
18. Budnick HC, Tyroch AH, Milan SA. Ethnic disparities in traumatic brain injury care referral in a Hispanic-majority population. *J Surg Res*. 2017;215:231–238.
19. Heron M. Deaths: leading causes for 2015. *Natl Vital Stat Rep*. 2017;66(5):1–76. https://www.cdc.gov/nchs/data/nvsr/nvsr66/nvsr66_05.pdf. Accessed June 1, 2018.
20. Linton KF. Interpersonal violence and traumatic brain injuries among Native Americans and women. *Brain Inj*. 2015;29(5):639–643.
21. Linton KF, Kim BJ. Traumatic brain injury as a result of violence in Native American and Black communities spanning from childhood to older adulthood. *Brain Inj*. 2014;29(8):1076–1081.
22. Krug EG, Powell KE, Dahlberg LL. Firearm-related deaths in the United States and 35 other high-and upper middle-income countries. *Int J Epidemiol*. 1998;27(2):214–221.
23. Resnick S, Smith RN, Eard JH, et al. Firearm deaths in America: can we learn from 462,000 lives lost? *Ann Surg*. 2017;266(3):432–440.
24. National Highway Traffic Safety Administration, US Department of Transportation. *Traffic Safety Facts 2003. Data: Pedestrians*. Washington, DC: National Highway Traffic Safety Administration; 2004.
25. Centers for Disease Control and Prevention. Child passenger deaths involving drinking and drivers—United States, 1997-2002 [published erratum appears in Morb Mortal Wkly Rep. 2004;53(5):109]. *Morb Mortal Wkly Rep*. 2004;53(4):77–79.
26. Emergency Nurses Association. *Trauma Nursing Core Course: Provider Manual*. 7th ed. Des Plaines, IL: Emergency Nurses Association; 2014.
27. National Association of Emergency Medical Technicians. *Pre-Hospital Trauma Life Support (PHTLS)*. 8th ed. Jones and Bartlett Learning; 2014.
28. Centers for Disease Control and Prevention. Nonfatal sports and recreational-related injuries treated in emergency departments—United States, July 2000-June 2001. *MMWR Morb Mortal Wkly Rep*. 2002;51(33):736–740.
29. Porter RS. Blunt trauma. In: Bledsoe BE, Porter RS, Cherry RA, eds. *Paramedic Care: Principles and Practice*. 5th ed. Upper Saddle River, NJ: Prentice-Hall; 2017.
30. National Highway Traffic Safety Administration, US Department of Transportation. *Traffic Safety Facts 2003*. Washington, DC: National Highway Traffic Safety Administration; 2004. 18;6(9):e523–e534. 6(6).
31. Centers for Disease Control and Prevention. Agriculture fact sheet. https://www.cdc.gov/niosh/topics/aginjury/, Published 2016. Accessed June 17, 2018.
32. US Coast Guard, Department of Homeland Security. *2017 Recreational Boating Statistics*. https://www.uscgboating.org/library/accident-statistics/Recreational-Boating-Statistics-2017.pdf, Published 2018. Accessed May 28, 2018.
33. Stevens JA, Dellinger AM. Motor vehicle and fall related deaths among older Americans 1990-1998: sex, race and ethnic disparities. *Inj Prev*. 2002;8(4):272–275.
34. Guskiewicz KM, Weaver N, Padua DA, Garrett Jr WE. Epidemiology of concussion in collegiate and high school football players. *Am J Sports Med*. 2000;28(5):643–650.
35. Howland J, Mangione T, Hingson R, et al. Alcohol as a risk factor for drowning and other aquatic injuries. In: Watson RR, ed. *Alcohol and Accidents, Drug and Alcohol Abuse Reviews*. Vol. 7. Totowa, NJ: Humana Press; 1995.
36. Kerr ZY, Wilkerson GB, Caswell SV, et al. The first decade of web-based sports injury surveillance: descriptive epidemiology of injuries in United States high school football (2005-2006 through 2013-2014) and National Collegiate Athletic Association Football (2004-2005 through 2013-2014). *J Athl Train*. 2018;53(8):738–751. https://doi.org/10.4085/1062-6050-144-17.
37. Fowler KA, Jack SPD, Lyons BH, Betz CJ, Petrosky E. Surveillance for violent death—National Violent Death Reporting system, 18 states, 2014. *MMWR Surveil Summ*. 2018;67(2):1–36.
38. American Burn Association. *Burn Incidence and Treatment in the United States*. 2016. https://ameriburn.org/who-we-are/media/burn-incidence-fact-sheet/. Accessed April 29, 2018.
39. Kochanek KD, Murphy SL, Anderson RN, Scott C. Deaths: final data for 2002?. *Natl Vital Stat Rep*. 2004;53(5): 1–115.
40. Ortiz AL, Jafri A, Hyder AA. Effective interventions for unintentional injuries: a systematic review and mortality impact assessment among the poorest billion. *Lancet Glob Health*. 20

35

Head Trauma

Beth Broering

Traumatic brain injury (TBI), a leading cause of death and permanent disability, is a major public health problem both in the United States and internationally. More than 2 million persons in the United States sustain a brain injury each year. In 2013, the Centers for Disease Control and Prevention (CDC) reported more than 50,000 deaths, more than 280,000 hospitalizations, and more than 2.5 million emergency department (ED) visits due to brain injury.[1] TBI has resulted in more than 5 million persons in the United States living with permanent disabilities, many requiring lifelong assistance with the activities of daily living.[2,3] Medical costs, both direct and indirect, for TBI, although difficult to determine, were estimated to be more than $60 billion in 2013.[3,4]

Mechanisms of injury include blunt, penetrating, and blast forces that disrupt the vascular and neuronal structures inside the cranial vault, leading to a complex cascade of cellular and biochemical processes. A small percentage of patients with severe TBI will have concomitant fracture of the cervical spine. Falls are the leading mechanism of injury in all age-groups, but particularly in the pediatric population and those older than 65 years of age. Persons of all ages sustain TBIs from motor vehicle crashes and crashes from other motorized vehicles (e.g., scooters, motorcycles, all-terrain vehicle); however, those 15 to 24 years of age are at greatest risk. Sports and recreation-related TBIs primarily affect males 19 years of age and younger.[5] Along with mechanisms, the forces of energy are important to understand. Brain injuries can result from acceleration, deceleration, rotational, or deformation forces. Table 35.1 provides an overview of the common energy forces associated with TBI.

Penetrating injuries occur most commonly from firearms, but they can also result from any sharp object that penetrates the scalp and skull. The extent of damage to brain tissue is determined by the point of entry, depth and angle of entry, and force of entry. Although all types of penetrating injuries are potentially lethal, gunshot wounds have the highest associated mortality rate. Blast injuries, the most common cause of TBI for military troops deployed to war zones, can occur in any type of explosion. Blast injury is often a combination of both blunt and penetrating forces. The impact of the blast waves moving through the victim's body causes shearing of neuronal structures, and flying debris might produce penetrating injuries.

It is important for the emergency nurse to have an understanding of the mechanisms of injury and forces involved to ensure appropriate management and minimize the potential for secondary brain injury, complications, and missed injuries.

This chapter begins with a brief review of anatomy and physiology. It also provides an overview of assessment techniques, focusing primarily on adult patients with TBI. Current management options for TBI are also discussed. For a more complete discussion on pediatric injuries, refer to Chapter 42.

ANATOMY AND PHYSIOLOGY

Anatomy

The hair, scalp, skull, meninges, and cerebrospinal fluid (CSF) protect the brain from injury (Fig. 35.1). Five layers of tissue form the scalp: skin, subcutaneous tissue, galea aponeurotica, ligaments, and periosteum. The cranium, composed of the frontal, parietal, temporal, and occipital bones, joins with the facial bones to form the cranial vault, a rigid, nonexpandable cavity that can hold a volume of approximately 1700 mL. Bones of the cranium consist of three layers (Fig. 35.2). The outer and inner tables are composed of hard cortical or compact bone. The diploë, or middle layer, is made up of soft, cancellous bone. The structure of the cranial bones provides significant protection to the brain parenchyma.

The skull is divided into the supratentorial and the infratentorial space. The cerebral hemispheres and the diencephalon are contained in the supratentorial space. The infratentorial space contains the cerebellum and the brain stem. Other bony structures of importance are depressions at the base of the skull called the anterior, middle, and posterior fossae. The frontal lobe is located in the anterior fossa. The deeper middle fossa contains the parietal, temporal, and occipital lobes. The posterior fossa is the largest and deepest and supports the brain stem and cerebellum.

Three layers of meninges surround the brain and provide additional protection. The outermost meninge is the dura mater (meaning "tough mother"), which consists of two layers of tough, fibrous tissue. The inner layer of the dura mater produces prominent folds that subdivide the interior of the cranial cavity. The largest of these folds forms the falx cerebri, which separates the brain into the right and left cerebral

TABLE 35.1 Energy Forces Associated With Traumatic Brain Injury.

Type of Force	Description	Result
Acceleration forces	When the head is struck by a moving object	Skull fractures Contusions Hematomas
Deceleration forces	When the head is moving and strikes a stationary object (e.g., head hits the steering wheel of a car, ejected occupant hits head on the ground)	Skull fractures Contusions Coup-contrecoup injuries Hematomas
Acceleration- deceleration forces	Combination of injuries due to rapid changes in the velocity of the brain	Coup-contrecoup injuries Diffuse axonal injuries Hematomas
Rotational forces	Side-to-side and twisting movement of brain tissue	Diffuse axonal injuries
Deformation forces	Direct blows or compression of the skull with resultant change in shape of the skull	Severity and extent of injury often determined by the velocity of blow or the length of compression

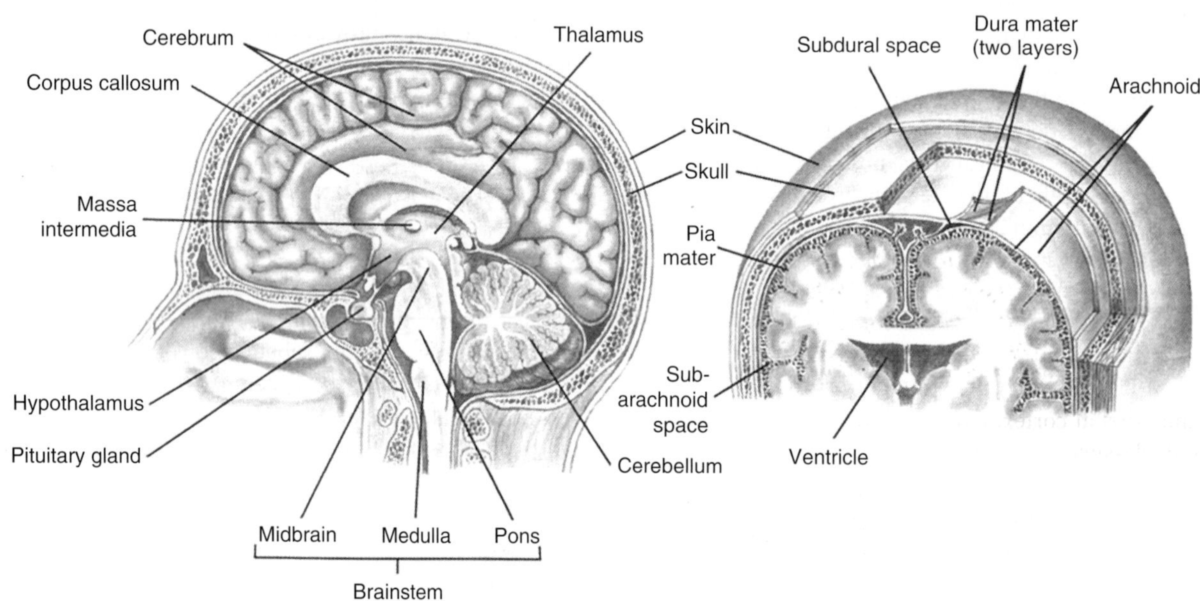

Fig. 35.1 Brain Structures. (From Thompson JM, McFarland G, Hirsch J, et al. *Mosby's Clinical Nursing*. 5th ed. St Louis, MO: Mosby; 2002.)

hemispheres. The next-largest fold is the tentorium cerebelli, which divides the posterior cranial fossa into the superior (supratentorial) and inferior (infratentorial) compartments. Potential spaces located above the dura mater (epidural) and below the dura mater (subdural) are at risk for hematoma formation because the middle meningeal artery lies in the epidural space, and bridging veins are located within the subdural space. The middle meningeal layer is the arachnoid (spiderlike) mater, a fine, elastic layer. Below the arachnoid mater, the subarachnoid space is a relatively large space that is normally filled with CSF and contains arachnoid villi, fingerlike projections forming channels for CSF absorption. Adhering to the surface of the brain is the pia mater (meaning "tender mother").

The cerebrum consists of two hemispheres separated by a longitudinal fissure. Each lobe of the cerebrum is responsible for specific functions. The frontal lobe coordinates voluntary motor movements and controls judgment, affect, and personality. Hearing, behavior, emotions, and dominant-hemisphere speech are controlled by the temporal lobe. Sensory interpretation occurs in the parietal lobe, whereas the occipital lobe is responsible for vision.

The cerebral hemispheres are connected with the midbrain by the diencephalon. The thalamus, hypothalamus, subthalamus, and epithalamus are located within the diencephalon (Fig. 35.3). The hypothalamus has numerous key roles in hormonal regulation and metabolic functions, including temperature regulation; release of hormones from the pituitary

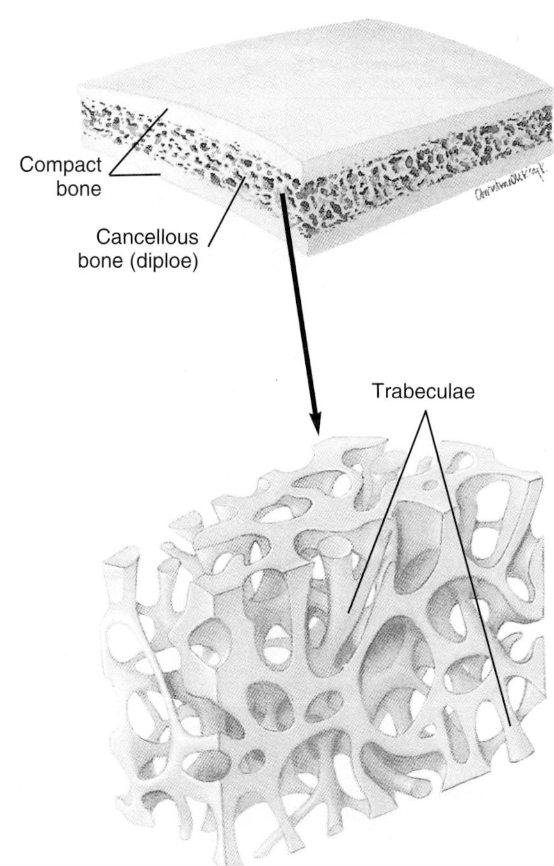

Fig. 35.2 The three layers of "skull bone": outer layer of compact bone surrounding cancellous bone. Note the fine structure of compact and cancellous bone. (From Thibodeau GA, Patton KT. *Anatomy and Physiology*. 6th ed. St Louis, MO: Mosby; 2007.)

gland and adrenal cortex; emotional behaviors such as fear, rage, and pleasure; and activation of the sympathetic and parasympathetic functions of the autonomic nervous system.

The cerebellum is located in the posterior fossa adjacent to the brain stem and separated from the cerebrum by the tentorium cerebelli. Primary functions of the cerebellum are integration of motor function, maintenance of equilibrium, and maintenance of muscle tone.

The brain stem consists of the midbrain, pons, and medulla. Although each structure has important pathway functions, the medulla contains the cardiac, respiratory, and vasomotor centers. The reticular formation, also located in the brain stem, is the central component of the reticular activating system and is responsible for arousal, the lowest level of consciousness, which is interpreted as wakefulness. Along with the primary cardiorespiratory centers, the brain stem contains many ascending and descending pathways carrying impulses between the spinal cord and the brain. In addition, all cranial nerves (CNs) except CN I and CN II originate in the brain stem. Table 35.2 describes the function of each CN.

The anatomic structure of the capillaries of the brain, the tight junctions between endothelial cells, and the surrounding neuroglia form the blood-brain barrier. The blood-brain barrier acts as a protective mechanism restricting the free movement of substances from the blood vessels into the interstitial spaces and CSF. The blood-brain barrier, although mainly protective in nature, can hinder the effectiveness of some drugs. In a brain injury, the breakdown of the blood-brain barrier may potentiate cerebral edema.

Physiology

In the adult patient, the skull is a closed box containing three volumes: the brain (80%), CSF (10%), and blood (10%). Intracranial pressure (ICP) is a dynamic state reflecting the pressure in the supratentorial space as exerted by the total of the three volumes, which under normal conditions is maintained in constant balance through multiple homeostatic mechanisms. Normal ICP is less than 10 mm Hg, with an upper limit of approximately 15 mm Hg. If one or more of the volumes of the cranial contents increases, ICP will rise and, if not immediately corrected, will compromise cerebral blood flow. The Monro-Kellie hypothesis describes the concept of reciprocal changes in volume as a means of compensation and maintaining ICP. As one of the volumes increases, there must be reciprocal decreases in the other two volumes, or ICP will rise. CSF is initially displaced out of the cranial compartment into the spinal subarachnoid space, and production of CSF is reduced. Once CSF is maximally displaced, there is vasoconstriction and compression of the cerebral venous system. Sustained ICP greater than 20 mm Hg represents intracranial hypertension. If ICP continues to rise, arterial blood flow is compromised. These compensatory mechanisms have a finite ability to reduce volume and maintain ICP. As the intracranial volume increases beyond the compensatory threshold, there are sharp increases in ICP (Fig. 35.4). Failure to reduce ICP may cause ischemia and necrosis of brain tissue.

The brain requires a constant supply of oxygen and nutrients, primarily glucose, to maintain function. It receives 15% of the cardiac output and consumes approximately 20% of the body's oxygen supply. Cerebral blood flow is maintained through highly sensitive and complex mechanisms of autoregulation. Cerebral autoregulation is the ability of the brain to maintain a constant blood flow over a wide range of metabolic demands and systemic mean arterial pressures (normally 50–150 mm Hg).[6-8] This is accomplished through vasoconstriction or vasodilation of the cerebral blood vessels. For example, if metabolic demands rise, the cerebral vessels will vasodilate to increase cerebral blood flow, oxygen, and glucose delivery. Cerebral blood flow also remains relatively constant with changes in systemic pressure. The cerebral vessels vasoconstrict when systemic pressure is high and vasodilate as systemic pressures begin to fall. Cerebral autoregulation can be impaired or lost, either locally or globally, after brain injury. When cerebral autoregulation is disrupted, cerebral blood flow becomes dependent on the systemic blood pressure.

Cerebral perfusion pressure (CPP) is the pressure gradient across the brain or the pressure difference between the arterial blood entering the brain and the venous blood exiting. Adequate delivery of oxygen and nutrients requires adequate CPP (i.e., CPP ≥50 mm Hg).[6,8] CPP plays an important role

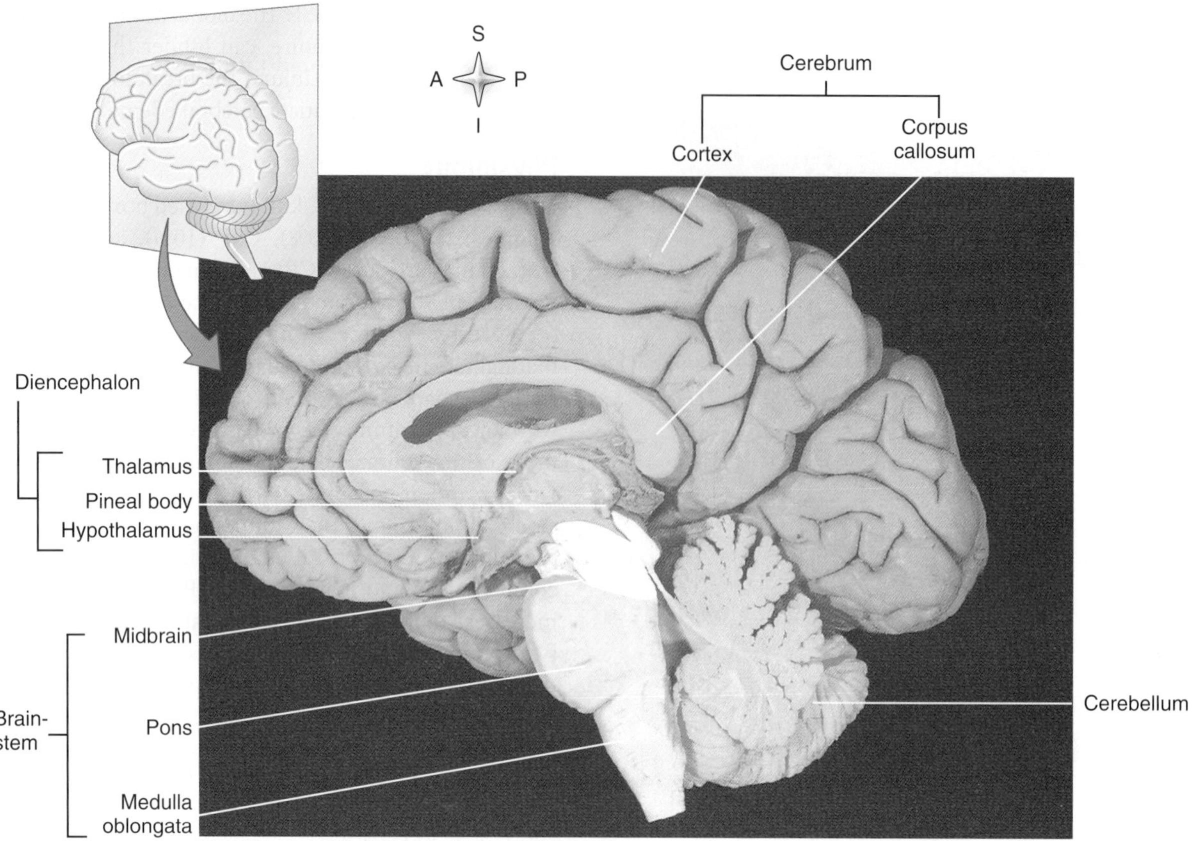

Fig. 35.3 Divisions of the Brain. A midsagittal section of the brain reveals features of its major divisions. (From Thibodeau GA, Patton KT. *Anatomy and Physiology*. 6th ed. St Louis, MO: Mosby; 2007.)

TABLE 35.2 Cranial Nerves and Their Functions.

Cranial Nerve	Function	Physiologic Effects
I. Olfactory	Sensory	Smell
II. Optic	Sensory	Vision
III. Oculomotor	Motor	Extraocular movement of eyes, raises eyelid, constricts pupils
IV. Trochlear	Motor	Allows eye to move down and inward
V. Trigeminal	Motor and sensory	Facial sensation, mastication, and corneal reflex
VI. Abducens	Motor	Allows eye to move outward
VII. Facial	Motor and sensory	Movement of facial muscles, closes eyes, secretes saliva and tears
VIII. Vestibulo-cochlear	Sensory	Hearing and equilibrium
IX. Glossopharyngeal	Motor and sensory	Gag reflex, swallowing, and phonation
X. Vagus	Motor and sensory	Voluntary muscles for swallowing, involuntary to visceral muscles (heart, lungs)
XI. Spinal accessory	Motor	Turns head, shrugs shoulders
XII. Hypoglossal	Motor	Tongue movement for swallowing

in regulating cerebral blood flow. As CPP falls, the cerebral vessels will vasodilate to maintain cerebral blood flow. If CPP drops too low, the cerebral vessels collapse, and cerebral blood flow will actually fall, resulting in ischemia and neuronal cell death. CPP is calculated by subtracting the ICP from the systemic mean arterial pressure (MAP; Box 35.1).

PATIENT ASSESSMENT

After ensuring adequate control of airway, breathing, and circulation (ABCs), the emergency nurse should perform a neurologic assessment. The goals of the neurologic assessment in brain-injured patients include detection of life-threatening

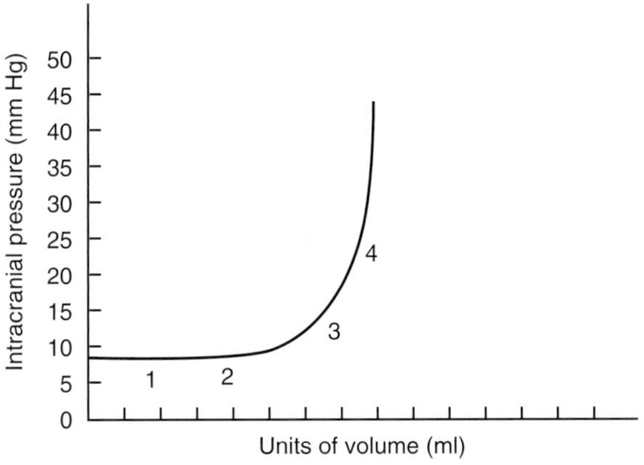

STAGES ON THE CURVE

Stage 1: There is a high compliance and low elastance. The brain is in total compensation, with accommodation and autoregulation intact. An increase in volume does not increase ICP.

Stage 2: The compliance is lower and elastance is increasing. An increase in volume places the patient at risk of increased ICP.

Stage 3: There is high elastance and low compliance. Any small addition of volume causes a great increase in pressure. There is a loss of autoregulation, and there may be symptoms indicating increased ICP, such as systolic hypertension with an increasing pulse pressure, bradycardia, and slowing of respiratory rate (Cushing's triad). With the loss of autoregulation and the rise in the systolic blood pressure as a result of the Cushing response, decompensation occurs. The ICP passively mimics the blood pressure.

Stage 4: Finally, when the patient is in stage 4, the ICP rises to terminal levels with little increase in volume. Herniation occurs as the brain tissue shifts from the compartment of greater pressure to the compartment of lesser pressure.

Fig. 35.4 Intracranial Volume-Pressure Curve. *ICP,* Intracranial pressure. (Modified from Lewis SM, Heitkemper MM, Dirksen RF, eds. *Medical-Surgical Nursing: Assessment and Management of Clinical Problems.* 7th ed. St Louis, MO: Mosby; 2007.)

BOX 35.1 Cerebral Perfusion Pressure.

MAP – ICF = CPP
Example: Mean arterial pressure = 90 mm Hg
Intracranial pressure = 15 mm Hg
90 mm Hg – 15 mm Hg = 75 mm Hg

CPP, Cerebral perfusion pressure; *ICP,* intracranial pressure; *MAP,* mean arterial pressure.

injuries and establishing a baseline assessment to be used as a comparison in subsequent examinations. A complete neurologic assessment, including mental status, level of consciousness or Glasgow Coma Scale (GCS) score, pupillary size and reactivity, CN assessment, reflexes, and motor symmetry and strength, can be performed in the awake and hemodynamically stable patient. In a patient with hemodynamic instability or with comorbid conditions preventing a complete neurologic examination, the patient's neurologic status should be described in as much detail as possible. A subtle change in

BOX 35.2 Signs and Symptoms of Increased Intracranial Pressure.

Early

Level of conscious deteriorates: Patient may become, restless, more confused, agitated, or combative
Headache
Nausea/vomiting
Slowed or slurred speech
Blurred vision or diplopia
Pupillary changes: Delayed/sluggish reactivity to light, pupil becomes ovoid, unilateral change in pupil size or shape
Decreased strength and sensation

Late

Progressive decline in level of consciousness to coma
Projectile vomiting (without nausea)
Speech significantly impaired, may only groan
Impaired brain-stem reflexes (corneal, gag)
Motor posturing
Unilateral or bilateral pupil that enlarges and becomes fixed
Irregular respirations
Cushing's response
Cardiac dysrhythmias
Abnormal reflexes (Babinski)

level of consciousness is often the earliest indication of deterioration in the head-injured patient. Box 35.2 describes the early and late signs and symptoms of increased ICP.

Table 35.3 lists the components of the GCS, an objective and universally accepted measure of a patient's neurologic status.[9] Assessment of level of consciousness should be directed toward acquiring the highest-level or best response with the least stimulus. Completing the GCS allows assignment of numeric values to clinical changes. Interpretation of the GCS must be correlated with other clinical assessment findings. Other physiologic conditions, such as hypotension, hypoxia, alcohol intoxication, or substance abuse, may falsely lower the initial GCS. Eye and facial trauma may make assessment of eye opening inaccurate or difficult. Motor response may be difficult to assess in patients with spinal cord injuries. In addition, the emergency nurse must also consider the accuracy of response in the non–English-speaking patient. However, in the acute resuscitation, a GCS score of 8 or less represents coma, and the nurse must assume the patient has sustained a severe head injury until further clinical and diagnostic studies can be completed.

Normal pupillary response to direct light examination is constriction. Consensual reaction (constriction of the opposite pupil) should occur with direct light examination. Anisocoria, or unequal pupils, is a normal finding in 15% to 17% of the population, so assessment of reactivity in the dilated pupil is critical. Sluggish pupillary response may be the first indication of increasing cerebral edema and rising ICP. An oval pupil is also commonly seen in patients with increasing ICP.[8] With aggressive intervention, the oval pupil will often return to normal size, shape, and reactivity as ICP is reduced. If ICP cannot be controlled, the pupil will become

TABLE 35.3 Glasgow Coma Scale.

Response	Score	Significance
Eye Opening		
Spontaneously	4	Reticular activating system is intact; patient may not be aware
To verbal command	3	Opens eyes when told to do so
To pain	2	Opens eyes in response to pain
None	1	Does not open eyes to any stimuli
Verbal Stimuli		
Oriented, converses	5	Relatively intact CNS, aware of self and environment
Disoriented, converses	4	Well articulated, organized, but disoriented
Inappropriate words	3	Random, exclamatory words
Incomprehensible	2	Moaning, no recognizable words
No response	1	No response or intubated
Motor Response		
Obeys verbal commands	6	Readily moves limbs when told to
Localizes to painful stimuli	5	Moves limb in an effort to remove painful stimuli
Withdrawal	4	Pulls away from pain in flexion
Abnormal flexion	3	Decorticate rigidity
Extension	2	Decerebrate rigidity
No response	1	Hypotonia, flaccid: suggests loss of medullary function or concomitant spinal cord injury

CNS, Central nervous system.
From Geegaard WG, Birow MH: Head. In: Marx J, Hockberger, Walls R: *Rosen's Emergency Medicine: Concepts and Clinical Practice,* 6th ed. St Louis, MO: Mosby; 2006.
Modified from Teasdale G, Jennett B. Assessment of coma and impaired consciousness: a practical scale. *Lancet* 2(7872):81, 1974.

dilated and nonreactive. CN III exits the brain stem and lies at the junction of the midbrain and the tentorial notch. Any increase in downward pressure at the tentorial notch compresses the third CN, resulting in unilateral pupil dilation (Fig. 35.5). Bilateral fixed and dilated pupils are indicative of impending transtentorial herniation.

The oculomotor (CN III), trochlear (CN IV), and abducens (CN VI) nerves control extraocular eye movements. In the conscious patient, extraocular movements should be assessed. Conjugate gaze is movement of both eyes simultaneously in the same direction. This indicates the brain stem and cerebral cortex are functioning. Disconjugate gaze is when one eye is deviated from the normal midposition with the patient at rest. Ask the patient to follow a finger through the

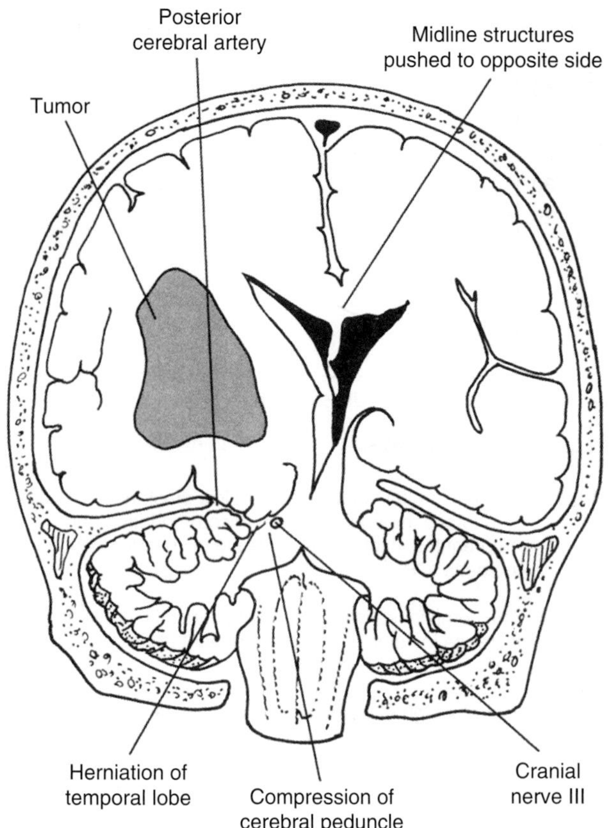

Fig. 35.5 Uncal Herniation With Oculomotor Nerve Compression. (From Barker E. *Neuroscience Nursing: A Spectrum of Care.* 3rd ed. St Louis, MO: Mosby; 2008.)

six directions of gaze. If any of the three CNs are injured, there will be paralysis or paresis of the extraocular muscles, leading to a disconjugate gaze. Ptosis (drooping eyelid) may also be observed with injury to the oculomotor nerve. Patients may also complain of diplopia as the eyes move through the different positions. Injuries can be unilateral or bilateral; therefore it is important to assess each eye separately and observe for consensual and/or conjugate response.

With severe brain injury, it is important to evaluate the integrity of brain-stem function. The oculocephalic (doll's eye) reflex tests the integrity of pontine centers. A doll's eye examination is performed only in an unconscious patient after the cervical spine has been cleared. To perform the doll's eye examination, briskly rotate the patient's head to the right and then to the left while holding the eyelids open and watching the eye movements. If the reflex is present (brain stem is intact), the patient's eyes deviate away from the direction the head is rotated. Loss of brain-stem integrity is presumed when eyes remain midline with rotation of the head or move in a disconjugate manner. The oculovestibular response (cold calorics) also assesses the integrity of the brain stem and is only evaluated in the unconscious patient. The head should be flexed to approximately 30 degrees, and 20 to 50 mL of cold saline is injected into the external auditory canal. Rapid nystagmus-like deviation of the eyes toward the irrigated ear is the normal response. No movement, disconjugate movement, or asymmetric movement indicates interruption in the functional connection between the medulla and the midbrain. Severe dizziness and vomiting occur with this test in a conscious patient, so the ice water test is contraindicated in semiconscious or conscious patients. Another contraindication is tympanic membrane rupture.

A patient's motor examination includes assessment for strength and symmetry when possible. Bilateral extremities should be assessed at the same time for comparison and to identify subtle abnormalities or differences. A central noxious stimulus should be used to elicit a motor response in the uncooperative or unconscious patient. Central stimulation (e.g., trapezius pinch or sternal rub) produces an overall body response. Peripheral stimulation (e.g., nail bed pressure) is also important to assess to differentiate between a spinal cord injury and brain or brain-stem injury. Voluntary purposeful movement should be distinguished from abnormal posturing. Abnormal motor responses include inequality in movement and strength from side to side and posturing. Posturing may be spontaneous or elicited by verbal or painful stimuli. Abnormal flexion posturing (previously called decorticate posturing) is rigid flexion with arms flexed toward the core and the lower extremities extended. This type of posturing is associated with lesions above the midbrain. Abnormal extension posturing (previously called decerebrate posturing) is rigid extension of the arms with wrist flexion and rigid extension of lower extremities and is associated with an insult to the brain stem. Fig. 35.6 illustrates abnormal flexion and extension posturing. Lateralization occurs when patients with TBI present with unilateral abnormal motor posturing. In a patient with hemiparesis contralateral to a fixed and dilated pupil, herniation should be suspected.[8,10]

A detailed CN examination may be delayed until the secondary or focused survey but should be completed in all patients who are awake and can cooperate. In the severely injured patient, the examination may be limited to pupillary responses (CN III) and corneal (CN V and VII) and gag reflexes (CN X).

Assessment of vital signs is an integral part of every initial assessment of a trauma patient. In the patient with brain injury, because of the significant influence the brain and brain stem have on cardiac and respiratory functions, changes in heart rate, blood pressure, and ventilatory rate may be indicators of neurologic deterioration. After major trauma and brain injury, the body frequently is in a hyperdynamic state. As ICP rises, the body's compensatory response is to increase systemic pressure in an attempt to maintain CPP. Hypertension is a common manifestation of severe brain injury. Increased heart rate and cardiac output are also part of the body's compensatory response. Increased ICP causes large amounts of catecholamines to be released both systemically and at the myocardial neuronal level, resulting in a variety of cardiac dysrhythmias and elevated creatine kinase levels. Along with ventilatory rate, the pattern of breathing, work of breathing, and auscultation of breath sounds should be assessed. Respiratory pattern changes are common after severe brain injury and can assist in determining the level of brain-stem dysfunction (Table 35.4).[7,8,10]

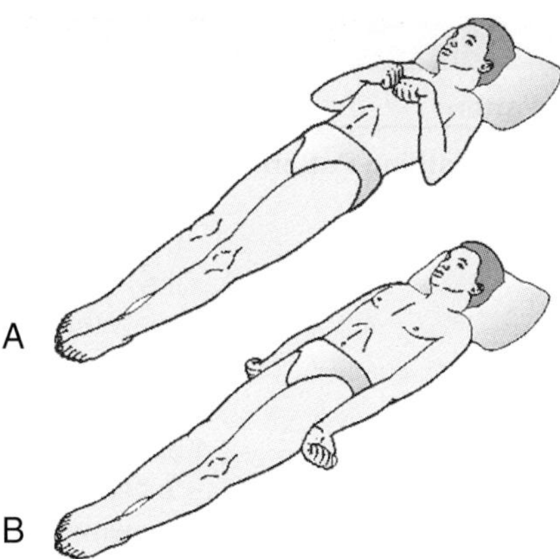

Fig. 35.6 Abnormal flexion (A) and extension (B). (Modified from Urden LD, Stacy KM, Lough ME. *Thelan's Critical Care Nursing: Diagnosis and Management.* 5th ed. St Louis, MO: Mosby; 2006.)

Temperature changes not only are common in brain injury but also may contribute to secondary injury if the temperature is not controlled. Hypothermia is frequently a result of environmental exposure and the infusion of cold or room-temperature intravenous fluids and blood products. Hypothermia is defined as a core temperature of less than 95°F (35°C). Hyperthermia may be seen with hypothalamic damage. Hyperthermia (core temperature >100.4°F [38°C]) increases the cerebral metabolic rate and oxygen requirements. To compensate, cerebral blood flow must increase, which results in increased ICP. In the acute resuscitation, one must also consider preexisting infection as a source of the hyperthermia if environmental factors have been eliminated. If cooling measures are necessary, shivering must be avoided because it further increases the metabolic demands.

With severe brain injury and progressive or uncontrolled intracranial hypertension, the body exhibits a syndrome of vital sign changes called the Cushing's reflex or Cushing's response. The presence of the Cushing's response is a late finding and indicates ICP has reached life-threatening levels. These changes include hypertension, widening pulse pressure, and bradycardia and are related to pressure on the medullary areas of the brain stem. The systolic pressure increases in an attempt to overcome the compression of the cerebral arteries and diminished flow to the brain (from ICP). Blood pressure that is decreased with brain injuries indicates a poor prognosis.

PATIENT MANAGEMENT

Management of a patient with a brain injury begins in the prehospital setting. In patients with suspected severe brain injury, hypoxemia should be corrected and ventilation supported to maintain oxygen saturations >90%.[11–13] Patients may benefit from early intubation and targeted ventilation to maintain normal breathing rates and end-tidal CO_2 ($EtCO_2$) 35 to 40 mm Hg.[11] In addition, it is important to ensure these patients are transported to trauma centers with neurosurgical and neurocritical care capabilities as early as possible to reduce morbidity and mortality.[11,14] Communication with

TABLE 35.4 Patterns of Breathing.

Breathing Pattern	Description	Location of Injury
Hemispheric Breathing Patterns		
Normal	After a period of hyperventilation that lowers the arterial carbon dioxide pressure ($Paco_2$), the individual continues to breathe regularly but with a reduced depth.	Response of the nervous system to an external stressor—not associated with injury to the CNS.
Posthyperventilation apnea (PHVA)	Respirations stop after hyperventilation has lowered the Pco_2 level below normal. Rhythmic breathing returns when the Pco_2 level returns to normal. (Usually an intact cerebral cortex will trigger breathing within 10 seconds, regardless of Pco_2.)	Associated with diffuse bilateral metabolic or structural disease of the cerebrum.
Cheyne-Stokes respirations (CSR)	The breathing pattern has a smooth increase (crescendo) in the rate and depth of breathing (hyperpnea), which peaks and is followed by a gradual smooth decrease (decrescendo) in the rate and depth of breathing to the point of apnea when the cycle repeats itself. The hyperpneic phase lasts longer than the apneic phase (represents an amplitude change).	Bilateral dysfunction of the deep cerebral or diencephalic structures, seen with supratentorial injury and metabolically induced coma states unrelated to neurologic dysfunction, also may be seen in CHF.
Brain Stem Breathing Patterns		
Central reflex hyperpnea (Central neurogenic hyperventilation [CNH])	A sustained deep, rapid, but regular pattern (hyperpnea) occurs, with a decreased $Paco_2$ and a corresponding increase in pH and increased Po_2	May result from CNS damage or disease that involves the midbrain and upper pons; seen after increased intracranial pressure and blunt level trauma.
Apneusis	A prolonged inspiratory cramp (a pause at full inspiration) occurs. A common variant of this is a brief end-inspiratory pause of 2 or 3 seconds often alternating with an end-expiratory pause.	Indicates damage to the respiratory control mechanism located at the pontine level; most commonly associated with pontine infarction but documented with hypoglycemia, anoxia, and meningitis.
Cluster breathing	A cluster of breaths has a disordered sequence with irregular pauses between breaths.	Dysfunction in the lower pontine and high medullary areas.
Ataxic breathing	Completely irregular breathing occurs, with random shallow and deep breaths and irregular pauses. Often the rate is slow.	Originates from a primary dysfunction of the lower pons or upper medulla.
Gasping breathing pattern (agonal gasps)	A pattern of deep "all-or-none" breaths is accompanied by a slow respiratory rate.	Indicative of a failing medullary respiratory center.

From Boss BJ: Concepts of neurologic dysfunction. In McCance KL, Huether SE: *Pathophysiology: The Biologic Basis for Disease in Adults and Children*, 5th ed. St Louis, MO: Mosby; 2006.
CHF, Congestive heart failure; *CNS*, central nervous system.

prehospital providers during transport allows ED and trauma personnel to be adequately prepared to receive and resuscitate the patient.

Once the patient is admitted into the ED, initial stabilization of the brain-injured patient is directed toward maintenance of oxygenation, ventilation, restoration of circulating blood volume, and maintenance of systemic blood pressure to ensure adequate cerebral perfusion. Patients with a GCS score of less than 8 are considered to have a significant brain injury and require endotracheal intubation to protect their airway to minimize the risk for aspiration and to ensure adequate ventilation. Because hypoxia has a significant contribution to the morbidity and mortality of the brain-injured patient, oxygen saturations should be maintained above 90% and PaO_2 levels greater than 60 mm Hg.[15] Circulatory management is directed at maintaining systolic blood pressure at greater than 100 mm Hg to ensure adequate CPP.

Fluid resuscitation should be based on estimated prehospital and ongoing blood loss. Often, patients with severe TBI have concomitant multisystem injuries and hemorrhagic shock. During the past decade, fluid resuscitation has shifted toward more blood products and less crystalloid.[16,17] Early use of plasma, packed red blood cells (PRBCs) and platelets in a 1:1:1 ratio, should be considered in these patients.[16,17] Hypotonic solutions should be avoided in the brain-injured patient because they can potentiate cerebral edema. Although a lower hemoglobin and hematocrit level is often considered acceptable in the

TABLE 35.5 Diagnostic Evaluation for Head Injury.

Diagnostic Examination	Purpose	Comments
Cervical spine radiographs	Visualization of all seven cervical vertebrae to rule out injury	Tomograms or CT scans of the cervical spine may be necessary to rule out injury.
CT scan	Detect intracranial injuries—bleeds, hematomas, cerebral edema	Patients may require sedation to obtain adequate CT scan.

CT, Computed tomography.

trauma patient, in the brain-injured patient, it is essential to maximize oxygen-carrying capacity and oxygen delivery.[15,18]

Once the patient is initially stabilized, diagnostic studies to evaluate the type, location, and extent of the brain injury are completed. Table 35.5 presents some of the diagnostic studies with regard to purpose and advantages. Currently, the primary radiographic study for the evaluation of brain injury in the ED phase of care is the computed tomography (CT) scan. Skull radiographs are no longer indicated because CT scanning has become much more efficient, as well as sensitive, for both skull fractures and intracranial lesions. Helical CT with multidetector technology allows for extremely rapid imaging and much higher-quality images, along with the ability to do three dimensional reconstruction. Other studies include cerebral angiography and magnetic resonance imaging (MRI). Cerebral angiography is useful when there is suspicion of cerebrovascular abnormality (aneurysm). MRI is beneficial to further delineate the extent of diffuse axonal injury and brain-stem injury; however, this is less commonly indicated as part of the acute evaluation. All patients with significant brain injury and alterations in level of consciousness must also be evaluated for cervical spine injury through spine radiographs or CT imaging.

TBI patients with or without multisystem trauma are at risk for coagulopathy. The frequent use of anticoagulant or antiplatelet agents, direct thrombin inhibitors (e.g., dabigatran) and direct factor Xa inhibitors (e.g., rivaroxaban), particularly in older adults, puts patients at risk for significant intracranial bleeding.[17,19,20] Traditional diagnostic studies (prothrombin time and international normalized ratio [PT/INR]) as well as thromboelastography and platelet assays should be done early in the resuscitative phase of care. Rapid anticoagulation reversal is associated with improved outcomes.[14]

After providing initial stabilization of the patient, the emergency nurse should consider other interventions to promote optimal neurologic recovery. In the remainder of this section, the emphasis will be directed toward the patient with a severe brain injury incorporating the Guidelines for the Management of Severe Traumatic Brain Injury published by the Brain Trauma Foundation and the American Association of Neurological Surgeons Joint Section on Neurotrauma and Critical Care.[15] Management of patients with mild TBIs will be discussed in the section on specific injuries. In addition, an integral component of caring for brain-injured patients is inclusion of the family or significant other in the plan of care. Brain injuries can be overwhelming for the family; psychosocial support and education regarding the injury cannot be overemphasized and should begin in the ED phase of care.

Hyperventilation

Traditionally, hyperventilation was used as a means of reducing ICP by vasoconstriction of cerebral vessels, which decreased cerebral blood flow and ultimately cerebral volume. However, now cerebral blood flow studies illustrate there is a substantial reduction in cerebral blood flow within the first few hours of injury.[15] Numerous studies have now concluded that hyperventilation can actually be more detrimental to the severely injured brain by causing further ischemia.[15] Hyperventilation reduces cerebral blood flow without consistently decreasing ICP. In addition, autoregulation may be interrupted, further compromising blood flow to the injured area. In the acute resuscitation with evidence of significant neurologic deterioration or when ICP is refractory to other measures, hyperventilation may be used as a temporizing measure; however, the Pco_2 should be maintained at greater than or equal to 30 mm Hg.[15] Prophylactic hyperventilation should be avoided.

Hyperosmolar Therapy

Hyperosmolar therapy is aimed at reducing ICP through several mechanisms: plasma expansion and reduced blood viscosity, improved cerebral blood flow with a concomitant decrease in cerebral blood volume, and finally by creating an osmotic gradient that pulls water from cerebral tissue into the vascular space.[21] Mannitol has been widely used as a method to control ICP. Along with its osmotic properties, mannitol has neuroprotective properties, including free radical scavenging. Mannitol should be administered at doses of 0.25 to 1 g/kg. Mannitol should only be administered in bolus doses, and the Guidelines for Severe Traumatic Brain Injury do not support the use of continuous infusions.[15] More recently, hypertonic saline in various strengths (3%, 7.5%, and 10%) has been used and studied as an additional hyperosmolar agent for the management of increased ICP. The principal effect of hypertonic saline on ICP is through the osmotic gradient created in the brain and subsequent reduction of water content. Along with an osmotic change, hypertonic saline has been shown to alter hemodynamics, including increased MAP and vasoregulatory and immunologic effects.[22] Some reported advantages of hypertonic saline over mannitol include a longer duration of therapeutic modification and immunomodulation.[22] Currently, there are no recommended

TABLE 35.6 Comparison of Intracranial Pressure Monitors.

Type	Site	Advantages	Disadvantages
Subarachnoid bolt or screw	Subarachnoid space	Can be used with small or collapsed ventricles; does not penetrate brain parenchyma; low infection rates; low cost; ease and safety of insertion that can be performed quickly	Does not allow CSF drainage or withdrawal; becomes occluded; may have dampened waveform to give unreliable readings after a few days; blood or brain tissue may herniate into bolt; less accurate at higher ICP elevations
Intraventricular catheter (IVC) or ventriculostomy	Ventricles	Ventricular site provides more accuracy; CSF cultures can be collected; allows CSF to be withdrawn to control ICP; contrast materials can be injected for radiologic studies	Risk for hemorrhage due to invasiveness; increased risk for infection; risk for CSF leak at site; artifacts may cause dampening of recordings; more difficult to insert, especially for collapsed, small or displaced ventricles
Epidural or subdural sensor	Epidural or subdural space	Ease of insertion; least invasive; recommended in case of meningitis and CNS infection; less risk for infection; does not require recalibration	Slower response time; fragile; can become wedged against skull; affected by heat or febrile patient; expensive; diaphragm can rupture; less accurate; unable to sample or drain CSF
Intraparenchymal	Brain parenchyma	Quick insertion, accurate, reliable approach when ventricular access is not an option	Unable to drain CSF; may become clogged

CSF, Cerebrospinal fluid; *ICP*, intracranial pressure.
From Barker E: *Neuroscience Nursing: A Spectrum of Care*, 3rd ed. St Louis, MO: Mosby; 2008.

doses or concentrations of hypertonic saline in adults. Use of 3% saline as a continuous infusion is recommended in children with severe brain injury.[15]

Intracranial Pressure Monitoring and Intracranial Pressure and Cerebral Perfusion Pressure Management

Recommended indications for invasive management of intracranial hypertension include abnormal admission CT scan with GCS score ≤8. Indications in the presence of a normal CT scan are two or more of the following: age older than 40 years, abnormal motor posturing, or systolic blood pressure less than 90 mm Hg. ICP monitoring aids in the detection of intracranial mass lesions, limits unnecessary use of adjunctive therapies to control ICP, facilitates drainage of CSF (through ventricular catheters), and helps guide therapy and predict outcome.[15] The ultimate goal of ICP monitoring is to optimize ICP and cerebral perfusion. There are several types of monitoring systems available. Table 35.6 describes the most common types of monitoring methods along with advantages and disadvantages. Studies have shown that ventricular catheters with an external strain gauge are the most accurate means of monitoring ICP. Many facilities use a fiberoptic monitor and an external strain gauge device simultaneously to ensure accurate ICP monitoring (Fig. 35.7).

Management of elevated ICP includes measures to ensure adequate cerebral blood flow. Scientific evidence has clearly established that maintaining ICP below 20 mm Hg improves outcomes. Treatment should be initiated when ICP is greater than 20 mm Hg for more than 5 minutes. Sedation with benzodiazepines and opioid analgesia (first-line agents) assists in minimizing the noxious effects of endotracheal intubation and other stimuli, pain from other traumatic injuries, and the control of ICP.[14,15] Common benzodiazepines include midazolam (Versed) and lorazepam (Ativan). Midazolam (Versed) has the advantage of being short acting with small intermittent dosing. Propofol has become widely used due to its rapid onset and short duration of action, allowing for repeat neurologic assessments in the brain-injured patient who requires sedation. Propofol may have additional beneficial properties of maintaining or improving cerebral autoregulation.[15] High-dose propofol is not recommended due to the risk for propofol infusion syndrome and increased mortality.[15]

In conjunction with management of intracranial hypertension, cerebral perfusion must be maximized. Current recommendations are to maintain cerebral perfusion between 50 mm Hg and 70 mm Hg.[15] Augmented CPP has demonstrated enhanced cerebral blood flow and may help maintain the autoregulatory mechanisms in the injured brain. CPP management is directed at keeping patients normovolemic and avoiding excessive hypotonic fluids. Vasopressors are widely used to augment systemic blood pressure and MAP and thus improve CPP. No clinical studies have compared the various vasopressors; however, phenylephrine (Neo-Synephrine), norepinephrine (Levophed), and vasopressin are the most frequently used agents. Along with fluids and pressures, maintaining a hematocrit level at 30% to 35% with administration of blood products improves oxygen delivery. Maintaining CPP at higher than 70 mm Hg with fluids and pressors is associated with increased risk for acute respiratory distress syndrome (ARDS).[15] Paralytic agents can also be used in conjunction with sedatives and analgesics to reduce

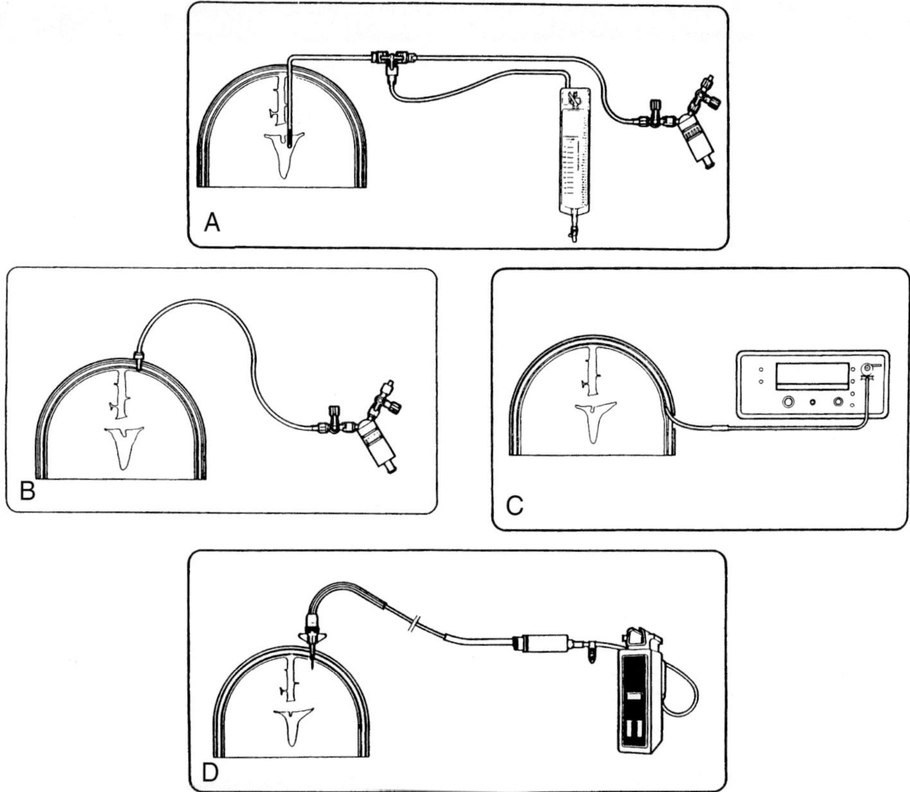

Fig. 35.7 (A) Ventricular pressure monitoring system. (B) Subarachnoid pressure monitoring system. (C) Epidural pressure monitoring system. (D) Intraparenchymal pressure monitoring system. (From Thelan LA, et al. *Critical Care Nursing: Diagnosis and Management.* 5th ed. St Louis, MO: Mosby; 1998.)

skeletal muscle activity, metabolic rate, and oxygen consumption. Short-acting paralytic agents are frequently part of institutional rapid sequence intubation protocols. Both short- and long-acting paralytics may be beneficial in the ED management of the brain-injured patient to facilitate diagnostic studies and help reduce the noxious stimuli associated with the acute resuscitation.

In the past decade, technology allowing for continuous monitoring of brain tissue oxygenation and temperature ($PbtO_2$) in conjunction with ICP has become available. The monitor is placed in the white matter of the brain 2 to 3 cm below the dura. Normal white-matter brain tissue oxygen is approximately 25 to 30 mm Hg.[15,23] Low values of $PbtO_2$ are associated with a poorer outcome. In conjunction with traditional ICP and CPP management, using the $PbtO_2$ levels to guide therapy may improve the outcomes of patients with severe brain injury. A full discussion of this technology is beyond the scope of this text.

Additional Treatment Modalities

Early seizure activity should be treated with appropriate anticonvulsants. Prophylactic use of anticonvulsants is not recommended for prevention of late postinjury seizure activity. Barbiturate therapy may be considered for patients with refractory intracranial hypertension. Hemodynamic stability should be confirmed before induction of barbiturate coma. No evidence exists to support routine use of glucocorticoids for a brain injury. Follow-up of patients who received steroids after a brain injury reveals no difference in outcomes. If cervical spine injury has been ruled out and the patient is hemodynamically stable, elevate the head of the bed to 30 to 45 degrees, which may decrease ICP. Maintaining the head in neutral alignment also facilitates venous drainage.

SPECIFIC INJURIES

Brain injuries can be classified by their mechanism (blunt or penetrating), by severity (mild, moderate, or severe), or by the type of injury (fracture, focal brain injury, diffuse brain injury). Patients with mild brain injuries have an initial GCS score of 14 to 15. Frequently, these patients are evaluated and treated in the ED and may be discharged home after a short period of observation. Moderate brain injuries are classified as those patients with initial GCS of 9 to13. Moderate brain injuries are associated with structural damage (e.g., contusions) and have a high potential for deterioration because of increasing cerebral edema and ICP. They require frequent neurologic assessments and a high index of suspicion for potential deterioration (Box 35.3). Severe brain injuries are found in patients who have an initial GCS score of 8 or less. These injuries are often associated with significant structural damage and have a high mortality rate, and patients who survive frequently have long-term or permanent cognitive and

BOX 35.3 Risk Stratification in Patients With Minor Head Trauma.

High Risk

Focal neurologic findings
Asymmetric pupils
Skull fracture on clinical examination
Multiple trauma
Serious, painful, distracting injuries
External signs of trauma above the clavicles
Initial Glasgow Coma Scale score of 14 or 15
Loss of consciousness
Posttraumatic confusion/anemia
Progressively worsening headache
Vomiting
Posttraumatic seizure
History of bleeding disorder/anticoagulation
Recent ingestion of intoxicants
Unreliable/unknown history of injury
Previous neurologic diagnosis
Previous epilepsy
Suspected child abuse
Age >60 y <2 y

Medium Risk

Initial Glasgow Coma Scale score of 15
Brief loss of consciousness
Posttraumatic amnesia
Vomiting
Headache
Intoxication

Low Risk

Currently asymptomatic
No other injuries
No focality on examination
Normal pupils
No change in consciousness
Intact orientation/memory
Initial Glasgow Coma Scale score of 15
Accurate history
Trivial mechanism Injury >24 h ago
No or mild headache
No vomiting
No preexisting high-risk factors

From Geegaard WG, Birov MH. Head. In: Marx J, Hoekberger R, Walls R: *Rosen's Emergency Medicine: Concepts and Clinical Practice*, 6th ed. St Louis, MO; Mosby: 2006.

physical disabilities. Aggressive management to ensure adequate oxygenation and prevention of hypotension is essential in these patients to prevent secondary brain injury.

Focal Injuries

Scalp Lacerations

The scalp protects the brain from injury by acting as a cushion to reduce energy transmission to underlying structures. Excessive force applied to the scalp often causes a laceration. The scalp has an extensive vascular supply with poor vasoconstrictive properties, causing lacerations to bleed profusely. Bleeding can be controlled with direct pressure to the affected area followed by wound repair and tetanus prophylaxis as indicated. Staples or clips may also be used for rapid closure.

Skull Fractures

Skull fractures occur when energy applied to the skull causes bony deformation. Clinical presentation of skull fractures is directly correlated to type of fracture, area involved, and damage to underlying structures. A linear skull fracture is nondisplaced and associated with minimal neurologic deficit (Fig. 35.8). Supportive care only is usually required for optimal neurologic recovery.

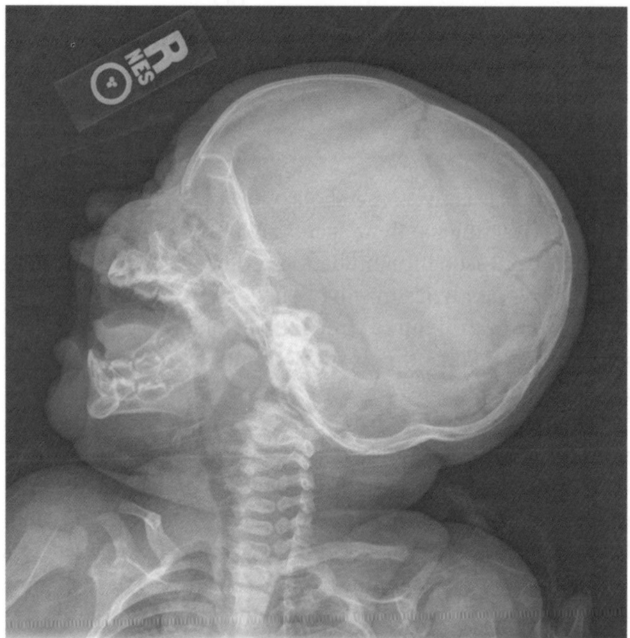

Fig. 35.8 Linear skull fractures in a 1-month-old child who was a victim of child abuse.

When energy displaces the outer table of bone below the inner table of the adjoining skull, a depressed skull fracture occurs (Fig. 35.9). Surgical elevation is required when depressed bone fragments become lodged in brain tissue. Open depressed skull fractures are surgically elevated and repaired as soon as possible because of increased risk for infection.

A basilar skull fracture develops when enough force is exerted on the base of the skull to cause deformity. The base of the skull includes any bony area where the skull ends and is not limited to the posterior aspect of the skull. A basilar skull fracture may be visualized on a radiograph; however, this is not always true. Approximately 25% of basilar skull fractures are not seen on radiographs; therefore diagnosis is usually made on the basis of clinical findings. Basilar skull fractures that overlay the middle meningeal artery may cause a subgaleal hematoma. Disruption of the middle meningeal artery is the cause of more than 75% of epidural hematomas. A basilar skull fracture may also cause intracerebral bleeding.

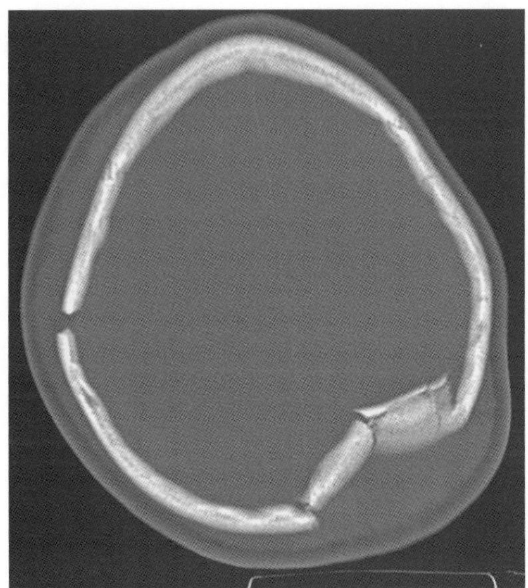

Fig. 35.9 Severely Depressed Skull Fracture in a Patient after a Fall.

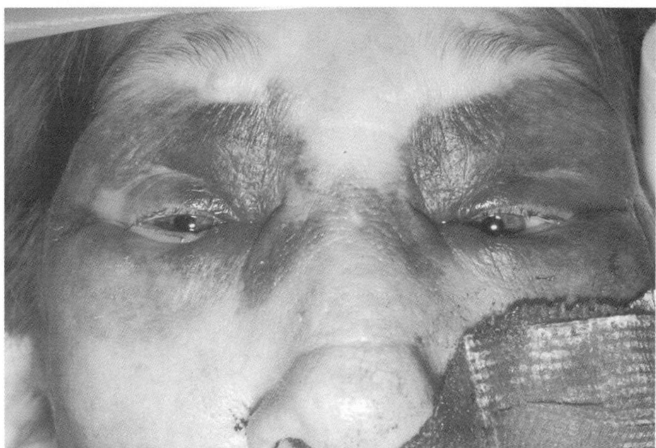

Fig. 35.10 Raccoon Eyes.

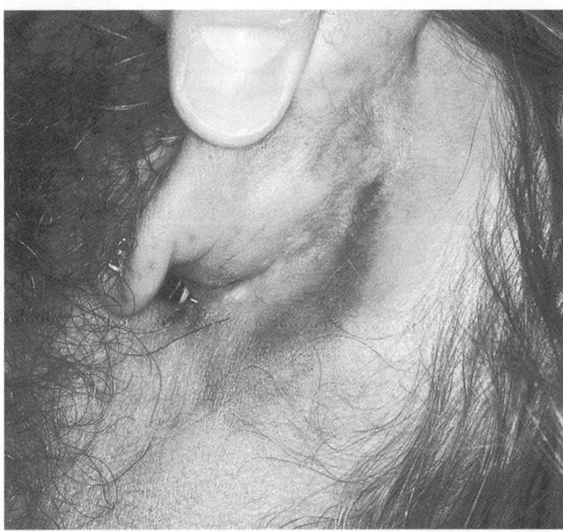

Fig. 35.11 Battle's Sign. (From London PS. *A Color Atlas of Diagnosis After Recent Injury*. London, England: Wolfe Medical Publications; 1990.)

Neurologic changes occurring with a basilar skull fracture range from mild changes in mentation to combativeness and severe agitation. Combative behavior is often considered a hallmark of a basilar skull fracture. Clinical manifestations of a basilar skull fracture include periorbital ecchymosis (raccoon eyes; Fig. 35.10) from intraorbital bleeding, Battle's sign (ecchymosis over the mastoid process; Fig. 35.11) 12 to 24 hours after initial injury, hemotympanum (blood behind the tympanic membrane caused by a fracture of the temporal bone), and CSF leak from the nose or ear caused by a temporal bone fracture. If the tympanic membrane is intact, fluid drains through the eustachian tube and appears as CSF rhinorrhea. However, absence of visible CSF does not eliminate the possibility of a basilar skull fracture. If a CSF leak is considered, test the fluid draining from the nose on filter paper. Formation of two distinct rings is called the "halo" or "ring" sign and indicates presence of CSF. Clear fluid should be tested for glucose, a normal finding in CSF.

Diagnostic interventions include CT scanning. Additional interventions focus on protecting the patient from injury, preventing infection, and using nasal drip pads as needed for rhinorrhea. Nasal packing is not recommended. Frequent neurologic assessment with ongoing reassessment is essential for early identification of deterioration in neurologic function.

Contusion

Cerebral contusion is a bruise on the surface of the brain, occurring from movement of the brain within the cranial vault (Figs. 35.12A–B). When an acceleration-deceleration injury occurs, two contusions may result, one at the initial site of impact (coup) and one on the opposite side of the impact (contrecoup). The clinical presentation varies with the size and location of the contusion. Commonly occurring symptoms include altered level of consciousness, nausea, vomiting, visual disturbances, weakness, and speech difficulty. Interventions focus on preservation of neurologic function, control of pain, and adequate hydration. Patients with cerebral contusions require admission and serial neurologic assessments. Contusions often increase in size over the first 12 to 24 hours, causing deterioration in neurologic status due to increased ICP. In patients with very large contusions at initial presentation, some neurosurgeons may elect to surgically evacuate the contusion and leave the bone flap off to allow for swelling of the brain.

Epidural Hematoma

Epidural hematoma is bleeding between the skull and dura mater (Fig. 35.13), usually resulting from a direct blow to the head. A torn middle meningeal artery with arterial bleeding leads to a rapidly forming hematoma, with associated morbidity and mortality of more than 50%. Approximately half of the patients with an epidural hematoma have no evidence of skull fracture. Signs and symptoms include a brief period of unconsciousness followed by a lucid period, then another loss of consciousness. This brief lucid period is considered a hallmark of an epidural hematoma; however, it does not occur in all patients. If alert, the patient with an epidural hematoma complains of severe headache and may exhibit hemiparesis

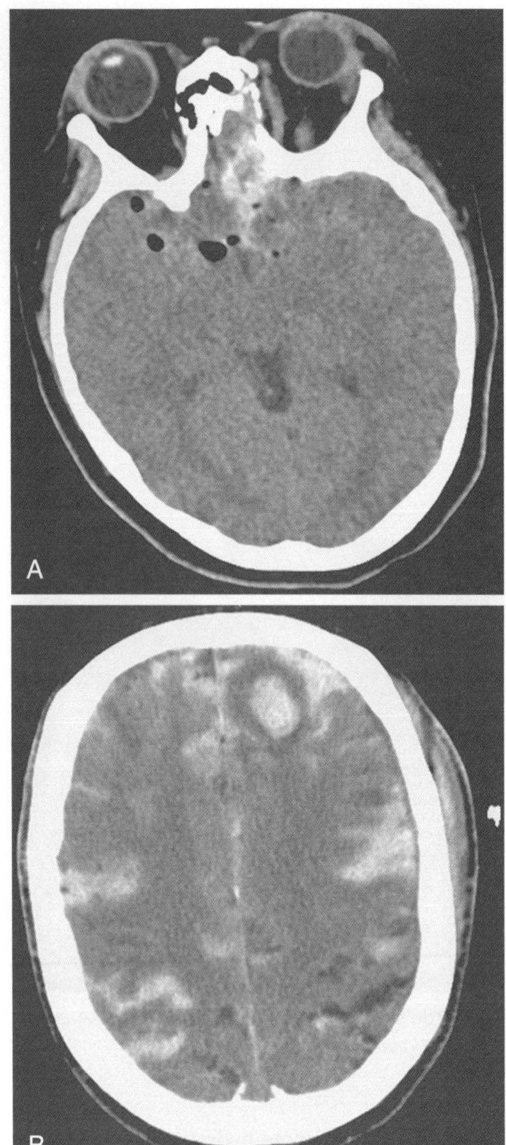

Fig. 35.12 (A) Right temporal contusion in a patient after motor vehicle collision. (B) Large left hemorrhagic contusion in a man who hit a deer. He also has a large amount of subarachnoid hemorrhage.

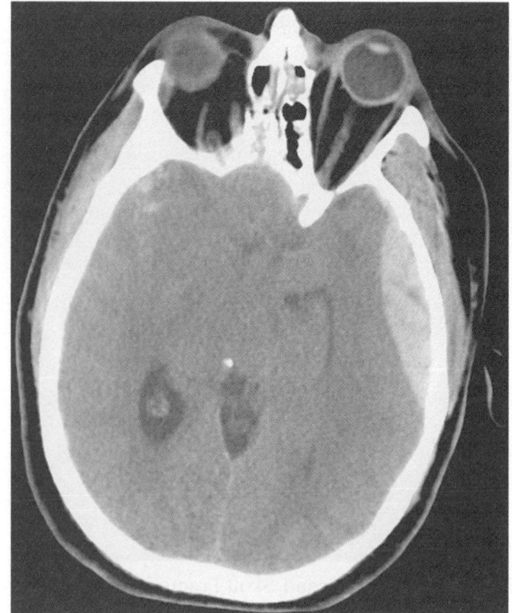

Fig. 35.13 Epidural Hematoma.

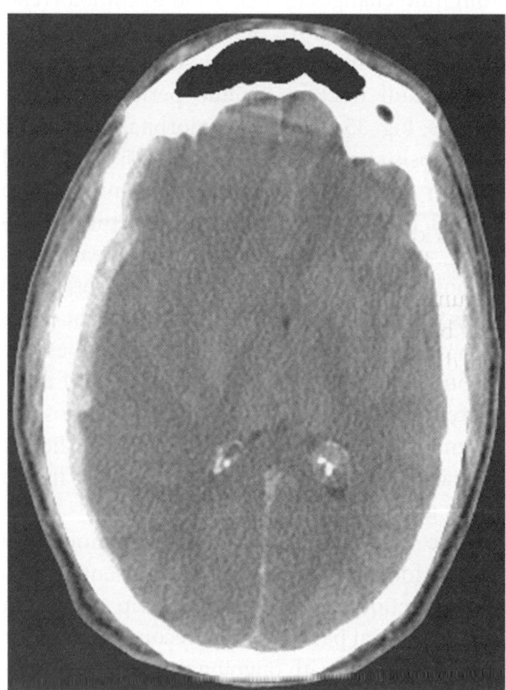

Fig. 35.14 Subdural Hematoma.

and a dilated pupil on the side of injury. Large epidural hematomas require emergent surgical evacuation; however, small hematomas may be managed conservatively with serial neurologic examinations and repeat diagnostic imaging, particularly in a patient who has minimal neurologic deficits on initial presentation to the ED.

Subdural Hematoma

Subdural hematomas occur more frequently than other intracranial injuries and have the highest morbidity and mortality of all hematomas. Bleeding into the subdural space between the dura mater and the arachnoid leads to subdural hematoma (Fig. 35.14). A subdural hematoma may be acute, subacute, or chronic. When acute, the hematoma usually results from dissipation of energy, rupturing bridging veins in the subdural space. Clinical features are loss of consciousness; hemiparesis; and fixed, dilated pupils. Surgical intervention within 4 hours of injury has the best potential for neurologic recovery.

Subacute subdural hematomas develop 48 hours to 2 weeks after injury. The clinical presentation is progressive decline in level of consciousness as the hematoma slowly expands. The brain compensates as a result of slow accumulation of blood over time, so a decline in neurologic function occurs gradually. After the subdural hematoma is drained, the patient improves quickly with little or no lasting neurologic deficit.

Chronic subdural hematomas, seen more frequently in older adults, progress slowly. Blood collects over weeks to months; by the time a person is examined, the causative mechanism may have been forgotten. Chronic subdural hematomas are initially tolerated by older adults because of brain atrophy associated with aging. As the brain decreases in size, the space within the cranial vault increases. A hematoma collects over time without obvious changes in neurologic status until its size is sufficient to produce a mass effect. Treatment of a chronic subdural consists of burr holes and a subdural drain. Patients often become more alert after the subdural is drained.

Other Focal Injuries

Intraventricular hemorrhage (Fig. 35.15) and intracerebral hematomas (Fig. 35.16) are types of focal injuries. Management depends on the size of the hematoma and source of bleeding. Surgical evacuation may be necessary in concert with medical management of increased ICP.

Diffuse Brain Injuries

Mild Traumatic Brain Injury (Concussion)

Previously called concussion, mild traumatic brain injury (mTBI) can occur as a result of a direct blow to the head or from an acceleration or deceleration injury in which the brain collides with the inside of the skull. Previously, mTBI was defined as a loss of consciousness without defined changes on initial diagnostic imaging. It is now known that there is some degree of neurochemical as well as axonal disruption associated with mTBI, and this is the basis for the persistence of symptoms known as postconcussive syndrome. In the past several years, there has been an increasing interest in measuring serum biomarkers in the diagnosis of mTBI.[24–26] An mTBI may be associated with cognitive, physical, emotional, and sleep disturbances (Table 35.7). Acutely, it is typically associated with a short period of impaired neurologic function, resolving spontaneously. Transient neurologic changes may include confusion, nausea, vomiting, temporary amnesia, headache, and possible brief loss of vision. In some cases, however, signs and symptoms may evolve over several hours.

Care for the patient with an mTBI includes observation, especially with prolonged loss of consciousness (greater than 2–3 minutes). With protracted nausea and vomiting, hospital admission may be considered to avoid dehydration. Nonnarcotic analgesia may be administered for headache. Narcotics affect the level of consciousness and interfere with ongoing patient assessment. Patients with an mTBI may be discharged with a responsible adult who will observe the patient overnight for possible complications, such as confusion, difficulty walking, altered level of consciousness, projectile vomiting, and unequal pupils. Discharge teaching includes instructions on how to assess neurologic status in the home and when to contact the primary care provider. Because mTBI is associated with some degree of structural changes, many experts in the field are now recommending periods of "brain rest" or cognitive rest along with physical rest after a brain injury.[27,28] Patients should not return to sports, work, school, or engage in high-risk activities until all symptoms of the brain injury are gone. A gradual return to work and school is recommended. With the increasing awareness and emphasis on mTBI in sports, in 2007 the CDC published several booklets for parents, athletes, coaches, and physicians on the diagnosis and management of mTBI.

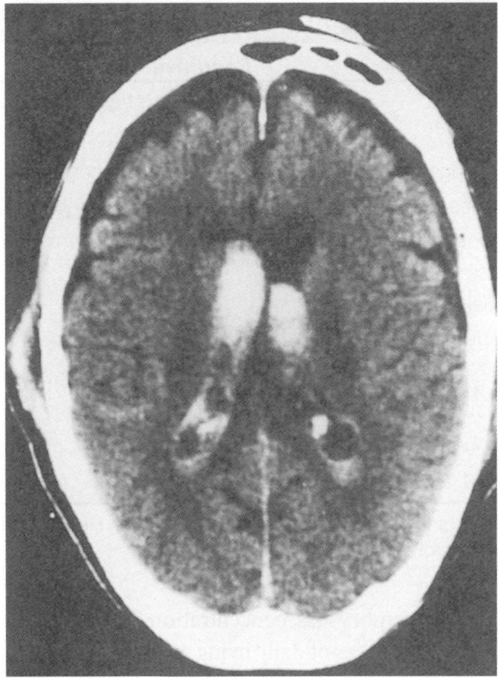

Fig. 35.15 Computed tomography scan of head showing intraventricular hemorrhage secondary to motor vehicle collision. (From Parrillo JE, Bone RC. *Critical Care Medicine: Principles of Diagnosis and Management.* St Louis, MO: Mosby; 1995.)

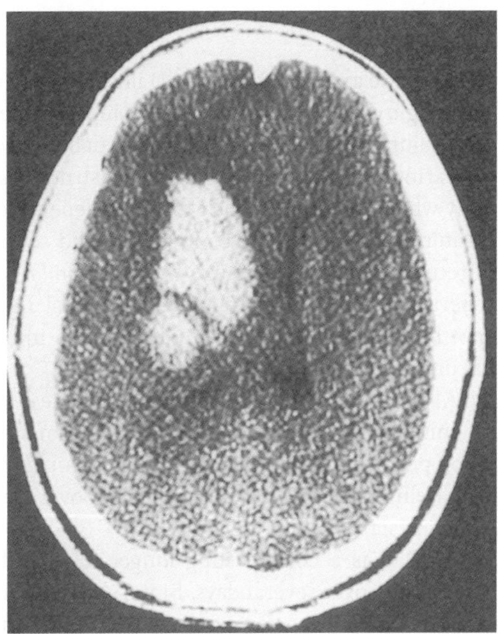

Fig. 35.16 Nonenhanced computed tomography scan showing large right hemispheric clot in 26-year-old male patient who sustained closed-head injury from a motor vehicle collision. Note mass effect on right lateral ventricle. (From Parrillo JE, Bone RC. *Critical Care Medicine: Principles of Diagnosis and Management.* St Louis, MO: Mosby; 1995.)

TABLE 35.7 Signs and Symptoms Associated With Mild Traumatic Brain Injury.

Physical	Cognitive	Emotional	Sleep
• Headache	• Feeling mentally "foggy"	• Irritability	• Drowsiness
• Nausea	• Feeling slowed down	• Sadness	• Sleeping less than usual
• Vomiting	• Difficulty concentrating	• More emotional	• Sleeping more than usual
• Balance problems	• Difficulty remembering	• Nervousness	• Trouble falling asleep
• Dizziness	• Forgetful of recent information or conversations		
• Visual problems			
• Fatigue	• Confused about recent events		
• Sensitivity to light	• Answers questions slowly		
• Sensitivity to noise	• Repeats questions		
• Numbness/Tingling			
• Dazed or stunned			

From Centers for Disease Control and Prevention. Heads up: fads for physicians about mild traumatic brain injury. Atlanta, GA: Centers for Disease Control and Prevention; 2007.

Headache, memory loss, concentration difficulties, and difficulty with the activities of daily living are characteristic of postconcussion syndrome. Clinical manifestations of this syndrome may persist for weeks or months and occasionally permanently after the patient's initial injury. Interventions include supportive treatment and recognition that this is a true physiologic consequence of what was perceived as a minor brain injury.

Diffuse Axonal Injury

The phrase "diffuse axonal injury" (DAI) illustrates the major pathophysiologic event associated with the most severe form of TBI. This injury is almost always the result of blunt trauma, causing shearing and disruption of neuronal structures, predominantly white matter. Prognosis for DAIs depends on the degree of injury (mild, moderate, or severe) and severity of damage from any secondary injury. The terms *mild, moderate,* and *severe* reflect the clinical presentation of DAI and should not be confused with the grading system indicating the actual underlying pathophysiology of DAI.

Mild DAI is characterized by loss of consciousness for 6 to 24 hours. Initially, the patient may exhibit abnormal flexion or extension posturing but improves rapidly within 24 hours. Return to baseline neurologic status may occur over days, but periods of amnesia may be present.

Moderate DAI is a coma lasting longer than 24 hours, possibly extending over several days. Brain-stem dysfunction (abnormal flexion or extension posturing) is evident almost immediately and may continue until the patient begins to awaken. Patients with moderate DAI usually recover but rarely return to full preinjury neurologic function.

Severe DAI is characterized by brain-stem impairment that does not resolve. Victims of severe DAI remain comatose for days to weeks. Autonomic dysfunction may also be present. Overall prognosis for severe DAI is extremely poor. Early CT scans may be unremarkable; however, serial examinations reveal areas of edema and microvascular hemorrhage (Fig. 35.17). Treatment for all degrees of DAI includes general supportive care, prevention of further brain injury, and support for the family.

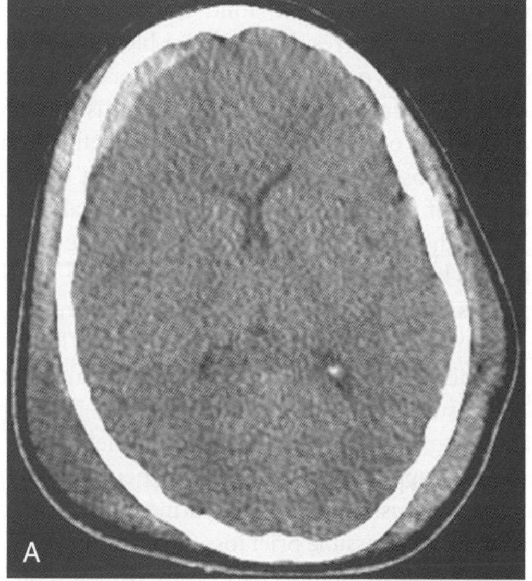

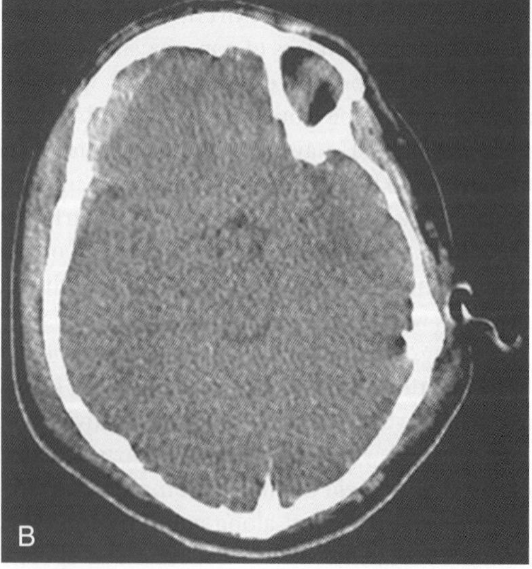

Fig. 35.17 (A) Severe diffuse axonal injury. (B) Severe diffuse axonal injury with right subdural hematoma.

SUMMARY

Despite advances in our understanding of the pathophysiologic changes of brain injury and advances in diagnostic technology and monitoring capabilities, TBI remains a major cause of death and long-term disability. Management of the severely injured patient in the acute resuscitation should focus on aggressive airway and ventilatory management to ensure adequate oxygenation along with restoring intravascular volume, preventing hypotension, and ensuring adequate cerebral perfusion. Maximizing outcomes for the severely brain-injured patient requires a collaborative multidisciplinary team from the time of injury throughout the continuum of care. Although there has been much research on managing severe brain injuries, the emergency nurse will care for many more patients with mild and moderate brain injuries. It is essential for emergency care providers to recognize the patient at risk for deterioration and ensure repeated neurologic assessments. Finally, there must be additional emphasis placed on patient education and the public's understanding of mTBI.

REFERENCES

1. Taylor CA, Bell JM, Breiding MJ, Xu L. Traumatic brain injury–related emergency department visits, hospitalizations, and deaths—United States, 2007 and 2013. *MMWR Surveill Summ.* 2017;66(No. SS-9):1–16. https://doi.org/10.15585/mmwr.ss6609a1.
2. Ling G. The need for VA leadership in advancing traumatic brain injury care. *Brain Inj.* 2017;319:1252–1255. https://doi.org/10.1080/02699052.2017.1359335.
3. Ma VY, Chan L, Carruthers KJ. The incidence, prevalence, costs and impact on disability of common conditions requiring rehabilitation in the US: stroke, spinal cord injury, traumatic brain injury, multiple sclerosis, osteoarthritis, rheumatoid arthritis, limb loss, and back pain. *Arch Phys Med Rehabil.* 2014;95(5):986–995.e1. https://doi.org/10.1016/j.apmr.2013.10.032.
4. The CDC, NIH, DoD, and VA Leadership Panel. *Report to Congress on Traumatic Brain Injury in the United States. Understanding the Public Health Problem among Current and Former Military Personnel. Centers for Disease Control and Prevention (CDC), the National Institutes of Health (NIH).* VA: the Department of Defense (DoD), and the Department of Veterans Affairs; 2013. https://www.cdc.gov/traumaticbraininjury/pubs/congress_military.html. Accessed May 27, 2019.
5. Coronado V, Haileyesus T, Cheng T, et al. Trends in sports- and recreation-related traumatic brain injuries treated in US emergency departments: the National Electronic Injury Surveillance System-All Injury Program (NEISS-AIP) 2001-2012. *J Head Trauma Rehabil.* n.d.;30(3):185-197.
6. Butterfield RJ. Structure and function of the neurologic system. In: McCance KL, Huether SE, eds. *Pathophysiology: The Biologic Basis for Disease in Adults and Children.* 8th ed. St Louis, MO: Mosby; 2018.
7. Boss BJ, Huether SE. Concepts of neurologic dysfunction. In: McCance KL, Huether SE, eds. *Pathophysiology: The Biologic Basis for Disease in Adults and Children.* 8th ed. St Louis, MO: Mosby; 2018.
8. Hickey JV, Kanusky JT. Overview of neuroanatomy and neurophysiology. In: Hickey JV, ed. *The Clinical Practice of Neurological and Neurosurgical Nursing.* 7th ed. Philadelphia, PA: Lippincott Williams & Wilkins; 2014.
9. Teasdale G, Jennett B. Assessment of coma and impaired consciousness: a practical scale. *Lancet.* 1974;2(7872):81.
10. Burke DM. Neurologic clinical assessment and diagnostic procedures. In: Urden LD, Stacy KM, Lough ME, eds. *Critical Care Nursing Diagnosis and Management.* 8th ed. Maryland Heights, MO: Elsevier; 2018.
11. Brain Trauma Foundation. Guidelines for the prehospital management of TBI. *Prehosp Emerg Care.* 2007;12(1).
12. Khormi YH, Gosadi I, Campbell S, Senthilselvan A, O'Kelly C, Zygun D. Adherence to Brain Trauma Foundation guidelines for management of traumatic brain injury patients: study protocol for a systematic review and meta-analysis. *Syst Rev.* 2015;4(1):149.
13. Spaite DW, Chengcheng H, Bobrow BJ, et al. The effect of combined out-of-hospital hypotension and hypoxia on mortality in major traumatic brain injury. *Ann Emerg Med.* 2017;69(1):62–72.
14. American College of Surgeons Committee on Trauma. *ACS TQIP Best Practice Guidelines in the Management of Traumatic Brain Injury*; 2015. https://www.facs.org/~/media/files/quality%20programs/trauma/tqip/traumatic%20brain%20injury%20guidelines.ashx. Accessed May 27, 2019.
15. Carney N, Totten AM, O'Reilly C, et al. Guidelines for the management of severe traumatic brain injury, fourth edition. *Neurosurgery.* 2017;80(1):6–15.
16. Holcomb JB, Tilley BC, Baraniuk S, et al. Transfusion of plasma, platelets and red blood cells in a 1:1:1 vs a 1:1:2 ratio and mortality in patients with severe trauma: the PROPPR randomized clinical trial. *JAMA.* 2015;313(5):471–482.
17. Rossaint R, Bouillon B, Cerny V, et al. The European guideline on management of major bleeding and coagulopathy following trauma: fourth. *Crit Care.* 2016;20:100.
18. American College of Surgeons Committee on Trauma. *ACS TQIP Massive Transfusion In Trauma Guidelines*; 2013. https://www.facs.org/~/media/files/quality%20programs/trauma/tqip/massive%20transfusion%20in%20trauma%20guildelines.ashx. Accessed May 27, 2019.
19. Nishijima D, Gaona S, Waechter T, et al. The incidence of traumatic intracranial hemorrhage in head-injured older adults transported by EMS with and without anticoagulant or antiplatelet use. *J Neurotrauma.* 2017. https://doi.org/10.1089/neu.2017.5232. Accessed May 27, 2019.
20. Zeeshan M, Jehan R, O'Keef T, et al. The novel oral anticoagulants (NOACs) have worse outcomes compared with warfarin in patients with intracranial hemorrhage after TBI. *J Trauma Acute Care Surg.* 2018;85(5):915–920.
21. Bales JW, Bonow RH, Ellenbogen RG. Closed head injury. In: Ellenbogen RG, Sekhar LN, Kitchen ND, eds. *Principles of Neurological Surgery.* 4th ed. Philadelphia, PA: Elsevier; 2018.
22. Aisiku IP, Silvestri DM, Roberson C. Critical care management of traumatic brain injury. In: Winn HR, ed. *Youmans and Winn Neurological Surgery.* 7th ed. Philadelphia, PA: Elsevier; 2017.

23. Rosenthal G, LeRoux PD. Physiologic monitoring for traumatic brain injury. In: Winn HR, ed. *Youmans and Winn Neurological Surgery*. 7th ed. Philadelphia, PA: Elsevier; 2017.
24. Peacock WF, Van Meter TE, Mirshahi N, et al. Derivation of a three biomarker panel to improve diagnosis in patients with mild traumatic brain injury. *Front Neurol.* 2017;8:641.
25. McCrea M, Meier T, Huber D, et al. Role of advanced neuroimaging, fluid biomarkers and genetic testing in the assessment of sport-related concussion: a systematic review. *Br J Sports Med.* 2017;51(12):919–929.
26. Lewis LM, Schloemann DT, Papa L, et al. Utility of serum biomarkers in the diagnosis and stratification of mild traumatic brain injury. *Acad Emerg Med.* 2017;24(6):710–720.
27. McCrory P, Meeuwisse W, Dvorak J, et al. Consensus statement on concussion in sport-the 5th international conference on concussion in sport held in Berlin, October 2016. *Br J Sports Med.* 2017;51(11):838–847. https://doi.org/10.1136/bjsports-2017-097699.
28. Brown AM, Twomey DM, Wong Shee A. Evaluating mild traumatic brain injury management at a regional emergency department. *Inj Prev.* 2018. https://doi.org/10.1136/injuryprev-2018-042865. Published online June 4. Accessed May 27, 2019.

36

Maxillofacial Trauma

Chris M. Gisness

Maxillofacial trauma, involving injury of the facial bones, neurovascular structures, skin, subcutaneous tissues, muscles, and glands, is a common presenting injury to the emergency department (ED). Patients with maxillofacial injuries require a thorough evaluation because damage to the anatomic structures can cause facial distortion. These injuries also have a close relationship to the head and neck, setting the stage for serious complications.

Currently, there are no evidence-based guidelines for the assessment and treatment of patients who sustain maxillofacial trauma; therefore Advanced Trauma Life Support guidelines are followed as the gold standard for assessment and treatment.[1] Maxillofacial trauma can be difficult to evaluate. Maintaining a patent airway is the most pressing of all goals, along with stabilization of the cervical spine. Cervical spine injury should be considered in all patients with facial trauma. The spine should be immobilized until a thorough evaluation of the spine is completed and the head and neck are cleared.[2] There can be significant blood loss from facial injuries due to vascularity of the face; therefore hemorrhage control is critical. Universal precautions should be followed, as with all patients, due to the vascularity of the face and head and the potential for hemorrhage. Facial trauma is frequently associated with other trauma occurring to the chest, abdomen, pelvis, and extremities. Therefore concomitant injuries must always be considered in patients with maxillofacial trauma. Once the life-threatening injuries are assessed and managed and the patient is stabilized, the management of facial trauma is then to restore occlusion, prevent loss of function and vision, and restore appearance.[1]

This chapter will address the common causes of maxillofacial trauma; anatomy and pathophysiology as it relates to the maxillofacial structures; assessment, including physical examination and diagnostic testing; and management of injuries.

COMMON CAUSES OF MAXILLOFACIAL TRAUMA

Motor vehicle crashes (MVCs), assault and personal violence, and falls are the major reasons for patients to present to the ED with maxillofacial trauma. Lack of and incorrect use of seat belts and helmets can cause injury to the maxillofacial area. The use of air bags and seat belt restraints in vehicles can save lives, but not without some risk. Maxillofacial injuries involving abrasions and chemical burns to the eye have occurred with the deployment of air bags. To avoid issues with air bags, children should be placed in the appropriate device and place in a vehicle, as recommended by the Centers for Disease Control and Prevention.

Domestic violence is responsible for some of the increase in the number of personal assaults. The use of handguns is also responsible for facial injuries. For the patient with a bullet trajectory above the mandible, intracranial injury should also be considered.

Facial injuries from falls are common among children and older adults. In children, skull and facial bone flexibility absorb energy associated with deceleration injuries, such as from MVCs and falls. Maxillofacial trauma in the pediatric patient is identified as "child's play," followed by sports injuries, traffic injuries, and violence. These injuries include bicycle injuries and falls, and as the child reaches adolescence, the injuries are caused by violence. For patients between the ages of 15 and 50 years, the leading cause of facial trauma is from MVCs, followed by sports injuries, violence, and falls.[3]

The incidence of facial trauma in the geriatric patient has increased in part due to the increased life span and active lifestyles. Falls and MVCs are two of the most common reasons that older adults sustain facial trauma.

ANATOMY AND PHYSIOLOGY

The principal facial bones include the frontal, nasal, maxilla, zygoma, and mandible. The frontal bone articulates with the frontal process of the maxilla and nasal bone and laterally with the zygoma. The orbital complex is composed of the frontal bone superiorly, the zygoma laterally, the maxilla inferiorly, and the processes of the maxilla and frontal bone medially. Paired nasal bones form the bridge of the nose and articulate with the frontal bone above and the maxilla below. The nasal cavity is divided by the nasal septum. The lateral wall of the septum has ridges, or conchae, which affect phonation. The nasal bone is largely supported by cartilage anteriorly and inferiorly and bone posteriorly and superiorly.

The midface, or maxilla, forms the upper jaw, anterior hard palate, part of the lateral wall of the nasal cavity, and part of the orbital floor. Below the orbit, the maxilla is perforated by the infraorbital foremen to allow passage of the infraorbital nerve and artery. Projecting downward, the alveolar process joins the opposite side to form the alveolar arch, which houses the upper teeth. Sinus cavities in the midface decrease weight and act as resonating chambers. Fractures to the maxilla usually result from high-energy blunt force.

The zygoma forms the cheek and the lateral wall and floor of the orbital cavity. Zygomatic fractures usually occur from motor vehicle injuries. The zygoma assists in maintaining the facial width and prominence of the cheek. The orbit comprises seven bones, which are the frontal, zygoma, maxilla, lacrimal, ethmoid, sphenoid, and palatine. Articulations with the maxilla, frontal bones, and zygomatic process of the temporal bone form the zygomatic arch.

The mandible is a horizontal horseshoe body with two rami, anterior coronoid processes, and posterior condyloid processes.[4] The mandibular notch lies medial to the zygomatic arch and separates the two processes. The mandible articulates with the temporal bone to form the temporomandibular joint (TMJ), whereas the upper body of the mandible, called the alveolar part, contains the lower teeth. The mandible is divided into the coronoid, condyle, ramus, angle, body, and symphysis (Fig. 36.1).

The facial nerve (cranial nerve VII) provides sensory and motor innervation to the side of the face. The cranial nerve originates in the brain stem, then divides into five branches to innervate the scalp, forehead, eyelids, facial muscles for expression, cheeks, and jaw. Specific functions for each nerve branch are listed in Table 36.1. Other cranial nerves possibly affected by facial trauma are the oculomotor, trochlear, and trigeminal. The function and testing for each cranial nerve are described in Table 36.2.

The parotid gland is located adjacent to the anterior ear and drains into the oral cavity through the parotid duct. These structures are located adjacent to branches of the facial nerve on top of the masseter muscle. Lacerations near this area can be concerning if they breach the parotid duct near the facial nerves. These types of injuries must be fully evaluated when there are injuries to the parotid duct and facial nerve (Fig. 36.2).

PATIENT ASSESSMENT

Assessment and management of a patient with maxillofacial trauma, regardless of severity, does not take priority over recognition and treatment of life-threatening injuries. It is essential to perform a rapid, thorough assessment using a systematic approach with emphasis on the patient's airway, breathing, circulation (ABCs), and cervical spine stabilization. Once the primary and secondary assessment have been completed, a focused assessment should be performed.

Airway and Breathing

The priority with facial injuries is to establish and maintain a clear and secure airway. Damaged facial structures can cause airway obstruction. If the mandible is displaced or fractured, the tongue loses anatomic support and may occlude the airway. Also, a displaced mandible fracture can cause a slow bleed, and bleeding can obstruct the airway. Foreign objects (e.g., dentures or avulsed teeth) can obstruct the airway, whereas fractures of the nasoorbital complex may compromise the airway due to hemorrhage. Gunshot wounds to the face can cause significant swelling and hematoma formation, which can obstruct the airway. When airway compromise is recognized, the chin lift–head tilt method should be used to open the airway unless cervical spine injury is suspected, in which case the jaw-thrust maneuver should be performed. Altered mental status from alcohol, drugs, or head injury can diminish the patient's gag reflex and leave the airway unprotected. Thus frequent reassessment of the airway is necessary. Suctioning of the oropharynx or nasopharynx is required when bleeding or excessive secretions are present. A tonsil-tip suction catheter can be provided to an alert patient to self-suction when secretions are present. If cervical spine injury is not a consideration or injury to the cervical spine has been ruled out, allow the patient to sit upright or elevate the head of the bed to promote drainage and decrease facial swelling.

Excessive bleeding and swelling of the mouth and facial structures, coupled with the inability to clear the airway, requires aggressive airway control. It is also essential to ascertain whether the patient is receiving anticoagulants or antiplatelets or has a past medical history of hemophilia. Supplemental oxygen and assisted ventilations can be provided by using a bag-mask device; however, in some patients, swelling and facial fractures can make use of a bag-mask device difficult. An oropharyngeal airway can be used in an unconscious patient who has obstruction from the tongue. A nasopharyngeal airway can be used in a conscious patient with no nasal or midface fractures. Noisy breathing suggests an obstructed airway. A patient who presents with fluctuating levels of consciousness may appear to have an intact airway, but alcohol or drugs may cause the patient to decompensate or experience inadequate ventilation. Also, attempt to find out when the patient had his or her last meal. A full stomach may lead to vomiting, with possible pulmonary aspiration and loss of a patent airway.[1]

Orotracheal intubation is preferred in the patient with facial injuries. Blind nasotracheal intubation should be avoided in facial fractures because this may cause further injury. Cribriform plate fractures increase the risk for cerebral penetration by an endotracheal tube. Gastric tubes placed after intubation should be placed through the orogastric method to avoid introduction into the brain. Significant mandible and midface fractures most often lead to airway edema and obstruction. A definitive airway is recommended.[3] Rapid-sequence induction facilitates intubation and has the added benefit of protecting the patient from increased intracranial pressure.[5] If rapid-sequence induction is used, equipment to perform a surgical airway opening must be available should cricothyrotomy or tracheostomy be needed. Pulse oximetry or capnography is an essential adjunct for monitoring the airway patency and breathing.

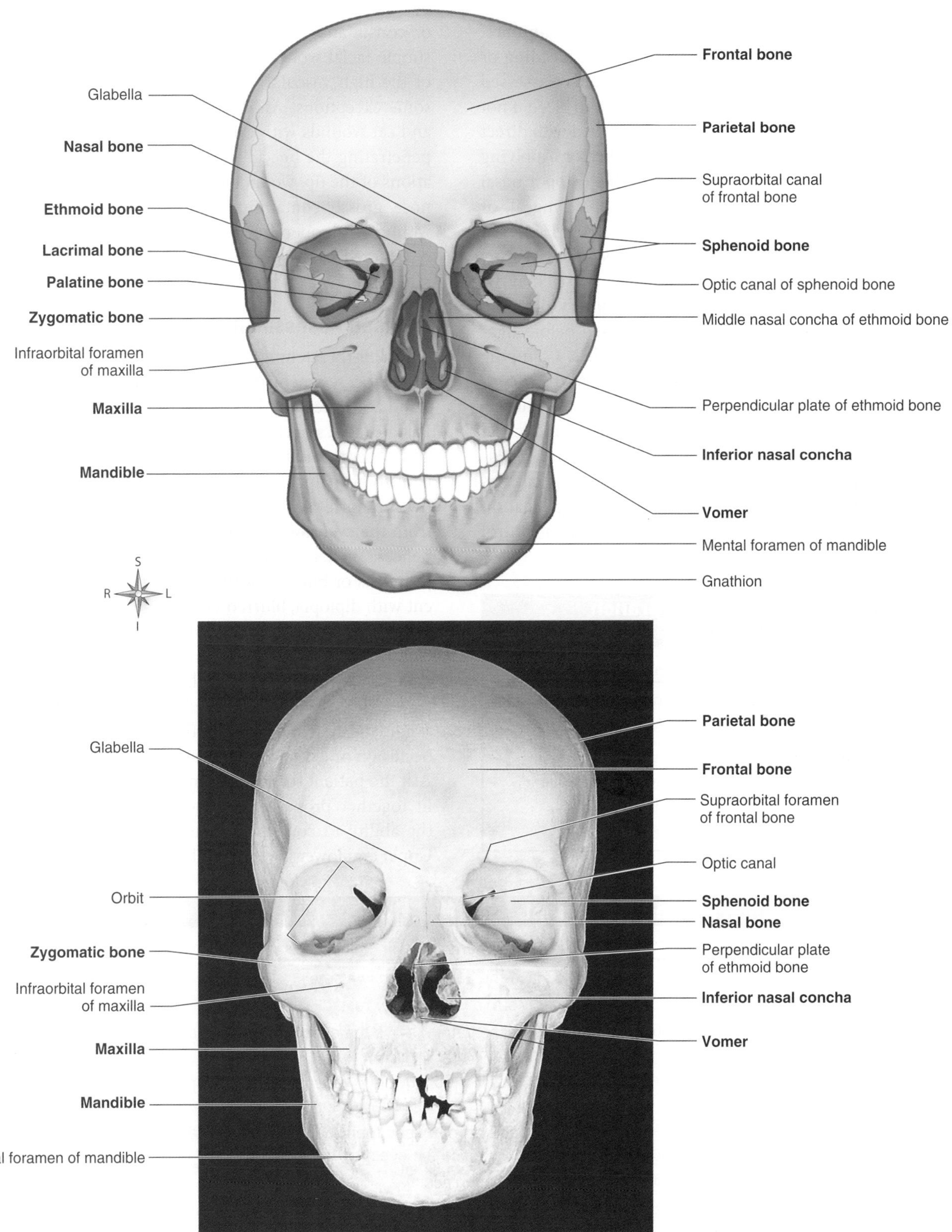

Fig. 36.1 Facial Bones. (From Patton KT. *Anatomy & Physiology*, 7th ed. St Louis, MO: Elsevier; 2010.)

Circulation

After a patent airway is established, the next priority is hemorrhage control. Bleeding is a frequent occurrence and can lead to compromise of the patient if it is not quickly controlled. The face is highly vascularized, and adult patients with maxillofacial injury can develop shock from profuse bleeding or from significant slow bleeding. The patient should be assessed for scalp lacerations because they may continue to bleed if not recognized early. Facial bleeding can be controlled with direct pressure, such as with a large cotton-tip applicator. Applying an ice pack and direct nasal pressure will help stop a nasal bleed. Compression through intranasal, nasopharyngeal, or oropharyngeal packing may also control bleeding. However, packing is a temporizing method. If compression fails, suturing, stapling, or a figure-eight ligation of a vessel may be required but must be done within 24 hours of injury. Bleeding vessels on the face should be carefully assessed before ligation to prevent damage to facial nerve branches. Clamping any facial wound is not recommended because of the potential for facial nerve damage or paralysis. Severe facial trauma, such as Le Fort II or III fractures, requires manual reduction of the face to control bleeding. With a closed fracture, bleeding from lacerated arteries and veins into the sinus cavities can cause significant posterior pharyngeal bleeding. Ligation of arteries and veins or embolization is necessary to control blood loss.

TABLE 36.1 Facial Nerve Branch Functions.

Branch	Function
Buccal	Wrinkle nose
Cervical	Wrinkle skin of neck
Mandibular	Purse and depress lips
Temporal	Raise eyebrows, wrinkle forehead
Zygomatic	Close eyelids

A facial wound with gross contamination from an embedded foreign body, such as gravel or glass, should be cleaned and irrigated with sterile saline solution as soon as possible.[5] Further debridement may be done by the ED provider or consultant.[2,5] Antibiotics are usually not indicated for a simple facial wound, which rarely become infected because of the high vascularization of the face. There are, however, some exceptions. Antibiotics may be prescribed for human and cat wounds with evidence of devascularization, wounds penetrating the buccal mucosa, through-and-through lacerations of the lip, wounds involving the cartilage of the ear or nose, grossly contaminated wounds requiring suturing, and wounds with open fractures.[6] Tetanus prophylaxis should be considered, and if the injury was caused by an animal bite, rabies prophylaxis may be indicated.

Focused Assessment

Once life-threatening conditions have been addressed, a more focused assessment of the face should be completed. First, stand at the head of the bed and observe for facial symmetry. Palpate facial structures before edema and hematomas worsen and obscure the bony landmarks. Use both hands simultaneously to palpate for step-off irregularities and crepitus of the supraorbital ridges and zygoma. Inspect the face, starting from the eyebrows, to compare the height of the malar eminences. Then, look up from below the chin. Make note for any proptosis or bulging of the eyes. Orbital fractures may present with diplopia, blurred vision, and periorbital ecchymosis. Suspect a blowout fracture with blunt trauma to the midface. Gently palpate nasal bones and look intranasally for a septal hematoma. Inspect intranasally for any potential cerebrospinal fluid (CSF) leaks. Palpate laterally for depressions in the zygomatic arch and visualize the mouth for gross dental malocclusion or dental avulsion, subluxations, or fractured teeth. Ask the patient to close the mouth and ascertain if the teeth fit together properly, as they did before the injury. Assess the ability to completely open the jaw. Assess for trismus. Upper and lower jaws should be carefully palpated intraorally

TABLE 36.2 Cranial Nerve Assessment.

Cranial Nerve(s)	Name	Assessment
I	Olfactory	Have the patient identify a smell.
II	Optic	Perform a visual acuity test.
III, IV, VI	Oculomotor, Trochlear, Abducens	Have the patient move the eyes through the various visual fields and test for pupil reactivity.
V	Trigeminal	Touch a wisp of cotton to various areas of the patient's face, looking for areas of altered sensation.
VII	Facial	Check symmetry and mobility of the face by having the patient frown, close the eyes, lift the eyebrows, and puff the cheeks.
VIII	Vestibulocochlear	Test hearing acuity.
IX, X	Glossopharyngeal	Listen to the sound of the patient's voice; it should be smooth. Assess for the presence of both the gag and swallowing reflexes.
XI	Accessory	Have the patient rotate the head and shrug the shoulders against resistance.
XII	Hypoglossal	Ask the patient to stick out his or her tongue or say the sounds of the letters L, T, and D.

From Sheehy S, Hammond B, Zimmermann P. *Sheehy's Manual of Emergency Care.* 7th ed. St. Louis: Mosby; 2013:442.
Maxillofacial Trauma

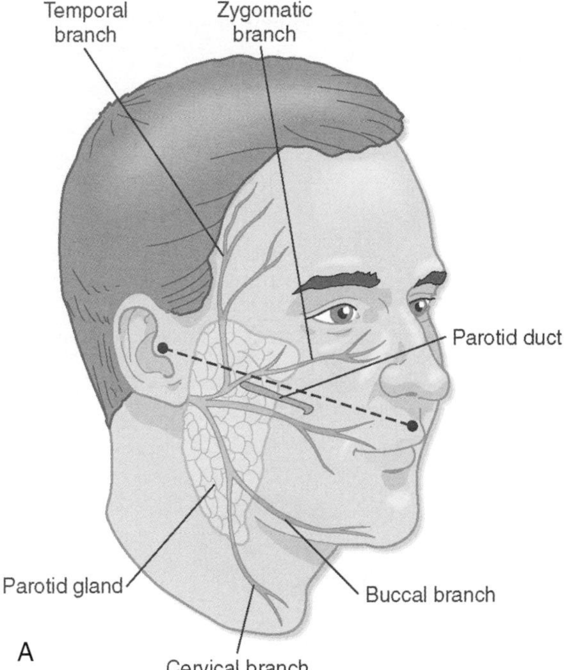

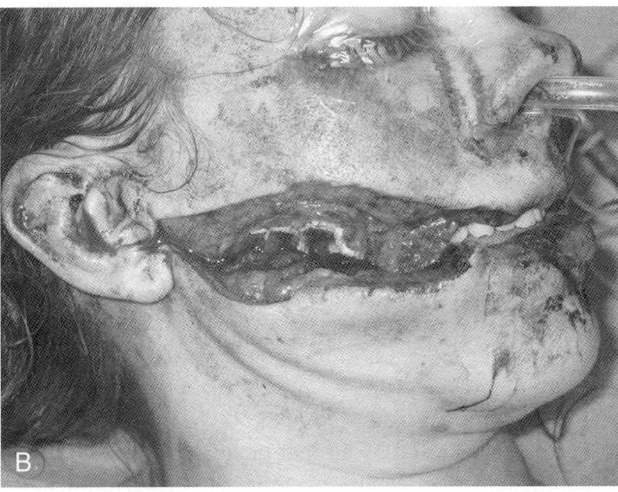

Fig. 36.2 (A) A line drawn from the tragus of the ear to the middle of the upper lip approximates the course of the parotid duct. Injury to the parotid gland duct is usually located at or distal to the anterior border of the masseter muscle along this line. (B) Facial laceration with high risk of injury to parotid gland and duct. (A, From Adams J, Barton E, Collings J, et al. *Emergency Medicine*. St Louis, MO: Saunders; 2008. B, From Fonesca RJ, Walker RV, Barber HD, et al. *Oral & Maxillofacial Trauma*. 4th ed. St Louis, MO: Elsevier Saunders; 2013.)

(wearing gloves). Check the patient's midface stability by attempting to move the upper teeth and hard palate. If they are unstable, a more thorough examination will be needed to assess for Le Fort fractures. During the intraoral examination, feel for signs of tenderness, look for mobility and lacerations, and assess the sensation of the upper and lower lip.[1] There may be some associated epistaxis. Dysphonia of the oropharynx may suggest a hematoma or fracture and indicate the risk for a potential airway problem.

Evaluate the facial nerve and its branches (Table 36.1). Loss of sensation over the upper lip, lateral nose, and anterior maxilla may indicate injury to the inferior alveolar nerve and a possible orbital floor fracture. Numbness over the upper lip occurs with fracture in the maxilla and injury to the infraorbital nerve. Evaluate extraocular movement to assess for entrapment of the inferior rectus muscle. Assessment of the eye should be done early and serially to look for subtle changes. The examination should be done before increasing lid edema will make it more difficult. Evaluate the supraorbital ridge and the infraorbital and inferior alveolar and mental nerves. Examine the eyes for any lacerations, hyphemia, subconjunctival hemorrhage, or infraorbital emphysema.

An eye examination is necessary for the complete assessment of a facial trauma to look for loss of vision or visual acuity. Visual acuity is determined with the use of the Snellen chart, handheld-card, or standard eye chart. If the patient is unable to count fingers, check for light perception and document findings before testing is done.[1] Assess for pupillary reactivity, symmetry, and extraocular movement and accommodation. Limited range of motion can be due to muscle entrapment associated with blowout fractures. Posttraumatic mydriasis may occur with direct blows to the eye. Check for the relevant afferent pupillary defect (RAPD). Ensure pupils are on the same facial plane. A teardrop-shaped pupil suggests a ruptured globe. Assess the position of the globe because exophthalmos or proptosis may indicate hemorrhage or an orbital fracture. Palpate the orbital rims for any tenderness or step-offs. Hyphema and subconjunctival injury can indicate a serious eye injury.

It is important to remember that intraocular injuries are a priority. A slit lamp examination should be used to assess for foreign bodies and to check the anterior chamber for red blood cells, which indicates a hyphema. A funduscopic examination is needed to assess the posterior chamber and retina for signs of retinal and vitreous detachment or hemorrhage. Fluorescein dye is used to check for any epithelial disruption from a foreign body and it is used for the Seidel test, which may indicate a globe rupture or vitreous leak. In some patients with periorbital injuries, widening of the distance between the medial canthus (referred to as telecanthus) may indicate a nasoorbital-ethmoid fracture. Raccoon eyes (i.e., periorbital ecchymosis) suggests a basilar skull fracture, Le Fort fracture, or nasoorbital-ethmoid fracture. Nasal or ear drainage may indicate a CSF leak, which can occur with fractures of the cribriform plate or basilar skull fracture. Appearance of a bull's-eye or halo when bloody or serous drainage from the nose or ear is placed on a white paper or sheet may indicate the presence of CSF. However, this test has a low sensitivity and other tests can be done, such as a β-2-transferrin electrophoretic examination.[3]

It is important to assess the stability of the maxilla and mandible, which is essential to maintain an open airway. To check for facial stability, grasp the teeth and hard palate and gently push horizontally and vertically to feel for movement or instability of the midface.[1,2] To assess the maxilla, grasp the alveolar ridge between the thumb and index finger with the other hand placed on the patient's forehead. Gently move the maxilla anteriorly and posteriorly to assess for movement.

It should not move if the maxilla is stable.[2] Malocclusion is evaluated by asking the patient to close his or her mouth and check to see if the teeth come together normally or if the bite is misaligned. Alternatively, have the patient bite down on a tongue blade as the examiner twists the blade in the patient's mouth, in an attempt to move it. If the patient is unable to bite down firmly, a fracture may be present in the mandible.

Soft-tissue injuries of the face can also be problematic. Lacerations near the parotid gland should raise suspicion for injury to the Stensen's duct. This can be assessed by having the patient open the mouth with the examiner looking intraorally near the second molar for bleeding. Three major salivary glands should be examined in facial trauma: the parotid, submandibular, and sublingual glands. Wharton's duct drains the submandibular and sublingual gland into the floor of the mouth near the frenulum of the tongue.[6]

The ears are examined by looking for any lacerations or damage to the tympanic membrane. Postauricular ecchymosis (Battle's sign) may indicate a basilar skull fracture but usually takes between 12 to 24 hours to develop. Otorrhea may be suggestive of a CSF leak.

DIAGNOSTIC TESTING

Visualization of facial fractures is best achieved by using computed tomography (CT), which is two-dimensional. The use of three-dimensional CT reconstruction improves diagnosis but is not available in all facilities. Bedside ultrasound, which can be used to evaluate patients with ocular and orbital injuries, helps detect vitreous hemorrhage, retinal detachment, and globe rupture.

Plain radiographs may be used as a screening tool if CT is unavailable. A Waters' view or occipitomental view can be used to look at the maxillary sinuses, frontal sinus, the zygomatic bones, arches, and the inferior orbital floor. A Caldwell or occipitofrontal view is used to look at the orbital rims, nasal septum, and ethmoid and frontal sinuses. A Towne view or angled antero-posterior axal view looks at the mandibular condyles and rami, nasal septum, maxillary ethmoid, and maxillary sinus. A Panorex is used to determine fractures of the mandible and is used in dental trauma. However, CT remains the preferred diagnostic test for evaluating facial trauma.[6,7]

SPECIFIC MAXILLOFACIAL INJURIES

Soft-Tissue Trauma

For soft-tissue injuries to the face, the goal is to retain function and have good cosmesis. It is important for repair of facial wounds to occur in a timely manner. Because of the highly vascular nature of the face, the length of time for wound closures can be extended to 24 hours from the time of injury, although it is preferable to delay no longer than 8 to 12 hours. In a healthy patient, the face is at low risk for infection. Deeper lacerations and lacerations associated with fractures can be conservatively debrided, irrigated, and closed before reduction. With tissue that is considered viable, excessive debridement should be avoided. Repair of facial lacerations in an uncooperative patient is extremely difficult and may injure other important structures. Delaying repair until the patient is more cooperative usually results in a better outcome. Fig. 36.3 shows contusions, abrasions, and lacerations of the face.

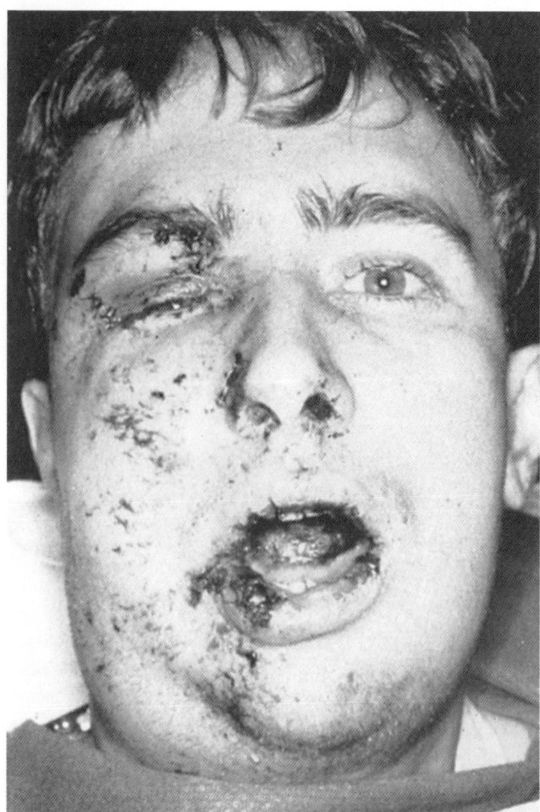

Fig. 36.3 Facial Injuries. (From Danis DM, Blansfield JS, Gervasini AA. *Manual of Clinical Trauma Care: The First Hour.* 4th ed. St Louis, MO: Mosby; 2007.)

Lacerations caused by animal or human bites are highly contaminated because of the bacterial and debris found in the mouth. All bites should be meticulously cleaned with soap and water and irrigated with warmed saline (preferred) because the warm temperature is more appealing to the patient. Tap water can be used because it is readily accessible and has a low cost.[7] Detergent, hydrogen peroxide, and concentrated povidone-iodine solutions should be avoided because they are considered toxic to the tissues and affect wound healing.[5,8] There are many factors to consider when deciding whether to close a facial laceration caused by a bite. Human and animal bite wounds on the face can be disfiguring, therefore suturing is more commonly done. However, cat bites, which are most often puncture wounds, are left open. Extensive or gaping wounds on the face present cosmetic problems, and consultation with a plastic surgeon is recommended. Most experts recommend closing the wound after meticulous irrigation and debridement. Both human and animal bites should be inspected for tooth fragments. Extensive animal bites, usually caused by large dogs, frequently require surgical exploration and repair. A helpful mnemonic for dealing with animal bites

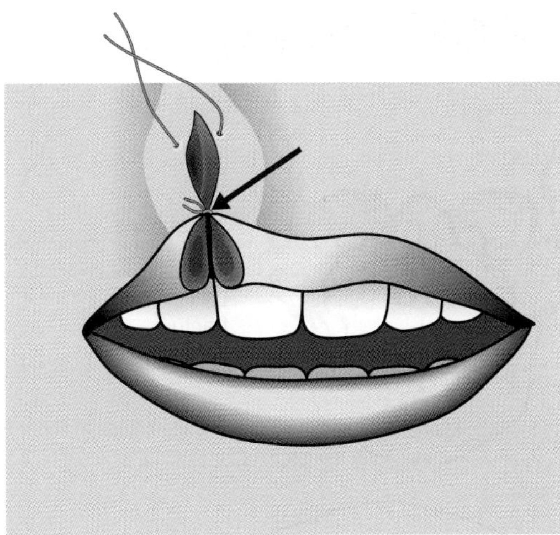

Fig. 36.4 Lip Laceration Through the Vermillion Border. Closure requires proper alignment with first suture placed at the vermillion-cutaneous border.

is RATS (Rabies, Antibiotics, Tetanus, and Soap). All patients should be covered for tetanus and rabies prophylaxis as indicated. Bite wounds tend to be polymicrobial.[8] General practice is to treat with a broad-spectrum β-lactam/β-lactamase inhibitor combination for animal bites to the face.[5]

Road rash, or friction injuries, present a unique problem because of potential tattooing or epidermal staining. Debridement should be done as soon as possible to avoid accidental, but permanent, tattooing from grease and asphalt. After the area has been injected with a local anesthetic, the skin should be vigorously scrubbed with a mild soap. Gunpowder can cause permanent discoloration of the skin with subsequent cosmetic disfigurement; therefore black powder fragments embedded in facial skin should be removed by using a local anesthetic and scrubbing with a hard brush or hard bristle toothbrush in the first hour wherever possible.[2] Gunpowder penetrating the skin is very hot and continues to burn epithelial and collagen layers. The longer it is allowed to remain, the greater the risk for permanent discoloration. When glass fragments are visible, tape applied to the face may help remove glass.

Lacerations of eyebrows and eyelids should be repaired before swelling occurs so that borders can be matched. Eyebrows should never be shaved because landmarks are eliminated and the brow is unlikely to grow back. When suturing the brow, hairs are aligned so they slant in a downward and outward direction.

Vermillion borders or margins are important anatomic landmarks in the repair of lip lacerations. Borders must be perfectly aligned to prevent development of step-off deformity of the lip. The philtrum of the lip is another area that must be closely aligned. Fig. 36.4 illustrates closure of this type of laceration. Tissue loss from the lip requires reconstructions by a plastic surgeon.

Intraoral injuries should be carefully inspected for debris, crushed tissue, and tooth fragments. Injuries should be meticulously cleaned and irrigated. Gaping intraoral lacerations tend to bleed and become infected, and they should therefore

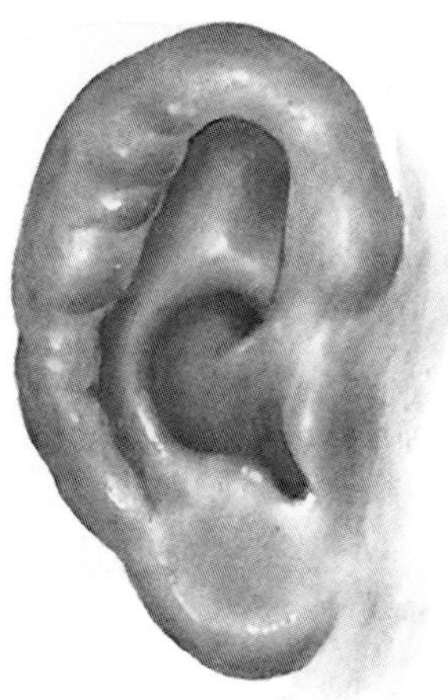

Fig. 36.5 Cauliflower Ear. (From Sheehy SB, Jimmerson CL. *Manual of Clinical Trauma Care.* 4th ed. St Louis, MO: Mosby; 2007.)

be closed. Antibiotics are usually prescribed.[3] Encourage the patient to use a mild antiseptic mouthwash to swish and spit several times a day.

When the tongue is lacerated, inspect the mouth carefully for other lacerations from teeth. Gaping or bleeding lacerations are sutured, and antibiotic therapy is indicated. Children are prone to hard and soft palate lacerations, usually from falling with a sharp object in the mouth.

Ear injuries are categorized into three groups: hematomas, lacerations, and avulsions. A perichondrial hematoma often results from blunt trauma and must be properly drained and dressed to prevent scar deformity resembling a cauliflower (Fig. 36.5). This can be complicated by avascular necrosis of the cartilage.[9] Follow-up with plastic surgery is necessary because hematomas tend to recur. Lacerations may involve skin or skin or cartilage. Pinna lacerations require repair, and the cartilage and overlying skin are approximated using absorbable suture. A pressure dressing is applied to prevent reaccumulation of blood.[9] Wounds to the ear require minimal debridement and are usually closed in two layers. However, avulsion injuries of the ear require skin preservation; otherwise, grafts from other body sites are required. Anesthetics containing epinephrine should not be used on the ear because of the deleterious effects of vasoconstriction. There has been recent controversary over the use of epinephrine when suturing the tips of the nose and earlobes, but most people are forgoing their use when these body parts are involved. Antibiotics are prescribed to prevent cartilage infection. Cartilage necrosis can occur if bandages are left unpadded or unchecked for long periods.

Deep cheek lacerations can damage the parotid gland, parotid duct, and branches of the facial nerve, a motor nerve governing muscle of facial expression. Injury to the temporal branch causes forehead asymmetry because the patient cannot wrinkle the forehead on the affected side. With injury to the temporal or zygomatic branch, the patient is unable to fully close the eyelids on the affected side. Buccal branch injury keeps the patient from pursing the lips to whistle, and injury to the mandibular branch causes the inability to lower or depress the lower lip. At rest, elevation of the lower lip

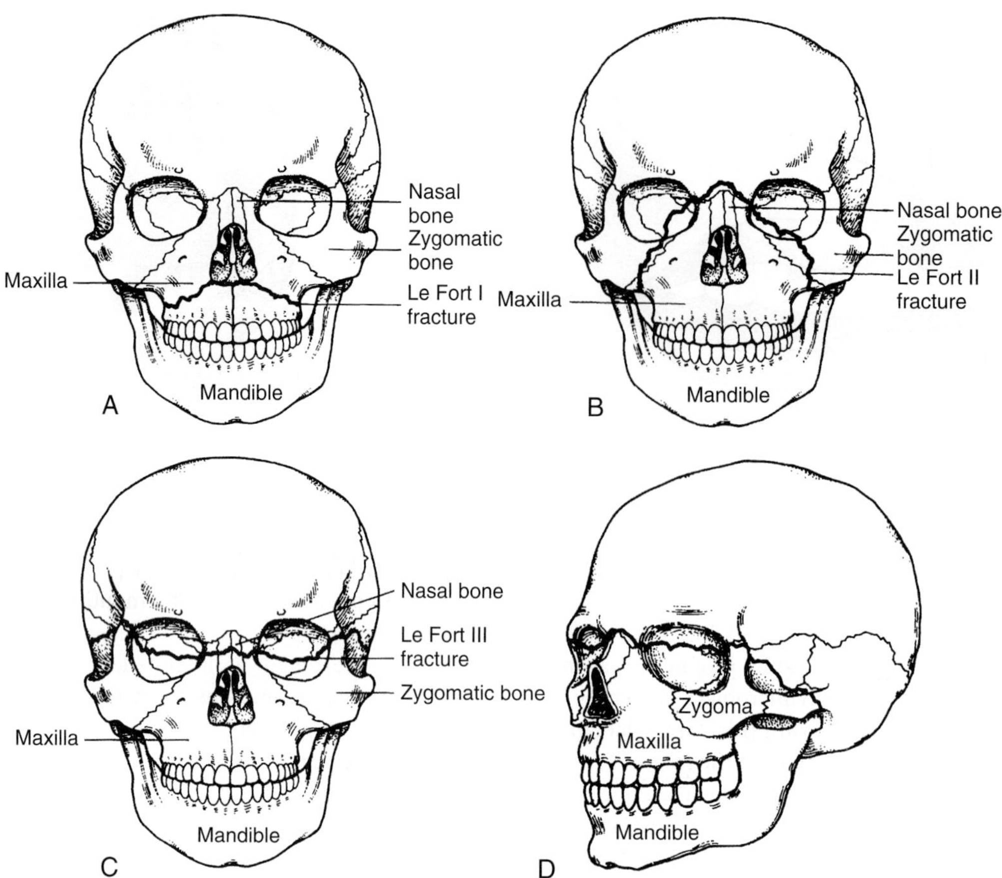

Fig. 36.6 (A) Le Fort I facial fracture. (B) Fort II facial fracture; (C & D) Le Fort III, lateral view. (From Sheehy S, Hammond B, Zimmermann P. *Sheehy's Manual of Emergency Care.* 7th ed. St Louis, MO: Mosby; 2013.)

occurs on the affected side. Injury to the facial nerves can be easily missed if the patient is unconscious or has numerous facial dressings. Facial paralysis after blunt facial trauma has a good prognosis for complete recovery if minimal soft-tissue damage occurs. Lacerations of the parotid duct or the parotid gland are an infrequent occurrence but must be considered.

Nasal Fractures

Nasal fractures are the most common type of facial fracture because the nose offers the least resistance. The mechanism of injury is usually blunt trauma associated with other injuries of the face. Overlooked nasal injury can lead to permanent deformity and airway obstruction. Clinical findings include swelling, deformity, bleeding, and crepitus, and the patient may have tenderness over the bridge of the nose. In children, the nose is more elastic and resistant to fractures; however, dislocations are more common. Nasal fractures can usually be diagnosed by the clinical examination. If radiographs are needed, the lateral view is usually the best. Unrecognized or untreated nasal fractures can lead to abnormal nasal bone growth affecting nasal contour.

Nasal bones are lined with mucoperiosteum. A nasal fracture with an overlying laceration is considered an open fracture. Fractures caused by a frontal blow can damage the ethmoid and frontal sinuses, lacrimal duct, and orbital margins. If the cribriform plate is affected and the dura is torn, CSF leak or rhinorrhea occurs. Thorough examination of each naris can identify septal hematomas, lacerations, and the ability of the patient to breathe through his or her nose.[3,4] A septal hematoma appears as a bulging, tense, bluish mass that feels doughy when palpated. Septal hematomas should be emergently drained to prevent airway obstructions and necrosis of septal cartilage. The patient should be receive an antistaphylococcal antibiotic. An untreated septal hematoma causes a permanent nasal deformity called a saddle deformity.[2]

Initial interventions focus on controlling bleeding with direct pressure. Bleeding may be intranasal and in the pharynx. Ice compresses applied to the bridge of the nose aid hemostasis and help relieve pain. Elevation of the head of the bed and the use of nasal decongestants help reduce swelling. Anterior or posterior nasal packing may be required to control bleeding. The packing should be removed in 3 to 4 days and antibiotics prescribed.[3] Splinting maintains position, ensures alignment, and prevents further edema and injury. In some cases, the physician may not set the fracture until the swelling subsides. When the fracture involves the nasal mucosa of the lacrimal system, blowing the nose causes intracranial air or subcutaneous emphysema, which can cause localized infection or meningitis. In the case of displaced nasal fractures, the physician will choose between closed nasal reduction (manipulation of the nasal bones) while the patient is alert and nasal reduction performed under general anesthesia, which is usually done when the nasal fracture is open. Both methods are being debated as to which provides better patient satisfaction.[5] The patient should be referred to a consultant in 3 to 5 days for close follow-up.

Nasoorbital-Ethmoidal Fracture

Nasoorbital-ethmoidal (NOE) fractures occur with a direct blow to the face that results in fractures of the medial orbital wall, nose, and ethmoid sinus. Most bones in this area are thin and fragile and have low tolerance to impact. Injury to this area can result in direct ocular injury. Fractures can extend through the cribriform plate and result in CSF leak (rhinorrhea) from the nose. This fracture is usually the result of high-impact motor vehicle crashes (MVCs). The presenting symptoms include pain and visual abnormalities.[6] The clinical presentation shows massive periorbital and upper facial edema with ecchymosis, epistaxis, traumatic telecanthus, foreshortening of the nose with telescoping, and associated intracranial injuries. Diagnostic findings on CT scan may include disruption of interorbital space and comminution of the nasal pyramid; frontal, zygomatic, orbital, and maxillary fractures are a common concomitant finding. Complications of NOE fractures are residual upper midface deformity ("dish face"); telecanthus; and frontal sinus—nasolacrimal system pathology with mucocele, mucopyocele, and dacryocystitis.

Maxillary Fractures

Maxillary, or midface, fractures are caused by significant force and are usually a combination of fractures involving several facial structures. Maxillary fractures are classified as Le Fort I, II, and III (i.e., lower third, middle third, and orbital complex). Plain radiographs of the face with emphasis on Waters' view have been used in the past, but CT is used for definitive diagnosis and identification of the fractures. Maxillary fractures are rarely seen in children because of the flexible and pliable nature of their maxillofacial structures.

Patients with maxillary fractures complain of severe facial pain, anesthesia, or paresthesia of the upper lip, and some visual disturbances, such as diplopia. Clinically, the patient has severe facial swelling, ecchymosis, periorbital or orbital swelling, subconjunctival hemorrhage, proptosis, elongation of the face, facial asymmetry, epistaxis, and malocclusion. The patient may have intraoral lacerations and dental trauma.[3] CSF may leak from the nose, which is a significant finding. CSF is usually clear but may have mucus when it leaks through the nasal passage. Many patients state it has a salty or sweet taste. The fluid can be sent for analysis to be checked for β-2-transferrin, which is characteristic of CSF leaks.[3]

Le Fort I, or lower third facture (Fig. 36.6A), is a horizontal fracture in which the body of the maxilla is separated from the base of the skull above the plate but below the zygomatic process attachment. Separation may be unilateral or bilateral. There is a free-floating segment of the upper teeth and the lower maxilla; however, the fracture may not be displaced. The hard palate and upper teeth are mobile when moved by grasping the alveolar process and anterior teeth. The presenting symptoms are pain in the upper jaw and numbness in the upper teeth. The midface fractures typically occur from high-energy blunt trauma events, such as from MVCs, falls, and physical altercations.[1] Clinical presentation includes midface edema and ecchymosis, epistaxis, malocclusion, and mobility of the maxillary dentition. Diagnosis is best determined by CT scan, but a Waters' and Panorex radiographic view may still be used. Findings demonstrate opaque maxillary sinus, displacement of fragments of alveolus if comminuted, and fracture through maxillary sinus and pterygoid plates. Complications of Le Fort I fracture include loss of teeth, infection, and malocclusion.

Le Fort II, or middle third fractures (see Fig. 36.6B), involves the pyramidal area, including the central maxilla, nasal area, and ethmoid bones. This portion of the face is a tripod shape with the apex at the nose. Grasping the front teeth and palate causes movement of the nose and upper lip with no movement of the orbital complex. Significant force is required to fracture this area, and the patient should be thoroughly evaluated for other injuries. The presenting symptoms are pain in the midface, numbness in the upper lip and lower lid, malocclusion, mobility of midface, nasal flattening, and anesthesia in the infraorbital nerve territory. The nose, mouth, and eyes are usually edematous, with subconjunctival hemorrhage and epistaxis frequently noted. The presence of rhinorrhea suggests an open skull fracture. A CT scan remains the diagnostic gold standard, although the Waters' radiograph view is still used. CT scan findings consistent with a midface fracture include opaque maxillary sinus and separation through frontal process, lacrimal bone, floor of orbits, zygomaticomaxillary suture line, lateral wall of maxillary sinus, and pterygoid plates. Complications of Le Fort II fractures include nonunion, malunion, lacrimal system obstruction, infraorbital nerve anesthesia, diplopia, and malocclusion. When the fracture involves the central portion of the ethmoid bone, this may also injure the first cranial nerve (olfactory nerve) causing anosmia.[6]

Le Fort III, or orbital complex fracture (see Fig. 36.6C and D), causes total cranial facial separation. The nose and dental arch move without frontal bone involvement. Massive edema, ecchymosis, epistaxis, and malocclusion are present with a spoonlike appearance of the face noted on side profile. Early ocular examination is necessary to prevent unrecognized ocular injuries secondary to extensive swelling.

Presenting symptoms of a Le Fort III fracture are facial pain and difficulty breathing. Clinical signs are "donkey-face" deformity and rhinorrhea. The CT scan findings demonstrate separation of the mid-third of the face zygomaticotemporal and nasofrontal sutures, and across the orbital floors; and opaque maxillary sinuses. Complications of Le Fort III include persistent CSF leakage, nonunion, malunion, malocclusion, lengthening of midface, and lacrimal system obstruction.[10]

Management of maxillary fractures includes aggressive airway control. Endotracheal intubation may be difficult because of edema and loss of normal anatomic contour. Nursing care should include anticipating potential cricothyroidotomy or tracheotomy. Excessive secretions and bleeding require frequent suctioning; therefore allow the patient to use a tonsil-tip suction when appropriate. Position the patient upright and leaning forward (once the cervical spine is cleared) to promote drainage and decrease swelling. Apply ice compresses to help relieve pain and decrease swelling. Administer prophylactic antibiotics and tetanus immunization as appropriate. Frequently assess for compromise to the airway, dyspnea, neck swelling, or voice changes. Notify the physician immediately if these signs are present.

Zygoma Fractures

Fractures of the zygoma usually occur in two patterns: zygomatic arch fracture and tripod fracture. The zygoma is frequently fractured during significant facial trauma due to its prominence and location on the face.[11] Fracture of the orbital floor may also be present with zygomatic fractures. Injury is usually caused by blunt trauma to the front and side of face. With a tripod fracture, the zygoma fractures in three places: zygomatic arch, posterior half of the infraorbital rim, and frontozygomatic suture. A step deformity is palpated at the infraorbital rim and frontozygomatic suture area with flattening of asymmetry of the check, periorbital edema, circumorbital or subconjunctival ecchymosis, and pain exacerbated by jaw motion. A zygoma fracture occurs at the arch and presents with pain in the lateral cheek and inability to close the jaw. There is swelling and crepitus over the arch and obvious asymmetry. Complications occurring with a zygomatic arch fracture are contour irregularities of the arch area and flattening of the arch. A fracture occurring at the body of the zygoma or a tripod fracture presents with pain, trismus, diplopia, and numbness of the upper lip, lower lid, and bilateral nasal area. Clinical signs include swelling, ecchymosis of malar and periorbital areas, palpable infraorbital rim step-off, entrapment of extraocular muscles with disconjugate gaze, scleral ecchymosis, lateral subconjunctival hemorrhage, and displacement of the lateral canthal ligament.

Patients with zygomatic arch fractures may present with trismus, secondarily to impingement of the temporalis muscle.[11] Epistaxis may also be present. Entrapment of the inferior rectus muscle causes double vision and asymmetry of ocular level and anesthesia of the upper lip, check, teeth, and gums. Interventions focus on controlling pain and decreasing swelling. Patients should be instructed to avoid blowing their nose when being treated for zygoma fractures.[1] Complications include residual malar deformity, enophthalmos (sunken appearance), diplopia, infraorbital nerve anesthesia, and chronic maxillary sinusitis.

A CT scan is the preferred diagnostic test, but a Waters' or submentovertex radiograph is acceptable. Diagnostic findings may show clouding, air/fluid level in the maxillary sinus, and separation of the zygomaticomaxillary, zygomaticofrontal, and zygomaticotemporal suture lines. Plain radiographs with a "bucket-handle" view demonstrate zygomatic arch and body fracture, whereas CT scans are often needed to demonstrate extent of a tripod fracture, which is more complex.[1]

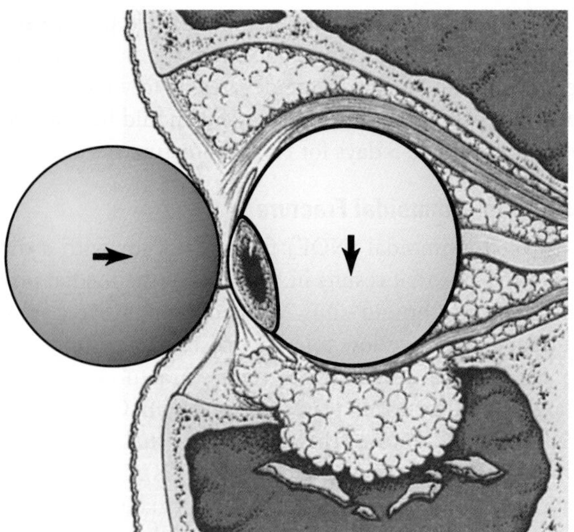

Fig. 36.7 Mechanism of a blowout fracture caused by the impact of a ball. The periorbital fat is forced through the floor of the orbit. (From Ragge N. *Immediate Eye Care*. London, England: Wolfe Medical Publications; 1990.)

Orbital Blowout Fractures

Zygoma fractures and orbital blowout fractures can occur independently but are often found in combination. The orbit consists of seven facial bones: frontal, zygoma, maxilla, lacrimal, ethmoid, sphenoid, and palatine.[12] Orbital blowout fractures occur when blunt trauma to the globe causes a downward displacement of the orbital floor with protrusion of contents into the maxillary sinus. This causes an abrupt rise in orbital pressure. The posterior medial orbital floor is the weakest part of the bony orbit, so increased pressure causes orbital contents to prolapse into the maxillary sinus (Fig. 36.7). Inferior rectus muscle, inferior oblique muscle, infraorbital nerve, orbital fat, and connective tissue become entrapped in the orbital floor, so extraocular movements should be thoroughly evaluated. The globe may also become entrapped. If there is damage to the infraorbital nerves, there may be numbness of the cheek and the area around the lateral nose. This fracture frequently results from MVCs, sports-related injuries, such as a baseball thrown at the eye, and altercations, such as violent fistfights. Golf balls can extend past the protective orbital rim and rupture the globe. If the globe is perforated, then manipulating the eyes or nose blowing can lead to intraorbital air. Forceful nose blowing should be avoided.

Presenting symptoms include binocular diplopia with an upward gaze, orbital pain, periorbital edema, and ecchymosis, enophthalmos, extraocular muscle entrapment, dysconjugate gaze, hyphema, subluxation of lens, retinal detachment, retinal tear, vitreous hemorrhage, secondary glaucoma, and rupture of the globe.

Subcutaneous orbital emphysema suggests a fracture in the sinus arch. Nose blowing, coughing, sneezing, vomiting, and straining can force air from sinuses through the fracture into the orbital space. Proptosis and limitation of extraocular motion suggest orbital involvement (Fig. 36.8). Double vision,

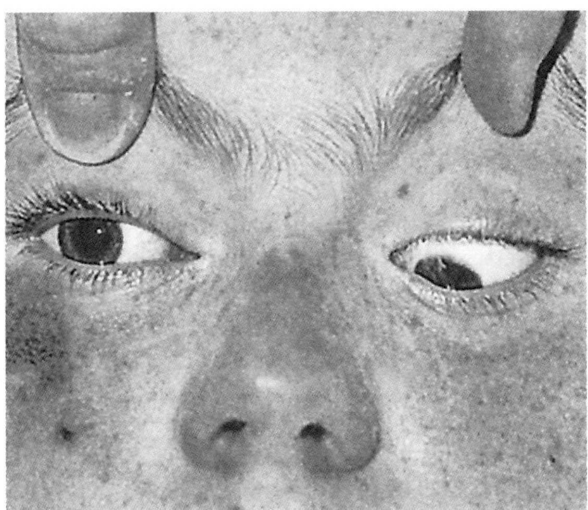

Fig. 36.8 Blowout Fracture. (From Zietelli BJ, Davis HW. *Atlas of Pediatric Physical Diagnosis.* 5th ed. St Louis, MO: Mosby; 2007.)

pupil asymmetry, enophthalmos, anesthesia of the cheek and upper lip, and ptosis (drooping of the lid) are clinical manifestations of blowout fracture. Extreme swelling may occur after a blowout fracture has occurred, making it difficult to obtain a good eye examination. It is important to remember to assess the eye early, before more swelling develops. Globe injuries may occur concurrently with blowout fractures, making it difficult to obtain a good eye examination. Patients who report bilateral visual acuity changes may have injury to the optic nerve.[12] Globe injuries may occur concurrently with blowout fractures. Ruptures usually occur at the weakest area of the globe or opposite the side of impact.[3,6,12] If a ruptured globe is suspected, an eye shield or plastic cup should be used over the eye to prevent further injury. A ruptured globe is an ophthalmologic emergency. Emergent ophthalmologic consultation is indicated. Complications of an orbital floor fracture are enophthalmos, diplopia, recurrent orbital cellulitis with implant (alloplastic), and extrusion.

CT scan without contrast is the preferred imaging method of choice. The CT scan is superior to magnetic resonance imaging (MRI) in evaluation or trauma to the orbit. But MRI has been found to be superior to CT when evaluating for soft-tissue injuries.[12]

Surgical intervention is usually postponed until swelling diminishes, usually several days. Using ice compresses and elevating the head of the bed help decrease swelling and relieve pain. Immediate surgery is indicated for retrobulbar hematoma, globe rupture, or any optic nerve compression causing vision impairment. Broad-spectrum antibiotics may be used to decrease the risk of infection from the orbital fracture. Nasal decongestants, steroids, pain medication, and ice are used to reduce swelling. The patient should be reminded to avoid straining and nose blowing. Complications from orbital floor fractures can occur from the oculocardiac reflex, such as nausea, vomiting, bradycardia, and vertigo. Follow-up with an ophthalmologist is necessary.[6]

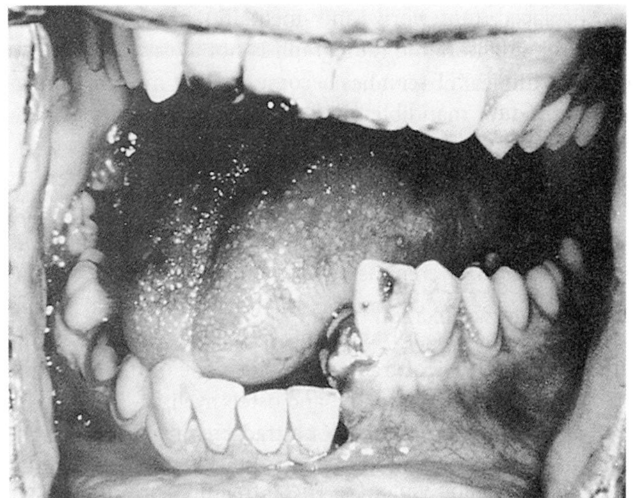

Fig. 36.9 Malocclusion Caused by Fracture. (From Danis DM, Blansfield JS, Gervasini AA. *Manual of Clinical Trauma Care: The First Hour.* 4th ed. St Louis, MO: Mosby; 2007; courtesy Dr. Daniel Cheney.)

Mandibular Fractures

Mandibular fractures are the second most common facial fracture. Blunt force, such as a severe blow to the face during contact sports, altercations, and MVCs, is the usual mechanism of injury. Mandibular fractures can be a significant life-threatening injury if loss of bony support displaces the tongue posteriorly and obstructs the airway. This may also cause difficulty swallowing. Malocclusion is a cardinal indication of mandibular fracture (Fig. 36.9). Signs and symptoms vary with fractures site; however, point tenderness and crepitus may be palpated and step-off deformity found. Trismus and decreased range of motion are usually noted. The face may be asymmetric and have swelling and ecchymosis. Paresthesia in the lower lip and chin imply injury to the inferior alveolar nerve. The oral cavity should be assessed for broken or loose teeth, lacerations, or ecchymosis. Sublingual hematoma can compromise the airway. Inspect both ears for tears in the external canal and tympanic membrane.

Mandibular fractures are classified according to their anatomic region in the mandible. The condyle is the most frequent site, followed by the angle of the mandible, symphysis coronoid, ramus, and alveolar ridge.[1] Reciprocal fractures can occur on the side opposite the point of impact. Specific symptoms related to a condyle fracture are pain at the fracture site with referred pain to the ear. Other symptoms might include crepitus, excessive salivation, swelling of the condylar region, deviation of the jaw toward the fracture, cross-bite, or open bite deformity. Any missing teeth that cannot be found should be assumed to be aspirated and the patient should have a chest radiograph to rule out aspiration. A patient with a mandibular fracture should always be assessed for trismus and malocclusion. An intraoral examination should be done to evaluate for bleeding, exposed bone, any injured teeth, or a sublingual hematoma. Plain radiographs with anteroposterior and oblique views or a Panorex can show a nondisplaced or displaced (anteriorly and medially) condyle fracture. However, a panoramic radiograph is not always available in every facility. A CT scan has become the best modality imaging method for mandible fractures, but the amount of radiation should be a consideration.

For a fracture at the angle of the mandible, there is pain at the fracture site and inability to close the mouth. Assessment finding may include swelling at the angle of the jaw, ecchymosis, crepitus, and malocclusion. Mandibular radiographic series or Panorex might reveal a nondisplaced fracture or a posterior fragment displaced upward and medially. Complications of fractures of the angle of the mandible include nonunion, malunion, and osteomyelitis.

The clinical presentation for a fracture of the body of the mandible includes pain at the fracture site and limitation of jaw movement with edema, ecchymosis, crepitus, and malocclusion. A mandibular radiographic series or Panoramic view might reveal a nondisplaced fracture, or a posterior fragment displaced upward and medially, anterior fragments rotated lingually. Complications of this type of fracture include osteomyelitis and infection of the tooth in the fracture line.

Finally, a fracture of the symphysis of the mandible might produce symptoms of pain, malocclusion, and soft-tissue wounds of the lower lip or tongue. A mandibular series or submentovertex view would find a nondisplaced or lingual rotation or anterior fragments and may be associated with angle or condyle fractures. Complications of this type of fracture include residual malocclusion, loss of chin projection, asymmetry, and osteomyelitis.

The management of mandibular fractures usually does not require urgent treatment, but treatment is likely to be done within 24 to 72 hours of injury. Depending on the location of the fracture, treatment may consist of surgical intervention with open reduction and internal fixation or wiring the jaw. Nursing care in the ED includes allowing the patient to sit upright as soon as the cervical spine is cleared and applying ice compresses to the face to minimize swelling and relieve pain. Oral saline rinses for the mouth may also be used. Intravenous antibiotics are indicated for open fractures, and repair of lacerations should occur as soon as possible. Antibiotics are commonly prescribed for mandibular fractures, but current evidence supporting their use is not highly rated for isolated mandibular fractures. Cephalosporins, clindamycin, metronidazole, and penicillin are commonly used for open fractures. Tetanus is also considered for open mandible fractures.

Conservative treatment for a nondisplaced mandible fracture is a soft diet and pain management. The patient is usually discharged. Mandibular fractures associated with any mucosal, gingival, or tooth disruption should be considered as open fractures. Definitive care usually consists of reduction and fixation and wiring. A patient with a potential for airway complication should be admitted. Follow-up with a maxillofacial surgeon usually occurs within 2 to 3 days.

Complications of mandibular fractures include ankylosis of the TMJ and chronic TMJ disorders.

SUMMARY

Maxillofacial injuries are a common occurrence in the ED. Special attention should be given to stabilizing the cervical spine, maintaining a patent airway, and controlling hemorrhage. Performing a thorough eye examination on a patient with maxillofacial injury must be thorough and done early in the evaluation to assess for any vision-threatening injuries. The goal of treatment is life, function, and esthetics.

It is important to remember to assess for blunt cerebrovascular injuries (BCVI) in patients who present with Le Fort II and III fractures and mandibular fractures due to the location of the significant structures. The preferred method for imaging facial injuries is the CT scan. Although radiographs are used, CT is the gold standard for identifying the degree of injury.

REFERENCES

1. Das D, Salazar L, Zaurova M. Maxillofacial trauma: managing potentially dangerous and disfiguring complex injuries. *Emerg Med Pract.* 2017;19(4).
2. Sheehy S, Hammond B, Zimmermann P. *Sheehy's Manual of Emergency Care.* 7th ed. St Louis, MO: Mosby; 2013.
3. Warta MH, Fakhro A. Maxillofacial trauma: critical aspects of management. *Trauma Reports.* 2014;15(1).
4. Snell R, Smith M. *Clinical Anatomy for Emergency Medicine.* St Louis, MO: Mosby; 1993.
5. Dougherty WM, Christophel JJ, Park SS. Evidence-based medicine in facial trauma. *Facial Plast Surg Clin North Am.* 2017;25(4):629–643.
6. Mayersak RJ. *Initial Evaluation and Management of Facial Trauma in Adults.* Waltham, MA: UpToDate; 2018. https://www.uptodate.com/contents/initial-evaluation-and-management-of-facial-trauma-in-adults. Accessed May 28, 2019.
7. Doerr TD. Evidence-based facial fracture management. *Facial Plast Surg Clin North Am.* 2015;23(3):335–345. https://doi.org/10.1016/j.fsc.2015.04.006.
8. Baddour L. *Soft Tissue Infections Due to Dog and cat Bites.* Waltham, MA: UpToDate; 2018. https://www.uptodate.com/contents/animal-and-human-bites-beyond-the-basics. Accessed May 28, 2019.
9. Huang C, Leetch A. Orofacial, eye, and ear trauma. *Pediatr Emerg Med Reports.* 2018;23(3).
10. Rogers L, ed. *Radiology of Skeletal Trauma.* 3rd ed. Philadelphia, PA: Churchill Livingstone; 2002.
11. Tollefson TT. Zygomaticomaxillary complex fractures. Medscape website. https://emedicine.medscape.com/article/867687-overview. Published March 13, 2019. Accessed May 28, 2019.
12. Ramponi DR, Astorino T, Bessetti-Barrett CR. Orbital floor fractures. *Adv Emerg Nurs J.* 2017;39(4):240–247.

37

Spinal Trauma

Jessie Balcom

Trauma to the spinal cord and spinal column can cause devastating and life-threatening injuries to the patient. A spinal column injury with or without neurologic deficits must always be considered in the trauma patient with multiple injuries. According to the National Spinal Cord Injury Association, as many as 450,000 people in the United States are living with a spinal cord injury (SCI). Each year there are approximately 11,000 SCIs occurring in the United States alone. The vast majority of these patients are 16 to 30 years of age, with males representing 80% of these injuries.[1] This percentage represents the number of SCIs that health care providers are faced with; thus precise management of these patients is key to optimize outcomes.

Trauma to the spinal cord and spinal column can result from both blunt force and penetrating trauma. Patients may sustain injuries from mechanisms from a motor vehicle crash, gunshot wounds, falls, high-risk sports, and motorcycle and diving accidents.[2] Motor vehicle crashes have been ranked the leading cause of vertebral injuries and SCIs in the United States for those aged 65 and younger.[1,2] The mechanism of injury in a motor vehicle crash is directly correlated with rollovers and ejections from unrestrained occupants. In patients 65 years and older, falls have been found to be the leading cause of SCIs and spinal column injuries.[2] The Centers for Disease Control and Prevention has estimated an overall cost of $9.7 billion each year for SCI care. Secondary injuries from SCI, such as pressure ulcers, cost an estimated $1.2 billion each year.[3]

Historically, many people with SCIs died of respiratory complications such as aspiration and pneumonia.[4] Establishment of SCI care systems has decreased complications from SCIs and improved outcomes and survivability. The initial care and treatment of those sustaining SCIs is stabilization.

Stabilization and treatment of those who have SCI or spinal column injury has improved over the years. The use of evidence-based practice guidelines has established improved care, outcomes, and survivability of the trauma patient. The care and stabilization of the trauma patient with a suspected SCI or spinal column injury often begins in the prehospital setting. Prehospital agencies have been trained to identify potential injuries sustained based on the assessment of the patient and appropriate triage guidelines. Spinal motion restriction guidelines have been developed to help determine the needs for spinal protection. Prehospital personnel have been trained to fully immobilize the trauma patient with suspected SCI or spinal column injuries and triage appropriately.[5] The utilization of rapid air transport agencies in the prehospital setting has improved time to definitive care for the trauma patient.[5]

Recent studies indicate that patients with head injuries are at higher risk for also having cervical spine injuries, particularly if the patient is unconscious or has a focal neurologic deficit.[2,6] On arrival in the emergency department (ED), the patient should be fully evaluated to rule out concomitant life-threatening injuries such as tension pneumothorax or intraabdominal bleeding while spine protection is continued.

Emergency care of the patient with spinal trauma requires an organized, multidisciplinary approach. Patient survival and quality of life after the acute injury depend on the emergency care a patient receives. This chapter discusses anatomy and physiology of spine trauma, mechanisms of injury, patient assessment and initial interventions, specific injuries, and current research related to management of an acute spinal injury.

ANATOMY AND PHYSIOLOGY

Vertebral Column

The vertebral column serves as bony support for the head and trunk and provides protection for the spinal cord. A total of 7 cervical vertebrae, 12 thoracic vertebrae, 5 lumbar vertebrae, 1 sacral vertebra (composed of 5 fused vertebrae), and 1 coccygeal vertebra (composed of 4 fused vertebrae) constitute the vertebral column. Each vertebra is composed of a body, a vertebral arch, and a vertebral foramen. The arch of the vertebra is composed of two pedicles, two laminae, four articular processes (facets), two transverse processes, and the spinous process, which can be felt when palpating the posterior spine.[7,8]

The cervical vertebrae are the most frequently injured because they are the most mobile part of the spine and are small and delicate.[7] The rib cage provides stability to the vertebrae from T1 to T10 and keeps this portion of the spine relatively immobile. Because the thoracic vertebrae are so strong, fractures, dislocations, or both at this level should increase suspicion for SCI.[8] The lumbar vertebrae are the largest and strongest in the vertebral column.[7,8]

Ligaments attach to the transverse and spinous processes to connect the vertebral bodies and provide support and stability to the vertebral column. They also limit the spinal column from excessive flexion and extension. Between the vertebral bodies are discs acting as shock absorbers and articulating surfaces for the adjacent vertebral bodies.[8,9]

Spinal Column

The spinal cord extends from the brain through the foramen magnum and down the vertebral column to the level of L2. This mass of nerve tissue regulates body movement and function through transmission of nerve impulses. The diameter of the spinal cord is largest in the cervical and lumbar regions and tapers in the lower thoracic area. In adults, it terminates in a cone-shaped structure, known as the conus medullaris, at the L1 or L2 level. Spinal nerve roots exiting below the conus medullaris are referred to as the cauda equina.[7-9]

The primary function of the spinal cord is to regulate bodily function and movement by transmitting nerve impulses between the brain and the body. Cross-sectional views of the spinal cord reveal a butterfly shaped core composed of gray matter, surrounded on the outer edges by white matter. The gray matter contains nerve cell bodies and is divided into three distinct regions, each with specific characteristics: the posterior (dorsal), intermediolateral (lateral), and anterior (ventral) horns. The posterior, or dorsal, horn contains sensory interneurons and axons whose cell bodies are located in the dorsal root ganglion. The intermediolateral, or lateral, horn contains cell bodies with autonomic nervous system function. The anterior, or ventral, horn contains somatic motor neurons that leave the spinal cord via the spinal nerves.[8,10]

The white matter of the spinal cord consists of multiple ascending and descending pathways (referred to collectively as "spinal tracts"), which are individually named based on their origins and terminations. These tracts run parallel to the spinal cord's vertical axis and transmit action potentials to and from the brain to other parts of the spinal cord. Table 37.1 lists some of these specific tracts and describes their functions.[7,10]

TABLE 37.1 Examples of Spinal Tracts and Their Functions.

Spinal Tract	Function
Dorsal column (ascending)	Proprioception, pressure, and vibration
Lateral spinothalamic tract (ascending)	Pain and temperature
Anterior spinothalamic tract (ascending)	Light touch, pressure, and itch sensation
Spinocerebellar tract (ascending)	Proprioception to the cerebellum
Pyramidal tracts (descending)	Voluntary control of skeletal muscle
Extrapyramidal tracts (descending)	Automatic control of skeletal muscle

Data from Seeley R, Stephens T, Tate P. *Anatomy and Physiology.* 6th ed. Boston, MA: McGraw-Hill; 2003.

Spinal Nerves

The spinal cord has 31 pairs of spinal nerves, which exit the spinal cord bilaterally and provide pathways for involuntary responses to specific stimuli. There are 8 cervical nerves, 12 thoracic nerves, 5 lumbar nerves, 5 sacral nerves, and 1 coccygeal nerve. The spinal nerves innervate voluntary striated muscle and are responsible for the majority of the communication between the spinal cord and the rest of the body. Each of these nerves has a posterior root transmitting sensory impulses from the periphery into the spinal cord and an anterior root transmitting motor impulses from the spinal cord out to the periphery. Table 37.2 lists the spinal nerve muscle innervations and their corresponding expected patient response. The dorsal root of these nerves innervates a distinct region of the body surface known as a dermatome.[8,9] Assessment of the 28 dermatomes provides information about function to sensory areas of the spinal cord. Fig. 37.1 illustrates the sensory dermatomes.

TABLE 37.2 Spinal Nerve Muscle Innervation and Patient Response.

Nerve Level	Muscles Innervated	Patient Response
C4	Diaphragm	Ventilation
C5	Deltoid	Shrug shoulders
	Biceps	Flex elbows
	Brachioradialis	
C6	Wrist extensor	Extend wrist
	Extensor carpi radialis longus	
C7	Triceps	Extend elbow
	Extensor digitorum communis	Extend fingers
	Flexor carpi radialis	
C8	Flexor digitorum profundus	Flex fingers
T1	Hand intrinsic muscles	Spread fingers
T2 to T12	Intercostals	Vital capacity
L1	Abdominal	Abdominal reflexes
L2	Iliopsoas	Hip flexion
L3	Quadriceps	Knee extension
L4	Tibialis anterior	Ankle dorsiflexion
L5	Extension hallucis longus	Ankle eversion
S1	Gastrocnemius	Ankle plantar flexion
		Big toe extension
S2 to S5	Perineal sphincter	Sphincter control

Vascular Supply

The vascular supply for the spinal cord comes from branches of the vertebral arteries and the aorta. The anterior and

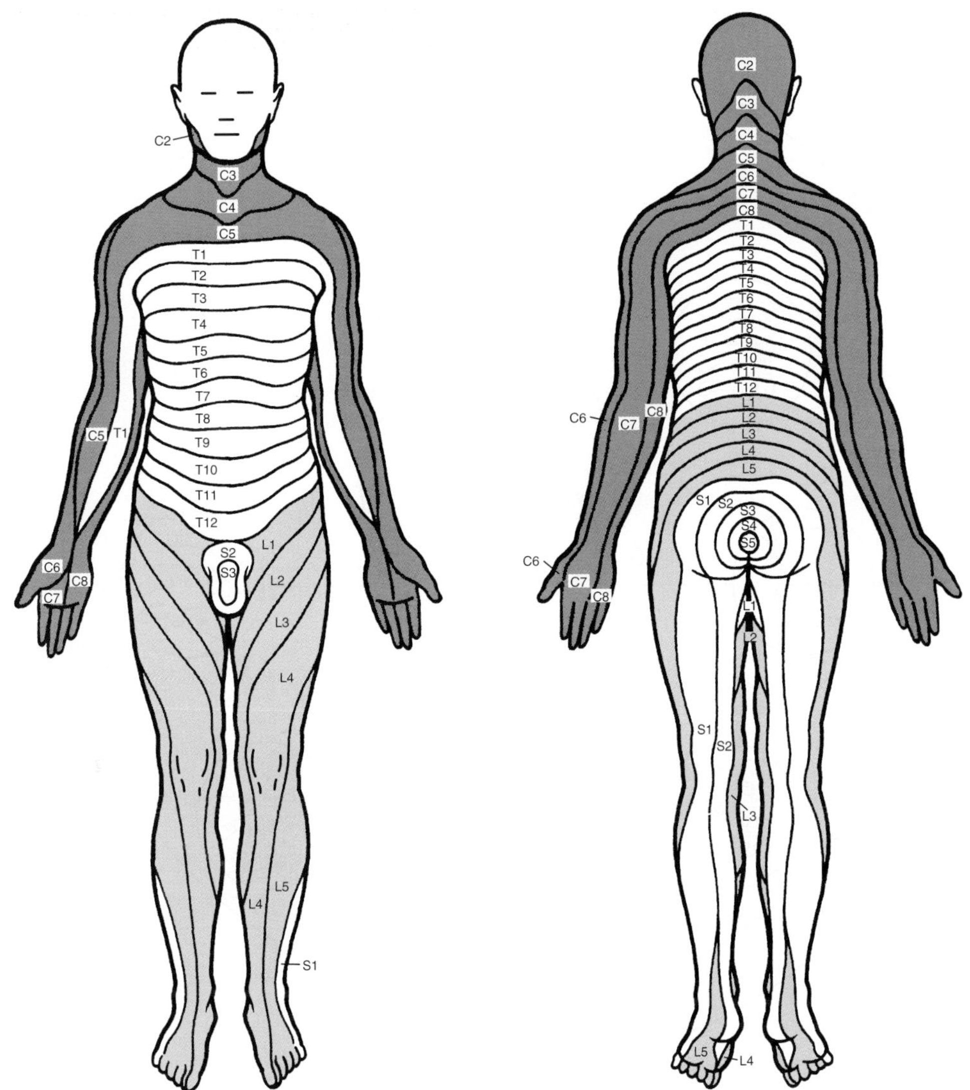

Fig. 37.1 Sensory Dermatomes. (From Marx JA, Hockberger RS, Walls RM, et al. *Rosen's Emergency Medicine: Concepts and Clinical Practice.* 6th ed. St Louis, MO: Mosby; 2006.)

posterior spinal arteries branch off the vertebral artery at the cranial base and descend parallel to the spinal cord.[10] Because spinal cord arteries cannot develop collateral blood supply, injuries to these arteries can be devastating.

PATIENT ASSESSMENT

The primary focus for any trauma patient is a primary survey. During the primary survey, the emergency nurse should assess the patient's airway, breathing, and circulation while simultaneously maintaining cervical spinal immobilization. Each trauma patient, especially those with multisystem injuries, should have his or her spine immobilization until an injury is ruled out. Cervical spinal immobilization during an assessment includes manual stabilization until a rigid cervical collar can be placed. The criteria for cervical immobilization will be discussed later in this chapter. In the prehospital setting, agencies may immobilize the spine with a rigid cervical collar, a lateral head block, and a backboard. The patient is fully immobilized on a backboard with the use of straps crossing the chest, abdomen, and knees.[5] After the primary survey has been completed and resuscitation measures have been initiated, the emergency nurse can proceed to the secondary survey.

The secondary survey consists of conducting a head-to-toe examination and obtaining a brief history. During this survey, assessment will determine whether there are any specific injuries sustained or suspected injures due to the mechanism.[11] After the secondary survey is completed, is essential to remove the patient from the long backboard, preferably within 2 hours from time of application.[12] Every effort should be made to remove the rigid spine board due to the risk of decubitus ulcer formation. Removal from the board should not be delayed solely for the purpose of obtaining definitive radiographic evaluation, especially if diagnostics may not be completed for hours.[12] Patients who have sustained spinal trauma, particularly those with sensory losses, are at great risk for developing skin breakdown, placing them at increased risk for additional injury and infection.[6,13]

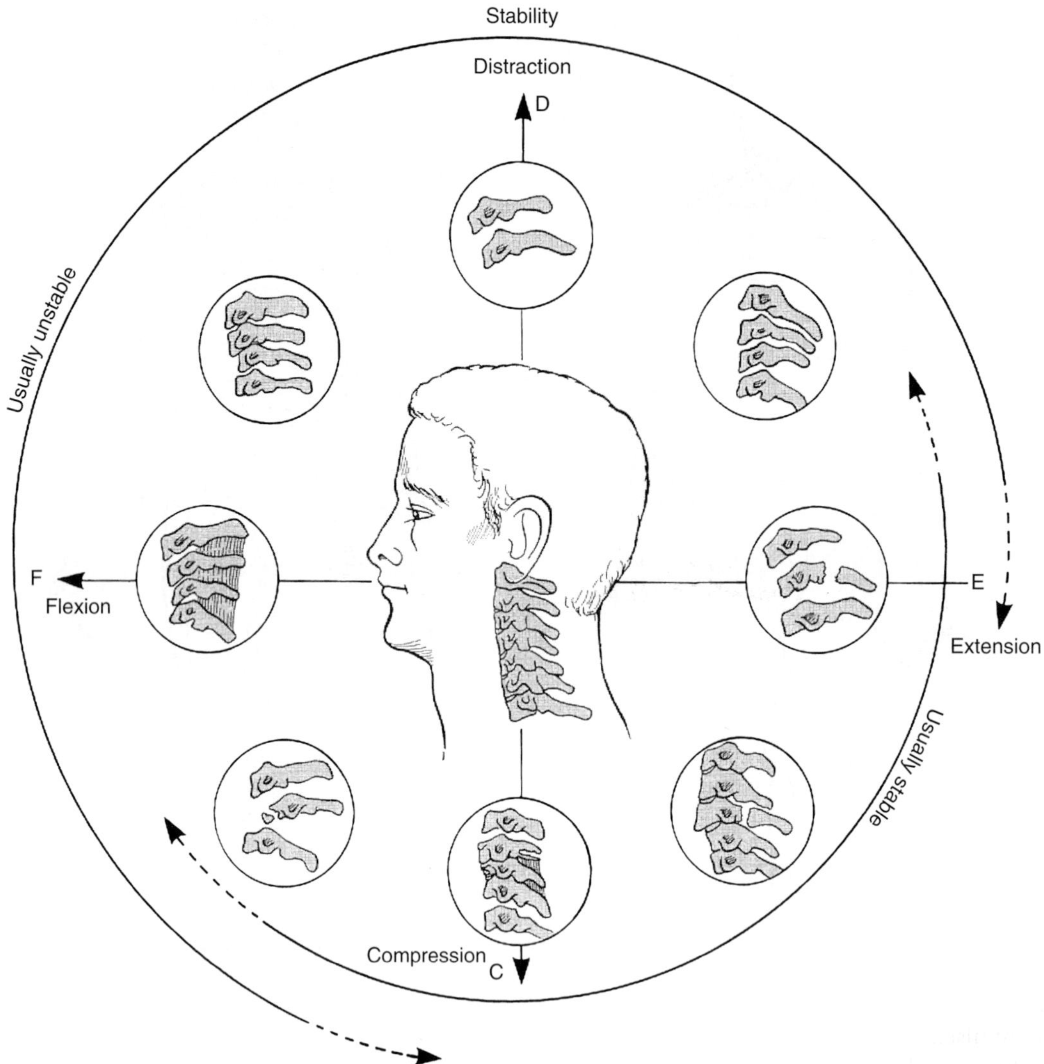

Fig. 37.2 Mechanisms of Injury to the Spine. The mechanism of cervical injury (flexion vs. extension) determines the type of cervical spine fracture or dislocation. (From Moore EE, ed. *Early Care of the Injured Patient.* 3rd ed. Philadelphia, PA: Decker; 1990.)

Mechanisms of Injury

Acute injuries of the spine are classified according to the mechanisms, location, and stability of the injury. Vertebral fractures often occur with or without SCI. The mechanism of the spinal injury can be caused by blunt force trauma or penetration. Cervical spinal injuries can be caused by mechanisms such as axial loading, flexion, extension, rotation, lateral bending, and distraction. These six types of movements can injure the spine and are illustrated in Fig. 37.2 and summarized in Table 37.3.

Special considerations should be focused on the older adult with osteoporosis. Osteoporosis in the older adult patient contributes to a high rate of spinal injury as a result of minimal trauma.[14] These patients are known to experience ground-level falls or a fall from a seated position. A high index of suspicion of a spinal injury or C1–C2 fracture should be considered in this population.[14]

History

In addition to the mechanism of injury, obtaining a thorough history and information on the present illness is key. The emergency nurse should careful when interviewing the patient, prehospital personnel, or the family (or all of these) to determine any "red flags." The following red flags should be noted in the presence of potential spinal trauma:

- complaints of neck or back pain with altered sensation in extremities
- back pain with loss of bowel or bladder control
- significant trauma with altered mental status from intoxication or drug impairment, neck tenderness, history of loss of consciousness, and injuries to the head or face.[11]

The history and present illness should include an assessment of any protective gear worn by the patient, such as seat belts, helmets, or off-road riding gear.

If the patient comes to the ED unresponsive or with altered mental status and cannot provide any details about the injury, the emergency nurse must rely on the prehospital personnel. It is important to obtain the prehospital personnel's initial presentation of the patient, whether extrication was needed, vehicle telemetry (for a motor vehicle crash), protective gear, whether seat belts were used, and treatment provided en

TABLE 37.3 Categories of Movement That May Result in Spinal Cord Injury.

Category	Mechanism of Injury
Hyperextension	The head is forced back, and the vertebrae of the cervical region are placed in an overextended position.
Hyperflexion	The head is forced forward, and the cervical vertebrae are placed in an overflexion position.
Axial loading	A severe blow to the top of the head causes a blunt downward force on the vertebrae and the spinal column.
Compression	Forces from above and below compress the vertebrae.
Lateral bend	The head and neck are bent to one side, beyond the normal range of motion.
Overrotation and distraction	The head turns to one side, and the cervical vertebrae are forced beyond normal limits.

route. Patients who are unconscious or have any altered mental status and those with distracting injuries are at a higher risk for missed cervical spine injury because their injuries are more easily overlooked, and they are unable to report any subjective symptoms.[14]

Inspection

SCIs can disrupt the ventilatory pattern of the patient, which should be addressed in the primary survey. If the patient has an uncompromised airway in the primary survey, then assessment continues with inspection of any abnormalities. The presence of cerebrospinal fluid (CSF) from the nose or ears should be noted for a potential head injury associated with a cervical injury. Due to the high incidence of simultaneous closed head injuries and cervical spine injuries, patients with CSF leaks raise even higher suspicion for serious spinal trauma.[4]

The emergency nurse should observe the patient for obvious signs of spinal injury, including deformity of the vertebral column; cervical edema; and ballistic wounds in the neck, chest, or abdomen. If any of these abnormalities are found, it is essential to maintain spinal restrictions until a spinal column injury or SCI is ruled out. An injury between C3 and C5 can result in progressive respiratory insufficiency secondary to significant respiratory muscle dysfunction. The respiratory muscle dysfunction is primary due to the disruption of the phrenic nerve.[15] Injuries below C5 can lead to decreased intercostal and abdominal muscle dysfunction, in turn altering the mechanics of ventilation and increases the work of breathing.[8,13,15]

Another key observation is the patient's ability to move and perceive pain. It would be concerning to see a patient with decreased movement to extremities, with diminished pain response during procedures such as intravenous and urinary catheterization, or both. This type of response can indicate a form of SCI. A normal response would be the ability to voluntarily follow commands or have pain response to interventions during resuscitation (or both). The presence of a continued penile erection (priapism) can occur with loss of sympathetic nervous system control and may indicate a cervical spine injury.[16]

Palpation

The patient's hemodynamic status should be assessed by the palpation of central pulses for rate and quality. A patient with SCI is at risk for developing neurogenic shock, a critical situation.[11] Neurogenic shock results from a temporary loss of autonomic function, which controls cardiovascular function. Marked hemodynamic and systemic effects are seen and typically result in hypotension, bradycardia, and hypothermia.[11] This condition is considered critical and the patient is managed with pharmacologic agents, which will be discussed later in this chapter.

Next, strength and symmetry of movement in all four extremities should be evaluated. A quick motor evaluation should include flexion and extension of the arms, flexion and extension of the legs, flexion of the foot, extension of the toes, and sphincter tone. In addition to strength and symmetry, sensation should be assessed. Sensory status may be assessed by evaluation of dermatomes (see Fig. 37.1). The patient should be able to distinguish between sharp and dull sensations when a safety pin or cotton swab is used. Testing should begin at the level of no reported sensation and proceed upward to identify the level at which feeling returns. The presence of sacral or perineal sensations should also be assessed.[7] If sacral sensations are present in patients with other focal deficits (termed "sacral sparing"), an incomplete SCI should be suspected.

Injuries above the T4 level usually disrupt the sympathetic nervous system, causing vasodilation below the level of the injury. If the patient is diaphoretic, sweat is present above rather than below the level of the injury. In addition, a patient with SCI becomes poikilothermic, assuming the temperature of his or her surroundings, due to the loss of sympathetic tone. This can leave the patient at great risk for becoming hypothermic.[7]

Finally, the patient's entire spinal column should be gently palpated for pain, tenderness, crepitus, and step-off deformity. Palpation requires the patient to be logrolled by at least four team members to maintain spinal alignment.[8] If the cervical collar is removed for this procedure, manual stabilization must be maintained.

Reflex Testing

The emergency nurse may perform an assessment of the patient's reflexes. Reflexes are summarized in Table 37.4.

Radiographic Evaluation

The diagnosis of SCI or spinal column injury is made with the use of radiographic imaging in conjunction with a clinical assessment. The diagnosis of SCI or vertebrae fracture

TABLE 37.4 Reflexes Tested in Spinal Trauma.

Reflex	Spinal Cord Level
Biceps	C5–C6
Brachioradialis	C5–C6
Triceps	C6–C7
Superficial abdominal (above umbilicus)	T8–T10
Superficial abdominal (below umbilicus)	T10–T12
Knee jerk	L2–L4
Ankle	S1
Anal wink	S2–S4
Plantar response	L5–S1

Data from Bickley L. *Bates' Guide to Physical Examination and History Taking.* 9th ed. Philadelphia, PA: Lippincott Williams & Wilkins; 2007.

traditionally began with the use of x-rays. Commonly a three-view x-ray film series of the cervical spine is obtained, and all seven cervical vertebrae, including the C7–T1 junction, must be visualized to rule out cervical spine injuries.[11,15] When all of the cervical vertebrae cannot be visualized, a swimmer's view (open-mouth series) may be used to evaluate integrity of the odontoid body and C1 and C2 vertebrae.

In trauma patients with a high risk for a spinal column injury or SCI, the provider may proceed directly to a computed tomography (CT) scan. The benefit of a CT scan versus an x-ray is that the CT scan is helpful in determining specific bone anatomy, including where a fracture is located. In addition to a CT scan of the cervical spine, the trauma patient with suspected SCI should have imaging to the thoracic and lumbar spine if indicated. Patients with altered mental status require complete spinal radiographic evaluation.[11] The use of a magnetic resonance imaging (MRI) scan of the spine is helpful for those determined to have SCI and who need more imaging to view the actual cord itself. The MRI scan can also detect any blood clots, herniated discs, or any other masses possibly compressing the spinal cord.[17] In addition, MRI is superior to CT in evaluating spinal cord injury without radiographic abnormality (SCIWORA).[18]

STABILIZATION

Initial stabilization of a patient with spinal trauma begins with recognition and treatment of life-threatening injuries such as airway and vascular compromise. The airway is evaluated while maintaining cervical spine control. Therapeutic interventions are directed at ensuring an adequate airway, maintaining ventilations, supporting adequate circulation, and preventing further injury.

Airway Management

Injuries to the cord at C3 to C5 can result in loss of phrenic nerve function, which results in paralysis of the diaphragm.[15] The patient with cervical spine trauma is at risk for hypoxia, respiratory arrest, and aspiration. SCIs may compromise muscles of respiration, and localized edema can cause airway obstruction, particularly in penetrating neck trauma. Injuries to T1 to T11 can result in loss of intercostal muscle function, which can cause hypoventilation.[15] Initial clearing of the airway may safely be done with a controlled chin lift or jaw thrust. Advanced airway management such as endotracheal intubation should be considered early, especially in patients with injuries at the C5 level or above. Any airway maneuvers require the cervical spine to remain adequately protected. The emergency care team must also initiate interventions to minimize postinjury edema.[8,11,13]

Cervical Spine Protection

Cervical spinal protection guidelines have changed with the establishment of evidence-based data collected by two recognized organizations. The Canadian C-Spine Rule and National Emergency X-radiography Utilization Study (NEXUS) created a criterion to establish clearing those at low risk for cervical injuries. These guidelines have been used in the field for first responders as well as ED staff for patients arriving by private vehicle. The criterion for each of these guidelines determines those at high risk for injury and whether cervical spinal immobilization is recommended. Fig. 37.3 summarizes those guidelines.

If cervical spinal immobilization is required, then the emergency nurse must ensure that spinal protection devices are appropriately applied to prevent further neurologic injury (Box 37.1).[16] The equipment required to protect the cervical spine includes a rigid cervical collar, a lateral head immobilizer, and a full backboard with straps.

A rigid cervical collar is applied to decrease head and neck movement. When applying a cervical collar, the emergency nurse should follow the manufacturer's instructions for size selection and application. Cervical collar application should occur only after the patient's head has been placed in a neutral in-line position, and in-line stabilization should be maintained throughout application. Rigid cervical collars should not obstruct the patient's mouth or airway or interfere with ventilations.

Placing the patient on a backboard does not completely protect the spine. The head must be stabilized laterally with a commercial head immobilizer, towel rolls and tape, or by taping the patient's head to the backboard. Tape or straps should never obstruct the patient's airway. The patient should be secured to the backboard at the chest, abdomen, and knees before the head is secured. Remember: patients should be removed from the backboard within 2 hours from time of application to prevent secondary injuries to the skin.

If the patient has a helmet in place, it should be removed before application of the cervical collar and before the patient is placed on the backboard. Fig. 37.4 illustrate this procedure.

Hemodynamic Management

Patients with spinal trauma may experience hypotension as a result of neurogenic or hypovolemic shock. Injuries to the spinal cord at the level of T6 or above may cause loss of

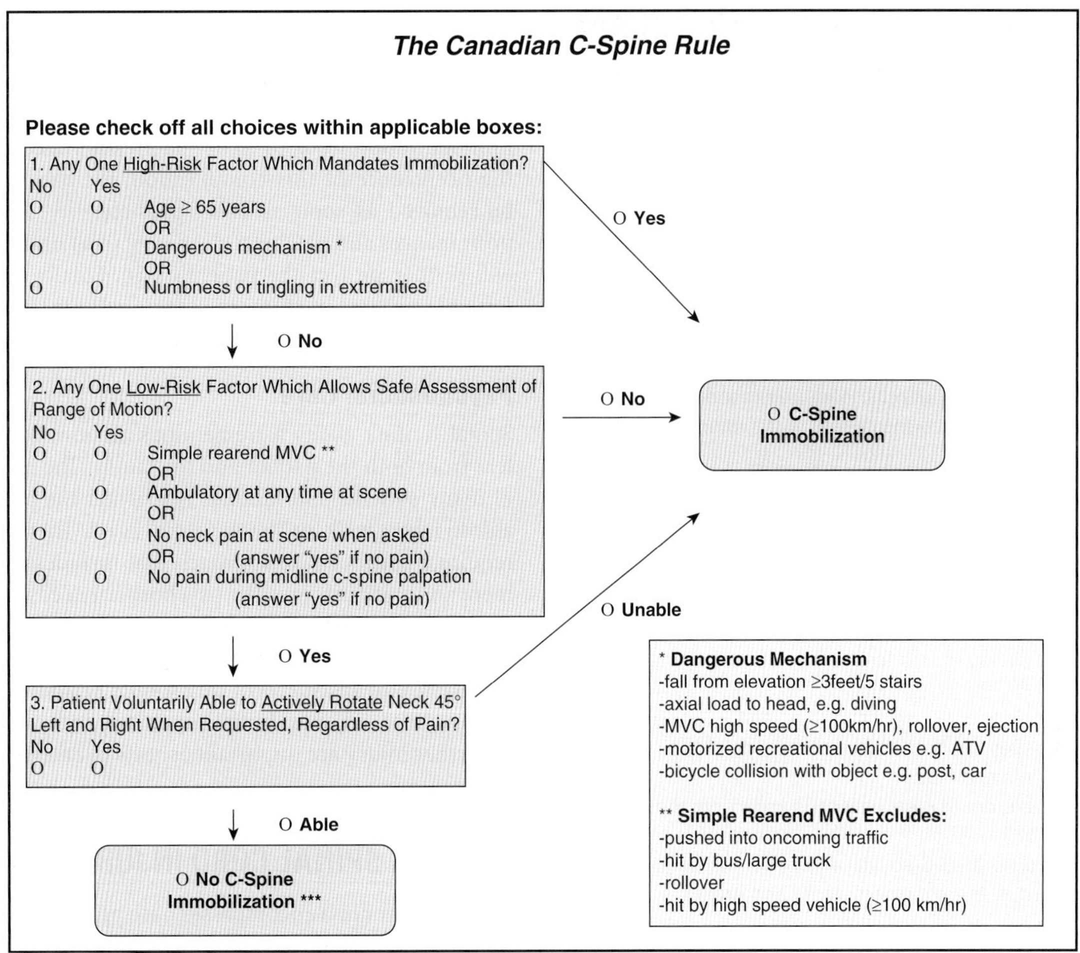

Fig. 37.3 The Canadian C-Spine Rule and NEXUS Criteria. *MVC,* motor vehicle crash. (From Clement WD, Stiell IG, Davies B, et al. Perceived facilitators and barriers to clinical clearance of the cervical spine by emergency department nurses: a major step towards changing practice in emergency department. *Int Emerg Nurs.* 2011;19(1):44-52, and Davenport M. Cervical spine fracture evaluation workup. Medscape website. https://emedicine.medscape.com/article/824380-workup. Updated August 18, 2017. Accessed June 9, 2019)

sympathetic vasomotor tone, leading to hypotension and bradycardia. This shock state (known as neurogenic shock) prevents a compensatory increase in the heart rate in response to hypotension.[5] Neurogenic shock assessment findings include bradycardia, hypotension, warm skin with normal color, and core temperature instability. This loss of sympathetic tone results in compromised perfusion to the spinal cord, which results in loss of function.

Spinal shock is another condition that can be caused by SCI. Spinal shock occurs when there is a disruption in the spinal cord that ceases impulses below the level of the injury. This results in complete loss of reflexes below the level of the injury. A transient episode of hypotension and inability for thermoregulation can be seen. Spinal shock may occur immediately after injury and can last up to 12 months after an injury.

Injuries possibly leading to hypovolemic shock (e.g., tension pneumothorax, hemothorax, or intraabdominal bleeding) should be ruled out. These types of injuries can identified through the use of a bedside ultrasound technique known as focused assessment sonography for trauma (FAST).

If hypotension occurs in the trauma patient with suspected SCI, isotonic crystalloids should be used judiciously to prevent pulmonary edema. If hypotension does not respond with isotonic fluid administration, vasopressor support should be considered.

Pharmacologic Management

The use of high-dose steroids has been controversial over the years, and studies have shown harmful effects with high-dose steroid administration. One study found evidence of significant adverse effects (including death) with administration of high-dose steroids.[19] The use of high-dose steroids such as methylprednisolone is no longer recommended.

Researchers are currently studying new pharmacologic treatment interventions to improve SCI care. Currently, the use of stem cells is being evaluated with regard to improved SCI outcomes.[20] Few human studies have been done, yet several animal studies have shown improved outcomes. One study found that the administration of intravenous bone marrow–derived mesenchymal stem cells (MSCs) can promote functional recovery in rodent models of contusive SCI

BOX 37.1 Spinal Protection Procedure.

Cervical spine stabilization should be performed as a team. Generally, four people should work together. Note that some patients (such as those with a compromised airway, neck deformities, or penetrating injuries) may not be able to tolerate lying flat. Massive neck swelling may result from a penetrating injury and may prohibit the use of a cervical collar. Towel rolls and tape may be a safer method of securing such patients to the board and allowing for evaluation of the patient's injury.

1. Leader is positioned at the head of the patient with hands on each side of the patient's head. Manual in-line stabilization is maintained throughout the entire procedure by placing the leader's hands on the patient with fingers along the mandible.
2. Assess the patient's motor and sensory level by asking the patient to wiggle his or her toes and fingers. Touch the patient's arms and legs to determine sensory response.
3. One assistant applies and secures an appropriately fitting cervical collar. Follow the directions for sizing that come with each collar. An ill-fitting collar can cause pain, occlude the patient's airway, or fail to give appropriate immobilization.
4. Straighten the patient's arms and legs, and position team members so they are both on the same side of the patient at the shoulders and hips.
5. On the leader's count, the patient is rolled on the backboard as a unit.
6. Straps should be placed so that the patient is secured to the backboard at the shoulders, hips, and proximal to the knees.
7. The patient's head should be further immobilized with head blocks or towel rolls. Tape or straps should not be placed across the chin.
8. Manual in-line stabilization is maintained until the head and neck are immobilized.
9. The patient's motor and sensory function should be reassessed after the patient is immobilized.

as well as accelerate the recovery of blood spinal cord barrier integrity.[20,21] The study of stem cell research is ongoing to find the maximal benefit for those with SCI.

Additional Interventions

The patient with acute SCI should have a urinary catheter to facilitate bladder emptying and to monitor urinary output during resuscitation. A gastric tube should be inserted to protect the patient from gastric distention and subsequent aspiration, which can result from decreased peristalsis.[5,12]

The emergency nurse must recognize that the patient with SCI has lost the ability to control body temperature.[22] The patient should be kept warm and protected from unnecessary exposure. Increasing the room temperature, applying warm blankets, and using a commercial warmer and warmed intravenous fluids are interventions to keep the patient normothermic.[23] These interventions are even more crucial in geriatric patients with SCI because older patients have a lower basal metabolic rate and are more prone to problems maintaining body temperature in the absence of injury.[22]

Finally, because patients with spinal injuries may lose the sensations of pain and pressure, skin care is crucial. Prolonged immobilization leads to ischemic pressure ulcers. To reduce the occurrence of this complication, the backboard should be removed as soon as safely possible.[8,13,17] Padding bony prominences and placing a clean, dry sheet under the patient will further protect the patient's skin. Finally, patients with unstable cervical fractures may require some type of external fixation or cervical tong support.

Psychosocial Care

Spinal trauma elicits a tremendous amount of anxiety and fear from both the patient and the family. The major concern of many patients and families is whether the patient will be able to move, walk, or "be the same" again. These patients will require a collaborative approach that includes case management and spiritual care. The psychosocial needs of the patient should be assessed to include spiritual or cultural preferences. The care of the SCI includes the use of a multidisciplinary approach, and all aspects of care should be addressed, including psychosocial ones. Initial supportive care and prevention of further injury are important aspects of emergency nursing interventions.

SPECIFIC SPINAL CORD INJURIES

Spinal cord trauma encompasses both primary and secondary injuries. The initial impact from blunt or penetrating forces results in the primary injury. Examples of primary injuries include vertebral fractures or dislocations, torn ligaments, and spinal cord transections. Fig. 37.5 identifies common fractures of the vertebral column. Secondary injuries to the spinal cord may develop within minutes of the initial injury. Microscopic hemorrhages and edema lead to spinal cord hypoperfusion (often complicated by hypotension in shock states), hypoxia, and endogenous biochemical responses. Secondary injuries extend the initial injury, increase morbidity, and limit future recovery. The emergency nurse must be alert to these and provide interventions to minimize their development.[5,11,21]

Injuries of the vertebral column may occur with or without associated SCI. Although they are the most devastating, not all SCIs involve transection (or severing) of the spinal cord. Contusions, lacerations, vascular damage, hemorrhage, and transection are all possible injuries to the spinal cord. When they do occur, spinal cord transections may be complete or incomplete. Complete spinal cord transections lead to loss of all motor and sensory function below the level of an injury and account for almost 50% of all SCIs.[24] Patients with incomplete spinal cord transections will have partial preservation of some motor or sensory tracts (or both).

Complications related to SCI are based on the location of the injury. An injury to the cervical spine puts the patient at risk for pulmonary and ventilatory problems. A low-thoracic spine injury causes loss of abdominal muscle functions,

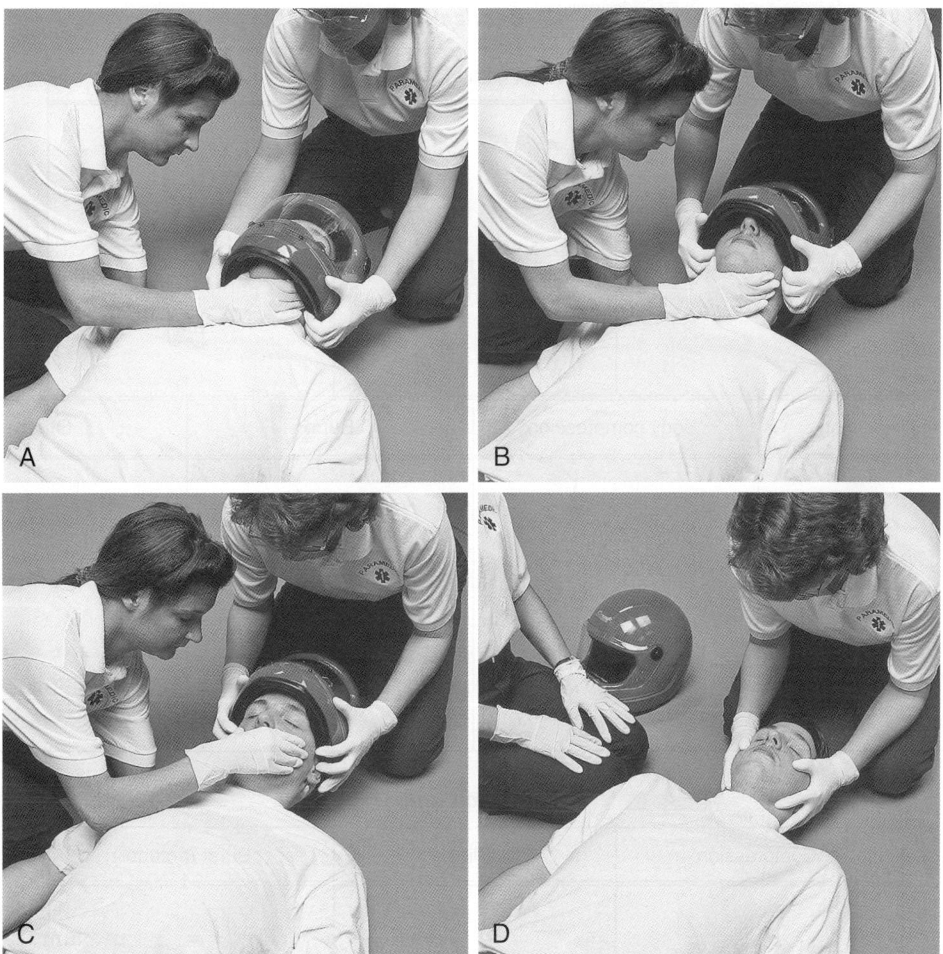

Fig. 37.4 Helmet Removal. (A) The helmet and the head are immobilized in an in-line position. The patient's mandible is grasped by placing the thumb at the angle of the mandible on one side and two fingers at the angle on the other side. The other hand is placed under the neck at the base of the skull, producing in-line immobilization of the patient's head. (B) The side of the helmet is carefully spread away from the patient's head and ears. (C) The helmet is then rotated to clear the nose and removed from the patient's head in a straight line. (D) After removal of the helmet, in-line immobilization is applied, as is a rigid cervical collar. (From Sanders M. *Mosby's Paramedic Textbook*. 2nd ed. St Louis, MO: Mosby; 2000.)

decreased respiratory reserves, and gastric distention. Injury to the lumbosacral area of the spinal cord may cause loss of temperature regulation and bowel and bladder function.[21] Injuries to the spinal cord at any level may lead to muscle flaccidity and the loss of reflexes below the level of injury. Because of decreased mobility from spinal injuries, all patients with SCI are at risk for developing deep vein thrombosis, decubitus ulcers, and pulmonary emboli.[21,22]

Spinal and Neurogenic Shock

When a complete SCI occurs, all motor and sensory functions cease below the level of the injury. Spinal shock is characterized by loss of reflexes and motor and sensory function below the level of the injury. The onset is usually immediate, and the intensity and duration are determined by the level of injury. Patients with spinal shock exhibit flaccid paralysis, areflexia, and bowel or bladder dysfunction. In addition, spinal shock disrupts the patient's ability to thermoregulate the body, causing the patient to assume the temperature of the surrounding air.[21]

Neurogenic shock, a form of distributive shock, may also be seen with injuries above the T6 level.[21] Temporary disruption of the sympathetic nervous system causes bradycardia and hypotension.[16,24] Neurogenic shock leads to further spinal cord hypoperfusion and must be recognized and treated early to prevent further damage to the spinal cord.

Incomplete Spinal Cord Injury

The many types of incomplete cord injuries are classified according to the affected spinal tracts. Regardless of the specific type of injury, patients with incomplete SCIs have asymmetric reflexes and flaccid paralysis, with some preserved sensations below the level of their injury. The specific types of incomplete cord syndromes are based on these characteristics and include central cord syndrome, anterior cord syndrome, posterior cord syndrome, Brown-Séquard syndrome, and nerve root injuries.[24] Confirmation of an incomplete lesion is based on evaluation of sensory and motor functions as defined by the American Spinal Injury Association.

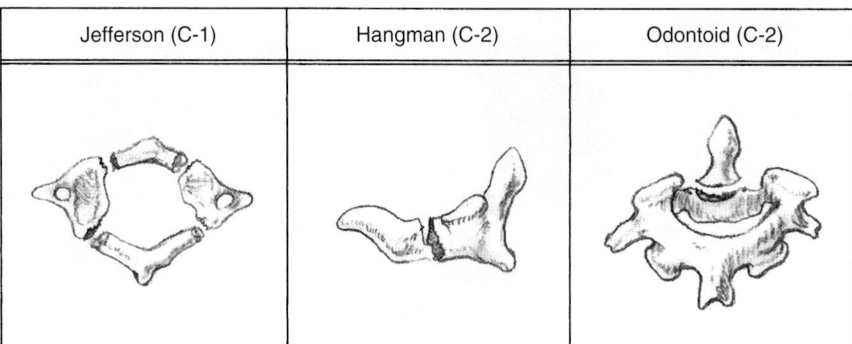

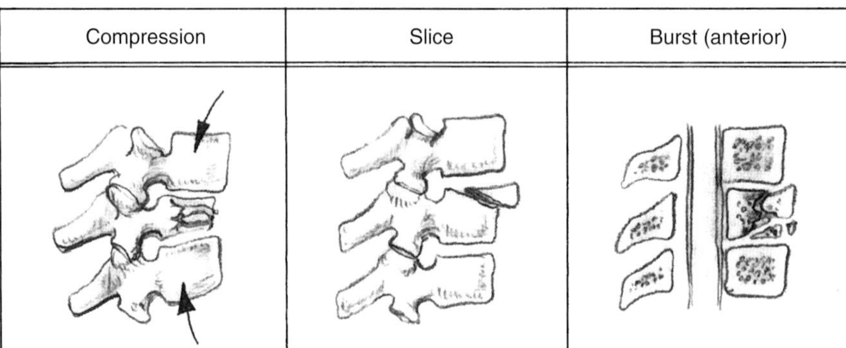

Fig. 37.5 Common Vertebral Column Fractures. (Modified from *Orthopaedic Knowledge: Update–I*. Chicago, IL: American Academy of Orthopaedic Surgeons, 1984.)

Central Cord Syndrome

Central cord syndrome (Fig. 37.6) is caused by hyperextension and results in swelling to the central portion of the spinal cord. This syndrome causes a greater loss of function in the upper extremities than in the lower extremities.[16,24] Bowel and bladder function typically are maintained.

Anterior Cord Syndrome

Anterior cord syndrome (Fig. 37.7) usually results from disruption of the anterior spinal artery, which supplies the motor and sensory pathways in the anterior portion of the spinal cord. The patient has a loss of motor function and pain and temperature sensations below the level of

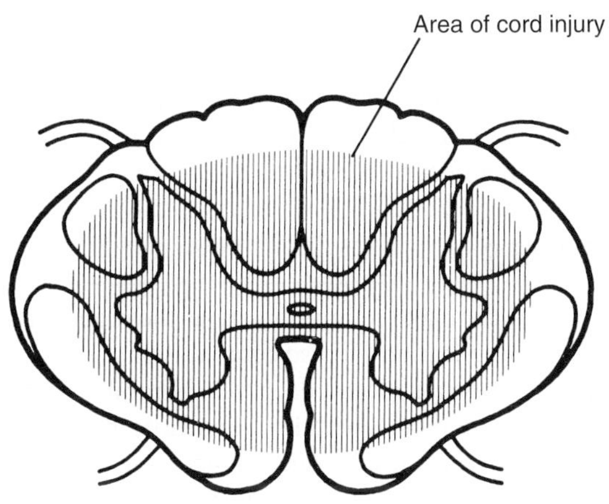

Fig. 37.6 Central Cord Syndrome. (Modified from Rosen P, Barkin RM, Hockberger RS, et al. *Emergency Medicine: Concepts and Clinical Practice.* 4th ed. St Louis, MO: Mosby, 1998.)

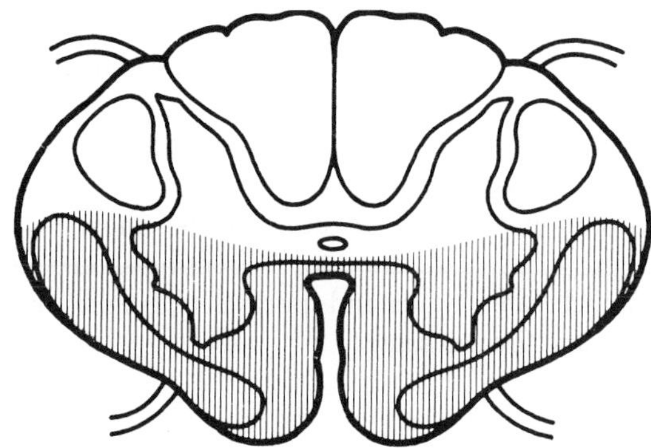

Fig. 37.7 Anterior Cord Syndrome. (Modified from Rosen P, Barkin RM, Hockberger RS, et al. *Emergency Medicine: Concepts and Clinical Practice.* 4th ed. St Louis, MO: Mosby; 1998.)

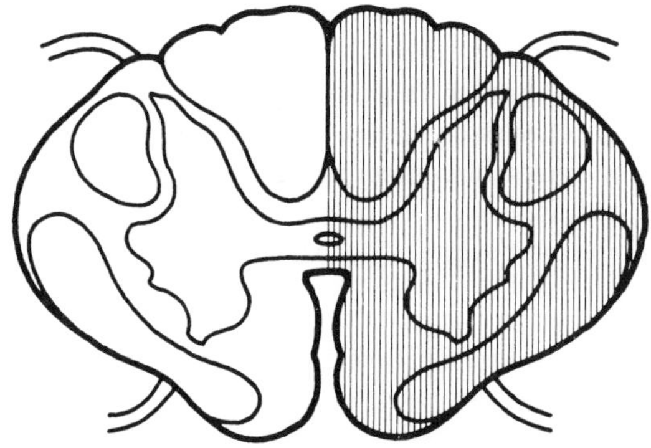

Fig. 37.8 Brown-Séquard Syndrome. (Modified from Rosen P, Barkin RM, Hockberger RS, et al. *Emergency Medicine: Concepts and Clinical Practice.* 4th ed. St Louis, MO: Mosby; 1998.)

the injury. Vibratory sense, touch, pressure, and proprioception remain intact because the posterior column is preserved.[16,24]

Posterior Cord Syndrome

Posterior cord syndrome is rare and results from hyperextension injuries that damage the dorsal column of the spinal cord. Light touch and proprioception are impaired but not completely lost.[24]

Brown-Séquard Syndrome

Brown-Séquard syndrome is an uncommon injury resulting from hemisection of the cord (Fig. 37.8). The most common cause is a penetrating injury such as a gunshot, knife, or missile-fragment penetration. Brown-Séquard syndrome is characterized by ipsilateral (same side) paresis or hemiplegia and loss of motor function, touch, pressure, vibratory sense, and proprioception. Contralateral (opposite side) losses include decreased sensation to pain and temperature changes.[16,24,25]

Nerve Root Injuries

Injuries to nerve roots may also occur as a result of spinal cord trauma. Common injuries include conus medullaris and cauda equina syndromes, both of which result from nerve root compression, most often secondary to other vertebral fractures or disk herniation. Conus medullaris syndrome occurs with compression at the level of T12 and results in flaccid paralysis of the legs with variable sensory deficits below the level of injury. Cauda equina syndrome occurs with compression of the nerve roots below the L1 level of the cord. Patients with cauda equina syndrome present with a triad of symptoms, including saddle paresthesia, bowel or bladder dysfunction, and lower extremity weakness. In both syndromes the patient loses anal sphincter tone.[4,16,24]

Penetrating Injuries

Penetrating injuries to the spinal cord are usually the result of gunshot wounds and stab wounds and account for at least one-fourth of all new SCIs. The emergency nurse should note the presence of any ballistic type of wounds or punctures. If possible, the emergency nurse should try to obtain the specific caliber of weapon to determine the possible number of fragments. For penetrating objects, the exact path is not known, and the visceral injuries must be suspected and ruled out. If the missile passes through the abdominal viscera into the spinal cord, the patient is at great risk for central nervous system infection, and antibiotic prophylaxis is required. If the patient is brought to the ED with a penetrating object in place, the emergency nurse should leave the object in place and stabilize it.[23,26,27] Bullets and wounding objects such as a knife are evidence and should be handled carefully to maintain integrity for investigation.

Spinal Cord Injury Without Radiographic Abnormality

SCIWORA is a condition in which neurologic deficits are present in the absence of identified radiographic abnormalities on plain films or on CT scans. Although most often seen in the pediatric population, SCIWORA is not uncommon in middle-aged or geriatric patients and accounts for up to 12% of SCI.[27] In children, the condition is often attributed to anatomic differences allowing for ligamentous laxity in the cervical spine. In adults, disc prolapse and cervical spondylosis have also been noted as causes in addition to ligamentous injuries. As previously discussed, MRI has been found invaluable in diagnosing this condition.[28]

Autonomic Dysreflexia

Autonomic dysreflexia is a complication of SCI above the T6 level occurring anytime after the resolution of spinal shock. This life-threatening emergency occurs when stimulation of the sympathetic nervous system leads to a massive, uncontrolled cardiovascular response. Multiple stimuli below the level of injury can trigger this response. Commonly, a full bowel or bladder is responsible for triggering the response, but stimulation of the skin or cutaneous pain receptors may also cause an autonomic dysreflexia crisis. Signs and symptoms of autonomic dysreflexia include sudden severe headache, hypertension, nausea, bradycardia, and sweating above the level of injury with coolness below the level of injury. The patient may also complain of nasal stuffiness and appear quite anxious.[26]

Treatment of autonomic dysreflexia begins with identifying the cause of the sympathetic response. Once the cause of the dysreflexia is identified, such as a full bladder or constipation, the nurse can begin to rapidly intervene. If the bladder is full, inserting a urinary catheter or irrigating an existing one may relieve the symptoms. Medications to relieve constipation or urinary retention, as well as antihypertensive medications, may be administered.[26] When medications are used to lower a patient's blood pressure, the patient must be closely monitored to prevent a precipitous drop in blood pressure and to quickly identify any serious complications. After the emergency is resolved, the emergency nurse should work with the patient and the family to develop interventions to prevent another occurrence.

OUTCOMES

Patients with complete tetraplegia are at the highest risk for secondary complications. These complications are known as pneumonia, pressure ulcers, deep vein thrombosis, pulmonary embolism, and postoperative wound infections. Pressure ulcerations are the most frequently observed complication seen during the first year after injury.[7] The most common pressure ulceration has been noted to the sacrum.

PREVENTION

The improvement in emergency care and rehabilitation has allowed many patients with SCI to survive. Although current research studies of decompression surgery, nerve cell transplantation, and nerve regeneration are being conducted to improve SCI outcomes, there is currently no cure. Ultimately, SCI prevention is crucial to decrease the impact of these injuries on society. Education for prevention should include motor vehicle safety, water and sport safety, fall prevention in the home, and firearm safety.

SUMMARY

Spinal trauma is not as common as other types of injury, but its consequences are devastating. Its impact is extremely expensive and far-reaching across the population. Patients are generally young and require extensive physical and psychosocial care, often for the remainder of their lives. Emergency care of these patients involves stabilization and resuscitation to decrease and prevent further injury to the spinal cord.

Current research focuses on preventing and treating the effects of secondary injuries occurring with spinal cord damage and regrowth of the damaged cells.[21] Techniques for regeneration of the injured spinal cord tissue through stem cell transplantation and gene therapy are also being studied.[21]

Regardless of advances in research and treatment, the most successful way to lessen the impact of spinal trauma is prevention. Some methods currently used to prevent spinal injury are using seat belts, air bags, improvements in new car construction such as reinforced side compartments, helmets, and other safety devices.[29] Teaching children, adolescents, and adults the consequences of risky behavior, extreme sports, and firearm safety may eventually help decrease the uncommon but devastating consequences of this injury.

REFERENCES

1. Hasler RM, Exadaktylos AK, Bouamra O, et al. Epidemiology and predictors of cervical spine injury in adult major trauma patients: a multicenter cohort study. *J Trauma Acute Care Surg*. 2012;72(4):975–981.
2. Clayton JL, Harris MB, Weintraub SL, et al. Risk factors for cervical spine injury. *Injury*. 2012;43(4):431–435.
3. Wilczweski P, Grimm D, Gianakis A, et al. Risk factors associated with pressure ulcer development in critically ill traumatic spinal cord injury patients. *J Trauma Nurs*. 2012;19(1):5–10.
4. Urdaneta F, Layon AJ. Respiratory complications in patients with traumatic cervical spine injuries: case report and review of the literature. *J Clin Anesth*. 2003;15(5):398–405.
5. Theodore N, Aarabi B, Dhall SS, et al. Transportation of patients with acute traumatic cervical spine injuries. *Neurosurg*. 2013;72(suppl 3):35–39.
6. Funk JR, Cormier JM, Manoogian SJ. Comparison of risk factors for cervical spine, head, serious, and fatal injury in rollover crashes. *Accid Anal Prev*. 2012;45:67–74.
7. Seeley R, Stephens T, Tate P. *Anatomy and Physiology*. 6th ed. Boston, MA: McGraw-Hill; 2003.
8. Morgan K, McCance K. Alterations of the reproductive system. In: McCance K, Huether S, eds. *Pathophysiology: The Biologic Basis for Disease in Adults and Children*. St Louis, MO: Mosby; 2006.
9. Waxman S, deGroot J. *Correlative Neuroanatomy*. Norwalk, CT: Appleton & Lange; 1995.

10. Sugerman R. Structure and function of the neurologic system. In: McCance K, Huether S, eds. *Pathophysiology: The Biologic Basis for Disease in Adults and Children*. St Louis, MO: Mosby; 2006.
11. Urden LD, Stacy KM, Lough ME. *Priorities in Critical Care Nursing*. 7th ed. St Louis, MO: Elsevier Health Sciences; 2015.
12. Martin AR, Aleksanderek I, Fehlings MG. Diagnosis and acute management of spinal cord injury: current best practices and emerging therapies. *Curr Trauma Rep*. 2015;1(3):169–181.
13. Harris MB, Sethi RK. The initial assessment and management of the multiple-trauma patient with an associated spine injury. *Spine (Phila Pa 1976)*. 2006;31(suppl 11):S9–S15.
14. O'Neill S, Brady RR, Kerssens JJ, Parks RW. Mortality associated with traumatic injuries in the elderly: a population-based study. *Archiv Gerontol Geriatri*. 2012;54(3):e426–e430.
15. Clement WD, Stiell IG, Davies B, et al. Perceived facilitators and barriers to clinical clearance of the cervical spine by emergency department nurses: a major step towards changing practice in emergency department. *Int Emerg Nurs*. 2011;19(1):44–52.
16. Michaleff ZA, Maher CG, Verhagen AP, Rebbeck T, Lin CWC. Accuracy of the Canadian C-spine rule and NEXUS to screen for clinically important cervical spine injury in patients following blunt trauma: a systematic review. *CMAJ*. 2012;184(16):E867–E876. https://doi.org/10.1503/cmaj.120675.
17. Chew BG, Swartz C, Quigley MR, Altman DT, Daffner RH, Wilberger JE. Cervical spine clearance in the traumatically injured patient: is multidetector CT scanning sufficient alone? Clinical article. *J Neurosurg: Spine*. 2013;19(5):576–581.
18. Cohen W, Giauque A, Hallam D, et al. Evidence-based approach to use of MR imaging in acute spinal trauma. *Eur J Radiol*. 2003;48(1):49–60.
19. Wang HT, Williamson J, Albert MA. Predictors of ventilatory outcome in cervical spinal injuries. *Crit Care*. 2014;18(suppl 1):450.
20. Schroeder GD, Kwon BK, Eck JC, Savage JW, Hsu WK, Patel AA. Survey of Cervical Spine Research Society members on the use of high-dose steroids for acute spinal cord injuries. *Spine*. 2014;39(12):971–977.
21. Ryu H-H, Kang BJ, Park SS, et al. Comparison of mesenchymal stem cells derived from fat, bone marrow, Wharton's jelly, and umbilical cord blood for treating spinal cord injuries in dogs. *J Vet Med Sci*. 2012;74(12):1617–1630.
22. Kanwar R, Delasobera BE, Hudson K, Frohna W. Emergency department evaluation and treatment of cervical spine injuries. *Emerg Med Clin North Am*. 2015;33(2):241–282.
23. Rahimi-Movaghar V, Sayyah MK, Akbari H, et al. Epidemiology of traumatic spinal cord injury in developing countries: a systematic review. *Neuroepidemiol*. 2013;41(2):65–85.
24. Boss B. Alterations of neurologic function. In: McCance K, Huether S, eds. *Pathophysiology: The Biologic Basis for Disease in Adults and Children*. St Louis, MO: Mosby; 2006.
25. Fehlings MG, Vaccaro A, Wilson JR, et al. Early versus delayed decompression for traumatic cervical spinal cord injury: results of the Surgical Timing in Acute Spinal Cord Injury Study (STASCIS). *PloS One*. 2012;7(2):e32037.
26. Kuster D, Gibson A, Abboud R, Drew T. Mechanisms of cervical spine injury in rugby union: a systematic review of the literature. *Br J Sports Med*. 2012;46(8):550–554.
27. McDonald JW, Becker D, Huettner J. Spinal cord injury. In: Lanza A, Atala A, eds. *Handbook of Stem Cells*. 2nd ed. St Louis, MO: Elsevier; 2013:723–738.
28. Boese CK, Lechler P. Spinal cord injury without radiologic abnormalities in adults: a systematic review. *J Trauma Acute Care Surg*. 2013;75(2):320–330.
29. Dididze M, Green BA, Dietrich WD, Vanni S, Wang MY, Levi AD. Systemic hypothermia in acute cervical spinal cord injury: a case-controlled study. *Spinal Cord*. 2013;51(5):395–400.

38

Thoracic Trauma

Nancy J. Denke

Thoracic trauma is a significant source of morbidity and mortality, accounting for 20% to 25% of trauma-related deaths in adults.[1] These life-threatening injuries occur due to major disruptions of the airway or impaired breathing, lethal alterations in circulation (injury to the heart and/or great vessels), or reactions of other organ functions as a secondary consequence of hypoxia or impaired circulation.[2] We can fix most of these life-threatening injuries occurring in the first 30 minutes to 3 hours by administering blood or using some type of tube (simple thoracotomy, endotracheal), or pericardiocentesis. The incidence of these injuries has increased markedly over the past 100 years due to high-speed vehicular travel and interpersonal violence. In children, thoracic trauma is comparatively uncommon and is often more devastating due to differences in a child's anatomy and physiology.[3]

Thoracic trauma can result from either penetrating or blunt trauma, causing a spectrum of injuries ranging from a simple rib fracture to severe vital organ injuries. Mechanism of injury, force, trajectory, type of weapon, angle of impact, proximity to the patient, secondary factors such as fire, and overall physical attributes of the patient determine the degree and type of injury. Understanding the mechanism of injury and energy transfer can help predict injuries and injury patterns. The physical nature of the chest wall allows for considerable elastic recoil; therefore the severity of thoracic trauma may need to be assessed. The focus should be on the potential for underlying damage based on mechanism of injury rather than on the initial appearance of the patient. The pediatric thorax is much more pliable than the adult thorax, allowing the chest to absorb a large amount of kinetic energy from any impact; this energy is then transferred to the intrathoracic structures, resulting in a child experiencing major intrathoracic injury with minimal or no injury to the structure of the chest.[3]

Blunt and penetrating injuries may be sustained in all types of trauma; therefore anticipation is key to the prompt management of patients with thoracic trauma. Blunt trauma is more common than penetrating injuries to the thorax, accounting for approximately 90% of all thoracic injuries, of which less than 10% require surgical intervention of any kind.[4] Blunt trauma may be caused by motor vehicle incidents, falls, exploding tires, or any mechanism where the force of impact (particularly sudden deceleration, compression, or a direct blow) causes internal structural damage to the chest wall, parenchyma, pleura, diaphragm, heart, trachea, and/or great vessels.

Penetrating thoracic trauma, although less common, brings with it a higher mortality. Penetrating injuries can be divided into low- and high-velocity injuries. Low-velocity injuries, such as those sustained from a hand-initiated "sharp force injury" (stab or puncture; incised/slash; or chopped wound), can produce localized tissue damage along the course of the object with a predictable pattern when the size, shape, and length of the object is known. Other factors that may influence the path are the position of and the distance between the victim and the assailant; the height, and strength of the assailant; and the angle of the weapon. The sex of the assailant is also important: women tend to stab downward, whereas men tend to stab upward with more force than women; subsequently, penetration is deeper.[5] High-velocity injuries are a direct consequence of a projectile's kinetic energy applied to any tissue or organs that may be in its path. These projectiles can rotate and create a permanent cavity; change shape when coming into contact with tissue; or shatter or ricochet within the chest cavity.

Another type of injury that can be classified as both blunt and penetrating is an injury sustained from kinetic-impact projectiles, commonly called rubber or plastic bullets. These projectiles are designed to incapacitate individuals by inflicting pain and limit kinetic energy on impact to prevent penetrating injury.[6] A review of 26 studies found that injuries from these types of projectiles can cause various degrees of injury (minor, permanent disability, or even death), with 27% of such injuries sustained to the abdomen and/or chest.[6]

Thoracic injury and treatment have been described for centuries; however, it was not until the end of World War II that a chest tube connected to underwater seal drainage became standard treatment for many thoracic injuries. Endotracheal intubation, anesthesia, and chest x-ray examinations developed in the 19th and early 20th centuries, and advances in the past 50 years, such as improved ventilatory assistance, antibiotics, blood gas analysis, and specialized nursing care, have increased survival in patients with thoracic injuries. Despite these advances, mortality rates for thoracic trauma remain high, making thoracic trauma the third most common cause of death after abdominal injury and head trauma in polytrauma patients.[7]

Thoracic trauma requires a systematic assessment for potentially lethal injuries followed by rapid intervention to prevent unnecessary complications and death. Ninety percent of patients with thoracic trauma can be managed by simple lifesaving treatments not requiring surgical interventions.[1] This chapter discusses assessment and treatment of various thoracic injuries. Understanding the anatomy and physiology is essential.

ANATOMY AND PHYSIOLOGY

The thoracic cavity skeleton includes the sternum, ribs, costal cartilages, and thoracic vertebrae, with the vital organs being protected by these bones. The thorax is fairly mobile and expands easily to accommodate respiratory efforts. The ribs are elastic arches of bone attaching posteriorly to thoracic vertebrae and anteriorly to the sternum. Seven upper ribs are joined directly to costal cartilages (CC), whereas ribs 8, 9, and 10 interface indirectly with the sternum through fusion of costal cartilage.[8] Ribs 11 and 12 do not interface with the sternum. (In other words, the CC of ribs 17 attach directly to the sternum, whereas those of ribs 1112 are floating).[9,10] The external intercostal muscles originate on the inferior surfaces of the proximal portions of the ribs and insert on the superior and distal portions of the next lower rib. Beneath each rib lies a neurovascular bundle, containing an intercostal nerve, artery, and vein. The sternum has three parts: the manubrium, the body (corpus), and the xiphoid process (tip). The diaphragm forms the inferior border of the thorax, whereas the superior border is continuous with structures of the neck.

Internal thoracic structures are composed of organs and structures of the pulmonary, cardiovascular, and gastrointestinal systems (Fig. 38.1).[8] Pulmonary structures are located in the pleural space, whereas cardiovascular structures are located in the mediastinum, a cavity between the two pleural spaces.

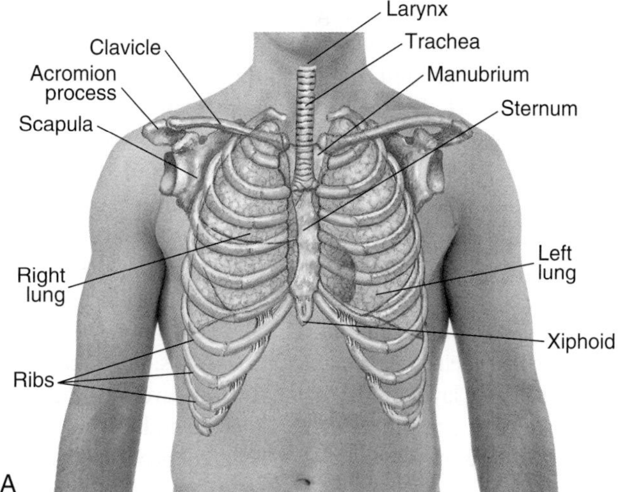

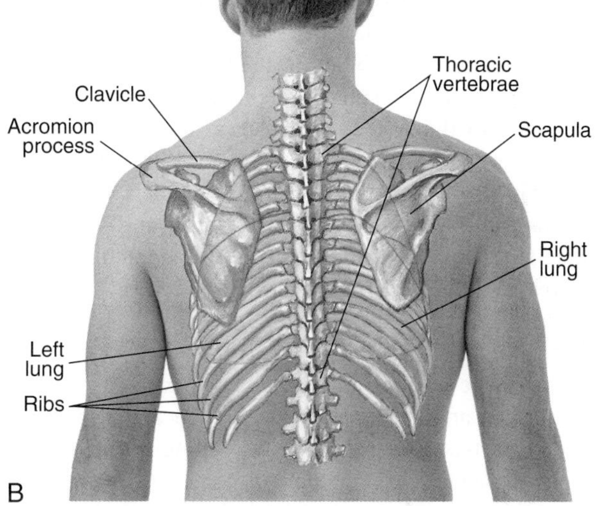

Fig. 38.1 Chest and Anatomic Landmarks (From Thompson JM, Wilson SF. Health assessment for nursing practice. St Louis, MO: Mosby; 1996. In: Ball JE, Dains JW, Flynn JA, Solomon B, Stewart RW. *Seidel's Guide to Physical Examination: An Interventional Approach.* 9th ed. St Louis, MO: Elsevier; 2017.)

Pulmonary System

Lungs are cone-shaped organs above the diaphragm extending approximately 1 inches above the clavicles. Each lung is located in a cavity lined with a serous membrane called the pleura. The visceral pleura covers the lungs, whereas the parietal pleura covers the rib cage, diaphragm, and pericardium. A potential space between these layers is the pleural cavity. Pleural cells secrete pleural fluid, which separates the lungs but allows membranes to remain in contact and move without creating friction.

Normal breathing occurs through the processes of ventilation, which moves air in and out of the lungs, and respiration, which exchanges gases across alveolar-capillary membranes. During inspiration, phrenic nerve stimulation causes the diaphragm to contract and pull downward. As the diaphragm pulls downward, it provides the force for expansion. This process is passive and requires no muscles. The external intercostals aid in the inspiration process by enlarging the thoracic cavity. The abdominal muscles and internal intercostals aid forceful expiration. These muscles move the chest wall and not the lungs, but the lungs follow because of the thin fluid in the pleura, which pastes the lungs to the chest wall.[11] The lungs have a surface tension that is reduced by surfactant, which stabilizes alveoli size while keeping the alveoli dry and reduces the work of breathing.[11] As lung capacity increases, intrathoracic pressure becomes negative (i.e., lower than atmospheric pressure). This negative intrathoracic pressure draws air into the lungs. During expiration, this process is reversed as the diaphragm relaxes and moves up. Intercostal muscles compress the chest so the lungs act as a spring and recoil passively and compress the lungs. Intrathoracic pressure becomes more positive as lung capacity diminishes.[11] These muscle movements and subsequent pressure changes cause air to either rush in or be forced out of the lungs.

Cardiovascular System

The heart is located in the mediastinum and is positioned with the right ventricle anteriorly beneath the sternum in the mediastinum. The pericardium is a fibroserous sac surrounding and protecting the heart. The outer fibrous (layer) pericardium securely anchors its connections within the thoracic cavity and maintains the general thoracic position of the heart. The serous (layer) pericardium, is divided into two layers, the *parietal pericardium,* which is fused to and inseparable from the fibrous pericardium, and the *visceral pericardium,* which is part of the epicardium. There is a narrow potential space between the two pericardial layers. Under normal circumstances, this potential space holds between 15 to 50 mL of fluid with its function consisting of lubrication of the heart to prevent friction during heart activity.[12]

The heart itself is composed of three layers: the epicardium (the outermost layer of the heart), the myocardium (the middle, voluminous muscular layer), and the endocardium (the innermost layer of tissue lining the chambers of the heart).

Four muscular chambers, two atria and two ventricles, contract rhythmically as they fill and empty with blood. The right atrium and ventricle receive deoxygenated blood from the body and pump the blood to the lungs for oxygenation. Oxygenated blood then enters the left side of the heart, which sends blood to the systemic circulation through the aorta. The left heart is a high-pressure system; the right heart a low-pressure system. Valves separate chambers to prevent regurgitation of blood back into the atria and ventricles. Cardiac function and output depend on contractility, heart rate, preload (volume achieved during diastolic filling of the ventricles), and afterload (force or resistance against which the heart must pump to eject blood).

The thoracic aorta carries oxygenated blood to various tissues. Three anatomic parts of the aorta are recognized: ascending aorta, aortic arch, and descending aorta. The aortic arch is attached to the pulmonary artery by the ligamentum arteriosum (a remnant of fetal circulation whose true function is unknown). Near the ligamentum, a portion of the aorta branches off to form the left subclavian artery. At this point the aorta, just distal to the ligamentum, is relatively immobile and carries with it an increased risk for disruption. More than 80% to 90% of aortic injuries caused by acceleration or deceleration forces occur at this site.[1]

The mediastinum also contains the trachea, located posterior to the heart; the esophagus, posterior to the trachea; the phrenic and vagus nerves; and the diaphragm. Other thoracic cavity structures include the thymus gland in the anterior mediastinum behind the sternum and the subclavian and common carotid arteries. The mediastinum is bordered by T4 (superior) to T9 (inferior).

PATIENT ASSESSMENT

The patient with obvious or suspected thoracic trauma must be promptly assessed. Fractures of the thoracic structures provide information concerning the dose of energy the patient received. Injury to thoracic structures may and can produce life-threatening alterations in ventilation and perfusion within minutes. Rapid assessment and intervention to support airway, breathing, and circulation (ABCs) are crucial. Protection of the cervical spine occurs simultaneously with assessment of airway patency. Assessment of rate, depth, and effort of breathing performed in conjunction with auscultation of breath sounds and inspection for symmetry and chest wall integrity is performed to identify overt and subtle injuries to the thorax. Recognizing changes in ventilation is of utmost importance in the care of the patient with thoracic trauma. Using various parameters such as end-tidal CO_2 and arterial CO_2 in conjunction with respiratory assessment can augment visual evaluation of the patient to improve outcomes.

Supplemental oxygen is administered with a 100% nonrebreather mask or bag-mask device to maintain adequate oxygenation and ventilation. Lifesaving interventions required during the initial patient assessment may include application of a three-sided occlusive dressing for an open pneumothorax and needle thoracentesis (decompression) for a tension pneumothorax. Assessment of circulation is performed by palpating the central and peripheral pulses for quality, rate, skin color/temperature, and capillary refill. Obvious external bleeding is controlled with direct pressure. Internal bleeding is initially managed with replacement of intravascular volume; two large-bore intravenous lines should be established and warmed crystalloids (0.9% normal saline or lactated Ringers solution), 1 L infused at a rapid rate, with the possible initiation of blood and blood products. Box 38.1 highlights initial assessment of the patient with thoracic trauma. Therapeutic interventions are listed in Box 38.2.

The focused assessment sonography for trauma (FAST) or extended FAST (eFAST)[13] examination has become an integral component of the initial assessment for patients with both blunt and penetrating trauma to the thorax. It is a rapid, noninvasive diagnostic study that can be performed at the bedside. Table 38.1 describes strengths and limitations of the FAST examination.) The subxiphoid view obtained in this four-view study allows for the most rapid identification of pericardial injury. The interpretation is straightforward: a positive subxiphoid examination is defined as detection of pericardial fluid on the cardiac window. The sensitivity of the FAST examination for detecting blood in the pericardial space has been reported at 96% to 100%.[13]

In the mid-2000s, the addition of ultrasound evaluation of the thorax to detect pneumothorax to the traditional FAST examination resulted in extended FAST (eFAST).[14] With eFAST, there have been several protocols developed for evaluation of shock, respiratory distress, and cardiac arrest. The RUSH (rapid US for shock and hypotension) protocol appears to be the most sensitive tool in evaluation of hypovolemia when added to the eFAST examination. It involves a three-part physiologic assessment of the **pump**; **tank**; and **pipes**[15,16] (See Fig. 38.2).

SPECIFIC THORACIC INJURIES

Thoracic injuries (Box 38.3) include injuries of the chest wall, pulmonary system, cardiovascular system, and esophagus. Fractures of the thoracic structures (ribs 13, scapula, posterior ribs, sternum, clavicle and T210 vertebral bodies)[17] provide information relating to the dose of energy received and the effects on ventilation and circulation.

BOX 38.1 Initial Assessment of Thoracic Trauma.

Airway Patency in Conjunction With Cervical Spine Protection
Any abnormal sounds
Hemoptysis
Level of consciousness

Effective Ventilation (Breathing): Any Loss of the Integrity of Lungs or Diaphragm may Compromise Ventilation
Spontaneous breathing
Symmetric rise and fall of the chest
Rate and pattern of breathing (such as shortness of breath, paradoxical chest wall movement, respiratory stridor, tachypnea)
Use of accessory muscles, diaphragmatic breathing, or both
Skin color (such as cyanosis)
Integrity of the soft tissues and bony structures of the chest wall and neck (such as sucking chest wound, impaled objects, subcutaneous emphysema, edema/hematomas, upper abdominal injury)
Bilateral breath sounds: equal, diminished, or absent
Tracheotomy

Circulation
Uncontrolled hemorrhage
Skin color, temperature, and moisture
Heart sounds: normal, rubs, distant or muffled
Heart rate and rhythm
Becks triad: hypotension, jugular venous distention (JVD), muffled heart tones
Blood pressure in upper extremities (equal or asymmetric)
Comparison of extremity pulses (equal, diminished, or absent)

Additional Considerations
Pattern of abrasions or bruising
Wound size and location

Chest Wall Injuries

Many thoracic injuries have associated chest wall injuries. An intact chest wall is essential to normal ventilation.

Costal Cartilage Injury

CC is important in the anatomy of the thorax. This chest cartilage allows movement of the rib cage during breathing. Although radiologic findings in chest trauma have been widely described in the literature, costal cartilage fractures are often overlooked in trauma patients (especially in the lower anterior ribs) despite being an indicator of severe thoracic trauma, contributing to rib cage instability as a part of flail chest and frequent association with injuries of other organs.[10,11] CC fractures are frequently seen with high-energy blunt trauma (motor vehicle crashes [MVCs] and falls). These fractures may manifest clinically as late as weeks or months after the acute trauma.[10,11] Computed tomography (CT), magnetic resonance imaging, and ultrasound scans have been the proven diagnostic tests and are treated conservatively.

BOX 38.2 Therapeutic Interventions for Thoracic Trauma.

Maintain Patent Airway
Promote adequate ventilation
Provide high-flow oxygen
Assist ventilations
Prepare for intubation
Cover open chest wound with a three-sided, nonporous dressing
Assist with chest tube insertion or needle thoracentesis (decompression)
Monitor bleeding from chest or drainage from chest tube
Prepare for autotransfusion
Initiate two large-bore intravenous lines

Facilitate Essential Imaging–ultrasonography, Radiography, Computed Tomography
Continuous monitoring of cardiac rhythm
Monitor blood pressure, respiratory rate and effort, pulse oximetry, and level of consciousness every hour or more often if indicated by patient condition
Document urine output and patient response to therapeutic interventions
Facilitate surgical intervention

TABLE 38.1 Strengths and Limitations of the eFAST (extended FAST) Examination.

Strengths	Limitations
• Rapid (2-3 minutes) • Portable • Noninvasive • Can be done serially • Sensitive and specific for free fluid is equal to a DPL or CT • Inexpensive • Minimal volume 100 mL for detection of free fluid	• Does not identify the source of bleeding or injuries not causing a hemoperitoneum • Operator dependent: accuracy improves after 25-50 examinations • Obesity and subcutaneous air may interfere with the examination • Detection of blunt mesenteric, bowel, diaphragmatic, and retroperitoneal injuries can be difficult • Volume of free fluid necessary to enable detection

CT, Computed tomography; *DPL*, diagnostic peritoneal lavage.

Rib Fractures

Rib fractures are the most common thoracic injury due to blunt injury and are associated with 20% of all thoracic traumas.[18] Fractures result from a direct or indirect blunt force or crush injury. MVCs and falls are the most common mechanisms of injury associated with rib fractures in the adult population. In the pediatric population, rib fractures are commonly the result of intentional injury in younger children, with recreational/athletic injuries being more common in the older pediatric population. Rib fractures in older adults are commonly seen with falls and MVCs and carry with them

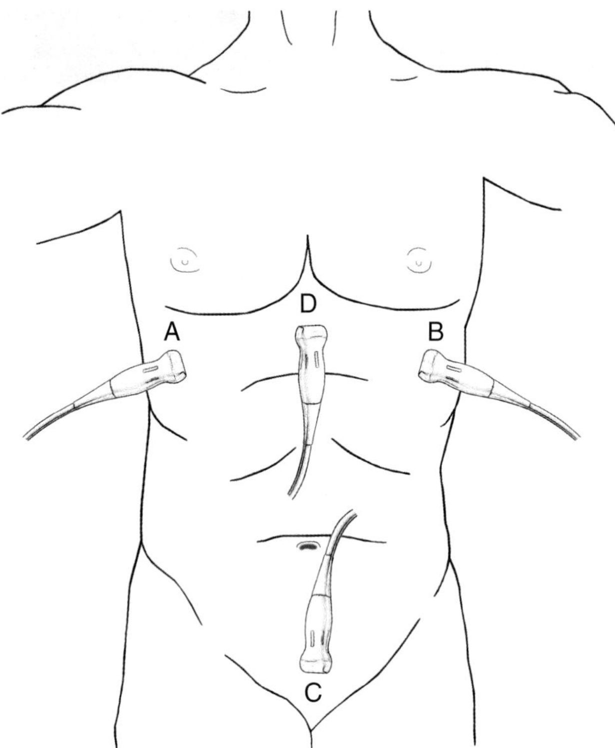

Fig. 38.2 **Extended FAST (eFAST) Landmarks** The four views for the original FAST scan are as follows: (A) right upper quadrant, (B) left upper quadrant, (C) suprapubic view, and (D) subxiphoid view of the heart. (From Richards JR, McGahan JP. Focused assessment with sonography in trauma (FAST) in 2017: What radiologists can learn. *Radiology.* 2017;283(1):30-48.)

BOX 38.3 Chest Injuries: Life-Threatening Versus Potential Lethal.

Life-Threatening Injuries	Potentially Lethal Injuries
Airway obstruction	Simple pneumothorax
Tension pneumothorax	Hemothorax
Open pneumothorax	Injury to tracheobronchial tree
Flail chest	Blunt cardiac trauma
Massive hemothorax	Traumatic aortic injury
Cardiac tamponade	Mediastinal traversing wound

From American College of Surgeons. *Advanced Trauma Life Support ATLS Student Course Manual.* 10th ed. Chicago, IL: American College of Surgeons; 2018.

an increased risk for pneumonia, acute respiratory distress syndrome (ARDS) and subsequent respiratory failure and prolonged hospital and intensive care unit lengths of stay (LOS).[19]

Rib fractures may occur in a single rib or multiple ribs, usually at the point of impact or in the back where structurally they are weakest.[20] Ribs 4 to 9 are the most common ribs to be fractured because they are long and thin and poorly protected.[17] These fractures may not be considered life-threatening but can be associated with potentially life-threatening injuries to the underlying organs (lungs or heart), with the potential for concomitant injuries to the head, neck and abdomen. (Note: At the end of expiration, the diaphragm is at the level of the fourth intercostal space. This raises the abdominal organs (liver and spleen) into the thoracic cavity, where they may come into contact with those pointy bone fragments, causing puncture wounds and lacerations to those organs).[17] Posterior ribs tend to be stubbier and protected by the muscles of the back, requiring more force to be fractured. Fractures to posterior ribs should be a red flag of concomitant thoracic spine injuries. Additionally, children have thin chest walls, and their bony thorax is more cartilaginous. Consequently, energy is easily transmitted to underlying thoracic structures without fracturing ribs. When rib fractures do occur in children, concurrent thoracic and abdominal injuries may be severe.

Patients often experience pain/tenderness at the fracture site, leading to shallow respirations to avoid movement of the chest wall. This splinting may lead to complications, such as atelectasis and pneumonia. Fragments of fractured ribs can also act as penetrating objects, leading to the formation of a hemothorax or a pneumothorax or even a laceration to the spleen or liver. Subcutaneous emphysema or crepitus may also be present. Chest radiographs are only 60% to 70% sensitive for detecting rib fractures and may not pick up simple, nondisplaced rib fractures.[21] Fractures separating the sternum from the costal cartilage are often not evident on a radiograph.

Fractures of the first and second ribs are rare due to the protection granted to them by the clavicle, but they are associated with significantly higher mortality and great vessel injury. Significant blunt force is required to fracture these ribs; therefore associated injuries to the underlying structures, the great vessels, and brachial plexus must be considered. Other injuries associated with upper rib fractures include injuries to the clavicles, scapulae, trachea, and lungs. Lower rib fractures (9 through 12) are associated with injuries to the spleen, liver, kidneys, or other abdominal contents, depending on location of the fracture(s).

Treatment of rib fractures is focused on the prevention of complications. Good pulmonary toilet, coughing, and deep breathing, in conjunction with use of an incentive spirometer and early mobilization, are recommended to prevent complications, including pneumonia or atelectasis. The use of binders or strapping is to be avoided in all patients. Patients with multiple rib fractures are frequently admitted for observation due to the mortality and complication risks of these injuries. In a recent National Trauma Data Bank (NTDB) study, patients with single rib fractures had only a 5.8% mortality. When the number of ribs fractured increased, so did the mortality rate; people with five fractured ribs had a 10% mortality; six fractured ribs carried a 11.4% mortality; seven fractured ribs had a 15% mortality; and eight or more rib fractures had a 34.4% mortality.[22]

Early management of pain is pivotal in the care of patients with rib fractures, to enhance early mobilization while allowing patients to better expand their chest wall and deepen their cough, and thus diminish the risk for atelectasis and pneumonia. A variety of analgesic modalities (oral, transdermal, or intravenous analgesia) is available for the treatment of pain. Isolated rib fracture pain may be achieved with a nonsteroidal antiinflammatory drug (NSAID). Use caution with the use of NSAIDs in older adults, if not contraindicated, due to the association with bleeding or renal disease. Lidocaine patches for pain control used with isolated rib fractures have been shown to alleviate pain and shorten LOS while reducing the dose of opioid pain-relieving medications.

As the number of rib fractures with or without displacement increases, so does the need for more aggressive pain management. (Remember that rib fracture displacement may suggest a higher force of kinetic energy absorbed by the chest wall during the initial impact, which leads to increased tissue damage and inflammation).[23] Opioids in the form of oral or parenteral medications may be used as part of a multimodal approach to pain. Monitoring the older adult patient for respiratory depression when giving opioids is also of utmost importance.

Intercostal blocks, also known as catheter-based analgesia-epidural and paravertebral nerve catheters, may be beneficial in patients with multiple rib fractures.[24] These catheters provide analgesia that allows normal inspiration and coughing without the risks of respiratory depression. These blocks may be placed in the thoracic or high-lumbar positions and typically provide relief for up to 12 hours; they can be repeated as needed. They are minimally invasive and provide a great deal of pain relief locally. Caution must be used when using epidural analgesia in the patient who may be hemodynamically unstable due to the sympathetic blockade associated with these epidural anesthetic agents, which may lead to hypotension.[24] Additionally, patients with concomitant thoracic spine injury may present a technical contraindication to epidural placement.[24]

Older adult patients with rib fractures are at greater risk for complications because of diminished vital capacity that occurs with aging. Impaired ventilation worsens in all patients during the first few days after injury secondary to increasing chest wall edema and decreasing compliance. In an older adult patient with rib injury and diminished capacity, serial assessment is essential to prevent complications. Patients with decreased pulmonary function from asthma or chronic obstructive pulmonary disease also require careful ongoing assessment, in conjunction with good pulmonary toileting, because vital capacity in this population is also decreased.

Providing ideal multimodal management of pain in these patients is of the utmost importance. A clinical pathway is an ideal way to accomplish this. Harborview Medical Center has devised such a pathway that is an excellent example of how to manage all patients with rib fractures. Their rib fracture management protocol applies to all patients admitted with acute rib and/or sternal fracture(s) who meet the following criteria: age >14 years, extubated or recently extubated, Glasgow Coma Scale score of 13 to 15, and absence of high spinal cord injury.[24] The protocol offers a guideline for all providers in the care and management of rib fractures (see Figs. 38.3 and 38.4).

Flail Chest

A flail chest is an unstable chest and is defined as fractures in two or more adjacent ribs at two or more sites, or bilateral detachment of the sternum from the CC[17] (Fig. 38.5A). Mechanically, a significant force is diffused over a large area (i.e., the thorax), creating multiple anterior and posterior rib fractures.[4] Flail chest is usually associated with a fall, a massive crush injury, or a high-speed MVC. A flail chest is relatively uncommon in children due to their pliable thoracic cage but commonly occurs in older adults due to their weakened structural components. A flail chest creates a free-floating, unstable segment moving in opposition to normal chest wall movement. Mechanically, the unattached flail segment moves inward rather than outward during inspiration, and outward motion with exhalation is then noted (Fig. 38.5BC). There is a loss of coordinated chest wall movement resulting in hypoventilation of both lungs, followed by atelectasis and, eventually, hypoxia. This injury is usually associated with an underlying pulmonary contusion further compromising ventilation because of loss of pulmonary compliance, increased airway resistance, and impaired gas exchange (decreased diffusion).

Diagnosis of flail chest is often made by direct observationthe affected area moves paradoxically from the rest of the chest. Paradoxical movement occurs due to two distinct physiologic factors: loss of anatomic continuity and the effects of negative intrapleural pressure acting on the detached segment.[25] Excessive shortening of the inspiratory muscles related to the flail segment increases the work of breathing, causing the mechanics of the chest was to become inefficient! Splinting may mask a flail chest until hours later, when intercostal muscles become fatigued and paradoxical movement becomes obvious, which causes a missed or delayed flail chest diagnosis.[25] Paradoxical chest wall movements are not visualized in patients who use mechanical ventilation; these may also lead to a delayed diagnosis. Palpation of the chest wall may demonstrate crepitus over the flail segment, step-off of the ribs and, in subtle cases, the paradoxical motion of the flail chest can be appreciated with inspiration. Respiratory dysfunction usually does not arise from the paradoxical chest motion but rather due to underlying contusions and splinting from pain and difficulties noted with breathing.

Plain chest radiographs may not be helpful because, many times, fractures are not visible. A three-dimensional reconstructed CT scan of the chest is more sensitive and will provide significant information re the number of ribs fractured and underlying pulmonary injuries. If there is any suspicion of involvement of the great vessels, a CT angiography (CTA) should be performed. Blood gas analysis illustrates the severity of the hypoventilation caused by both a pulmonary contusion and the pain associated with the rib fractures. It can be helpful as a baseline in assessing the need for mechanical ventilation. Use of the rib fracture protocol noted earlier can be helpful also in managing this type of patient.[24]

Treatment consists of ensuring adequate oxygenation, judicious fluid administration, and pain management. Fluids are limited because a flail chest is almost commonly accompanied with a pulmonary contusion and potential development of ARDS. Intubation and mechanical ventilation are not required for all patients, but patients should be monitored

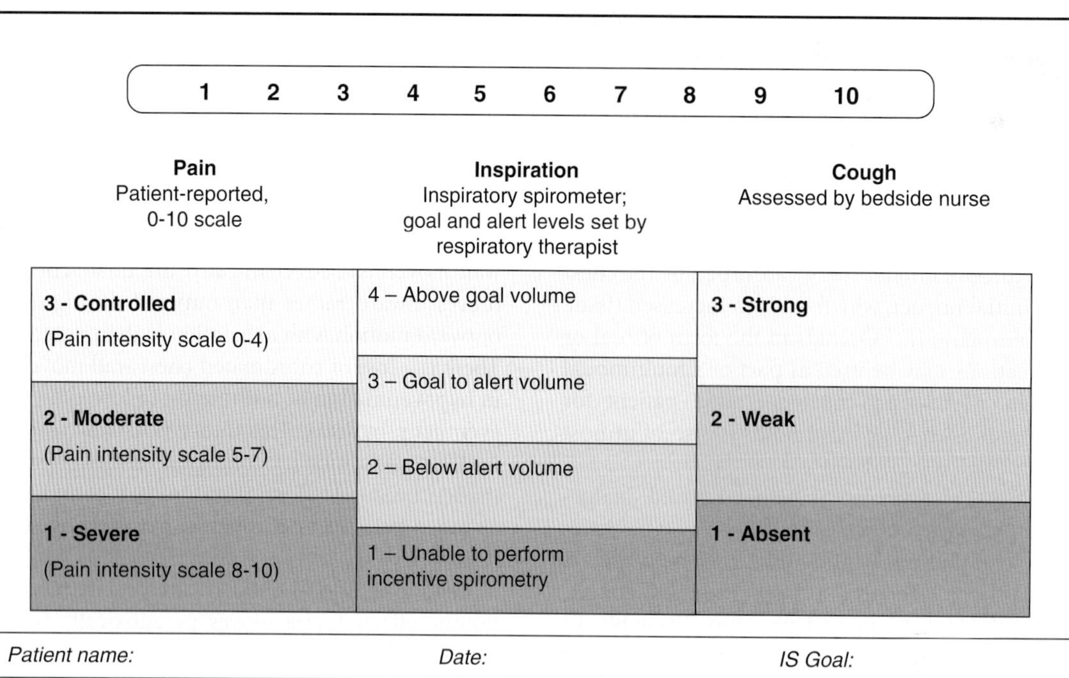

Fig. 38.3 Pain-Inspiration-Cough Scoring Tool (From Witt CE, Bulger EM. Comprehensive approach to the management of the patient with multiple rib fractures: a review and introduction of a bundled rib fracture management protocol. *Trauma Surg Acute Care Open.* 2017;2:1-7. doi:10.1136/tsaco-2016-000064.)

carefully for any change in respiratory status indicating a need for more aggressive management (i.e., changes in respiratory rate, arterial oxygen tension, and work of breathing).[24] Patients who require mechanical ventilation can usually managed with continuous positive end-expiratory pressure (PEEP); continuous positive airway pressure (CPAP) may successfully be used for some patients. Patient-controlled analgesia (PCA) pumps, oral/transdermal/intravenous pain medications, intercostal blocks, and indwelling epidural catheters form the multimodal pathway of pain management.

Traumatic disruption of the chest wall can seriously affect the mechanics of respiration, increasing morbidity and mortality in these patients.[26] Improving structural integrity must be considered in those individuals with five or more fractured ribs with a flail segment to improve outcomes.[18] Other possible indications for operative rib fracture repair include severe displaced and painful rib fractures resistant to sufficient pain management, chest wall deformity, rib fracture nonunion, and during a thoracotomy due to associated intrathoracic injury[26] (Fig. 38.6).[18]

Sternal Fracture

With the increased use of seat belts, shoulder restraints, and air bags in motor vehicles, there has been a decrease in the number of sternal fractures. Sternal fractures occur when tremendous force is applied to the mediastinum, which occurs in approximately 3% of blunt thoracic trauma cases.[27] Sixty percent to 90% of these cases occur due to seat belts, and a lesser extent occur due to direct impact with the steering wheel or front console of the car (due to air bags both on the drivers side and passengers side).[27] Sternal fractures due to cardiac compressions during basic life support measures, or even stress fractures (as in weight lifters) do occur, but rarely. Occurrence is more common in the older adult population due to their inelastic or weakened bony thorax. The most common site of fracture is the body or the manubrium. Chest wall ecchymosis, sternal deformity, or crepitus may also occur. Sternal fractures are frequently associated with other injuries. Fracture location can provide information regarding concomitant injuries, such as fractures of the manubrium sterni having a high incidence of accompanying cervical spine injuries.[28]

Poor outcomes in patients with sternal fracture are associated with the severity of other injuries (pulmonary contusion, blunt cardiac injury, and pericardial tamponade), complications, and preexisting comorbidities.[29] Of note, 12.5% of patients with sternal fracture may develop a delayed hemothorax. If these patients are discharged from the emergency department (ED), instructions must be given as to when to return to the ED (e.g., if the patients has increasing shortness of breath, chest pain, or fever).[30]

The patient may experience dyspnea and localized pain with movement and may hypoventilate to avoid chest wall movement. Primary treatment is adequate analgesia with NSAIDs, acetaminophen, and/or opiates. Other management includes a baseline ECG and cardiac markers to evaluate potential blunt cardiac injury, and serial patient assessments. If the fracture is displaced, operative reduction may be required. If cardiac symptoms are present, an echocardiogram may be obtained to evaluate myocardial performance.

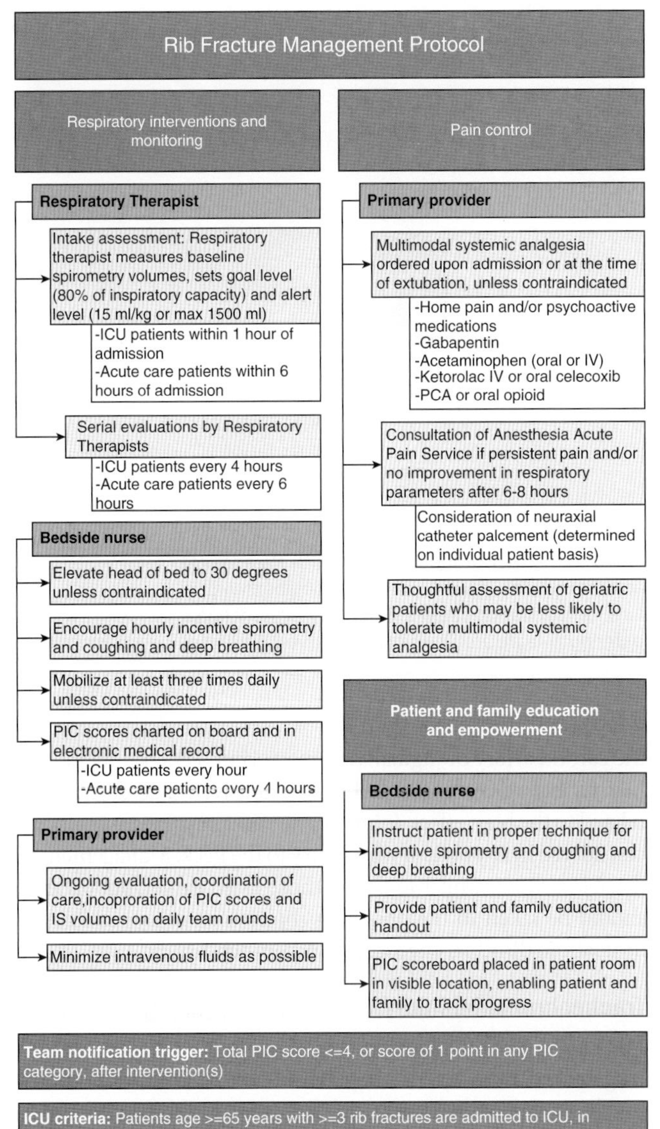

Fig. 38.4 Rib Fracture Management Protocol *ICU,* Intensive care unit; *IS,* incentive spirometry; *IV,* intravenous; *PCA,* patient-controlled analgesia; *PIC,* pain-inspiration-cough. (From Witt CE, Bulger EM. Comprehensive approach to the management of the patient with multiple rib fractures: a review and introduction of a bundled rib fracture management protocol. *Trauma Surg Acute Care Open.* 2017;2:1-7. doi:10.1136/tsaco-2016-000064.)

No surgical intervention is usually required. Patients are treated symptomatically and may be discharged from the ED.

UPPER AIRWAY INJURIES

Traumatic Asphyxia

Traumatic asphyxia (also known as Perthes syndrome), is a clinical syndrome that results from a sudden severe crush/compression injury to the thorax or thoracoabdominal region and is preceded by deep inspiration. The exact pathophysiology of traumatic asphyxia is still not fully understood, but we know it involves alveolar disruption, interstitial emphysema, and pneumothorax if the glottis is closed when the compression occurs.[31] Some theories note there is an increased intrathoracic pressure, driving blood from the right atrium and superior vena cava into the innominate (brachiocephalic) and jugular veins, where the valves prevent backflow when encountering this excessive pressure. Also, compression against a closed glottis (Valsalva maneuver), also known as the fear response, may contribute to the increased intrathoracic pressure. Patients will present with a moon-shaped face with cyanosis (violet/black) of the face and neck, petechiae, and subconjunctival and retinal hemorrhage. Sore throat, hoarseness, dizziness, numbness, and headaches are also common. Neurologic symptoms such as loss of consciousness, seizure, or even blindness are generally transient. The diagnosis is made primarily from the history and physical examination, with a chest radiograph (CXR) being essentially normal.

Treatment is focused on supporting airway and ventilation and preventing secondary cerebral injury. If no cervical injury is suspected, the head of the bed should be elevated to 30 degrees to decrease the edema of the head. Serial neurologic examinations are required to monitor the patient. Outcomes are dependent on the degree of hypoxia, duration, and magnitude of the compressive force, and the extent of anoxic neurologic injury.[32] Skin discoloration resolves within 3 weeks, but complete resolution of subconjunctival hemorrhage can take up to 1 month.

Laryngeal Injury

Fracture of the larynx is a rare, life-threatening injury due to the high mobility of the larynx and the protection it receives from the surrounding bony structures of the sternum, mandible, and cervical spine.[33] Common mechanisms of injury include striking the extended anterior neck on the steering wheel or dashboard, karate blows, and clothesline injuries suffered when a snowmobiler or motorcycle rider comes into contact with a clothesline, wire, or tree limb.[35] Fortunately, the frequency of these injuries has declined due to air bags, increased use of seat belts, and improved dashboard designs.[35] Females tend to have slimmer, longer necks, predisposing them to a higher susceptibility to laryngeal injury. Blunt laryngotracheal injuries can be frequently overlooked; therefore history must guide assessment and treatment, even if the symptoms are subtle.[34]

The patient with laryngeal injury commonly will present with either no symptoms or one or more of the following clinical features: hoarseness, dysphagia, odynophagia, anterior neck pain, dyspnea, hemoptysis, stridor, hematoma, ecchymosis, laryngeal tenderness, subcutaneous emphysema, or loss of anatomic landmarks. The cornerstone of diagnostic evaluation in suspected laryngeal trauma is a CT scan[33,34]; any patient with a laryngeal injury must be evaluated for a concomitant cervical injury, and patients with cervical injury must be assessed for laryngeal injury.

In minor injuries to the larynx, close observation is essential for the first 24 to 48 hours, but if penetrating trauma is present, hemodynamic and neurologic status should always be monitored closely for at least 48 to 72 hours.[34] Maintaining airway patency is the primary treatment. Keeping the head of the bed elevated 30 to 45 degrees in conjunction with the use

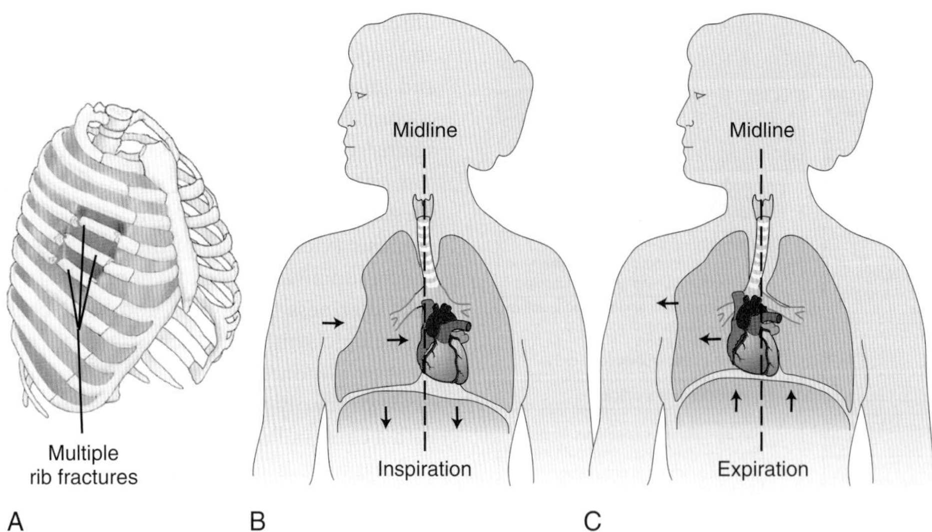

Fig. 38.5 Flail Chest (A) Fractured rib sections are unattached to the rest of the chest wall. (B) Paradoxical breathing occurs when instability (i.e., from multiple rib fractures) causes inward motion of the chest wall in response to the generation of negative intrathoracic pressure. (C) Expiration causes a similarly dysfunctional expansion of the unstable chest wall. (From Shiland B. *Mastering Healthcare Terminology.* 5th ed. St Louis, MO: Mosby, 2016.)

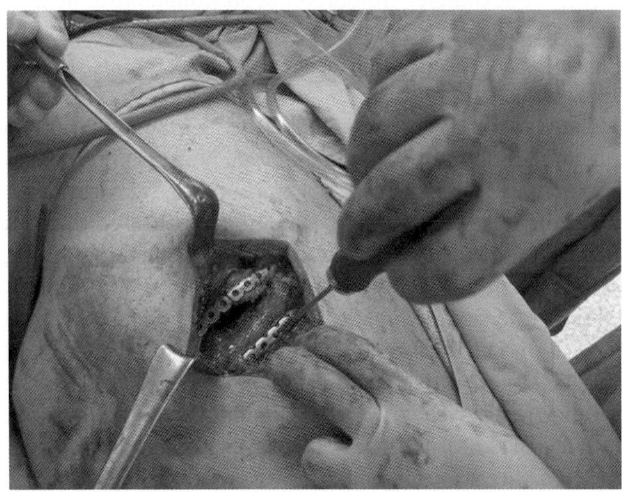

Fig. 38.6 Thoracotomy with rib fixation. (From de Moya M, Nirula R, Biffl W. Rib fixation: who, what, when? *Trauma Surg Acute Care Open.* 2017;2(1):1-4. doi:10.1136/tsaco-2016-000059.)

of humidified air and keeping the patient NPO and on voice rest will minimize edema and subcutaneous emphysema. Intubation may be difficult due to distorted anatomy and poor visualization.[33] Numerous references have been made that cricothyroidotomy can be a reasonable alternative in the patient with a compromised airway.[33] Special consideration must be given to pediatric patients with laryngeal injuries and an unstable airway because local tracheotomy is not usually a viable option. It is suggested these patients be managed in a manner similar to that of epiglottitis, using inhalation anesthesia with spontaneous respirations, followed by rigid endoscopic intubation. Once the airway has been evaluated and secured in this manner, tracheotomy can be performed if needed.

Penetrating trauma to the larynx is readily apparent and requires immediate surgical intervention. Associated injuries to the carotid artery or jugular vein may occur. Penetrating missile injuries have been associated with extensive tissue destruction related to the blast effect. Injury to the cervical spine must also be considered in any patient with injury to the neck. Management of these injuries is similar to that of those listed earlier, but patients should be taken to the operating room as soon as possible for intubation, direct laryngoscopy, and bronchoscopy.

Tracheobronchial Injury

Traumatic tracheobronchial injuries are uncommon, occurring in less than 1% of all patients, and therefore often are overlooked. These injuries involve trauma (blunt and penetrating) to the airway, between the cricoid cartilage and the right and left main stem bronchial bifurcations. The majority of injuries to this area are most commonly encountered in the situation of penetrating neck trauma in the proximal trachea, and many patients die at the scene. Blunt trauma to the chest causing bronchial injury has a high mortality because of delayed or missed diagnosis of the injury. Clinical manifestations include hemoptysis, dyspnea, hoarseness/dysphonia, anterior neck swelling and bruising, major air leaks in the chest tube, subcutaneous emphysema, or tension pneumothorax with mediastinal shift. If air accumulates in the mediastinum, a crunching sound called Hamman sign occurs. With bronchial disruption into both pleural spaces, bilateral tension pneumothoraces occur. Persistent emphysema or air leak after chest tube insertion should increase the index of suspicion for this injury; bronchoscopy confirms the diagnosis.

CXR is the most useful initial imaging study. Deep cervical emphysema and pneumomediastinum will be seen in 60% and pneumothorax occurs in 70% of patients with tracheobronchial injuries.[36] CT scan is valuable, but ultimately bronchoscopy is the most definitive assessment and therapeutic tool.[36] Maintaining a stable airway is the cornerstone of management until inflammation and edema resolve; however, surgical intervention is required for patients with a significant tear.

PNEUMOTHORAX

Injury in the parietal pleura leads to paradoxical lung movement. This section will describe the different types of pneumothorax: simple, open (communicating or sucking); tension; and hemothorax.

Simple

Pneumothorax refers to accumulation of air in the pleural space, resulting in partial or complete collapse of the lung as negative intrapleural pressure is lost (Fig. 38.7). Pneumothorax may most commonly result from blunt injuries when the impact occurs at full inspiration, when the glottis is closed, thereby increasing intraalveolar pressure, which results in subsequent rupture of the alveoli. Laceration of lung tissue, often associated with rib fractures, also commonly occurs.[37]

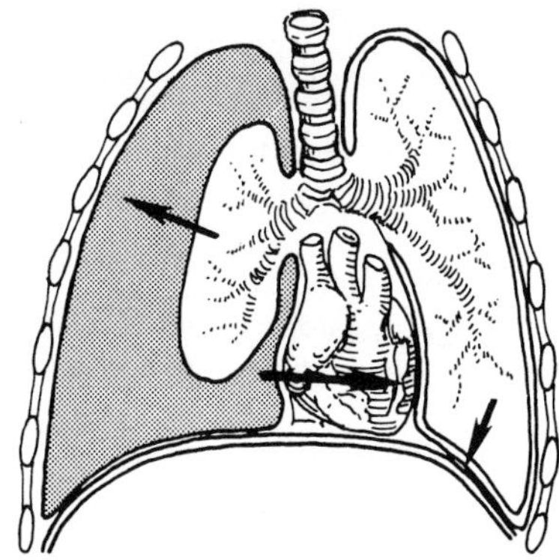

Fig. 38.7 Closed Pneumothorax Simple pneumothorax is present in the right lung with air in the pleural cavity and collapse of the right lung.

A patient with a pneumothorax complains of chest pain and shortness of breath. Auscultation of the chest on the injured side demonstrates decreased or absent breath sounds; percussion demonstrates hyperresonance. Normal breath sounds can occur as a result of resonance within the thoracic cavity. Tachycardia and tachypnea are usually present. An upright CXR has been the preferred diagnostic study until recently, when several studies found a chest ultrasound scan to have greater sensitivity and expose the patient to less radiation.[37,38] (Fig. 38.8).

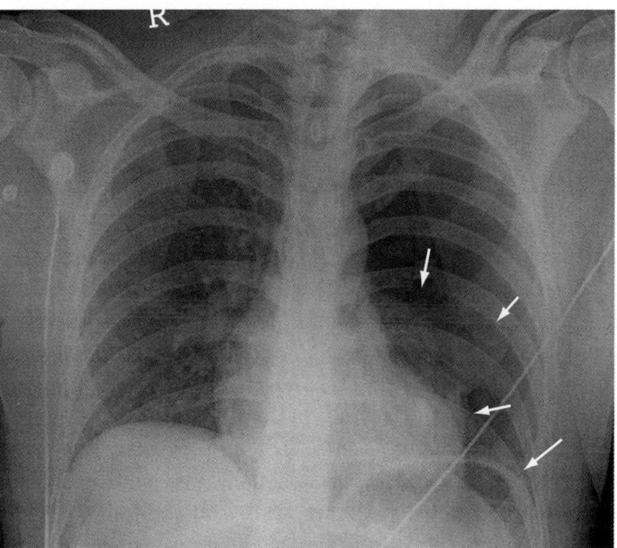

Fig. 38.8 Large Left-Sided Pneumothorax on Plain Chest Radiograph The *arrows* identify the lateral border of the collapsed lung. (From Martin RS, Meredith JW. Management of acute trauma. In: Townsend CM Jr, Beauchamp DM, Evers M, Mattox KL. *Sabiston Textbook of Surgery*. 12th ed. Philadelphia, PA: Elsevier; 2017:428.)

The size of the pneumothorax will determine the treatment. For example, if it is <20%, no treatment may be indicated; we would simply observe this patient and provide supplemental O_2. If it is >50%, a chest tube is placed (a pigtail or small-bore catheter), depending once again on the patients symptoms and the clinical presentation.[39] Individuals who are asymptomatic (with <3 cm pneumothorax on x-ray) and who do not require a chest tube) may only require observation (as little as 36 hours).[40] If a subsequent CXR is without progression of the pneumothorax, the patient may be safely discharged with instructions to have a follow-up CXR within 48 hours.[40]

The optimum drain size in the management of various pleural diseases remains controversial, with current guidelines recommending small-bore catheters. It must be remembered that the optimum drain size must be specific to the pleural disease in question, the intended treatment outcome, and the drainage to be managed.[41,42] Pigtail catheters have become a more common method of relieving both spontaneous and traumatic pneumothorax due to ease of placement, less pain to the patient, and fewer complications.[40] These small-bore catheters can be attached to a Heimlich valve, and patients are able to be discharged directly from the ED. The optimal insertion site lies within the safety triangle: the lateral edge of the pectoral muscle, the lateral edge of the latissimus dorsi, and a line along the fifth intercostal space at the nipple line. Insertion here minimizes the risk of damage to nerves, vessels, and organs.[40] These small-bore catheters are usually attached to a Heimlich valve, which does not require suction, and allow for greater mobility and less discomfort.

Large-bore catheters are most generally commonly placed in the fourth or fifth intercostal space, along the anterior axillary line required for moderate to large pneumothoraces, for patients who are symptomatic regardless of size of the pneumothorax and patients requiring mechanical ventilation[37] (Box 38.4). The chest tube is then connected to an underwater drainage system with 20 to 30 cm H_2O for more rapid suction to facilitate lung reexpansion[37] (Box 38.5). Once either tube has been inserted, a CXR must be completed to confirm tube placement. Oxygen administration, good pulmonary hygiene (use of an incentive spirometer), pain management, and serial chest radiographs to monitor lung reexpansion are standard treatment plans for all patients with a chest tube.

BOX 38.4 Indications for Tube Thoracostomy.

Indications for Tube Thoracostomy

Traumatic cause of pneumothorax (except asymptomatic, apical pneumothorax)
Moderate to large pneumothorax
Respiratory symptoms regardless of size of pneumothorax
Increasing size of pneumothorax after initial conservative therapy
Recurrence of pneumothorax after removal of an initial chest tube
Patient requires ventilator support
Patient requires general anesthesia
Associated hemothorax
Bilateral pneumothorax regardless of size
Tension pneumothorax

From Raja AS. Thoracic trauma. In: Walls RM, Hockberger RS, Gauche-Hill M. *Rosens Emergency Medicine: Concepts and Clinical Practice.* 9th ed. Philadelphia, PA: Elsevier; 2018:388.

Open (Communicating) Pneumothorax (Sucking Chest Wound)

Open pneumothorax, or sucking chest wound, occurs when there is an opening in the chest wall. This injury is usually the result of penetrating trauma to the chest wall. However, blunt trauma may also cause an open chest wound. An open chest wound causes loss of the negative intrathoracic pressure required for effective ventilation (Fig. 38.9).

Presenting symptoms may include chest pain, shortness of breath, hemoptysis, and occasionally, hypotension. Breath sounds may be decreased or absent on the affected side, and a sucking or hissing sound may be heard with inspiration. Bubbles, or froth, often may be observed as air escapes through the bloodied wound. Immediate treatment consists of placing a sterile, nonporous, three-sided occlusive dressing or a commercially available vented chest seal (which have drainage channels perform facing away from the wound).[43,44] Using a three-sided dressing allows air to escape but prevents air from entering through the wound. A totally occlusive dressing carries with it the danger of the development of a tension pneumothorax. Therefore, after placement of any dressing, the patient should be carefully monitored for development of a tension pneumothorax. If symptoms suggesting a tension pneumothorax, the taped dressing must be removed immediately. Definitively, a chest tube should be inserted to facilitate reexpansion of the lung, and the patient may be taken to the operating room for treatment (operative closure of the open chest wound). If the injury is caused by penetrating trauma with an impaled object, the object must be stabilized and left in place. **Never remove** the object in the ED. It should be removed only in a controlled environment.

Tension Pneumothorax

Tension pneumothorax is a life-threatening condition occurring when accumulation of air in one pleural space forces thoracic contents to the opposite side of the chest (Fig. 38.10). Initial lung injury allows air into the pleural space with inspiration; however, air cannot escape with expiration. Air continues to accumulate and intrathoracic pressure increases, forcing thoracic contents away from the injured side. Eventually the lung on the opposite side, the heart, and great vessels are compressed as mediastinal shift occurs.

Auscultation reveals decreased or absent breath sounds on the affected side and possibly decreased sounds on the unaffected side as that lung is compressed. If the patient is alert and able to speak, he or she may complain of chest pain, severe shortness of breath, and a feeling of impending doom. Compression of the heart causes cardiac dysrhythmias, decreases diastolic filling, and decreases cardiac output. The vena cava becomes compressed, impairing venous return to the heart, which worsens diastolic filling and further decreases cardiac output. Neck vein distention occurs as venous return is impaired by compression of the heart; however, neck veins may remain flat if concurrent hypovolemia exists. The trachea

BOX 38.5 Chest Drainage Systems: Components and Management.

Fluid Collection Chamber

Fluid drains from the patient through a long tube to a collection chamber, marked for assessment of drainage.

Water Seal Chamber

With the water seal chamber, during spontaneous respirations, the water level should rise during inhalation and fall during exhalation.

Suction Control Chamber

Improves drainage and helps overcome the air leak. Keep suction control at −10 to −20 cm H_2O.

Nursing Responsibilities

Secure all connections.
Monitor catheters to prevent kinking.
Monitor drainage output.
Assess for air leaks.
Maintain unit in upright position.

Assessing for Air Leaks

Look at the underwater seal. Leaks may originate with the patient or the drainage system.
For a patient receiving mechanical ventilation with positive end-expiratory pressure (PEEP), leaking causes continuous bubbling.
Note the pattern of the bubbling. If it fluctuates with respirations (i.e., occurs on exhalation in a patient breathing spontaneously), the most likely source is the lung.

Indications of Patency

Water level in the water seal should fluctuate with breathing, rising with inspiration and falling with expiration, and is an indicator of chest tube patency.
Fluctuations stop when the lung is fully reexpanded or when the tube is kinked or compressed.

No Milking or Clamping Tube!

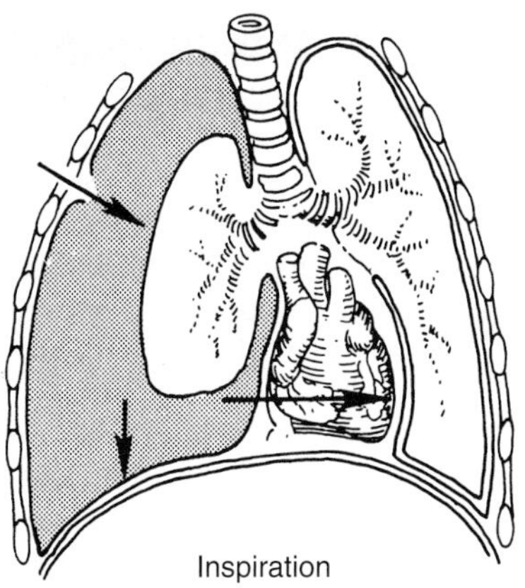

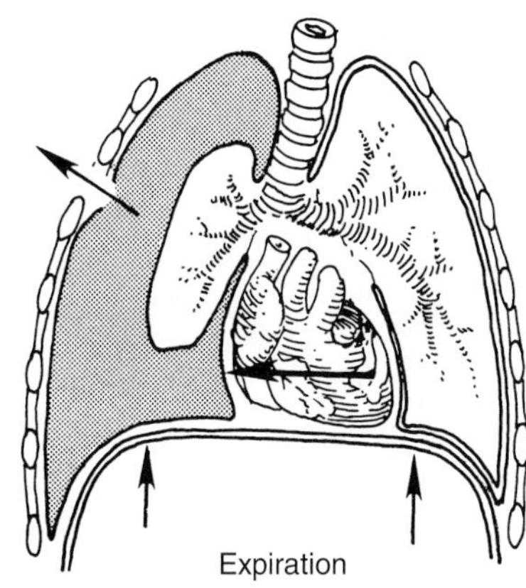

Fig. 38.9 Open Pneumothorax Inspiration *(left):* The diaphragm contracts, causing negative intrathoracic pressure *(arrow 1)* that draws air through the sucking chest wound in the pleural cavity *(arrow 2)* and causing the mediastinal structures to shift to the patient's left *(arrow 3)*. Expiration *(right):* The diaphragm recoils *(arrow 1)*, causing air to exit the chest *(arrow 2)* and allowing the mediastinum to shift back to normal position *(arrow 3)*. The collapsed lung paradoxically shrinks on inspiration and expands on expiration. (From Marx J, Hockberger RS, Walls R: *Rosen's Emergency Medicine: Concepts and Clinical Practice.* 6th ed. St Louis, MO: Mosby; 2006.)

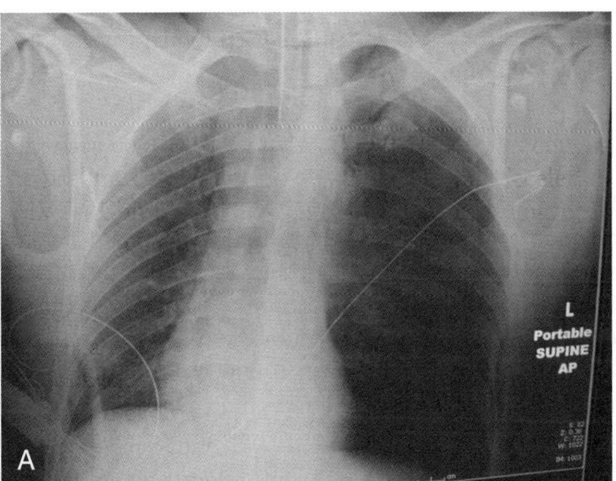

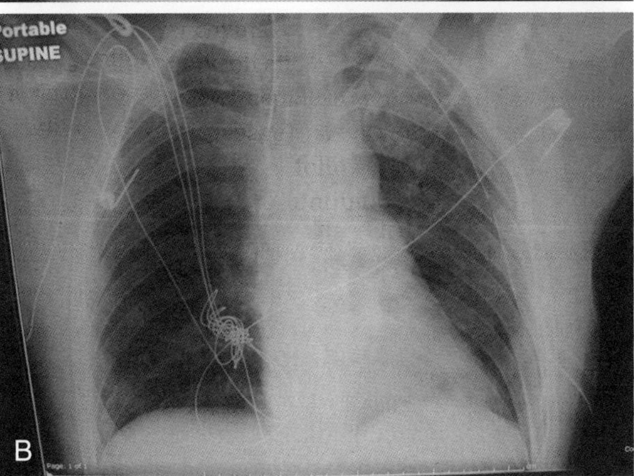

Fig. 38.10 (A) Tension pneumothorax seen in intubated patient. (B) Resolution of the tension pneumothorax shown in *A* with placement of a left-sided tube thoracostomy. (From Raja AS. Thoracic trauma. In: Walls RM, Hockberger RS, Gauche-Hill M. *Rosen's Emergency Medicine: Concepts and Clinical Practice.* 9th ed. Philadelphia, PA: Elsevier;2018:382-403.)

eventually deviates to the unaffected side as mediastinal shift worsens. The most common radiographic manifestations of tension pneumothorax are mediastinal shift, diaphragmatic depression, and rib cage expansion.[37]

Immediate needle decompression is the recommended emergent procedure to relieve increased intrapleural pressure found with a tension pneumothorax. Decompression failure has been reported, and it has been found to be due to insufficient needle length in proportion to the chest wall thickness. Therefore it has been recommended that a 14- or 16-gauge (7 cm in length)[45,46] catheter be inserted into the second intercostal space at the midclavicular line on the injured side. New evidence from observational studies suggests that the fourth/fifth intercostal space anterior axillary line be used because it has the lowest failure rate of needle decompression in multiple populations (Fig. 38.11). Hearing a rush of air upon needle insertion, with a rapid improvement in symptoms, confirms the diagnosis. Definitive therapy is chest tube insertion.

Hemothorax

A hemothorax is accumulation of blood in the pleural space resulting from blunt or penetrating trauma that inflicts injury to the lung parenchyma, heart or major vessel injury, or injury to an internal mammary artery. The most common cause is an injury to the intercostal vein or arteries (small vessels lying beneath each ribs), resulting in bleeding into the pleural space. Bleeding from an intercostal vessel is usually minimal and will usually taper off over a few hours when a clot forms in the small vessels. In addition to chest pain, shortness of breath, and decreased or absent breath sounds on the affected side, the patient has dullness on chest percussion. Signs and symptoms of hypovolemic shock and respiratory distress may often be present. FAST examination is used in the initial evaluation of hypotensive patients with thoracic trauma in which a hemothorax is suspected.

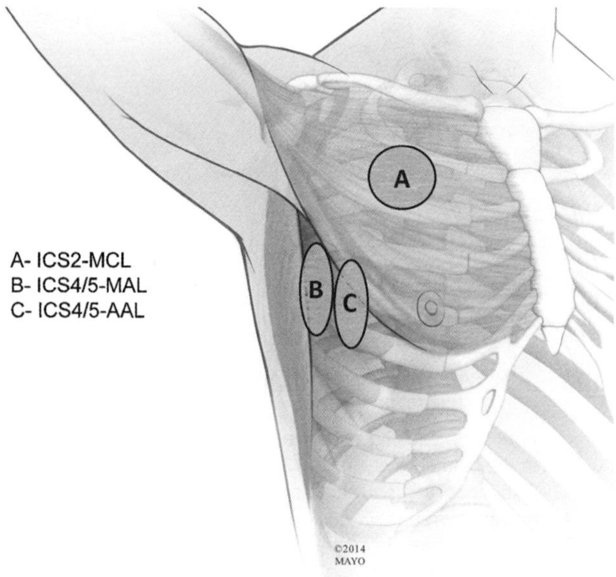

Fig. 38.11 Needle thoracostomy (decompression) site with anatomic locations for needle thoracostomy decompression. (A) The currently recommended second intercostal space midclavicular line (ICS2-MCL); (B) the fourth and fifth intercostal spaces midaxillary line (ICS4/5-MAL); and (C) the fourth and fifth intercostal spaces anterior axillary line (ICS4/5-AAL). (From Laan DV, et al. *Injury.* 2016;47(4):797-804. Used with permission of Mayo Foundation for Medical Education and Research.)

BOX 38.6 Indications for OR Thoracotomy.

Initial thoracostomy tube drainage is more than 20 mL of blood per kilogram.
Persistent bleeding at a rate greater than 7 mL/kg/h is present.
Increasing hemothorax seen on chest x-ray films.
Patient remains hypotensive despite adequate blood replacement, and other sites of blood loss have been ruled out.
Patient decompensates after initial response to resuscitation.

Treatment consists of early identification and intervention to decrease morbidity and mortality associated with hemothoraces. Key interventions include restoring or maintaining circulation with large-bore intravenous lines for fluid replacement and possible operative repair of bleeding vessels or injured parenchyma maintenance of the airway (usually with high-flow oxygen via a nonrebreather mask); possible operative repair of bleeding vessels or injured parenchyma; and evacuating accumulating blood with insertion of a large-bore chest catheter (usually size 32 Fr or 36 Fr in an adult) inserted into the fifth intercostal space midaxillary line.[37] Immediate blood return with chest tube insertion of 1000 to 1500 mL or blood loss of 200 mL/hour for 3 to 4 hours are indications for surgical intervention[37] (Box 38.6). Persistent hypotension or massive air leak are additional indicators for surgery.[37] Chest drainage should be carefully monitored to assess the need for autotransfusion or clots occluding the tube. Chest radiography may confirm the diagnosis; a CT scan may be used to identify and quantify the hemothorax.

BOX 38.7 Advantages of Autotransfusion.

1. Immediately available–no delay in crossmatching and no storage required
2. Blood compatibility and allergic reaction not an issue
3. Autologous blood usually normothermic
4. No risk for transfusion transmissible disease
5. No risk for hypocalcemia or hyperkalemia[a,b]
6. Decreased risk for acute respiratory distress syndrome
7. Higher levels of 2,3-diphosphoglycerate than in banked red blood cells[c]
8. Decreased use of banked blood; more available for subsequent patients in need[d]
9. Decreased cost of medical care[d-f]
10. May be acceptable to religions opposed to homologous blood transfusions[a,g,h]
11. May be a valuable alternative to banked blood in developing countries where infected donor blood is a problem

From Neavyn MJ, Pena ME, Babcock C. Autotransfusion. In: https://www.clinicalkey.com/#!/browse/book/3-s2.0-C20140019958. *Roberts and Hedges Clinical Procedures in Emergency Medicine and Acute Care.* 7th ed. Philadelphia, PA: Elsevier; 2019:493.

Autotransfusion

Autotransfusion, collecting and reinfusing the patients own blood, is a valuable tool during resuscitation of select hypovolemic trauma victims. Noncontaminated blood shed into the thoracic cavity from blunt trauma may be easily collected and infused via most chest drain collection systems connecting to a large-bore chest tube. Significant intrathoracic blood loss (more than 350 mL) and wounds that are less than 4 to 6 hours old are potential indications for autotransfusion. Autotransfusion is also useful when homologous blood is not available or the patients religious convictions forbid homologous transfusion. Box 38.7 highlights specific advantages of autotransfusion. Autotransfusion is not appropriate when enteric contamination has occurred or is suspected (e.g., ruptured diaphragm), infection is present, a patient has established coagulopathies or hepatic/renal insufficiency, or the blood has been in the autotransfuser for more than 6 hours. In some situations, emergency autotransfusion may pose more risk than benefit due to complications such as coagulopathy and/or disseminated intravascular coagulopathy (DIC).

Autotransfusion requires a chest drainage unit and autotransfusion device as well as user competence with the process and collection device. In the ED, an anticoagulant may be added before blood collection to prevent clotting during the collection phase and plugging of the blood filter and intravenous line during reinfusion. Citrate dextrose solution-A and citrate phosphate dextrose are the most common anticoagulants used; however, many trauma centers elect not to add an anticoagulant[47] (Box 38.8). Continuous monitoring of respiratory and cardiac status in conjunction with serial laboratory assessments must be performed.

BOX 38.8 General Autotransfusion Information.

1. Use each liner bag only once.
2. Insert a new filter for each autotransfusion bag used.
3. To minimize risk for bacterial overgrowth, blood collected must be reinfused within 6 hours from the time of injury.[a]
4. After reinfusing a total of 3500 mL (approximately 7 units) of autologous blood, it has been suggested that 1 unit of fresh frozen plasma be given for every 2 units (approximately 1000 mL) of autotransfused blood.[b]
5. If some or all the collected blood becomes clotted in the liner bag, the blood should be discarded.
6. To reduce the risk for air embolism, remove all the air from the bag with the collected blood before hanging it for reinfusion.[c]

From Neavyn MJ, Pena ME, Babcock C. Autotransfusion. In: https://www.clinicalkey.com/#!/browse/book/3-s2.0-C20140019958. *Roberts and Hedges Clinical Procedures in Emergency Medicine and Acute Care.* 7th ed. Philadelphia, PA: Elsevier; 2019:498.

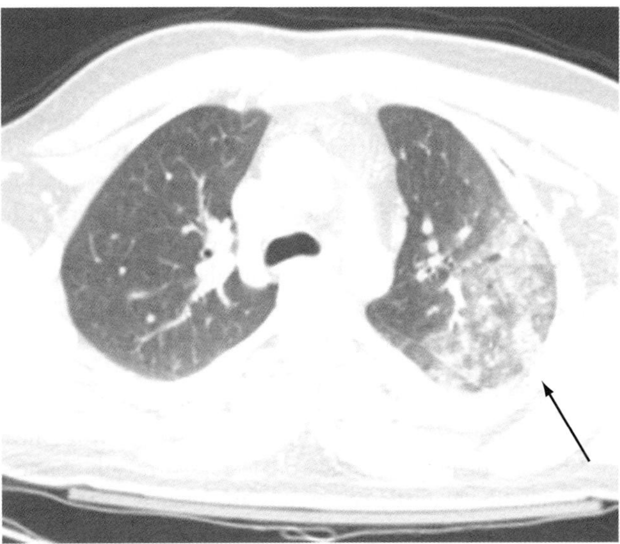

Fig. 38.12 Left Pulmonary Contusion on Thoracic Computed Tomography Scan The *arrow* identifies contused lung, which appears as higher-density tissue because of air space hemorrhage and associated edema. (From Martin RS, Meredith JW. Management of acute trauma. In: Townsend CM Jr, Beauchamp D, Evers M, Mattox KL. *Sabiston Textbook of Surgery.* 12th ed. Philadelphia, PA: Elsevier; 2017:429.)

PULMONARY INJURY OR INJURIES TO THE LUNG PARENCHYMA

Pulmonary Contusion

Pulmonary contusion is seen in up to 75% of patients who sustain blunt chest trauma secondary to rapid deceleration in MVCs. Contusions occur when underlying lung parenchyma is damaged, causing edema and hemorrhage (in other words, a large, edematous bruise of the lung tissue). This edematous, fluid-filled tissue causes breathing difficulties as a result of impaired gas exchange diffusion at the alveolar level. Injury to the lung parenchyma progressively worsens and evolves over time. Thoracic injuries associated with pulmonary contusion include rib fractures, flail chest, hemothorax, pneumothorax, and scapular fractures. Injury to the lung parenchyma, without pulmonary laceration, causes ruptures of alveoli and consolidation of small airways as a result of damaged capillaries (increased capillary permeability and hemorrhage). As a result, airways collapse, reducing lung compliance, followed by loss of ventilation, pulmonary right-to-left shunting, hypercarbia, increased work of breathing, and hypoxia.[48] The subsequent inflammatory response impairs gas exchange and diffusion and worsens the clinical picture. Diagnosis is based on the index of suspicion.

Clinical features that may be present include dyspnea, hemoptysis, increasing restlessness, hypoxia, cyanosis, hypotension, increased work of breathing, and possible chest wall abrasions or ecchymosis. (Note: hypoxemia, increased work of breathing, and agitation indicate respiratory decompensation). Many patients with pulmonary contusion have no external physical findings. Auscultation rarely detects abnormalities, but a baseline blood gas measurement may be helpful.

The chest radiograph is usually not helpful during initial evaluation, but changes may be seen within 6 hours.[37] The contused areas do not fully blossom and become noticeably apparent until 24 to 48 hours after the injury.[47] CT scan of the chest may be used to quantify the contusion because it is a more sensitive indicator of tissue injury[48] (Fig. 38.12)[38]. Contusions change rapidly, usually improving within 72 hours and resolving within 5 to 7 days.[48] Treatment initially consists of supportive by maintaining euvolemia with judicious infusion of or no intravenous fluids; placing the patient in the semi-Fowlers position to facilitate lung reexpansion, and providing pulmonary hygiene with incentive spirometry, early mobilization, and nasotracheal suctioning.[47] Consideration of noninvasive ventilation (i.e., CPAP or BiPAP) before endotracheal intubation and mechanical ventilation should be made.

Cardiac and Great Vessel Injuries

Diaphragmatic Injury

The diaphragm is a bidomed structure that separates the contents of the thorax from the abdominal cavity. Diaphragmatic injuries are seen in 1% to 6% of major thoracic trauma,[37] with a mortality of 26.3% as a result of injury to adjacent vital organs.[38] Blunt diaphragmatic injuries occur in only 1.6%[38] of blunt thoracic injuries and result from an abrupt increase in intraabdominal pressure during an anterior impact, which causes a diaphragmatic tissue to explode. Approximately 75% of diaphragmatic injuries occur on the left side of the diaphragm; the right side is protected by its proximity and coverage by the liver. When injuries do occur on the right, they may be difficult to identify because of the liver. Diaphragmatic injuries rarely occur alone. They are most commonly seen in conjunction with other blunt thoracic injuries, such as trauma to the intraabdominal organs, mainly the liver or spleen; rib fractures; or other thoracic injuries and pelvic or long-bone fractures.

Diaphragmatic injuries are frequently not easily recognized due to other distracting and possibly life-threatening injuries. They can be a diagnostic challenge. Delayed diagnosis is common and, if not made in the first 4 hours, injuries may be undiagnosed for months or years. It is important to understand that lateral impact injuries from an MVC are three times more likely to cause a rupture, causing the chest wall to become distorted and shearing the ipsilateral diaphragm. Frontal impacts can cause an increase in intraabdominal pressure, causing tears also.

Physical findings can vary and may have thoracic and/or abdominal components to them. The presence of dyspnea, the absence of breath sounds or decreased breath sounds, in conjunction with bowel sounds auscultated in the chest (think diaphragmatic rupture), represents the thoracic signs. Abdominal signs include abdominal pain radiating to the left shoulder (Kehr sign) due to phrenic nerve irritation; guarding and abdominal rigidity, and the absence of bowel sounds.

Normal or nonspecific findings on radiographs are seen in 10% to 40% of all patients with diaphragmatic injuries and masked if the patient is intubated.[49] The chest radiograph may demonstrate an elevated diaphragm, loss of the diaphragmatic shadow, irregularity of the diaphragm, or an abnormal mediastinum.[50] In the stable patient, the CT scan of the chest is the diagnostic tool of choice but is not 100% sensitive.[49] Segmental loss of the normal diaphragm contour is the most common finding, seen in about 96% of cases.[51] Blood on both sides of the diaphragm is strongly suggestive of a ruptured diaphragm.[51]

Treatment focuses on early identification (both in blunt and penetrating injuries) and involves control of hemorrhage and other life-threatening injuries along with gastrointestinal spillage. An exploration of the abdominal cavity and the diaphragm, in suspected injuries, is indicated to avoid morbidity and mortality from visceral herniation/strangulation and even cardiopulmonary compromise.

Blunt Cardiac Injury

Blunt cardiac injury was once known as cardiac contusion, cardiac concussion, or *commotio cordis (agitation of heart).* Blunt cardiac injury describes a spectrum of potential injuries to the myocardium resulting from deceleration injuries sustained from blunt trauma to the anterior chest. Such injuries cause the heart to be stunned when crushed between the sternum and the spine in 15% to 75% of patients, causing a nonperfusing rhythm.[52] Any patient sustaining trauma to the anterior chest should lead to a high index of suspicion for blunt cardiac injury. Common mechanisms of injury include impact with the steering wheel, falls, assaults, and direct blows from an object or a large animal (e.g., a kick from a horse). These common mechanisms may cause blunt cardiac injury resulting in disruption of the valves, myocardial contusion, or cardiac chamber rupture.[52]

The signs and symptoms of blunt cardiac injury are nonspecific, and often these patients present with arrythmias.[37] The spectrum of clinical presentations ranges from asymptomatic to cardiogenic shock; many times, the only information to suggest the patient has blunt cardiac injury is the patients history of blunt anterior chest trauma. Some common presentations seen are chest pain, crepitus, abrasions/ecchymosis, or visible flail segments noted to the anterior chest. Chest pain associated with blunt cardiac injury mimics ischemic chest pain. Unlike ischemic pain, however, pain with blunt cardiac injury does not respond to coronary vasodilators such as nitroglycerine. One of the most sensitive but least specific signs of myocardial contusion is sinus tachycardia with premature ventricular contractions (PVCs), occurring in approximately 70% of patients.[37,53] Other dysrhythmias observed are atrial fibrillation/flutter, atrial and ventricular extrasystoles, and even ventricular tachycardia/fibrillation. Conduction disturbances such as right bundle branch block are also identified.[53] This presentation should not be surprising given the relatively anterior location of the right-sided heart structures.[53] Most of the lethal dysrhythmias and cardiac failures occur within 24 to 48 hours of the injury.

Treatment begins with the current recommendations found in the Eastern Association for the Surgery of Trauma Guidelines (EAST).[54] These guidelines recommend that an ECG should be completed on all patients with suspected cardiac injury. It must be noted a standard ECG may not be as sensitive to right ventricular damage and cannot be used as a gold standard for diagnosing injury. An echocardiogram may be useful for differentiating cardiac dysfunction and to visualize cardiac structures or abnormalities such as pericardial tamponade, valve rupture, and pericardial effusion but should not be used as a screening tool. However, transesophageal echocardiogram (TEE) is thought to be the more sensitive test.

A mild injury can cause cardiac dysrhythmias, yet the echocardiogram may be normal. Extensive myocardial injury is characterized by 12-lead ECG changes, dysrhythmias, and some evidence of myocardial dysfunction on the echocardiogram. Serial ECGs and continuous cardiac monitoring are essential. Cardiac isoenzymes or cardiac biomarkers (especially troponin) in combination with ECG findings have been found to have a 100% sensitivity for the detection of clinically significant blunt chest trauma when both are found to be abnormal. Atrial and septal ruptures are generally less dramatic, present with just a murmur, and should be treated accordingly. Treatment of dysrhythmias is of utmost importance.

Penetrating Cardiac Injuries

Most penetrating cardiac injuries are caused by person-against-person violence or industrial incidents. Most victims of penetrating cardiac injuries arrive in the ED in cardiac arrest or with significant hypotension due to cardiac tamponade or hemorrhage. The right ventricle is the most frequently injured chamber because of its anterior

BOX 38.9 Indications for Emergency Thoracotomy.

Penetrating Traumatic Cardiac Arrest

Cardiac arrest at any point with initial signs of life in the field
Systolic blood pressure below 50 mm Hg after fluid resuscitation
Severe shock with clinical signs of cardiac tamponade

Blunt Trauma

Cardiac arrest in the emergency department

From Raja AS. Thoracic trauma. In: RM Walls, Hockberger RS, Gauche-Hill M. *Rosens Emergency Medicine: Concepts and Clinical Practice*. 9th ed. Philadelphia, PA: Elsevier; 2018:395.

position.[37] Other chambers injured are the left ventricle and right atrium. Penetrating injuries are associated with a high mortality (80%); only 20% to 25% of the victims reach the hospital alive.[37,38] Patients who arrive with stable cardiac injuries have the best chance for survival with early diagnosis and treatment. Patients with injuries to the chest between the midclavicular lines, clavicles, and costal margins should be aggressively evaluated for cardiac involvement. According to Raja (2018), two conditions may occur after penetrating heart injury: (1) exsanguinating hemorrhage if the cardiac lesion communicates freely with the pleural cavity, or (2) cardiac tamponade if the hemorrhage is contained within the pericardium (p. 395).[37]

Stabilization of the ABCs followed by echocardiography is recommended if the patient has cardiac activity. Use of the FAST examination has led to earlier diagnosis and definitive surgical intervention, with a specificity of 99.3% and sensitivity of 100% for identifying penetrating cardiac injury.[55] Positive findings indicating tamponade suggest the need for a subxiphoid window.

Immediate thoracotomy in the ED may be indicated for selected patients presenting with penetrating chest trauma. The best results are obtained in patients with a single penetrating injury to the anterior or precordial thoracic area and in patients who had a witnessed cardiac arrest in the ED. Holes in the myocardium, lungs, or great vessels can be temporarily plugged with the balloon of a urinary catheter, sutures, staples, clamps, or a finger while an operating room is readied. Box 38.9 describes considerations of the emergency thoracotomy.

Cardiac Tamponade

Cardiac tamponade occurs when rapid accumulation of blood in the pericardial sac decreases ventricular filling. As the pericardial sac fills, blood presses on the ventricles and impairs ventricular filling and the hearts pumping ability, and then cardiac output decreases. Classic signs of cardiac tamponade are a complex of symptoms called Beck triad: hypotension, muffled heart tones, and distended neck veins (Fig. 38.13).[56] Hypotension is due to myocardial compression and decreased cardiac output as more blood accumulates in the pericardium. Muffled heart sounds are caused by the insulating ability of blood in the pericardium, whereas neck vein distension occurs because the heart cannot expand normally to accommodate blood return to the heart. Classic symptoms may not always be evident because of associated injuries such as hypovolemia. As the tamponade worsens, the patient exhibits air hunger, agitation, and deterioration in level of consciousness.

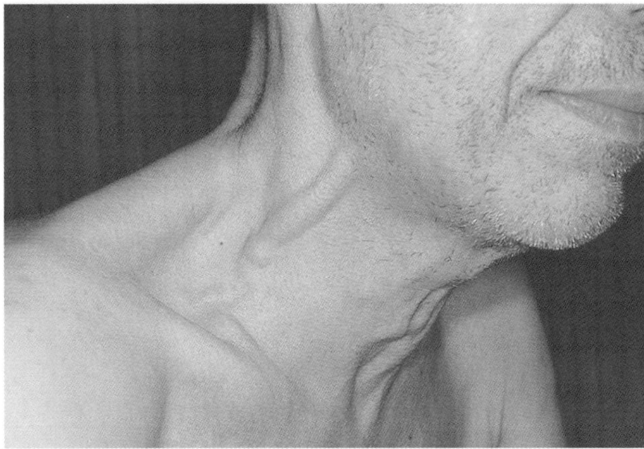

Fig. 38.13 Jugular Venous Distension (JVD) With Pericardial Tamponade The neck veins might be markedly distended with cardiac tamponade, but this finding is not universal, especially in patients with hypovolemic trauma. (From Swartz M: *Textbook of Physical Diagnosis*. 5th ed. Philadelphia, PA: Saunders; 2005.)

Knowing mechanisms of injury and location of the wounds is crucial for accurate assessment. Gunshot wounds and stab wounds to the chest are the most suggestive for this condition. Hemodynamically unstable patients with injuries to the chest should be immediately evaluated for tamponade using bedside sonography (FAST/eFAST examination). In a stable patient, an echocardiogram and subxiphoid pericardial window are diagnostic tools of choice. Pericardiocentesis (Fig. 38.14) may be lifesaving for some patients with pericardial tamponade who are in extremis.[56] It is a temporizing procedure performed to improve cardiac function while waiting for operative management with a pericardial window. ECG has acceptable specificity but poor sensitivity in diagnosing pericardial effusion and tamponade.[56] Pulsus alternans (the beat-to-beat alternation in the voltage in the P-QRS-T) may develop in patients with pericardial effusion and cardiac tamponade. Pulsus alternans may also reveal low QRS voltage and sinus tachycardia.[56] Early identification and prompt intervention are essential for patient survival.

Aortic Disruption

The majority (60%90%)[37] of victims with aortic rupture caused by blunt trauma die at the scene of the injury. For patients who survive to hospital arrival, 50% will die within 24 hours.[57]

Aortic injury is commonly associated with sudden horizontal or vertical acceleration or deceleration injuries such as high-speed MVCs and falls from a great height. The use of seat belts and air bags does not protect against this type

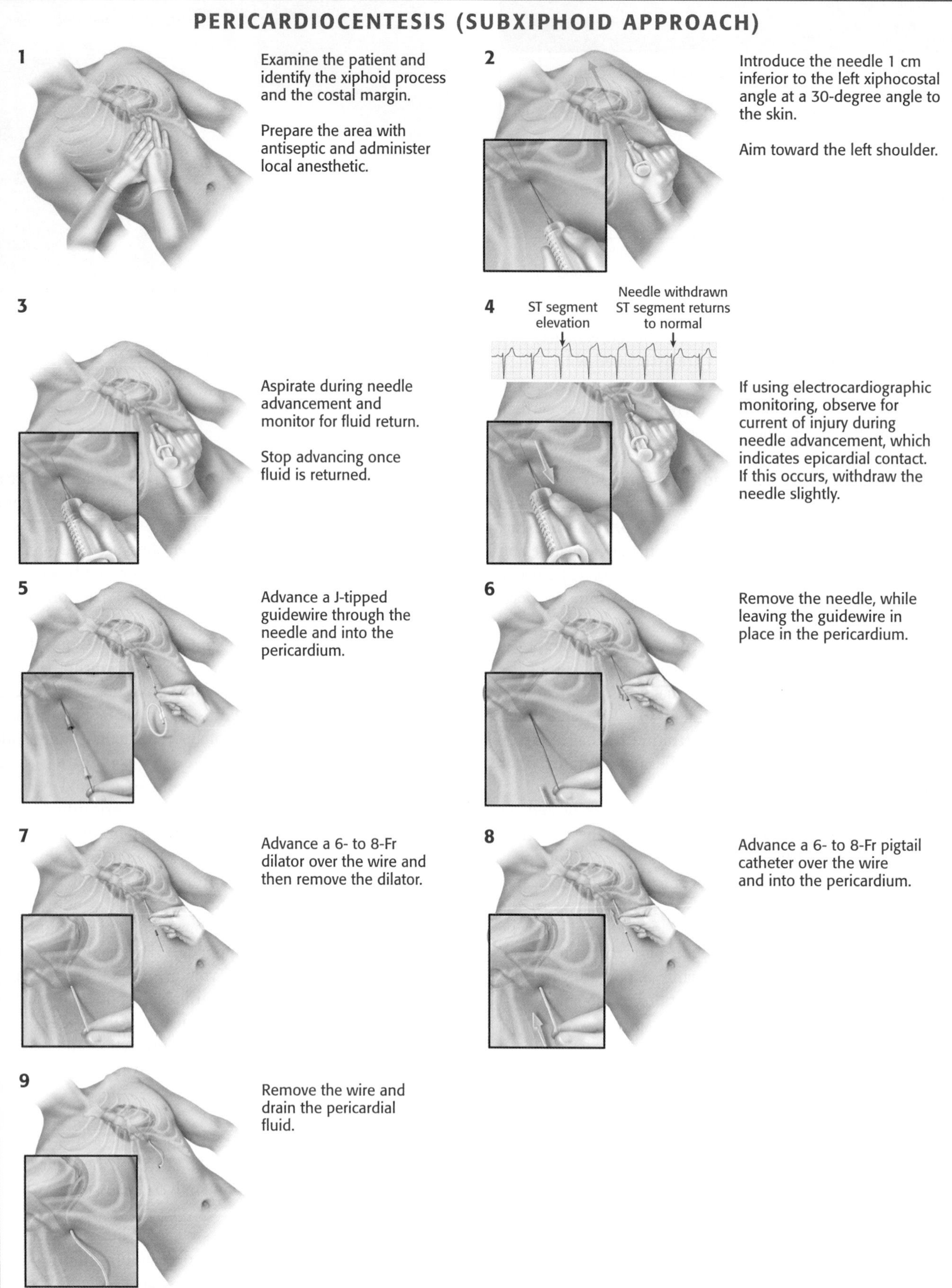

Fig. 38.14 Pericardiocentesis (From Custalow CB: *Color Atlas of Emergency Department Procedures.* Philadelphia, PA: Saunders: 2005. In: Roberts JR, Custalow CB, Thomsen TW, eds. *Roberts and Hedges, Clinical Procedures in Emergency Medicine and Acute Care.* 7th ed. Philadelphia, PA: Elsevier; 2019.)

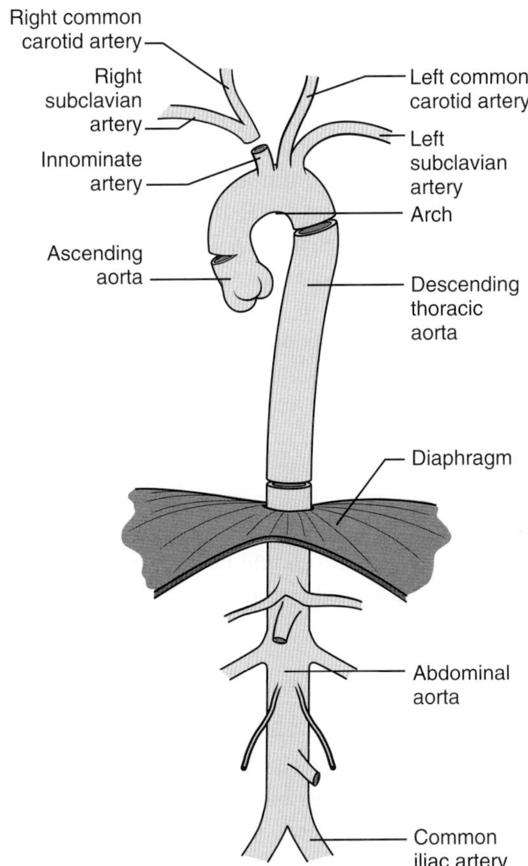

Fig. 38.15 Anatomy of the Descending and Abdominal Aorta (From Day MW. Thoracic and neck trauma. In: Emergency Nurses Association. *Trauma Nursing Core Course: Provider Manual.* 7th ed. Des Plaines, IL: Emergency Nurses Association. 2014;138.)

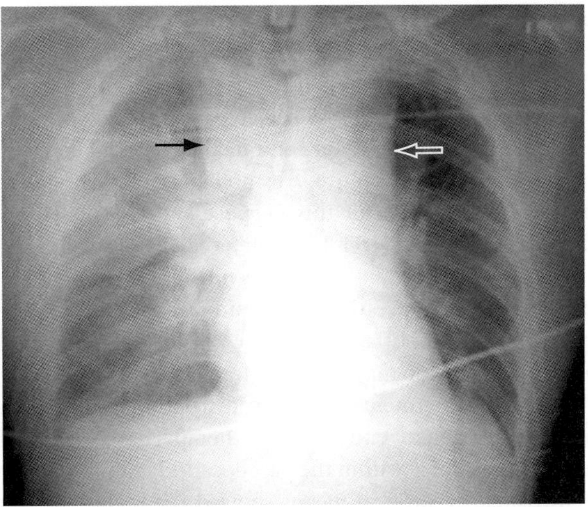

Fig. 38.16 Radiograph of Chest *Arrows* demonstrate widened mediastinum. (From Raja AS. Thoracic trauma. In: Walls RM, Hockberger RS, Gauche-Hill M. *Rosens Emergency Medicine: Concepts and Clinical Practice.* 9th ed. Philadelphia, PA: Elsevier; 2018:399.)

BOX 38.10 Chest X-Ray Findings for Blunt Aortic injury.

- Widened mediastinum (more than 8 cm when supine, or more than 6 cm when upright)
- Indistinct or abnormal aortic contour–obscured aortic knob
- Deviation of trachea L with a displaced nasogastric (NG) or orogastric (OG) tube
- Depression of left main bronchus
- Loss of the anterior-posterior (AP) window
- Widened paraspinal and/or paratracheal stripe
- Left apical pleural cap
- Large left hemothorax/pleural effusion

From Hapugoda S, D'Souza D. Thoracic aortic injury. https://radiopaedia.org/articles/thoracic-aortic-aortic-injury?lang=us Published 2018 Accessed June 7 2019.

of injury.[58] A combination of shearing forces, compression of the aorta against the vertebral column, and an increase in intraluminal pressure inside the vessel at the time of the injuring event are responsible for disrupting aortic integrity. The most common sites of injury are at sites of aortic tethering, the aortic root, the isthmus, and at the diaphragmatic hiatus. The most common injury is associated with a tear across the intima and media just distal to the takeoff of the left subclavian artery, where the proximal thoracic aorta is tethered at the ligamentum arteriosum. Fig. 38.15 describes the anatomy of the descending and abdominal aorta.

The possibility of aortic disruption should be considered in every patient who sustains a severe deceleration injury.[37] Patients may complain of chest pain or pain between the scapulae, often described as unrelenting and severe. Other symptoms include dyspnea and hemoptysis. A loud systolic murmur may be heard over the precordium if aortic valve integrity has been lost. Signs of hemorrhagic shock may be present. Hypertension can be an important clinical sign. A discrepancy between blood pressure (BP) values and pulse strength in the right and left arms may occur: BP and pulse quality in the upper extremities are elevated, whereas pulses and BP in the lower extremities are decreased or absent.[37] Lower extremity paralysis may also be seen.

The most common diagnostic test used to detect aortic disruption is a chest radiograph; the most common finding is mediastinal widening (Fig. 38.16). A supine chest radiograph may not adequately demonstrate mediastinal widening or may demonstrate one falsely in the bariatric patient. Other chest film findings are described in Box 38.10. The diagnostic standard for identification of aortic injury is CT scan of the chest, which has resulted in an earlier and more frequent diagnosis of traumatic aortic injuries. This, too, carries with it false-positive readings. There are multiple anatomic mimics found on CT scan for an acute aortic injury. Therefore it is important to be aware of these potential mimics to assure accurate diagnosis and subsequent appropriate therapy for these patients.

Stabilization and management in the ED include insertion of large-bore intravenous catheters and collection of blood for type and crossmatch. Careful regulation of BP is mandatory until definitive surgical repair can be performed. Consideration for delay of any surgical procedure should be made for patients who present with life-threatening intracranial or intraabdominal injury or profuse retroperitoneal hemorrhage or who are at high risk for infection. Careful regulation of BP (systolic BP should be maintained between 100 and 120 mm Hg) is mandatory until definitive surgical repair can be performed.[37] The objective of BP management is to decrease the possibility of continued adventitial dissection and subsequent free rupture.[37] Esmolol, a short-acting titratable -blocker, is ideal for this purpose and is initiated with a bolus of 0.5 mg/kg over 1 minute, followed by an infusion of 0.05 mg/kg per minute. Unlike nitroprusside sodium, it decreases the pulse pressure and minimizes the shearing effect on the intact adventitia of the aorta.[37] If the BP remains elevated, nitroprusside may be added for additional BP control.

Definitive treatment for aortic disruption is immediate surgical repair, and endovascular therapy has become the treatment of choice within the past decade. Patients who have been treated by surgical means showed the highest survival rate. Endovascular therapy (thoracic endovascular aortic repair, or TEVAR) has especially shown a favorable low mortality rate.

Esophageal Injury

Injury to the esophagus is rare and often lethal, almost universally the result of penetrating trauma. The increased mortality of this injury is due to its anatomic location in which any area of the esophagus that is perforated has direct access to the mediastinum. The continued drainage from this injury causes a chemical and bacterial mediastinitis.[37] The most dependable symptom is pleuritic pain focused along the path of the esophagus and is exacerbated by swallowing or neck flexion.[37] Dyspnea occurs as the inflammatory process worsens. Subcutaneous air in the neck and mediastinum is present in only approximately 60% of patients.[37] A crunching sound (Hamman crunch) may be heard during systole as mediastinal air surrounds the heart.[37]

Management of the airway is done with either intubation or cricothyroidotomy. Diagnosis is confirmed by esophagoscopy on the stable patient. Urgent repair is indicated in >90% of esophageal injuries and should be performed to avoid the formation of a fistula, mediastinitis, or abscess.[37]

SUMMARY

Thoracic injuries are challenging, chaotic to manage, and potentially life-threatening due to compromises in breathing and circulation. Changes in diagnostic technology (i.e., FAST/eFAST examinations) have made early identification of many of these serious injuries easier. With more research, management of chest injuries may change significantly. The patient with a thoracic injury requires rapid assessment and intervention. The emergency nurse must anticipate potentially lethal thoracic injuries and rapidly intervene.

REFERENCES

1. Eckstein M, Henderson SO. Thoracic trauma. In: Marx JA, Hockberger RS, Walls RM, eds. *Rosens Emergency Medicine: Concepts and Clinical Practice*. 8th ed. St Louis, MO: Elsevier; 2014:431–458.
2. Bouzat P, Raux M, David JS, Tazarourte K, Vardon F. Chest trauma: First 48 hours management. *Anaesth Crit Care Pain Med*. 2017;36(2):135–145. org/10.1016/j.accpm.2017.01.003.
3. Pearson EG, Fitzgerald CA, Santore MT. Pediatric thoracic trauma: current trends. *Semin Pediatr Surg*. 2017;26(1):36–42.
4. Ludwig C, Koryllos A. Management of chest trauma. *J Thorac Dis*. 2017;9(suppl 3):S172–S177.
5. Sleightholm K. *Knife Wounds*. *ProTrainings Website*; 2018. https://www.profaw.co.uk/wiki/knife-wounds/. Published January 27. Accessed June 7, 2019.
6. Haar RJ, Iacopino V, Ranadive N, Dandu M, Weiser SD. Death, injury and disability from kinetic impact projectiles in crowd control settings: a systematic review. *BMJ Open*. 2017;7(12):e018154. https://doi.org/10.1136/bmjopen-2017-018154.
7. Chrysou K, Halat G, Hoksch B, Schmid RA, Kocher GJ. Lessons from a large trauma center: impact of blunt chest trauma in polytrauma patients—still a relevant problem? *Scand J Trauma Resusc Emerg Med*. 2017;25(1):42. https://doi.org/10.1186/s13049-017-0384-y.
8. Ball JE, Dains JW, Flynn JA, Solomon B, Stewart RW. *Seidels Guide to Physical Examination: An Interventional Approach*. 9th ed. St Louis, MO: Elsevier; 2017.
9. Kaewlai. Costal Cartilage Fractures are Common in Multi-Trauma Patients. Radprompt website http://radprompt.com/en/2018/01/03/costal-cartilage-fractures-are-common-in-multi-trauma-patients-2/ Published January 3, 2018. Accessed June 8, 2019.
10. Nummela MT, Bensch FV, Pyhlt TT, Koskinen SK. Incidence and imaging findings of costal cartilage fractures in patients with blunt chest trauma: a retrospective review of 1461 consecutive whole body CT examinations for trauma. *Radiology*. 2018;286(2):696–704.
11. Feher J. The mechanics of breathing. In: *Quantitative Human Physiology. An Introduction*. 2nd ed. London, England: Academic Press; 2017:623–632. org/10.1016/B978-0-12-800883-6.00060-4.
12. Phelen D, Collier P, Grimm RA. Pericardial disease. Cleveland Clinic website. http://www.clevelandclinicmeded.com/medicalpubs/diseasemanagement/cardiology/pericardial-disease/. Published July 2015. Accessed June 7, 2019.
13. Savatmongkorngul S, Wongwaisayawan S, Kaewlai R. Focused assessment with sonography for trauma: current perspectives. *Open Access Emerg Med*. 2017;9:57–62.
14. Richards JR, McGahan JP. Focused assessment with sonography in trauma (FAST) in 2017: what radiologists can learn. *Radiology*. 2017;283(1):30–48.

15. Weingart SD, Duque D, Nelson B. Rapid ultrasound for shock and hypotension. EMCrit 2009. https://emcrit.org/RUSH-exam/. Accessed June 7, 2019.
16. Seif D, Perera P, Mailhot T, Riley D, Mandavia D. Bedside ultrasound in resuscitation and the rapid ultrasound in shock protocol. *Crit Care Res Pract.* 2012;2012:503254. https://doi.org/10.1155/2012/503254.
17. American College of Surgeons. *Advanced Trauma Life Support ATLS Student Course Manual.* 10th ed. Chicago, IL: American College of Surgeons; 2018.
18. de Moya M, Nirula R, Biffl W. Rib fixation: who, what, when? *Trauma Surg Acute Care Open.* 2017;2(1):1–4. https://doi.org/10.1136/tsaco-2016-000059.
19. Shenvi C. Rib fractures in older adults—Whats the big deal? Aliem website. https://www.aliem.com/2015/06/rib-fractures-in-older-adults-whats-the-big-deal/. Published June 3, 2015. Accessed June 7, 2019.
20. American Association for the Surgery of Trauma. Rib fractures. 2018. http://www.aast.org/rib-fractures. Accessed June 7, 2019.
21. Murphy CEIV, Raja AS, Baumann BM, etal. Rib fracture diagnosis in the Panscan era. *Ann Emerg Med.* 2017;70(6):904–909. org/10.1016/j.annemergmed.2017.04.011.
22. Chen YJ. Lidocaine skin patch (Lidopat 5%) is effective in the treatment of traumatic rib fractures: a prospective double-blinded and vehicle-controlled study. *Med Principles Pract.* 2016;25:36–39. https://doi.org/10.1159/000441002.
23. Bugaev N, Breeze JL, Alhazmi M, etal. Magnitude of rib fracture displacement predicts opioid requirements. *J Trauma Acute Care Surg.* 2016;81(4):699–704. https://doi.org/10.1097/TA.0000000000001169.
24. Witt CE, Bulger EM. Comprehensive approach to the management of the patient with multiple rib fractures: a review and introduction of a bundled rib fracture management protocol. *Trauma Surg Acute Care Open.* 2017;2:1–7. https://doi.org/10.1136/tsaco-2016-000064.
25. Thoracic Key. The pathophysiology of flail chest injury. https://thoracickey.com/the-pathophysiology-of-flail-chest-injury/. Accessed June 7, 2019.
26. Michelitsch C, Acklin YP, Hssi G, Sommer C, Furrer M. Operative stabilization of chest wall trauma: single-center report of initial management and long-term outcome. *World J Surg.* 2018;42(12):3918–3926. https://doi.org/10.1007/s00268-018-4721-8.
27. Guthrie K. Sternal fractures. Life in the Fastlane website. https://lifeinthefastlane.com/sternal-fractures/. Updated May 3, 2017. Accessed June 7, 2019.
28. Scheyerer MJ, Zimmermann SM, Bouaicha S, Simmen HP, Wanner GA, Werner CM. Location of sternal fractures as a possible marker for associated injuries. *Emerg Med Int.* 2013;2013:407589. https://doi.org/10.1155/2013/407589.
29. Yeh DD, Hwabejire JO, DeMoya MA, etal. Sternal fracture-An analysis of the National Trauma Data Bank. *J Surg Res.* 2014;186(1):39–43.
30. Racine S, Émond M, Audette-Côté JS, et al. Delayed complications and functional outcome of isolated sternal fracture after emergency department discharge: a prospective, multicentre cohort study. *Can J Emerg Med.* 2016;18(5):349–357. https://doi.org/10.1017/cem.2016.326.
31. Crawford TC, Kemp CD, Yang SC. Thoracic trauma. In: Sellke FW, del Nido PJ, Swanson SJ, eds. *Sabiston and Spencer Surgery of the Chest.* 9th ed. St Louis, MO: Elsevier; 2016:100–130.
32. Richards CE, Wallis DN. Asphyxiation: a review. *Trauma.* 2005;7:37–45.
33. Schaefer N, Griffin A, Gerhardy B, Gochee P. Early recognition and management of laryngeal fracture: a case report. *Ochsner J.* 2014;14(2):264–265.
34. Horn DB, Maisel RH. *Penetrating and blunt trauma to the neck. Cummings Otolaryngology.* 6th ed. Philadelphia, PA: Elsevier; 2015:1872–1883Horn DB, Maisel RH. Penetrating and blunt trauma to the neck. Cummings Otolaryngology. 6th ed. Philadelphia, PA: Elsevier; 2015:1872-1883.
35. Moonsamy P, Sachdeva UM, Morse CR. Management of laryngotracheal trauma. *Ann Cardiothoracic Surg.* 2018;7(2):210–216.
36. Jennings A, Joe M, Karmy-Jones R. Tracheobronchial trauma. *JSM Burns Trauma.* 2017;2(1):1011.
37. Raja AS. Thoracic trauma. In: Walls RM, Hockberger RS, Gauche-Hill M, eds. *Rosens Emergency Medicine: Concepts and Clinical Practice.* 9th ed. Philadelphia, PA: Elsevier; 2018:382–403.
38. Martin RS, Meredith JW. Management of acute trauma. In: Townsend Jr CM, Beauchamp D, Evers M, Mattox KL, eds. *Sabiston Textbook of Surgery.* 12th ed. Philadelphia, PA: Elsevier; 2017:407–448.
39. EMCORE. How big is that pneumothorax? https://www.resus.com.au/2014/08/01/how-big-is-that-pneumothorax/. Published January 8, 2014. Accessed June 7, 2019.
40. EPmonthly. Pigtail catheter. http://epmonthly.com/article/pigtail-insertion/. Published 2014. Accessed June 7, 2019.
41. Chang SH, Kang YN, Chiu HY, Chiu YH. A systematic review and meta-analysis comparing pigtail catheter and chest tube as the initial treatment for pneumothorax. *Chest.* 2018;153(5):1201–1212.
42. McCracken DJ, Psallidas I, Rahman NM. Chest drain size: does it matter? *Eurasian J Pulmonol.* 2018;20(1):1–6.
43. Kheirabadi BS, Terrazas IB, Koller A, et al. Vented versus unvented chest seals for treatment of pneumothorax and prevention of tension pneumothorax in a swine model. *J Trauma Acute Care Surg.* 2013;75(1):150–156.
44. Kotora Jr JG, Henao J, Littlejohn LF, Kircher S. Vented chest seals for prevention of tension pneumothorax in a communicating pneumothorax. *J Emerg Med.* 2013;45(5):686–694.
45. Hecker M, Hegenscheid K, Vlzke H. Needle decompression of tension pneumothorax: population-based epidemiologic approach to adequate needle length in healthy volunteers in Northeast Germany. *J Trauma Acute Care Surg.* 2016;80(1):119–124.
46. Laan DV, Vu TDN, Thiels CA, etal. Chest wall thickness and decompression failure: a systematic review and meta-analysis comparing anatomic locations in needle thoracostomy. *Injury.* 2016;47(4):797–804. https://doi.org/10.1016/j.injury.2015.11.045.
47. Neavyn MJ, Pena ME, Babcock C. Autotransfusion. In: Roberts JR, Custalow CB, Thomsen TW, eds. *Roberts and Hedges Clinical Procedures in Emergency Medicine and Acute Care.* 7th ed. Philadelphia, PA: Elsevier; 2019:491–499.
48. Pharaon KS, Marasco S, Mayberry J. Rib fractures, flail chest, and pulmonary contusion. *Curr Trauma Rep.* 2015;1:237–242.
49. Welsford M. Diaphragmatic injuries. Medscape website. https://emedicine.medscape.com/article/822999-overview#a5. Updated October 8, 2015. Accessed June 7, 2019.
50. Bocchini G, Guida F. Diaphragmatic injuries after blunt trauma: are they still a challenge? https://www.semanticscholar.org/paper/Diaphragmatic-injuries-after-blunt-trauma%3A-are-they-Bocchini- Guida/0159be3097c72e100abd83d34be33a6099db1acd. Published 2012. Accessed June 7, 2019.
51. Newbury A, Dorfman JD, Lo HS. Imaging and management of thoracic trauma. *Semin Ultrasound CT MRI.* 2018;39(4):347–354.

52. Fallouh H, Dattani-Patel R, Rathinam S. Blunt thoracic trauma. *Surgery*. 2017;35(5):262–268.
53. Brewer B, Zarzaur BL. Cardiac contusions. *Curr Trauma Rep*. 2015;1(4):232–236.
54. Clancy K, Velopulos C, Bilaniuk J, etal. Screening for blunt cardiac injury: an Eastern Association for the Surgery of Trauma practice management guideline. *J Trauma*. 2012;73(5 supp 4):S301–S306.
55. Tayal VS, Beatty MA, Marx JA, Tomaszewski CA, Thomason MH. FAST (Focused Assessment With Sonography in Trauma) accurate for cardiac and intraperitoneal injury in penetrating anterior chest trauma. *J Ultrasound Med*. 2004;23(4):467–472.
56. Mallemat HA, Tewelde SZ. Pericardiocentesis. In: Roberts JR, Custalow CB, Thomsen TW, eds. *Roberts and Hedges Clinical Procedures in Emergency Medicine and Acute Care*. 7th ed. Philadelphia, PA: Elsevier; 2019:309–331.
57. Fox N, Schwartz D, Salazar JH, Haut ER, Scalea TM, Fabian TC. Evaluation and management of blunt traumatic aortic injury: a practice management guideline from the Eastern Association for the Surgery of Trauma. *J Trauma Acute Care Surg*. 2015;78(2):136–146.
58. Di Marco L, Pacini D, Di Bartolomeo R. Acute traumatic thoracic aortic injury: considerations and reflections on the endovascular aneurysm repair. *Aorta*. 2013;1(2):117–122.
59. Day MW. Thoracic and neck trauma. In: Emergency Nurses Association. *Trauma Nursing Core Course Provider Manual*. 7th ed. Des Plaines, IL: Emergency Nurses Association; 2014:138.
60. Hapugoda S, DSouza D. Thoracic aortic injury. https://radiopaedia.org/articles/thoracic-aortic-injury. Published 2018. Accessed June 7, 2019.

39

Abdominal and Genitourinary Trauma

Vicki Bacidore

Abdominal injuries are a significant source of morbidity and mortality. Abdominal injuries after blunt (80%) or penetrating (20%) trauma cause a significant number of traumatic fatalities. Motor vehicle crashes (MVC) and falls are the common cause of blunt trauma, whereas gunshot and stab wounds are the most common causes of penetrating trauma.[1]

Resulting massive hemorrhages from abdominal trauma and infection both lead to the high rates of mortality and morbidity.[2] One of the most frequent causes of preventable death is an abdominal injury unrecognized or missed by the emergency care provider.[3] The emergency nurse should initially manage patients with abdominal trauma in the same manner as all other trauma patients. Identifying the mechanism of injury and understanding kinetic injury forces (which raise the suspicion of specific organ involvement) and the hemodynamic status of the patient determine the prioritization of care.[4] Evaluation should begin with a rapid assessment and concurrent emergency management of any airway, breathing, circulation, and disability.

Blunt injury occurs most often from MVCs. These injuries are often related to mechanisms of shearing, tearing, or direct-impact forces. Blunt abdominal trauma has a higher mortality rate than penetrating injuries because blunt injuries are more difficult to detect and are often associated with other concomitant injuries to the head, chest, and extremities. Multiple abdominal organ injuries are associated with higher mortality. Penetrating injuries are often caused by gunshots or stabbings but can be due to any sharp object. Stab injuries occur almost three times more often than gunshot injuries, are usually less destructive, and have a much lower mortality rate. Penetrating trauma is more likely to involve vascular structures. Gunshot wounds can be deceiving because there is almost always some blast effect, and the dissipation of kinetic energy can damage structures not in direct contact with the bullet. Also, because of the force involved, the wound tract can close in on itself, making an accurate estimate of tissue damage difficult.[5] Chapter 34 will discuss mechanism of injury in more detail.

ANATOMY AND PHYSIOLOGY

Knowledge of the anatomic boundaries of the abdomen is important as one considers injury patterns, such as hollow-organ injury, vascular injury, solid-organ injury, or injuries to the retroperitoneal area (Fig. 39.1). The oval-shaped abdominal cavity extends from the dome-shaped diaphragm, a large muscle separating the thoracic cavity from the abdomen, to the pelvic brim. The pelvic brim stretches at an angle from the intervertebral disk between L5 and S1 to the pubic symphysis.

The abdomen is divided into three sections: the anterior abdomen, the flanks, and the posterior abdomen or back. The outer boundary of the abdominal cavity is the abdominal wall on the front of the body and the peritoneal surface on the back of the body. The abdomen extends upward into the lower thorax at about the level of the nipples or the fourth intercostal space. The anterior part of the abdomen extends inferiorly to the inguinal ligaments and symphysis pubis, and laterally to the front of the axillary line. The flanks include the regions between the anterior and posterior axillary lines from the sixth intercostal space to the iliac crest. The back extends posteriorly between the posterior axillary lines, from the scapula to the iliac crests. The flanks and the back are protected by thick abdominal wall muscles protecting the region from low-velocity penetrating trauma.

Peritoneum

The peritoneum is a smooth, serous membrane providing cover to the abdominal structures and allows the viscera to move within the abdomen without friction. The parietal peritoneum lines the abdominal wall, and the visceral peritoneum surrounds the organs of the abdomen. The mesenteries are double layers of the peritoneum. They surround, supply blood, and attach organs like the large and small bowel to the abdominal wall. Organs in the retroperitoneal space (e.g., kidneys, parts of the colon, duodenum, pancreas, aorta, and inferior vena cava [Fig. 39.2]) are only partially covered by the peritoneum. In men the peritoneum is closed, but in women it is open where the ends of the fallopian tubes communicate with the peritoneum.

Solid Organs

The liver is a solid organ and is the largest organ in the abdomen. It is located in the right upper quadrant (RUQ) with extension into the midline and is extremely vascular. Circulation is through the hepatic artery and portal vein and represents about 30% of the total cardiac output. Aside from its metabolic functions, the liver releases bile to aid in fat

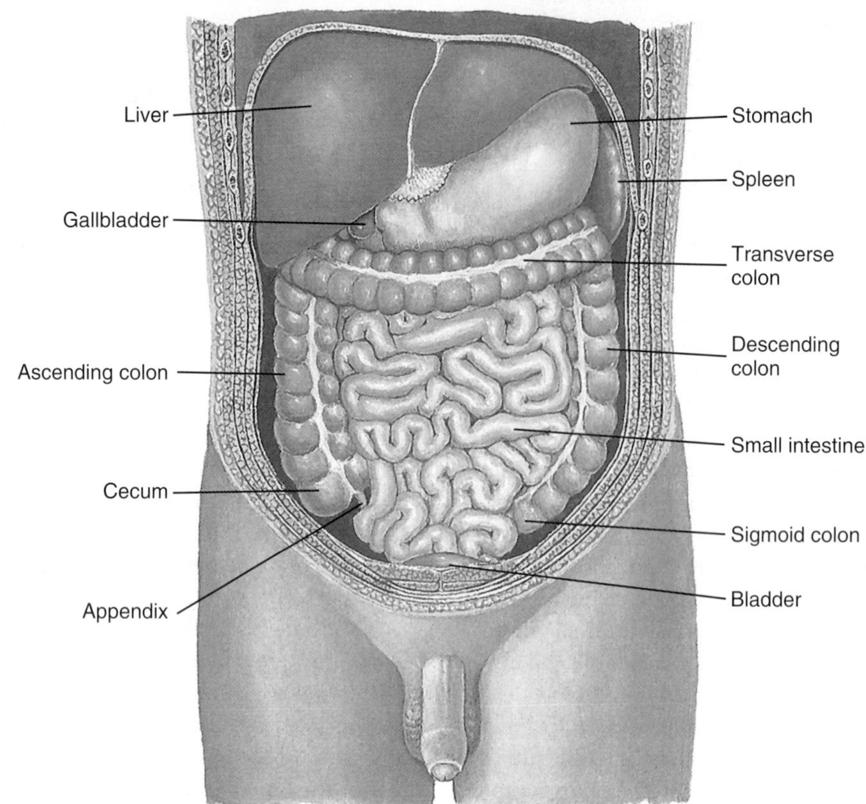

Fig. 39.1 Abdominal Viscera (From Seidel HM, Ball JW, Dains JE, Benedict, GW. *Mosby's Guide to Physical Examination.* 6th ed. St Louis, MO: Mosby; 2006.)

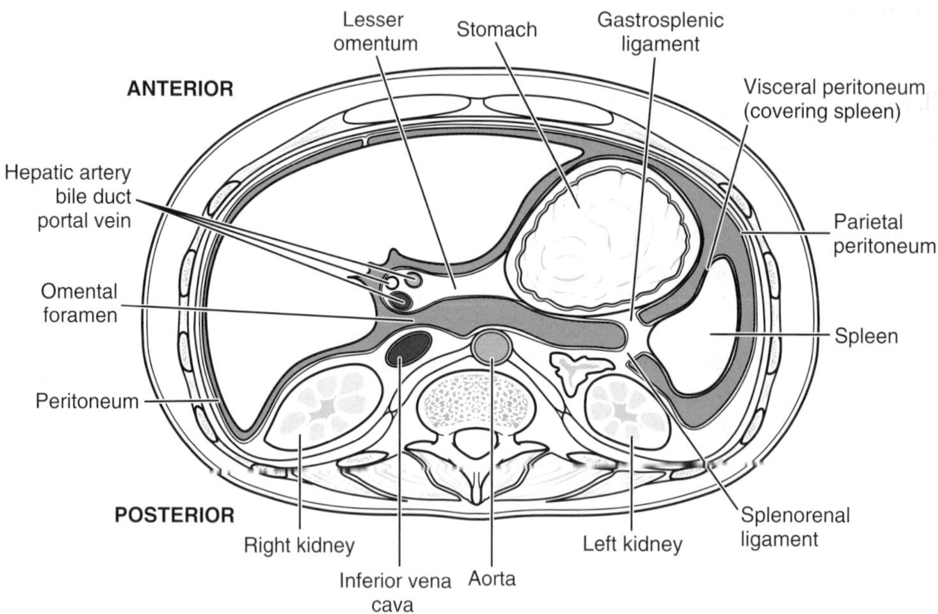

Fig. 39.2 Retroperitoneal Structures.

emulsification and the absorption of fatty acids. It also filters and stores up to 500 mL of blood at any given time.

The spleen is also a large vascular organ located in the left upper quadrant (LUQ), beneath the diaphragm at the level of the ninth through the 11th ribs. The spleen is important in the body's immune function for its clearance of bacteria. It also filters and stores up to 200 mL of blood.

The gallbladder is a saclike organ located on the lower surface of the liver acting as a reservoir for bile, one of the digestive enzymes produced by the liver. The liver continually secretes bile, and the gallbladder stores it until it is released through the cystic duct during the digestive process.

The kidneys are retroperitoneal organs that lie at the level of the 12th thoracic vertebra to the third lumbar vertebra. The kidneys lie posterior to the stomach, spleen, colonic flexure, and small bowel. They are enclosed in a capsule of fatty tissue and a layer of renal fascia, which maintains their position. They are well protected by the vertebral bodies, the back muscles, and the abdominal viscera. They are protected because of their deep location in the retroperitoneal space and by abdominal contents, muscles, and the vertebral spine. They filter blood and excrete body wastes in the form of urine.

The pancreas is located behind the stomach along the abdomen's posterior wall in the retroperitoneum. Its exocrine cells produce enzymes, electrolytes, and bicarbonate to assist in the digestion and absorption of nutrients. Its endocrine cells produce insulin, glucagon, and somatostatin, which are involved in carbohydrate metabolism.

Hollow Organs

The stomach is located in the LUQ between the liver and spleen at the level of the seventh and ninth ribs. Entry to the stomach is controlled by the lower esophageal sphincter (sometimes referred to as the cardiac sphincter), and exit is controlled by the pyloric sphincter. The stomach stores food, makes acidic gastric secretions, mixes food with the secretions, and then propels the mixture into the duodenum.

The small bowel connects to the pyloric sphincter and fills most of the abdominal cavity because it is approximately 7 m long. It is composed of three sections: duodenum, jejunum, and ileum, and it is held in position by the adjacent viscera, the peritoneal membrane attachments to the posterior abdominal wall, and ligaments. It functions by releasing enzymes and aiding in digestion and absorption.

The large bowel is about 1.5 m long; it connects with the ileum proximally and ends distally at the rectum. Its divisions consist of the ascending colon, transverse colon, descending colon, and sigmoid colon. The primary functions of the large bowel are to absorb water and nutrients and store fecal matter until it can be eliminated.

The urinary bladder is an extraperitoneal organ for storage of urine. When empty, it lies in the pelvic cavity, and when full, it can expand into the abdomen. Its blood supply is large and derived from branches of the iliac artery. The ureters are a pair of thick-walled, hollow tubes carrying urine from the kidneys to the urinary bladder. The female urethra is short and well protected by the symphysis pubis, whereas the male urethra is about 20 cm long and lies mostly outside of the body.

Reproductive Organs

The abdomen also contains organs of the reproductive system. The female reproductive system contains the uterus, a pear-shaped organ allowing implantation, growth, and nourishment of a fetus during pregnancy. The nongravid uterus is in the pelvis, and the gravid uterus is in the midline of the lower abdomen. The female ovaries, located in the pelvis, one on each side of the uterus, produce the precursors to mature eggs and produce hormones regulating female reproductive function.

The male reproductive system contains the penis, the male external reproductive organ, as well as the testes. The penis has three vascular bodies (erectile tissue): the paired corpora cavernosa and the corpus spongiosum. A testis and epididymis lie in each scrotal compartment. Testicular blood supply is obtained via the spermatic cord and the testicular artery, the artery to the vas deferens, and the cremasteric artery. The scrotum is covered by a thin layer of skin and obtains its blood supply via the branches of the femoral and internal pudendal arteries.

Vascular Structures

The abdominal aorta lies left of the midline and bifurcates into the iliac arteries, which supply blood to the lower extremities. Three unpaired arteries originating from the abdominal aorta (the celiac trunk and the superior and inferior mesentery arteries) supply the abdominal organs. The celiac trunk branches into the hepatic, left gastric, and splenic arteries. The inferior vena cava is the major vein in the abdomen.

PATIENT ASSESSMENT

History

Because the patient with abdominal trauma may not exhibit any obvious injuries, abdominal trauma should be suspected based on the patient's chief complaint and mechanism of injury. Abdominal trauma should also be considered in a patient with multisystem trauma or history of injury with unexplained hypotension or tachycardia. Complaints of pain, rigidity, guarding, or spasms in the abdominal musculature are classic signs of intraabdominal injury. Peritoneal membranes may be irritated due to free blood, air, or gastric or intestinal contents within the peritoneal cavity. Irritation of the inferior surface of the diaphragm and phrenic nerve can cause referred pain to the left shoulder. This finding, known as the Kehr sign, should alert the nurse to a possible splenic injury. Patient history and assessment triggers requiring further evaluation include the following[2]:

1. Presence of abdominal pain, tenderness, or distention
2. Mechanism of injury and prehospital details suggest potential for injury
3. Lower chest or pelvic injury
4. High-speed collisions or collisions in which there has been substantial deformity to the vehicle (particularly if the patient was unrestrained)
5. MVCs with fatalities or those in which there were others with substantial injuries
6. Unprotected injury (i.e., motorcycle crashes)
7. Inability to tolerate a delayed diagnosis (e.g., older adults, those with significant comorbid diseases)
8. Presence of distracting injuries (e.g., long-bone fractures)
9. Decreased level of consciousness/altered sensorium
10. Pain-masking drugs (e.g., ethanol, opiates)

Mechanisms of Injury

Understanding the mechanism of injury, the type of force applied, and the tissue density of the injured organ (solid, hollow) aids the trauma team by focusing the assessment and having a high index of suspicion regarding specific organ involvement. Blunt and penetrating abdominal trauma can cause extensive injury to the viscera, resulting in massive blood loss, spillage of intestinal contents into the peritoneal space, and peritonitis.

Blunt

The diffuse injury patterns from blunt trauma place all abdominal organs at risk for injury. The organs most often injured from a blunt trauma mechanism are the spleen, liver, and small bowel.[4] The biomechanics of blunt injury involve a compression or crushing by direct energy transmission. If the compressive, shearing, or stretching forces exceed tissue tolerance limits, they are disrupted. This may result in injury to solid viscera (liver, spleen) or rupture of hollow viscera (gastrointestinal tract). Injury also can result from the movement of organs within the body. Some organs are rigidly fixed in place, whereas others are semifixed by ligaments, such as the mesenteric attachments of the intestines. During energy transfer, longitudinal shearing forces may cause rupture of these organs at their attachment points or where the blood vessels enter the organ. Examples of structures semifixed in place and therefore susceptible to injury include the mesentery and small bowel, particularly at the ligament of Treitz or at the junction of the distal small bowel and right colon. Falls from a height produce a unique pattern of injury. In this case injury severity is a function of distance and the surface on which the victim lands. Intraabdominal injuries are uncommon from vertical falls. Hollow visceral rupture is most frequent. Retroperitoneal injuries with significant blood loss, however, are common because force is transmitted up the axial skeleton.

Penetrating

Stab wounds and low-velocity gunshot wounds result in damage to the tissue by laceration. Stab wounds pass through adjacent abdominal organs and most commonly involve the liver, small bowel, diaphragm, and colon.[4] External examination of a stab wound may underestimate internal damage and cannot define the trajectory of the blade. Any stab wound in the lower chest, pelvis, flank, or back has caused abdominal injury until proven otherwise. Gunshot wounds most commonly involve the small bowel, colon, liver, and the abdominal vasculature[4] and cause injury in several ways. Bullets may injure organs directly, via secondary missiles such as bone or bullet fragments, or from energy transmitted from the bullet. Bullets designed to break apart once they enter a victim cause much more tissue destruction than a bullet remaining intact. Tissue disruptions presumed to be entrance and exit wounds can approximate the missile trajectory. Plain radiographs help localize the foreign body, allowing prediction of organs at risk. Unfortunately, bullets may not travel in a straight line. Thus all structures in any proximity to the presumed trajectory must be considered injured.[2]

Motor Vehicle Crashes

In MVCs, there are five typical patterns of impact: frontal, lateral, rear, rotational, and rollover. Each of these different mechanisms, with the exception of rear impact, has the potential to cause significant injury to the abdominal organs. In a rear-impact collision, the patient is less likely to have an abdominal injury if proper vehicular restraints are used. However, if restraints are improperly worn or not used at all, the potential for injury is great. Rollover impacts present the greatest potential to inflict lethal injuries. Unrestrained occupants may change direction several times with an increased risk for ejection from the vehicle. The occupants involved in a rollover may collide with each other, as well as with the vehicle interior, producing a wide range of potential injuries.

Inspection

Observe the lower chest for asymmetric chest wall movement, which may indicate lower rib fractures and liver, spleen, or diaphragmatic injury. Look at the contour of the abdomen: distention may be due to massive bleeding, pneumoperitoneum, gastric dilation, or ileus produced by peritoneal irritation; a flat or concave abdomen may be indicative of a ruptured diaphragm with herniation of abdominal organs into the thoracic cavity. Assess for bruising, abrasions, or lacerations. Ecchymosis in the left upper quadrant may indicate soft-tissue injury or a splenic injury. Bruising or patterning over where the seat belt would be located or steering wheel–shaped contusions suggest a significant mechanism of injury, and other intraabdominal injuries should be suspected. A seat belt sign is associated in 20% of mesenteric, bowel, and lumbar spine injuries.[6] Cullen sign (i.e., periumbilical ecchymosis) may indicate intraperitoneal hemorrhage; however, this symptom usually takes several hours to develop. Flank bruising, Grey Turner sign, may raise suspicion for retroperitoneal injury and bleeding. Old surgical scars should be noted because this may help narrow the search for injured organs. Inspect for gunshot or stab wounds, and inspect the pelvic area for soft-tissue bruising.

Percussion and Auscultation

Percussion has been used to detect the presence of free fluid in the abdomen. With the ready availability of more sensitive, noninvasive diagnostic techniques (e.g., ultrasonography and computed tomography [CT]), listening to percussion sounds to diagnose abdominal injury may seldom be done.

All four quadrants of the abdomen should be auscultated for the presence and frequency of bowel sounds. The presence of bowel sounds is a reassuring indicator of peristalsis, but it is not reliable for ruling out visceral injuries. Up to 30% of patients have active bowel sounds in the presence of intraperitoneal bleeding or rupture of hollow viscera. Conversely, about 30% of patients who have absolutely no bowel sounds after careful listening for at least 5 minutes have no visceral damage.[7] An abdominal bruit may indicate underlying vascular disease or traumatic arteriovenous fistula. Auscultation of bowel sounds in the thoracic cavity, especially on the left side, may indicate the presence of a diaphragmatic injury.

Palpation

Beginning in an area where the patient has not complained of pain, palpate the abdomen for pain, rigidity, tenderness, and guarding in all four quadrants. To determine the presence of rebound tenderness, press on the abdomen and quickly release. Fullness and doughy consistency may indicate intraabdominal hemorrhage. Crepitus or instability of the lower thoracic cage indicates the potential for splenic or hepatic injuries associated with lower rib injuries. Pelvic instability indicates the potential for lower urinary tract injury, as well as pelvic and retroperitoneal hematoma.

Initial Stabilization

Initial stabilization of the patient with abdominal or genitourinary (GU) trauma follows the same sequence as for any patient with major trauma and begins by securing airway, breathing, and circulation. Two large-bore intravenous (IV) catheters should be secured for administration of crystalloids (e.g., lactated Ringer's solution or normal saline), blood products, and medications. Baseline laboratory studies are obtained, as well as a pregnancy test for any woman of childbearing age. Efforts should be made to limit hypothermia, including use of warm blankets and prewarmed fluids.

Medications

Analgesia

Pain relief is appropriate for most injuries. Morphine sulfate 2 to 5 mg or 0.1 mg/kg IV is commonly used, but fentanyl 50 to 100 mcg IV may be used as a first-line agent for pain control due to its advantageous hemodynamic profile. It has less histamine release than morphine and thus causes less hypotension; its shorter duration of action may be advantageous in trauma situations in which serial examinations are required.[8] Avoid medications with antiplatelet activity potential, such as nonsteroidal antiinflammatory drugs.

Antibiotics

Anaerobes and coliforms are the predominant organisms found in cases of intestinal perforation, and antibiotics active against these organisms should be given to decrease the incidence of intraabdominal sepsis.

Emergency Department Interventions

Urinary Catheter

A urinary catheter should be inserted to monitor urine output in all patients with major trauma. Before inserting a urinary catheter in patients with severe blunt trauma, a rectal examination must be performed to check the position of the prostate, look for any rectal blood, and check sphincter tone. If there is any suspicion of damage to the urethra, as evidenced by blood at the urethral meatus, penile or perineal hematomas, a displaced prostate, or a severe anterior pelvic fracture, a retrograde urethrogram should be performed before a urinary catheter is inserted.[4]

Gastric Decompression

Early gastric decompression with a gastric tube is particularly important when there is a possibility of intraabdominal visceral damage or when the patient may have eaten or drunk recently. All trauma patients should be assumed to have full stomachs, even if they deny recent ingestion of food or liquids. The gastric tube may be a valuable diagnostic tool for revealing injury to the upper gastrointestinal tract. Oral rather than nasal insertion of the tube is recommended in patients with concurrent head injury (i.e., basilar skull fracture) or midface injuries. Injured patients tend to swallow air, especially if they have any respiratory distress. Patients resuscitated with a bag-mask device can also have large amounts of air forced into their stomachs. The resulting distention of the stomach not only increases the chances of vomiting and aspirating but also raises the diaphragm, increasing the resistance to ventilation.

Wound Care

Penetrating wounds should be covered with sterile dressings. In cases of traumatic eviscerations, the intraabdominal contents extrude through the abdominal wall and are exposed to the environment. To prevent further injury and to keep the exposed organs viable for surgical replacement, the extruded contents must be kept moist at all times with sterile saline–soaked dressings. Eviscerated organs, especially the small bowel, should never be allowed to dry out. Never attempt to push the eviscerated contents back into the peritoneal cavity, which may further injure the tissue.[9]

Disposition

A trauma surgeon should be consulted for any patient suspected of having an abdominal or GU injury. The patient should be transferred to another facility if a trauma surgeon is unavailable. All patients with intraabdominal injuries require admission for emergent surgery or for observation. Stable and reliable patients with no identifiable injury can be discharged to home, as well as patients with stab wounds to the abdominal cavity found to be superficial after wound exploration. Discharged patients should be provided with detailed instructions describing signs of undiagnosed injury. Patients should be advised to return if they experience increased abdominal pain or distention, nausea and/or vomiting, light-headedness, syncope, or new or increased bleeding in urine or feces. All patients require close follow-up and repeat evaluation.

Diagnostic Evaluation

Diagnostic evaluation of a patient with abdominal trauma is based on the patient's hemodynamic stability. If the patient is or becomes hemodynamically unstable secondary to intraperitoneal injury, transfusion with fluids or blood is begun and the patient is prepared for surgery. If the patient's condition permits, major diagnostic tools, including radiology, CT, focused assessment sonography for trauma (FAST) examination, magnetic resonance imaging (MRI), angiography,

TABLE 39.1 Comparison of Diagnostic Tests.

Procedure	Advantages	Disadvantages	Results
FAST (focused assessment sonography for trauma)	Noninvasive Provides rapid evaluation of hemoperitoneum	Operator dependent Hollow viscus injury rarely identified	As accurate as DPL Free fluid appears as black stripe Sensitivity/specificity of 85%–95%
CT (computerized tomography)	Provides most detailed images Useful in determining nonoperative management of solid injuries	Expensive Time consuming Use only on hemodynamically stable patients May miss injuries to diaphragm and gastrointestinal tract	High specificity
DPL (diagnostic peritoneal lavage)	Provides rapid evaluation of intraperitoneal blood Useful in unstable patients, patients with unreliable history, or inability to perform serial abdominal examinations	Invasive procedure Complications of bleeding, infection	Can have false-positive results leading to unnecessary laparotomy

From Emergency Nurses Association. *Emergency Nursing Core Curriculum.* 7th ed. St Louis, MO: Elsevier; 2018.

diagnostic peritoneal lavage (DPL), and laparoscopy, may be used. Table 39.1 provides a comparison of DPL, FAST, and CT scans in blunt abdominal trauma.

Imaging

Computed tomography scan of the abdomen and pelvis. CT with IV contrast is the gold standard study for abdominal injury. A CT scan is noninvasive but requires a hemodynamically stable patient. It can reveal intraperitoneal injury, retroperitoneal injury, the source of intraabdominal hemorrhage, and, occasionally, active bleeding. A CT scan can aid in evaluating the vertebral column and can be extended to visualize the thorax and pelvis. One advantage of the CT scan is the reduction of nontherapeutic laparotomies for self-limited injuries to the liver and spleen. Unfortunately, the CT scan is not accurate enough to detect injury to the pancreas, diaphragm, small bowel, and mesentery. Oral contrast is not routinely used at many trauma centers—the risk for aspiration is increased with administration of oral contrast, and the delay in imaging is potentially harmful. IV contrast is essential to increase the ability of CT scans to identify hemorrhage.[2]

Focused assessment sonography for trauma/ultrasonography. FAST is a portable (bedside), rapid, accurate, and inexpensive diagnostic tool used to detect the presence of hemoperitoneum in patients primarily with blunt abdominal trauma. Four areas are examined: the hepatorenal fossa, the splenorenal fossa, the pericardial sac, and the pelvis (Fig. 39.3). FAST is considered to be extremely sensitive, with the ability to detect as little as 100 mL of fluid. However, FAST is typically not considered positive until at least 200 to 500 mL of fluid is detected in the abdomen.[5] The disadvantage of FAST is its inability to diagnose hollow visceral and retroperitoneal injuries or intraperitoneal injuries not associated with hemoperitoneum. Ultrasonography can be used to rapidly outline kidney parenchyma and provide evidence of intraperitoneal fluid. It is operator dependent and is not accurate in distinguishing blood from other intraperitoneal fluids, such as ascites. The FAST scan is being increasingly used in the initial assessment of trauma patients and has been incorporated into the recommendations for investigations of blunt trauma by the American College of Surgeons.[4]

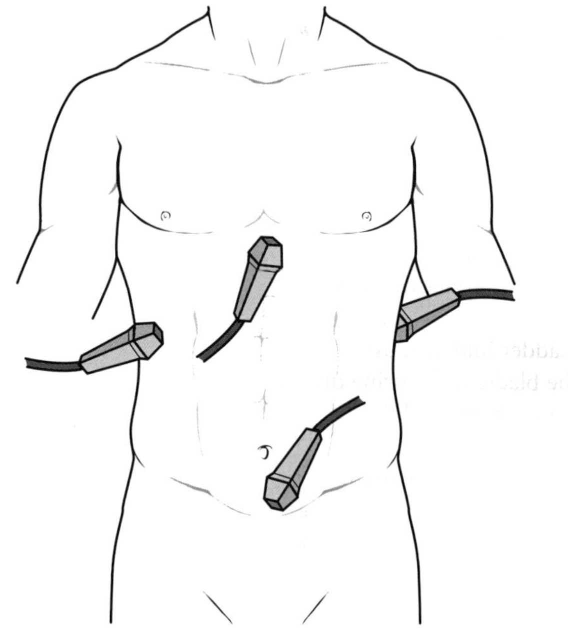

Fig. 39.3 Four sites viewed in focused assessment sonography for trauma (FAST) examinations. (From Emergency Nurses Association. *Trauma Nursing Core Course Provider Manual.* 6th ed. Des Plaines, IL: Emergency Nurses Association; 2007.)

Diagnostic peritoneal lavage. Although regarded as less useful than the FAST examination, DPL in blunt trauma is primarily indicated in the hemodynamically unstable patient who has multiple injuries. In the attempt to aspirate free peritoneal blood, the retrieval of 10 or more milliliters of frank blood (100,000/mm red blood cells) from the peritoneum is a strong indicator of intraperitoneal injury, and the procedure is then concluded. For lower-chest stab wounds and gunshot wounds, the cutoff for red blood cells is 5000/mm. If aspiration findings are negative, lavage is conducted in which the peritoneal cavity is washed with saline. This fluid is introduced by catheter, recovered by gravity drainage, and analyzed. The sole absolute contraindication to DPL is the established need for laparotomy. Relative contraindications include prior abdominal surgery or infections, coagulopathy, obesity, and second- or third-trimester pregnancy. Patients with equivocal findings should be observed for at least 24 hours. Many injuries will be to hollow viscera, and clinical manifestations should develop within that period. Elevated levels of peritoneal amylase may be indicative of small bowel or pancreatic injury. Other positive but less commonly documented DPL results include food fibers or the presence of fecal matter in the lavage fluid. As a precaution to minimize the risk for inadvertent injury to the stomach or bladder, a gastric tube and urinary catheter should be inserted before performing a DPL.[5]

Retrograde urethrography. Retrograde urethrography is indicated for any suspected urethral injury and should be performed before catheterization to prevent possible further urethral injury. Twenty to 30 mL of contrast is injected in the urethra and a radiograph is obtained. Any extravasation will identify the location of a tear. A CT scan of the abdomen and pelvis should be completed before this study because it can interfere with CT diagnosis and embolization treatment of pelvic arterial extravasation from pelvic fractures.[2]

Cystography. Cystography is indicated for any suspected bladder injury. A urinary catheter can be placed directly into the bladder, the urine drained, and the bladder refilled with contrast material. It is important to fully distend the bladder to avoid missing small injuries. Images are then obtained under retrograde urethrography.

Arteriography. Arteriography is needed if the mechanism of injury suggests a renal artery injury, because it can provide detailed information regarding vascular injury.

Laboratory Studies

Initial hemoglobin and hematocrit levels do not reflect the amount of recent hemorrhage that may have occurred, but these values can serve as a baseline and are important if the patient will be going to surgery. In the absence of hypotension, a progressive decrease in hemoglobin and hematocrit levels can serve as a warning of continued bleeding, but this finding tends to be relatively late. Serum amylase levels must be interpreted in conjunction with other clinical findings; however, an increasing level or a persistently high amylase level is suggestive of pancreatic injury.[7]

A urinalysis should be performed on any patient with suspected abdominal or pelvic damage as a guide to possible injury of the urinary tract and to detect diabetes mellitus or concomitant renal parenchymal disease. A urine dipstick alone is not sensitive or specific enough to predict abdominal injury.[9,10] If the urine dipstick is positive for hemoglobin but has few or no red blood cells, one should suspect myoglobinuria. With minor microscopic hematuria, a detailed urologic workup is not generally indicated, but a repeat urinalysis is appropriate. Microscopic hematuria, heme-positive dipstick, and gross hematuria are the strongest indicators of GU injury. However, the degree of hematuria does not necessarily correlate with the degree of injury. Furthermore, blunt injury to the renovascular pedicle or penetrating ureteral injury may not produce gross or even microscopic hematuria. The best urine sample for the assessment of hematuria in the trauma patient is the first voided or catheterized specimen because a later sample can often be diluted by diuresis. A urine pregnancy test should be done in all women of reproductive age.

SPECIFIC INJURIES

Abdominal Injuries

Spleen

Falls and MVCs commonly injure the spleen. However, less obvious injury patterns in activities such as sports (tackling in football or checking in lacrosse) can also cause injury. The spleen, which stores 200 to 300 mL of blood,[6] is one of the organs most often injured by blunt trauma. Its small size makes it a difficult target, so it is injured less often with penetrating trauma. Due to the spleen being encapsulated, injury may damage only the capsule or can actually fracture the spleen. Table 39.2 summarizes grading of splenic injury. Injury is suggested when the patient has sustained blunt trauma to the LUQ. The patient should be assessed for LUQ pain and tenderness, pain referred to the left shoulder (Kehr sign), peritoneal irritation, and hypotension.

When assessing for bruising or pain in the LUQ, the presence of the Kehr sign suggests diaphragmatic irritation by peritoneal blood. Splenic injuries may cause significant hemodynamic instability. Shock and hypotension are present in as few as 30% of patients with splenic trauma.[11] Not all patients with splenic injury require surgery; those who are hemodynamically stable may be managed nonoperatively, focusing on serial abdominal examinations, vital signs, and laboratory values. Nonoperative management ranges from observation and monitoring to angiography/angioembolization to preserve the spleen and its function.[12] Operative management is reserved for unstable patients, gunshot wounds, or injuries violating all layers of the splenic capsule. The CT scan is noninvasive and sensitive in stable patients. The FAST examination can be used for unstable patients.

Liver

The liver's size and anterior location make it an easy target for blunt and penetrating forces. The liver is one of the most commonly injured abdominal organs in blunt trauma. A healthy liver filters 1.7 liters of blood per minute and can hold 13% of the body's blood supply, resulting in serious sequelae if it is injured. Overall mortality for liver injuries is 10%. MVCs still account for the majority of hepatic injuries.[6] Like the spleen, the liver is encapsulated, so injuries can affect only the capsule

TABLE 39.2 Splenic Injuries.

Grade	Category	Description
I	Hematoma	Subcapsular; involves less than 10% surface area; hematoma does not expand
	Laceration	Nonbleeding capsular tear; less than 1 cm deep
II	Hematoma	Subcapsular hematoma covering 10%–50% surface area Hematoma does not expand; intraparenchymal hematoma less than 2 cm wide
	Laceration	Capsular tear with active bleeding; intraparenchymal injury 1–3 cm deep
III	Hematoma	Subscapular hematoma involving more than 50% surface area or one that is expanding; intraparenchymal hematoma ≥5 cm or expanding; ruptured subscapular hematoma with active bleeding
	Laceration	More than 3 cm deep or involving intracellular vessels
IV	Hematoma	Ruptured intraparenchymal hematoma with active bleeding
	Laceration	Segmental laceration or one that involves hilar vessels Devascularization of more than 25% of spleen
V	Laceration	Shattered spleen
	Vascular	Hilar vascular injury; spleen is devascularized

From Pearl WS, Todd KH. Ultrasonography for the initial evaluation of blunt abdominal trauma: a review in prospective trials. *Ann Emerg Med.* 1996;27(3):353-361.

TABLE 39.3 Liver Injuries.

Grade	Category	Description
I	Hematoma	Nonexpanding subcapsular hematoma less than 10% of liver surface
	Laceration	Nonbleeding capsular tear less than 1 cm deep
II	Hematoma	Nonexpanding subcapsular hematoma covering 10%–50% surface area; less than 2 cm deep
	Laceration	Less than 3 cm parenchymal penetration; less than 10 cm long
III	Hematoma	Subcapsular hematoma more than 50% of surface area or one that is expanding; ruptured subcapsular hematoma with active bleeding; intraparenchymal hematoma more than 2 cm wide
	Laceration	More than 3 cm deep
IV	Hematoma	Ruptured central hematoma
	Laceration	15%–25% hepatic lobe destroyed
V	Laceration	More than 75% hepatic lobe destroyed
	Vascular	Major hepatic veins injured
VI	Vascular	Avulsed liver

From Pearl WS, Todd KH. Ultrasonography for the initial evaluation of blunt abdominal trauma: a review in prospective trials. *Ann Emerg Med* 1996;27(3):353-361.

or fracture the liver itself. Table 39.3 summarizes graded liver injuries. Liver injuries are suggested when the patient has a direct blow to the RUQ from the eighth rib to the central abdomen. Clinical indications include RUQ pain and tenderness, bruising over the RUQ, or referred pain to the right shoulder. Hemodynamic instability is almost always present when the liver sustains major damage. The trauma team should consider acute hepatic injury if the patient remains hypotensive despite aggressive IV fluid resuscitation. The CT scan is noninvasive and sensitive in stable patients, and the FAST examination can be used for unstable patients. Surgical repair of liver injuries is determined by the extent of the injury and the patient's hemodynamic status. Nonoperative management of blunt liver injuries is now the standard in the majority of hemodynamically stable patients.[13]

Stomach

The stomach is a hollow organ that can be easily displaced, so it is rarely injured with blunt trauma. Gastric and esophageal injuries occur more with multiorgan and multisystem injuries and are most commonly associated with penetrating trauma because of their size and anterior location.[3] Physical signs and symptoms associated with stomach injuries include LUQ pain and tenderness. Diagnosis is based on patient assessment, aspiration of blood via the gastric tube, and presence of free air on the abdominal radiograph. All patients with gastric injury require surgical exploration.

Large and Small Intestine

The intestines are hollow, highly vascular organs fixed at various points in the peritoneal cavity. Their anterior location, relative lack of protection, vascularity, and fixed points of attachment make the intestines vulnerable to both blunt and penetrating injuries. Penetrating trauma, particularly stab wounds, can eviscerate the bowel or omentum. Management includes covering the evisceration with sterile saline–soaked pads, taking care not to pour saline directly onto pads on the wound. Wounds should then be covered with an occlusive dressing. Examine the back, because organs can eviscerate from penetrating injury to the posterior surface as well. Establish IV access, and prepare the patient for surgery. The intestines are frequently injured by inappropriately worn seat belts. Injury to the intestines usually causes rupture, followed by spillage of chemical and bacterial contamination into the peritoneum. Initial signs and symptoms of intestinal injury include tenderness and rigidity. As time progresses and more peritoneal contamination occurs, the patient may develop fever, elevated white blood cell count, abdominal distention, and hypoactive bowel sounds. Reassessments are important because peritoneal signs may be delayed and injuries can be missed on initial plain radiographs and CT scans.

Pancreas

The pancreas, a semisolid organ in the retroperitoneal space, is well protected by the liver and stomach, so it is more likely to be injured by penetrating trauma. Pancreatic injury from blunt trauma is more unusual but does occur. Children sustain pancreatic injury in bicycle crashes when the handlebars are driven into the abdomen. Patients with pancreatic injury may present with epigastric or back pain. Cullen sign is often associated with pancreatic injury and pancreatitis. The retroperitoneal location of the pancreas makes DPL an unreliable indicator of pancreatic injury. Elevated serum amylase level is also an unreliable indicator of pancreatic injury because up to 40% of all patients with pancreatic injury initially have a normal serum amylase level. Lipase is considered a better indicator of pancreatic injury.[14] CT scan is noninvasive and sensitive to detect pancreatic injury. Endoscopic retrograde pancreatography has proven useful in identifying injury to the pancreatic duct. When surgery is required, every effort is made to preserve the pancreas because of its essential endocrine and exocrine functions. The majority of patients with pancreatic injury have other injuries, with associated hemorrhage being the major cause of death.

Diaphragm

Diaphragmatic rupture may be due to blunt or penetrating mechanisms. Rupture almost always occurs on the left side because the liver protects the right hemidiaphragm. Rupture should be suspected in all patients with thoracoabdominal injuries. In diaphragmatic rupture, abdominal organs herniate into the thoracic cavity, causing respiratory compromise secondary to lung compression. Bowel sounds may be auscultated in the chest cavity. Loss of negative pressure in the chest and inability of the diaphragm to function normally further compromise respiratory function. Cardiac output also decreases because of cardiac compression. Diagnosis is usually confirmed by a CT scan of the chest showing abdominal contents or the gastric tube in the left chest or laparoscopy. These patients require immediate surgical repair. Mortality increases with delay in identification and treatment (see also Chapter 38, Thoracic Trauma).

Vascular Structures

Major vascular structures in the abdomen include the abdominal aorta, inferior vena cava, iliac artery, and hepatic veins. Vessels can be injured by blunt or penetrating mechanisms—injury of major abdominal vessels occurs in 5% to 10% of patients with blunt abdominal trauma. Disruption of vascular structures causes severe hemorrhage and death if damage is not repaired. Hemorrhagic shock from intraabdominal hemorrhage often leads to metabolic acidosis accompanied by coagulopathy and hypothermia—often referred to as the "lethal triad of trauma."[15] Identification of injuries is often made in surgery, particularly in an unstable patient. A CT scan and arteriography may be used for the stable patient. Emergency management of patients with vascular injuries includes establishing IV access and providing rapid transport to the surgical suite.

Foreign Bodies

Abdominal injuries may result from foreign bodies in the stomach and rectum. This may be the result of ingestion, masturbation, autoeroticism, assault, confusion, or psychiatric illness. Body packing (i.e., drug-filled condoms or plastic bags swallowed or placed in the rectum) has been increasing as drug smugglers attempt to bring opium, heroin, cocaine, amphetamines, or other drugs into various countries. The substance most frequently carried is cocaine. Often these drugs will be wrapped in capsules, condoms, balloons, plastic bags, or latex glove fingers and swallowed or placed in the rectum, where they are prone to rupture. Not only may the patient suffer from the toxic effects of the drugs, but there have been some reports of gastrointestinal hemorrhage caused by prolonged pressure of the packets on the gastric mucosa. Body packing should be considered in patients who show signs of drug-induced toxic effects after recent international travel. Many patients do not acknowledge the presence of a foreign body during initial evaluation. Complaints are often vague and relate to pain or discomfort. Diagnosis is usually made using radiography. Removal of the foreign body may be done in the emergency department or may require surgical intervention, depending on the size, shape, and location of the foreign body.[16]

Genitourinary Injuries

Most GU injuries occur from blunt force and are usually not immediately life-threatening. Red flags suggesting GU injury include the following[17]:

- flank, abdominal, rib, back, or scrotal pain
- inability to void spontaneously
- hemodynamic instability
- gross hematuria or blood at the urethral meatus or vaginal introitus
- perineal ecchymosis
- high-riding prostate
- Pelvic Fracture

In patients with GU trauma, symptoms are nonspecific and may be masked by or attributed to other injuries.

Renal Injuries

Renal injuries account for approximately 3% of all trauma cases and occur in up to 10% of abdominal trauma cases. The majority of renal injuries are due to blunt trauma forces, as in MVCs. The patient should be assessed for abdominal pain and tenderness over the kidneys, denoting significant force transfer. There may be a large flank ecchymosis,

TABLE 39.4 Renal Injury Scale.

Grade	Injury Description
I	Contusion: Microscopic or gross hematuria; normal urologic studies Subscapular hematoma, nonexpanding, no laceration
II	Laceration of renal parenchyma <1 cm; no extravasation Perinephric hematoma, nonexpanding
III	Laceration of renal parenchyma >1 cm No urinary extravasation; no collecting system involvement
IV	Laceration involving collecting system Perinephric and paranephric extravasation Thrombosis of segmental renal artery Main renal artery or vein injury; hemorrhage controlled
V	Fractured kidney Thrombosis of main renal artery Avulsion of main renal artery or vein

Grades I and II are minor; Grades III, IV, and V are major.
From Dixon MD, McAninch JW. American Urological Association update series, traumatic renal injuries, part 1: assessment and management. Houston, TX: American Urological Association; 1991.

palpable mass, or hematoma. Unfortunately, it is possible to have significant renal injury without any physical findings. Obtain a urinalysis, complete blood count, and chemistry panel to assess for hematuria, baseline hematocrit, and renal function. CT scan is the imaging study of choice because it can also reveal other abdominal injuries. Ultrasonography has a limited role but can reveal free fluid in the abdomen. Arteriography is most useful in showing injuries of the renal artery. Renal injuries can be graded from I to V depending on the location (Table 39.4); grades I to III will usually not require operative management. Higher-grade lesions may require nephrectomy, especially in hemodynamically unstable patients.

Penetrating renal injury results in a higher renal loss than blunt injury. Evidence of penetrating trauma to the flank should be obvious on examination; however, gunshot trajectories with known entry points not involving the flank can still involve the kidney and should be managed by the trauma surgeon along with a urologist. Surgical exploration of the abdomen is required for most gunshot wounds regardless of the grade of the injury, with selective operative management for stab wounds.[18]

Ureteral Injuries

The ureter is the least commonly injured part of the GU tract. The most common mechanism of ureteral injury is penetrating trauma. The patient should be assessed for this type of injury when there is an appropriate mechanism with or without abdominal pain. Penetrating injury can cause partial or complete ureteral transection. Hematuria may be detected on urinalysis, and a CT scan or arteriogram should be obtained. Surgical repair is primarily done by direct reanastomosis or stenting and temporary diversion. Because of the high rate of missed ureteral injuries, the possibility should be considered in trauma patients with worsening abdominal pain, fever, leukocytosis, or an unexplained fluid collection, possibly representing a urinoma.[19]

Bladder Injuries

The likelihood of bladder injury varies by the severity of the mechanism and also by the degree of bladder distention at the time of the injuring event. The fuller the bladder is, the greater the opportunity for injury. The majority of bladder injuries are usually associated with pelvic injuries from MVCs, falls from heights, and physical assaults to the lower abdomen.[2] These mechanisms may cause a pelvic fracture to perforate the bladder. Signs and symptoms of bladder injuries are generally nonspecific but may present as gross hematuria, suprapubic pain and tenderness, difficulty voiding, bruising and ecchymosis around the bladder/thighs, and abdominal distention, guarding, or rebound tenderness. The presence of signs of peritoneal irritation may also indicate the possibility of an intraperitoneal bladder rupture. Urinalysis typically shows gross hematuria. Gunshot wounds to the bladder may result in microscopic hematuria. Rupture of the bladder can be seen on routine abdominal CT and more accurately with a CT cystogram. Intraperitoneal bladder rupture requires exploratory laparotomy and repair through a layered closure, whereas extraperitoneal injuries can be managed with bladder drainage alone. Urologic follow-up and antibiotics are needed to prevent long-term complications, including strictures, fistulas, infection, and delayed healing.

Urethral Injuries

Most urethral injuries occur as a result of blunt trauma and occur primarily in men because the male urethra is longer and found mostly outside the body, whereas the female urethra is shorter and more protected. Injuries are usually a result of high-energy impact or straddle mechanisms and should be considered with any pelvic fracture. For classification of male injuries, the urethra is divided into a posterior segment (prostatic and membranous) and anterior segment (bulbous and pendulous). Posterior-segment injuries are associated with pelvic ring fractures, whereas anterior injuries are the result of external blunt or straddle mechanisms.[20] Evaluate the patient for blood at the urethral meatus (a contraindication to inserting a urinary catheter), a high-riding prostate, and pain, swelling, and ecchymosis in the penis or perineum. Gross hematuria is common. A retrograde urethrogram reveals extravasation of contrast anywhere along the course of the urethra, confirming the presence of disruption. If bladder filling is noted, then the lesion is considered partial, whereas no contrast ending up in the bladder is indicative of a complete tear. Minor injuries can be managed conservatively with passage of a catheter. Most injuries require suprapubic cystostomy and delayed repair of the urethral injury.

Foreign bodies of the urethra are usually the result of self-insertion and more recently as a result of retention of external equipment from minimally invasive surgeries (guidewires, tubes, laser fibers, clips, surgical instruments). Other complaints are suprapubic or perineal pain, urethral discharge, hematuria, difficulty urinating, swelling, or abscess formation. Clinical diagnosis is based on history and should always be considered in patients with chronic urinary tract infections. Radiographic studies, including plain radiographs, are usually helpful for detecting radiopaque objects. Management is focused on removing the foreign body and treating complications. Foreign bodies below the urogenital diaphragm can usually be palpated and readily removed endoscopically. When they are above the urogenital diaphragm, greater manipulation is required; perineal urethrostomy or suprapubic cystostomy is performed.[21]

Penile Injuries

Penile fracture and possible urethral injury typically occur when the corpus cavernosum ruptures after being bent by force, usually during vigorous sexual intercourse. The patient may report a popping sound as the tunica tears, followed by pain, swelling, visible deformity, and discoloration. Urinalysis will show microscopic and often gross hematuria. Retrograde urethrography should be performed to rule out a urethral injury, particularly in the presence of gross hematuria, inability to void, or blood at the urethral meatus. Early surgical treatment is essential to prevent complications such as deformity, impotence, erectile dysfunction, and urethral stenosis. Penile amputations are rare and are usually due to self-mutilation or from clothing trapped by heavy machinery. Penile rings used to enhance erection can cause constricting strangulation. Emergent urologic consultation is required for immediate reimplantation. Successful reimplantation has been accomplished up to 24 hours after amputation. The penis should be preserved in saline-soaked gauze, placed within a sterile plastic bag, and then placed on ice.[2]

Testicular Injuries

The testicles may be injured by a direct blow, MVCs, or sports-related activities. The right testicle, due to its higher lying position, is more commonly injured than the left. Injuries include contusion, hematocele, rupture, dislocation, or traumatic torsion. Testicular injury can be difficult to distinguish on examination alone, and imaging is required to assess the extent of the damage. Findings can include significant pain, swelling, and ecchymosis in the scrotal area. An ultrasound study should include Doppler flow studies to assess arterial flow. Ice and adequate analgesia should be used while obtaining urologic consultation. Do not delay consultation for imaging studies if the testicle appears ruptured. Complications of testicular trauma include testicular atrophy, infection, infarction, and infertility.

Straddle Injuries

Straddle injuries occur when a patient falls and takes the brunt of the fall on the perineum. These injuries commonly occur in young patients as they fall onto bicycle bars, motorcycles, and fences. On examination of the female patient, a vulvovaginal laceration with extensive ecchymosis of the perineum may be evident. Straddle injuries are often accompanied by vulvar hematomas that can extend into the retroperitoneal space. Associated urethral injuries and rectal tears should be ruled out. Treatment for straddle injuries involves repair of the laceration with evacuation and drainage of hematomas. The most common complication of the immediate postoperative period is infection. Sexual dysfunction may also result.

SUMMARY

Abdominal trauma is very common but often missed because other injuries distract attention from the abdomen. The delay in the development of signs and symptoms further confounds the ability to identify problems. Moreover, the bulk of injuries are seen in young people, whose compensatory capacities are high. An objective evaluation of the abdomen is often necessary with ultrasonography, followed by imaging studies dependent on the patient's stability. Penetrating injuries, especially high-velocity gunshot wounds, carry an extremely high chance of internal injury, so virtually all of these patients will require laparotomy. Blunt injuries are more difficult to recognize and require a higher level of suspicion based on the mechanism of injury. The emergency nurse who understands anatomy and recognizes injury patterns and pathophysiologic consequences of injury as a basis for signs and symptoms will contribute significantly to the effective management of the patient with abdominal and genitourinary trauma.

REFERENCES

1. Nishijima DK, Simel DL, Wisner DH, Holmes JF. Does this adult patient have a blunt intra-abdominal injury? *JAMA*. 2012;307(14):1517–1527.
2. French LK, Gordy S, Ma OJ. Abdominal trauma. In: Tintinalli JE, Stapczynski JS, Ma OJ, Yealy DM, Meckler GD, Cline DM, eds. *Tintinalli's Emergency Medicine: A Comprehensive Study Guide*. 8th ed. New York, NY: McGraw-Hill; 2016:1761–1775.
3. Todd SR. Critical concepts in abdominal injury. *Crit Care Clin*. 2004;20(1):119–1134.
4. American College of Surgeons. Abdominal and pelvic trauma. In: *Advanced Trauma Life Support for Doctors*. 9th ed. Chicago, IL: American College of Surgeons; 2012:122–147.
5. Puskarich MA, Marx JA. Abdominal trauma. In: 8th ed. Marx JA, Hockberger RS, Walls RM, eds. *Rosen's Emergency Medicine: Concepts and Clinical Practice*. Vol. 1. St Louis, MO: Saunders; 2013:459–478.

6. Emergency Nurses Association. *Trauma Nursing Core Course: Provider Manual.* 7th ed. Des Plaines, IL: Emergency Nurses Association; 2014.
7. Wilson RF. *Handbook of Trauma: Pitfalls and Pearls*. Philadelphia, PA: Lippincott Williams & Wilkins; 1999.
8. Levine MD, Gilmore WS. Traumatic emergencies: Abdomen. In: *The Washington Manual of Emergency Medicine*. Philadelphia, PA: Wolters Kluwer; 2018.
9. Criss E. Many elements involved in penetrating abdominal wounds: Do you know what to look for? *JEMS*. 2011;36(4). https://www.jems.com/articles/print/volume-36/issue-4/patient-care/many-elements-are-involved-pen.html?c=1. Published March 31, 2011 Accessed June 8, 2019.
10. Moustafa F, Loze C, Pereira B, et al. Assessment of urinary dipstick in patients admitted to an ED for blunt abdominal trauma. *Am J Emerg Med*. 2017;35(4):628–631.
11. Stone CK, Humphries RL. *Current Emergency Diagnosis and Treatment*. 8th ed. New York, NY: Lange Medical Books/McGraw-Hill; 2017.
12. Coccolini F, Montori G, Catena F, et al. Splenic trauma: WSES classification and guidelines for adult and pediatric patients. *World J Emerg Surg*. 2017;12(40). https://doi.org/10.1186/s13017-017-0151-4.
13. Barbier L, Calmels M, Lagadec M, et al. Can we refine the management of blunt liver trauma? *J Visc Surg*. 2018;156(1):23–29.
14. Cheng-Shyuan R, et al. Identification of pancreatic injury in patients with elevated amylase or lipase level using a decision tree classifier: a cross-sectional retrospective analysis in a level I trauma center. *Int J Environ Res Public Health*. 2018;14(277):1–12.
15. Dyer M, Neal MD. Defining the lethal triad. In: Pape HC, Peitzman AB, Rotondo MF, Giannoudis PV, eds. *Damage Control Management in the Polytrauma Patient*. 2nd ed. Cham, Switzerland: Springer; 2017:41–56.
16. Alvarez Llano L, Rey Valcalcel C, Al-Lal YM, Pérez Díaz MD, Stafford A, Turégano Fuentes F. The role of surgery in the management of "body packers." *Eur J Trauma Emerg Surg*. 2014;40(3):351–355.
17. Blair M. Overview of genitourinary trauma. *Urol Nurs*. 2011;31(3):139–146.
18. Zabkowski T, Skiba R, Saracyn M, Zielinski H. Analysis of renal trauma in adult patients: a 6-year own experiences trauma center. *Urol J*. 2015;12(4):2276–2279.
19. Shewakramani S, Reed KC. Genitourinary trauma. *Emerg Med Clin North Am*. 2011;29(3):501–518.
20. Campbell MR. Abdominal and urologic trauma. In: *Emergency Nurses Association. Emergency Nursing Core Curriculum*. 7th ed. St Louis, MO: Elsevier; 2018.
21. Alkan A, Basar MM. Endourological treatment of foreign bodies in the urinary system. *JSLS*. 2014;18(3). https://doi.org/10.4293/JSLS.2014.00271.

Orthopedic and Neurovascular Trauma

Mary Jo Cerepani

Musculoskeletal injury is one of the most common types of trauma seen in the emergency department (ED) and is a significant cause of disability. Primary mechanisms for these injuries include motor vehicle crashes (MVCs), assaults, falls, sports and recreation, and injuries sustained at work or home. Bone, soft-tissue, and associated neurovascular injuries are rarely emergent unless accompanied by a life-threatening hemorrhage, as in certain amputations and pelvic fractures. Fractures and soft-tissue injuries are primarily designated as urgent because of potential neurovascular injury with resultant limb disability and pain. Early intervention enhances preservation of limb and function. This chapter focuses on common orthopedic and neurovascular extremity injuries and appropriate therapeutic interventions. Related anatomy and physiology are briefly reviewed.

ANATOMY AND PHYSIOLOGY

The musculoskeletal system and related neurovascular structures consist of bones, joints, tendons, ligaments, muscles, vessels, and nerves. The skeletal system contains 206 bones, which provide support, strength, movement, and protection to the body and organs. Bones store a number of minerals, including calcium and phosphorus, and are involved in blood cell production. Bones are characterized by shape, such as long, short, flat, or irregular, with the shape of a particular bone suited for a unique function or purpose. The skeleton is composed of two types of bones: cancellous and cortical. Cancellous (spongy) bone is found in the skull, vertebrae, pelvis, and long-bone ends. Cortical (dense) bone is found in the long bones. Bones are supplied by blood vessels, nerves, and lymphatic vessels that nourish bone tissue and allow the bone to repair injuries. The periosteum covers the bones and provides a point for the attachment of muscle, as well as the blood supply for underlying bone tissue.

A bone is connected to other bones by stabilizing bands of elastic, fibrous connective tissue called ligaments. Nonelastic fibrous cords connecting muscle to bone are tendons. Dense connective tissue found between the ribs, in the nasal septum, ear, larynx, trachea, bronchi, between vertebrae, and on articulating surfaces is known as cartilage. Cartilage has a limited vascular supply, whereas bone tissue has abundant vascular structures.

Joints are classified as nonsynovial (immovable and slightly immovable) and synovial (freely movable). Synovial joints have two articulating surfaces covered with cartilage and are surrounded by a two-layered synovial membrane sac. The entire joint is encapsulated by dense, ligamentous material. Joints provide mobility and stability, flexion and extension, medial and lateral rotation, and abduction and adduction. Joint movement is enhanced by muscles and ligaments that overlie the joint.

Nerves and arteries lie in close proximity to bones and muscle groups, with arterioles distributed throughout the periosteum to provide nutrients. Nerves provide sensation and movement. The closeness of arteries and nerves to bone structures increases their risk for injury with trauma to soft tissue, muscles, bones, or joints.

PATIENT ASSESSMENT

Assessment of orthopedic trauma begins with assessment of the airway, breathing, and circulation (ABCs). Rapid assessment identifies major injuries of the head, cervical spine, chest, and abdomen and prioritizes essential interventions. After ensuring no life-threatening injury has been left unattended, the nurse assesses and stabilizes any extremity injuries. Assessment of orthopedic injuries includes inspecting for edema, obvious deformity, presence of contusions, abrasions, lacerations, or puncture wounds and palpating for crepitus and point tenderness. A focused neurovascular evaluation is conducted for any injuries identified, noting the presence and/or absence of pain, pulses, paralysis, paraesthesia, pallor, temperature, and capillary refill.[1]

Before immobilization, open fractures should be stabilized and bleeding controlled. Open fractures with obvious bone protrusion or a deep laceration should be rinsed with sterile normal saline to remove gross contamination and be covered with a dry sterile dressing.

Puncture wounds over a fracture site should not be irrigated because this can force bacteria deeper into the wound. Reduction of an open fracture should not be attempted in a prehospital setting because this may force contaminants into the wound, increasing risk for infection.

To control bleeding, apply pressure directly to the injury site, edges of the wound, or an adjacent pressure point. Use of a tourniquet for hemorrhage control should be considered only as a last resort (life over limb) because of potential neurovascular compromise.

Immobilization

Immobilization should be accomplished as soon as possible to minimize further damage or complications secondary to bone fragments or neurovascular injury and to reduce pain in the injured limb. A splint should include the joints above and below the injury. Neurovascular status must be checked before and after immobilization. If neurovascular status is initially compromised, gradual traction may be used to promote return of neurologic or vascular function before splinting. If neurovascular status is compromised after splinting or traction, the splint should be removed and reapplied or the traction should be decreased. Angulation should be corrected only if it prevents immobilization or if neurovascular compromise is present. Splinting is best accomplished with an assistant to support the limb while a padded splint is placed and wrapped with a noncompressive bandage. Neurovascular status is rechecked after splinting.

Four basic types of splints exist, including soft splints such as pillows; hard splints such as padded board, cardboard, aluminum, plaster, fiberglass, or a ladder splint; inflatable air splints or vacuum splints; and traction splints, which reduce angulation and provide support.[2] Common splints used to immobilize the thumb/finger, wrist/forearm, elbow, and lower extremities are thumb spica, volar splint, boxer splint, sugar tong, and posterior splints (Fig. 40.1).

Air splints were used extensively when first developed because they conformed well and provided visualization of the injured extremity. However, an air splint that is not open on the distal end does not allow for neurovascular checks without deflating or unzipping the splint (Fig. 40.2). An air splint should be inflated only to the point where a finger can be slipped between the splint and the skin. Excessive pressure in the splint can compromise circulation. Air splints also stick to the skin, cause irritation, and are difficult to remove in patients with excessive diaphoresis.

Several types of traction splints are available and are usually applied by prehospital providers. The Thomas ring splint, Sager splint, and Hare splint (Fig. 40.3) are used for fractures of the midshaft of the femur or upper third of the tibia but should not be used for the hip, lower tibia or fibula, ankle, or a femur fracture with associated tibial-fibular fractures.

After immobilization, the limb should be elevated and an ice pack applied to minimize swelling. Caution is advised because overzealous elevation may compromise arterial circulation and excessive, prolonged cold may damage tissues.

The patient should be completely disrobed and examined for anterior injuries and then logrolled to identify posterior injuries while maintaining adequate cervical spine protection. Rings should be removed if the injury involves the hand, arm, foot, or toes. Elevation and cooling measures should be maintained, and neurovascular status should be checked periodically.

Taking a careful history should include discussing circumstances of the injury (time and mechanism) and significant medical history, including acute and chronic alcohol use, medications, allergies, and tetanus immunization status. Time of last oral intake should be recorded, and the patient should be allowed nothing by mouth (NPO) if procedural sedation or surgical intervention is a possibility.

SOFT-TISSUE INJURIES

Soft-tissue injuries generally accompany orthopedic trauma and can involve skin, muscles, tendons, cartilage, ligaments, veins, arteries, and nerves; circulation and function can be compromised from soft-tissue injury. Common injuries to the skin include abrasions, avulsions, contusions, hematomas, lacerations, and puncture wounds.

Principles of nursing care are generally the same for various soft-tissue injuries. Inspection involves checking for wounds, swelling, hematomas, and bleeding, then assessing neurovascular status. A soft, bulky dressing is applied, and swelling can be minimized with elevation and cooling measures. Radiographs are used to rule out foreign bodies and fractures. Analgesia is administered as prescribed for isolated injuries, and antibiotics are administered for significant, contaminated wounds. Written discharge instructions discuss RICE: rest, ice (e.g., apply a covered ice bag to the injury for 20 minutes every 2–3 hours for 24–48 hours), compression, and elevation. (See Chapter 11 for more specific information.)

Fingertip Injuries

Fingertip injuries are frequently seen in the ED, with the most common type being a crush injury to the distal phalanx occurring when a heavy object falls on the finger or the digit is caught in a door. Crush injuries can also be associated with a fracture. If a hematoma forms under the fingernail, it may cause a subungual hematoma (Fig. 40.4), which requires nail trephination by penetrating the fingernail over the hematoma with a nail drill, scalpel, pencil cautery, or superheated paper clip to release blood under the nail and relieve pressure.[3]

Fingertip injuries caused by a high-pressure paint or grease gun have increased in recent years. This injury occurs when a person is cleaning the gun tip and a stream of paint or grease is released into the fingertip or hand under high pressure. A pressure greater than 7000 pounds per square inch has been associated with a high amputation rate.[4] Particular attention to history and time of injury is crucial; the injury appears as a small pinhole in the fingertip but represents a serious, limb-threatening surgical emergency because material has been injected into the soft tissue of the involved limb. Treatment must not be delayed. Therapeutic intervention requires debridement of the paint- or grease-injected limb under general anesthesia.

Traumatic Amputations

Traumatic amputations occur among farm workers secondary to heavy farm machinery, in factory workers when a limb is caught by a heavy machine and in motorcyclists when the motorcycle and driver collide with another vehicle. Other causes include snow blowers and lawn mowers. Body parts frequently amputated are digits (fingers, toes), the distal half

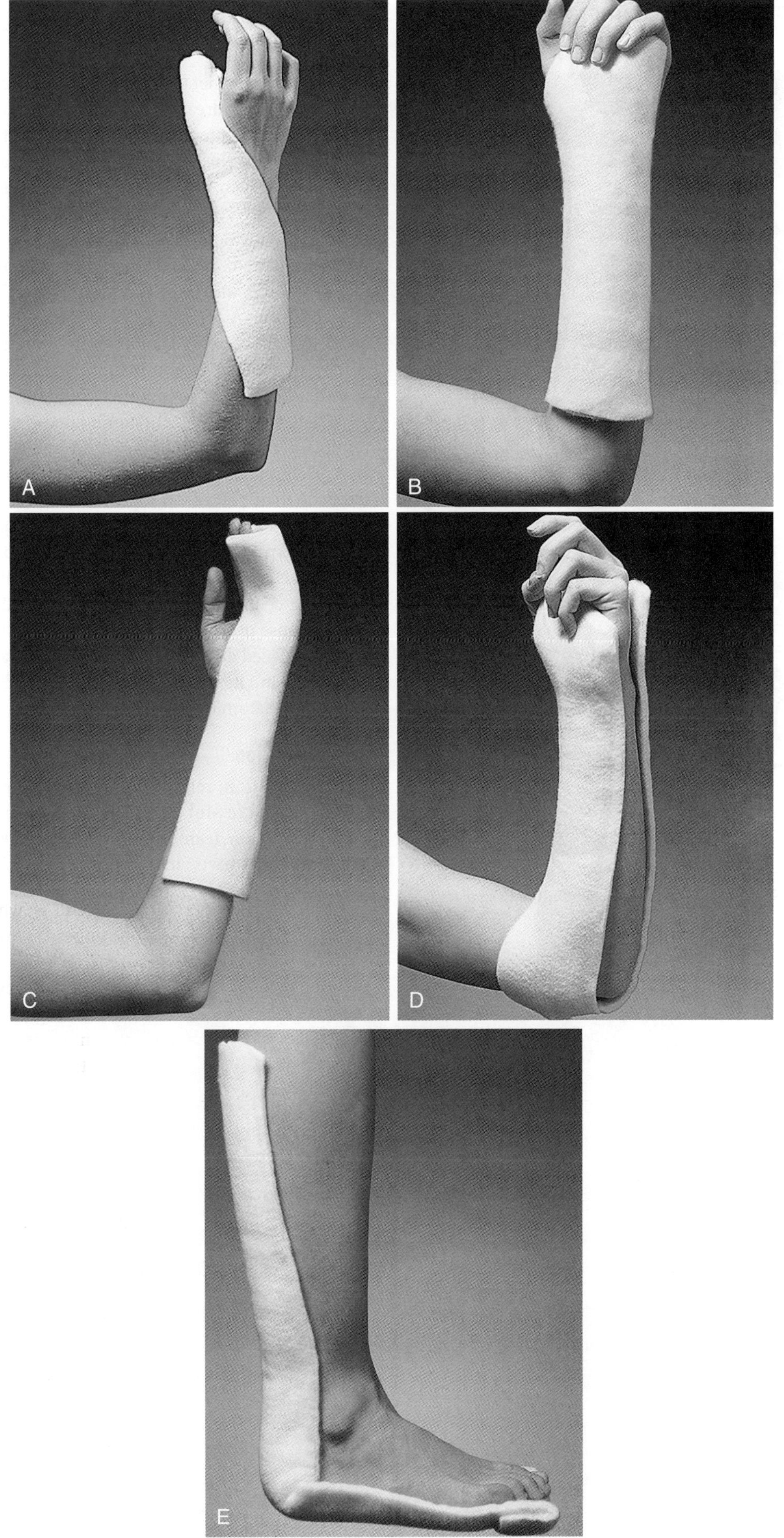

Fig. 40.1 Types of Splints and Their Indications. (A) Thumb spica splint. (B) Volar splint. (C) Boxer splint. (D) Sugar tong splint. (E) Posterior splint. (Courtesy BSN Medical, Inc.)

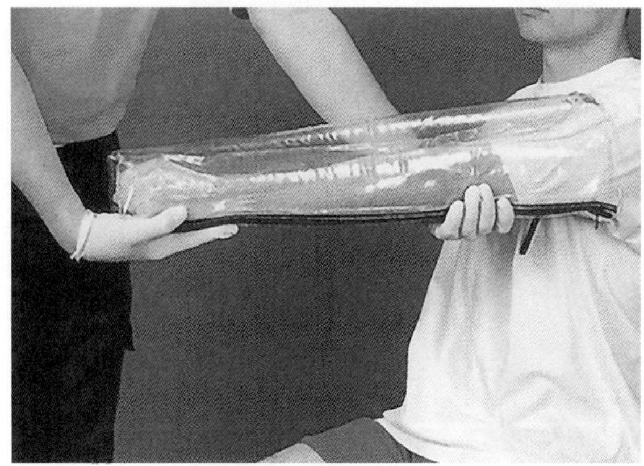

Fig. 40.2 Air Splint. (From Stoy W. *Mosby's EMT: Basic Textbook.* 2nd ed. St Louis, MO: Mosby; 2007.)

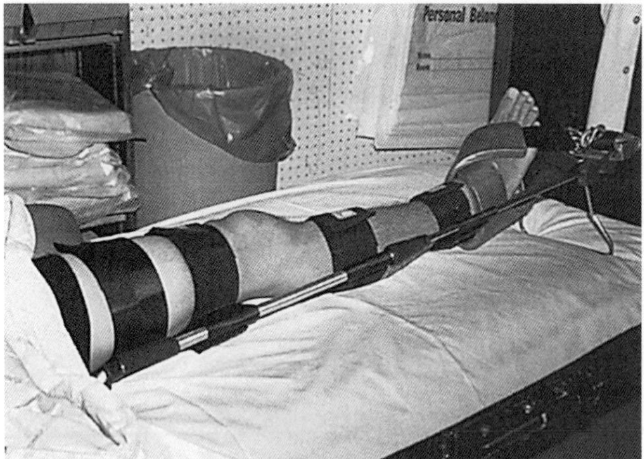

Fig. 40.3 Hare Traction Splint. (From Marx JA, Hockberger RS, Walls RM. *Rosen's Emergency Medicine: Concepts and Clinical Practice.* 6th ed. St Louis, MO: Mosby: 2006.)

of the foot (transmetatarsal), the leg (above, at, or below the knee), the hand, forearm, arm, ears, nose, and penis.

Therapeutic interventions for amputations begin with stabilization of the ABCs, including the administration of high-flow oxygen, the initiation of two large-bore intravenous (IV) lines, control of bleeding, and rapid transportation to a facility for definitive care. If the body part is only partially amputated, the limb should be supported and splinted in a position of anatomic function. Fig. 40.5 shows anatomic hand position. A completely amputated stump should be irrigated to remove gross contamination, dressed, and elevated. Antibiotics, a tetanus booster, and tetanus immune globulin, as indicated, should be initiated in the ED.

Whenever possible, the amputated part is preserved for reimplantation by wrapping it in saline-moistened gauze and placing it in a plastic bag or container. The sealed container is then placed on top of crushed ice and water. This cools the part without causing direct damage to tissue. If the amputated part is placed directly in water or on ice, cells can be damaged by water moving across the cellular membranes, including cellular freezing and death. Distilled water is not used because of its deleterious effect on tissue. Iodine should never be placed directly on the amputated part because of discoloration and its effects on tissue viability. Maintain the limb in correct anatomic position.

Reimplantation

After amputation, reimplantation may be possible. Limiting factors for successful reimplantation include availability of a reimplantation team, amount of damage to the attached and amputated parts, method of preservation of the amputated part, and time elapsed since the accident. Sharp, guillotine-like cuts have a better outcome than crush or avulsion

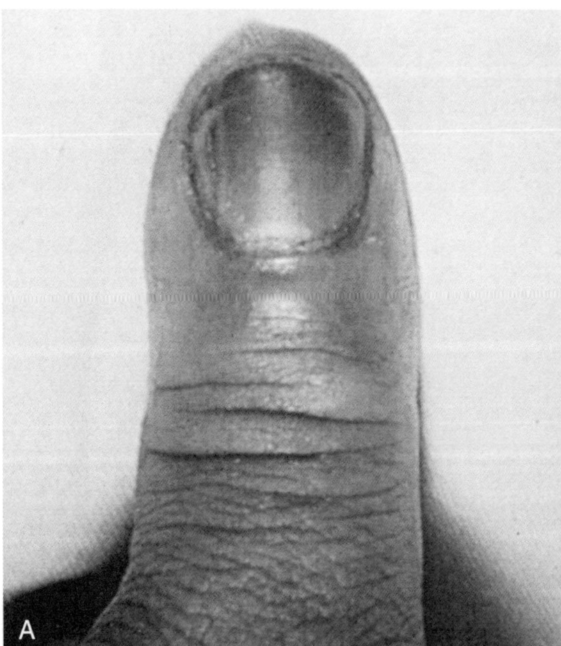

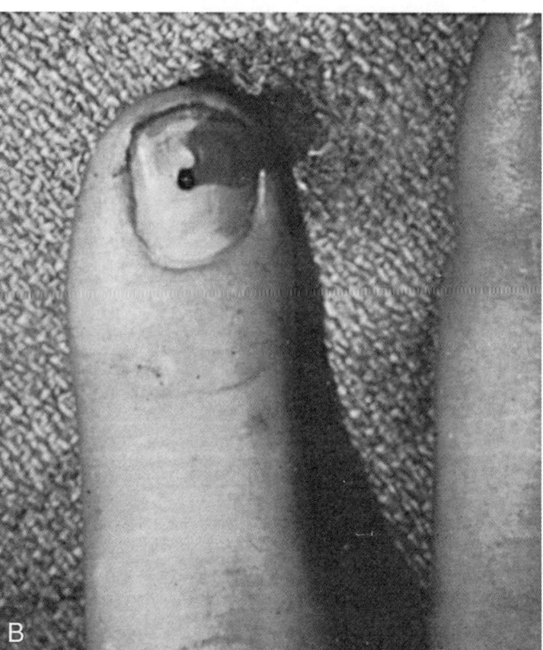

Fig. 40.4 (A) Subungual hematoma. (B) Subungual hematoma after trephination. (From Roberts JR, Hedges JR. *Clinical Procedures in Emergency Medicine.* 4th ed. Philadelphia, PA: Saunders; 2004.)

injuries. Muscles can survive 12 hours of cold ischemia; bone, tendon, and skin can survive 24 hours; warm survival time is much less.[5] The predicted outcome of reimplantation is further determined by age, occupation, motivation, and general physical condition of the victim. Historically, upper extremity reimplantations are more successful than lower extremity reimplantations, and children typically have a better outcome with this type of reimplantation.

Impaling Injuries

Impaling injuries usually result from an industrial accident in which the victim falls onto a sharp, immobile object. Injuries with nails from a powered nail gun are also common. Nails used in these guns are coated with a special adhesive that can stick to tissue. Impaled objects should not be immediately removed; surgical removal may be required. Complications from this type of injury include infection and problems specific to the structures in which the object is impaled. Biologic substances such as wood carry an increased risk of infection.

Gunshot Wounds

Gunshot wounds usually result from hunting or acts of violence. Tissue damage depends on the type of weapon, size of ammunition used, distance from the weapon, and part of the body injured (Fig. 40.6). Tissue, bones, organs, and vessels away from the bullet's unpredictable path may also be injured. Appearance of the entrance wound does not always reflect the amount of destruction beneath. An extremity injury may be associated with a truncal injury because of a projectile path through the chest into the arm or through the arm into the chest or because of multiple bullet wounds. (See Chapter 34 for further discussion of gunshot wounds.) Careful assessment, including neurovascular assessment of all limbs, is critical so that other wounds are not overlooked; immunization status must be verified. With gunshot wounds, evidence surrounding the wound site or powder burns on the hand should be carefully protected until the police can perform requisite testing. (See Chapter 48 for a detailed discussion of evidence collection and preservation.)

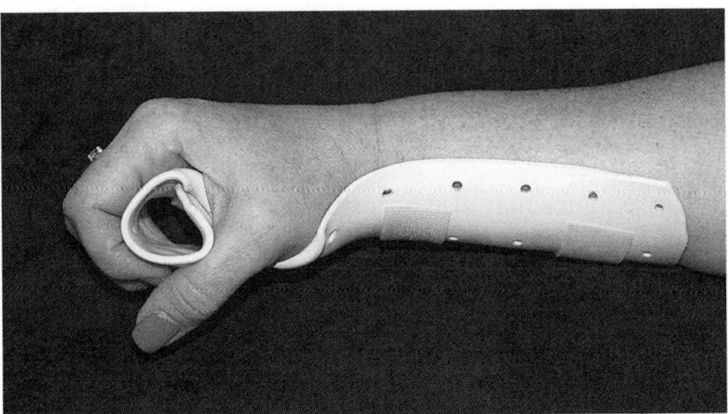

Fig. 40.5 Anatomic Positioning of Hand. (From Canale TS, Beaty JH. *Campbell's Operative Orthopedics.* 11th ed. St Louis, MO: Mosby; 2007.)

Tendon and Muscle Rupture

Tendon and muscle ruptures are generally related to sports or recreation; however, metabolic disease and age may be causative factors. Runners may experience a quadriceps tear, whereas a biceps tear can occur with minimal effort in middle-age or older individuals. Surgery may be required to restore function for complete tears. For an incomplete injury, treatment usually consists of rest and intermittent application of ice for 24 to 48 hours followed by heat.

An Achilles tendon rupture can occur in start-and-stop sports in which a person steps off abruptly on the forefoot with the knee forced in extension. The patient may also report hearing a loud crack or snap or sensation of something striking their posterior ankle. This causes sharp pain extending from the heel into the back of the leg, sudden inability to use the foot, and obvious deformity. A clinical tool to assist in the diagnosis is the Thompson test: the patient lies supine on the examination table with the feet hanging off the edge; the examiner squeezes each calf bilaterally and observes for plantar flexion. If a complete rupture has occurred, there is minimal or no foot movement (a positive Thompson's sign). A splint in plantar flexion should be applied and the patient prepared for surgery.[6]

Crush Injuries

Crush injuries frequently occur in industrial settings (e.g., when an arm is caught in the wringer of an industrial washing machine, press, or conveyor; or when limbs or the trunk is caught between equipment). Injury may involve only the distal end of a digit or large areas of the body. Depending on the extent of damage, orthopedic, surgical,

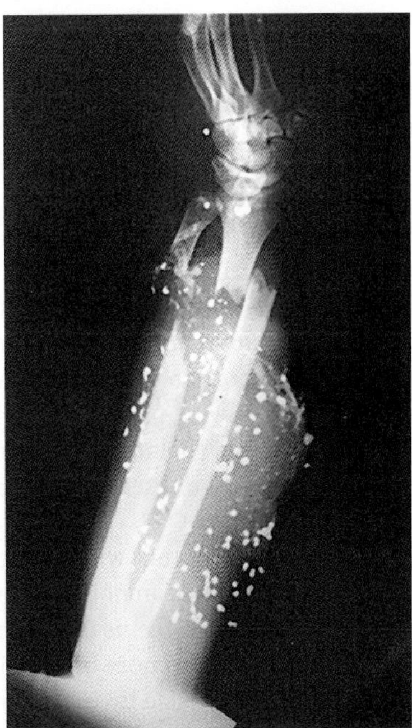

Fig. 40.6 Gunshot wound fracture of radius and ulna with extensive soft-tissue damage. (From Frank ED, Long BW, Smith BJ. *Merrill's Atlas of Radiographic Positioning and Procedures.* 11th ed. St Louis, MO: Mosby; 2007.)

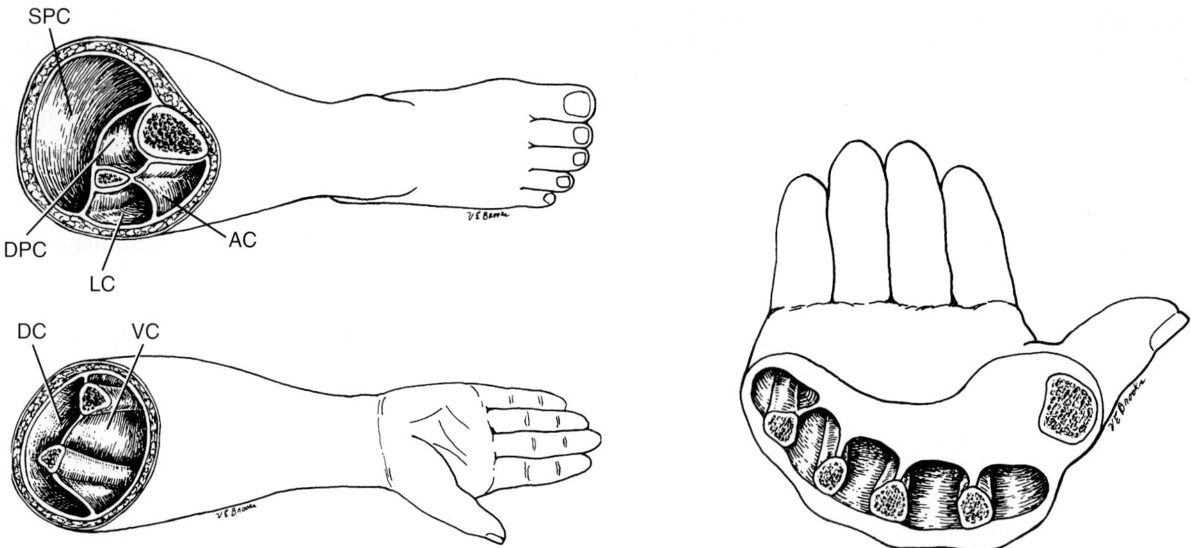

Fig. 40.7 Cross-section anatomy of calf, forearm, and hand showing fascial compartments. *AC*, Anterior compartment; *DC*, dorsal compartment; *DPC*, deep posterior compartment; *LC*, lateral compartment; *SPC*, superficial posterior compartment; *VC*, volar compartment. (From Matsen FA III. *Compartmental Syndromes.* New York, NY: Grune & Stratton; 1980.)

neurosurgical, or vascular-surgical intervention may be required.

Complications from crush injuries depend on the mechanism of injury and extent of tissue damage. With significant tissue necrosis, systemic crush syndrome can develop, characterized by myoglobinuria, extracellular fluid loss, acidosis, increased potassium, renal failure, shock, and cardiac disruption.[3]

Compartment Syndrome

Compartment syndrome occurs when swelling or compression-restriction causes pressure in the muscle compartment to rise to the point that microvascular circulation is interrupted. The resulting tissue ischemia threatens limb survival. Compartment syndrome is associated with severe soft-tissue injuries and fractures, casts, or a pneumatic antishock garment (PASG). Prolonged pressure directly on a limb, frostbite, or snakebite can also lead to compartment syndrome. It usually occurs in compartments of the lower leg and forearm (Fig. 40.7). Symptoms develop 6 to 8 hours after injury but may be delayed 48 to 96 hours. Symptoms include deep, throbbing pain out of proportion to the original injury not relieved by narcotics, pain with passive flexion, decreased mobility of digits, paresthesia, coolness, pallor, and tenseness of overlying skin. Pulses may be absent, decreased, or palpable with compartment syndrome.

Irreversible tissue damage occurs within 4 to 6 hours of ischemia; therefore prompt physician notification is essential. The limb is positioned level with the heart, and neurovascular function is assessed hourly, or more often if indicated, to identify changes. Diagnosis is made by measuring compartment pressure with a syringe or catheter device (Fig. 40.8). Pressures greater than 30 to 60 mm Hg usually require fasciotomy.[7] A high index of suspicion is necessary when caring for injured comatose patients who cannot verbalize increasing pain or paresthesia.[8]

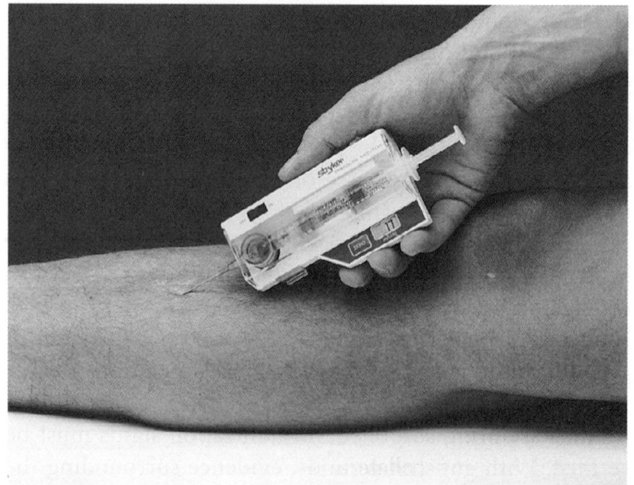

Fig. 40.8 The Stryker 295 Intracompartmental Pressure Monitor. (Courtesy Stryker Surgical, Kalamazoo, MI.)

Peripheral Nerve and Artery Injury

The most common causes of peripheral nerve and artery injuries are lacerations, penetrating wounds, fractures, and dislocations. Joints are well innervated and vascularized, so they are especially prone to nerve or artery damage. Familiarity with major nerves and arteries is necessary for assessment of tissue injuries.

Nerve injury may also occur from compression caused by prolonged PASG use or skeletal traction. Resolution of symptoms depends on the type of injury and length of time before compression is corrected. Partial nerve injury may be caused by a contusion, leading to temporary paralysis and sensory deficit. Complete and total disruption of the nerve causes loss of all functions and usually requires surgical repair. Nerve evaluation and repair of an isolated injury may be done on an outpatient basis. Table 40.1 describes the assessment of common peripheral nerve injuries.

TABLE 40.1 Assessment of Common Peripheral Nerve Injuries.

Nerve	Frequently Associated Injuries	Assessment Findings
Radial	Fracture of humerus, especially middle and distal thirds	Inability to extend thumb in "hitchhiker's sign"
Ulnar	Fracture of medial humeral epicondyle	Loss of pain perception in tip of little finger
Median	Elbow dislocation or wrist or forearm injury	Loss of pain perception in tip of index finger
Peroneal	Tibia or fibula fracture; dislocation of knee	Inability to extend great toe or foot; may also be associated with sciatic nerve injury
Sciatic and tibial	Infrequent with fractures or dislocations	Loss of pain perception in sole of foot

Axillary, brachial, radial, and ulnar arteries are the major arteries in the arms. Femoral, popliteal, anterior tibial, posterior tibial, and peroneal arteries are the major arteries in the leg. High-impact and rapid-deceleration mechanisms are most likely to cause arterial injury. Assessment should evaluate pulse quality, skin color and temperature, capillary refill, bleeding, hematoma formation, and presence of bruits.

Arterial injuries may be difficult to discover; 10% to 15% of significant arterial disruptions can have detectable distal pulses.[9] A Doppler ultrasound should be used for pulses that are difficult to palpate. Evaluation may require angiography; however, injury in association with an open fracture may be evaluated during surgery. Arterial injuries may not require repair if existing collateral circulation prevents ischemia. Complications of undiagnosed arterial disruptions include thrombosis, arteriovenous fistula, aneurysm, false aneurysm, and tissue ischemia with resultant limb dysfunction.[5]

Strains

A strain is a weakening or overstretching of a muscle at the point of attachment to the tendon. Strains may occur as a result of almost any type of movement, from twisting the ankle to wrenching forces caused by an MVC or violent muscle contraction. Strains are most often associated with athletic injuries.

A patient with a first-degree or mild strain complains of local pain, point tenderness, and slight muscle spasms. Therapeutic interventions include a compression bandage, intermittent elevation of the limb above heart level for 12 hours, application of a cold pack for the same period, and light weight bearing on the injured part.

With a second-degree strain the patient has local pain, point tenderness, swelling, discoloration, and inability to use the limb for prolonged periods. Therapeutic interventions include a compression bandage, elevation, and intermittent cold pack application for 24 hours; analgesia; and light weight bearing.

Severe strains (third-degree) cause complete disruption of the muscle or tendon. This disruption can cause a small avulsion fracture seen on x-ray films. The patient complains of local pain, point tenderness, swelling, and discoloration. The patient often describes a "snapping noise" at the time of injury. Therapeutic interventions include a compression bandage or splints, elevation, and cold pack application for 24 to 72 hours; analgesia; and no weight bearing for 48 hours. Surgery may be required if a complete rupture occurs at the tendon-bone attachment site.

Sprains

Mechanism of injury for sprains may be the same as for strains, but a sprain is usually the result of more traumatic force. A sprain occurs when a joint exceeds its normal limit and damages ligaments. The patient may have a history of a popping or snapping sound. Sprains often occur in ankles, knees, and shoulders. In children, epiphyseal disruption is more common than ligamentous injury. A mild sprain (first-degree) produces slight pain and slight swelling. Therapeutic interventions include a compression bandage, elevation, intermittent cold pack application for 12 hours, and light weight bearing. A moderate sprain (second-degree) causes pain, point tenderness, swelling, and inability to use the limb for more than a brief period. Therapeutic interventions include compression bandage, elevation, intermittent cold pack application for 24 hours, and light weight bearing with crutches. A stirrup ankle brace is commonly applied to the ankle to prevent inversion and eversion of the ankle but to allow flexion and extension.

A severe sprain (third-degree) involves torn ligaments, which cause pain, point tenderness, swelling, discoloration, and inability to use the limb. Therapeutic interventions include a splint or cast, elevation, intermittent cold pack application for 48 hours, and light to no weight bearing with crutches (lower extremity injury).

Knee Injuries

Knee injuries are a common form of soft-tissue injury in which rotation or excess flexion strains or tears the medial meniscus, collateral ligament, or cruciate ligament. Symptoms include swelling, ecchymosis, effusion, pain, and tenderness. Therapeutic interventions include a compression bandage, knee immobilizer, or cylinder cast; elevation of the injured limb; intermittent cold pack application to the injured area for the first 24 hours; and non–weight bearing with crutch walking. If the injury is a ligament tear, surgical repair within 24 to 48 hours of injury is recommended.

FRACTURES

A fracture is a disruption or break in the bone. Patients may arrive in the ED with angulation, deformity, pain, regional and point tenderness, swelling, immobility, and/or crepitus.

TABLE 40.2 Causes of Different Types of Fractures.

Type	Etiology
Transverse fracture	Sharp, direct blow
Oblique fracture	Twisting force
Spiral fracture	Twisting force while foot is firmly planted
Comminuted fracture	Severe direct trauma causes more than two fragments
Impacted fracture	Severe trauma, causes bone ends to jam together
Compression fracture	Severe force to top of head, sacrum, or os calcis (axial loading) forces vertebrae together
Greenstick fracture	Compression force; usually occurs in school-age children
Avulsion fracture	Forceful contraction of a muscle mass; causes a bone fragment to break away at the insertion point
Depressed fracture	Blunt trauma to a flat bone; usually associated with significant soft-tissue damage

Other findings might include bony fragment protrusion, impaired neurovascular status, and occasionally shock.

Fractures are divided into two general categories: closed and open. With closed or simple fractures, the bone is broken but the skin is intact. Open or compound fractures are characterized by bone protrusion or puncture wounds in which the bone punctures the skin or a foreign object penetrates the skin and bone, causing a fracture. Table 40.2 describes the etiology for various types of fractures; illustrations for each type are found in Fig. 40.9.

Open fractures are considered contaminated and require prophylactic antibiotic therapy. These fractures are graded by severity, then further categorized by wound size, amount of soft-tissue damage, injury to the periosteum, and vascular damage. Most open fractures require surgical debridement. A greater potential for shock exists with open fractures because of the potential for significant blood loss; closed injuries are more likely to tamponade and limit blood loss.[8] General nursing care includes fracture immobilization and establishing IV access for fluid replacement, antibiotics, analgesia, and anesthesia. Wound care includes irrigation with normal saline, covering with a dry sterile dressing, and verification of tetanus immunization status.

After evaluation of ABCs, specific limb injury assessment should be completed, followed by immobilization, elevation, and ice packs. Repeated neurovascular assessments are essential for identifying changes secondary to swelling. History should be obtained to determine the mechanism of injury. The emergency nurse should also be alert for signs of abuse when the injury does not match the history. Understanding patterns of injury also facilitates assessment and identification of less obvious injuries.

When a limb suffers significant trauma, a fracture should be suspected until proven otherwise by radiologic studies. Radiography should include both anterior and lateral views because fractures may appear from only one angle.[10] Joints above and below the injury should be included in all radiographic evaluations.

Open fractures and certain closed fractures require surgical intervention. Ideally, patients with open fractures should have surgery within 8 hours of the injury.[2] The patient should be kept NPO and prepared for surgery. IV lines are inserted, and consent should be obtained before narcotics are administered. Prophylactic broad-spectrum antibiotics are given as soon as possible for open fractures and vascular injuries.

Fractures are associated with numerous complications. Jagged bone ends may lacerate vital organs, arteries, and nerves, causing hemorrhage and neurovascular compromise. Open fractures can result in serious infections leading to permanent limb dysfunction or limb loss. Long-term complications of fractures include nonunion, deformity, disability, avascular necrosis from decreased blood supply, and Volkmann's contracture (contracture in a group of muscles caused by ischemia) secondary to untreated compartment syndrome.[2]

Fat embolism is a relatively uncommon, but life-threatening sequela of bone injury and usually presents 24 to 48 hours after injury. Seen most often with pelvic, femoral, or tibial fractures, this complication has a high mortality rate. A fracture causes release of fat particles into the bloodstream that embolize to end organs, particularly the pulmonary vasculature. The patient suddenly develops tachycardia accompanied by elevated temperature, altered level of consciousness, tachypnea, cough, shortness of breath, cyanosis, petechiae over the upper half of the body—particularly in the axillae—and pulmonary edema leading to adult respiratory distress syndrome. Immediate therapeutic interventions include high-flow oxygen, support of ABCs, and possible administration of a corticosteroid.[8]

Fractures occur frequently among children 6 to 16 years old and older adults. Children's bones are softer and more porous and therefore more likely to have a partial or greenstick fracture.[11] Epiphyseal or growth plate (Salter-type) fractures may affect future bone growth because of early closure of the epiphyseal plate and resultant limb shortening (Fig. 40.10). Angulation may occur with partial growth plate fractures because bone growth continues in the noninjured area. Epiphyseal fractures require close orthopedic follow-up for several months to monitor healing and identify growth abnormalities.[12] Another concern with pediatric fractures is bleeding. A child with a femur fracture can lose 300 to 1000 mL of blood, a significant amount given the child's body size and circulating blood volume.[13]

Older adult patients have brittle bones because of calcium loss associated with aging. This physiologic change combined with problems older adults have with balance increases the risk for falls and fractures. These patients may also have multiple medical problems complicating recovery. Planning home care may be difficult for the older adult patient with a

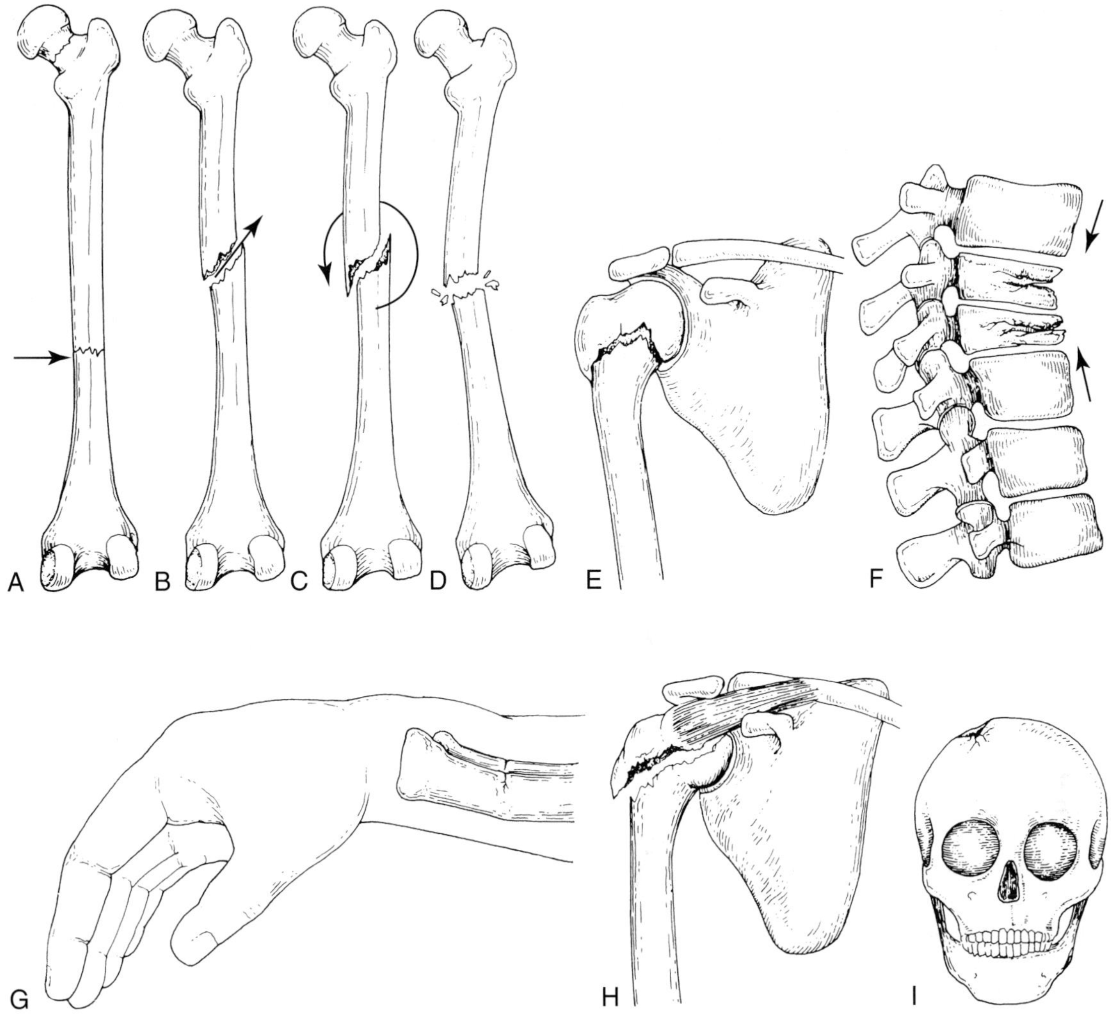

Fig. 40.9 Types of Fractures. (A) Transverse fracture. (B) Oblique fracture. (C) Spiral fracture. (D) Comminuted fracture. (E) Impacted fracture. (F) Compression fracture. (G) Greenstick fracture. (H) Avulsion fracture. (I) Depressed fracture.

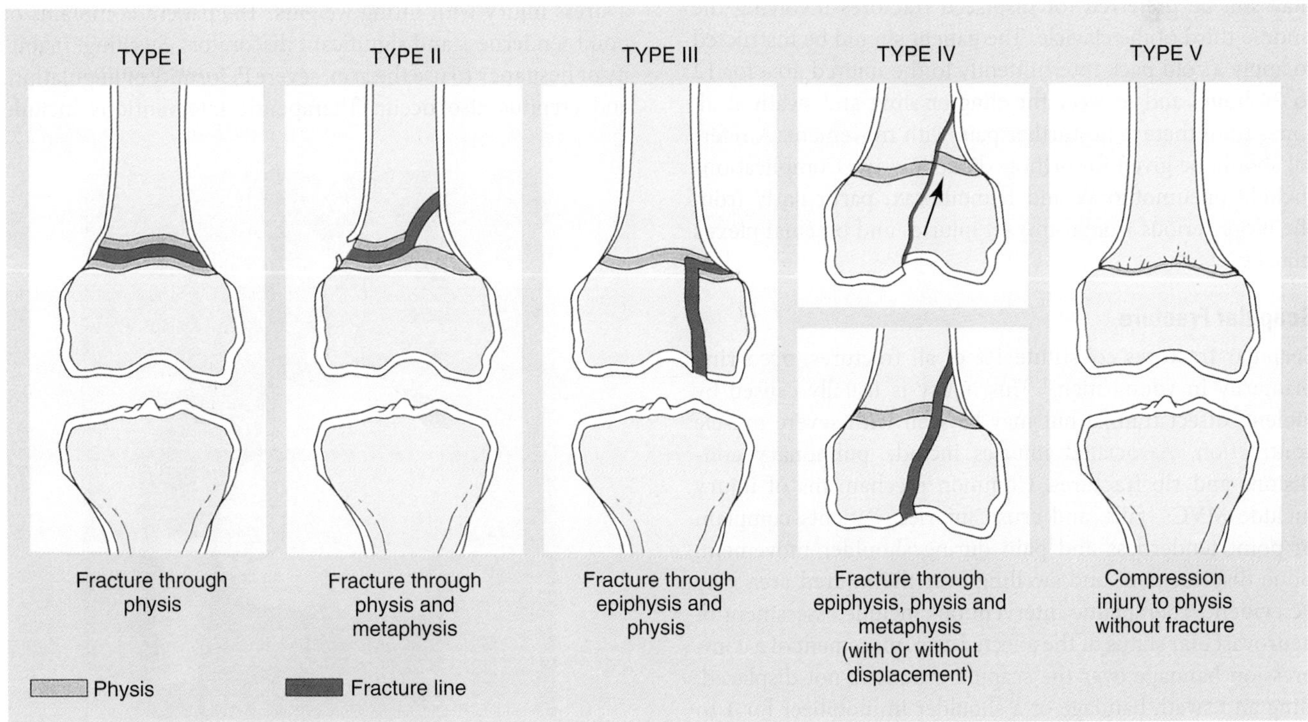

Fig. 40.10 Salter-Harris Classification. (From Zitelli BJ, Davis HW. *Atlas of Pediatric Physical Diagnosis.* 4th ed. St Louis, MO: Mosby; 2002.)

fracture who may be already challenged by normal activities of daily living. A cast and crutches cause greater loss of balance and impaired mobility.

Fracture Healing

Bone healing occurs over weeks or can take several months. Fracture healing is determined by the type of bone, type of fracture, degree of opposition, immobility, and general state of health.[8] Infection and decreased neurovascular supply hamper healing, as does chronic hypoxia. Conversely, exercise promotes bone healing. Alterations in healing are described as delayed, malunion (residual deformity), and nonunion (failure to unite).

Upper Torso Fractures

Bones in the upper torso communicating with the upper extremities include the clavicle and the scapula.

Clavicular Fracture

Fracture of the clavicle occurs in all age-groups but is particularly common in children and adolescents.[11] A fall on an arm or shoulder, such as a contact injury when athletes run into each other or with direct frontal impact, is a frequently reported mechanism of injury. Eighty percent of fractures occur in the middle third of the clavicle. Patients complain of pain in the clavicular area with point tenderness, swelling, deformity, and crepitus found on assessment. The patient will not raise the affected arm and tilts the head toward the side of injury with the chin directed toward the opposite side. Neurovascular status of the arm should be assessed, including the axillary, median, ulnar, and radial nerve; distal pulses; and capillary refill. The arm should be supported and a sling or a sling and a swath applied; a figure-eight splint or clavicle strap may still be preferred for displaced fractures involving the middle third of the clavicle. The patient should be instructed to apply a cold pack intermittently to the injured area for 12 to 24 hours and to wear the sling or sling and swath at all times until there is no further pain with movement. A referral should be given for orthopedic follow-up. Complications include pneumothorax and hemothorax, particularly from the more serious frontal-impact injuries and brachial plexus injuries.

Scapular Fracture

Scapular fractures constitute 1% of all fractures, occurring primarily in young men.[3] This injury is usually caused by violent, direct trauma but may be seen with severe muscle contraction. Associated injuries include pulmonary contusions and rib fractures. Common mechanisms of injury include MVCs, falls, and crush injuries. Patients complain of point tenderness and pain during shoulder movement. Bone displacement and swelling over the injured area may be evident. Therapeutic interventions include assessment of neurovascular status of the affected arm, placement of a compression bandage over the scapula if bone is not displaced, sling and swath bandage or a shoulder immobilizer for 1 to 2 weeks (Fig. 40.11), and intermittent application of a cold pack for the first 24 hours. Complications include injuries to underlying ribs or viscera from the force required to cause the fracture.

Upper-Extremity Fractures

Shoulder Fracture

A shoulder fracture is a fracture of the glenoid, humeral head, or humeral neck. Shoulder fractures occur frequently in older adult patients, resulting from a fall on an outstretched arm or direct trauma to the shoulder. When this same mechanism of injury occurs in a younger person, shoulder dislocation usually occurs. Fracture occurs in an older adult because of the weaker bone structure.

The patient arrives with pain in the shoulder area, point tenderness, immobility of the affected arm, gross swelling, and discoloration. Most injuries are impacted or nondisplaced fractures and require only a sling and swath or a shoulder immobilizer. A Velpeau immobilizer (i.e., a sling with a strap attached to the elbow end that comes around the patient's back and attaches to the sling near the fingers) may also be used. A significantly displaced fracture may require open reduction or skeletal traction but is generally reduced with closed traction. This injury can complicate activities of daily living and requires extra planning for home care, particularly for an older adult patient living alone. Complications include neurovascular compromise (axillary nerve injury) and possible adhesive capsulitis or "frozen" (stiff) shoulder.

Upper-Arm Fractures

Fractures of the upper arm (humeral shaft) are commonly seen in children and older adults (Fig. 40.12). This type of fracture results from a fall on the arm or direct trauma or in association with dislocation of the shoulder and may also occur as a stress injury with lifting weights. The patient complains of point tenderness and significant discomfort. Swelling, inability or hesitancy to use the arm, severe deformity or angulation, and crepitus also occur. Therapeutic interventions include

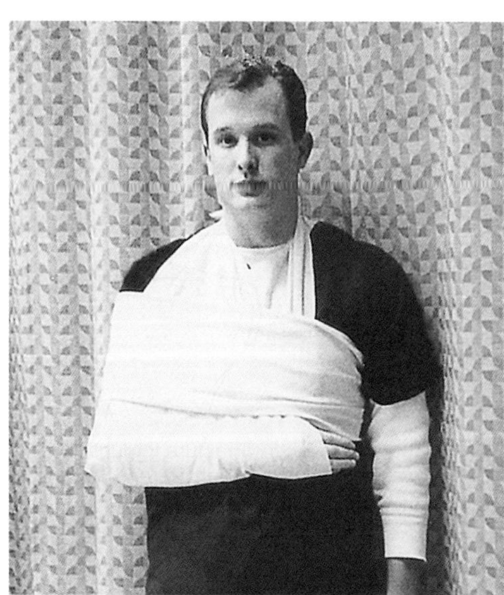

Fig. 40.11 Sling and Swath.

assessment for other injuries (e.g., chest trauma) and fracture management. The fracture is usually reduced by closed reduction with mild, steady, downward traction. Fractures of the proximal humerus are generally treated with a sling and swath; midshaft fractures are casted with a Y-shaped (sugar tong) splint applied from the axilla, around the elbow, and back to the shoulder (acromial process).[7] The patient should sit and lean forward during this procedure. The arm may be secured to the chest for additional stabilization. In addition to routine cast-care instructions, the patient should be given instructions to exercise the wrist and fingers frequently. Radial nerve damage commonly accompanies fracture of the middle or distal portion of the humeral shaft.

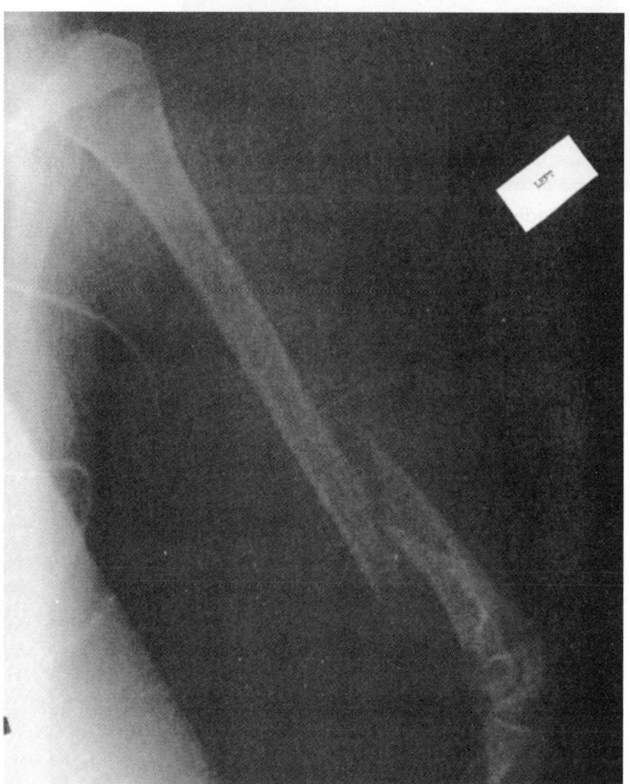

Fig. 40.12 Radiograph of Humerus Fracture.

Elbow Fractures

Elbow fractures (Fig. 40.13) are seen most often in young children and athletes. These injuries occur with a fall on an extended arm or flexed elbow, such as a fall from a skateboard. Fractures of the elbow involve the distal humerus or head of the ulna or radius. Typically, supracondylar fractures of the humerus are extension injuries and are more likely to damage the brachial artery. Ulnar head fractures are generally the result of a direct blow and are usually comminuted.

Elbow fractures are associated with considerable swelling and potential neurovascular compromise. The arm should be splinted as found and a sling applied. Prompt initial neurovascular assessment should be followed by serial assessment every 30 to 60 minutes. If compromise is present, the arm may be flexed at a greater angle. When closed reduction is used, the arm is casted and placed in a sling. Sling immobilization is usually sufficient for radial head fractures. Open reduction and fixation are required for comminuted or intraarticular fractures. Complications associated with elbow fractures include brachial artery laceration, nerve (median, radial, or ulnar) damage, and Volkmann's contracture.

Volkmann's contracture is due to ischemia of the muscles and nerves from untreated compartment syndrome. The patient presents with the inability to move his or her fingers, severe pain with manipulation, severe pain in forearm flexor

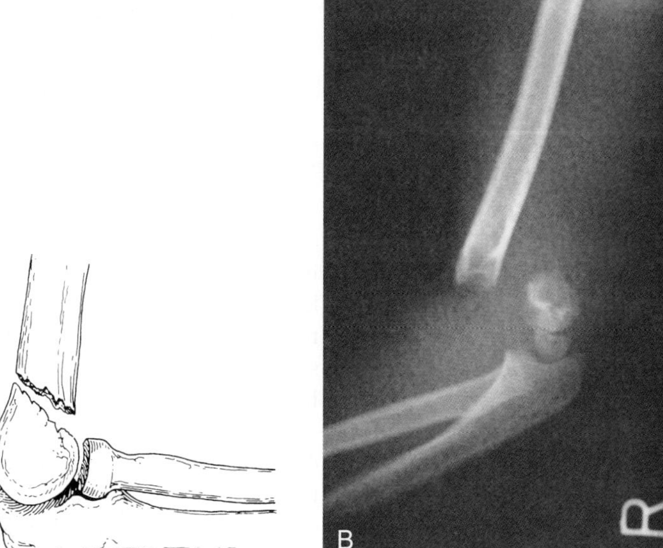

Fig. 40.13 (A) Elbow fracture. (B) Radiograph.

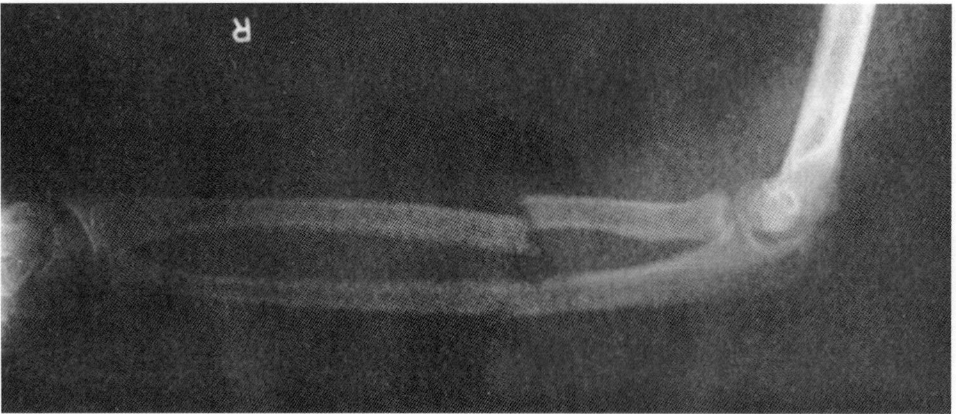

Fig. 40.14 Radiograph of Fracture of Radius and Ulna.

muscles even after reduction, pulse deficit, swelling, extremity coolness, cyanosis, and decreased sensation. Temporary therapeutic intervention includes cast removal, extension of the forearm, and possible cold pack application. Prompt orthopedic consultation is essential for further therapeutic interventions. Nonintervention leads to atrophy and a claw-like deformity.

Forearm Fractures

Forearm fractures include fractures of the radius and ulna. Common in adults and children, forearm fractures usually result from a fall on an extended arm or a direct blow (Fig. 40.14). The patient presents with pain, point tenderness, swelling, deformity, and angulation and, occasionally, shortening of the extremity. Therapeutic interventions include a splint to immobilize the fracture and a sling. Many fractures can be manipulated by closed reduction and then casted with the elbow flexed 90 degrees. The shoulder and fingers should be free of the cast. If a sling is used, the entire arm and hand should be supported. The hand should not become dependent or droop at the wrist. Complications of forearm fractures include neurovascular compromise leading to Volkmann's contracture.

Wrist and Hand Fractures

Carpal fractures. The scaphoid is the carpal bone most prone to fracture (Fig. 40.15). The patient complains of tenderness over the depression in the wrist on the thumb side of the hand (anatomic snuffbox). A specific navicular-view radiograph demonstrates scaphoid fractures best; however, fractures may not appear on radiographs for 2 to 4 weeks. If symptoms are present, a cast is placed regardless of negative results from radiographs. Complications include avascular necrosis or tissue death of the scaphoid from loss of blood supply.

Wrist fractures. Fractures of the wrist include the distal radius, distal ulna, and carpal bones of the hand (Fig. 40.16). The most common mechanism is a fall onto an extended arm and open hand, causing swelling and deformity. Fractures of the distal radius and ulna are the most common fracture, typically seen in older adults. A Colles fracture may also occur in association with a calcaneus and vertebral fracture sustained in a fall from a height. Wrist fractures are generally manipulated with closed reduction and then casted. Some physicians may not prescribe a sling because it can hinder elevation; some prefer a hanging apparatus, such as an IV pole for the first 2 days of elevation, even for home care.

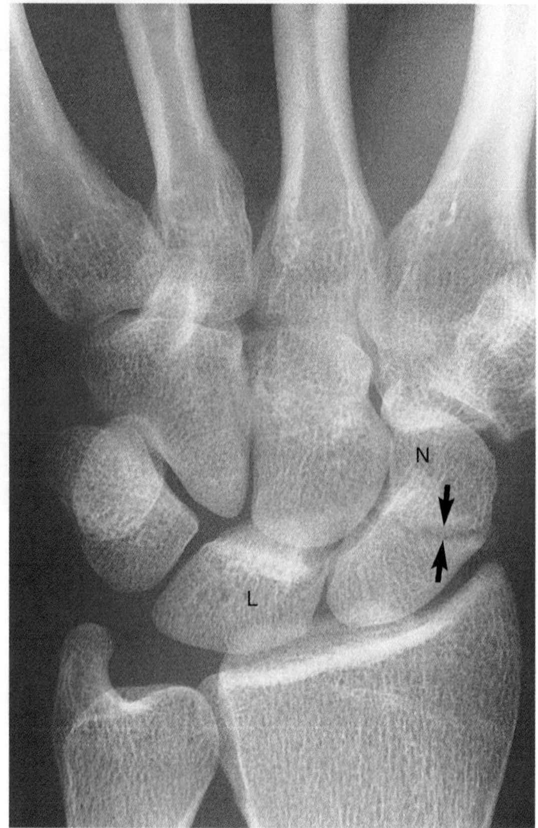

Fig. 40.15 Scaphoid Fracture. (From Mettler FA. *Essentials of Radiology*. 2nd ed. Philadelphia, PA: Saunders; 2005.)

Metacarpal fractures. Fractures of the metacarpals (Fig. 40.17) are common athletic injuries, particularly during contact sports. Striking a person or a wall with a closed fist causes a boxer's fracture, a midshaft fracture of the fifth metacarpal. Throwing a baseball may cause the distal attachment of the extensor tendon to tear loose along with a segment of bone,

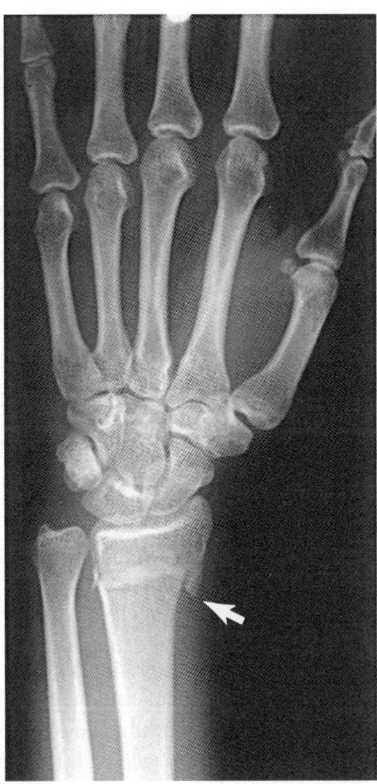

Fig. 40.16 Wrist Fracture (Radius). (From Ballinger PW. *Merrill's Atlas of Radiographic Positions and Radiologic Procedures.* 8th ed. St Louis, MO: Mosby; 1995.)

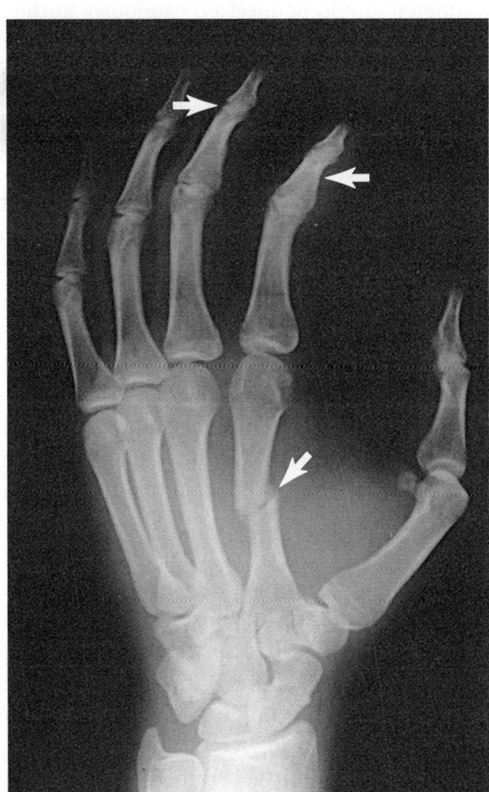

Fig. 40.17 Metacarpal Fracture. (From Frank ED, Long BW, Smith BJ. *Merrill's Atlas of Radiographic Positioning and Procedures.* 11th ed. St Louis, MO: Mosby; 2007.)

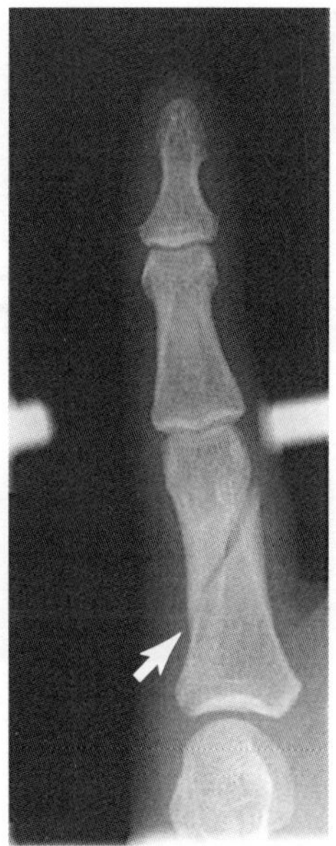

Fig. 40.18 Fractured Fifth Digit. (From Frank ED, Long BW, Smith BJ. *Merrill's Atlas of Radiographic Positioning and Procedures.* 11th ed. St Louis, MO: Mosby; 2007.)

resulting in an avulsion fracture. Industrial crush injuries to the hand can also fracture metacarpals. If an open fracture occurs, a compression bandage is used to control bleeding.[14] Rings are removed before swelling increases and makes removal difficult. Metacarpal fractures are seldom displaced to any degree and are generally casted in the ED.

Phalanx fractures. Fractured phalanges (fingers) are common in all age-groups (Fig. 40.18). Symptoms are similar to those for carpal and metacarpal fractures with therapeutic interventions basically the same. Sometimes a phalanx fracture is associated with a hematoma beneath the fingernail (subungual hematoma), causing severe, throbbing pain. Therapeutic intervention for phalanx fractures is usually splinting the finger. Occasionally, surgical reduction is necessary to realign fractured segments. Subungual hematoma is treated with nail trephination.

Pelvic Fractures

Pelvic fractures (Fig. 40.19) occur most frequently in middle-aged and older adults and have a mortality rate of 8% to 13%. An estimated 65% of patients with pelvic fractures have sustained other concurrent injuries.[5] Mortality increases to 50% when the patient has an open pelvic fracture. Open fractures into the rectum or vagina constitute approximately 3% of pelvic injuries but have a 40% to 60% mortality.[4] Vehicular trauma, particularly in pedestrians, accounts for almost two-thirds of pelvic fractures. Other causes are direct trauma, falls from a height, sudden contraction of a muscle against a resistance, and even doing splits while waterskiing. Pelvic fractures are classified as stable or unstable, depending on disruption of the pelvic ring (Fig. 40.20). A particularly unstable fracture results from vertical-shear force, which causes significant bone and tissue damage. Specific neurovascular structures at risk for injury with pelvic fractures include the iliac artery,

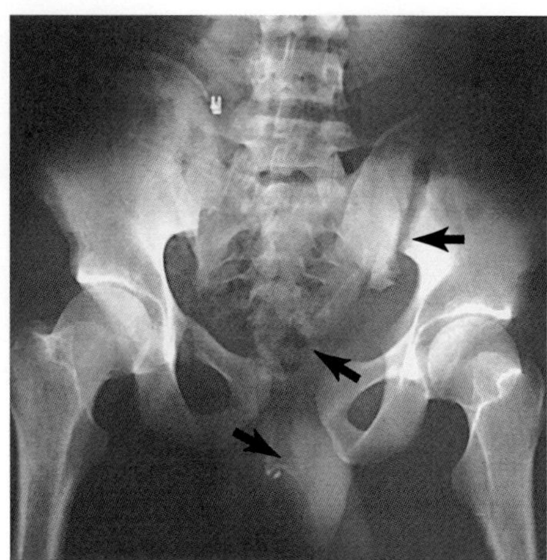

Fig. 40.19 **Pelvis Fracture.** (From Frank ED, Long BW, Smith BJ. *Merrill's Atlas of Radiographic Positioning and Procedures.* 11th ed. St Louis, MO: Mosby; 2007.)

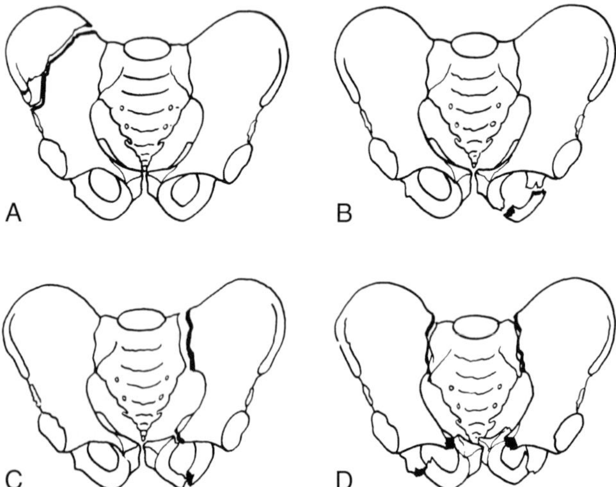

Fig. 40.20 **Types of Pelvic Fractures.** (A) Stable fracture of the iliac, without disruption of the pelvic ring. (B) Stable fracture of the ischial tuberosity. (C) Unstable fracture of pubis symphysis involving the ischial tuberosity and pelvic ring. (D) Unstable fracture involving the pubis symphysis and ischial tuberosity. (From Danis DM, Blansfield JS, Gervasini AA. *Handbook of Clinical Trauma Care: The First Hour.* 4th ed. St Louis, MO: Mosby; 2007.)

venous plexus, and sciatic nerve. Large-volume blood loss from lacerated pelvic veins, arteries, or the fracture itself can occur as well as injury to the genitourinary system.[13]

Compression of the iliac wings causes tenderness over the pubis in the patient with a pelvic fracture. These patients can also have paraspinous muscle spasm, sacroiliac joint tenderness, paresis or hemiparesis, pelvic ecchymosis, and hematuria. Hemorrhagic shock resulting from associated blood loss should be suspected in the patient with tachycardia and hypotension.

Therapeutic interventions include high-flow oxygen, serial vital signs, and two large-bore IV lines for volume replacement titrated to blood pressure and pulse rate. The spine and the legs are usually immobilized with a long spine board before the patient's arrival at the ED. After the long board is removed, the pelvis may be wrapped tightly with a sheet and secured with towel clips or a pelvic binder splint. This is done temporarily to assist in tamponading the bleeding from the pelvic fracture(s). Patients with pelvic fractures can bleed profusely because the pelvis is supplied with major arteries and a rich venous plexus, so a type and crossmatch for at least 4 to 5 units of blood should be done. Average blood loss for a closed fracture is 1500 to 3000 mL[15]; exsanguinating hemorrhage can occur with both closed and open fractures. A urinary catheter should be inserted cautiously in the patient with pelvic trauma because of the potential for associated urethral injury. Never insert a urinary catheter when a patient has blood at the meatus or if there is penile deformity in a male patient.

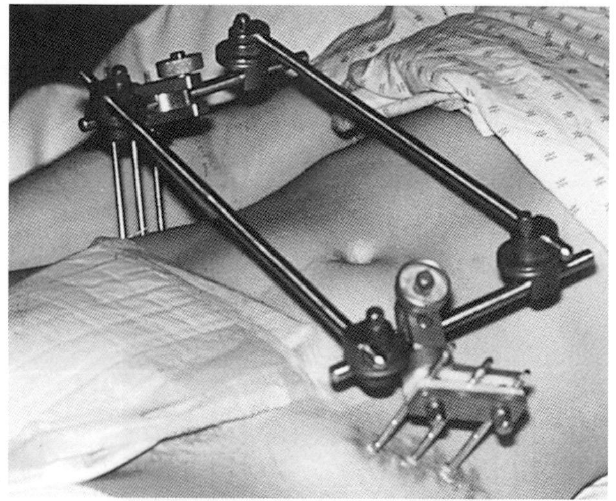

Fig. 40.21 **External Fixator: Pelvis.** (From Maher AB, Salmond SW, Pellino TA. *Orthopedic Nursing.* 3rd ed. Philadelphia, PA: Saunders; 2002.)

Definitive interventions depend on the severity of the fracture. Less severe, non–weight-bearing injuries are treated with bed rest and traction. Unstable, weight-bearing fractures are treated with external fixation devices (Fig. 40.21) or with open reduction using internal fixation devices. Hemorrhage from lacerated pelvic vessels may require an angiogram with embolization.

Complications from pelvic fractures include bladder trauma, genital trauma, lumbosacral trauma, ruptured internal organs, sepsis, shock, and death. Long-term complications include thrombophlebitis, fat embolism, chronic pain, and loss of function.

Hip Fractures

Hip fractures are common in older adults and are usually caused by falls or minor trauma (Fig. 40.22). Conversely, major trauma accounts for most hip fractures in younger patients. Fractures can occur in the femoral head, femoral neck (intracapsular), and intertrochanteric region. Femoral head fractures are rare but generally are associated with a high-speed MVC. Symptoms associated with hip fractures include pain in the groin, hip, or knee; severe pain with leg movement; and immobility. Patients with greater trochanteric

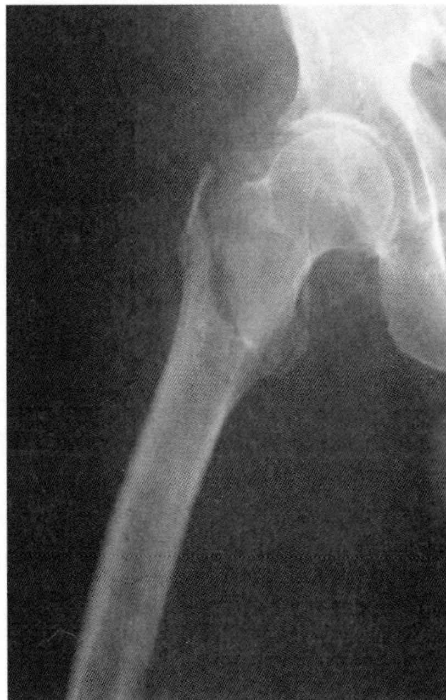

Fig. 40.22 Hip Fracture.

fractures can be ambulatory. Extracapsular trochanteric fractures are associated with pain in the lateral hip, shortening of the extremity, and a greater degree of external rotation.

Immediate therapeutic interventions include minimizing movement of the affected leg (e.g., splinting the hip to a long spine board or to the opposite leg). Monitoring serial vital signs is recommended because of the potential for blood loss. Early immobilization with Buck's traction or surgical intervention is often necessary. Complications of hip fracture include hypovolemia, shock, avascular necrosis with femoral head and neck fractures, and nonunion. These patients are generally at a greater risk for developing postoperative complications related to age and immobility.

Lower Extremity Fractures

Femoral Fracture

Femoral fractures (Fig. 40.23) occur in all age-groups, usually secondary to major trauma. The patient has severe pain, inability to bear weight on the injured leg, deformity, swelling, and angulation. Severe muscle spasms cause significant pain and also cause the limb to shorten. Crepitus occurs over the fracture site as bone pieces move.

Initial therapeutic interventions include the use of a traction splint (e.g., Hare, Sager, or Thomas) for immobilization. A long air splint with an enclosed foot or using the other leg as a splint is not recommended because these methods do not provide adequate stability. Associated injuries such as knee trauma are assessed. IV access is established, ideally in two sites, and vital signs are monitored frequently. Analgesia and volume replacement should be determined based on individual patient assessment. The patient should be prepared for traction, pin placement in the ED, or surgery.

The greatest complication of femoral fracture is shock secondary to hypovolemia. Average blood loss from a closed fracture is 1000 mL[15] and can exceed 3000 mL.[13] Severe muscle spasms can move bone ends, causing further soft-tissue injury, muscle damage, and pain. Neurovascular structures that can be damaged include the peroneal nerve, sciatic nerve, and popliteal artery.

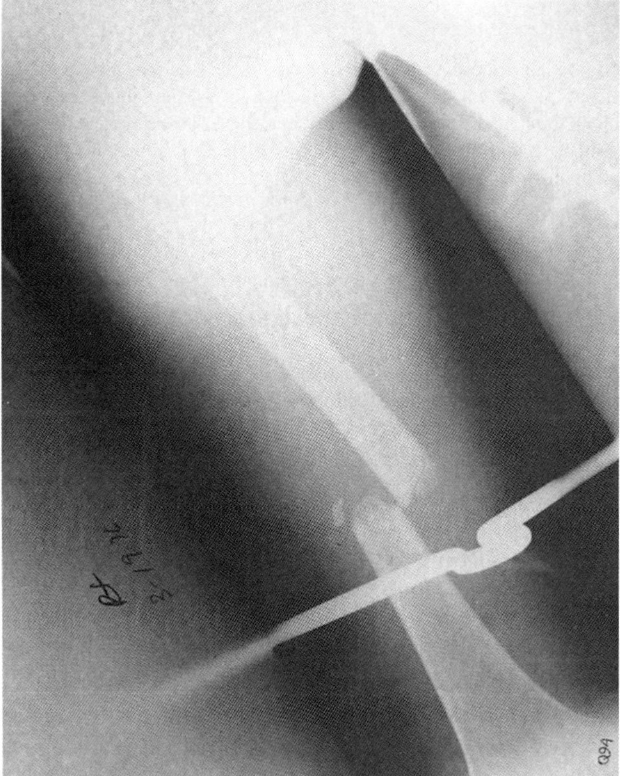

Fig. 40.23 Femur Fracture.

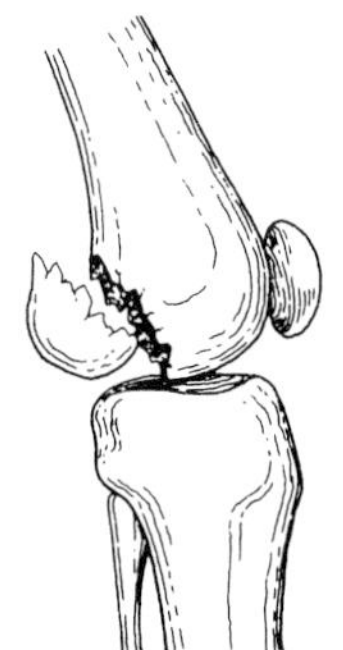

Fig. 40.24 Knee Fracture.

Knee Fractures

Knee fractures may be supracondylar fractures of the femur or intraarticular fractures of the femur or tibia (Fig. 40.24). This type of injury occurs in all age-groups and is usually the result of automobile, motorcycle, or automobile-pedestrian collisions causing direct trauma to the knee. Patients complain of knee pain, inability to bend or straighten the knee (depending on the position of the knee at the time of injury), swelling, and tenderness. Therapeutic interventions include a long leg splint or securing one leg to the other. Depending on the extent of injury, the patient may require surgical repair.

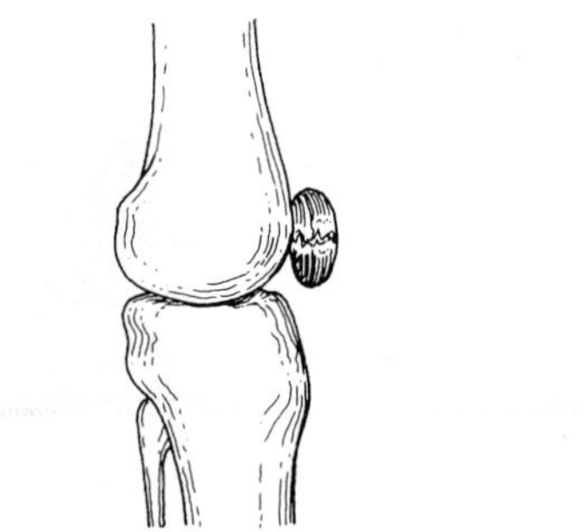

Fig. 40.25 Patella Fracture.

The knee will most likely be casted. The most common complication of knee fracture is neurovascular compromise of the peroneal or tibial nerve or the popliteal artery.

Patellar Fractures

Patellar fractures are seen in all age-groups (Fig. 40.25) usually after direct trauma from a fall or impact with the dashboard. Indirect trauma such as a severe muscle pull can also cause fracture of the patella. The patient presents with knee pain and often has an obvious deformity of the patella. Open patellar fractures also occur. Therapeutic interventions include covering any open wounds and applying a long leg splint. Radiographs of the affected limb should be obtained to determine the extent of the fracture. Treatment for a nondisplaced patellar fracture is use of a long leg cylinder cast. If the fracture is displaced, reduction is attempted, with surgery if appropriate, to realign fractured parts. The patella is an important part of the knee aiding in leverage and protection of the knee joint. Complete disruption of leg extension warrants surgery.

Tibial and Fibular Fractures

Tibial and fibular fractures are seen in all age-groups (Fig. 40.26) secondary to direct trauma, indirect trauma, or rotational force. The patient has pain in the leg, point tenderness, swelling, deformity, and crepitus. Many tibial and fibular fractures are open. Open and closed tibial injuries should be splinted as they are found; realignment of an open fracture should not be attempted unless neurovascular compromise is present. Any open wounds should be covered with a dry sterile dressing. The patient with a stable, nondisplaced tibial fracture may be discharged in a long leg splint or cast. Open or closed reduction may be necessary when the fracture is unstable or displaced. Reduction of these fractures is followed by application of a splint or cast. Use of a cast or splint immediately after reduction is determined by the degree of edema and the potential for swelling to increase.

An isolated fibular fracture is unusual. A walking cast is usually applied because the fibula is not a weight-bearing bone. Complications of tibial and fibular fractures include blood loss up to 2 L, infection, soft-tissue damage, neurovascular compromise, compartment syndrome, and Volkmann's contracture.

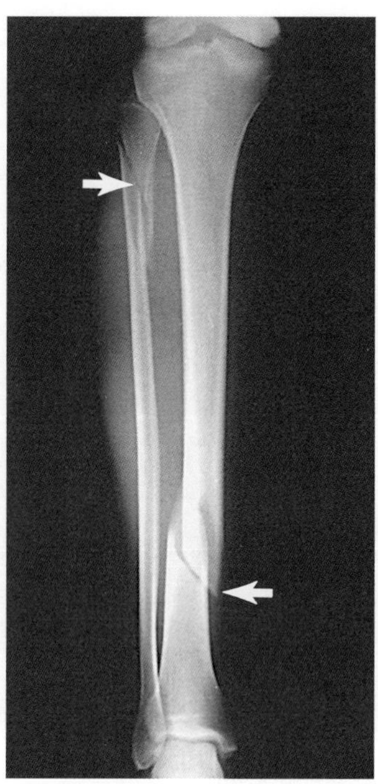

Fig. 40.26 Fracture of Tibia and Fibula. (From Frank ED, Long BW, Smith BJ. *Merrill's Atlas of Radiographic Positioning and Procedures*. 11th ed. St Louis, MO: Mosby; 2007.)

Ankle Fractures

Fractures of the ankle involve the distal tibia, distal fibula, or talus and occur in all age-groups (Fig. 40.27). Direct trauma, indirect trauma, or torsion can lead to open or closed ankle fractures. The patient complains of pain in the injured area, inability to bear weight on the extremity, point tenderness, swelling, and deformity. After closed reduction, the patient is placed in a walking cast. Depending on the extent of injury, the patient may require open reduction and pinning. The most frequent complication is neurovascular compromise, particularly of the peroneal nerve.

Foot Fractures

Tarsal and metatarsal fractures. Fractures of the tarsals and metatarsals (Fig. 40.28) occur in all age-groups, usually from MVCs, athletic injuries, crush injuries, or direct trauma. Fifth metatarsal fractures can occur with inversion injuries of the foot. The patient complains of pain in the foot and hesitates to bear weight. Therapeutic intervention includes a compression dressing and a soft splint. Minimally displaced fractures are treated with open-toed walking shoes or casts. With significant displacement, open reduction may be required. Crutches may be used to assist with weight bearing or non–weight bearing. Complications from this type of fracture are rare.

Calcaneus fractures. Fractures of the calcaneus are usually seen in young adults secondary to a fall in which the victim lands on his or her feet (Fig. 40.29). The patient complains of pain in the heel, point tenderness, and swelling. Dislocation may also occur. Management includes reduction of the

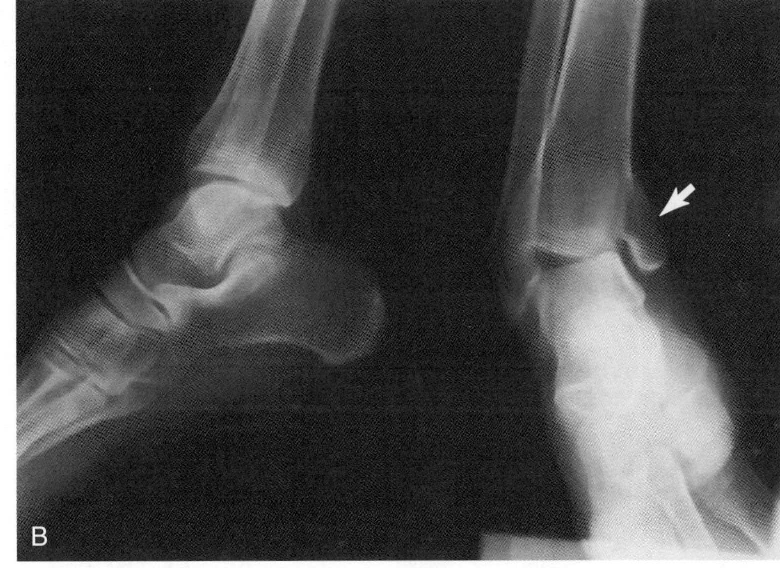

Fig. 40.27 (A) Ankle fracture. (B) Radiograph.

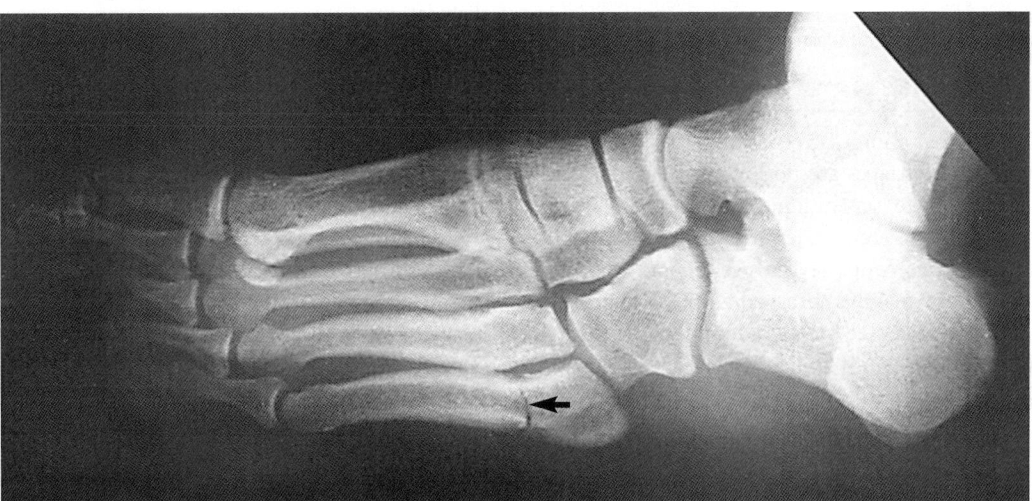

Fig. 40.28 Foot Fracture. (From Marx JA, Hockberger RS, Walls RM. *Rosen's Emergency Medicine: Concepts and Clinical Practice.* 6th ed. St Louis, MO: Mosby; 2006.)

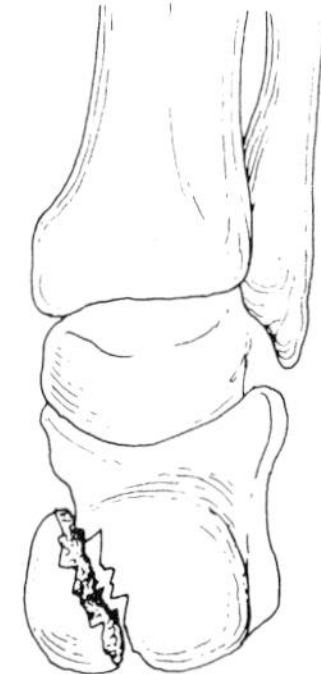

Fig. 40.29 Calcaneus Fracture.

fracture when necessary and application of a below-the-knee, weight-bearing cast. Open reduction is occasionally necessary. Associated injuries seen with calcaneus fractures include lumbosacral compression fracture and Colles fracture.

Toe (phalangeal) fractures. Fractures of the toes (Fig. 40.30) occur in all age-groups secondary to kicking a hard object or running into an immovable object. The patient has pain in the toe, swelling, and discoloration. Felt or cotton is placed between the fractured toe and the adjacent toe, and then both toes are taped together (buddy taped) so the uninjured toe acts as a splint. The patient may bear weight as tolerated and is instructed to wear hard-soled shoes, such as wooden or hard-soled, open-toed shoes, which do not put pressure on the toes. Complications are rare, but nail injury may occur.

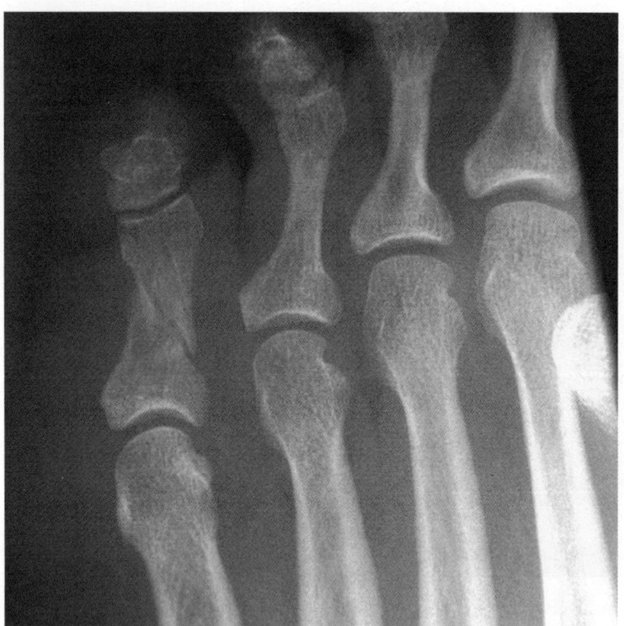

Fig. 40.30 Phalangeal Fracture. (From Browner BD, Jupiter JB, Levine AM, et al. *Skeletal Trauma: Basic Science, Management, and Reconstruction.* 3rd ed. Philadelphia, PA: Saunders; 2003.)

DISLOCATIONS

Dislocations occur when a joint exceeds its normal range of motion such that joint surfaces are no longer intact. Partial (subluxation) or complete separation of both articulating surfaces can occur. Soft-tissue injuries within the joint capsule and surrounding ligaments; severe swelling; and nerve, vein, and artery damage may be observed with dislocations. Diagnosis can often be predicted before radiographs are taken by soliciting information about the mechanism of injury and noting clinical assessment findings.

In general, dislocations produce severe pain, joint deformity, inability to move the joint, swelling, and point tenderness. Potential for vascular compromise also exists, so the distal pulse should be assessed carefully. Initial interventions include careful palpation of the joint and splinting the joint as it is found. Analgesia and sedation are given before reduction by the ED physician or orthopedist. Significant sedation (e.g., morphine, fentanyl, midazolam, methohexital, etomidate, propofol) may be required to reduce dislocations, so the patient requires careful monitoring. Nitrous oxide is used in some institutions. Complications related to dislocations include ischemia, aseptic necrosis, and recurrent dislocations.

Acromioclavicular Dislocation

Acromioclavicular separations (Fig. 40.31) are commonly seen in athletes secondary to a fall or direct force on the point of the shoulder. The patient complains of great pain in the joint area and cannot raise the affected arm or bring the arm across the chest. Deformity, point or area tenderness, swelling, and hematoma over the injury site are also noted. The injury is classified in degrees of separation; third-degree injuries involve a complete separation of the joint. Treatment for first- and second-degree injuries involves reducing the separation, regaining anatomic alignment, and immobilizing the affected limb with a sling and swath. More involved third-degree injuries often require surgery for open reduction and wiring. The patient may experience painful range of motion after reduction.

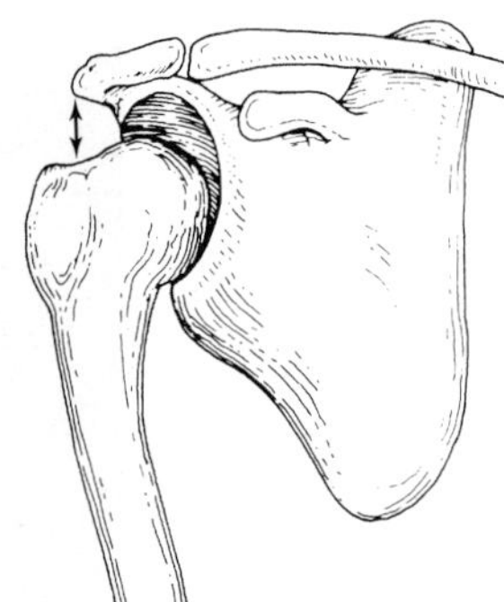

Fig. 40.31 Acromioclavicular Separation.

Shoulder Dislocation

Dislocations of the shoulder usually occur in children and athletes. Two general categories are anterior and posterior dislocations.

Anterior shoulder dislocations occur as an athletic injury when the athlete falls on an extended arm which is abducted and externally rotated. The force pushes the head of the humerus in front of the shoulder joint (Fig. 40.32). Posterior dislocations are rare and usually occur in patients with seizures when the arm is abducted and internally rotated. In all shoulder dislocations, the patient complains of severe pain in the shoulder area, inability to move the arm, and deformity. Deformity is sometimes difficult to see in posterior dislocation. An estimated 55% to 60% of shoulder dislocations seen in the ED are recurrent. The extremity is placed in the position of greatest comfort, then distal pulses are checked, followed by evaluation of skin temperature and moisture and neurologic status. Radiographs are obtained before the joint is relocated unless neurovascular compromise has occurred. After the joint is relocated, it is immobilized with a sling and swath or shoulder immobilizer. Postreduction radiographs are obtained to confirm placement. The patient should be referred to an orthopedic surgeon. Complications from this type of injury are neurovascular compromise of the brachial plexus and axillary artery and associated fractures.

Elbow Dislocation

Dislocations of the elbow are seen most often in children, teenagers, and young adults. Elbow dislocation is a common athletic injury caused by a fall on an externally rotated arm or when a young child is jerked or lifted by a single arm (known as nursemaid's elbow). The patient complains of pain in the joint, which may feel "locked." Any movement can produce severe pain. Swelling, deformity, and displacement are also noted. The arm is immobilized in the position of greatest comfort. The joint is relocated, then immobilized after radiographs are obtained. The most common complication of this injury is neurovascular compromise to the median nerve or brachial artery.

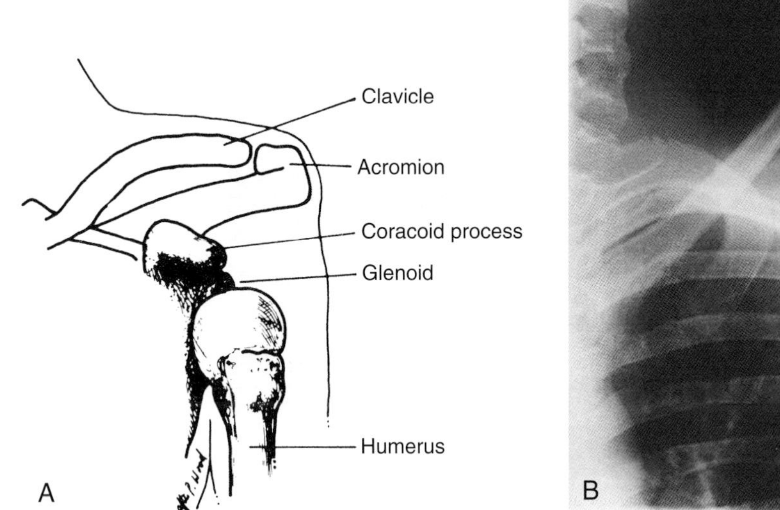

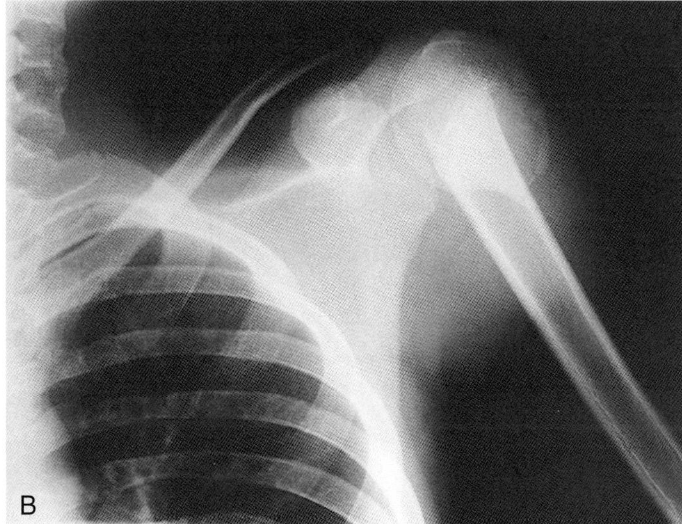

Fig. 40.32 (A) Anterior shoulder dislocation. (B) Radiograph. (B, From Marx JA, Hockberger RS, Walls RM. *Rosen's Emergency Medicine: Concepts and Clinical Practice.* 6th ed. St Louis, MO: Mosby; 2006.)

Radial head subluxation (nursemaid's elbow) accounts for about 20% of upper extremity injuries in children and is seen in children ages 6 months to 5 years, most often in 1- to 3-year-olds. History of a pull on the arm or a fall is reported. The child refuses to use the arm but does not seem in pain or distress. The injury does not require radiographic studies if the dislocation can be easily relocated with good return of function; immobilization after reduction is not necessary. Reduction of a nursemaid's elbow is accomplished by positioning the child with the elbow flexed 90 degrees, hypersupinating the wrist, and placing the thumb on the radial head. Upon hypersupination, a click will be felt on the radial head, confirming the reduction was successful (Fig. 40.33).

Wrist Dislocation

Dislocation of the wrist (Fig. 40.34) is seen most frequently in athletes but does occur in all age-groups from a fall on an outstretched hand. The patient complains of severe pain in the wrist with swelling, deformity, and point tenderness. The wrist is placed in a splint in the position of comfort and then a cold pack is applied. Radiographic studies are obtained, the joint is relocated, and a cast is applied. Complications include neurovascular compromise, especially median nerve damage.

Hand or Finger Dislocation

Hand or finger dislocations (Fig. 40.35) are usually seen in athletes secondary to a fall on an outstretched hand or finger and may also result from direct trauma to the tip of the finger. The patient presents with pain in the area of the injury, inability to move the joint, deformity, and swelling. The patient is sent for radiographs of both the anterior and lateral view of the dislocated finger. After reviewing the films and making certain a fracture is not present, the patient is given a digital block and reduction is done by emergency care providers. A postreduction film is obtained to confirm successful reduction. The injured area is splinted to immobilize the joint.

Hip Dislocation

Hip dislocations occur in all age-groups, usually when the leg is extended before an impact. The injury is common with head-on, frontal impact MVCs when the leg is extended with the foot on the brake pedal just before impact or when the knee jams into the dashboard. Injury also occurs with falls and crush injuries. Hip dislocations can also result from a failed or displaced implant in patients who have previously undergone surgical interventions for joint replacement or hip fracture (Fig. 40.36). Dislocation may be anterior or posterior. The patient complains of pain in the hip and knee and arrives with the hip flexed, adducted, and internally rotated (posterior dislocation) or flexed, abducted, and externally rotated (anterior dislocation). The joint feels locked, and the patient cannot move the leg.

The extremity is splinted in the presenting position or position of greatest comfort. Other injuries are assessed. Necrosis of the femoral head may occur if the joint is not relocated within 4 to 6 hours. After the hip joint is relocated, the patient begins a period of bed rest with traction. Children may be placed in a spica cast. Complications from this type of injury are femoral artery and nerve damage.

Knee Dislocation

Knee dislocations are common in all age-groups and are usually caused by major trauma. The patient complains of severe pain in the knee, inability to move the leg, swelling, and deformity (Fig. 40.37). Immediate therapeutic intervention includes splinting the limb in a position of comfort or the presenting position. A fractured tibia is frequently associated with a knee dislocation. Almost all people with dislocation of the knee joint have associated damage to the joint capsule.

After reduction, the patient is admitted to the hospital for bed rest with the knee elevated and intermittent cold packs

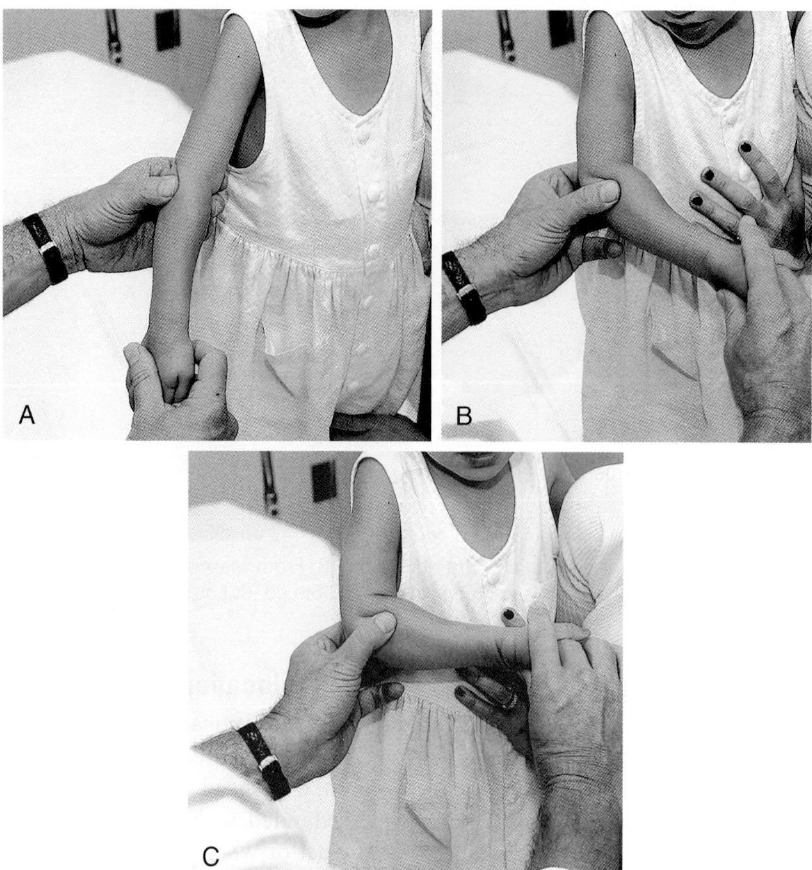

Fig. 40.33 Technique for Reducing Nursemaid's Elbow. (A) Applying pressure to the radial head. (B) Supinating the forearm. (C) Flexing elbow, in one continuous motion. (From Marx JA, Hockberger RS, Walls RM. *Rosen's Emergency Medicine: Concepts and Clinical practice.* 6th ed. St Louis, MO: Mosby; 2006.)

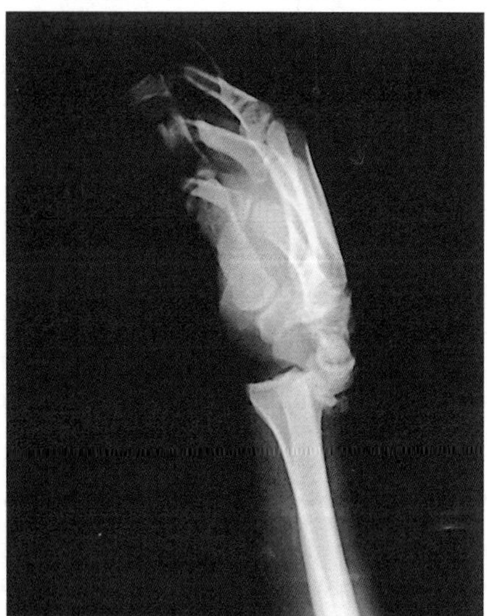

Fig. 40.34 Wrist Dislocation. (From Ballinger PW. *Merrill's Atlas of Radiographic Positions and Radiologic Procedures.* 8th ed. St Louis, MO: Mosby; 1995.)

for 24 to 48 hours. A cast is usually applied after this time. Knee dislocations are associated with a high incidence of injury to the popliteal artery; vascular integrity must be evaluated. Other complications include peroneal and tibial nerve damage.

Patellar Dislocation

Dislocation of the patella occurs in all age-groups, usually during athletic events secondary to direct trauma to the lateral aspect of the knee or rapid rotation on a planted foot. Patients usually have severe pain, keep the affected knee in a flexed position, and are unable to use the knee (Fig. 40.38). Significant tenderness and swelling in the patellar area are evident. The patella can usually be observed or palpated outside of its normal position. The leg is splinted in the presenting position and a cold pack applied. After radiographs, if spontaneous reduction does not occur with extension of the leg, the patella is reduced. After relocation, the knee is placed in a compression bandage and knee immobilizer or cylinder cast.

Ankle Dislocation

Ankle dislocation is usually the result of athletic injury and is commonly associated with a fracture. Dislocation results from lateral stress motion when normal range of motion for the ankle is exceeded (Fig. 40.39). Patients complain of severe pain in the ankle, inability to move the joint, swelling, and deformity. The ankle and foot are splinted in a position of comfort, and an ice pack is applied. The ankle may be relocated by a closed or open method, depending on the degree of

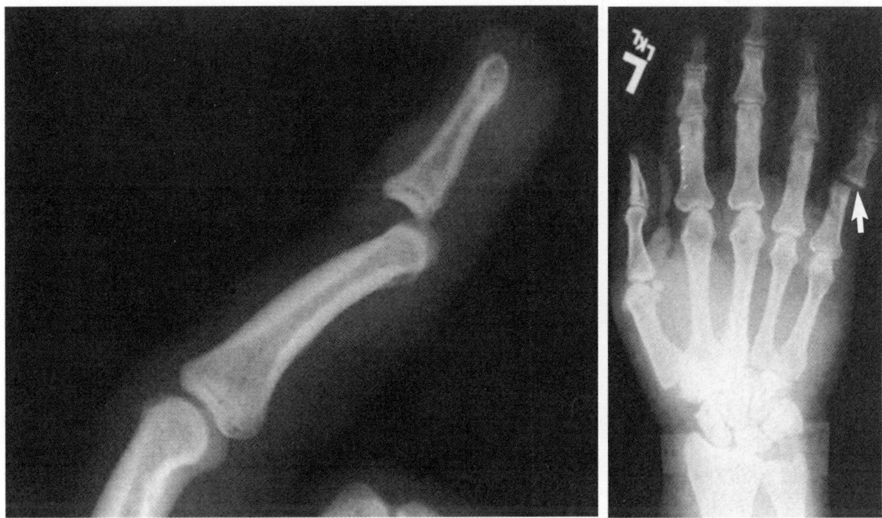

Fig. 40.35 Finger Dislocation.

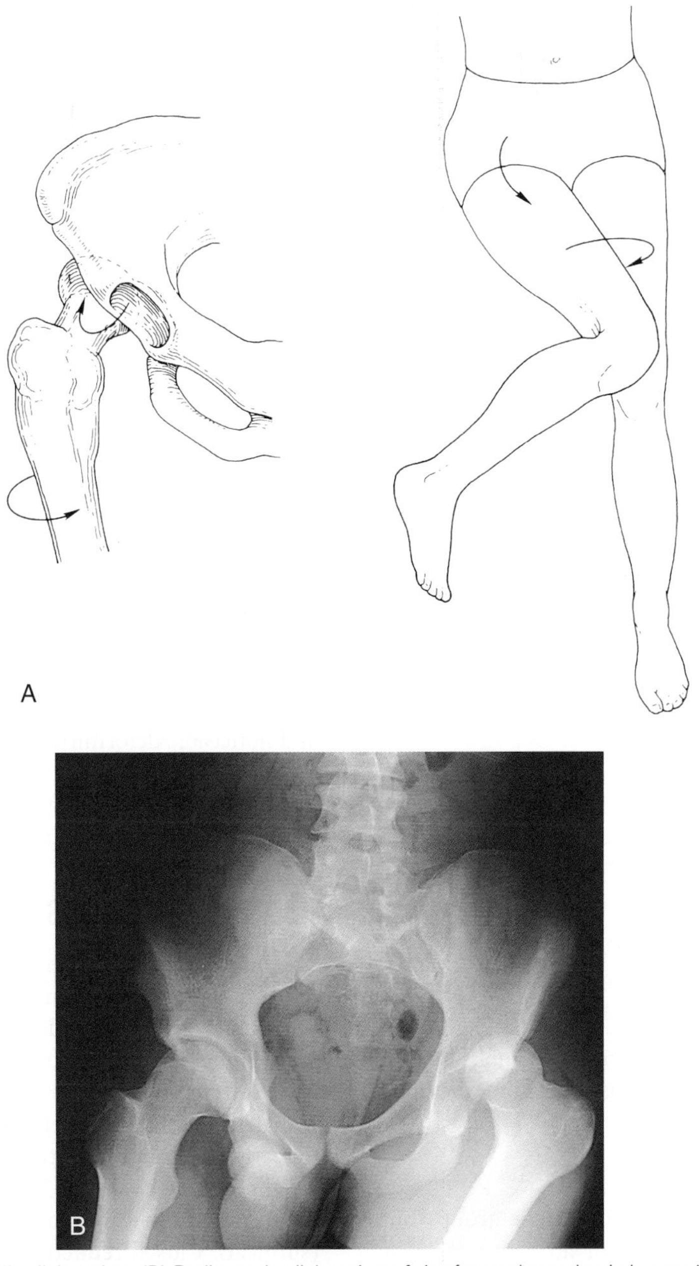

Fig. 40.36 (A) Hip dislocation. (B) Radiograph: dislocation of the femoral prosthesis in a patient with a total hip arthroplasty. (From Marx JA, Hockberger RS, Walls RM. *Rosen's Emergency Medicine: Concepts and Clinical practice.* 6th ed. St Louis, MO: Mosby; 2006.)

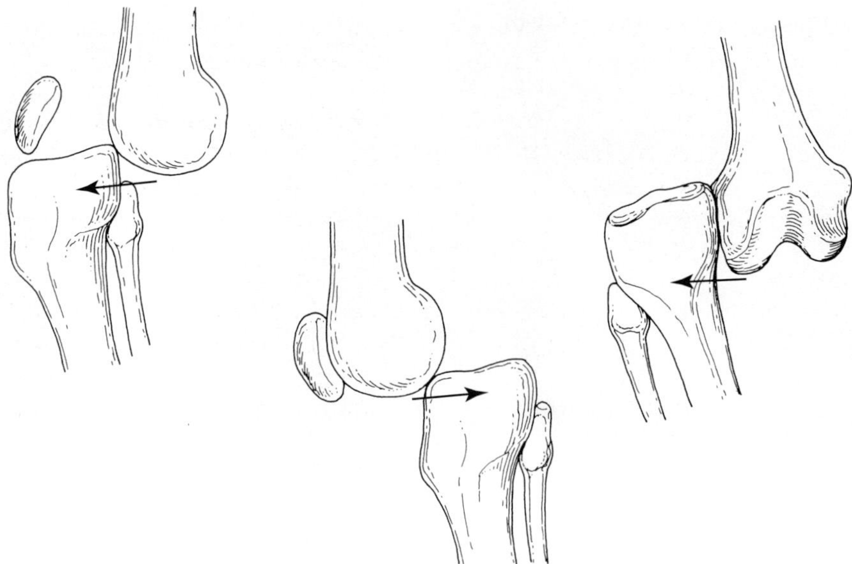

Fig. 40.37 Knee Dislocation.

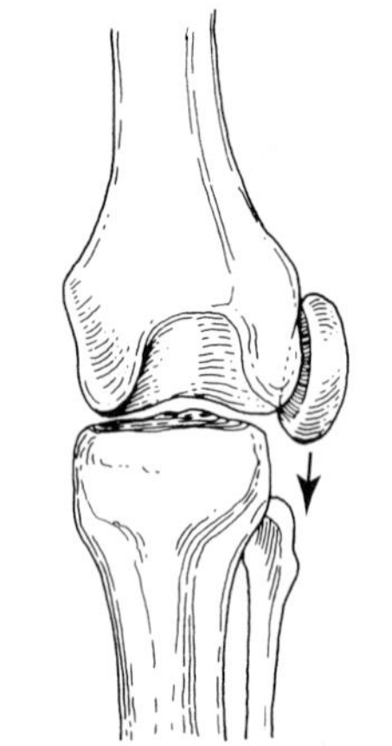

Fig. 40.38 Patella Dislocation.

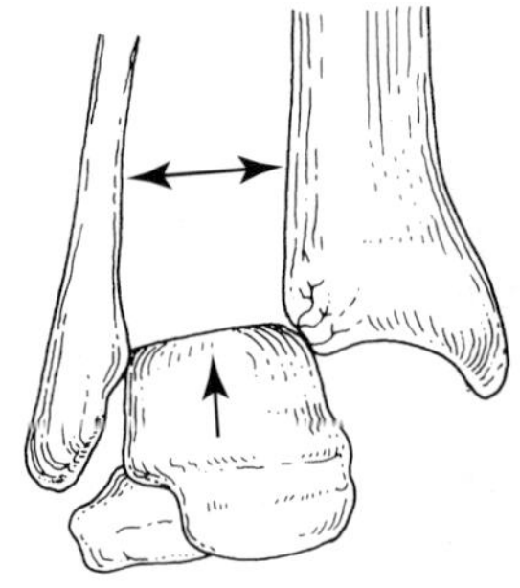

Fig. 40.39 Ankle Dislocation.

injury and associated fractures. The primary complication of this injury is neurovascular compromise, including the tibial artery.

Foot Dislocation

Dislocations of the foot can occur in all age-groups but are rare. Injury is often the result of an automobile or motorcycle collision in which a combination of forces occurs simultaneously. Foot dislocation is almost always associated with an open wound. The patient complains of severe pain in the foot with point tenderness and inability to use the foot. Significant swelling and deformity are evident. If present, an open wound is covered with a sterile dressing before a soft splint is applied. After the foot is relocated, a cast is applied. The patient is instructed to elevate the limb and apply cold packs for 24 hours. No weight bearing is permitted.

Toe (Metatarsophalangeal) Dislocation

Dislocations of the metatarsophalangeal joints (toes) are rare; when they do occur, they are often associated with open fractures. Toe dislocations should be reduced immediately because delay can result in swelling, making closed reduction more difficult to perform. The patient complains of pain and point tenderness in the joint area with significant swelling and noticeable deformity. The area should be covered with a bulky dressing to prevent further damage. After radiographs have been obtained, the dislocation is reduced and then the foot and toes are immobilized.

REDUCTION ISSUES

The goal for reduction of fractures and dislocations is to restore anatomic alignment, allow bone healing, and preserve function. Fractures that do not require anatomic alignment for healing include an impacted fracture of the humeral neck, a fractured clavicle (particularly in children), and a pediatric nonangulated femur. Conversely, reduction is particularly important for intraarticular fractures, especially for weight-bearing bones.

Reduction methods are described as closed or open (surgical). Closed reduction uses traction-countertraction,

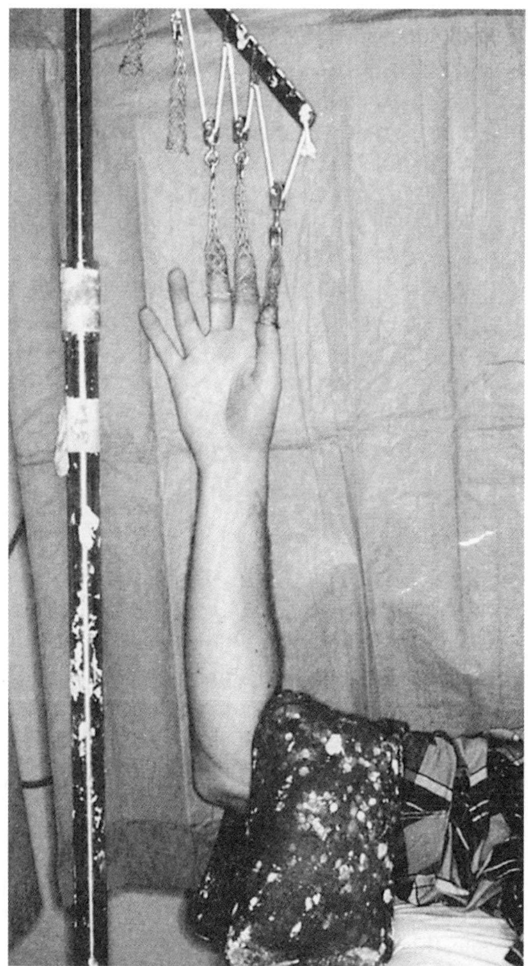

Fig. 40.40 Finger traps and distal traction at the elbow to distract and reduce fracture dislocations. (From Rosen P, Barkin RM, Rockberger RS at al. *Emergency Medicine: Concepts and Clinical Practice.* 4th ed. St Louis, MO: Mosby; 1998.)

angulation, and rotation (i.e., the reverse force of what caused the injury). A finger trap and weights may be used for forearm reduction (Fig. 40.40). Manipulation may require local anesthesia, IV sedation, pain medications, or general anesthesia. Reduction should be accomplished as soon as possible after stabilization of other injuries because swelling can impede successful reduction. Postreduction radiographs are done after casting to verify acceptable bone alignment.

Open reduction is used for open fractures; multiple injuries; major fractures; and fractures involving intraarticular joints, the epiphysis, or the femoral neck. Surgical reduction is also used for soft-tissue entrapment; major nerve, arterial, or ligament injuries; pathologic fractures; unsatisfactory or failed closed reduction; or delayed union. Open reduction uses internal fixation or external fixation devices.

TRACTION

Skin or skeletal traction may be initiated in the ED. A traction splint (e.g., Hare or Sager) can be used until more definitive stabilization is available. Buck's traction uses a wrapped dressing or boot to provide temporary immobilization before surgery for a hip or femur fracture and to reduce muscle spasm. Traction is set up on a hospital bed brought to the ED. This eliminates painful and possibly injurious removal of traction with transfer of the patient from the ED stretcher.

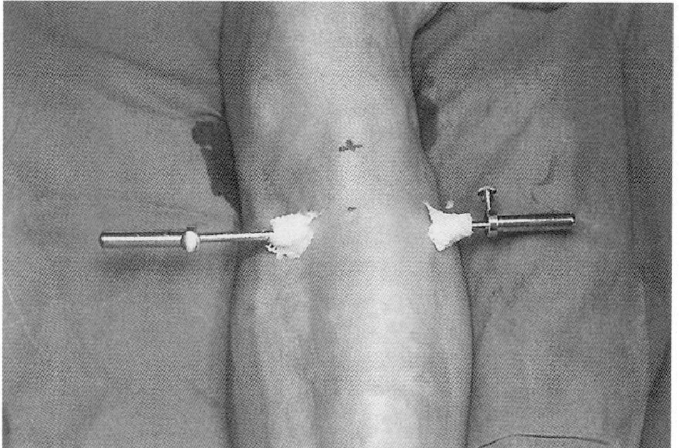

Fig. 40.41 The pin is passed through the tibia to project equally medially and laterally. Points are protected with covers. (From Mills K, Morton R, Page G. *Color Atlas and Text of Emergencies.* 2nd ed. London, England: Times Mirror International; 1995.)

Steinman Pin

Skeletal traction may be applied in the ED with a Steinman pin (Fig. 40.41). This provides temporary reduction of long-bone fractures until open reduction and internal fixation can be done. The pin is a round, stainless steel rod drilled perpendicularly into the distal femur or proximal tibia for connection to a stirrup with traction (15–40 pounds). After pin placement, sterile dressings are placed around insertion sites. Osteomyelitis is a potential complication of pin insertion.

Casts

In the ED, the decision to immobilize an injury with a cast versus a splint or fiberglass mold is based on the actual amount of edema and potential swelling likely to occur. The goal is to prevent neurovascular compromise (and compartment syndrome) from a restrictive immobilization device. A brief overview of casting and care of casts is presented here. An orthopedic or medical-surgical text should be consulted for a complete description of techniques and types of casts/molds.

Before a cast is applied, any particulate matter is removed and the skin is completely dried. Any skin abnormalities are documented. Casting equipment includes plaster or fiberglass, stockinette and padding, a bucket of cool-to-warm water, gloves, and a gauze or elastic bandage if a splint is applied.

After the cast is applied, the patient should remain immobile with the limb placed on a plastic-coated pillow for at least 20 minutes to avoid pressure and indentations

BOX 40.1 Aftercare Instructions for Patients With Casts

Keep cast dry and elevated above the heart 24 hours after injury.
Apply cold packs or sealed ice bags over the injured area for 30 minutes every 2 to 3 hours for 1 to 2 days.
See your physician immediately if you have a change in temperature of fingers or toes (digits are very cold or very hot), a change in color of fingers or toes (they are blue), or loss of feeling in fingers or toes.
Wiggle fingers or toes at least once each hour.
See a physician immediately if a foreign object is dropped into the cast.
Do not put anything inside your cast.
If swelling returns or a foul odor is present, see your physician.
Make an appointment to see a private physician or orthopedic physician for follow-up care.

and to allow the cast to set. A plaster cast generally requires 24 hours or more to dry thoroughly; a fiberglass cast dries in about an hour. Box 40.1 lists aftercare instructions for a patient with a cast.

Complications associated with casting include compartment syndrome, pressure sores, and infection. Symptoms of compartment syndrome include severe pain disproportionate to the injury with accompanying neurovascular compromise. An elevated temperature accompanied by a foul odor from the cast suggests infection from a possible pressure sore. Interventions include immediate cast removal. Cast removal or a bivalve procedure is accomplished with an electric cast saw. The saw blade cuts by vibrating rapidly back and forth. The patient should be reassured the blade does not cut the skin, but heat, vibration, or pressure may be felt. Burns secondary to the blade are rare. After the cast is cut, a cast spreader is used to widen the split and allow removal. Padding beneath the cast should be cut with bandage scissors.

ASSISTED AMBULATION: CRUTCHES, CANE, AND WALKER

When a patient is fitted for crutches, a cane, or a walker, measurement is ideally taken with the patient wearing shoes worn for ambulating. The shoes should be sturdy, fit well, have low heels, and fasten with a tie, buckle, or Velcro.

Axillary Crutches

Axillary crutches should fit so that each arm piece is 2 inches or two to three fingerwidths below the axilla with no weight placed on the axilla. Tips of the crutches should be placed 6 inches to the side (or with enough room for the patient's hips to swing through) and 6 inches to the front. Taller individuals require a broader base, so crutches may be placed up to 12 inches to the side for these patients. Each hand piece should be fitted so that the elbow is flexed 30 degrees. For most people, this can be accomplished by having the patient place the crutch in the correct position and extend the arm along the crutch—the hand piece should hit at the level of the wrist.

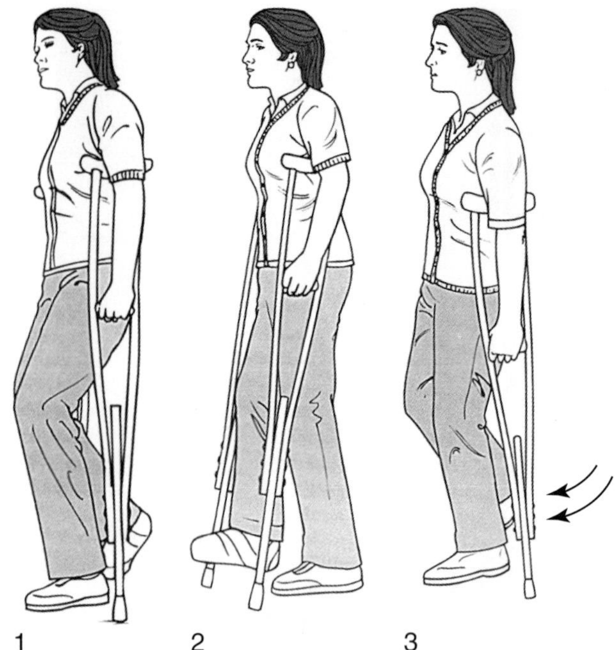

Fig. 40.42 Three-Point Gait. *1,* Standing with crutches, with all weight on the good leg. *2,* Move crutches and the injured leg forward simultaneously. *3,* Bearing weight on the palms of the hands, step forward onto the good leg. (From Proehl JA, Jones LM. *Mosby's Emergency Department Teaching Guides.* St Louis, MO: Mosby; 1997.)

Cane

A cane should be fitted so that when it is held next to the heel, the elbow is at a 30-degree angle of flexion. A cane should be used for minimal support during ambulation and to assist with balance and stability. A cane should be used on the side opposite the injury.

Walker

A walker may be chosen for patients who are unsteady on crutches and those who can bear full weight on at least one leg. A walker is measured to fit with the arms bent at 30 degrees. Patients having difficulty ambulating with assist devices may require physical therapy for training, using a wheelchair temporarily until able to ambulate safely. A walker is not ideal for use on stairs.

Gait Training

A three-point gait is used when minimal or no weight bearing is desired, making this gait ideal for ED patients. Fig. 40.42 shows this gait. Figs. 40.43 and 40.44 illustrate movement on stairs and changing from a sitting to standing position using crutches.

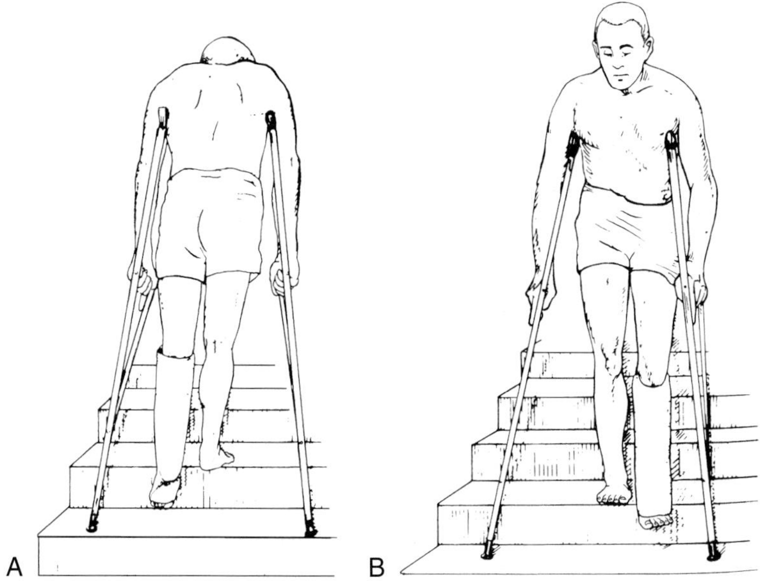

Fig. 40.43 (A) Going up stairs. (B) Going down stairs with crutches. (From Barber J, Stokes L, Billings D. *Adult and Child Care*. 2nd ed. St Louis, MO: Mosby; 1977.)

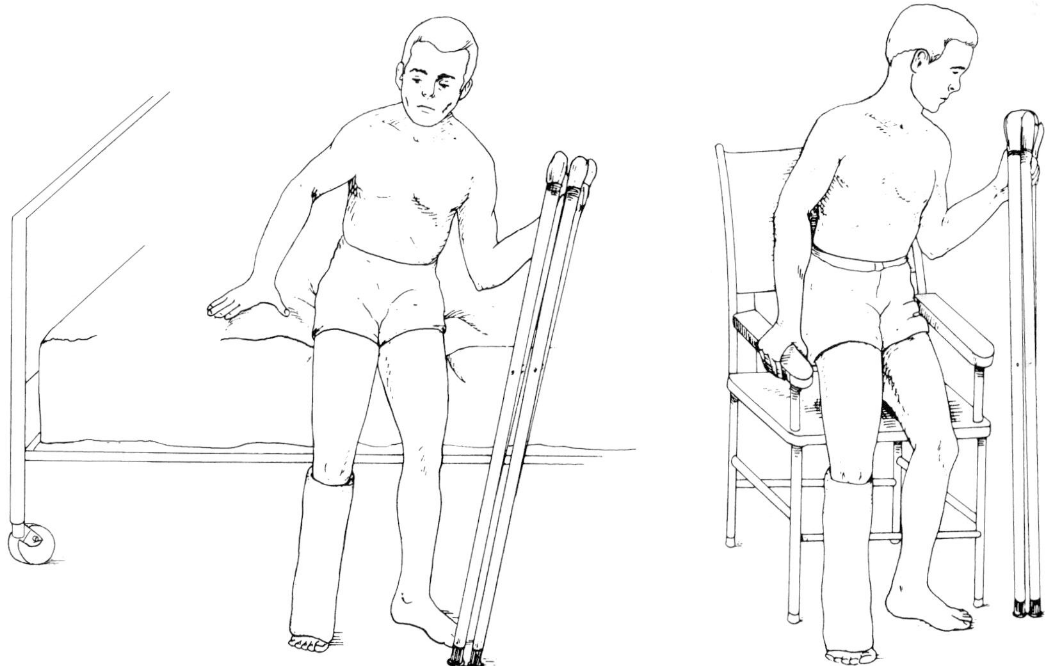

Fig. 40.44 Transferring from sitting to standing with crutches. (From Barber J, Stokes L, Billings D. *Adult and Child Care*. 2nd ed. St Louis, MO: Mosby; 1977.)

SUMMARY

Advances in surgical and orthopedic treatments have improved outcomes for patients with soft-tissue injuries and fractures. However, the best outcomes occur if injury never happens. Trauma prevention through education and legislation should be the primary goal of overall trauma management.

The main objective for nursing care of the patient with an orthopedic or soft-tissue injury is to preserve or restore normal neurovascular status and motor function. Attention to these injuries is a secondary priority to ABCs. The emergency nurse must assess and intervene as soon as possible and monitor for developing complications to prevent further harm to the extremity.

REFERENCES

1. Cerepani MJ, Emergency Nurses Association. Orthopedic emergencies. In: *Emergency Nursing Core Curriculum*. 7th ed. St Louis, MO: Elsevier; 2018:387–397.
2. Armstrong A, Hubbard MC. *Essentials of Musculoskeletal Care*. 5th ed. Rosemont, IL: American Academy of Orthopaedic Surgeons; 2016.
3. Simon RR, Sherman SC. *Koeningsknecht: Emergency Orthopedics*. 5th ed. New York, NY: McGraw-Hill; 2007.
4. Maher AB, Salmond SW, Pellino T. *Orthopaedic Nursing*. 3rd ed. Philadelphia, PA: Saunders; 2002.
5. Magee DJ. *Orthopedic Physical Assessment*. 6th ed. St Louis, MO: Elsevier Saunders; 2014.
6. Crowther CL. *Primary Orthopedic Care*. 2nd ed. St Louis, MO: Mosby; 2004.
7. Moore WH, Smith T. Salter-Harris fracture imaging, 2006. *eMedicine*. http://www.emedicine.com/radio/topic613.htm. Published October 25, 2006. Accessed June 13, 2019.
8. Edmunds-Winterton M. *Procedures for Primary Care Practitioners*. 3rd ed. St Louis, MO: Elsevier; 2017.
9. Pope Jr TL, Harris JH. *Harris & Harris' The Radiology of Emergency Medicine*. 5th ed. Philadelphia, PA: Lippincott Williams & Wilkins; 2013.
10. Frank ED, Long BW, Smith BJ. *Merrill's Atlas of Radiographic Positioning and Procedures*. 11th ed. St Louis, MO: Mosby; 2007.
11. Schnell ZB, Leeuwen AVM, Kranpitz TR. *Davis's Comprehensive Handbook of Laboratory and Diagnostic Tests With Nursing Implications*. Philadelphia, PA: FA Davis; 2003.
12. Moore EE, Feliciano DV, Mattox KL. *Trauma*. 8th ed. New York, NY: McGraw-Hill; 2017.
13. American College of Surgeons. Committee on Trauma: Shock. *Advanced Trauma Life Support for Doctors: Instructor Course Manual*. 9th ed. Chicago, IL: American College of Surgeons; 2012.
14. Black JM, Hawks-Hokanson J. *Medical-Surgical Nursing*. 7th ed. St Louis, MO: Saunders; 2005.
15. Roberts JR, Hedges JR. *Clinical Procedures in Emergency Medicine*. 5th ed. Philadelphia, PA: Saunders/Elsevier; 2010.

41

Burns

Cheryl Wraa

Burn trauma continues to be an immense challenge to caregivers in the emergency department (ED). Every year in the United States, an estimated one million patients seek treatment for burn injury, and approximately one-third are treated in EDs. In 2016 it was estimated that 486,000 patients received treatment for burn injuries. Approximately 40,000 patients were admitted to an acute care facility, with 60% admitted to 128 burn centers. Approximately 15,000 pediatric burn-injured patients were also admitted. Decreases in burn incidence and hospitalization are attributed to fire and burn prevention education, regulation of consumer products, and implementation of occupational safety standards. The decline in mortality is attributed to early care of the burn wound. Other factors contributing to the decline are management of patients with burns in specialty burn units, improved resuscitation, control of infection, and support of the hypermetabolic response. The survival rate at burn centers is reported as 96.8%. A significant portion of morbidity and mortality associated with burn injuries is caused by associated injuries. Pulmonary pathology from inhalation injury is the major cause of burn trauma death, with the majority of deaths at the extremes of age.[1–7]

More than 90% of all burns are considered preventable. Education, particularly in the school-age population, combined with legislative efforts, is helping decrease the number of burn injuries. The American Burn Association has developed effective public education programs. Legislation has been enacted requiring smoke alarms and sprinkler systems in public buildings, hotels, apartments, and new homes. For the caregiver, an accurate classification of injury, timely intervention, and rapid transport to an appropriate burn facility significantly reduces burn injury mortality and morbidity.[1]

ETIOLOGY

Not all burns are caused by fire. Tissue damage may be secondary to chemicals, hot liquids, tar, electricity, lightning, or frostbite. The location and duration of exposure to the source affects outcome, regardless of the specific source of burn injury. Specific mechanisms of burn injury are described in the following sections.

Thermal Burns

Thermal injuries represent the majority of all burns. They may result from flame, flash, steam, or scalding liquid. Fig. 41.1 presents an example of one cause of burn injury.

Scald Burns

Scalds from hot liquids are the most common cause of all burns. Exposure to water at 140°F (60°C) for 3 seconds can cause a deep partial-thickness or full-thickness burn. If water is 156°F (69°C), the same type of burn occurs in only 1 second. As a comparison, freshly brewed coffee is about 180°F (82°C). Tap water scalds occur within seconds and often happen during routine activities, involve large body surface area (BSA) burns, and are the most common source of scald-related deaths.[8] Soups and sauces, which are a thicker consistency, remain in contact longer with the skin and cause deeper burns. Other liquids causing scalds are cooking oil and grease. When used for cooking, oil and grease may reach 400°F (204°C). Immersion burns are usually deep and severe because of prolonged contact with a scalding liquid.

Specific groups of patients at risk for scald burns include those with preinjury comorbidities such as neurologic impairment, diabetes, and the extremes of ages. Adults older than 60 years disproportionately suffer burns from hot liquids.[8] It is well documented that older patients are at high risk for burn injury and experience worse prognoses than younger patients. This has been attributed to their compromised physical health status with chronic, debilitating conditions that increase the risk, exacerbate the extent of the injury, and impair recovery.[10,11]

Flame Burns

Burns from flames are the next most common cause of burns. Fortunately, the number of house fires has decreased with increased use of smoke detectors. Most flame burns are caused by careless smoking, motor vehicle crashes, and clothing ignited from stoves or space heaters. Flame burns occurring outdoors are usually caused by misuse of cooking stoves fueled by white gasoline, lanterns in tents, smoking in a sleeping bag, and gasoline or kerosene used in a charcoal fire.[6,7]

Flash Burns

Explosions of natural gas, propane, gasoline, or other flammable liquids cause flash burns—the third most common type of thermal burn. The explosion causes intense heat for a very brief time. Flash burns are usually partial thickness, although depth is dependent on the amount and kind of exploding fuel.

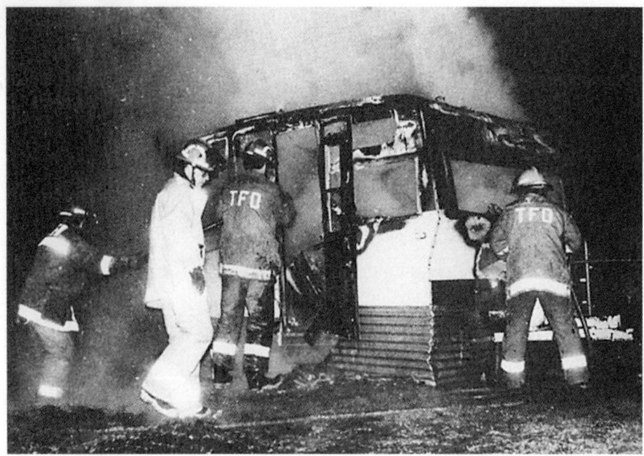

Fig. 41.1 Burn injuries occur as a result of exposure to flame and smoke. (Courtesy Tacoma Fire Department, Tacoma, WA.)

Flash burns can be large and are often associated with significant thermal damage to the upper airway.[11]

Contact Burns

Contact with a hot object such as metal, plastic, glass, or hot coals results in contact burns. The burns are usually not extensive but tend to be deep. People involved in industrial accidents often have contact burns associated with crush injuries from machine presses or hot, heavy objects. An increased incidence of contact burns has been seen in toddlers owing to the increased use of wood-burning stoves. The most common injury is to the palm when a child falls against the stove with hands outstretched.[8,11]

Electrical Burns

As electricity passes through the body and meets resistance from body tissues, it is converted to heat in direct proportion to amperage and the body's electrical resistance. It initially passes through the skin, causing an external burn at the entry and exit sites, with extensive damage internally between these sites. Nerves, blood vessels, and muscle are less resistant and more easily damaged than bone or fat. The heart, lungs, and brain can sustain immediate damage. The nervous system is particularly sensitive to electrical burns. Damage to the brain, spinal cord, and myelin-producing cells causes devastating transverse myelitis. Autonomic dysfunction can cause pupils to appear fixed and dilated, but this finding should not cause resuscitation efforts to stop. The smaller the body part through which the electricity passes, the more intense the heat and the less it is dissipated. Consequently, extensive damage can occur in the fingers, hands, forearms, toes, feet, and lower legs. If the path is near or through the heart, damage to the heart's electrical conduction system can cause spontaneous ventricular fibrillation or other dysrhythmias. Alternating current is more likely to induce ventricular fibrillation than direct current.

Most lightning injuries do not traverse the body but flow around it, creating a shock wave capable of causing fractures and dislocations. Approximately 74% of patients who survive a lightning strike may have a permanent disability.[9]

Chemical Burns

Chemicals cause a denaturing of protein within the tissues or a desiccation of cells. Chemical concentration and duration of exposure determine extent of the burn. Alkali products usually cause more tissue damage than acids. A wet chemical should be removed as soon as possible by flushing with copious amounts of water. Dry substances should be brushed off the skin before the area is flushed. Care must be taken not to expose the caregiver to the chemical during this procedure. All fluids used to decontaminate the patient should be contained; the fluid should not be allowed to drain into the general drainage system. Chemical burns can be deceiving as to depth; appearances can be similar in surface discoloration until tissue begins to slough days later. Consequently, all chemical burns should be considered deep partial thickness or full thickness until proven otherwise. After removal of chemicals, wounds are managed in the same manner as thermal burns.[8,9]

E-Cigarette Burns

Electronic cigarette (EC) use has increased, as have battery explosions causing burn injury. EC use has significantly increased among adolescents, with use reported up to 40% among middle and high school students. ECs have rechargeable lithium-ion batteries that provide the thermal energy, transforming the liquid nicotine into the inhalable vapor. Most EC explosions are caused by the battery. Lithium batteries can generate massive amounts of thermal energy, causing spontaneous explosion. When the battery explodes, the contents, lithium-cobalt and lithium-manganese oxides, are released and may leak onto the skin and be absorbed by the body. The absorption of these elemental metals may lead to heavy metal poisoning. Toxicity from cobalt can affect the heart, skin, and nervous system and cause dysfunction of vision and hearing. Removal of the contents from the wound will decrease the incidence of toxicity. Burns from elemental metals can worsen when exposed to water. Before irrigation and debridement, a litmus test to identify alkali pH should be done and, if positive, the elemental metals should be removed with mineral oils or other nonaqueous solutions.[12]

Frostbite

Frostbite is actual freezing of tissue from exposure to freezing or below-freezing temperatures. In a cold environment, the body attempts to maintain heat by vasoconstriction of peripheral blood vessels to reduce heat exchange. The longer the period of exposure, the more peripheral blood flow is reduced. When extremities are left unprotected, intracellular and extracellular fluids can freeze, forming crystals that damage local tissues. Blood clots may form and impair circulation to the area.

Signs, symptoms, and classification of frostbite are the same as thermal burns. The affected extremity should be rapidly rewarmed using warm water. Use of excessive heat such as steam is dangerous and can cause unnecessary damage. Dress the rewarmed extremity and immobilize it with a padded splint. As with flame burns, frostbite can be very painful, so pain management is needed.[12] See also Chapter 30, Environmental Emergencies.

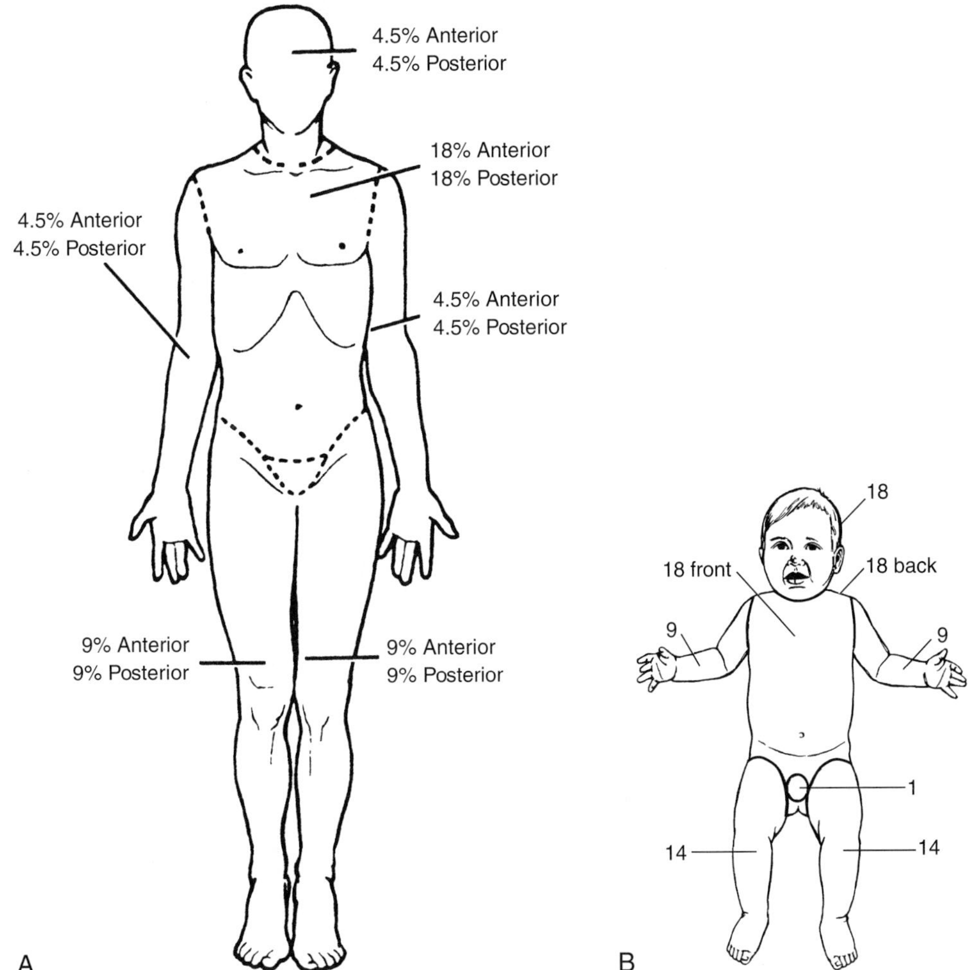

Fig. 41.2 Rule of Nines. (A) Adult. (B) Child. (A, From Ignatavicius DD, Workman LM. *Medical-Surgical Nursing: Critical Thinking for Collaborative Care.* 5th ed. Philadelphia, PA: Saunders; 2006. B, From Sole ML, Klein DG, Moseley MJ. *Introduction to Critical Care Nursing.* 4th ed. Philadelphia, PA: Saunders; 2005.)

Cold immersion of the foot or hand is a nonfreezing injury, occurring from chronic exposure to wet conditions at temperatures just above freezing. The extremity may appear black, but deep tissue destruction may not be present. Initially there is an alternating arterial vasospasm and vasodilation with the tissue first cold and numb, progressing to hyperemia in 24 to 48 hours. As the injury progresses to hyperemia, the patient experiences an intense burning sensation and dysesthesia. Tissue damage occurs with resultant edema, blistering, redness, ecchymosis, and ulcerations. Attention to hygiene will prevent local infection, cellulitis, or gangrene.[13]

Patients who have exposure to chronic, repetitive, damp cold may develop chilblain, or pernio. This is a dermatologic condition, usually occurring on the face, dorsum of the hands and feet, or any area chronically exposed to a cold environment. Signs and symptoms include pruritic, reddened skin lesions. These lesions, with continued exposure, ulcerate or develop hemorrhagic lesions progressing to scarring, fibrosis, or atrophy with itching, tenderness, and pain. Symptoms are controlled by protection from further exposure and the use of antiadrenergics or calcium channel blockers.[13]

BURN ASSESSMENT

Burn depth and extent are assessed to determine the severity of burn injury. In many cases, final determination is not made for several days.

Depth of Burn

Burns are described as partial thickness or full thickness. Identification of the depth of injury may be difficult initially because depth may actually increase over time as edema forms and circulation to the area of injury is compromised. This process usually peaks at 48 hours; therefore a more accurate determination of depth can be made between 48 and 72 hours. Depth determination is not a priority during initial resuscitation.

Extent of Burn

Extent of injury for thermal and chemical injuries is assessed by using formulas such as the rule of nines (Fig. 41.2), Berkow formula, or Lund and Browder table (Figs. 41.3 and 41.4). The caregiver should remember to modify the rule of nines for children. As noted in Fig. 41.2B, the head and neck of an

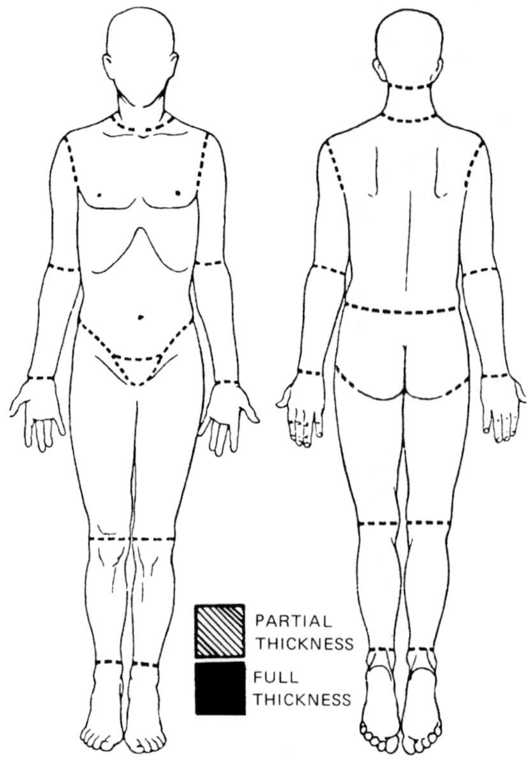

Percent Surface Area Burned

AREA	1 YEAR	1-4 YEARS	5-9 YEARS	10-14 YEARS	Y 15 YEARS	ADULT	2°	3°
Head	19	17	13	11	9	7		
Neck	2	2	2	2	2	2		
Ant. Trunk	13	13	13	13	13	13		
Post Trunk	13	13	13	13	13	13		
R. Buttock	2½	2½	2½	2½	2½	2½		
L. Buttock	2½	2½	2½	2½	2½	2½		
Genitalia	1	1	1	1	1	1		
R. U. Arm	4	4	4	4	4	4		
L. U. Arm	4	4	4	4	4	4		
R. L. Arm	3	3	3	3	3	3		
L. L. Arm	3	3	3	3	3	3		
R. Hand	2½	2½	2½	2½	2½	2½		
L. Hand	2½	2½	2½	2½	2½	2½		
R. Thigh	5½	6½	8	8½	9	9½		
L. Thigh	5½	6½	8	8½	9	9½		
R. Leg	5	5	5½	6	6½	7		
L. Leg	5	5	5½	6	6½	7		
R. Foot	3½	3½	3½	3½	3½	3½		
L. Foot	3½	3½	3½	3½	3½	3½		
TOTAL								

Fig. 41.3 Lund and Browder Formula. (From Cornwell P, Gregory C. Management of clients with burn injury. In: Black J, Hawks J, eds. *Medical-Surgical Nursing.* 7th ed. St Louis, MO: Elsevier; 2005.)

infant represent 18% of BSA, whereas the legs represent 14% for each lower extremity. To correct for age, 1% is subtracted from the head for each year of age through 10 years, and 0.5% is added to each lower extremity. To estimate scatter burns, the size of the patient's palm (including the fingers) is used to represent 1% of the total BSA (TBSA). The palm is visualized over the burned areas. To obtain a more accurate estimate of the extent of burns, both burned and unburned areas are calculated. The two estimates should then be compared. If the total is more or less than 100%, the areas should be reestimated. Assessing extent of injury in electrical burns is more difficult because surface damage is minimal compared with underlying damage. When discussing an electrical injury, describing the injury anatomically is more important than calculating percentage of BSA burned.

Severity of Burn

The severity of burn injury is based on assessment of extent and depth of injury, patient age, presence of concomitant injuries, smoke inhalation, and preexisting diseases. Care of patients with burns of different severity is determined by availability of specialized care facilities. Initial stabilization of

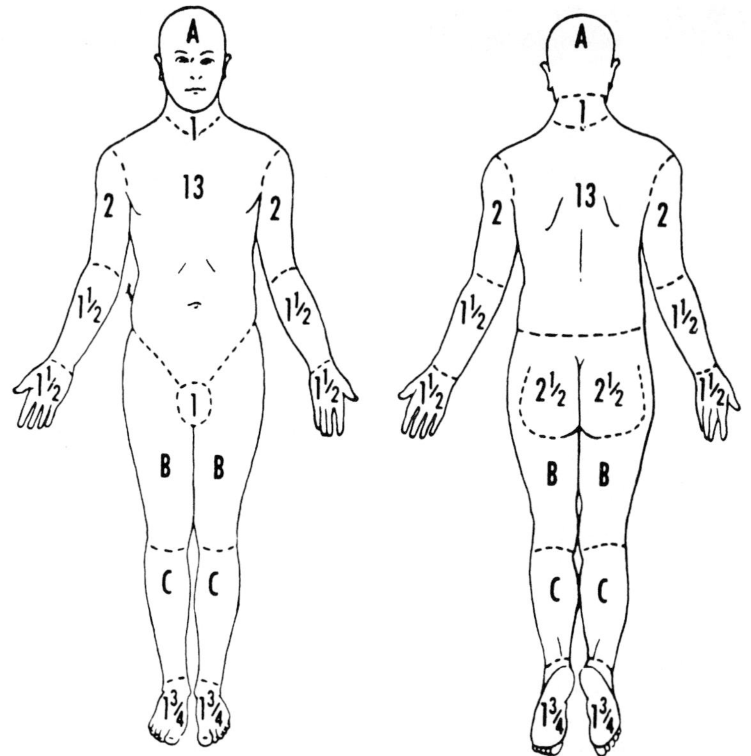

Relative Percentage of Areas Affected by Growth

	Age in Years					
	0	1	5	10	15	Adult
A—½ of head	9½	8½	6½	5½	4½	3½
B—½ of one thigh	2¾	3¼	4	4¼	4½	4¾
C—½ of one leg	2½	2½	2¾	3	3¼	3½

Fig. 41.4 Lund and Browder Formula. (From Artz CP, Moncrief JA. *The Treatment of Burns*. 2nd ed. Philadelphia, PA: Saunders; 1979.)

the patient with a burn should be available in any community hospital with 24-hour emergency capabilities. Patients with minor burns may be treated as outpatients or admitted to the community hospital. Patients with moderate burns may be treated in a community hospital with appropriate staff and facilities to deliver burn care or transferred to a specialized burn care facility. Patients with major burns require care in a specialized burn care facility. Transfer agreements with special-care units should be developed in advance to facilitate timely and uneventful transfer.[6,7,14] Box 41.1 summarizes criteria for transfer to a burn center. Any patient with concomitant trauma is at increased risk for morbidity or mortality and should be treated in a trauma center until he or she is stable and then transferred to a burn center as appropriate.

PATHOPHYSIOLOGY

Burn injury occurs when skin is exposed to more energy than it can absorb. The cause of the burn may vary, but local and systemic responses are generally similar. To understand the pathophysiology of burns, one must first understand the functions of the skin, which consists of two layers: the epidermis and the dermis. The epidermis, the outer layer of the basement layer of cells, consists of cells that migrate upward to become surface keratin. The dermis, or inner layer, consists of collagen and elastic fibers and contains hair follicles, sweat and sebaceous glands, nerve endings, and blood vessels. The skin is the largest organ of the body and acts as an infection barrier, vapor barrier, and a heat regulator.[5,6]

Three zones of tissue damage occur at the burn site. First is the central zone of coagulation, an area of irreversible damage. Concentrically surrounding this area is the zone of stasis, where capillary and small vessel stasis occurs. The ultimate fate of the burn wound depends on resolution or progression of the zone of stasis. Edema formation and prolonged compromise of blood flow to this area cause a deeper, more extensive wound; therefore depth and severity of burn wounds may not be known for 2 or more days after the initial injury. The third zone of damage is the zone of hyperemia, an area of superficial damage that heals quickly on its own.[8]

The body responds to the burn injury with varying degrees of tissue damage, cellular impairment, and fluid shifts. A brief decrease in blood flow to the affected area is followed by a marked increase in arteriolar vasodilation. Damaged tissues

BOX 41.1 Criteria for Transfer to a Burn Center.

1. Partial-thickness and full-thickness burns greater than 10% total body surface area (TBSA) in patients less than 10 years or over 50 years of age.
2. Partial-thickness and full-thickness burns greater than 20% TBSA in other age-groups.
3. Burns that involve the face, eyes, ears, hands, feet, genitalia, perineum, or major joints.
4. Full-thickness burns greater than 5% TBSA in any age-group.
5. Electrical burns, including lightning injury.
6. Significant chemical burns.
7. Inhalation injury.
8. Burn injury in patients with preexisting medical disorders that could complicate management, prolong recovery, or affect mortality.
9. Any patient with a burn injury that has concomitant trauma has an increased risk of morbidity or mortality and may be treated initially in a trauma center until stable before being transferred to a burn center.
10. Children with burn injuries in hospitals without qualified personnel or equipment for the care of children.
11. Burn injury in patients who will require special social, emotional, or long-term rehabilitative intervention, including cases involving suspected child abuse and neglect.

Data from American College of Surgeons. *Advanced Trauma Life Support Student Manual.* Chicago: The College; 2008.

release mediators that initiate an inflammatory response. Histamine, serotonin, prostaglandin derivatives, and the complement cascade are all activated. Release of proinflammatory mediators combined with vasodilation causes increased capillary permeability, leading to intravascular fluid loss and wound edema. For burn injuries of less than 20% TBSA, these actions are usually limited to the burn site, with 90% of the edema present by 4 hours. The edema tends to reside within the dermis, and resorption is complete by 4 days. As the affected TBSA goes beyond 20%, local response becomes systemic. With large burns, the overwhelming inflammation, coagulation, and fibrinolysis can continue and constantly be reactivated. The cytokine activity creates a state of exaggerated or reactivated inflammation that includes organ involvement such as acute respiratory distress syndrome (ARDS), systemic inflammatory response syndrome (SIRS), and multiple organ dysfunction syndrome (MODS). Large burns cause a hypermetabolic state that has multiple harmful physiologic derangements associated with it. Derangements noted are muscle catabolism, hepatic dysfunction, and immunosuppression.[8,14] Basal metabolic rate increases from insensible fluid loss, which, along with fluid shift, produces hypovolemia. Hypoproteinemia resulting from increased capillary permeability aggravates edema in nonburned tissue. Capillary permeability increases for 2 to 3 weeks, with the most significant changes occurring in the first 24 to 36 hours.[8,14]

Initially, blood viscosity increases when hematocrit rises secondary to vascular fluid shifts into the interstitium. Because of a marked increase in peripheral vascular resistance, decreased intravascular fluid volume, and increased blood viscosity, cardiac output falls. Capillary leakage and depressed cardiac output can depress central nervous system function, causing restlessness, followed by lethargy, and finally coma. Decreased cardiac output, decreased blood volume, and intense sympathetic response cause a decreased perfusion to the skin, viscera, and kidneys. Levels of thromboxane A2, a potent vasoconstrictor, are significantly increased in burned patients and contribute to mesenteric vasoconstriction and decreased splanchnic blood flow. Decreased flow can convert a zone of stasis to a zone of coagulation, which increases depth of the burn. Decreased circulating plasma with increased hematocrit can cause hemoglobinuria, which can lead to renal failure. Immediate hemolysis of red blood cells occurs, with the life span of remaining red cells reduced by approximately 30% of normal. Platelet count and platelet survival time initially drop drastically and then continue to decrease for 5 days after injury. This period is followed by a rebound increase in platelets over the next 2 to 3 weeks.[8,14]

Cardiovascular changes begin immediately after a burn. The extent varies with burn size and presence of additional injuries. Patients with an uncomplicated burn of less than 15% TBSA can usually be treated with oral fluid resuscitation. Patients with burns of the TBSA that surpass 20% have massive shifts of fluid and electrolytes from intravascular to extravascular spaces. This shift begins to resolve in 18 to 36 hours; however, normal extracellular volume is not completely restored until 7 to 10 days after the burn injury. If intravascular volume is not replenished, hypovolemic shock occurs. If untreated, the patient can die of cardiovascular collapse. Inadequate treatment may lead to renal failure from acute tubular necrosis.

The vasoconstriction of the mesentery mentioned previously predisposes the patient to gastric distention, aspiration, and ulceration (Curling's ulcer). A patient with a burn of greater than 20% TBSA should have a gastric tube placed to decompress the stomach and avoid aspiration. Admission orders will include medication to reduce gastric secretion and early enteral feedings (within 24 hours of injury) to meet basic energy needs.[6,14]

The hypermetabolic response after burn trauma far exceeds the response seen in other forms of trauma. The patient's metabolic rate can increase as much as two to three times the normal rate. Release of catabolic hormones, including catecholamines, cortisol, and glucagon, initiates a persistent hypermetabolic response. This response causes accelerated breakdown of skeletal muscle, decreased protein synthesis, increased peripheral lipolysis, and increased utilization of glucose, which rapidly depletes glycogen stores. It manifests clinically as severe muscle wasting, decreased muscle strength, and increased liver fat with hepatomegaly and functional impairment. The hypermetabolic response is commensurate with the size of the burn. The adverse effects of the response are managed through nutritional and pharmacologic intervention to improve net nitrogen balance, preserve lean body mass, decrease cardiac work, and decrease hepatic fatty infiltration.[8,14]

Inhalation injury or smoke inhalation is a syndrome comprising three distinct problems: carbon monoxide intoxication, upper airway obstruction, and chemical injury to the lower airways and lung parenchyma. The majority of deaths from fires are caused by smoke inhalation rather than the burn injury or its sequelae. A burn injury with associated inhalation injury increases the mortality rate. Pulmonary complications associated with inhalation injury directly contribute to death in up to 77% of patients with combined cutaneous and inhalation injury.[6–8,14]

Carbon monoxide intoxication is the most common killer of victims of fire.[6] Most people who die in a fire have been overcome by carbon monoxide before they sustain a burn injury. In the body, carbon monoxide has a 240 times greater affinity for hemoglobin than oxygen, which causes inadequate oxygen delivery to the tissues. Carbon monoxide combines with myoglobin in muscle cells, causing muscle weakness. Tissue hypoxia and the resultant confusion and muscle weakness may be the major reasons for most fire fatalities. Carbon monoxide poisoning is characterized by pink to cherry-red skin, tachypnea, tachycardia, headache, dizziness, and nausea. An arterial blood gas sample is drawn to measure the carboxyhemoglobin level. Levels below 15% are rarely associated with symptoms of carbon monoxide poisoning and can be normal for a heavy smoker. Levels of 15% to 40% are associated with varying disturbances such as headache and confusion. Levels greater than 40% are associated with coma. Reliance on pulse oximetry or an oxygen saturation of arterial blood (Sao_2) that is calculated from the partial pressure of oxygen (Po_2) rather than measured on a CO oximeter may result in failure to diagnose carbon monoxide poisoning. Most pulse oximeters cannot reliably differentiate between oxygenated hemoglobin and hemoglobin with carbon monoxide and will give a false high measurement. All patients with suspected carbon monoxide poisoning should receive 100% oxygen.[5–8,10,14]

Cyanide poisoning may also occur during a fire and can rapidly result in death. Hydrogen cyanide is highly toxic and can be formed in high-temperature combustion from materials such as polyurethane, acrylonitrile, wool, cotton, and nylon. Cyanide binds to a variety of iron-containing enzymes, one of which plays a critical role in electron transport during oxidative phosphorylation. Even minute amounts of bound cyanide can inhibit aerobic metabolism and rapidly result in death.

The patient with cyanide poisoning will rapidly develop coma, apnea, cardiac dysfunction, and severe lactic acidosis. Diagnosis can be difficult when combined with carbon monoxide poisoning, and the patient can have sublethal levels of carbon monoxide and cyanide and still die owing to the combination. The two are synergistic because carbon monoxide primarily affects oxygen delivery and cyanide affects oxygen utilization.

Thermal injury to the upper airway is usually associated with facial burns. Upper airway obstruction is the result of intrinsic or extrinsic edema that may lead to airway occlusion at or above the vocal cords. Edema progresses rapidly, totally occluding the airway in minutes to hours (Fig. 41.5). This injury is primarily a thermal injury, resulting in tissue damage in the posterior pharynx. Fig. 41.6B shows radiographic evidence of epiglottitis secondary to thermal/chemical injury. Upper airway edema will usually manifest within 24 hours of the injury. Management for airway edema is early intubation or tracheostomy if intubation is not possible. If the patient exhibits dyspnea, stridor, or cyanosis, suspect impending airway obstruction and be prepared to assist with intubation that may be difficult.

Thermal injury below the vocal cords is rare because the posterior pharynx is such an efficient heat exchange system. True thermal injury below the vocal cords is usually the result of superheated steam in which water vapor carries heat into the lungs. Injuries that occur in an oxygen-enriched atmosphere or one in which the person was inhaling explosive gases (e.g., during inhalation anesthesia) also cause true thermal injury below the vocal cords. True thermal injury to the lungs is almost always fatal.

Chemical injury to the lower airway is a common problem with inhalation of smoke. Many lower-molecular-weight constituents of smoke are toxic to the mucosa and alveoli because of their pH or the ability to form free radicals. Chemical injury, from acids and aldehydes in the smoke, may damage the lung parenchyma. These chemicals, attached to carbon particles in the smoke, are heavier than air, so they are readily inhaled and find their way down the bronchi into alveoli. This chemical injury causes hemorrhagic tracheobronchitis, increased edema formation, decreased surfactant levels, and decreased pulmonary macrophage function. Although the compounds produce acute neutrophilic airway inflammation, the symptoms (cough, bronchorrhea, dyspnea, and wheezing) may not appear for 12 to 26 hours. Many centers perform early bronchoscopy to determine whether there is injury to the lower airways. The bronchoscopy will reveal erythema, edema, carbonaceous debris, and ulceration of the airways. This condition may lead to rapid development of ARDS over 24 to 48 hours. Severe inhalation injury may increase the patient's fluid needs in the first 24 hours by as much as 50% of calculated values.[8,14]

PATIENT MANAGEMENT

The patient with burns may have other injuries in addition to the burn; therefore the patient should be initially evaluated using the ABCDE survey for trauma.[5–7] The cervical spine is protected while assessing for an adequate airway. Assessment of specific burn injuries should be done after the primary assessment is completed. A history is obtained as time and patient condition permit. How did the injury occur? What caused the injury—flame, scald, or other factors? Was smoke involved? Did injury occur in a confined space? What was the patient doing before the injury? Did the patient have a stroke or myocardial infarction before the injury? Does the patient have any medical problems or allergies? General assessment and interventions for the burn patient are described in this section.

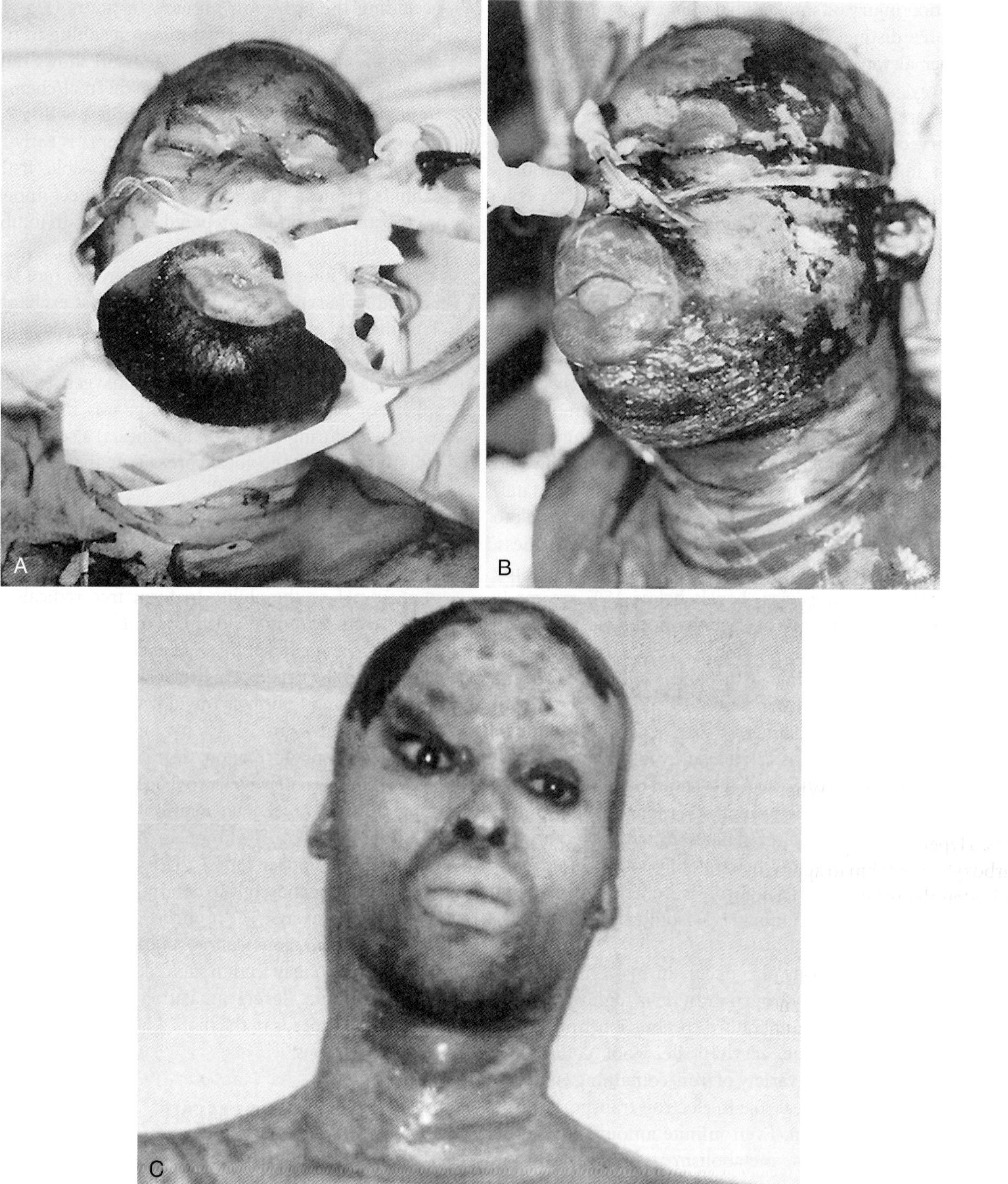

Fig. 41.5 Facial Edema. (A) Four to 5 hours after burn. (B) Thirty hours after burn, showing distortion of facial features and necessity of intubation before the full extent of burn edema development. (C) Facial contour 3 months after burn. (Courtesy Anne E. Missavage, MD, UC Davis Regional Burn Center, Sacramento, CA.)

Airway

A primary trauma survey should be performed with appropriate management. Look for evidence of respiratory distress and smoke inhalation injury. A high index of suspicion for smoke inhalation is essential for these patients. Burns that occur in small spaces are often associated with smoke inhalation. Administration of high-flow oxygen should be started in an attempt to reverse tissue hypoxia resulting from a low fraction of inspired oxygen (Fio_2) at the fire and to begin displacing carbon monoxide and cyanide from their protein-binding sites. If the patient has a history of chronic obstructive pulmonary disease and is a suspected carbon dioxide retainer, immediate intubation is recommended to prevent progressive carbon dioxide retention.

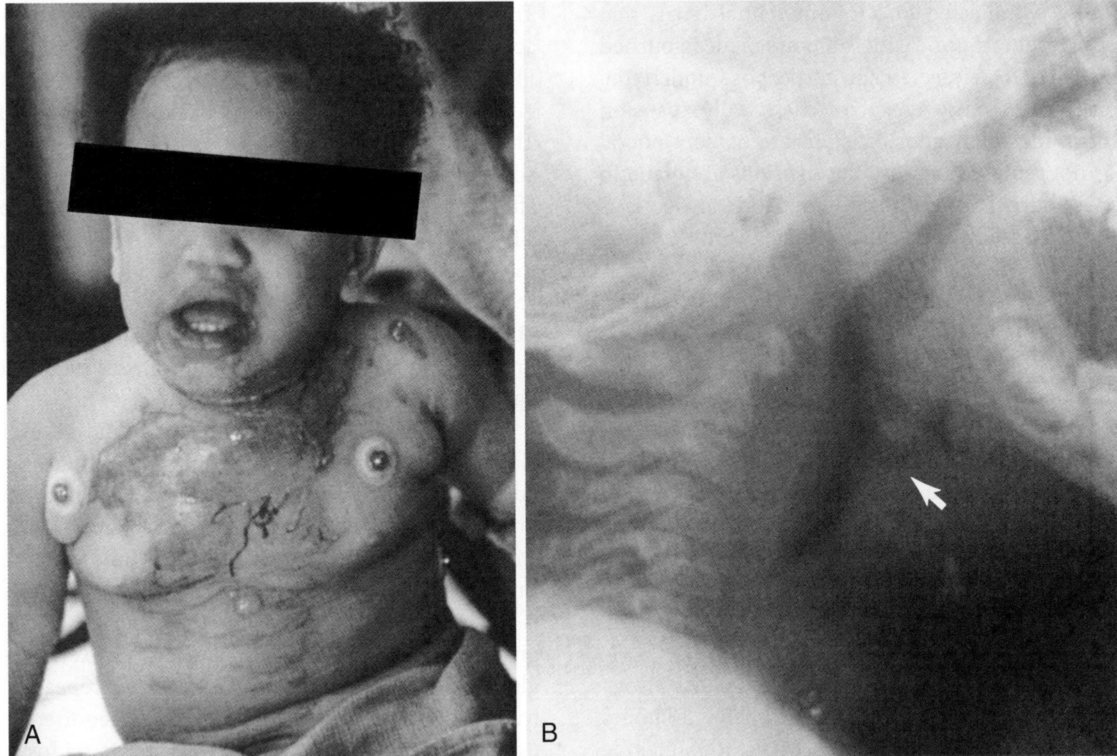

Fig. 41.6 (A) Photograph of a 22-month-old child showing a burn primarily to the anterior chest wall. (B) Lateral airway radiograph of the same child demonstrating effects of thermal or chemical epiglottitis. (From Barkin RM. *Pediatric Emergency Medicine: Concepts and Clinical Practice.* 2nd ed. St Louis, MO: Mosby; 1997.)

The half-life of carboxyhemoglobin on room air is approximately 240 minutes. When the patient is placed on 100% Fio_2, the half-life is reduced to approximately 75 to 80 minutes. Hyperbaric oxygen at 2.0 atm decreases the half-life of carboxyhemoglobin to approximately 20 minutes and appears to hasten the resolution of symptoms. The use of hyperbaric oxygen in the treatment of carbon monoxide poisoning is controversial. Centers that advocate hyperbaric oxygen use it for patients with a carboxyhemoglobin level greater than 40%, for loss of consciousness, or in pregnant women with a carboxyhemoglobin level greater than 20% or evidence of fetal distress.

Hyperbaric chambers are limited in availability and most are small and hold only the patient. Larger multiplace chambers allow an attendant to dive with the patient, but even then, complex medical interventions are difficult to perform in this setting. Therefore an unstable patient who may require intensive therapy should not be placed in a chamber. A complication of hyperbaric therapy is barotrauma to the ear caused by the inability of the patient to equalize the pressure within the ear as the atmospheric pressure increases. Myringotomy with tube placement has been used as a preventative measure because the pressure difference that leads to barotrauma cannot occur with a hole in the tympanic membrane.[6,8]

If the patient has suspected cyanide poisoning, antidotal treatment includes induction of methemoglobinemia, use of sulfur donors, and binding of cyanide. Outside the United States, the combination of sodium thiosulfate and hydroxocobalamin has been successful in the treatment of severe poisoning. In the United States, the Taylor cyanide antidote package is used and includes amyl nitrate and sodium nitrite to induce methemoglobinemia and sodium thiosulfate to act as a sulfur donor. The kit will treat two adult patients. If the patient also has carbon monoxide poisoning, the treatment with amyl nitrite or sodium nitrite is contraindicated until normal carbon monoxide levels can be confirmed. Pending test results for carboxyhemoglobin, sodium thiosulfate may be given intravenously.[8]

The oropharynx and vocal cords should be inspected for redness, blisters, and carbonaceous particles. The patient is observed for increasing restlessness, dyspnea, difficulty swallowing, increasing hoarseness, and rapid, shallow respirations. The patient may have increasing difficulty managing secretions, with a significant risk for impending airway obstruction. Early intubation is recommended before complete obstruction occurs. Tracheostomies should be avoided initially because edema of the neck makes this procedure difficult.

Breathing

Circumferential full-thickness burns of the chest can impair breathing by limiting chest wall excursion and preventing adequate gas exchange. The chest should be visually inspected for tight, leathery eschar that circles the chest. Evidence of breathing compromise includes inadequate chest expansion, restlessness, confusion, decreased oxygenation, decreased tidal volume, and rapid, shallow respirations.

Escharotomy is indicated for circumferential burns that compromise breathing. Surgical incisions are made in burned tissue on the chest to release eschar and expose underlying subcutaneous tissue. Improvement in chest wall expansion should occur immediately after incisions are made. General anesthesia is not required because the incisions are made in a full-thickness burn. Intravenous (IV) narcotic analgesia is usually adequate to relieve any pain associated with escharotomy.

The patient with a burn injury is also at risk for carbon monoxide poisoning. Altered breathing patterns such as decreased respirations or apnea may be evident, as may the characteristic cherry-red skin, or the skin can appear slightly cyanotic. Confusion, irritability, or coma may be present. Carboxyhemoglobin level and chest radiograph are obtained to assess for carbon monoxide poisoning and the presence of pulmonary damage or associated injuries. High-flow oxygen with a nonrebreather mask or bag-mask device is administered as appropriate. If the patient does not respond after 1 to 1½ hours of regular oxygen therapy, hyperbaric oxygen therapy may be used.

ARDS occurs in patients with carbon monoxide poisoning but is usually not a problem until approximately 18 hours after injury. Clinical findings associated with ARDS include decreased oxygenation, increased secretions, rapid respirations, confusion, and increasing patchy infiltrates on the radiograph. Treatment includes intubation and ventilation with positive end-expiratory pressure (PEEP). Bronchodilators may be indicated; however, corticosteroids are not. Giving corticosteroids to patients with burns and smoke inhalation can increase morbidity and mortality.

The patient with a burn injury should be assessed for other injuries that can affect breathing, such as pneumothorax, hemothorax, tension pneumothorax, and flail chest. These problems can occur with a burn injury from a motor vehicle crash or explosion. Additional injuries may be present when a patient has jumped to escape the fire. Preexisting health problems that may affect respiratory functions (e.g., chronic obstructive pulmonary disease, asthma) should be noted.

Circulation

The patient with a burn injury is at significant risk for hypovolemia from actual fluid loss and fluid movement from increased capillary permeability and vasodilation. Assess the patient for increased respirations, increased pulse, decreased blood pressure, decreased urine output, diminished capillary refill, restlessness, confusion, nausea, and vomiting. Additional indications of volume compromise include central venous pressure less than 3 cm H_2O, hematocrit greater than 50 mg/dL, presence of an ileus, and urine output less than 0.5 mL/kg per hour.

One or two large-bore IV catheters should be started. A single IV catheter is adequate for a burn of less than 40% TBSA. Two peripheral access sites are established if the burn is greater than 40% TBSA, or the patient will be transferred. Leg veins are avoided because of increased risk for thrombophlebitis. The IV catheter can be inserted into burned tissue if no other access is available, but this should be considered a last resort. Fluid volume requirements are calculated using an accepted guideline such as the Parkland or modified Brooke formulas. The Parkland Formula is the most commonly used guideline, advising estimated fluid replacement for the first 24 hours after injury to be 4 mL/kg of body weight for each percent of TBSA burned. These formulas are guidelines for fluid replacement type and volume and should be adjusted to the patient's response to the fluid. Ideally, fluid resuscitation is adequate if pulse and blood pressure are within normal limits for age and urine output is 0.5 mL/kg per hour for adults and 1 to 1.5 mL/kg per hour for infants.

No formula exists for calculating fluid resuscitation in electrical injuries. An infusion of lactated Ringer's solution is administered at 1 to 2 L/hour in the average adult until he or she shows signs of adequate resuscitation. Urine output should be maintained at two to three times the normal volume to facilitate excretion of myoglobin. After urine output is established, an osmotic diuretic such as mannitol may be given to increase urine flow and aid in excretion of myoglobin. Significant acidosis can occur, so repeated administration of sodium bicarbonate may be required to prevent dysrhythmias. Once fluid therapy corrects acidosis, repeated administration may not be necessary.

Disability and Exposure

If not yet done, all clothing and jewelry should be removed and a head-to-toe assessment done to check for any concomitant trauma and to estimate burn depth and size. Refer to the earlier section on burn assessment for estimate of burn depth and size. Because the burn-injured patient has lost the ability to control body temperature, it is important to increase the temperature in the room and to monitor the patient. Body temperature below 35°C should be avoided.

Diagnostic Procedures

Diagnostic procedures that may assist during the resuscitation of the burn patient are the following:

Laboratory

1. complete blood count with differential
2. serum electrolytes
3. carboxyhemoglobin
4. type and crossmatch/screen blood
5. urinalysis, pregnancy test in females of childbearing age
6. arterial blood gas

Radiography

1. chest
2. other x-ray examinations as indicated for associated trauma

Other special studies as indicated for associated trauma

1. focused assessment sonography for trauma (FAST)
2. computed tomography (CT) scan as indicated by assessment findings
3. possible peritoneal lavage
4. 12-lead electrocardiogram (ECG) if electrical or lightning injury

Protection Against Infection

The patient with a burn injury has lost the greatest protection against invasion by various pathogens and must be protected with scrupulous aseptic technique. Gloves, masks, caps, and gowns must be worn. Sterile technique is necessary for all procedures. Wounds are kept covered with clean sheets while other care is provided. If the patient is transferred, sterile sheets are used to cover the patient. If treatment is followed by discharge, the nurse should debride the burn, apply a topical antibiotic, and cover the wound with a fluffy dressing. Systemic antibiotics are rarely indicated even in severe burns until infection is confirmed by culture. Exceptions to this guideline may include young children, older adult patients, diabetic patients, or those with immune system compromise.

For minor or moderate burns, tetanus immunization is given if the patient has not been immunized within the past 10 years. In major burns or grossly contaminated burns, tetanus immunization is given if previous immunization has occurred within 5 years. If the patient has never been immunized or no clear history of immunization exists, tetanus hyperimmune globulin (HyperTET) and tetanus immunization is given.

Pain Management

Burn wounds are exquisitely painful and deserve special consideration. The pain of primary tissue damage and nerve damage may be worsened by primary and secondary hyperalgesia. Intravenous opioid administration should be the prime treatment for burn pain. During initial resuscitation, analgesics or anesthetics should be titrated to effect.[6,7,10] After 24 hours, decreased plasma protein levels increase bioavailability of free drugs, especially those that are protein bound. Giving pain medication as needed may increase the patient's awareness of pain and other symptoms. Administering opioids on a schedule, based on drug half-life or by continuous infusion, can facilitate the patient's ability to cope with the pain. The opioid of choice has been IV morphine at 25 to 50 mcg/kg per hour, titrating to avoid respiratory depression. Fentanyl may also be used for some patients. For the burn-injured patient, pain can be made worse by fear of pain or disfigurement, anxiety related to loss of control, and distress over losing family members or material possessions at the time of injury. Anxiety decreases pain tolerance. Reducing anxiety minimizes interplay between acute pain and sympathetic arousal. For the burn-injured patient, anxiolytics may help decrease anxiety and improve pain tolerance. They are especially helpful during painful procedures. The most commonly used anxiolytics are benzodiazepine drugs. Diazepam has a long half-life and high lipid solubility. After repeated use in the patient with burns, prolonged mental impairment may occur when the drug is stopped. Therefore short-term administration of lorazepam and midazolam is preferred.

Patients with burn-induced or traumatic nerve injury may develop neuropathic pain. Pain is usually described as tingling, burning, shooting, or numbing. When a postburn patient comes to the ED with this type of pain, it is because the pain did not respond to opiate analgesics. Drugs that decrease neuronal excitability by mechanisms other than opiate receptors are useful for this type of pain. Tricyclic antidepressants in low doses are often successful in relieving neuropathic pain. Sodium channel–blocking drugs such as IV lidocaine, carbamazepine, phenytoin, and mexiletine have also produced successful analgesia.[8]

Wound Care

Wound care should be delayed until the patient's condition is stabilized; however, initial management must include removal of jewelry and constrictive clothing. Wounds must be kept covered with clean sheets until more definitive care can be provided. All patients with full-thickness burns are assessed for circulatory problems. Capillary refill and the presence of paresthesia are evaluated with distal pulses checked by Doppler ultrasonography. Because burn tissue does not stretch, swelling beneath burned tissue compromises circulation because of lack of elasticity. If the patient has signs of compromise, escharotomy is indicated. Fig. 41.7 illustrates placement of these surgical incisions. Significant bleeding that occurs with escharotomy can be controlled with an electrocautery unit or small hemostats (Fig. 41.8). After the procedure is completed, a topical antibacterial agent is applied to the open wound, a light pressure dressing is applied, and the extremity is slightly elevated.

Thermal burns may be secondary to flame, flash, scalds, or hot objects. Fig. 41.9 shows an example of a thermal burn. Thermal burns are cleaned with mild soap and water. The use of skin disinfectant, such as povidone-iodine (Betadine), has been shown to inhibit the healing process and is discouraged. Ruptured blisters should be removed, but intact blisters may

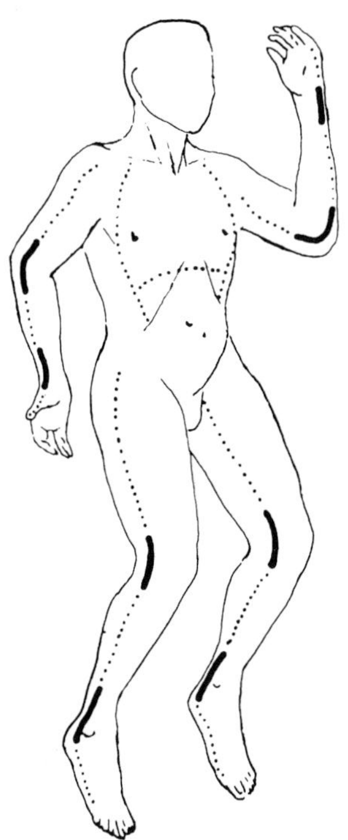

Fig. 41.7 Placement of Escharotomies.

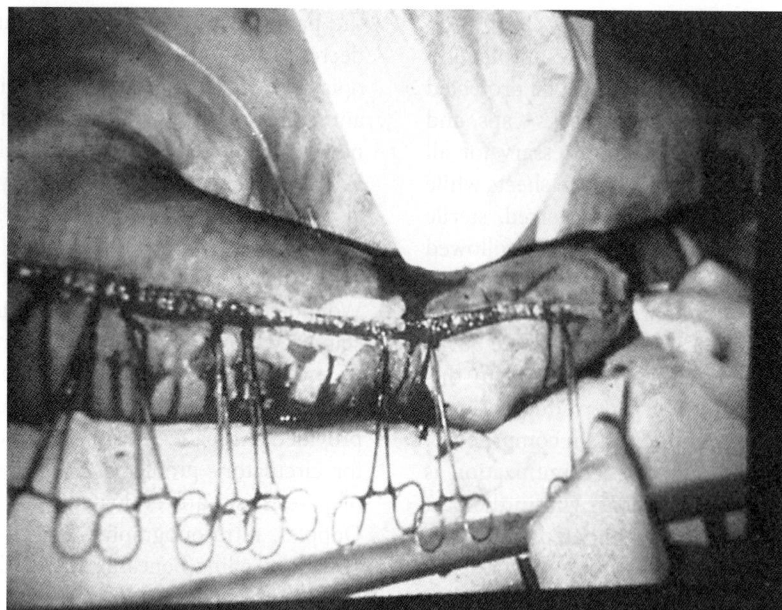

Fig. 41.8 Control of Bleeding From Escharotomy.

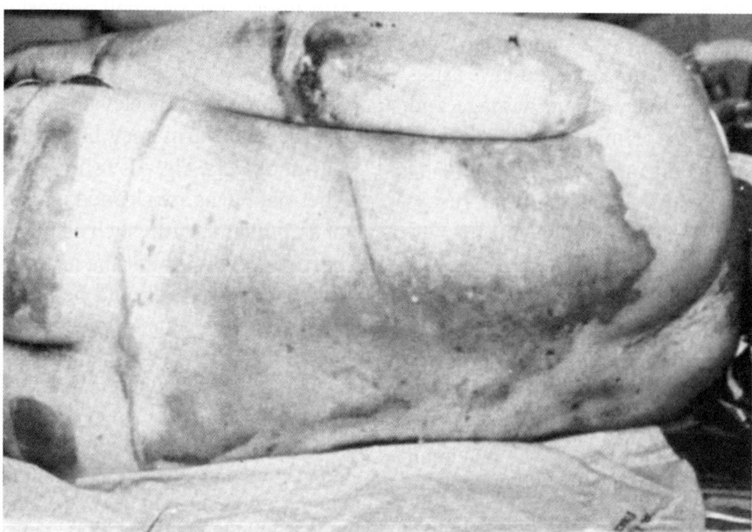

Fig. 41.9 Flame Burns to Back.

be left alone and should never be aspirated with a needle because this increases the chance of infection. The wound is covered immediately with a topical antibacterial agent such as silver sulfadiazine (Silvadene) or bacitracin. Burns of the face should be left open and covered by a topical antibiotic ointment such as bacitracin, which is reapplied every 6 hours after gently washing the skin.

Chemical burns should be immediately irrigated with tap water or normal saline for at least 5 to 10 minutes to remove the chemical. Clothing and jewelry are removed, and unburned areas adjacent to the burned areas are rinsed. These areas can be injured but may not hurt, blister, or turn red immediately. If the chemical is dry, it can be brushed from the patient before irrigating. After the wound is thoroughly irrigated, it is treated like a thermal burn. Chemical burns of the eye are an ophthalmologic emergency. The eye must be irrigated thoroughly with copious amounts of water or saline. (Refer to Chapter 33 for additional discussion of chemical eye injuries.)

Electrical injuries are different from thermal and chemical burns. These wounds may have little superficial tissue loss; however, massive muscle injury may be present beneath normal-looking skin or minor to severe exit wounds (Figs. 41.10 and 41.11). Wounds should be cleaned gently with a 0.25% povidone-iodine solution using sterile water or 0.9% sodium chloride; they rarely need immediate debridement. Topical agents such as mafenide acetate (Sulfamylon) solution that deeply penetrate tissue are used to cover the wound. Light dressings may be applied to cover these often grotesque wounds; however, dressings must not interfere with assessment for circulatory compromise and possible compartment

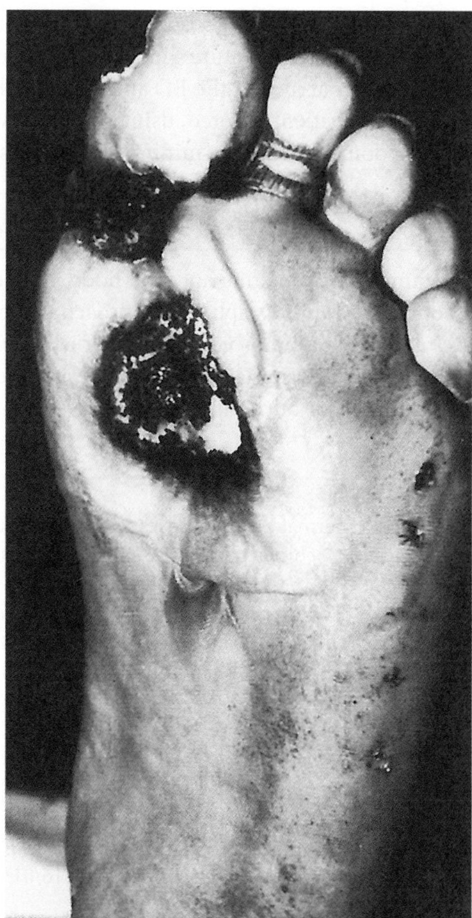

Fig. 41.10 Exit Wound From Direct Current. (From Air & Transport Nurses Association. *Air & Surface Patient Transport: Principles and Practice*. 4th ed. St Louis, MO: Mosby; 2019.)

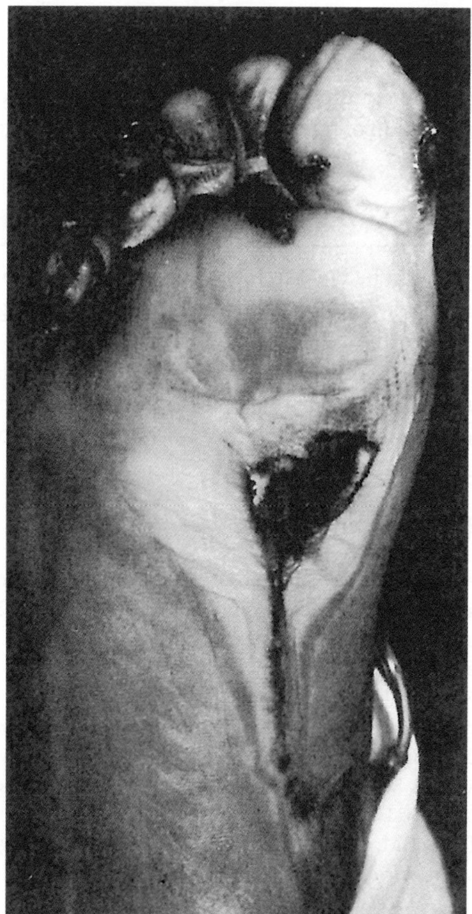

Fig. 41.11 Exit Wound From Alternating Current. (From *Air & Surface Patient Transport: Principles and Practice*. 4th ed. St Louis, MO: Mosby; 2019.)

syndrome. High-voltage injuries are associated with severe muscle contractions, so radiographs of the cervical spine may be indicated.

Electrical injuries of the extremities cause significant damage that leads to tissue swelling. Consequently, these patients are at risk for compartment syndrome. Symptoms associated with this condition include pain, pallor, paresthesia, pulselessness, paralysis, and pressure in the affected area. Fasciotomies are used to relieve compartment syndrome.

Tar or asphalt burns may be deep or superficial depending on the temperature of the tar, which may range from 150°F to more than 600°F, as well as the length of time the skin was in contact with it. Fig. 41.12 shows a tar burn before tar removal. Immediate treatment of a tar burn is to cool the tar, but do not try to peel it off the patient's skin. Using mineral oil, petroleum jelly, or a solvent such as Medi-Sol loosens the tar. In areas where the burn is not circumferential, oil or ointment is applied and the burn is covered with a light dressing. Dressings are removed in 4 to 12 hours, oil or ointment is reapplied, and a new dressing is applied. For areas with circumferential tar, oil or ointment can be applied with light dressings and changed every 20 to 30 minutes until tar is removed. After the tar is removed, the burn is treated as a thermal injury.

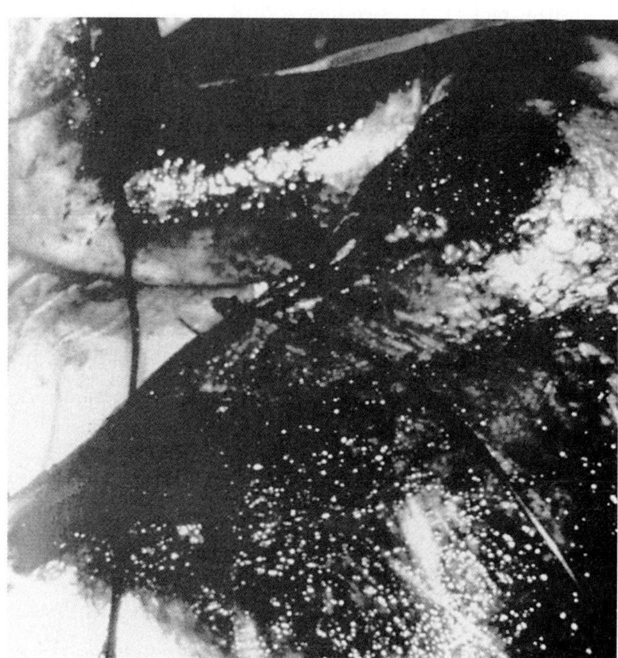

Fig. 41.12 Tar Burns of Chest Before Removal of Tar.

Temperature Regulation

The patient with a burn injury has lost a major control mechanism for temperature regulation. This heat loss is worsened by administration of room temperature IV fluids, irrigation of burned tissue, and environmental coolness often encountered in the ED. The patient's temperature should be documented as soon as possible after arrival in the ED and rechecked within 1 hour. Keeping the patient covered, using warmed IV fluids, and increasing room temperature minimizes heat loss.

SUMMARY

Burn injury can be devastating to the patient and family; for the caregiver, it can also be visually disturbing. Regardless of how severe the burn may be, a primary survey should be performed for potentially life-threatening injuries. Resuscitation of the burn patient includes evaluation of the burn, replacement of fluid losses, wound care, protection against contamination, maintenance of body temperature, and pain control. A multidisciplinary approach to burn care can reduce mortality and morbidity. Appropriate application of burn center transfer criteria ensures the best outcome for the patient with a major burn injury.

REFERENCES

1. American Burn Association. Burn Incidence and Treatment in the United States. https://ameriburn.org. Published 2016. Accessed July 1, 2018.
2. American Burn Association. Burn Injury Fact Sheet. https://ameriburn.org. Accessed July 1, 2018.
3. Burn Foundation. Pediatric Burn Fact Sheet. https://www.burnfoundation.org. Accessed July 1, 2018.
4. Capek KD, Sousse LE, Hundeshagen G, et al. Contemporary burn survival. *J Am Coll Surg*. 2018;226(4):453–463.
5. Heffernan JM, Comeau OY. The ABCDEs of emergency burn care. *Am Nurse Today*. 2015;10(10). https://americannursetoday.com. Accessed March 12, 2018.
6. Rice PL Jr, Orgill DP. Emergency care of moderate and severe thermal burns in adults. UpToDate website. https://www.uptodate.com/contents/emergency-care-of-moderate-and-severe-thermal-burns-in-adults?search=rice%20PL,%20Orgill%20DP.%20Emergency%20care%20of%20moderate%20andsevere%20thermal%20burns%20%20adults&source=search_result&selectedTitle=1~150&usage_type=default&dispaly_rank=1. Accessed June 2, 2018.
7. Schraga ED. Emergent Management of Thermal Burns. Medscape website. https://emedicine.medscape.com/article/769193-overview. Accessed March 12, 2018 Updated August 10, 2017.
8. Vorstenbosch J. Thermal Burns. Medscape Website. http://emedicine.medscape.com/article/1278244-print. Updated December 29, 2017. Accessed June 28, 2018.
9. Pinto DS, Clardy PF. Environmental and weapon-related electrical injuries. UpToDate website. https://www.uptodate.com/contents/environmental-and-weapon-related-electrical-injuries?search=Environmental%20and%2020weapon-related%20electrical%20injuries&source=search_result&selectedTitle=1~150usage_type=default&display_rank=1. Accessed June 2, 2018.
10. Texas EMS Trauma & Acute Care Foundation (TETAF) Trauma Division. Burn Clinical Practice Guideline. TETAF Website. http://tetaf.org/wp-content/uploads/2016/01/Burn-Practice-Guideline.pdf. Accessed June 14, 2019.
11. Valles LJ, Plourde BD, Wentz JE, Nelson-Cheesemon BB, Abraham JP. A review of scald burn injuries. *Int Med Rev*. 2017;3(3):1–17. http://internalmedicinereview.org/index.php/imr/article/download/372/pdf. Accessed June 28, 2018.
12. Maraqa T, Mohamed AT, Salib M, Morris S, Mercer L, Sachwani-Daswani GR. Too hot for your pocket! Burns from E-cigarette lithium battery explosions: a case series. *J Burn Care Res*. 2018;39(6):1043–1047. https://doi.org/10.1093/jbcr/irx015.
13. Stoppler MC. Frostbite. https://www.emedicinehealth.com/frostbite/article_em.htm. Accessed June 15, 2019.
14. ISBI Practice Guidelines Committee. ISBI practice guidelines for burn care. *Burns*. 2016;42(5):953–1021.

Pediatric Trauma

Amy Waunch, Kimberly Zaky

Despite scientific advances in injury prevention and treatment, traumatic injury continues to be the leading cause of death in children older than 1 year of age. Each year approximately 7.4 million children, aged 1 to 17 years, are treated in emergency departments (EDs) for nonfatal injuries, and 70,000 die as a result of unintentional injury.[1] Although children have significantly lower mortality after traumatic injury compared with adults (11.39 vs. 75.97 per 100,000), the associated morbidity, primarily related to traumatic brain injury (TBI) and risk for neurologic sequelae, can lead to lifelong disabilities.[2] More than one-third of US pediatric trauma patients use nonemergency medical services transport to arrive at EDs.[1]

Several factors influence childhood injuries, including age, sex, behavior, and the surrounding environment. Of these, age and sex are the most important factors affecting the patterns of injury. Male children younger than 18 years have higher injury and mortality rates, most likely due in part to their more aggressive behavior and exposure to contact sports. In the infant and toddler age-group, falls are a common cause of severe injury. The most common scene of pediatric injuries is the home environment. The frequency of childhood injuries compels the emergency nurse to participate in primary, secondary, and tertiary prevention of pediatric injuries. This chapter highlights anatomic and physiologic differences in pediatric patients, describes patient assessment, reviews essential interventions, discusses treatment of selected traumatic injuries, and identifies specific injury-prevention strategies.

EPIDEMIOLOGY

Blunt force trauma is the most common mechanism of pediatric morbidity and mortality, with motor vehicle collisions and falls being the leading mechanism of injury for all age groups.[3] In 2015 motor vehicle crashes (MVCs) killed 1065 occupants younger than 20 years of age. Penetrating trauma accounts for injury in 7.5% of children 0 to 18 years and 12.7% of children aged 13 to 18 years. It is the second most frequent mechanism of injury for adolescents aged 16 to 18 years and is the cause of 20% of traumatic deaths in children.[4] Gunshot wounds are responsible for most penetrating injuries and carry a significantly higher mortality compared with blunt mechanism injury. In 2014, 106 children died of unintentional firearm-related injuries.[4] Access to unsecured firearms in the home increases the risk for unintentional firearm-related death and injury among children.[4] Additionally, a 22% prevalence rate of mental illness during childhood and adolescence places affected youth at a higher risk of self-inflicted and impulsive firearm injury.[49] These two mechanisms of injury, blunt and penetrating, are interrelated in that blunt mechanical force can result in penetrating injury, such as injuries caused by fender edges, door handles, or shrapnel.

For children between ages 4 and 14 years, unintentional injury-related deaths occur most often when riding in a car. Although child passenger safety has evolved over the past decade, MVCs continue to be the leading cause of death for children 4 years of age and older.[5] In 2016, 1430 children aged 15 years and younger lost their lives in MVCs.[6]

Children are most often injured, suffer more severe injuries, or die in MVCs when they are not properly restrained. Safety seats are the most effective protection against fatal injury for child passengers in motor vehicles; they reduce the risk of injury by 71% to 82% and reduce the risk of death by 28% compared with children of similar ages who use seat belts.[5] According to the National Highway Traffic Safety Administration, 248 children younger than age 5 years were saved by car seats in 2015.[7] Rear-facing infant safety seats reduce the risk for death in an MVC by 71%, forward-facing seats for toddlers reduce the risk for death by 54%, and safety belts reduce the risk for death by 45%.[8]

However, parents must know how to correctly install and use child safety seats to achieve the most protection for their children. As many as 85% of child safety seats are found to be improperly installed. Infants and toddlers should be placed in rear-facing seats until they reach the highest weight or height allowed by the safety seat manufacturer because they have large heads, proportionally, and weak neck muscles, which place them at risk for cervical distraction and dislocation during frontal crashes.[5] Once a child has outgrown the rear-facing weight or height limit, he or she should be placed in a forward-facing safety seat with a harness for as long as possible, up to the highest weight or height allowed by the manufacturer.[8] Children do not fit in adult shoulder and lap belts until they are 58 inches tall, usually between ages 8 and 12 years. Therefore they should use a belt-positioning booster seat until that time.

Children restrained with a lap belt and shoulder harness are susceptible to certain injuries. Young children have a shorter sitting height than adults and a higher center of gravity above the lap belt. A greater proportion of body mass is located above the safety belt, which may cause more forward motion and increase the risk for head and neck injury. Children can "jackknife" over restraints, causing an airway or hanging injury. Similarly, a child can "submarine" under the restraint system, leading to neck and airway injuries. The lap belt itself can also cause injuries. During sudden deceleration, children are thrown forward with their full body weight going into the lap belt. Resulting injuries include lumbar spine fractures, small-bowel injuries, and abdominal bruising.

All children younger than 13 years should be restrained with a lap and shoulder seat belt in the rear seats of vehicles for optimal protection. Parents must be encouraged to restrain children with proper child-safety devices in the vehicle's rear seat for optimal protection in the event of an MVC.

Other high-risk motor vehicle situations are trunk entrapment and leaving children unattended in cars. When left unattended, children may be able to start the vehicle or put the vehicle in neutral. They can also suffer from hypothermia or hyperthermia, depending on the environmental temperature. Additionally, in 2016, a total of 1430 children younger than age 16 years were killed because of a driver impaired by alcohol.[5]

MVCs are the leading cause of death for teens in the United States. Graduated driver's licensing programs, which place restrictions on new drivers, have reduced the incidence of fatal crashes among 16- and 17-year-olds by 8% to 14%. In addition, limiting driving at night or with teenaged passengers had greater reductions in overall crash rates involving teen drivers than graduated licensing laws alone.[9]

Children and adolescents sustain injuries as passengers or operators of all-terrain vehicles, two-wheeled off-road vehicles, and go-carts/buggies. These children had a mean age of 12.7 years, and 77% were male. Most injuries occur from disruptions in the driving surface, such as bumps, holes, and uneven terrain.[10] Young children riding as passengers can be crushed by the adult driver on impact with a stationary or moving object. Older children who are not the appropriate size or weight to operate such vehicles can flip vehicles onto themselves and sustain serious multisystem injuries.

Falls are the most common mechanism of injury in children and the leading cause of nonfatal injuries in children younger than age 14.[11] Many serious falls among children occur on playgrounds and during sports and recreational activities. For children aged 0 to 2 years, falls from furniture, beds, and parents' arms were most common. For children aged 3 to 9 years, falls from playground equipment were most frequent.[3] Children also fall while running, playing, and participating in sports. Injuries sustained from falls vary from mild to severe single-system or multisystem trauma.

Pedestrian injuries are a common cause of morbidity and mortality in the pediatric population. As pedestrians, children are struck by moving vehicles while playing, walking, running, crossing the street, or entering or exiting a school bus. Most pedestrians younger than age 15 years are struck by the front of the vehicle. In 2016, 281 pedestrians younger than 16 years of age were killed.[6] Most injuries occur in the afternoon and early evening hours on urban streets outside of an intersection area.

Children are also injured when struck by a motor vehicle while riding a bicycle. In 2016, 59 pedal cyclists younger than age 15 years were killed by a motor vehicle. Of these 59 fatalities, only 12% occurred in riders wearing helmets. The environmental characteristics of pediatric pedal cyclist fatalities are consistent with the previously mentioned pedestrian fatalities.[5]

Young children struck by motor vehicles in driveways are at risk for severe injury and death. In 2017, 44 children died as a result of motor vehicle "back-overs." This number has decreased significantly since 2008, when a federal law went into effect requiring all vehicles sold or leased in the United States to come with a rearview camera as standard equipment.[12]

Bicycle crashes are a common mechanism of fatal and nonfatal injuries. Approximately 501 per 100,000 children aged 5 years to 14 years are treated in EDs for bicycle-related injuries each year in the United States. Lower socioeconomic status, which may be a proxy for more dangerous environments, is associated with increased injury risk, and child and adolescent bicyclists incur more severe injuries when exposed to motor vehicle traffic.[13] It has been reported that approximately 75% of all bicycle-related mortality is secondary to head injuries, 85% of which could have been prevented by wearing a bicycle helmet, according to The Center for Head Injury Statistics, 2014.[51] Other injuries associated with bicycle crashes are long-bone fractures and abdominal, thoracic, and facial injuries. Visits at which children present after a minor injury provide an opportunity for educating the child and the family on the importance of proper helmet use.

Children can sustain injuries from skateboards and scooters. Compared with adults, children have a high center of gravity, less development, and poor balance, which limit their ability to break a fall. The American Academy of Pediatrics recommends that children younger than age 10 years should not use skateboards without close supervision by an adult or a responsible adolescent. Children younger than 5 years should not use skateboards. Skateboards should not be ridden in traffic. Proper protective wear, including helmets, elbow pads, and knee pads, should be worn. Approximately 70,000 skateboard injuries require a visit to the ED each year, almost half of which involve children younger than age 15 years. Injuries to the arms, legs, neck, and trunk range from cuts and bruises to sprains, strains, and broken bones, with wrist fractures being very common. Facial injuries, such as a broken nose, are also common.[15] Nonpowered scooter–related injuries accounted for an estimated 9400 ED visits; 90% of these were for children younger than age 15 years.[15] Proper protective gear for scooter safety includes a helmet, knee pads, and elbow pads; wrist guards are not recommended because they make it difficult to grip the handle and steer the scooter. Children younger than 8 years of age should not use scooters without close adult supervision. Children should not ride scooters in streets, in traffic, or at night.

Annually, approximately 2100 children younger than 15 years are treated in EDs for nonfatal drownings. There were 351 reported fatal child drownings in pools and spas in 2015 in children; with 76% of those involving children younger than 5 years.[16] Bathtub drowning is most common in children younger than 1 year of age. In the preschool-aged child, drowning occurs most commonly in residential swimming pools. Young adults typically drown in ponds, lakes, rivers, and oceans. Children should never be unsupervised when in or around water. Additional water safety education for parents and caregivers includes designating a "water watcher"; learning cardiopulmonary resuscitation (CPR); and installing proper barriers, covers, and alarms on and around pools and spas.

ANATOMY AND PHYSIOLOGY

Children differ from adults developmentally, anatomically, and physiologically. Recognizing differences and implementing appropriate interventions to support these differences can result in increased survivability of the pediatric trauma patient.

Respiratory System

Crucial anatomic and physiologic differences exist between adult and pediatric airways. The child's oropharynx is relatively small; therefore the airway is easily obstructed by the large tongue. The U-shaped epiglottis protrudes into the pharynx, with the tonsils and adenoids often enlarged. Vocal cords are short and concave, with the larynx relatively cephalad and easily collapsible if the neck is hyperflexed or extended. In a child younger than 10 years of age, the narrowest portion of the airway is the cricoid cartilage.[17] Lower airways are smaller and supporting cartilage is less developed in infants and small children, so airways are easily obstructed by small amounts of blood, mucus, edema, and foreign objects.[18] Ribs are pliable and do not provide adequate protection and support for the lungs; therefore blunt trauma to the chest causes pulmonary contusions rather than rib fractures. If rib fractures are present, a high index of suspicion for severe internal trauma should be raised.[19] The mediastinum is more mobile, causing greater susceptibility to great-vessel damage. Retractions are more likely when the child is in respiratory distress. These can be suprasternal, supraclavicular, infraclavicular, intercostal, or substernal.

Breathing is primarily diaphragmatic or abdominal in children younger than 7 or 8 years of age. Crying children are more prone to swallowing air, which causes gastric distention and hampers respiratory excursion. A thin chest wall transmits breath sounds easily from one location or side of the thorax to another, which can make an accurate respiratory assessment difficult. It is challenging to detect the presence of a pneumothorax by auscultation alone in younger children. Respiratory rates are higher in children because of higher metabolic rates and contribute to overall insensible fluid losses, resulting in greater risk for hypovolemia.[18] Oxygen consumption in infants is 6 to 8 mL/kg per minute compared with 3 to 4 mL/kg per minute in adults; therefore hypoxemia can occur rapidly due to limited oxygen reserves.[18]

Cardiovascular System

The child's estimated blood volume is 80 mL/kg. Although this absolute blood volume is small, it is larger than an adult's on a milliliter-per-kilogram basis. Seemingly small amounts of blood loss can impair perfusion and decrease circulating blood volume. Because of their large cardiac reserve and catecholamine response, children can maintain a high to normal blood pressure even with significant blood loss. Hypotension is not observed until the child has lost 20% to 25% of circulating blood volume.[17] Hypotension is a late sign of hypovolemia in children and signals imminent cardiac arrest. The best assessment of perfusion is skin parameters (color, temperature, moisture) and capillary refill—normal is 2 seconds or less on all four extremities, and this should be checked at frequent intervals. Other assessment factors include the presence of bradycardia or tachycardia with decreased urinary output.

Children have a less compliant myocardium than adults do. As a result, tachycardia is the initial compensatory response to decreased oxygenation. However, when this compensatory mechanism is exhausted, decompensation, often manifested as bradycardia, is sudden and rapid.[18] Children can present with a variety of congenital heart defects (e.g., etralogy of Fallot, large ventricular septal defect), which may impair circulatory status. If a child has had a shunting surgical procedure to redirect blood flow, blood pressure readings are unattainable in the arm from which the subclavian artery was used because that arm is perfused by collateral circulation. Children may also have functional or nonfunctional heart murmurs. Children with congenital heart defects may also experience heart failure and dysrhythmias.

Neurologic System

An infant's head is larger in proportion to the rest of the body than an adult's is. The skull is more malleable, providing less protection to the brain.[17] The posterior fontanel closes at age 4 months; the anterior fontanel is normally closed by age 18 months. Although open fontanels allow for release of increased intracranial pressure (ICP), they may allow direct injury to the brain or cause extensive bleeding. Additionally, larger amounts of blood can be lost in the cranial vault before signs of increased ICP develop.[18] Infants bleed significantly from a scalp laceration because of the large surface area and increased vascularity. Finally, a young child has a higher center of gravity, which, together with the larger head, makes the child prone to head injuries.

Children's cerebral tissues are thin, soft, and flexible compared with those of adults. Sulci are still deepening during childhood, and myelinization is still occurring. These differences make brain tissues more easily damaged, especially from shearing injuries. Several features make the cervical spine vulnerable to injury in children younger than 9 years of age[17]:

- The head is disproportionately large, making the child vulnerable to flexion-extension injury.
- The neck muscles are underdeveloped.
- The vertebral bodies are wedge shaped.
- The articulating facets are angled horizontally, resulting in subluxation from minimal force.
- The end plates are cartilaginous.
- The interspinous ligaments are elastic and lax, leading to increased spinal mobility.

Gastrointestinal and Genitourinary Systems

Young children have protuberant abdomens as a result of underdeveloped abdominal musculature.[20] Because solid abdominal organs are relatively larger in children compared with adults, there is an increased risk for direct organ injury after blunt and penetrating kinetic forces.[20] A pliable rib cage does not afford adequate protection to abdominal organs and can predispose children to further internal injuries.[19] The large size of the organs in a relatively small space predisposes children to have multiple-organ injury with trauma. Although it is partially protected by the flexible rib cage, the liver is still vulnerable to injury because of its large size and fragility. The transverse diameter of the abdomen is small, and lower abdominal organs are not well protected by the pelvis.[20]

Renal injuries occur because the relatively large kidneys are not protected by the small amount of perinephric fat, weak abdominal muscles, and elastic rib cage.[21] The kidneys also retain fetal lobulations, which may predispose these organs to separation and fracture. Congenital abnormalities such as hydronephrosis, horseshoe kidneys, and ectopic kidneys make the child more susceptible to renal trauma.

Many congenital anomalies are not diagnosed until abdominal trauma has occurred. Greater elasticity makes ureteral tearing rare. Ureteral injuries are suspected with penetrating trauma to the abdomen or flank area. The bladder is an abdominal organ and not well protected. In girls, the bladder neck is also less protected. Tissues of a prepubescent girl are more rigid because of a lack of estrogen; they do not become more pliable until adolescence, when estrogen is released.

Musculoskeletal System

The periosteum in a growing child is stronger, thicker, and more osteogenic compared with the periosteum in an adult, which results in decreased fracture displacement and fewer open fractures.[22] Consequently, four unique, bone-fracture patterns are found in children: plastic deformity (the bone is deformed but not broken); torus (buckle) fracture (compression forces applied at the metaphysis and diaphysis cause bone to buckle rather than break because of its porous nature); greenstick fracture (an incomplete fracture in which the compressed side's cortex and periosteum are intact); and physis fractures (injury to the growth plate, which can lead to angulation deformities if not diagnosed and treated properly).[22] Bone osteogenicity allows rapid callus formation, permitting bones to heal quickly. Even though bone is strong, fractures occur more frequently than muscle sprains or ligament tears because these structures are stronger than the bones themselves.

Another unique feature of the pediatric musculoskeletal system is the presence of a physis, or growth plate. This area of bone, which is responsible for longitudinal bone growth, is found between the epiphysis and metaphysis. The physis is cartilaginous and does not ossify until puberty; therefore treatment to attain proper anatomic alignment is critical to optimize bone growth and reduce the risk for deformity.[22]

Integumentary System

Children have a larger ratio of body surface area to weight, which makes them prone to convective and conductive heat loss. Having less subcutaneous fat for insulation can increase heat loss through radiation, convection, conduction, and evaporation. Children do not have the fine-motor coordination to shiver and are unable to keep themselves warm. Nonshivering thermogenesis does occur in infants; in this process, brown fat is broken down slowly to produce warmth. Shivering is a high-energy-consuming, nonproductive muscular activity initiated for thermogenesis.[23] Shivering may not be possible in injured children receiving sedation or neuromuscular blocking agents.

PATIENT ASSESSMENT

Each ED should be equipped with personnel and supplies necessary to treat an injured child effectively and efficiently. Equipment should be readily available and prepared before patient arrival.

Initial assessment and stabilization of the pediatric trauma patient requires knowledge of developmental and physiologic differences among infants, children, and adolescents. Injured children are frightened—strange, painful things are happening. The patient may feel that he or she is being punished for a real or imagined wrongdoing. Talking with the child in language he or she understands is essential for relieving anxiety and developing trust.

Initial assessment consists of a primary and secondary assessment by inspection, auscultation, and palpation. During primary assessment, airway with cervical spine protection, breathing, circulation, and disability (neurologic status) are assessed. Life-threatening injuries are identified and treated. Table 42.1 describes the primary survey in the preferred order. During secondary assessment, all other body

TABLE 42.1 Primary Survey of the Pediatric Trauma Patient

Component	Actions
Airway	Assess for patency; look for loose teeth, vomitus, or other obstruction; note position of head. Suspect cervical spine injury with multiple trauma; maintain neutral alignment during assessment; evaluate effectiveness of cervical collar, cervical immobilization device, or other equipment used to immobilize the spine. Open cervical collar to evaluate neck for jugular vein distention and tracheal deviation.
Breathing	Auscultate breath sounds in the axillae for presence and equality. Assess chest for contusions, penetrating wounds, abrasions, or paradoxical movement.
Circulation	Assess apical pulse for rate, rhythm, and quality; compare apical and peripheral pulses for quality and equality. Evaluate capillary refill; normal is 2 seconds or less. Check skin color and temperature.
Disability	Assess level of consciousness; check for orientation to person, place, and time in the older child. In a younger child, assess alertness, ability to interact with environment, and ability to follow commands. Is the child easily consoled and interested in the environment? Does the child recognize a familiar object and respond when you speak to him or her? Check pupils for size, shape, reactivity, and equality. Remove clothing to allow visual inspection of entire body.
Expose	Note open wounds or uncontrolled bleeding.

systems are assessed and other injuries are treated. Table 42.2 details the secondary survey. Throughout the initial assessment and stabilization, airway, breathing, and circulation are continually reassessed.

Initial Stabilization

Airway/Cervical Spine

The tongue is the most common cause of airway obstruction in the child. Opening the airway with the jaw-thrust technique to prevent hyperextension of the cervical spine is the initial step in relieving airway obstruction. Suction the oropharynx with a tonsil suction device if vomitus, blood, or loose teeth are present.

Place an oropharyngeal airway to help maintain airway patency in the child with an altered level of consciousness who does not have an intact gag reflex. Oropharyngeal airways are measured from the corner of the mouth to the tragus of the ear. An oropharyngeal airway that is too small or too large will obstruct the airway, so having the correct size is critical. Use a tongue depressor to insert the airway directly. Do not rotate 90 degrees as in the adult patient because a child's oropharyngeal tissues can be damaged and the tongue inadvertently pushed posteriorly, causing obstruction. A nasopharyngeal airway may be used for airway patency if there is no evidence of head and midface trauma. This airway is measured from the nares to the tragus of the ear.

In a child who requires continuous airway maintenance, endotracheal intubation using rapid-sequence intubation (RSI) is necessary. RSI is defined as "the combination of preoxygenation with the administration of sedative and neuromuscular blockings medications in rapid succession to optimize conditions for efficient endotracheal tube placement in critically ill or injured patients while limiting the risk of patient harm."[24] This procedure must be undertaken by a health care professional skilled in pediatric intubation. The orotracheal route is preferred because the nasotracheal route can be difficult or contraindicated in severe facial trauma or basilar skull fracture.

Before the intubation attempt, cardiac and pulse oximetry monitoring devices are placed on the child. Sedating medications followed by paralyzing agents are administered while the child's lungs are ventilated with 100% oxygen. After the trachea is intubated, observe for rise and fall of the chest; auscultate breath sounds bilaterally in the midaxillary line, then over the epigastrium; listen high in the axilla because breath sounds are easily transmittable across the thin chest wall. Right mainstem bronchus intubations are a common complication with pediatric intubation; therefore bilateral chest wall movement should be observed during ventilation with a bag-mask device. Movement is best assessed by standing at the foot of the bed and watching the chest rise and fall during ventilation.

Correct endotracheal tube placement is determined through auscultation of equal, bilateral breath sounds in all fields; observation of condensation in the endotracheal tube; and assessment of end-tidal carbon dioxide measurements with pediatric-specific equipment while evaluating the child's response. Final confirmation is made by chest radiograph. The tube must be secured with commercially available holders, tape, or ties and the measurement of the tube at the lip line should be documented. The tube should not press on the corner of the mouth (or the nares for nasotracheal intubation) because of the potential for tissue breakdown. Frequent suctioning may be necessary if aspiration is suspected or injury to the airway or lung tissue has occurred.

Children are diaphragmatic breathers, so compression on the diaphragm impedes lung expansion. A gastric tube is inserted to relieve gastric distention. The preferred method is to insert the tube orally. The tube should not be inserted nasally if the child has obvious facial trauma or signs of a

TABLE 42.2 Secondary Survey of the Pediatric Trauma Patient

Component	Actions
Head, eye, ear, nose	Assess scalp for lacerations or open wounds; palpate for step-off defects, depressions, hematomas, and pain. Reassess pupils for size, reactivity, equality, and extraocular movements; ask the child if he or she can see. Assess nose and ears for rhinorrhea or otorrhea. Observe for raccoon eyes (bruising around the eyes) or Battle's sign (bruising over the mastoid process). Palpate forehead, orbits, maxilla, and mandible for crepitus, deformities, step-off defect, pain, and stability; evaluate malocclusion by asking the child to open and close the mouth; note open wounds. Inspect for loose, broken, or chipped teeth as well as oral lacerations. Check orthodontic appliances for stability. Evaluate facial symmetry by asking the child to smile, grimace, and open and close the mouth. Do not remove impaled objects or foreign objects.
Neck	Open cervical collar, and reassess anterior neck for jugular vein distention and tracheal deviation; note bruising, edema, open wounds, pain, and crepitus. Check for hoarseness or changes in voice by asking the child to speak.
Chest	Obtain respiratory rate; reassess breath sounds in anterior lobes for equality. Palpate chest wall and sternum for pain, tenderness, and crepitus. Observe inspiration and expiration for symmetry or paradoxical movement; note use of accessory muscles. Reassess apical heart rate for rate, rhythm, and clarity.
Abdomen/pelvis/genitourinary	Observe abdomen for bruising and distention; auscultate bowel sounds briefly in all four quadrants; palpate abdomen gently for tenderness; assess pelvis for tenderness and stability. Palpate bladder for distention and tenderness; check urinary meatus for signs of injury or bleeding; note priapism and genital trauma such as lacerations or foreign body. Have rectal sphincter tone assessed, usually by physician.
Musculoskeletal	Assess extremities for deformities, swelling, lacerations, or other injuries. Palpate distal pulses for equality, rate, and rhythm; compare with central pulses. Ask the child to wiggle the toes and fingers; evaluate strength through hand grips and foot flexion/extension.
Back	Logroll as a unit to inspect back; maintain spinal alignment during examination; observe for bruising and open wounds; palpate each vertebral body for tenderness, pain, deformity, and stability; assess flank area for bruising and tenderness.

basilar skull fracture. After the tube is inserted, it is taped to the child's face and connected to low intermittent suction.

Cricothyrotomy and tracheostomy are reserved for severe cases of airway instability from facial, head, and neck trauma. Fortunately, these procedures are rarely required in children.

Strategies to protect the cervical spine in the child with multiple injuries include application of a rigid cervical collar and cervical immobilization devices. Care must be taken to prevent cervical spine flexion from the cervical collar or backboard (Fig. 42.1). Movement can worsen spinal cord injury (SCI) and compromise the airway. Spinal protection is maintained until radiographic and clinical evidence demonstrates that SCI is not present.

Use of an appropriately sized cervical collar is essential to prevent SCI and airway compromise. A collar that is too large pushes the jaw backward, causes airway obstruction, and allows the child to move the head from side to side, which prevents cervical spine control. A collar that is too small does not provide appropriate alignment and may cause airway compromise from constriction. A cervical collar fits properly if the chin rests securely in the chin holder, the collar is beneath the ears, and the upper part of the sternum is not covered.

Infants and young children may arrive in the ED secured in their car safety seat. Children can initially remain in their car seats if there are no signs of distress and the car seat is intact.[18] Cervical protection with a collar, if possible, and towel rolls should be completed.[18] Although no evidence-based guidelines indicate car-seat immobilization is effective, it may be an option for emergency medical services personnel to transport stable, injured children.[18]

Cervical spine radiographs from C1 through T1 are obtained in the anterior-posterior and lateral views to evaluate for vertebral fractures. The radiograph is assessed for

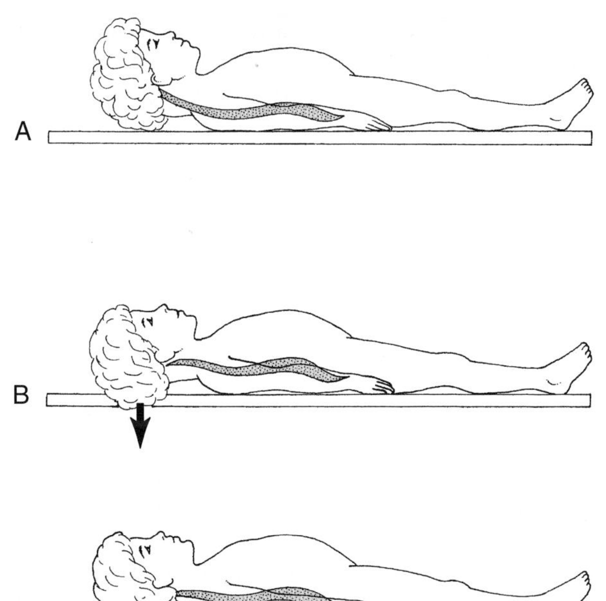

Fig. 42.1 (A) Young child immobilized on a standard backboard; note how the large head forces the neck into flexion. Backboards can be modified by an occiput cutout (B) or a double mattress pad (C) to raise the chest. (From Roberts JR, Hedges JR. *Clinical Procedures in Emergency Medicine.* 4th ed. Philadelphia, PA: Saunders; 2004.)

vertebral symmetry, alignment, and spacing. Spinal protection can be discontinued if there is no radiographic evidence of cervical spine injury, the child is alert with no distracting injuries, and the child has normal neurologic findings.

Breathing

Assess the adequacy of breathing and look for signs of ineffective ventilation, such as noisy or decreased breath sounds, retractions and accessory muscle use, nasal flaring, pallor of skin, use of abdominal muscles, tracheal deviation, and unilateral absence of breath sounds. Supplemental oxygen is administered to any child with multiple trauma. Hypoxia/hypoventilation is the most common cause of bradycardia and cardiac arrest in children.

Flow rate for a nasal cannula should be no more than 6 L/min of oxygen; higher flow rates will irritate the nasopharynx. A nasal cannula is used in children with minimal oxygen requirements. With infants and young children, it is important to secure the cannula in the nares and then initiate oxygen flow. Nonrebreather oxygen masks are used for a child with greater oxygen requirements; flow rate is set at 10 to 12 L/min. A properly fitting face mask fits snugly on the face, covering the nose and mouth without covering the eyes or cheeks. In the child who is not breathing spontaneously or effectively, ventilations are assisted with a bag-mask device set at 15 L/min, which allows oxygen delivery up to 90%.[25] A bag-mask device must be self-inflating in case there is no oxygen source available. Bag-mask devices are equipped with pop-off valves to avoid delivery of high pressures while bagging the patient.[25] Abdominal distention may occur with bag-valve-mask ventilation, resulting in diminished tidal volume. Decompression with a gastric tube is recommended early. In patients with unilateral absence of breath sounds, the nurse should anticipate needle decompression of the affected side to relive the tension pneumothorax. This will be followed by placement of a chest tube.[25]

A pulse oximeter sensor is applied to the child's finger, earlobe, or toe to determine oxygen saturation. Pulse oximetry readings should be 95% or more (at sea level).

Circulation

To assess adequacy of circulation, palpate central versus peripheral pulses for quality and assess capillary refill and skin temperature. Continuous cardiopulmonary and blood-pressure monitoring devices are connected to the child immediately in a trauma situation. Vital signs should be measured every 5 minutes until the child's condition stabilizes. Blood-pressure readings should be evaluated against other vital signs. A properly fitting blood-pressure cuff fits two-thirds of the upper arm. A cuff that is too small gives false-high readings, whereas a cuff that is too large gives false-low readings.

Hemorrhage is the leading preventable cause of death in trauma. Therefore recognition and control of uncontrolled external bleeding with direct pressure must occur immediately. Any patient with external bleeding that cannot be controlled with direct pressure should be considered a candidate for the use of a tourniquet.[26]

Two large-bore intravenous (IV) catheters are inserted, preferably in the antecubital fossae, for venous access and fluid replacement. Catheter size is determined by the size of the child's veins. If peripheral venous access is not readily available, the intraosseous route should be used.[25] Central venous access through the jugular, subclavian, or femoral vein may be obtained by an experienced practitioner. It is important to obtain blood for laboratory analysis and initiate crystalloid fluid replacement. Central venous pressure monitoring or arterial pressure monitoring is reserved for severely injured children and should be performed only under controlled circumstances by experienced providers.

Hypovolemic shock is suspected in the child with tachypnea, tachycardia, decreased level of consciousness, decreased urinary output, and prolonged capillary refill. Isotonic crystalloid fluid bolus of 20 mL/kg normal saline or lactated Ringer's solution should be administered rapidly, with effectiveness determined by reassessment. Stopcocks connected to IV tubing allow easy administration of fluid boluses. If there is no improvement, a second bolus can be administered, followed by a third bolus. Warmed O-negative blood may be given at 10 mL/kg if there is no improvement after two boluses.[17] Excessive fluid administration in the child with a head injury may increase ICP; therefore strict intake and output of trauma patients should be documented.

Damage control resuscitation is a strategy used to attempt to avoid the lethal triad of hypothermia, acidosis, and coagulopathy. It consists of immediate hemorrhage control, limited use of crystalloid fluids, early use of warmed blood products, balanced massive transfusion protocols (MTPs), permissive hypotension, use of hemostatic agents, and damage-control surgery.[27] Judicious crystalloid resuscitation (10–40 mL/kg) in the injured and bleeding child is appropriate for patients in compensated shock. Children in decompensated hemorrhagic shock require blood immediately. Massive transfusion in pediatrics, which had not been clearly defined before 2015, is a balanced transfusion ratio of plasma, platelets, and packed red blood cells (PRBCs) mimicking whole blood and minimizing clotting factor hemodilution and coagulopathy. Although routinely accepted in the adult trauma practice, permissive hypotension in young children is still controversial due to differences in physiologic responses.[27]

Routine blood tests include complete blood count (CBC) and differential, electrolytes, blood urea nitrogen, creatinine, glucose, venous blood gas, type and screen, prothrombin time, partial thromboplastin times and, less frequently, toxicology screening. If abdominal trauma is suspected, amylase, lipase, and liver enzymes may be obtained. In suspected cardiac or muscle damage, creatine phosphokinase levels are also obtained. Urine may be sent for complete urinalysis and toxicology testing. Pregnancy testing should be considered in the postmenarcheal female.

An indwelling urinary catheter is placed if there is no sign of genitourinary trauma (e.g., no blood at the meatus). A urimeter on the urine collection bag allows monitoring of hourly urinary output. Decreased output can indicate hypovolemic shock. Hematuria suggests genitourinary trauma; however, the first urine specimen may test negative for blood because of urine in the bladder before injury. Therefore a subsequent urine specimen may be necessary. 1 mL/kg/hr is optimal urinary output for the pediatric setting. Urine output of 0.5ml/kg/h or less indicates hypoperfusion.[28]

Children may arrive in the ED after a traumatic arrest. Children with traumatic injuries who are found to be asystolic or hypotensive by prehospital personnel have a poor prognosis. If the patient survives to hospital discharge, there are almost always neurologic side effects.

Disability

Serial neurologic assessments are necessary to identify changes in mental status. Changes in level of consciousness can indicate hypovolemia or increased ICP. Early signs of increased ICP are vomiting and irritability. In infants, a bulging fontanel is a late sign of increasing ICP. Another important assessment finding during disability is the pupil examination. Check pupils for symmetry, size, reactivity, and shape.

In older children, the first sign of increased ICP is disorientation to time, place, and familiar people, then to self. This description is not applicable to the younger child, who has no concept of time or place. The Glasgow Coma Scale (GCS) can be slightly modified for children (Table 42.3). Children as young as 3 months old should recognize their parents/caregivers; toddlers should know the names of their pets and may also recognize popular cartoon or television characters or favorite toys.

TABLE 42.3 Pediatric Modification of Glasgow Coma Scale

GCS Score		Pediatric Modification
Eye Opening		
≥1 year	0–1 year	
4 Spontaneously	4 Spontaneously	
3 To verbal command	3 To shout	
2 To pain	2 To pain	
1 No response	1 No response	
Best Motor Response		
≥1 year	0–1 year	
6 Obeys	5 Localizes pain	
5 Localizes pain	4 Flexion—withdrawal	
4 Flexion—withdrawal	3 Flexion—abnormal (decorticate rigidity)	
3 Flexion—abnormal (decorticate rigidity)	2 Extension (decerebrate rigidity)	
2 Extension (decerebrate rigidity)	1 No response	
1 No response		
Best Verbal Response		
0–2 years	2–5 years	>5 years
5 Cries appropriately, smiles, coos	5 Appropriate words and phrases	5 Oriented and converses
4 Cries	4 Inappropriate words	4 Disoriented and converses
3 Inappropriate crying/screaming	3 Cries/screams	3 Inappropriate words
2 Grunts	2 Grunts	2 Incomprehensible sounds
1 No response	1 No response	1 No response

From Barkin RM, Rosen P. *Emergency Pediatrics: A Guide to Ambulatory Care.* 6th ed. St Louis, MO: Mosby; 2003.

In a child with severe head trauma, ventilation with 100% oxygen is initiated. Hypertonic saline should be considered for patients with severe TBI in whom intracranial hypertension is suspected. Mild hyperventilation may be considered to maintain arterial carbon dioxide pressure ($Paco_2$) between 30 and 35 mm Hg if herniation is impending.[29]

Exposure/Environmental Control

The child's temperature is recorded initially and monitored throughout initial stabilization to detect and treat hypothermia. Common temperature measurement routes are tympanic, temporal artery, oral, rectal, and bladder. Factors to consider when selecting a route for temperature measurement in pediatric trauma patients include safety, accuracy, and compliance.

Numerous factors during the child's initial ED care increase the risk for hypothermia, including transfusion of large amounts of unwarmed IV fluids or blood products[17]; clothing removal during assessment and treatment; large, open wounds; neurologic or multisystem injuries; administration of paralytic or sedative agents; and treatment in cold trauma rooms and diagnostic suites. Therefore measures to prevent heat loss and promote thermoregulation should be initiated. Passive warming measures include increasing ambient temperature by using overhead lights and applying warm blankets. Active warming measures include administering warmed IV fluids and blood products.

Full Set of Vital Signs

Vital signs (temperature, heart rate, respiratory rate, blood pressure) are measured on ED arrival and throughout initial ED treatment. Vital signs should be measured continuously and recorded every 5 minutes in unstable patients and every 15 minutes in stable patients. Documenting patient care on a trauma flowsheet allows visual inspection of trends in patient vital signs and permits rapid interventions as needed. Weight should be determined through actual measurement or by estimation with a length-based resuscitation tape (Fig. 42.2).

Family Presence

The presence of a supportive parent does wonders for a frightened child. Allow parents to see the child as soon as possible after stabilization is complete. Explain to the parents beforehand what they will see and why because this allows them to look at the child and not become overwhelmed with the medical equipment involved in the care of their child. Parents may believe they must have permission to touch or talk to their child, so encourage them to do so.

Controversy exists as to whether parents should be present during resuscitation. If parents are present, a designated support person must stay with them and explain what is happening to their child. The Emergency Nurses Association advocates parental presence during resuscitation. Such presence may be beneficial to the child and the family members. A designated emergency nurse or social worker can stay with the family and explain treatment that is taking place.

While parents are waiting to see their child, a social worker, emergency nurse, or designated patient advocate should keep them apprised of the situation and serve as a support person. If the decision is made to transfer the child to another facility, parents should see their child before departure. If the child dies before parents arrive at the accepting institution, they may feel guilty because they were not able to see the child or agreed to have their child transferred elsewhere. When the child leaves, say "Mommy will see you later" rather than "goodbye" because "goodbye" implies they may never see each other again. Most flight programs have policies in place for transport of a family member with a patient. Many factors influence the decision to have a parent or other family member accompany a child in a helicopter, so the decision to do so ultimately rests with the pilot and flight crew and should be respected.

Give Comfort Measures

The injured child has several fears—mutilation, losing control, getting in trouble with his or her parents for engaging

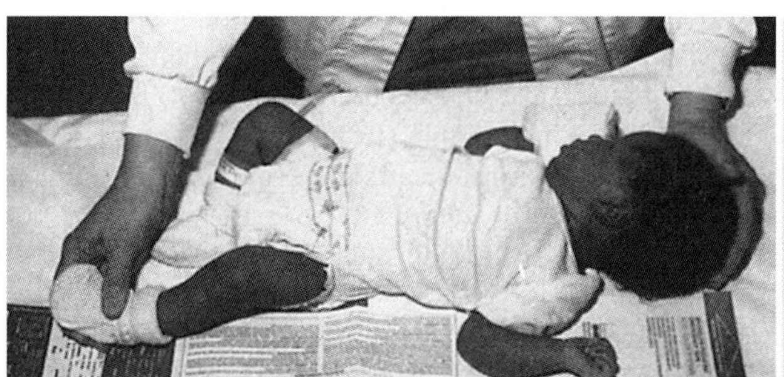

12 kg

INFUSIONS

ISOPRO 1.4 mg fill
EPI to 100 ml
NOREPI at 5-25 ml/hr

DOPA 72 mg fill to
DOBUT 100 ml at 5-20 ml/hr

LIDO 144 mg fill to 100 ml at 10-25 ml/hr

FLUIDS

Volume Expansion

Crystalloid 240 ml

Colloid / blood 120 ml

Maintenance Fluids

46 ml/hour D5W + 1/4NS with 20 meq KCl/L

PARALYZING AGENTS

Succinylcholine 24 mg

Pancuronium 1.2 mg

Vecuronium 1.2 mg

Fig. 42.2 The Broselow tape can be used as a rapid method for generating drug and fluid doses and endotracheal tube and suction catheter sizes. The tape uses the principle that length correlates with body surface area and weight. The patient is measured with the tape in the supine position, and the line on which the foot of the patient reaches contains the precalculated drug doses and equipment sizes appropriate for the patient. (From Barkin R, et al. *Pediatric Emergency Nursing*. 2nd ed. St Louis, MO: Mosby; 1997.)

in a forbidden activity, death, disfigurement, and pain. It is the responsibility of the emergency nurse to help the child cope effectively with these fears during trauma resuscitation. Children who are hearing impaired or require a translator should have an interpreter other than a family member present during the examination.

Assign one nurse as the child's support person. While the child remains in cervical protection, the nurse should stand at the child's side and down from his or her face, about chest level, so the child is able to see the person. Standing directly over the child's face is frightening, especially when different faces keep appearing and reappearing. Hold the child's hand or stroke his or her hair to provide tactile comfort. Talk softly and slowly, using words he or she can understand (e.g., "The doctor is going to listen to your heartbeat," "You will feel a pinch in your right arm. You can scream, but you must keep your right arm still."). Avoid words such as "take" or "cut out" because they imply mutilation. Use words such as "make it better." If the child requires general anesthesia, avoid telling the child he or she will "be put to sleep." If the child had a pet that was "put to sleep," this statement may create death fears. Instead, tell the child he or she will get "special medicine to help you take a short nap." The child understands "nap" is a short time. Tell the child what will happen before it happens. Children do not like surprises any more than adults do. Prepare them by using feeling terms, such as, "This will feel cold; this will feel heavy; this will smell sweet." If a procedure will hurt, tell the child. Lying will only cause him or her to mistrust you. A child life specialist is a professional trained to work with children in medical settings. They serve as a resource to help patients and families adjust and understand the hospital and medical situation.

Children cope in a variety of ways. Because young children are mobile, crying and kicking are ways for them to cope. Being restrained removes one of their coping mechanisms, which can increase their fear. School-aged children and adolescents cope by seeking information; they may ask the same questions over and over again. Be patient. Scolding or threatening the child is fruitless and will only increase fear and resistance.

Severe injuries should be shielded from the child's visual field. Refrain from discussing the magnitude of an injury in the child's presence. It is not known whether unconscious children remember discussions in their presence, so it is best to avoid talking about other family members or the child's condition in his or her presence. Talk to the child who is comatose or unresponsive just as if he or she were awake.

Pain management is of utmost importance when treating the injured child; however, it may be neglected. Recent requirements from The Joint Commission strive to ensure that all patients receive pain assessment and appropriate pain-relief measures. The awake child may be able to use a pain scale to rate the pain.

Various pain scales are available to measure pain in preverbal and verbal children. The appropriate pain scale should be used according to the age and development of the child. The most common pain scales are FACES, FLACC (face, legs, activity, cry, and consolability), and the number scale for older children (see Chapter 10).

Analgesics may be administered after all injuries are identified and the child is determined to be physiologically and neurologically intact. Pharmacologic management of pain includes narcotic and nonnarcotic analgesics. Nonpharmacologic management of pain includes comfort measures such as distraction techniques, progressive relaxation, positive self-talk, and deep-breathing exercises. Allowing an infant to suck a pacifier promotes comfort, whereas allowing a toddler to hold a transitional object such as a blanket or toy promotes security. Reevaluation is necessary after any pain relief measures are initiated.

Head-to-Toe-Assessment

The secondary survey is outlined in Table 42.2. Each body area is inspected and palpated to identify signs of injury; auscultation is performed while the nurse is assessing the chest and abdomen. In addition, frequent monitoring of the neurovascular status of an injured extremity is necessary to identify impairment of circulation or possible compartment syndrome. An injured extremity can be splinted for protection and comfort until definitive care is provided. After the extremity is splinted or casted, frequent reevaluation is necessary because edema may develop and impede circulation.

Inspect the Posterior Surface

The child is logrolled as a unit to inspect the posterior surface for contusions, abrasions, open wounds, and impaled objects; the spine and flank are palpated for tenderness and pain. The child is logrolled back into the supine position, with spinal protection resumed or removed at that time.

History

History allows the trauma team to prepare for the patient and anticipate required interventions. However, this information is not always available because the injury may not have been witnessed. The awake, nonverbal child cannot relate circumstances surrounding the injury. Such situations require special attention because child neglect or abuse may be involved (see Chapter 49). In all injuries, it is important to ascertain whether loss of consciousness occurred.

The AMPLE mnemonic (Box 42.1) is helpful for organizing and obtaining an adequate patient history. This information may be obtained from the parent, a family member, or an awake, older child or adolescent. In

BOX 42.1 History: AMPLE Mnemonic

A Allergies
M Medications
P Past health history
L Last meal eaten
E Events leading to the injury

addition to this information, it is important to determine the need for vision or hearing aids, such as eyeglasses, contact lenses, or hearing aids. These may or may not be with the child on arrival.

Additional Interventions

Additional interventions undertaken during emergency management of the injured child include radiologic testing, medication administration, laboratory testing, management of pain, and provision of emotional support.

Radiologic testing. Along with cervical spine radiographs, other radiographic testing may be undertaken relative to suspected injuries. A head computed tomography (CT) scan is indicated for a child with suspected brain injury; an abdominal CT scan may be indicated in a child with abdominal trauma; and chest, spine, and pelvis films may be indicated for the child with multiple injuries. Specific radiographs with views of injured extremities before definitive treatment is administered may also be performed. Radiographs may be obtained in the trauma room, or the child may be transported to the radiology department. A nurse should remain with the child to explain procedures and monitor the child's condition.

A CT scan of the abdomen and the pelvis is performed as indicated and serves as the gold standard imaging technique to verify presence or absence of free fluid in the abdomen. The focused assessment sonography for trauma (FAST) examination currently cannot replace CT scanning in the pediatric patient.[29] Although detection of free fluid in the abdomen may be possible using sonography, additional research is needed to validate the usefulness of this diagnostic tool in the initial care of children with abdominal injuries.

A CT scan is indicated in children with head, chest, spinal, or abdominal trauma. Mechanism of injury should also be used in determining the need for radiologic testing. In the absence of identifying injuries, type of injury should factor into the need for further studies. Again, a nurse must accompany the child for continuous monitoring. Appropriate equipment should be readily available in case there is a change in the child's status. Sedation may be required for stable children undergoing a CT scan of the head after head injury. Sedation practices vary widely among health care providers. Emergency nurses should follow hospital policies for sedation for all trauma patients undergoing diagnostic procedures.

Medications. Antibiotics may be administered to the child who has large, open, contaminated wounds; open fractures; or arterial injury. Determine the child's immunization status to ensure appropriate tetanus prophylaxis. Children bitten by domestic or wild animals may require rabies prophylaxis, in which case local health department guidelines should be followed.

Laboratory testing. Baseline tests are a routine component of the trauma evaluation. A type and screen, CBC, serum chemistries, and urinalysis are typically obtained, and liver function tests and pancreatic enzymes may be included for abdominal organ injuries.

SPECIFIC CONDITIONS

Traumatic Brain Injuries

TBI is the leading cause of death and disability in children older than 1 year of age.[30] The central nervous system is the most commonly injured isolated system and is the principal determinant of outcome. Most children with multiple trauma have TBI, and most trauma deaths are associated with TBI.[18] TBI often results from blunt trauma from MVCs, bicycle crashes, falls, and maltreatment. Children are susceptible to brain injury because of their larger head-to-body ratio, thin cranial bones providing less protection to the intracranial contents, and less-myelinated brain, leading to a greater incidence of diffuse axonal injury and cerebral edema compared with adults.[30] Furthermore, cranial sutures remain open in early infancy, with the anterior fontanel open until 18 months. These features increase the child's susceptibility to head injury but also serve as an outlet for swollen cerebral tissues, allowing greater tolerance for increases in ICP.

When one is determining the severity of brain trauma, the GCS score is used to differentiate between mild, moderate, and severe injuries. A GCS score of 13 to 15 indicates mild head injury, a GCS score of 9 to 12 indicates moderate head injury, and a GCS score of less than 8 indicates severe head injury.[31] Mild to moderate head injuries are more common than severe head injuries. Brain injuries are divided into primary and secondary injuries. Primary injury results from mechanical damage from traumatic forces applied to the brain where the brain contacts the interior skull or from foreign bodies causing direct brain injury. Diffuse axonal injury, skull fractures, contusions, and hemorrhage can result. Secondary injury occurs from the resultant changes in the brain caused by the initial injury; for example, cerebral edema, hypoxia, ICP, and decreased cerebral blood flow.[29]

Mild to Moderate Traumatic Brain Injury

Mild to moderate TBI may cause persistent vomiting, posttraumatic seizure, and loss of consciousness. CT is the imaging of choice for the evaluation and diagnosis of a child who has experienced a traumatic head injury exhibiting neurological symptoms.[31] Persistent vomiting (over a few hours) warrants further observation and evaluation with possible hospital admission. Children who experience posttraumatic seizures require a CT scan and hospital admission, especially children older than 5 years of age when seizures occur late after the injury, reoccur, persist, or if other symptoms suggest severe injury. Loss of consciousness immediately after injury may not be known because no witnesses may have been present. The child may arrive in the ED awake and alert or unconscious. In either situation, further assessment and evaluation are warranted.

Children with mild to moderate TBI must receive serial neurologic evaluations to determine whether ICP is increasing. Serial evaluations include measurement of level of consciousness, pupillary response, motor and sensory response, and vital signs. Making a game of assessment may elicit cooperation from the young, awake, and frightened child. Having the awake child touch the nose and move the heels down the shins tests cerebellar function, whereas having the child squeeze the nurse's fingers and "push on the gas pedal" tests motor strength. The awake infant or toddler should be able to focus on and reach for a toy or object. This child should recognize the parent and be easily consoled. Any changes in the child's level of consciousness should be reported immediately to avoid subsequent deterioration and possible brain-stem herniation from increased ICP. The child should be evaluated for clinical signs of TBI, including hemotympanum, cerebrospinal fluid (CSF) otorrhea, CSF rhinorrhea, orbital bruising (raccoon eyes), or mastoid bruising (Battle's sign), because these may indicate a basilar skull fracture.[28] Other clinical findings that may be evident are an altered level of consciousness, altered pupillary responses, speech deficits, and sensory motor deficits.

A CT scan without contrast may be obtained if intracranial pathology is suspected. Skull radiographs may be obtained to detect the location and extent of skull fractures in infants and young children. Toxicology screening is considered in children with altered level of consciousness. In general, children with mild to moderate TBI are admitted to the hospital for observation if they have any neurologic deficits, seizures, vomiting, severe headache, fever, prolonged loss of consciousness, skull fracture, altered level of consciousness, or suspected child maltreatment.[28]

Children with mild TBI may be discharged home if parents or guardians understand the required home care. Parents should be instructed to return to the ED if the child has persistent vomiting, changes in vision, unequal pupil size, persistent headache or drowsiness, changes in level of consciousness, unequal strength or gait, or seizures. Be sure parents understand that the child may sleep and that sleeping is not an indication of a problem. They should be instructed to observe for nose or ear drainage on the pillow and to return to the ED if this is observed. Acetaminophen may be administered for headache.

Among children who undergo neuroimaging, an isolated skull fracture is the most common traumatic finding. Many children with isolated skull fractures are admitted for 24-hour observation, although the risk of emergency neurosurgery or death is extremely low.[32] Reasons for hospital admission include evaluation for nonaccidental trauma, treatment for persistent symptoms, or observation for clinical decompensation. However, children with isolated skull fractures may not require hospitalization if they can be cared for by reliable parents, child maltreatment is not suspected, and neurologic symptoms are not present.[32]

Skull fractures occurring in one of the suture lines should create a high index of suspicion for epidural hematomas. A complication of these fractures is growth of the fracture. This expansion of the fracture is usually observed in infants and children younger than 3 years of age and is thought to result from cerebral tissue or arachnoid membrane herniation through a dural laceration[28] causing a pulsatile mass. Surgery may be indicated for these situations; therefore infants and young children with this type of fracture must receive follow-up treatment. Infants can sustain significant blood loss from scalp lacerations, so they require close observation for development of hypovolemic shock.

Severe Traumatic Brain Injury

Severe TBI is defined as a brain injury resulting in loss of consciousness for more than 6 hours and a GCS score of 3 to 8. These TBIs are characterized by decreased level of consciousness, posturing, combative behavior, and abnormal neurologic findings. This catastrophic injury can be caused by severe shaking, falls, or MVCs.

In severe TBI, the airway is secured using RSI and followed by controlled ventilation. A quick neurologic assessment should be completed before administering sedative and paralytic agents. Because carbon dioxide is a potent cerebral vasodilator, $Paco_2$ should be maintained between 35 and 40 mm Hg to allow adequate cerebral blood flow.[29] Arterial oxygen saturation should be maintained at greater than 90% with mean arterial pressure slightly higher than age-appropriate norms. Current treatment of elevated ICP includes CSF drainage, sedation, neuromuscular blockade, mannitol, and hypertonic saline. The only recommended role for hyperventilation is in the setting of acute herniation, to briefly assist while definitive measures are being pursued.[29]

Laboratory analyses, including type and crossmatch, toxicologic testing, and clotting times (prothrombin time and partial thromboplastin time) should be performed in the event surgery is required. A CT scan without contrast is performed emergently as soon as the patient is stabilized, to determine location and extent of the injury. Operative management may be indicated, followed by admission to an intensive care unit for ongoing nursing and medical care.

Generally, children have better outcomes than adults after TBI, although the reasons are not clear. Neurologic deficits are the most common complications of TBI and are relative to the area of brain injury. For example, frontal brain injury results in cognitive deficits. Children may require rehabilitation for speech, motor, and cognitive improvements.

Maxillofacial Injuries

The incidence of maxillofacial injuries in children occurs less frequently as compared to the adult population.[17] MVCs account for the largest proportion of maxillofacial injuries.[33] The most frequently fractured facial area is the mandible, followed by the midface and upper face.[33] One concern in the young pediatric population is damage to growing facial structures, such as incomplete calcification of bone or developing dentition, as well as injury to cartilaginous and soft tissue. Facial injuries are diagnosed by clinical assessment and confirmed by diagnostic tests such as CT scan.[33] Plain or panoramic radiographs are not effective in detecting facial injuries because of the aforementioned composition of facial structures.

Dental injuries are the most common orofacial injuries sustained during sports activities.[34] More than 5 million teeth are avulsed annually. Avulsed primary teeth should not be replaced, but avulsed adult (permanent) teeth should be reimplanted within 2 hours (preferably 30 minutes).[34] The avulsed tooth should be handled by the crown and placed in milk, saline, or tooth preservative solution. Tissues attached to the teeth are left in place and not scrubbed away.[34] Consultation with a maxillofacial surgeon should be considered for children with severe facial injuries. It is important to pay close attention to potential airway compromise in patients with facial injuries.

Spinal Cord Injuries

SCIs are relatively uncommon in the pediatric population, with an overall incidence in the United States of 7.41 per 100,000. When these injuries do occur, rapid acceleration-deceleration forces and hyperflexion-hyperextension forces are suspected. Cervical spine is the most common level (60%–80%) for pediatric SCI, with 25% to 44% of injuries involving ligamentous disruption.[35] Children younger than 9 years of age are susceptible to cervical spine injuries because of their larger head size, which acts as a fulcrum, and their weaker neck muscles, ligaments, and horizontal facets.[31] Laxity of the pediatric spine contributes to SCI without radiographic abnormality (SCIWORA). This phenomenon occurs because of inherent elasticity of the pediatric spine, shaping of vertebral bodies, and level of flexion in the cervical spine.[36] Hyperflexion or hyperextension of the spinal cord can lead to injury or transection. The spinal cord then returns to normal length and the vertebrae to normal alignment. The child may exhibit signs of SCI, such as numbness, tingling, or weakness; however, subsequent radiographs show no evidence of bony abnormality. Although SCIWORA is most often diagnosed at the cervical level, thoracic SCIWORA is also possible. The most common mechanism of injury for SCI in children is MVCs. The second most common cause in children younger than 8 years of age is falls, whereas older children are more likely to sustain SCI from sports-related injuries.[36]

Signs and symptoms of SCI are the same in children as in adults. The classic triad of symptoms includes pain, muscle spasm, and restricted neck movements, which may be accompanied by varying degrees of neurologic symptoms such as numbness, tingling, weakness, and spasticity or flaccidity. Priapism suggests neurogenic shock. Spinal injuries should always be suspected in children with head injury or multiple injuries. Precautions must be taken to limit the motion of the spine until the injury is excluded. Previously this was described as "spinal immobilization." However, full spinal immobilization has been reported to cause substantial pain, which may last well beyond the immediate period of immobilization. Furthermore, pain caused by spinal immobilization may be confused with pain caused by injury, leading to unnecessary diagnostic evaluations and exposure to ionizing radiation. Recent trauma experts have adopted the term "spinal motion restriction" because true immobilization of the spine is unattainable.[35]

A clinical decision on clearing the cervical spine (without additional imaging) can be made in children older than 3 years of age who have experienced trauma and are alert, have no neurologic deficit, have no midline cervical tenderness, have no painful distracting injuries, do not have unexplained hypotension, and are not intoxicated. In children younger than 3 years of age, cervical spine imaging may not be required for patients with the following characteristics:

- have experienced trauma and have a GCS score of more than 13
- have no neurologic deficit
- have no midline cervical tenderness
- have no painful distracting injuries
- do not have unexplained hypotension
- are not intoxicated
- do not have motor vehicle accident (MVA) as a mechanism of injury.[37]

Endotracheal intubation and mechanical ventilation are indicated in children with high cervical SCIs. Children with lower cervical injuries require close observation for changes in their respiratory status. IV fluids should be administered at one-half to two-thirds of maintenance requirements. The use of high-dose steroids continues to be a controversial treatment in SCI. Pediatric patients are more likely to experience more complications than those patients who did not receive steroids.[38] There is limited research in children younger than 13 years of age; however, these patients may benefit from this protocol. If used, steroids are administered within 8 hours of injury: methylprednisolone 30 mg/kg IV is administered over 15 minutes, followed by normal saline over the next 45 minutes. A continuous infusion of 5.4 mg/kg per hour is then run for 23 hours if the injury occurred within 8 hours. Lateral, anterior-posterior, and open mouth (odontoid) radiographic views of the cervical spine are obtained. Anterior-posterior views of the thoracic or lumbar spine are obtained as needed. Serial neurologic assessments are performed to identify changes in neurologic function, such as level of sensation and movement resulting from increasing cord swelling.

Unconscious children with suspected SCI should remain in spinal protection until they are awake and able to complete a neurologic examination. Advanced diagnostic tests, such as magnetic resonance imaging and somatosensory evoked potentials, may be indicated to determine the presence or extent of SCI. Operative management may be required for children with unstable vertebral fractures or dislocations.

Complications or sequelae of SCI range from mild neurologic deficits to complete hemiplegia, paraplegia, or quadriplegia. Autonomic areflexia, bowel and bladder incontinence, and ventilator dependence occur relative to the level of the cord lesion. Rehabilitation assists the child to maximize his or her potential for recovery.

Thoracic Injuries

Thoracic injuries are the second leading cause of accidental death in the pediatric population, with the number of cases slightly less than those for traumatic brain injury.[39] Most thoracic injuries are caused by blunt trauma. In infants and young children, these injuries are usually caused by falls, whereas older children sustain these injuries as pedestrians or passengers in motor vehicles. Penetrating chest trauma is seen in adolescents as a result of violence—intentional or self-inflicted. Common thoracic injuries in the pediatric population are pulmonary contusion, hemothorax, and pneumothorax.[19]

Children are susceptible to transmission of blunt forces to underlying thoracic structures (heart, lungs, great vessels) because soft cartilage and developing bones make the thorax pliable.[19] Rib fractures should raise a high index of suspicion for severe blunt forces. Similarly, when flail segments are present, severe parenchymal pulmonary injury should be suspected.[19] The mediastinum is easily displaced by air or fluid. As the mediastinum shifts, venous return, cardiac output, and lung volume are severely compromised.[19]

Rib Fractures

Rib fractures are less common in the pediatric population compared with the adult population. This is attributed to the compliancy of a child's rib cage and the ability of the cartilaginous frame to absorb blunt force trauma more adequately than the older population. Infants and children with rib fractures should be closely evaluated for underlying organ injuries.[19] Flail segments lead to paradoxical chest wall movement during respiration. Changes in pulse oximetry and respiratory rate and effort may occur. Children should receive supplemental oxygen as needed and analgesics for pain relief. A chest radiograph is obtained to determine the location and extent of fractures. Evaluate carefully for spleen or liver injury with lower rib fractures. It is also imperative for the clinician to consider nonaccidental trauma in infants and children with rib fractures. It has been noted that children younger than age 3 years are found to have a correlation of nonaccidental trauma history with associated rib fractures.[40]

Pneumothorax and Hemothorax

Pneumothorax may be open, closed, or tension. The goal of treating pneumothorax injury is to restore optimal ventilation in a patient experiencing ventilation/perfusion mismatch due to bleeding, edema, or structural degradation.[19] Clinical signs and symptoms vary with severity of injury but can include respiratory distress, crepitus, decreased or absent breath sounds on the affected side, and anxiety. In a tension pneumothorax, these symptoms are combined with hypotension and tracheal deviation (a late sign) away from the affected side; jugular vein distention may be observed, although this sign is difficult to detect in young children with short necks.[19] A small percentage of the pediatric population sustaining blunt thoracic trauma is subject to pneumomediastinum. Although treatment of pneumomediastinum alone remains conservative, it is pertinent to rule out associated tracheobronchial and esophageal injuries, which require more aggressive interventions.[19]

Pneumothoraces are treated relative to severity. Chest radiographs confirm the presence of air in the pleural space as well as structural changes to lung anatomy.[19] Interventions directed toward restoring ventilation should not be delayed to complete imaging in a symptomatic patient. Children in no acute distress with a small pneumothorax receive supplemental oxygen and are observed for worsening symptoms. Large pneumothoraces/hemothoraces require chest tube placement. Tubes are usually inserted at the fourth intercostal space midaxillary line, attached to water seal drainage and suction. In tension pneumothoraces, needle decompression is the immediate treatment: a large IV catheter is inserted into the second intercostal space, midclavicular line, and left in place until a chest tube has been inserted. Needle decompression precedes chest radiograph because this situation is an immediate threat to life. After needle decompression, chest tubes are inserted and a chest radiograph is obtained. Similarly, in hemothoraces, chest radiographs may be delayed until chest tubes are inserted. Autotransfusion may be considered for these patients when there are no contraindications, such as enteric contamination or a wound more than 6 hours old. Surgical intervention is indicated for ongoing blood loss into the chest drainage system greater than 25% of the child's estimated circulating blood volume.[44] A local anesthetic, and preferably sedatives, should be administered before insertion of chest tubes.

Pulmonary Contusion

Pulmonary contusions are the most frequently diagnosed injury found in the pediatric population sustaining blunt force thoracic trauma.[20] Pulmonary contusions should be suspected in children with respiratory distress after blunt chest trauma without abnormal radiographic findings. Pulmonary contusion is usually not diagnosed until after hospital admission. Signs and symptoms include increasing respiratory distress, hemoptysis, and decreased pulmonary function.[20] Chest radiographs show changes from the initial film. Management of these patients in the ED begins with supplemental oxygen and pain management to support optimal respiratory effort. Endotracheal intubation and subsequent ventilation with positive end-expiratory pressure is usually reserved for severe injuries. Fluids may be limited if the child is not hypovolemic.[19]

Tracheobronchial Injury

Tracheobronchial rupture, although rare, can occur with blunt or penetrating forces to the neck and chest.[41] Up to one-third of traumatic tracheobronchial injuries are fatal within the first hour of occurrence. The child may exhibit respiratory distress, subcutaneous emphysema, and difficulty swallowing. Severe tracheobronchial rupture causes massive subcutaneous emphysema, persistent air leak, mediastinal air, tension pneumothorax, and failure of the lung to expand after chest tube insertion. Airway management with endotracheal intubation or tracheostomy is imperative. Chest tubes may also be required. Ongoing reassessment is essential in this fragile situation.[19]

Diaphragmatic Injury

Diaphragmatic rupture can occur after blunt trauma. In this case diminished breath sounds are auscultated (usually on the left side), bowel sounds are heard within the chest cavity, and significant respiratory distress is present. CT imaging often identifies injuries to the diaphragm that may be missed by plain films. Diaphragmatic rupture requires early identification, operative management, and repair—mortality increases with delayed identification and treatment.[19]

Cardiac Injury

In general, cardiac injuries are suspected in children with chest bruising, upper body cyanosis, unexplained hypotension, and dysrhythmias. Injuries include cardiac tamponade, blunt cardiac injury (formerly termed cardiac contusion), and great vessel injuries. Children with rib fractures and lung contusions must be evaluated for concomitant cardiac injuries.[19] Management of cardiac injuries includes initial and ongoing evaluations of ECGs.[19] Cardiac enzymes and echocardiographic studies are not recommended as routine diagnostic testing in the pediatric population.[19]

Abdominal Injuries

Blunt force is the most common cause of abdominal trauma in children, with subsequent hemorrhaging a common cause of traumatic death. Because of the child's smaller abdomen, injuries can occur to multiple organs.[28] The spleen is the most commonly injured abdominal organ in blunt trauma,[28] followed by the liver. Trauma can result from pedestrian MVCs, falls or forces applied to the abdomen, bicycles, and child maltreatment. Penetrating abdominal trauma usually results from acts of violence and require an emergent evaluation by a surgeon.[28] Penetrating injuries can be treated conservatively in hemodynamically stable children or by emergent laparotomy, depending on the clinical severity of the situation. The lap belt complex—small-bowel contusion/laceration, lumbar flexion-distraction injury (Chance fracture), and cutaneous bruising—may occur in restrained passengers in an MVC.[42]

The alert child who sustains abdominal trauma may complain of tenderness with palpation, may have tachypnea, and may exhibit signs of compensated shock.[28] Deep palpation should be avoided to prevent guarding. For young infants and toddlers, placing a warm hand on the abdomen for a few seconds before palpation may avoid startling or frightening the patient. Abdominal distention, abrasions, or contusions may be noted. Hypovolemic shock suggests internal hemorrhaging. CT is considered the gold standard and can identify injury to solid abdominal organs.[29]

Children with blunt abdominal trauma are treated according to their hemodynamic stability. A gastric tube (nasogastric tubes should be avoided in the child with TBI) is inserted to decompress the stomach and avoid aspiration. Serial CBCs are obtained to monitor for ongoing blood loss. A CT scan with contrast is used to determine the extent of injuries in the hemodynamically stable child. This test is preferred over a FAST examination in the pediatric population because of accuracy in detecting specific abdominal organ involvement and retroperitoneal injury. Diagnostic peritoneal lavage has fallen out of favor due to the reliability of CT and ultrasound screening.[29] Many injuries are treated conservatively with serial reevaluation; however, approximately 5% require surgical intervention for persistent hemorrhaging or peritonitis.[29] Embolization of extravasation visualized on CT in solid organs (liver and spleen) should be considered in hemodynamically stable children: however, successful nonoperative outcomes are seen in the majority of the cases.[43] The hemodynamically unstable child who does not respond to fluid and blood boluses must be prepared for immediate surgery.[29] The American Pediatric Surgery Association standardized management guidelines for solid-organ injury and favors nonoperative management in the pediatric population, reserving surgery for the most severe cases.[44]

Splenic injury is suspected in children with tenderness in the left upper quadrant. Pain in the left shoulder may be elicited with abdominal palpation (Kehr sign).[28] Splenic injury is suspected in children with altered level of consciousness, altered vital signs, low blood count, left lower rib fractures, abdominal pain, or grunting. Children with splenic injuries who are hemodynamically stable are admitted to the hospital and managed with bed rest and serial reevaluation. Hemodynamically unstable patients (those who are hypotensive even with fluid and blood administration) require an emergent surgical consult.[28]

Liver injuries are suspected in children who sustain any blunt force trauma to the abdomen. Right upper quadrant pain, tenderness, or diffuse pain are symptoms of liver injury.[28] Levels of serum aspartate aminotransferase and serum alanine aminotransferase are obtained and evaluated in consideration with clinical examination findings and imaging results to assess the seriousness of hepatic injury. Large liver lacerations cause significant blood loss and require immediate surgical repair, whereas smaller lacerations without signs of hypovolemia can be managed conservatively with serial abdominal examinations and timed hemoglobin level monitoring.[28]

Children sustaining pancreatic injuries can elicit vague abdominal pain cues such as pain that radiates to the back and persistent epigastric tenderness or vomiting[28]; however, it is not uncommon that these injuries are only noted several days after injury. Serum amylase and lipase levels are monitored, and the patient is hospitalized for further evaluation.

Intestinal injury is suspected in MVC passengers with abdominal bruising from the seat belt, bicycle riders who strike the handlebars, and those sustaining penetrating trauma. Pain can be the only symptom, but free air may be noted on radiographs in some patients. These patients require a CT scan, hospitalization, and observation for possible intestinal perforation and subsequent surgical repair. Intestinal perforation should be suspected in children with lap belt injuries. Delayed symptoms include fever, increasing pain, hypotension, and peritoneal signs.[44]

Genitourinary Injuries

Genitourinary injuries result from pedestrian or passenger MVCs, sports activities, falls, and all-terrain accidents.[21] Bladder and urethral injuries result mostly from blunt trauma and are often associated with pelvic fractures. Blunt and penetrating injuries to the kidneys and ureters also occur. Renal injuries may be minor or so severe that surgical intervention is necessary.

Renal Injury

Renal injury should be considered in children sustaining blunt abdominal trauma. The kidney is the most frequently damaged organ in the pediatric population who have sustained blunt trauma. This is due to the location where the kidneys rest in the abdomen and the lack of protection the abdomen offers in this age-group.[21] In such cases, there may be direct flank trauma or rapid deceleration forces, crushing the kidney against the rib cage or vertebral column. Symptoms of renal trauma include abdominal, back, or flank tenderness. The awake, stable child may be able to provide a urine specimen by voiding spontaneously, or an indwelling bladder catheter can be inserted to measure urine output and obtain urine specimens for testing. A catheter should not be passed in suspected urethral trauma. Hematuria is an important indicator of both severe and nonsevere renal injury, with the degree of hematuria correlating with a higher risk for renal injury. Hematuria may also occur without substantial renal injury resulting from capillary disruption after blunt force trauma. In the presence of gross hematuria, CT scan of the abdomen is indicated because there is an association between gross hematuria and severe intraabdominal injury.[21] Bedside urine screening may be performed to identify blood in the urine. Urinalysis testing with a threshold of more than 50 red blood cells (RBCs) per high-power field (hpf) indicates the need for further genitourinary tract evaluation.[21]

A CT scan with contrast dye is usually obtained. Treatment is specialized relative to the type of injury and may range from observation and bed rest to surgical exploration for patients. Hemodynamic stability, not imaging studies, ultimately guides the surgical team's decision-making process.[21]

Ureteral Injury

Ureteral injuries are rare, so recognition may be delayed unless the possibility for this injury is entertained.[45] Hematuria or urinary leak may present as a flank mass; iliac pain may be present. Symptoms may not be noted until 7 to 10 days after the initial injury. Urine may appear at entrance or exit wounds or on a surgical dressing. If no wound is present, signs of retroperitoneal abscess such as chills, fever, lower abdominal pain, palpable mass, pyuria, and frequency may occur. Surgical repair is indicated for ureteral injuries, with a ureteral stent required in some patients.

Bladder Injury

Symptoms of bladder injuries vary with sustained injury. Suprapubic tenderness, urgency to void, inability to void, hematuria, and palpable abdominal mass may be observed with a ruptured bladder. Children with an extraperitoneal rupture may be able to pass small amounts of sanguineous urine but with significant discomfort. If severe hemorrhaging is present, signs of shock are observed. Most bladder contusions are minor and managed conservatively with observation and reevaluation. Large extraperitoneal injuries and intraperitoneal bladder ruptures with pelvic fractures necessitate surgical intervention for most patients.[46]

Urethral Injury

Urethral injury should be suspected in patients with vaginal bleeding; penile, scrotal, perineal, and prostate trauma; or the inability to advance an indwelling bladder catheter.[46] No attempt should be made to insert a urinary bladder catheter when there is blood at the meatus because the child may have a partial urethral tear. Inserting a catheter may convert a partial tear to a complete tear. Urethrography is indicated with cystography, and CT cystography/CT scan of the abdomen and pelvis may be performed for some patients.[46] Partial urethral tears are managed conservatively with a suprapubic catheter or an indwelling urethral catheter inserted under fluoroscopy. Complete urethral tears require surgical repair.

Genital Injuries

Injuries to female genitalia can result from falls, straddle type of injuries (e.g., falls on monkey bars, chairs), and sexual abuse or assault. Testicular trauma can also result from straddle type of injuries. The most common cause of penile injuries is direct forces such as zipper injuries and trauma from toilet seats.[47] Infants can sustain a tourniquet injury from threads, bands, rings, or human hair lodged in the coronal groove, which forms a constricting ring and lacerates the penile shaft. Sexual abuse must be considered in any child with genital trauma, particularly when injuries are inconsistent with the history. In children with suspected sexual abuse or assault, proper evidence collection is critical (see Chapter 49).

Musculoskeletal Injuries

Musculoskeletal injuries are common occurrences in the pediatric population. Long-bone fractures occur from falls, sports activities, and motor vehicle and pedestrian crashes. Strong ligaments account for the prevalence of fractures rather than ligamentous injury.

The most unique feature of the child's musculoskeletal system is the epiphyseal growth plate (physis) located at the articulating ends of bones between the epiphysis and metaphysis. The epiphyseal growth plate is responsible for longitudinal bone growth; therefore injury can cause growth disturbance or arrest.[48] In general, growth is completed in boys by age 16 years and in girls by 14 years of age. If a patient has tenderness along the physis concurrent with examination, the provider

TABLE 42.4 **Salter-Harris Classification, Fracture Descriptions, and Outcome**

Type	Description of Fractures	Treatment and Outcome
Type I	Horizontal separation of epiphysis and metaphysis; point tenderness; radiographs may be normal; mild soft-tissue swelling produced by shearing forces	No disturbance in growth if properly diagnosed; favorable prognosis; treated with closed reduction and casting
Type II	Separation of epiphysis and metaphysis with some avulsion of the metaphysis produced by shearing forces	No disturbance in growth if properly diagnosed; favorable prognosis; treated with closed reduction and casting
Type III	Produced by intraarticular shearing forces; intraarticular fracture; fracture extends through epiphyseal plate into the metaphysis	Angular deformities may occur; requires good reduction; variable-poor prognosis
Type IV	Fracture starts at the articular surface and extends through the epiphysis, epiphyseal plate, and metaphysis; intraarticular fracture produced by shearing forces	Open reduction and external fixation is needed; variable-poor prognosis; angular deformity may result
Type V	Epiphyseal plate is crushed without fracture or displacement; radiographic diagnosis virtually impossible; produced by crushing force	Poor prognosis, even when correctly identified and treated

From Bernardo LM, Trunzo R. Pediatric trauma. In: Kitt S, Selfridge-Thomas J, Proehl J, et al, eds. *Emergency Nursing: A Physiologic and Clinical Perspective.* 2nd ed. Philadelphia, PA: Saunders; 1995.

should consider the injury to be a fracture versus a sprain in this population.[48] Growth plate fractures are categorized with the Salter-Harris classification (Table 42.4).

Signs of musculoskeletal trauma include point tenderness; soft-tissue swelling; discoloration; limitations in range of motion; loss of function; altered sensory perception; and changes in pulses, temperature, or capillary refill distal to the injury.[48] Administering analgesics should be considered to help ease the child's pain. An obvious deformity may be noted, or an actual open fracture may be observed. The child may complain of pain and splint the injured extremity by holding the broken arm with the other hand, for example.

Musculoskeletal trauma is rarely life-threatening, so the child's airway, breathing, circulation, and neurologic status are usually intact. The injured extremity is elevated, and ice is applied. A splint or sling and swath can be applied if neurovascular status is assessed before and after splint application. A sterile dressing is applied to any open fracture. Prophylactic antibiotics are given for open fractures, and tetanus prophylaxis is administered as needed. Analgesia is required during splinting and during any reduction measures.

Radiographs of the anteroposterior and lateral views of the injured extremity should be obtained.[49] Comparative views of the injured and uninjured extremities may be obtained, although they are not usually necessary.[49] Child maltreatment should be investigated in nonambulatory children with fractures, toddlers with femur fractures, young children with multiple fractures, fractures with different stages of healing, or in circumstances in which the injury does not match the history. A complete skeletal film should be obtained on infants and toddlers when the provider suspects nonaccidental trauma.[49]

Most children require a simple cast when the fracture is nondisplaced. Casting may be performed in the ED or deferred until swelling has subsided. The injury may be stabilized in a splint or fiberglass mold. Parents or guardians are given discharge instructions to observe for swelling of the toes or fingers, odor from the cast/splint/mold, and changes in skin color and temperature. Parents should contact the ED with any of these complaints or if the child complains of sharp pain or numbness.

Displaced fractures require manipulation to realign the fractured bone(s). In such situations, the ED physician or orthopedic surgeon may attempt closed reduction in the ED. Procedural sedation is administered using analgesics and sedatives such as midazolam, fentanyl, or ketamine. The nurse must carefully monitor the child throughout the procedure for adverse effects of the sedation. After the fracture is reduced, sedatives are stopped, the cast/splint/mold is applied, and postreduction radiographs are obtained. If reduction is not successful, the child may require open reduction and internal fixation in the operating room.

Treatment for femoral fractures varies with age. Infants are placed in spica casts, often in the ED. Reamed- and nonreamed-intramedullary rodding used in older children allows early mobilization. Tibial skeletal traction, external fixation, and plating techniques are also used depending on the type of fracture and the child's age. Children with pelvic fractures require admission to the hospital and subsequent bed rest and weight-bearing limitations.[50] Older children with unstable pelvic fractures may require surgical fixation.[50]

SUMMARY

Pediatric trauma patients provide a unique challenge for the emergency nurse. The ability to identify potentially life-threatening conditions is essential. Emergency nurses are in a unique position to offer anticipatory guidance to families concerning primary injury prevention.

Becoming actively involved in trauma prevention and safety education is another opportunity for emergency nurses to promote safety through education, engineering, and enforcement strategies. Educating parents and children during ED visits using posters, pamphlets, one-on-one discussions, and videos provides families with opportunities for discussion with nurses and with each other regarding their safety practices. Volunteer to speak with students and parent-teacher groups about safety on such topics as wearing bicycle helmets, practicing firearm safety, or wearing safety belts.

Engineering efforts include becoming a car seat safety inspector with the National Safe Kids Campaign to check proper installation and security of car safety seats. Write to manufacturers to express concerns about product safety. Report unsafe products or patients injured by products to the Consumer Product Safety Commission.

Enforcement includes promoting safety laws in one's community. Become politically aware and support legislators who favor legislation aimed at reducing injuries (e.g., mandatory bicycle, motorcycle, and skateboard helmet use). Educate legislators and government officials about unsafe road conditions, traffic problems, and other community hazards that may cause injuries in children.

Emergency nurses can become involved in organizations such as the National Safe Kids Campaign and the Emergency Nurses Association's Injury Prevention Institute. Emergency nurses can minimize the effects of pediatric trauma by providing high-quality patient care to injured children and their families. Participating in injury prevention activities helps reduce the incidence of pediatric trauma and enhances the professional image of nursing.

REFERENCES

1. Corrado MM, Shi J, Wheeler KK, et al. Original contribution: emergency medical services (EMS) versus non-EMS transport among injured children in the United States. *Am J Emerg Med*. 2017;35:475–478. https://doi.org/10.1016/j.ajem.2016.11.059.
2. Flynn-O'Brien K, Fallat ME, Rice TB, et al. Pediatric trauma assessment and management database: leveraging existing data systems to predict mortality and functional status after pediatric injury. *J Am Coll Surg*. 2017vol. 224(5):933–944.
3. Tracy ET, Englum BR, Barbas AS, Foley C, Rice HE, Shapiro ML. Pediatric injury patterns by year of age. *J Pediatr Surg*. 2013;48:1384–1388. https://doi.org/10.1016/j.jpedsurg.2013.03.041.
4. Schaechter J, Alvarez PG. Growing up – or not – with gun violence. *Pediatr Clin North Am*. 2016;63:813–826. https://doi.org/10.1016/j.pcl.2016.06.004.
5. Traffic safety facts 2016 data. Retrieved September 24, 2018 from http://www.nhtsa.gov.
6. Leonard JC, Mao J, Jaffe DM. Potential adverse effects of spinal immobilization in children. *Prehosp Emerg Care*. 2012;16(4);513–518. https://doi.org/10.3109/10903127.2012.689925.
7. National Highway Traffic Safety Administration. Car seats and booster seats. Retrieved on October 3, 2018 from: https://www.nhtsa.gov/equipment/car-seats-and-booster-seats#age-size-rec.
8. Dennis R. Durbin, Benjamin D. Hoffman, Child Passenger Safety: COUNCIL ON INJURY, VIOLENCE, AND POISON PREVENTION Pediatrics Aug 2018, e20182460; https://doi.org/10.1542/peds.2018-2460
9. *Graduated drivers licensing programs reduce fata teen crashes, November 4, 2011*, National Institutes of Health. Retrieved October 3, 2018 from https://www.nih.gov/news-events/news-releases/graduated-drivers-licensing-programs-reduce-fatal-teen-crashes.
10. Committee on Injury and Poison Prevention. All-terrain vehicle injury prevention: two-, three-, and four-wheeled unlicensed motor vehicles. *Pediatrics*. 2000;105:1352.
11. Durbin DR, Hoffman BD. Child passenger safety. *Pediatrics*. 2018. https://doi.org/10.1542/peds.2018-2460.
12. KidsAndCars.org database. Retrieved October 3, 2018 from http://www.kidsandcars.org/wp-content/uploads/2018/05/National-Stats-Table-5-8-18.png .
13. Embree TE, Romanow NTR, Djerboua MS, Morgunov NJ, Bourdeaux JJ, Hagel BE. Risk factors for bicycling injuries in children and adolescents: a systematic review. *Pediatrics*. 2016;138(5). https://search.ebscohost.com/login.aspx?direct=true&db=mdc&AN=27940760&site=eds-live&scope=site. Accessed October 12, 2018.
14. Duncan P, Hagan J. *Maximizing Children's Health: Screening, Anticipatory Guidance and Counseling*. Nelson Textbook of Pediatrics. 20th ed. Chapter 5, 2016;37–47.
15. American Fischer, SJ. American Academy of Orthopedic Surgeons. Skateboarding Safety - January 2018. Retrieved October 3, 2018 from https://orthoinfo.aaos.org/en/staying-healthy/skateboarding-safety
16. Pool or Spa Submersion: Estimated Non-Fatal Drowning Injuries and Reported Drownings, 2018 Report. Retrieved on October 3, 2018 from https://www.poolsafely.gov/2018
17. Kenefake ME, Swarm M, Walthall J. Nuances in pediatric trauma. *Emerg Med Clin North Am*. 2013;31:627–652. https://doi.org/10.1016/j.emc.2013.04.004.
18. *Trauma Nursing Core Course Provider Manual*. 7th ed. Des Plaines, IL: Emergency Nurses Association; 2014.
19. Reynolds SL. Pediatric thoracic trauma. Recognition and management. *Emerg Med Clin North Am*. 2018;36:473–483. https://doi.org/10.1016/j.emc.2017.12.013 19-4.
20. Mikrogianakis A, Grant V. The Kids are alright. Pediatric trauma pearls. *Emerg Med Clin North Am*. 2018;36:237–257. https://doi.org/10.1016/j.emc.2017.08.015.

21. Ishida Yuichi, Tyroch Alan H, Emami Nader, McLean Susan F. Characteristics and management of blunt renal injury in children. Journal of Emergencies, Trauma and Shock. 2017;10(3):140–145. https://doi.org/10.4103/JETS.JETS-pass:[_]93_16.
22. Rosendahl K, Strouse PJ. Sports injury of the pediatric musculoskeletal system. *La Radiologia Medica*. 2016;121(5):431–441. https://doi.org/10.1007/s11547-015-0615-0.
23. Hamer DH, Lunze K. Thermal Protection of the Newborn in resource-limited Environments. *J Perinatol*. May 2012;32(5):317–324.
24. Walls R, Murphy M. *Manual of Emergency Airway Management*. Phildelphia, PA: Wolters Kluwer Health; 2012.
25. Canzian S, Glenn M, Henn R, et al. *Advanced Trauma Care for Nurses*. Lexington, KY: edition. Society of Trauma Nurses; 2013.
26. Cunningham A, Auerbach M, Cicero M, Jafri M. Tourniquet usage in prehospital care and resuscitation of pediatric trauma patients-Pediatric Trauma Society position statement. *The Journal Of Trauma And Acute Care Surgery*. 2018;85(4):665–667. https://doi.org/10.1097/TA.0000000000001839.
27. Gilley M, Beno S. Damage control resuscitation in pediatric trauma. *Curr Opin Pediatr*. 2013;30(3):338–343.
28. Rosen's Emergency Medicine: Concepts and Clinical Practice 9th ed.
29. Lynch T, Kilgar J, Al Shibli A. Pediatric abdominal trauma. *Curr Pediatr Rev*. 2018;14(1):59–63. https://doi.org/10.2174/1573396313666170815100547.
30. Kannan N, Ramaiah R, Vavilala MS. Pediatric neurotrauma. *Int J Crit Illn Inj Sci*. 2014;4(2):131. https://search.ebscohost.com/login.aspx?direct=true&db=edb&AN=96545995&site=eds-live&scope=site. Accessed October 2, 2018.
31. Pinto PS, Poretti A, Meoded A, Tekes A, Huisman TAGM. The unique features of traumatic brain injury in children. Review of the characteristics of the pediatric skull and brain, mechanisms of trauma, patterns of injury, complications and their imaging findings--part 1. *J Neuroimaging*. 2012;22(2):e1–e17. https://doi.org/10.1111/j.1552-6569.2011.00688.x.
32. Bressan S, Marchetto L, Lyons TW, et al. A systematic review and meta-analysis of the management and outcomes of isolated skull fractures in children. *Ann Emerg Med*. 2018;71(6):714–724.
33. Streubel S-O, Mirsky DM. Craniomaxillofacial Trauma. *Facial Plast Surg Clin North Am*. 2016;24:605–617. https://doi.org/10.1016/j.fsc.2016.06.014.
34. American Academy of Pediatric Dentistry. *Guideline on Management of Acute Dental Trauma*; 2011. http://www.aapd.org/media/Policies_Guidelines/G_trauma.pdf.
35. Gopinathan NR, Viswanathan VK, Crawford AH. Cervical spine evaluation in pediatric trauma: a review and an update of current concepts. *Indian J Orthop*. 2018;52(5):489. https://search.ebscohost.com/login.aspx?direct=true&db=edb&AN=131650863&site=eds-live&scope=site. Accessed October 2, 2018.
36. Knox J. Epidemiology of spinal cord injury without radiographic abnormality in children: a nationwide perspective. *J Childs Orthop*. 2016;10(3):255. https://search.ebscohost.com/login.aspx?direct=true&db=edb&AN=116170475&site=eds-live&scope=site. Accessed October 12, 2018.
37. McLaughlin C, Zagory JA, Fenlon M, et al. Basic Science: timing of mortality in pediatric trauma patients: a National Trauma Data Bank analysis. *J Pediatr Surg*. 2018;53:344–351. https://doi.org/10.1016/j.jpedsurg.2017.10.006.
38. Caruso MC, Daugherty MC, Moody SM, Falcone Jr RA, Bierbrauer KS, Geis GL. Lessons learned from administration of high-dose methylprednisolone sodium succinate for acute pediatric spinal cord injuries. *J Neurosurg Pediatr*. 2017;20(6):567–574. https://doi.org/10.3171/2017.7.PEDS1756.
39. Tovar JA, Vazquez JJ. Management of chest trauma in children. *Paediatr Respir Rev*. 2013;14(2):86–91. https://doi.org/10.1016/j.prrv.2013.02.011.
40. Darling SE, Done SL, Friedman SD, Feldman KW. Frequency of intrathoracic injuries in children younger than 3 years with rib fractures. *Pediatr Radiol*. 2014;44(10):1230–1236. https://doi.org/10.1007/s00247-014-2988-y.
41. Shemmeri E, Vallières E. Blunt tracheobronchial trauma. *Thorac Surg Clin*. 2018;28:429–434. https://doi.org/10.1016/j.thorsurg.2018.04.008.
42. Schonfeld D, Lee LK. Blunt abdominal trauma in children. *Curr Opin Pediatr*. 2012;24(3):314–318. https://doi.org/10.1097/MOP.0b013e328352de97.
43. Notrica DM, Linnaus ME. Nonoperative management of blunt solid organ injury in pediatric surgery. *Surg Clin North Am*. 2017;97:1–20. https://doi.org/10.1016/j.suc.2016.08.001.
44. Deleted as per review
45. K.P. Debbink, D.B. Tashjian, M.V. Tirabassi, R. Gaffey, J. Nahmias. Ureteric transection secondary to penetrating handlebar injury. Trauma Case Reports, Vol. 10, Iss , Pp 16-18 (2017). 2017;(16-18):16. https://doi.org/10.1016/j.tcr.2017.07.002.
46. Lumen N, Kuehhas FE, Djakovic N, et al. Guidelines: review of the current management of lower urinary tract injuries by the EAU trauma guidelines panel. *Eur Urol*. 2015;67:925–929. https://doi.org/10.1016/j.eururo.2014.12.035.
47. Tasian GE, Bagga HS, Fisher PB, et al. Pediatric Urology: pediatric genitourinary injuries in the United States from 2002 to 2010. *The Journal of Urology*. 2013;189:288–294. https://doi.org/10.1016/j.juro.2012.09.003.
48. Thornton MD, Della-Giustina K, Aronson PL. Emergency department evaluation and treatment of pediatric orthopedic injuries. *Emerg Med Clin North Am*. 2015;33:423–449. https://doi.org/10.1016/j.emc.2014.12.012.
49. Ho-Fung VM, Zapala MA, Lee EY. Musculoskeletal traumatic injuries in children. characteristic imaging findings and mimickers. *Radiol Clin North Am*. 2017;55:785–802. https://doi.org/10.1016/j.rcl.2017.02.011.
50. Sawyer, J. and Spence, D: Fractures and Dislocations in Children. Campbell's Operative Orthopaedics. 13th Ed. Chapter 36, 2017;1423–1569.
51. Kaushik R, Krisch IM, Schroeder DR, Flick R, Nemergut ME. Pediatric bicycle-related head injuries: a population-based study in a county without a helmet law. *Inj Epidemiol*. 2015;2(1):16. https://doi.org/10.1186/s40621-015-0048-1

FURTHER READING

McLean S, Tyroch A. Abdominal Trauma in Pediatric Critical Care. *Pediatr Crit Care*. 2017. Chapter 21 1644-1654 5th ed.

Liller KD: Unintentional Injuries in children, APHA 2006, 2006. Retrieved September 2, 2007, from http://www.medscape.com/viewarticle/553273?rss.

Ludwig S. Resuscitation—pediatric basic and advanced life support. In: Fleisher G, Ludwig S, eds. *Textbook of Pediatric Emergency Medicine*. 4th ed. Philadelphia: Lippincott Williams & Wilkins; 2000.

Moulton S. Early management of the child with multiple injuries. *Clin Orthop Relat Res*. 2000;376(6).

Partrick D, Bensard D, Moore E, et al. Driveway crush injuries in young children: a highly lethal, devastating, and potentially preventable event. *J Pediatr Surg*. 1998;33:1712.

Dietrich A, Shaner S, Campbell J. *Pediatric Basic Trauma Life Support*. Oakbrook Terrace, Ill: Basic Trauma Life Support International; 2002.

43

Obstetric Trauma

Terri McGowan Repasky

The actual incidence of obstetric trauma is unknown; however, it has been estimated that injuries complicate 1 in 12 pregnancies.[1,2] In women of childbearing age, trauma is the leading cause of maternal death from nonobstetric causes. Most obstetric trauma involves minor injury to the mother. Severity of injury is the major predictive factor of maternal death,[3,4] yet minor trauma may account for up to 50% of fetal deaths.[5] Priorities for the pregnant and nonpregnant trauma patient are the same; however, interventions are intended to benefit two patients: the mother and the fetus.

Like their nonpregnant counterparts, pregnant patients sustain blunt, penetrating, burn, and submersion injuries as well as toxic exposures. Blunt trauma is the most common, often due to motor vehicle crashes (MVCs), falls, and assaults.[1,3,4,6] Even low-speed MVCs can result in significant trauma. Pregnant women are more likely to experience violent intentional trauma.[4] The most common form of intentional trauma is domestic or intimate partner violence, which increases with advancing gestational age.[1,6,7] One source reported that trauma from domestic violence is the most frequently reported mechanism of trauma in pregnant women.[8] Overexertion and instability may also lead to injuries during pregnancy.

Most maternal deaths from trauma are secondary to head injury or hemorrhagic shock. Fetal morbidity and mortality are usually related to direct and indirect consequences of maternal trauma, although direct fetal injury may occur. Pelvic fracture is the most common maternal injury that results in fetal death. Placental abruption and premature delivery are the most common trauma-related causes of fetal demise.

Primary and secondary assessment and initial nursing priorities for the pregnant trauma patient are essentially the same as for a nonpregnant patient. The best initial treatment of the fetus is to provide optimal resuscitation of the mother;[6,7,9] however, anatomic and physiologic differences related to the gravid state must be considered during all stages of the trauma nursing process.

ANATOMY AND PHYSIOLOGY

Pregnancy alters anatomic relationships of organs and causes major physiologic changes involving nearly every organ system in the body. Normal respiratory and circulatory changes during pregnancy can mask the typical signs and symptoms that emergency nurses rely on to guide care of a trauma patient. Attaining the optimal outcome for the mother and the fetus depends on a sound knowledge of maternal anatomy and physiology and implications for interventions.

Uterine

Uterine size and blood flow are a concern in the gravid trauma patient. The uterus enlarges from a 7-cm and 70-g structure to a 36-cm and 1100-g walled organ (similar in size and weight to a bowling ball). As the uterus grows, its wall becomes thinner. Through the first 12 weeks of pregnancy, the uterus remains a small, self-contained intrapelvic organ protected from abdominal injury by the bony pelvis.[7] After 12 weeks, the uterus becomes an intraabdominal organ as it enlarges and ascends, encroaching on the peritoneal cavity and confining the intestines to the upper abdomen. Fig. 43.1 shows the uterine size for various gestational periods. During the second trimester the uterus is susceptible to abdominal injury, although the fetus remains small and relatively cushioned by large amounts of amniotic fluid. By the third trimester, the uterus is large and thin walled. During the last 2 to 8 weeks' gestation, the fetus descends and the fetal head engages in the pelvis. The fetus occupies most of the intrauterine and abdominal space when the head becomes fixed in the pelvis. Maternal pelvic fractures during this trimester may be associated with fetal skull fractures, intracranial hemorrhage, and significant maternal blood loss.

Uteroplacental blood flow increases from a baseline of about 60 mL/min to close to 1000 mL/min during the third trimester.[9] Uterine blood flow has no autoregulation and depends solely on maternal perfusion pressure. Uterine veins may dilate up to 60 times their prepregnant state; uterine injury may be a major source of blood loss. In response to trauma, maternal catecholamines are released by the sympathetic nervous system and cause uteroplacental constriction, which shunts blood to the mother and away from the fetus and leads to fetal distress. By the third trimester, vessels of the uterus and the placenta have reached maximum vasodilatation and cannot increase blood flow in response to decreased perfusion.

Cardiovascular

Anatomically, the heart is elevated and rotated forward by the ascending diaphragm and pushed up by the enlarging uterus. This cardiac displacement causes a 15- to 20-degree left axis deviation that is considered a normal change of pregnancy. An ECG may also show a flattened or inverted T wave in lead III and Q waves in III and aV_F. Ectopic beats are also common during pregnancy.[3,7]

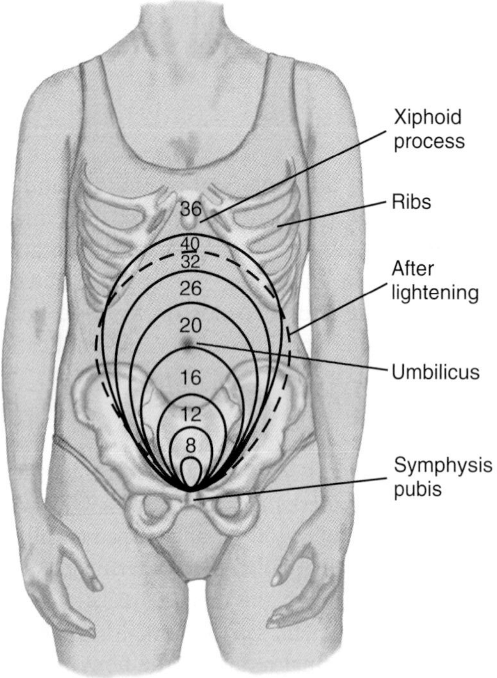

Fig. 43.1 Uterine Growth Patterns During Pregnancy. (From Murray SS, McKinney ES. *Foundations of Maternal-Newborn Nursing.* 4th ed. Philadelphia, PA: Saunders; 2006.)

Cardiovascular physiology is profoundly altered during pregnancy. Maternal blood volume increases by the 10th week of gestation and increases 40% to 50% by the 28th week, remaining at that level until delivery. Uteroplacental blood flow increases to almost 1000 mL/min by the end of pregnancy. Increased blood flow and volume increase maternal cardiac output significantly.

Blood flow may be compromised by compression from the gravid uterus and the fetus when the mother is in a supine position. Both the aorta and the inferior vena cava may be compressed as early as 12 to 14 weeks of gestation, leading to decreased cardiac return and increased afterload.[9] After approximately 20 weeks' gestation, cardiac output can significantly decrease owing to this compression. This event is referred to as inferior vena cava syndrome or supine hypotensive syndrome. Compression of the vena cava by the uterus/fetus may decrease cardiac output by 25% to 30% and systolic blood pressure by 30 mm Hg. Sequestering blood in the venous system and deceasing preload may decrease perfusion to the uterus; when maternal systolic blood pressure is below 80 mm Hg, the uterus and the fetus will not be perfused. Displacing the gravid uterus to the side by placing the pregnant patient in a lateral decubitus position or with manual uterine displacement reverses aortocaval compression (Fig. 43.2). Maternal resting heart rate increases until the second trimester and remains 10 to 20 beats/min above baseline for the duration of the pregnancy. Systolic and diastolic blood pressures decrease in the first trimester, reach their lowest levels in the second trimester, then rise toward prepregnancy levels during the final 2 months of gestation. A decrease of

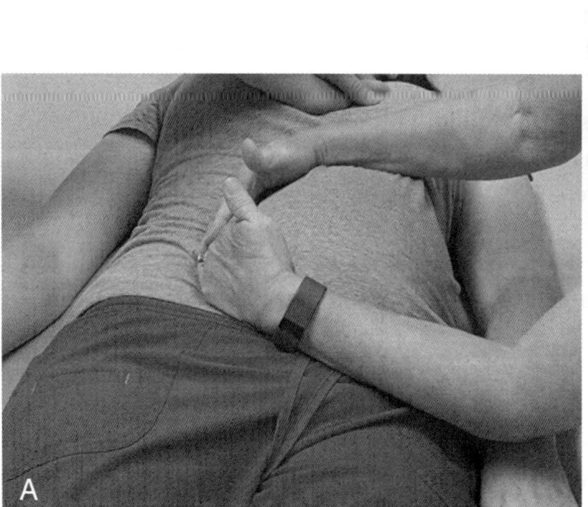

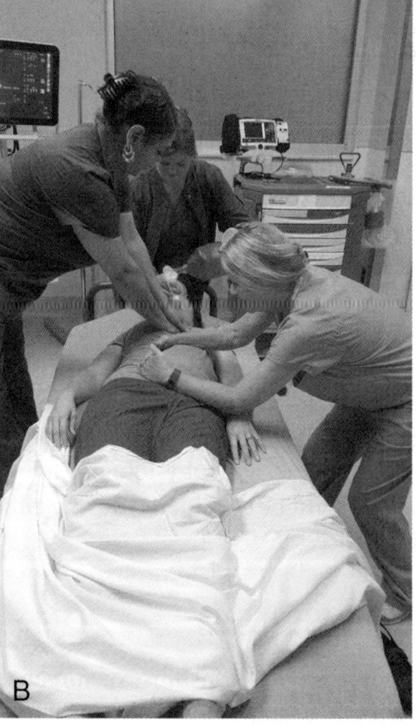

Fig. 43.2 Photo of Manual Displacement of Uterus.

15 mm Hg for systolic and diastolic pressure is normal in the second trimester.[7]

Hemodynamic measurements and assessments may be misleading. Signs of shock such as tachycardia and hypotension may be normal physiologic changes of pregnancy. Conversely, "normal" findings may mask an underlying shock state. Hypervolemia of pregnancy enables a woman to tolerate acute blood loss of 10% to 15% or gradual loss of 30% to 40% (~1500 mL) without a change in vital signs.[9] The pregnant patient may lose a significant amount of circulating blood volume before a significant drop in blood pressure occurs. Gravid women in shock may not have the cool, clammy skin typical of shock because of maternal vasodilatation during the first and second trimester.

Vasoconstriction in response to stress occurs predominantly in the third trimester. Pregnant patients with a heart rate over 100 beats per minute should be carefully assessed for causes of the tachycardia and possible hypovolemic shock.[5,10] Signs of fetal distress may be the first indication of maternal hypovolemia. Uterine hypoperfusion and fetal hypoxia can occur before evidence of maternal shock.[8-10] Catecholamine release, caused by maternal hypovolemia, leads to vasoconstriction of peripheral and uterine vascular beds and shunting of blood to vital maternal organs. A 15% to 30% reduction of uterine blood flow can occur without obvious change in maternal blood pressure. Signs of fetal distress include fetal bradycardia, fetal tachycardia, and decreased or increased fetal movement. The nurse should monitor fetal heart rate (FHR) and maternal urinary output as indicators of perfusion along with maternal pulse and blood pressure.[10]

Hematologic

Cautious interpretation of laboratory values is required. Dilutional anemia in pregnancy is caused by the disproportionate increase of plasma volume relative to erythrocyte volume. Dilutional states can decrease the hematocrit level to the low 30% range and reduce hemoglobin to 11.0 g/dL.[7,10] Platelet levels may be normal or slightly decreased. Physiologic leukocytosis occurs during the second and third trimesters. An increase in white blood cells of 15,000/mm^3 may occur by term and rise even higher during stress or labor. Sedimentation rate also increases during pregnancy. These increased levels may mask or falsely indicate an infectious process.

Fibrinogen levels start to rise in the third month and double by term; levels greater than 200 are desirable.[3] The average fibrinogen level in pregnancy is 450 mg/dL.[10] Normal fibrinogen levels may indicate early disseminated intravascular coagulopathy (DIC).[3,7,10] An increase in clotting factors VII, VIII, IX, X, and XII produces hypercoagulability and increased thromboembolic risk. Deep vein thrombosis and pulmonary embolism are a significant risk, especially when the gravid woman is inactive. The pregnant woman who sustains trauma is at a high risk for DIC if placental abruption or amniotic fluid embolism occur; DIC should be suspected if fibrinogen levels are less than 100 mg/dL.[3,7]

Pulmonary/Respiratory

Significant anatomic and physiologic alterations occur in the pulmonary system during pregnancy. Capillary engorgement of the mucosal lining of the respiratory tract predisposes gravid women to nosebleeds and airway obstruction. Complications of pregnancy such as pregnancy-induced hypertension (PIH) and gestational diabetes exacerbate normal airway engorgement, making intubation more difficult. The gravid uterus leads to diaphragmatic elevation, flaring of the ribs, and decreased residual capacity.[9] Reduction is associated with increased maternal oxygen consumption and diminished oxygen reserve. Respiratory rates will increase. Arterial oxygen pressure (PaO_2) levels increase to 101 to 108 mm Hg.[2,5] Arterial carbon dioxide pressure ($Paco_2$) levels decrease to 25 to 30 mm Hg by the end of the second trimester and remain at this level until delivery. It is important to recognize that a $Paco_2$ of 35 to 40 may indicate impending respiratory failure.[7]

The maternal respiratory center is especially sensitive to minute changes in $Paco_2$ levels. Although normal arterial and venous pH levels are maintained because of increased renal excretion of bicarbonate, partially compensated respiratory alkalosis occurs during pregnancy, making the pregnant patient less able to cope with respiratory distress and acidosis associated with trauma. A diminished maternal oxygen reserve makes the gravid uterus and fetus vulnerable to hypoxia. Because maternal hypoxia affects fetal oxygenation, fetal compromise may occur with minimal maternal distress. FHR changes are frequently the first indicator of maternal hypoxia. Maternal trauma may require blood gas analysis to determine hypoxia and acidosis. Adequate maternal oxygenation may require early intubation. Caution should be used owing to increased risk of edema and aspiration.[3,9,10]

Gastrointestinal/Abdominal

Various anatomic and physiologic gastrointestinal (GI) and abdominal changes occur during pregnancy. The small bowel is pushed up into the upper abdomen by the uterus, and the large bowel moves posteriorly. Diminished bowel sounds may be a normal finding in pregnancy or indicate intraperitoneal injury. The spleen and the liver are displaced upward toward the rib cage and are thus at increased risk from blunt trauma. Stretching of the abdominal wall due to uterine growth can impair maternal sensitivity to peritoneal irritation; muscle guarding, rigidity, or rebound tenderness may be dulled or absent.[10]

Increased progesterone and estrogen affect the GI tract, reducing motility and tone and relaxing the gastric sphincter. Gastric emptying may be delayed, and gastroesophageal reflux occurs frequently. The lower esophageal sphincter is displaced into the thorax. These changes along with increased intraabdominal pressure increase the risk of aspiration. As with all trauma patients, the pregnant patient is always considered to have a full stomach.

Genitourinary

Maternal susceptibility to traumatic bladder injury increases as the bladder moves from a pelvic organ to an intraabdominal position by 12 weeks' gestation. Urinary frequency increases in the third trimester secondary to uterine compression of the bladder. Dilation of the ureters, renal calyces, and the pelvis from compression by the ovarian plexus can result in urinary stasis. Renal blood flow is increased by about 40% and glomerular filtration rate increases, causing a decrease in blood urea nitrogen and creatinine. Glycosuria is common.[7,9]

Musculoskeletal

The pelvis becomes more flexible during pregnancy in preparation for fetal delivery. Hormonal changes loosen ligaments of the symphysis pubis and sacroiliac joints. By 7 months' gestation, there is considerable widening of the pelvis. Practitioners must consider these changes when interpreting x-rays of the pelvis. An unsteady gait, usually caused by the widening pelvis and heavy abdomen, predisposes the gravid female to falls. Pelvic fractures may be associated with massive retroperitoneal bleeding, even more so than in the nonpregnant patient.

Neurologic

Changes in the central nervous system (CNS) related to pregnancy are abnormal findings. Altered mentation, seizures, and hypertension may indicate traumatic head injury, eclampsia, or both. PIH, formerly referred to as preeclampsia, may occur after 20 to 24 weeks' gestation and is characterized by hypertension, proteinuria, hyperreflexia, and peripheral edema. The CNS irritability associated with PIH can lead to seizures (eclampsia). Increased intracranial pressure associated with traumatic head injury can also lead to seizures. Hypoxia from seizure activity, whether it be from PIH or head injury, places the mother and the fetus at risk. PIH must be differentiated from head injury; thus meticulous neurologic assessment of the pregnant trauma patient is essential.

Endocrine

The pituitary gland doubles in size and weight by term, requiring a greater blood supply. Hypoperfusion causes ischemia and can lead to pituitary necrosis. Hemorrhage within the gland can occur with reperfusion. Sheehan's syndrome, which is necrosis of the anterior pituitary gland, produces long-term complications related to decreased hormone levels. Aggressive and rapid treatment of shock is required to prevent these serious complications.

PATIENT ASSESSMENT AND EARLY INTERVENTIONS

The anatomic and physiologic changes of normal pregnancy can obscure the pregnant woman's response to trauma. Maternal compensatory mechanisms preserve vital maternal functions at the expense of the fetus. Fetal survival depends on adequate gas exchange and uterine/placental perfusion. Rapid and efficient assessment and appropriate interventions provide for an optimal maternal-fetal outcome.

The primary survey focuses on airway, breathing, and circulation. Repositioning the airway by chin-lift or jaw-thrust maneuvers may be enough to establish patency and should not interfere with cervical spine protection. Airway adjuncts should be used as needed to prevent secondary injury from hypoxia; nasal airways should be used with caution because the mother may be predisposed to nasopharyngeal bleeding that can lead to further airway obstruction. Gentle suction and intubation may be necessary to control epistaxis and prevent airway compromise.

Cervical spine protection is maintained until the neck is cleared. If injury is suspected, spinal protection should be maintained with a rigid cervical collar; the patient should be logrolled off the backboard as soon as possible. To reverse aortocaval compression, the pregnant patient should be placed in a lateral decubitus position, or pillows or foam wedges should be used to tilt the patient 15 to 30 degrees laterally to deflect the uterus from the great vessels.[3,5,7,9,10] When spinal injury is suspected, spinal protection should be maintained and the patient tilted 15 to 30 degrees (4–6 inches) laterally or, preferably, the uterus should be manually displaced[1,3,6-10] (see Fig. 43.2). Manual displacement can be performed from the left or right of the patient; the uterus is cupped and lifted or pushed up and leftward to relieve pressure on the maternal great vessels.[9] Care must be taken not to push downward and cause increased pressure on the vessels.

Hypoxia can develop quickly during pregnancy; maternal oxygen saturation should be maintained at greater than 95%.[3] Injury can exacerbate existing pulmonary alterations related to pregnancy, such as decreased pulmonary reserve and increased maternal oxygen consumption, compromising the mother and the fetus. Oxygen is critical for fetal survival because of fetal inability to tolerate hypoxia. If rapid sequence intubation (RSI) is done, induction agents and neuromuscular blockade may be used in conventional doses.[10] Often a smaller-than-expected endotracheal tube is required, and video-assisted laryngoscopy may be beneficial. A gastric tube should be considered early to minimize risk for aspiration; nasal insertion of gastric tubes should be performed cautiously (to minimize the risk for epistaxis) using a smaller-sized tube. During the third trimester, chest tubes, when needed, should be inserted in the third or fourth intercostal space to avoid diaphragm and possible intraabdominal injury.[1,3,7,8]

Assessment and intervention for external and internal hemorrhage is necessary to ensure maternal-fetal survival. Control of bleeding along with adequate and appropriate fluid replacement is necessary to restore maternal and uteroplacental perfusion. Direct pressure should be applied to sites of uncontrolled external bleeding. The mother can lose 1500 mL of blood before signs of shock are evident. Retroperitoneal and uteroplacental injury can be sources of occult blood loss.

Intravenous (IV) access with two large-bore catheters and aggressive fluid volume replacement optimize maternal blood volume and oxygen-carrying capacity. IVs should be established above the level of the diaphragm to ensure that flow is not restricted by the gravid uterus.[9] Blood replacement with Rh-compatible blood should be initiated if crystalloids do not stabilize circulatory status. O-negative or type-specific blood is acceptable. Aortocaval compression should be relieved by displacing the uterus and can increase cardiac output by 20%. Topical hemostatic agents such as chitosan-impregnated gauze have been shown to be effective in pregnancy. Tranexamic acid is considered safe for the fetus and may be used.[8] Initiation of massive transfusion protocols may be indicated; the goal is to maintain hematocrit at 25% to 30% and urine output greater than 30 mL/hour.[10] Administration of large amounts of fluid containing dextrose 5% should be avoided because it may cause problems with neonatal glucose regulation should delivery be imminent; lactated Ringer's solution is more appropriate for initial resuscitation.[10] Some centers are using thromboelastography (TEG) to test efficiency of coagulation and to help guide intervention during trauma resuscitation. Vasopressors are not indicated for initial management of hypovolemic shock because they further reduce uterine blood flow and fetal hypoxia. Vasopressors may be used in management of cardiogenic shock secondary to cardiac contusion or distributive shock resulting from spinal cord injury. Insertion of an arterial line or a central venous line provides accurate monitoring of circulation and response to treatment and may be used in some centers.

Primary assessment includes a brief neurologic assessment. If neurologic deficits are found, both PIH and trauma should be considered as potential causes. Magnesium sulfate is considered a safe intervention for PIH.[10] Although seizures may result from head trauma, the seizing patient should be evaluated for eclampsia as well.[3]

Secondary assessment involves identification of other injuries; pain interventions, tetanus or tetanus-diphtheria booster and administration of antibiotics may be indicated. Local anesthesia and narcotics may be used. A thorough history includes a standard trauma history and an obstetric history—last menstrual period (LMP), expected date of delivery, parity, problems and complications of current or past pregnancies, presence of uterine contractions, and current fetal activity.

Focused obstetric assessment in the secondary survey includes evaluation of the abdomen, uterus, and fetus. Most women who develop adverse obstetric outcomes have symptoms such as abdominal pain, contractions, or vaginal bleeding. Pain that seems to be out of proportion to physical findings may be an indication for admission. Digital vaginal examination may be performed to assess for source of pain, bleeding, presence of amniotic fluid, and evidence of labor but should be avoided until placenta previa has been ruled out. Disturbing the placenta can lead to massive bleeding.[3]

Abdomen

The abdomen may be difficult to assess because clinical signs of peritoneal irritation are less evident. The gravid uterus lifts and stretches the abdominal wall and may impede contact between the parietal peritoneum and area of irritation.[3,7] Severe occult intraabdominal hemorrhage may occur without signs of impending shock. Liver and splenic injuries are common in MVCs and may be a source of intraperitoneal hemorrhage.

The abdomen should be inspected for signs of injury, including ecchymosis, abrasions, and contusions. The shape and contour should be noted because irregularity or deformity may indicate uterine rupture. Inspect and palpate for masses, abdominal tenderness, contractions, and fetal movement. Abdominal rigidity, guarding, and rebound tenderness may be blunted by the stretched abdominal wall.

Ultrasonography is beneficial in determining intraabdominal injury and fetal status. Some centers use focused assessment sonography for trauma (FAST) examinations routinely in the initial assessment of each trauma patient. Abdominal computed tomography (CT) is used to determine abdominal injuries in the stable trauma patient. Diagnostic peritoneal lavage (DPL) has been safely and accurately used to detect intraperitoneal hemorrhage in obstetric trauma.

Fetus and Uterus

Assessment of the fetus and the uterus should occur early in the secondary survey. Signs of abdominal pain, uterine tenderness, or contractions may indicate uteroplacental injury and maternal-fetal compromise.

Determining gestational age is critical because this guides fetal assessment and intervention. The best indicator of gestational age is LMP. If the woman is unsure about LMP or is unresponsive about LMP, she is assumed pregnant until a negative result from a human chorionic gonadotropin (hCG) level test is documented. Normal gestation is 40 weeks, with the uterus usually palpable by 12 to 14 weeks' gestation. The fundus generally reaches the umbilicus by 20 weeks' gestation (see Fig. 43.1). Fundal height just below the xiphoid indicates a term fetus. Fetal gestational age is frequently estimated by ultrasonography.

If emergency ultrasonography is not available, an estimate of gestational age of a single fetus can be accomplished by measuring the fundal height. A measurement midline from the symphysis pubis to the top of the uterus correlates gestational age with the height of the fundus in centimeters. A fundal height of 25 cm corresponds to a gestational age of 25 weeks. Fetal viability is generally considered to be 24 to 25 weeks' gestation, although fetal survival has occurred earlier with advanced neonatal resuscitation and treatment in a neonatal intensive care unit. Serial fundal measurements every 30 minutes are beneficial[5]; increased fundal height may indicate occult intrauterine bleeding, placental abruption, or uterine injury. It is possible for fundal height to be skewed by abdominal distention.[9]

The fetus should be assessed as soon as possible, but this assessment should not interfere with maternal resuscitation and stabilization. Evaluation of fetal well-being begins with a baseline FHR or evaluation of fetal heart tones (FHTs). FHTs are audible with Doppler testing by 10 to 12 weeks' gestation. FHR is a sensitive indicator of both maternal blood volume and fetal well-being. Normal FHR ranges from 100 to 160 beats/min at term and postterm (gestational age of 37 weeks or more) and 120 to 160 beats/min in a preterm fetus (less than 37 weeks).[3] FHR will initially increase in response to hypoxia or hypotension; however, severe hypoxia is associated with fetal bradycardia (less than 100–120 beats/min). Fetal bradycardia indicates serious fetal stress and decompensation. Another indicator of fetal well-being is fetal movement and activity. Maternal report of approximately 10 "kicks" in 2 hours may be considered a sign of fetal well-being.[11,12]

The gravid trauma patient may require continuous fetal monitoring or cardiotocography based on the gestational age of the fetus. Cardiotocography consists of continuous electronic monitoring of FHR, patterns, and uterine contractions. When possible, early continuous monitoring should be initiated for patients at greater than 20 weeks' gestation.[7] Fetal tachycardia (rate greater than 160 beats/min), bradycardia (rate less than 100–120 beats/min), and decreased variability in FHR or FHR decelerations associated with contractions (or both) are indicators of fetal distress. Fetal and maternal heart rates should be compared and ensure that FHR is being monitored. Significant FHR patterns such as late deceleration are ominous signs of fetal distress. The minimum duration of monitoring FHR and contractions is controversial; most sources recommend 4 to 6 hours in the absence of uterine tenderness, vaginal bleeding, fetal distress, or serious maternal injury or complications.[1,3,6,7,10]

Indications for continued monitoring are maternal heart rate greater than 110, an Injury Severity Score (ISS) greater than 9, evidence of placental abruption, FHR greater than 160 or less than 120, ejection during a MVC, and motorcycle or pedestrian collisions.[7] If FHR abnormalities or maternal complications are detected, monitoring should continue for at least 24 hours or until fetal well-being is established.[3] Fetal monitoring should be performed and interpreted by a clinician skilled in the use of the equipment, interpretation of the data, and requisite interventions; ideally a nurse from the labor and delivery unit should perform this monitoring. Box 43.1 summarizes signs of fetal distress.

Assessment includes inspection of the perineum for blood or amniotic fluid in addition to presenting parts and injury. Presence of amniotic fluid indicates a leaking or ruptured amniotic membrane and places the fetus at risk for infection and early delivery. Patient report of a "sudden gush of fluid" may indicate rupture of amniotic membrane or a spontaneous bladder void.[5]

BOX 43.1 Signs of Fetal Distress.

- Fetal heart rates consistently below 100 beats/min in known term or postterm fetus (37 weeks or greater gestational age)[13]
- Fetal heart rates consistently below 120 beats/min in a preterm fetus (gestational age less than 37 weeks)
- Fetal heart rates consistently above 160 beats/min
- No fetal movement reported by mother or per nursing examination (approximately 10 "kicks" in 2 hours may be considered a sign of fetal well-being)
- Bloody or meconium-stained amniotic fluid

Microscopic examination of vaginal fluid can determine the presence of amniotic fluid. Fluid is placed on a slide and allowed to air dry; if the specimen contains amniotic fluid, a fern pattern appears on the slide. Some centers use point-of-care tests that use vaginal swabs and color cards to detect amniotic fluid. In the absence of blood or urine, nitrazine paper can be used to differentiate amniotic fluid from vaginal fluid. Fluid should be obtained as close to the cervical os as possible to avoid a false-positive test. Normal vaginal fluid has a pH of 4.5 to 5.5. Amniotic fluid has a pH of 7.0 to 7.5, which turns nitrazine paper blue. The presence of vaginal fluid with a pH greater than 4.5 to 5.5 suggests ruptured membranes.[7] If blood is detected, the source of bleeding must be determined.

A general pelvic examination identifies crowning, fetal presentation, blood, and fluids. The necessity for speculum examination is determined by the trauma physician and may be deferred to the attending obstetrician. Direct visualization allows assessment of cervical dilation, locates the source of blood or fluids, and may identify uterine or fetal injury. Bimanual examination is avoided unless delivery is imminent or genital tract injury is present. Urinary catheter placement may be indicated to empty the bladder and to assist in monitoring fluid resuscitation. Return of blood or hematuria suggests genitourinary (GU) injury.

Diagnostics

Ultrasonography

Ultrasonography, and in some centers FAST, is used to identify acute problems with the pregnant trauma patient. Ultrasonography can determine fetal cardiac activity, body movement, placental location, estimated gestational age, volume of amniotic fluid, and intraperitoneal bleeding. Although a FAST examination can provide essential information, it should not be relied on to determine placental abruption; many abruptions are not visualized with ultrasound.[2] Fetal death may also be diagnosed by ultrasonography. Maternal intraabdominal and intrapericardial fluid can be detected during a FAST examination.

Laboratory

Laboratory studies include standard trauma profiles; however, results should be interpreted cautiously because of hematologic changes with pregnancy. Standard laboratory studies include complete blood count, serum electrolytes, amylase, coagulation profile, arterial blood gas, type and screen or type and crossmatch, and urinalysis. Hospital policy and the attending physician determine the need for toxicology screen, hepatitis B, and human immunodeficiency virus screening. Levels of hCG, which can confirm pregnancy as early as 1 to 2 weeks after conception, should be obtained for all women of childbearing age if the LMP is unknown or has occurred more than 4½ weeks before admission.[6]

Special attention to antibody screening is needed for Rh immune status because maternal Rh sensitization can occur when an Rh-negative mother carries an Rh-positive fetus. As little as 0.01 mL of Rh-positive blood will sensitize most

Rh-negative patients,[7] and about 40% of pregnant trauma patients will experience this maternal fetal mixing.[10] Rh_O (D) immune globulin (RhoGAM or Rhophylac) can prevent maternal sensitization, and administration to all Rh-negative trauma patients is recommended unless there is isolated injury remote from the uterus.[7] If maternal Rh status is unknown and administration of blood is anticipated, administration of immune globulin should be considered. A Kleihauer-Betke (KB) test, which measures the percent of red blood cells containing fetal hemoglobin in maternal blood, is used to identify the mixing of fetal blood in maternal circulation and should be performed on Rh-negative women at more than 12 weeks' gestation.[1,3,6] KB test results may be useful in predicting the risk for preterm labor after maternal trauma.[10] and can be used to determine whether additional doses of Rh immune globulin are indicated, which is often the case with blunt abdominal trauma.[8] A positive test result may be used as an indication for admission.[8] Some hemoglobinopathies such as sickle cell disease can result in a positive KB test. The presence of a positive KB test result alone does not necessarily indicate pathologic trauma and should not be used to diagnose placental abruption.[2,3,8,10]

Radiographic Evaluation

Radiodiagnostic procedures necessary for trauma evaluation should not be omitted in the presence of a gravid uterus. Studies should be performed with a vigilant attempt to minimize fetal irradiation. The need for radiographic studies is determined by clinical examination and provider suspicion of injury.

Every effort should be made to minimize fetal risk. An expert radiology technician can avoid duplicate films, shield the uterus whenever possible, and perform only essential radiodiagnostics. Consulting with an obstetrician or a geneticist may be beneficial when fetal radiation exposure is a concern and if there is time.[6] Although magnetic resonance imaging (MRI) scans are generally more detailed and involve no ionizing radiation,[10] MRI is less commonly used in the emergency setting and is not recommended for use in the first trimester.[6]

Diagnostic Peritoneal Lavage

Although DPL can effectively assess abdominal injury for hemoperitoneum and is considered safe and accurate for the gravid trauma patient, it is rarely used since the development of FAST and helical CT scanning. DPL does not assess retroperitoneal or intrauterine injury, and CT assessment is used more often. If CT is not available, DPL may be indicated in a symptomatic patient after blunt or multiple traumatic injury. Before the procedure, an indwelling urinary catheter should be inserted to decompress the bladder and decrease the risk for perforation. Decompression of the stomach with an orogastric or nasogastric tube decreases the risk for perforation and aspiration. Criteria for a "positive tap" are the same of those for nonpregnant patients.[3] Further diagnostics are required to locate the source and extent of injury. Immediate, delayed, or deferred laparotomy is determined by the maternal and fetal conditions.

INJURIES

Blunt Trauma

Blunt abdominal trauma can cause minor or severe life-threatening injuries to the mother and the fetus. The most common causes of abdominal trauma are MVCs, falls, and assaults.[1] Hormonal changes soften joints and relax pelvic ligaments, which decreases stability in balance and gait. These changes in combination with a protruding abdomen and easy fatigue increase the mother's susceptibility to falls. Many falls occur during the third trimester and are the second most common cause of maternal injury.[1] During the secondary assessment and history, the nurse should inquire regarding the height of the fall and the surface on which the patient landed in addition to which body structure was affected.

Blunt injury to the abdomen can result from direct force during an MVC as the abdomen impacts the dashboard, steering wheel, or air bag, or from a direct blow to the mother during an assault. Abdominal injury can also be secondary to organ displacement and hemorrhage from a coup-contrecoup event. Injury to the uterus can cause severe complications for the fetus, including premature labor, placental abruption, uterine rupture, fetal head injury, and fetal-maternal hemorrhage. Treatment varies depending on the injuries sustained and the status of the mother and the fetus.

Seat Belt–Related Injuries

MVCs are one of the most common causes of maternal injury or mortality, and unrestrained pregnant women have a higher risk of premature delivery and fetal death than other passengers.[7] Ejection from the vehicle with resulting head trauma accounts for most maternal deaths. Fetal death rates are also high when the mother is ejected. During the secondary assessment and history, it is important to ascertain whether a safety restraint device was worn and how it was positioned. Combined lap and shoulder restraints (i.e., three-point restraints) reduce maternal ejection and risk for fetal injury. Lap belts without shoulder harnesses also decrease ejection from the vehicle; however, the lap restraint alone can cause intraabdominal injuries. A lap belt worn too high over the uterus may lead to uterine rupture.[7] Elevation of the small bowel during pregnancy exposes the protuberant uterus and increases the risk for uterine or fetal injury from the lap belt. The two-point shoulder harness without lap restraint does not prevent ejection. Proper use of three-point restraints is an important component of patient education to reduce maternal mortality and fetal risk. The lap belt should be worn snugly across the pelvis below the abdomen and uterus; the shoulder harness should be worn in the normal position across the chest and between the breasts.

Premature Uterine Contractions

A frequently occurring complication of obstetric trauma is uterine contractions, or "preterm labor." Common causes include placental abruption, hypoxia, and hypovolemia. Damage to myometrial (muscular layer of the uterus) and decidual (epithelial lining of the uterus) cells releases prostaglandins, which stimulate the uterus. The extent of uterine damage, release of prostaglandins, and fetal age determine labor progression. More than six to eight uterine contractions per hour may indicate preterm labor, and they may go undetected in unconscious or intubated patients. Conscious patients may report abdominal or low back pain, pressure, or cramping. Usually contractions are self-limiting if the underlying cause is addressed and tocolysis is not indicated. Tocolysis, pharmacologic suppression of contractions, may be effective in halting preterm labor of the injured but hemodynamically stable gravida. Pharmacology is determined by provider discretion.

Adequate fluid volume replacement and positioning the mother in the lateral tilt position can minimize uterine irritability. Cardiotocographic monitoring should be initiated early to assess uterine activity and fetal response.

Placental Abruption

Placental abruption is premature separation of the normally implanted placenta from the uterine wall. Major abruptions may cause fetal anoxia, exsanguination, or premature delivery and are the most common cause of fetal death with a surviving mother.[1,3,6] As illustrated in Fig. 43.3, the abruption may be partial, marginal, or complete. Hemorrhage may be concealed. Blood trapped behind the separating placenta is old blood and appears dark when expelled. Fresh bleeding is usually bright red, whereas a port-wine color is seen when blood is mixed with amniotic fluid. Abruption may occur after even minor injuries.[7] In addition to blunt trauma, predisposing factors for placental abruption are related to PIH, glomerulonephritis, diabetes, increased maternal age, cigarette smoking, alcohol consumption, or possible dietary deficiencies.

Abdominal trauma is a direct force that can trigger placental abruption. Energy from a blunt force is dissipated to the elastic uterus, causing the placenta, which is relatively inelastic, to shear away from the uterine lining. Risk for placental abruption is usually immediately after injury; however, abruption may occur up to 48 hours later.[6] Bleeding can be severe enough to cause immediate maternal circulatory shock. Lack of oxygenation from impaired maternal-fetal gas exchange can lead to infant mortality resulting from hypoxia or intracranial hemorrhage. DIC may develop as late as 48 hours after the initial trauma.[5]

Classic signs of abruption include vaginal bleeding, uterine tenderness, abdominal pain, back pain, and uterine hyperactivity with poor relaxation between contractions, uterine tetany, or rigidity. Presentation may be vague or severe, and a high degree of suspicion is important.[8] Other indications of abruption include preterm labor, maternal shock, increasing fundal height, and fetal distress. Vaginal bleeding may be absent with concealed retroplacental bleeding. Fetal distress may be the first indication of uteroplacental injury and potential abruption. Rapid deterioration can occur in both the mother and the fetus, so intensive monitoring of both is essential. A small abruption may be compatible with fetal survival; however, a viable fetus in distress requires immediate surgical delivery.

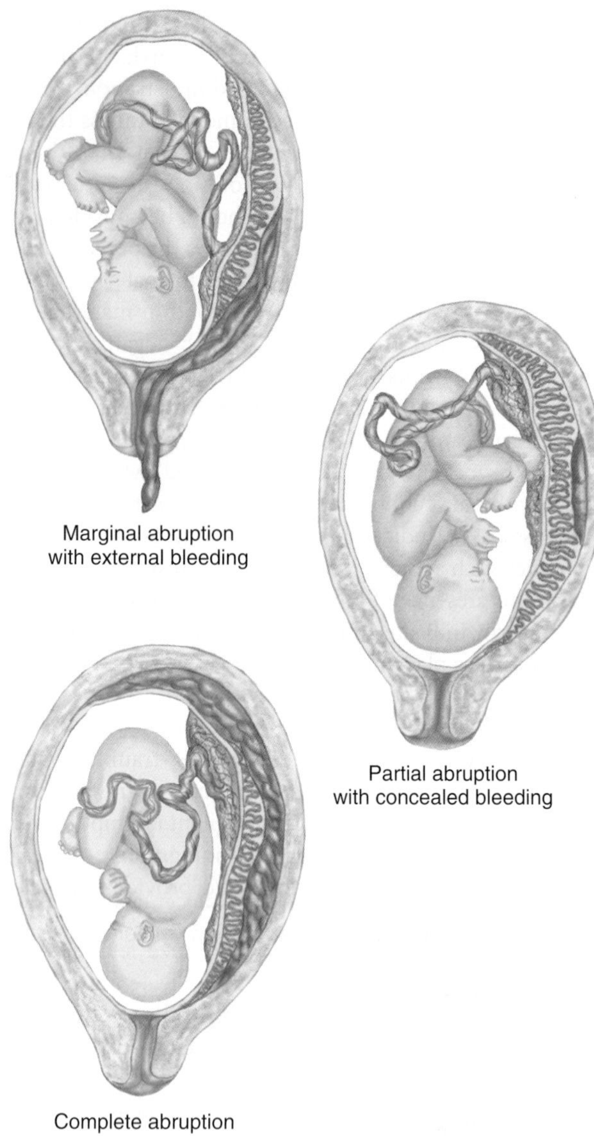

Fig. 43.3 Types of Placental Abruption (From Murray SS, McKinney ES. *Foundations of Maternal-Newborn Nursing.* 4th ed. Philadelphia, PA: Saunders; 2006.)

Uterine Rupture

Rupture of the uterus is an uncommon catastrophic injury resulting from blunt abdominal trauma. Previous cesarean section is a predisposing factor because rupture can occur at the healed incision site. Rupture of the posterior aspect of the uterus usually occurs in an unscarred uterus and is likely to involve bladder injury; urine may contain blood or meconium. Increased maternal blood volume and perfusion increase the risk for maternal hypovolemic shock with uterine rupture. The patient may initially have acute pain followed by no pain. The uterus will be tender, and fetal parts may be palpated outside the uterine borders with uterine rupture. Uterine contour may be abnormal and fundal height difficult to assess. There may be vaginal bleeding. Fetal distress may be evident. Early detection and repair of minor lacerations may prevent maternal hemorrhage and fetal compromise, but rarely can the uterus be repaired; hysterectomy is indicated for almost all patients with uterine rupture. Fetal mortality is almost 100%.

Direct Fetal Injury

The potential for direct fetal injury increases with each trimester. Blunt trauma infrequently results in direct fetal injury, with fetal skull fractures and intracranial hemorrhage the most common injuries noted.[5] Injuries most often occur in association with maternal pelvic fractures. Later in pregnancy, when the head is engaged in the pelvis, the fetal skull can become trapped and injured by the fractured pelvis. Compression of the fetal skull may occur between the maternal spine and restraining lap belt or a striking object. Other fetal fractures from direct injury may include clavicle and long-bone injury.

Penetrating Injury

Increasing size and position make the gravid uterus susceptible to penetrating trauma. Fetal injury after penetrating trauma to the mother is a frequent occurrence, with a high rate of fetal mortality. Gunshot wounds to the abdomen are more common than stab wounds. The degree of injury depends on the type, caliber, and range of the weapon. Upper abdominal wounds involve bowel perforation or retroperitoneal injuries to the mother caused by compartmentalization by the gravid uterus. Lower abdominal entry wounds cause direct injury to the fetus. Indirect injury to the fetus may be caused by trauma to the umbilical cord, placenta, or amniotic membrane. All abdominal gunshot wounds require exploratory laparotomy.

Stab wounds have a better prognosis for the mother and the fetus. Visceral organs can slide away from the penetrating object, so fewer organs are injured. Surgical exploration is usually required in cases of upper abdominal trauma from a bullet or a stab wound. Conservative management of lower abdominal injuries is indicated if the patient is stable or there is no evidence of GI or GU trauma. Diagnostic options include local exploration of wounds and CT, ultrasonography, or DPL of the abdomen. Emergency exploratory laparotomy is indicated for the pregnant patient with penetrating trauma and unstable vital signs or fetal distress. The decision to deliver the fetus depends on (1) gestational age, (2) evidence of penetration of the amniotic sac, (3) evidence of fetal death or distress, and (4) maternal injuries requiring abdominal exploration. Otherwise, vaginal delivery can be anticipated as the fetus continues to grow and mature.

Burns

Most burn injuries in pregnant women occur in the home, with the extremities, face, and neck burned most often. Injury can be thermal, associated with inhalation of toxic substances, or both. Fortunately, most burn injuries are minor. Pregnancy does not appear to affect maternal outcome; however, fetal outcome is affected by maternal condition. Total body surface area (BSA) involved and the severity of the burn affect maternal outcome, premature delivery, and fetal death. Fetal mortality is close to 90% when maternal burns are greater than 50% and, for a viable fetus, urgent cesarean delivery is recommended for maternal burns of 55% or more.[3,8] Fetal mortality results from hypoxia, hyponatremia, sepsis, and prematurity. Spontaneous abortion usually occurs within the first week after a severe burn event.[1] Occasionally, delivery of a healthy term infant is possible.

One potential complication associated with burn injury and smoke exposure is carbon monoxide (CO) poisoning. Fetal hemoglobin has a higher affinity for CO than maternal hemoglobin; when measuring maternal carboxyhemoglobin, it must be kept in mind that the fetus's level will be higher. Hyperbaric oxygen therapy should be considered if elevated carboxyhemoglobin levels are detected in the gravid patient.[8]

Immediate care of the burned pregnant woman is the same as that of the nonpregnant patient. Severe burns require treatment at a burn center. Aggressive and appropriate fluid resuscitation, electrolyte therapy, supplemental oxygen, ventilation, and prevention of infection are critical. Sterile, dry dressings should be applied; wet or cool dressings should be avoided. Antibiotics should be used if necessary; however, silver sulfadiazine cream should be avoided because it can displace bound bilirubin in fetal plasma, resulting in an increase in circulating fetal bilirubin. Elevated fetal bilirubin can cross the fetal blood-brain barrier and interfere with neuronal development, leading to fetal kernicterus or brain damage.

Electrical Injury

Few cases of electrical injury during pregnancy are reported; however, fetal mortality has been associated with even minor electrical shock. Most electrical incidents occur at home. Alternating current found in the home usually follows a hand-to-foot route. Consequently, the fetus lies in the direct path of the current. Fetal injury can result from cardiac conduction changes or uteroplacental lesions. If the fetus survives, oligohydramnios or growth retardation can develop. Pregnant women should report all incidents of electrical shock to the obstetrician. Baseline fetal monitoring and close, frequent follow-ups are necessary to evaluate fetal well-being.

SPECIAL CONSIDERATIONS

Maternal Cardiac Arrest

Objectives for cardiopulmonary resuscitation (CPR) during pregnancy are to sustain circulation and perfusion for both patients—the mother and the fetus. Basic and advanced life support should be initiated early, and manual displacement of the uterus should be maintained throughout the resuscitation if the uterus is palpated at or above the umbilicus (see Fig. 43.2). Occasionally, displacing the uterus may be all that is needed to restore maternal pulses. High-quality CPR with chest compressions of at least 100 per minute at a depth of at least 2 inches (5 cm) while allowing full recoil between compressions and with minimal interruptions is essential. Previous guidelines recommended placing the hands slightly higher on the sternum in the pregnant patient, but there is no evidence to support this, and the American Heart Association

(AHA) has removed this recommendation from its guidelines. Mechanical chest compression during pregnancy is not recommended. There are no contraindications to external defibrillation during pregnancy; however, if an internal fetal monitor has been inserted, it should be removed before use of electrical intervention.

Because oxygen reserves are lower and demands higher in the pregnant patient, hypoxemia should always be considered as a cause for arrest. Aggressive ventilation with supplemental oxygen and fluid loading with isotonic crystalloids and possibly blood products are necessary for resuscitation. Prompt, gentle intubation can facilitate ventilations and may reduce risk for nasoesophageal or oroesophageal bleeding and aspiration. Medical therapy during cardiac arrest is the same as that for nonpregnant patients, but careful attention must be directed toward the cause of the arrest. In the presence of maternal hypoxia and acidemia, vasoconstriction occurs in the uteroplacental vascular bed. Monitoring blood gas levels and serum pH levels is vital to determining maternal acidosis and response to treatment. Renal excretion of sodium bicarbonate increases during pregnancy; bicarbonate administration is determined by blood gas results. Vasopressors should be used with caution because of uteroplacental vasoconstriction and deleterious effects on the fetus. Targeted Temperature Management (TTM)/Therapeutic Hypothermia is usually not used on posttraumatic arrest because of the associated coagulopathies and potential for increased bleeding. The AHA recommends that TTM should be considered during pregnancy on an individual basis and that the same protocol be followed as with the nonpregnant patient.[9] At gestation greater than 24 weeks, fetal viability and survival must be considered. Perimortem cesarean section (PMCS) promotes survival of the mother and the fetus; however, there are few documented cases of maternal recovery with return to the preresuscitation state after cesarean delivery. After the need for cesarean section is determined, the procedure must be performed quickly, with a neonatal resuscitation team immediately available.

Emergency and Perimortem Cesarean Section

PMCS should be differentiated from emergency cesarean (EMCS). The injured mother may require emergency delivery of a potentially viable fetus.[6,9] EMCS may be indicated for fetal or maternal distress; indications may include premature rupture of membranes, placental abruption, uterine rupture, or unstable pelvic or lumbosacral fracture during labor. EMCS may be performed to provide adequate surgical exposure for management of maternal injuries or when a displaced pelvic fracture precludes vaginal delivery. Pelvic fracture is not, however, an absolute contraindication to vaginal delivery.[8] If preterm delivery is anticipated, corticosteroids may be ordered to decrease the risk of newborn respiratory distress syndrome.[3]

Perimortem cesarean delivery (PMCD) is delivery of the neonate at the time of maternal arrest or death. The purpose is twofold: first, to facilitate resuscitation of the mother by relieving aortocaval compression and second, to decrease the risk of permanent neurologic damage to a viable fetus. Fetal survival depends on the interval between maternal arrest and fetal delivery, gestational age, fetal condition, and cause of maternal arrest. When considering a PMCD, the American College of Obstetricians and Gynecologists (ACOG) recommends attaining a gestational age of at least 24 weeks.[6] Gestational age and due date are best determined by LMP. The nurse should count backward from the first day of the LMP and add 7 days; however, measurement of fundal height can be used to estimate fetal age. A fundal height above the umbilicus suggests a viable fetus.

The interval between maternal arrest and fetal delivery is the most important factor predictive of fetal survival. Most infants who survive are delivered within 5 minutes of maternal arrest;[3,7-9] however, neonate survival has been documented even when delivery occurred 30 minutes after maternal arrest.[9] As the interval increases, neonatal survival decreases. PMCS should be initiated while maternal CPR is performed to ensure uteroplacental perfusion. The "4-minute rule" (that is, PMCS should be initiated within 4 minutes after maternal cardiac arrest and the infant delivered by the fifth minute; the "5-minute rule") promotes the best maternal and fetal outcome.[1,3,6,9]

Maternal recovery may occur after cesarean section secondary to release of aortocaval compression, increased cardiac output, and increased tissue perfusion.[1,9] Two resuscitation teams should be in attendance, one for the mother and one for the infant. Optimally, the procedure should be performed in the emergency department (ED; or location of the arrest in the hospital) as opposed to transporting the patient to the operating room (OR). Research has shown that the quality of CPR decreases during transport to the OR and that time should not be wasted to move the patient.[9] Evidence of FHTs and viability is often considered as primary indications for PMCS; however, PMCS is sometimes completed in an attempt to resuscitate the mother even if the fetus is not viable. PMCS is recommended if maternal death is imminent, regardless of presence or absence of FHTs. After the uterus is emptied, there can be a 25% to 56% increase in maternal circulating blood volume. Releasing the weight of the gravid uterus off the maternal great vessels may restore maternal vital signs.[9] Fetal death is not usually an indication for PMCS, except in some cases of placental abruption that have resulted in maternal hemodynamic instability and coagulopathy.

Neonatal Resuscitation

Emergency delivery of a neonate is performed because of maternal or fetal distress, or both. Compromised fetal condition secondary to maternal arrest or other stressors may necessitate aggressive resuscitation. A neonatal team skilled in assessment and treatment of the newborn should be prepared with equipment necessary to resuscitate the fetus. Ideally, a neonatal team will include a neonatologist/pediatrician, neonatal nurses, and a respiratory therapist, but at times the emergency nurse may have to resuscitate the neonate. Management of the neonate should follow the most current AHA guidelines. Assessment and resuscitation should be performed simultaneously in a stepwise fashion. Drying, warming, positioning, suctioning, and providing tactile stimulation are the first interventions and are required of all neonates. The apneic neonate will require positive-pressure ventilation with a bag-mask device. Oxygen is needed by a compromised neonate if central cyanosis is present. Chest compressions should be initiated when heart rate is absent or the neonate has a heart rate less than 60 beats/min after 30 seconds of adequate assisted ventilation. Intubation may be performed at various steps in the resuscitation effort; medication administration is the final phase of neonatal resuscitation and is rarely needed by most newborns. Apgar scoring, an objective method of quantifying the newborn's condition based on the newborn's color, heart rate, reflex irritability, muscle tone, and respirations, is calculated at 1 minute after delivery and repeated at 5 minutes. Resuscitation should not be delayed to await the 1-minute Apgar score.

Patient Transport

Prehospital care and transport of the pregnant woman are influenced by several factors. As with any trauma patient, the initial focus is on spinal integrity, basic life support assessment, and emergency interventions. Supplemental oxygen may benefit the mother and the fetus because the pregnant woman is at higher risk for respiratory compromise than a nonpregnant woman and because the fetus cannot tolerate hypoxia. Supplemental oxygen should be administered to maintain maternal oxygenation saturation greater than 95%.[2,3,7] IV access is needed for fluid replacement to treat maternal hypovolemia and ensure uterine perfusion. To avoid serious maternal-fetal complications, appropriate maternal positioning during transport is vital. The left lateral decubitus position or manual displacement is advocated to avoid aortocaval compression in gestation greater than 20 weeks. If spinal protection is needed, a cervical collar and a backboard with a lateral tilt should maintain spinal protection and minimize compression of the great vessels.

SUMMARY

Obstetric trauma, although rare, can be a catastrophic event because two patients, the mother and the fetus, must be considered during assessment and treatment. Clinical management requires a team approach. All pregnant patients with major injuries should be admitted to a facility with trauma and obstetric capabilities.[7,8] The emergency physician, emergency nurse, trauma surgeon, obstetrician, perinatologist, labor and delivery nurse, and neonatal nurse may be key members of the trauma team during resuscitation of an obstetric trauma patient. Members must be aware of and assess for conditions unique to the injured pregnant patient, such as blunt or penetrating uterine trauma, placental abruption, amniotic fluid embolism, isoimmunization, premature labor, and premature rupture of membranes. Ideally, all indicated team members can respond to the ED. Although telemedicine is being used more often in trauma care, there is limited information related to telemedicine for obstetric trauma.[8]

Optimal fetal outcomes are dependent on maternal survival. Aggressive resuscitation and stabilization of the mother promotes the best maternal and fetal outcomes. Concern for the conditions of both the mother and the fetus produces elevated stress levels in the patient and the family. Keeping the family informed and providing emotional support for the patient and the family are essential during trauma intervention.

Prevention efforts can decrease the incidence and severity of obstetric trauma. Public and private education about properly using seat belts, not turning off air bags, and avoiding accidental poisoning and overexertion during pregnancy can reduce maternal and fetal injury. Violence, especially intimate partner violence, should be assessed in the ED. Appropriate intervention may prevent a repeat attack and avoid maternal injury. Education and discharge teaching that the fetal condition basically depends on the maternal condition may help the mother choose actions that promote fetal well-being.

Staff preparation for this rare event is important. Standardized order sets and drills have been shown to improve resuscitation skills.[9] The Emergency Nurses Association and other expert references recommend specialized education, training, and competencies that support emergency nurses in providing evidence-based care.[5,8,9] One recommended course for nurses that provides education on obstetric trauma is the *Trauma Nursing Core Course* (courses may be found on www.ENA.org).

Postevent debriefing and feedback are important for all health care providers involved, and inclusion of those not directly involved in the event can promote learning and preparation for the next encounter with a pregnant trauma patient.

REFERENCES

1. Mendez-Figueroa H, Dahlke JD, Vrees RA, Rouse DR. Trauma in pregnancy: an updated systematic review. *Am J Obstet Gynecol.* 2013;209(1):1–10.
2. Jain V, Chari R, Maslovitz S, et al. Guidelines for the management of a pregnant trauma patient. *J Obstet Gynaecol Can.* 2015;37(6):553–574.
3. Kilpatrick SJ. Initial evaluation and management of pregnant women with major trauma. UpToDate website. https://www.uptodate.com/contents/initial-evaluation-and-management-of-pregnant-women-with-major-trauma, Updated February 11, 2019. Accessed June 13, 2019.
4. Deshpande NA, Kucirka LM, Smith RN, Oxford CM. Pregnant trauma victims experience nearly 2-fold higher mortality compared to their nonpregnant counterparts. *Am J Obstet Gynecol.* 2017;217(5):590.e1–e9. https://doi.org/10.1016/j.ajog.2017.08.004.

5. Emergency Nurses Association. Special populations: the pregnant trauma patient. In: *Trauma Nursing Core Course: Provider Manual*. 7th ed. Park Ridge, IL: Emergency Nurses Association; 2014.
6. Barraco R, Chiu W, Clancy T, et al. Practice management guidelines for the diagnosis and management of injury in the pregnant patient: the EAST management guidelines work group. *J Trauma*. 2010;69(1):211–214. https://doi.org/10.1097/TA.0b013e3181dbe1ea.
7. Trauma in pregnancy and intimate partner violence. In: Henry S, ed. *ATLS Advanced Trauma Life Support: Student Course Manual*. 10th ed. Chicago, IL: American College of Surgeons; 2018.
8. Huls CK, Detlefs C. Trauma in pregnancy. *Semin Perinatol*. 2018;42(1):13–20. https://doi.org/10.1053/j.semperi.2017.11.004.
9. Jeejeebhoy FM, Zelop CM, Lipman S, et al. Cardiac arrest in pregnancy: a scientific statement from the American Heart Association. *Circulation*. 2015;132(18):1747–1773.
10. American College of Emergency Physicians. Trauma in the obstetric patient: a bedside tool. https://www.acep.org/Clinical—-Practice-Management/Trauma-in-the-Obstetric-Patient—A-Bedside-Tool. Accessed June 13, 2019.
11. American Pregnancy Association. Kick counts. http://americanpregnancy.org/while-pregnant/kick-counts, Updated April 3, 2017. Accessed April 9, 2018.
12. *Fetal movement counts: interactive patient education*. https://www.elsevier.com/solutions/interactive-patient-education. Revised May 22, 2017.
13. Murray M. *Antepartal and Intrapartal Fetal Monitoring*. New York: Springer; 2007.

44

Geriatric Trauma

Patricia Weismann

Individuals 65 and older comprise one of the fastest-growing segments of the population worldwide. This significant shift in demographics can be attributed largely to longer life expectancies, decreased birth rates, and advances in medicine. By 2060 the number of Americans aged 65 years and older is projected to double, to nearly 98 million, from 49.2 million[1] in 2016. Although health care and health and wellness programs are becoming more accessible, many older Americans are living longer with chronic conditions such as diabetes, hypertension, heart disease, and disability. Americans are also working longer in the labor force and are leading more active lifestyles, which can increase the risk of injury and visits to the emergency department (ED). In 2010 alone, 19.6 million visits to the ED were attributed to adults older than 65 years.[2]

Trauma is the seventh leading cause of death in adults 65 years and older.[3] This demographic accounts for 10% of all trauma-related injury and 28% of deaths due to traumatic injury.[3] In 2016 alone, more than 62,000 deaths for adults older than 65 years were related to unintentional injury.[4] Falls accounted for 47.4% of unintentional deaths, 11.8% of deaths were related to motor vehicle crashes (MVCs) and traffic injuries, and 10% were firearm related. The ED visit rate related to injury for adults aged 65 to 74 years was 9 per 100 persons in 2013 and increased significantly with age. The ED visit rate related to injury for adults aged 85 years and older was 25 per 100 persons, with a greater percentage of older adult patients presenting via ambulance than those of similar age for illness.[5]

Although mechanisms of injury are similar to those experienced by younger age-groups, geriatric trauma patients experience an estimated six times higher rate of mortality.[3] Complicating factors such as physiologic age-related changes, disabilities, polypharmacy, and concomitant comorbidities must be considered and can often add complexity to the assessment and medical management of the geriatric trauma patient.[1] Trauma in the older adult population can also lead to an overall decrease in quality of life and mobility, a higher rate of hospital readmission, and death. Providing early identification of the geriatric trauma patient, using prioritization, initiating rapid treatment, and ensuring prompt delivery to the appropriate level of care are important measures leading to improved patient outcomes for this at-risk population.[6]

TRIAGE

Accurate and expedited triage is critical to the outcome of the geriatric trauma patient. Undertriage of the older population occurs far too often and is linked with increases in morbidity and mortality.[7] Studies suggest older adults are undertriaged at a significantly greater rate than younger age-groups, and of undertriaged individuals, older adults are at four times greater the risk of mortality than the younger age-groups.[7] Factors contributing to undertriage include trauma criteria that are not specific to a certain age-group, delayed or decreased pain response, altered vital signs due to polypharmacy, and delayed physiologic response to trauma.[7] Research indicates that trauma criteria should be expanded to be more accommodating of advanced age. Recommendations include increasing the systolic blood pressure trauma parameter from 90 mm Hg to 110 mm Hg for older adults because this has been shown to be promising in identifying geriatric trauma patients who otherwise would have not met trauma criteria.[7] Rapid identification of the trauma patient, accurate triage, and expedited trauma team notification are critical steps in the older adult patient's healthcare continuum patient.

MEDICATIONS

Home medication usage in the older adult population can contribute to injury and can be a complicating factor both in compensating for the injury and progressing to health. Frequently prescribed medications in the geriatric population include anticoagulants, cardiac medications, and opioids.

Anticoagulants

Anticoagulant therapy is widely prescribed to the older adult population for prevention of complications such as venous thromboembolism (VTE), pulmonary embolus (PE), deep vein thrombosis (DVT), and for patients diagnosed with atrial fibrillation, to reduce their risk of thromboembolic stroke.[8] The widespread use of anticoagulants can pose significant complications in the geriatric trauma patient, such as an increased risk of bleeding, hemorrhage, and intracranial bleeding.[8]

Cardiac Medications

Cardiac medications, such as β-blockers, are commonly prescribed to treat hypertension and heart disease in a large portion of the older adult population and can add complexity to the triage process and identification of shock. Vital signs may not be an accurate predictor of the severity of injury or shock in this population because certain cardiac medications can blunt the body's overt response to trauma.[9,10] Although preinjury use of β-blockers has been linked to improved outcomes for the older adult population presenting with head trauma, increased rates of mortality have been associated with preinjury use of β-blockers for other forms of trauma.[9] Along with obtaining a detailed history and a physical examination, it is important to identify the name and dosage of preinjury home medications to assist in the medical management and treatment of geriatric trauma.

Opioids

Opioids are frequently prescribed for the treatment of both acute and chronic pain and can pose significant complications for the geriatric patient with trauma. Complications of opioid use in this age cohort include decreased sensorium, decreased respiratory rate, oversedation, overdose, vomiting, and immunologic dysfunction.

MECHANISMS OF INJURY

A growing number of older adults present to EDs for the treatment of both intentional and unintentional injuries each year. Frequent mechanisms of injury include falls, burns, self-harm, MVCs, assault, and abuse.

Blunt Trauma

Blunt trauma can affect multiple organ systems, resulting in a greater risk of morbidity and mortality for older adults compared with their younger counterparts.[11] Factors increasing the risk of mortality from blunt trauma in the older adult population include malnutrition, anticoagulant use, risk of hemorrhage, and decreased cardiopulmonary reserve.[1] Blunt trauma is caused by a transfer of force and can result from the following[12]:

- falls
- assault
- MVCs
- auto versus pedestrian collisions
- motorcycle/bicycle crashes
- crush injuries

Blunt chest trauma accounts for approximately 25% of trauma deaths, 80% of which are attributed to MVCs.[13] Blunt trauma related to assault most often involves injuries to the head and neck, and a traumatic brain injury (TBI) should be suspected.

Penetrating Trauma

Although penetrating trauma occurs less frequently in the older adult population, the in-hospital mortality rate for penetrating trauma is higher than for blunt trauma for the older population.[14] Penetrating trauma injuries more often are inflicted to the abdomen, neck, and thorax and lead to a higher number of mortalities in the hospital setting as compared with bunt trauma injuries.[14]

Falls

Falls in the older adult population are frequent occurrences, often with fatal outcomes. Falls are reported by approximately one of every four Americans every year, with an estimated 3 million fall-related ED visits annually.[15] Fall-related injuries are the cause of an estimated 750,000 hospital admissions, with $34 billion in directly related medical costs per year.[15] In 2016 nearly 30,000 unintentional deaths in adults older than 65 years of age were related to falls—a significant increase[4] from the 18,334 fall-related deaths in 2007. Factors increasing the risk of falls in the older population include the following[4]:

- polypharmacy
- substance abuse
- reduced activity
- age-related physiologic changes,
- pain/discomfort
- confusion/delirium
- arthritis
- reduced strength
- disability
- impaired gait
- previous fall(s)

Falls continue to pose a significant health risk to older adults, and the prevalence is increasing annually. Although more older adult men are injured as a result of falls due to increased activity and mobility, older adult women are nearly twice as likely to fracture a hip as a result of a fall, with osteoporosis being a contributing factor.[16] Other factors associated with a high risk for injury after a fall include the ABCs: Age over 85 years old, Bone fragility, Coagulopathy, or Surgery recently.[17]

Complications related to falls could include massive internal or external bleeding, intracerebral hemorrhage, rhabdomyolysis, PE/DVT or infection, such as pneumonia or uremia. Additional long-term complications related to a fall can include an increase in subsequent falls, depression, and an increased fear of falling leading to immobility, decreased motor function, and quality of life.

Burns

As the population of older Americans continues to rise, so does the rate of traumatic injuries and deaths related to burns. Factors predisposing older adults to burn injuries include the following:

- sensory impairment
- cognitive decline
- decreased mobility
- slower reaction times
- smoking
- dementia

Ninety-three percent of burn-related deaths for older adults in 2016 were reported to be unintentional, and although many of those deaths were attributed to house fire injuries and smoke inhalation,[18] scalding and contact injuries can also cause significant harm to the older adult. This population is also at a greater risk of hospital readmission and late mortality due to complications resulting from delayed healing and infection, coupled with comorbidities. Age-related factors contributing to an increased rate of complications and mortality for older adult burn victims include delayed responses to injury, weakened immunity, malnutrition, and difficulty in responding to the physiologic stress and hypermetabolic state occurring as a result of burn injuries.[19] After sustaining significant burn injuries, nearly half of adults older than 75 years of age are discharged to skilled nursing facilities (SNFs), further increasing their risk of death after discharge.[20] Even with advances in medicine, older adults are more likely to die within a year of significant burn injuries due to complications, compared with their younger counterparts. Geriatric burn survivors may develop unanticipated complications such as pneumonia, sepsis, delayed healing, skin breakdown, neuropathy, hypertrophic scars, or contractures.[21]

Rapid identification of critically ill patients, appropriate treatment and fluid resuscitation, along with monitoring and transfer to the appropriate level of care, are measures significantly improving patient outcomes.[19]

Self-Harm

Although the rate of self-harm for many adult age-groups is on the rise, older adults have a greater suicide mortality rate than younger adults.[22] In the older adult population in 2016, 13% of deaths were attributed to suicide, and 45% to 75% of these individuals had been evaluated by a physician a few months previously.[23] Seventy percent of the deaths were firearm related, 10.5% were linked to suffocation, and 10% of deaths occurred as a result of drug poisoning.[18] Older adults do not heal from major injury as well or as quickly as their younger counterparts,[22] and if a self-inflicted traumatic injury is survived, it can often leave the older adult disabled, requiring extended care services, or both. Several predisposing factors can increase the risk of self-harm:

- history of depression
- history of suicide attempts
- mental illness/abuse
- thoughts of hopelessness
- chronic comorbidities
- financial stressors
- lack of support structure
- alcohol or substance abuse
- being male

In addition to performing a thorough physical assessment and obtaining a medical history of the older adult patient, as with all patients, it is crucial for nurses to also consider the risk factors predisposing the patient to self-harm.

Motor Vehicle Crashes

MVCs are the second leading cause of trauma-related death for the older population. The causes of MVCs in this age-group may be attributed to physiologic age-related changes such as decreased reaction time, hearing and vision impairment, and cognitive decline. Due to a decreased physiologic reserve and impaired compensatory mechanisms, older adults are at an increased risk of morbidity and mortality as a result of MVC injuries, regardless of speed and severity of vehicle impact.[24]

Assault

Assault is a common cause of trauma-related injury for the older adult population. Approximately 6.5% of hospital admissions occur as a result of assault-related injuries for the older adult.[14] Although mortality rates are similar for both assault and unintentional trauma injuries, assault injuries correlate with an increased length of stay in the intensive care unit (ICU) and increased surgical intervention.

Assault can be physical or sexual. Men are more likely to be the victim of assault compared with geriatric women, and victims often screen positive for drugs and or alcohol when presenting for emergency care.[14] Older adults are also at an increased risk of sustaining a TBI as opposed to a younger population of assault victims.[14]

TBI occurs in approximately 1.4 million Americans every year. This injury can be catastrophic in older adults due to the use of anticoagulants, an increased risk of hemorrhage, and the decreased ability to compensate and recover from injury.[25] TBI in the older adult can be difficult to assess due to complications such as an indeterminable baseline mental status, cognitive impairment, Alzheimer's disease, dementia, or age-related changes such as delayed response or a decrease in sensation.

Abuse

Elder abuse can occur at the hands of a trusted caregiver, a family member, or even a close loved one. (See also Chapter 49, Abuse and Neglect.) Cases of elder abuse occur all too frequently, although they are often underreported, and can lead to injury, hospital admission, an unsafe discharge, and an increased risk of mortality.[14] Special consideration must be given to the precipitating circumstances leading to traumatic injury and the corresponding injuries for this at-risk population. Although a staggering 1 of 10 older adults reported experiencing abuse, a greater number of occurrences go unnoticed or unreported. An estimated two-thirds of abuse cases are not reported to authorities and, with the growth in the older adult population, the prevalence of abuse is expected to rise.[14,26]

Abuse can occur in any setting, in any socioeconomic category, and to any race or gender. See Table 44.1 for types of abuse and associated signs.[27] Studies show that women are abused at a higher rate than men, older adults with disability or dementia are at greater risk of being abused, and neglect is the most often reported method of abuse.[28] Abuse can be inflicted by any individual, although immediate caregivers and family represent a large population of offenders.[28] If abuse is suspected in any case, it is imperative that the suspicion be escalated and reported.

GERIATRIC TRAUMA ASSESSMENT

Airway

The older adult may present with dentures, secretions, blood, or foreign bodies obstructing the airway. Physiologic

TABLE 44.1 Spotting Potential Types of Abuse.

Type	Definition	Signs
Physical	Use of physical force to knowingly or unknowingly cause injury	Pinching, pushing, striking, biting, and/or burning, visible bruising (sometimes in various stages of healing), skin tears, unexplained injury, untreated fractures, and/or behavior such as an older adult withdrawing from or exhibiting fear of an individual (or both)
Sexual	Unwanted sexual interaction of any kind, either physical or harassment	Unexplained sexually transmitted infections, pain, bruising, and/or bleeding
Emotional or Psychological	Nonverbal acts and/or behaviors causing emotional responses such as mental anguish, emotional pain, humiliation and/or fear	Controlling behaviors, such as name calling, threatening, isolating, degrading and/or devaluing another, expressions of fear from the older adult, such as withdrawing from another individual
Neglect	Basic needs, such as food, water, medical care, and/or shelter are withheld by a caregiver	An older adult who presents as emaciated, dehydrated, with single or multiple pressure injuries, in poor health and/or hygiene
Financial or Material Exploitation	Unauthorized or forced use of materials, finances, or benefits	Making unauthorized modifications to a will, using credit cards, cars, or property, and/or writing unauthorized checks

Adapted from National Center for Injury Prevention and Control. *Understanding elder abuse: fact sheet* (2016). https://www.cdc.gov/violenceprevention/pdf/em-factsheet-a.pdf. Published 2016. Accessed 3 June 2019.

changes in cranial nerves may affect tongue control, resulting in obstruction, and increased incidence of neurologic events, such as strokes, in the geriatric population may cause altered level of consciousness and further compromising of the airway.[6] If the patient requires ventilatory support, age-related changes such as neck and back stiffness, thinning of the oral mucosa, and changes in bones and joints could potentiate a difficult intubation.[29] (See also Chapter 9, Patient Assessment.)

Breathing

Dentures that do not compromise the airway may be left in place to enhance the seal of a bag-mask device needed to supplement breathing.[6] A respiratory rate of 10 or less in the older adult population has been linked to an increased risk of mortality and, with age-related decreases in respiratory reserve, administering high-flow supplemental oxygen can be a critical intervention.[30] Early intubation for ventilatory support should always be considered for geriatric patients.

Circulation

Geriatric patients' ability to respond to physiologic stressors by increasing heart rate and cardiac output declines with age. Cardiac medications further blunt the response to trauma and shock in the older adult population. Decreasing cardiac reserves reduces the ability to tolerate hypoperfusion states.[6] Fragile venous structures may complicate central or peripheral access for fluid resuscitation.

Disability

Brain tissue atrophy leads to stretched bridging veins, increasing the risk of tearing or shearing, and general atrophy allows for additional space in the cranial vault, allowing for significant blood collection before onset of symptoms related to increased intracranial pressure.[6] Age-related cognitive decline can prove challenging in accurate assessment of baseline status and can add a level of complexity when assessing a patient for a TBI. Signs of a TBI may also present in a delayed manner in this population. If possible, try to obtain a baseline assessment of cognitive function from an individual or a family member who is present. Natural conductive nerve slowing that occurs with advanced age can slow reflexes, reduce sensation, and affect perception of pain and control of movement.[6]

Exposure/Environment

Hypothermia directly correlates to morbidity and mortality in the trauma patient, and geriatric trauma patients are at increased risk of hypothermia due to a loss of the subcutaneous fat layer, thinner skin, and a decreased ability to sweat. Nutrition status, underlying chronic conditions, and some medications may also compromise thermoregulation.[6]

Trauma Resuscitation Monitoring

The following can assist in trauma resuscitation

- *Laboratory studies:* Coagulation studies, such as prothrombin time (PT), partial thromboplastin time (PTT), or international normalized ratio (INR), help set a patient's baseline, because anticoagulants are commonly prescribed. Chronic use of alcohol may affect the liver and, subsequently, clotting times. Alcohol use may also lead to withdrawal, which could go undetected for prolonged periods if baseline levels are not obtained.
- *Monitoring:* An ECG can help determine whether a myocardial infarction (MI) was associated with the traumatic event. Telemetry monitoring may be appropriate for patients with underlying cardiac conditions.[6] Poor peripheral circulation may affect the accuracy of pulse oximetry, so nurses should be aware of patient condition and changes from known or suspected baseline.

- *Gastric tube placement:* Friable tissues associated with aging, as well as increased use of anticoagulants, may increase complications experienced with insertion of nasogastric or orogastric tubes. Relaxation of pharyngeal muscles, specifically in the oropharynx, does increase the risk of aspiration, so the emergency nurse should consider early gastric tube placement, when appropriate.
- *Oxygen and ventilation considerations:* Due to decreased pulmonary reserves and endurance, geriatric patients may not be able to compensate as well as younger populations. Loss of recoil in airways and alveoli increases the risk of airway collapse and ventilation/perfusion (V/Q) mismatches.[6] Consider supportive oxygenation and early intubation to support oxygenation and ventilation.
- *Pain assessment:* Pain is often underreported and undertreated in the geriatric population, which could lead to complications such as delirium, precipitating additional falls.[2,6] Anxiety, confusion, and dementia may also affect accurate reporting of pain in the geriatric patient. Due to risk for respiratory compromise, low initial doses of pain management medications and frequent reassessments are recommended.

History

Along with assessment and interventions, it is important to identify the actions or event(s) preceding the injury, medications the patient is currently taking or has been prescribed, and a comprehensive health and surgical history. Because older patients may have more than one provider, asking specific questions about medical and medication history and about providers is essential for safe care. Asking about compliance with taking prescribed medications and obstacles to taking medications as prescribed can provide insight into the patient's ability to provide self-care after discharge after a traumatic event. A comprehensively documented history adds to the systematic assessment of the geriatric patient, assisting to determine disposition.

TRANSFER TO A HIGHER LEVEL OF CARE

Geriatric patients with trauma can present to any facility, at any time, regardless of trauma designation. Older adults presenting with traumatic injury are at greater risk for developing complications such as multiorgan failure and a higher rate of morbidity and mortality. Due to the profound physiologic response to injury, combined with preexisting health states and polypharmacy, the older adult can benefit greatly from treatment at a designated trauma center. To obtain improved outcomes, it is critical to rapidly identify and triage these at-risk patients, aggressively treat them, and initiate transfer to a higher level of care.[21]

END-OF-LIFE CARE

Even with early identification, accurate triage, and aggressive treatment, the mortality rate for older adults as a result of traumatic injury is nearly 28%.[3] Advance directives may be in place and can help guide the clinical teams to carry out the wishes of patients. Transparency between the clinical teams and the family members can assist in decision-making processes when it comes to ethical issues and circumstances surrounding outcomes and quality of life.[31] At these critical moments, as in all other patient interactions, compassion, kindness, empathy for both the patient and family are crucial to the process of healing. (See also Chapter 14, Palliative and End-of-Life Care in the Emergency Department.)

SUMMARY

Individuals aged 65 years and older comprise one of the fastest-growing segments of the population worldwide, and trauma is the seventh leading cause of death for this age-group. Undertriage of a geriatric trauma patient increases the risk of mortality from the traumatic injury. Outcomes can be improved through rapid identification, thorough assessments, and aggressive treatment.

Home medication usage in the older adult population can contribute to injury and be a complicating factor, both in compensating to injury and progressing to healing. Other common mechanisms of injury for the older adult population include falls, burns, self- harm, MVCs, and assault, although suspicion of abuse must be also be investigated and, if found, escalated and reported. As with any patient, delivery of compassionate, patient-centered care, will assist with the process of healing.

REFERENCES

1. Hranjec T, Sawyer RG, Young JS, Swenson BR, Calland JF. Mortality factors in geriatric blunt trauma patients: creation of a highly predictive statistical model for mortality using 50,765 consecutive elderly trauma admissions from the national sample project. *Am Surg*. 2012;78(12):1369–1375.
2. Emergency Nurses Association, Institute for Quality, Safety, and Injury Prevention. *ENA Topic Brief: Screening Tools for Older Adults in the Emergency Care Setting*. https://www.ena.org/docs/default-source/resource-library/practice-resources/topic-briefs/screening-tools-for-older-adults-in-the-emergency-care-setting.pdf?sfvrsn=979a0c8f_10 Published 2017 Accessed 3 June 2019.
3. Wiles L, Day M, Harris L. Delta Alerts: changing outcomes in geriatric trauma. *J Trauma Nurs*. 2016;23(4):189–193.
4. Burns E, Ramakrishna K. Deaths from falls among persons aged ≥65 years—United States, 2007-2016. *MMWR Morb Mortal Wkly Rep*. 2018;67(18):509–514. Centers for Disease Control and Prevention website https://www.cdc.gov/mmwr/volumes/67/wr/mm6718a1.htm. Accessed 3 June 2019.

5. Albert M, Rui P, McCaig LF. *Emergency Department Visits for Injury and Illness Among Adults Aged 65 and Over: United States, 2012-2013. NCHS Data Brief, no 272.* Hyattsville, MD: National Center for Health Statistics; 2017.
6. Emergency Nurses Association. *Trauma Nursing Core Course: Provider Manual.* 8th ed. Des Plaines, IL: Emergency Nurses Association; 2020.
7. Brown J, Gestring M, Forsythe R, et al. Systolic blood pressure criteria in the National Trauma Triage Protocol for geriatric trauma: 110 is the new 90. *J Trauma Acute Care Surg.* 2015;78(2):352–359.
8. Office of Disease Prevention and Health Promotion, US Department of Health and Human Services. *National Action Plan for Adverse Drug Event Prevention.* Washington, DC: Office of Disease Prevention and Health Promotion; 2014.
9. Evans DC, Khoo KM, Radulescu A, et al. Pre-injury beta blocker use does not affect the hyperdynamic response in older trauma patients. *J Emerg Trauma Shock.* 2014;7(4):305–309. http://doi.org/10.4103/0974-2700.142766.
10. Cliche J, Bourque JSC, Daoust R, Chauny J, Paquet J, Piette E. Effect of β-blockers and calcium channel blockers on shock index predictability in patients suffering from urosepsis. *Crit Care.* 2013;17(suppl 2):P225. http://doi.org/10.1186/cc12163.
11. Louis F. The lived experience of suffering males after blunt trauma: a phenomenological study. *J Trauma Nurs.* 2017;24(3):193–202.
12. Fox N, Schwartz D, Salazar J, et al. Evaluation and management of blunt traumatic aortic injury: a practice management guideline from the Eastern Association for the Surgery of Trauma. *J Trauma Nurs.* 2015;22(2):99–110.
13. Stewart D. Blunt chest trauma. *J Trauma Nurs.* 2014;21(6):282–284.
14. Rosen T, Clark S, Bloemen EM, et al. Geriatric assault victims treated at U.S. trauma centers: five-year analysis of the national trauma data bank. *Injury.* 2016;47(12):2671–2678. http://doi.org/10.1016/j.injury.2016.09.001.
15. Centers for Disease Control and Prevention. *WISQARS: Fatal Injury Data Visualization Tool.* Centers for Disease Control and Prevention website. https://wisqars-viz.cdc.gov. Published 2016. Accessed 3 June 2019.
16. Crandall M, Duncan T, Mallat A, et al. Prevention of fall-related injuries in the elderly: an Eastern Association for the Surgery of Trauma Practice Management Guideline. *J Trauma Acute Care Surg.* 2016;81(1):196–206.
17. Quigley PA, Hahm B, Collazo S, et al. Reducing serious injury from falls in two veterans' hospital medical-surgical units. *J Nurs Care Qual.* 2009;24(1):33–41.
18. Centers for Disease Control and Prevention. *WISQARS: Overall Injury-Related Death Statistics.* Centers for Disease Control and Prevention website. https://www.cdc.gov/injury/wisqars/index.html. Published 2016. Accessed 3 June 2019.
19. Abu-Sittah GS, Chahine FM, Janom H. Management of burns in the elderly. *Ann Burns Fire Disasters.* 2016;29(4):249–245.
20. Duke JM, Boyd JH, Rea S, Randall SM, Wood FM. Long-term mortality among older adults with burn injury: a population-based study in Australia. *Bull World Health Organ.* 2015;93(6):400–406. https://doi.org/10.2471/BLT.14.149146.
21. Jain S, Bhamidipati C, Cooney R. Trauma transfers to a rural level 1 center: a retrospective cohort study. *J Trauma Manag Outcomes.* 2016;10(1). https://doi.org/10.1186/s13032-016-0031-z.
22. Fantus R, Sakai L. Guns and the golden years. Bulletin of American College of Surgeons website. http://bulletin.facs.org/2016/11/guns-and-the-golden-years/#printpreview. Published November 1, 2016. Accessed 3 June 2019.
23. Steele I, Thrower N, Noroian P, Saleh F. Understanding suicide across the lifespan: a United States perspective of suicide risk factors, assessment & management. *J Forensic Sci.* 2018;63(1):162–169.
24. Gabel A, Keiser M. Challenges in the management of geriatric trauma: a case report. *J Trauma Nurs.* 2017;24(4):245–250.
25. Adoni A, McNett M. The pupillary response in traumatic brain injury: a guide for trauma nurses. *J Trauma Nurs.* 2007;14(4):191–196.
26. Acierno R, Hernandez MA, Amstadter AB, et al. Prevalence and correlates of emotional, physical, sexual, and financial abuse and potential neglect in the United States: the National Elder Mistreatment Study. *Am J Public Health.* 2010;100(2):292–297. http://doi.org/10.2105/AJPH.2009.163089.
27. National Center for Injury Prevention and Control. Understanding elder abuse: fact sheet. https://www.cdc.gov/violenceprevention/pdf/em-factsheet-a.pdf. Published 2016. Accessed 3 June 2019.
28. Evans CS, Hunold KM, Rosen T, Platts-Mills TF. Diagnosis of elder abuse in US emergency departments. *J Am Geriatr Soc.* 2017;65(1):91–97. http://doi.org/10.1111/jgs.14480.
29. Colwell C. Geriatric trauma: initial evaluation and management. 2018. UpToDate website. https://www.uptodate.com/contents/geriatric-trauma-initial-evaluation-and-management. Updated August 2, 2017. Accessed 3 June 2019.
30. Lee S-Y, Shih S-C, Leu Y-S, Chang W-H, Lin H-C, Ku H-C. Implications of age-related changes in anatomy for geriatric-focused difficult airways. *Int J Gerontol.* 2017;11(3):130–133.
31. Stevens C. Geriatric trauma: a clinical and ethical review. *J Trauma Nurs.* 2016;23(1):36–41. https://doi.org/10.1097/JTN.0000000000000179.

UNIT VI

Special Populations

45

Pediatric Emergencies

Katherine Logee

Sick children present distinctive challenges to many health care professionals. Assessment and treatment of children is unique because of the developmental, anatomic, and physiologic differences between adults and children. Understanding and appreciating these differences is the foundation for providing appropriate care for children. Being able to quickly recognize a sick child is an acquired skill requiring time and practice to develop. A child's fear and anxiety of being ill and in a hospital, as well as the parent's fear and anxiety, can at times make simple communication a challenge.

Parents or guardians should be encouraged and allowed to remain with their child during care delivered in the emergency department (ED). Fear and uncertainty surrounding the child's condition, coupled with a loss of control of the situation, add to the stress that both the parent and child may be experiencing. Begin the assessment as soon as the child enters the ED; approaching the child slowly while interviewing the parent is the best way to start the interaction with the child. Calling the child by name, making direct eye contact, using simple understandable terms, and offering choices when appropriate are all basic guidelines to be used with patients and families of all ages.

Most emergency nurses, regardless of practice area, will encounter a sick child at some point in their career. The ability to intervene in critical situations requires a strong foundation of knowledge and assessment skills. This chapter provides an overview of pediatric assessment and common pediatric emergencies.

TRIAGE

Pediatric patients, defined by the Centers for Disease Control and Prevention (CDC) as individuals younger than 15 years of age, account for 19.8% of annual ED visits nationally.[1] The triage nurse must have outstanding assessment, communication, and organization skills. The emergency nurse who becomes skilled at triage will also develop a "sixth sense" for identifying the "sick" infant or child.

A sick child in the ED can make nurses who are unfamiliar with children uneasy, just as an adult with chest pain can generate alarm in a pediatric nurse. Triage of a child does not require familiarity with every childhood disease or medication. Pediatric triage does require understanding of concepts related to pediatric emergencies, including the following:

- anatomic, physiologic, and developmental differences between children and adults
- recognition of conditions leading to pediatric arrest (hypoxia and shock) and appropriate interventions
- effective communication with parents
- "rules" of pediatric triage

Children are a challenge to evaluate compared with adults for several reasons. Children often have nonspecific symptoms, such as fever, and communication can be difficult. In the younger infant, because of limited vocabulary and verbal skills, the nurse must depend on the parent and subtle clues from the child for history. A child's response to illness or injury depends on his or her current developmental stage. Toddlers cling to parents, whereas adolescents are more independent. Children compensate physiologically for longer periods in the face of illness; therefore they may not be outwardly symptomatic despite the presence of a life-threatening condition. Normal vital signs do not always indicate stability in the pediatric patient.

Special Pediatric Considerations

Some of the most significant differences between children and adults are found in the respiratory and circulatory systems. One of the most obvious anatomic differences is infants and young children have larger tongues in proportion to the size of their mouths. This means the tongue can easily obstruct the airway; proper positioning is often all that is necessary to provide airway patency. Because of the smaller diameter of their airway, children have increased airway resistance compared with an adult; small amounts of mucus or swelling exacerbate this difference and can easily obstruct the airway. Infants younger than 4 months of age are obligatory nasal breathers; any process obstructing the nose can lead to respiratory distress. Cartilage of a child's larynx is softer than in an adult. It is becoming increasingly common to use cuffed endotracheal tubes in neonates, infants, and young children. It is now believed that cuffed tubes can provide better ventilating conditions while also minimizing trauma to a child's delicate airway.[2] The sternum and ribs of the pediatric patient are cartilaginous, the chest wall is soft, and intercostal muscles are poorly developed, leading easily to fatigue. All of these factors contribute to a more inefficient respiratory system and the cause of frequent respiratory distress.

Some specific differences in the cardiovascular system of the pediatric patient have clinical significance. Infants and children have a higher cardiac output than adults (200 mL/kg per minute vs. 100 mL/kg per minute).[3,4] Cardiac output is the volume of blood ejected by the heart each minute; it is defined by the following equation: heart rate × stroke volume = cardiac output. A higher cardiac output is required because the pediatric patient has a higher oxygen demand as a result of a higher metabolic rate and greater oxygen consumption (6–8 mL/kg per minute compared with 3–4 mL/kg per minute in adults). In pediatric patients, the myocardial fibers are shorter and less elastic, which means the myocardium has poorer compliance and less ability to adjust stroke volume in an altered cardiac output state. This is why heart rate is such an important and sensitive indicator of cardiac output in pediatric patients.[3,5]

Children have a greater percentage of total body water than adults (80 mL/kg vs. 70 mL/kg in adults) and are more susceptible to volume depletion with even small unreplaced losses. This is why children are at a greater risk for dehydration than adults. However, part of the challenge with pediatrics is that children can maintain an adequate cardiac output for a long time by compensating for fluid loss with an increased heart rate (tachycardia) and peripheral vasoconstriction.[3,5] Because of their strong compensatory mechanisms, 25% to 30% of circulating volume may be lost before a decrease in systolic blood pressure (SBP) occurs, indicating the child has progressed to a decompensated shock state.[3,5] By the time the shock state is recognized, the child may already be in critical condition.

Neonates, term infants from birth to 28 days of age, and particularly preterm neonates, possess unique physiologic characteristics and should be assessed and treated very carefully. The thermoregulatory system is very immature in the neonatal period, and thus keeping newborns warm without overheating them can be a challenge. There can be serious consequences of hypothermia and hyperthermia. Hypoglycemia, apnea, metabolic acidosis, and poor feeding can result from cold stress. Warm stress can also lead to poor feeding, lethargy, hypotonia, and hypotension.

Simply taking care to not leave the newborn undressed or unwrapped for long periods of time during the ED visit is a simple way to avert problems. Other methods used to keep the newborn warm include using warmed intravenous (IV) fluids, covering the head of the newborn, or using an overhead radiant warmer or even warm blankets. An effortless way to ensure thermoregulation of the newborn in the ED is to maintain a higher temperature in the room where the newborn will be examined. As a rule of thumb, if an adult in short sleeves is feeling warm, the room temperature should be about right for the newborn. However, as mentioned, overheating can become an issue for the newborn as well, so it is important not to overdo the heating methods. Temperature monitoring should not be overlooked. The neonatal immune system is also immature; therefore a fever of 100.4°F (38°C) is considered significant for a newborn. The inability to localize infections makes neonates even harder to assess for infectious processes because they have fewer signs and symptoms.[6] Newborns, young infants, and children have limited glycogen stores and are vulnerable to hypoglycemia when stressed by an illness, injury, or cold stress.

Guidelines for Pediatric Triage

The following guidelines for pediatric triage may assist triage nurses in evaluating children.

- Parents know their children better than you do—listen to them. Parents' history can give clues to the cause of an illness or injury and help triage nurses determine urgency.
- Remember airway, breathing, and circulation (ABCs)—children are different. Do not always focus on the obvious; a subtle, more serious problem can be overlooked.
- Some children can talk, walk, and still be in shock; do not depend solely on the child's appearance. Consider history and vital signs, but do not allow normal vital signs to give you a false sense of security.

Pediatric Triage Evaluation

Depending on the facility, the triage assessment may be brief, limited to determining the chief complaint and looking at the child, or it may be more comprehensive and include obtaining vital signs and providing treatment such as antipyretics, splinting, or ice packs. Whatever triage protocols or pathways exist, the first and most important aspect is prompt assessment with observation. This first assessment is sometimes referred to as the "across-the-room assessment," or the "looks good–looks bad" assessment using the Pediatric Assessment Triangle (PAT).[3,7] The PAT uses three physiologic parameters reflecting severity of illness or injury: the child's general appearance, work of breathing, and circulation to skin (Fig. 45.1). General appearance refers to the child's tone, interactiveness, consolability, look/gaze, and speech/cry. Work of breathing is evaluated by signs such as airway sounds, positioning, retractions, and nasal flaring. Circulation to the skin is obtained by assessing skin color. With experience and practice, a triage nurse can look at a room of children and quickly sort out who needs to be triaged first.[8]

Primary Assessment

Primary assessment consists of evaluation of the ABCs and neurologic status of the child. ABCs may be the only part of the assessment performed in triage if the child has an emergent condition. The primary survey includes assessment of level of consciousness; respiratory effort, rate, and quality; skin color, temperature, and capillary refill; and pulse rate and quality.[4]

Secondary Assessment

Secondary assessment consists of vital signs and a head-to-toe survey. During triage, secondary assessment is usually limited to evaluating the area of chief complaint or focused examination. The rest of the examination is performed later in a treatment area. When performing a secondary assessment on

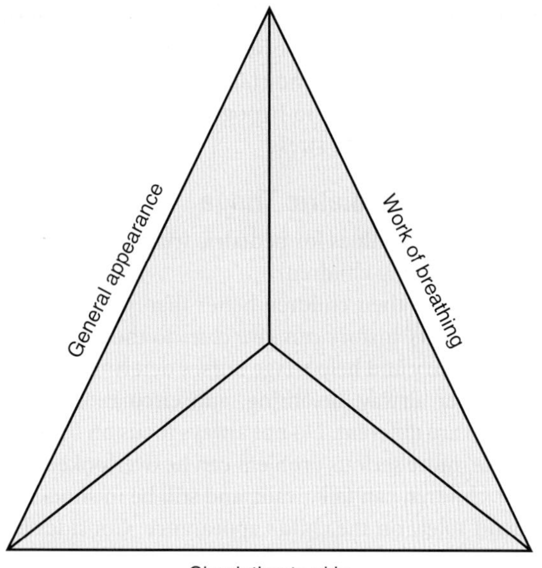

Fig. 45.1 Pediatric Assessment Triangle. (From *Emergency Nursing Pediatric Course: Provider Manual (ENPC)*. 5th ed. Des Plaines, IL: Emergency Nurses Association; 2020.)

a child, do not focus only on the obvious injury. Do not forget to take into account the patient's chronic condition(s) or any significant past medical history.[3,4]

History

Obtaining a standardized history of the child's illness is an important part of the pediatric assessment. If the triage nurse identifies a life-threatening condition during the PAT assessment, the standardized history can be obtained by the patient's primary nurse. In infants younger than 1 year of age, and especially with neonates, history may be vague, nonspecific, and limited by the parents' ability to communicate their concern for their child. Past medical history is also important in determining whether the child has a prior condition affecting assessment (e.g., congenital heart disease, chronic respiratory condition, prematurity). The CIAMPEDS mnemonic is a standardized tool describing components of a basic pediatric history (Table 45.1).[8]

Vital Signs

Obtaining accurate vital sign measurements on children is one of the more challenging aspects of pediatric assessment. Temperature, pulse rate, respiratory rate, blood pressure, weight, and pain scores should be obtained on every patient. Vital signs vary with age (Table 45.2); therefore alterations from normal must be viewed in light of the child's history and other symptoms.[8] Infants localize infections poorly because of their immature immune system; therefore any child younger than 3 months of age should be evaluated for possible bacterial infection when the child has fever greater than 100.4°F (38.0°C). Temperatures less than 96.8°F (36.5°C) in this age-group can be a sign of infection as well.

An accurate weight (in kg) should be obtained as early in the patient visit as possible. This will be done ideally during the triage assessment. Weight, measured only in kilograms, reduces the chance of error in medication calculations and improves the overall safety of patient care while in the ED.[8,9] A length-based resuscitation tape (e.g., Broselow tape) may be used in situations in which a measured weight cannot be readily obtained. Birth weight should be documented for infants younger than 8 weeks of age.

Pulse and respirations can be measured consecutively while the nurse is evaluating airway and breathing. An apical pulse can be obtained with the stethoscope on the child's chest, and a full minute of respirations can also be counted while the stethoscope is on the chest. Temperatures may be obtained by a variety of routes, including oral, tympanic, temporal artery, axillary, or rectal. The method chosen will depend on the age of the child, medical history of the child, institutional preference, and the needed reliability of the measurement. When an accurate temperature is required to make a treatment decision, a measurement strategy that approaches core temperature is desired—rectal temperature is considered the gold standard.[8]

Obtaining a blood pressure can be a bit more difficult in the younger child. Beginning with the correct size cuff is the first priority. The cuff must cover two-thirds of the area being used.[5] A cuff that is too small gives a false high reading, whereas an oversized cuff gives a false low reading. Having a wide variety of cuff sizes is very important when caring for pediatric patients. Using the lower extremity on younger infants and toddlers while distracting them during the procedure is often an alternative way to obtain an accurate blood pressure reading. If the noninvasive blood pressure monitor will not record a blood pressure, it is important to document signs describing the patient's perfusion status, including level of consciousness, pulses, and capillary refill.

RESPIRATORY EMERGENCIES

Recognition of respiratory distress and failure in the pediatric patient is crucial because unrecognized or undertreated respiratory compromise is almost always the precursor to cardiac arrest in children.[4,7] A child having difficulty breathing can display a variety of symptoms. Upper airway conditions can cause the child to be apprehensive, restless, and stridorous and exhibit intercostal and sternal retractions. Sudden onset of respiratory distress may suggest foreign body obstruction or laryngeal spasms. Airway obstruction in children results from a myriad of causes, including congenital anomalies, peritonsillar abscess, laryngeal obstruction, drug intoxication, and foreign bodies such as coins or toy parts.

Gradual onset of respiratory distress with coughing and an increased work of breathing that includes wheezing, retractions, hypoxia, and nasal flaring is more suggestive of a lower airway problem.[10] Viruses cause 80% to 90% of childhood respiratory infections with respiratory syncytial virus (RSV), rhinovirus, parainfluenza, influenza, and adenovirus the most common ones in the pediatric population. An individual virus can cause several different patterns of illness (e.g., RSV can cause bronchiolitis, croup, pneumonia, or the common cold).

TABLE 45.1 Components of Basic Pediatric Assessment (CIAMPEDS).

C	Chief complaint	Reason for the child's ED visit and duration of complaint (e.g., fever lasting 2 days).
I	Immunizations	Evaluation of the child's current immunization status: • The completion of all scheduled immunizations for the child's age must be evaluated. The most current immunization recommendations are published by the American Academy of Pediatrics. • If the child has not received immunization because of religion or cultural beliefs, document this information.
	Isolation	Evaluation of the child's exposure to communicable diseases (influenza, chickenpox, shingles, mumps, measles, whooping cough, tuberculosis): • A child with active disease or who is potentially infectious, based on a history of exposure and the disease incubation period, must be placed in respiratory isolation on arrival in the ED. • Immunosuppressed or immunocompromised children can develop active disease even when previously immune. These children must also be protected from inadvertent exposure to viral and bacterial illness while in the ED and placed in *protective* or *reverse* isolation. • Other exposures that may be evaluated include exposure to meningitis (with or without evidence of purpura), pneumonia, and scabies.
A	Allergies	Evaluation of the child's previous allergic or hypersensitivity reactions: • Document reactions to medications, foods, products (e.g., latex), and environmental allergens. The type of reaction must also be documented.
M	Medications	Evaluation of the child's current medication regimen, including prescription and over-the-counter medications: • Dose administered. • Time of last dose. • Duration of medication use.
P	Past medical history	A review of the child's health status, including prior illnesses, injuries, hospitalizations, surgeries, and chronic physical and psychiatric illnesses. Use of alcohol, tobacco, drugs, or other substances of abuse must be evaluated, as appropriate: The medical history of an infant must include the prenatal and birth history: • Complications during pregnancy or delivery. • Number of days infant remained in hospital post birth. • Infant's birth weight. • The medical history of the menarcheal female includes the date and description of last menstrual period.
	Parent's/caregiver's impression of the child's condition	• Identification of the child's primary caregiver. • Consider cultural differences that may affect the caregiver's impressions. • Evaluation of the caregiver's concerns and observations of the child's condition. Especially significant in evaluating the special needs child.
E	Events surrounding the illness or injury	Evaluation of the onset of the illness or circumstances and mechanism of injury: • Illness: • Length of illness, including date and day of onset and sequence of symptoms. • Exposure to others with similar symptoms. • Treatment provided before ED visit. • Examination by primary care provider. • Injury: • Time and date injury occurred. • M: Mechanism of injury, including the use of protective devices such as seat belts and helmets. • I: Injuries suspected. • V: Vital signs in prehospital environment. • T: Treatment by prehospital providers. • Description of circumstances leading to injury. • Witnessed or unwitnessed.
D	Diet	Assessment of the child's recent oral intake and changes in eating patterns related to the illness or injury: • Changes in eating patterns or fluid intake. • Time of last meal and last fluid intake. • Regular diet: Breast milk, type of formula, solid foods, diet for age, developmental level, and cultural differences. • Special diet or diet restrictions

Continued

TABLE 45.1 Components of Basic Pediatric Assessment (CIAMPEDS).—cont'd

	Diapers	Assessment of the child's urine and stool output: • Frequency of urination over last 24 hours (number of wet diapers); changes in frequency. • Time of last void. • Changes in odor or color of urine. • Last bowel movement; color and consistency of stool. • Change in frequency of bowel movements.
S	Symptoms associated with the illness or injury	Identification of symptoms and progression of symptoms since the onset of the illness or injury event.

ED, Emergency department.
From Brady K. Acute gastroenteritis: evidence-based management of pediatric patients. *Pediatr Emerg Med Pract.* 2018;15(2):1-25.
From Bernardo L, Thomas D, eds. *Core Curriculum for Pediatric Emergency Nursing.* 2rd ed. Boston, MA: Jones & Bartlett; 2009.

TABLE 45.2 Normal Vital Signs by Age.

Age	Heart Rate (beats/min)	Respiratory Rate (breaths/min)	Systolic Blood Pressure (mm Hg)	Weight (kg)
Preterm	120–180	55–65	40–60	2
Term newborn	90–170	40–60	52–92	3
1 month	110–180	30–50	60–104	4
6 months	110–180	25–35	65–125	7
1 year	80–160	20–30	70–118	10
2 years	80–130	20–30	73–117	12
4 years	80–120	20–30	65–117	16
6 years	75–115	18–24	76–116	20
8 years	70–110	18–22	76–119	25
10 years	70–110	16–20	82–122	30
12 years	60–110	16–20	84–128	40
14 years	60–105	16–20	85–136	50

Modified from Barken RM, Rosen P. *Emergency Pediatrics.* 6th ed. St Louis, MO: Mosby; 2003.

Assessment

When a child first arrives in the ED with any respiratory problem, rapid assessment should be completed using a systematic approach with the least-intrusive methods first. Observe the child quickly to obtain vital information on respiratory effort and level of consciousness. Inspect the child's bare chest for structural abnormalities, symmetry of movement, and use of accessory muscles. Note the child's position. A child in respiratory distress finds a position of comfort with the body leaning slightly forward and the head in the "sniffing" position; this position allows maximum airway opening.

Respiratory Rate and Pattern

The young child's respiratory muscles are not well developed, so the diaphragm plays a critical role in breathing. Chest auscultation and observation of the rise and fall of the abdomen are the best methods for assessing respiratory rate in patients younger than 2 years. Respiratory rates are often irregular in small children, so the rate should be carefully assessed for 1 full minute.

Normal respiratory rates vary by age. A neonate has a normal respiratory rate from 40 to 60 breaths/min, which slows as the child gets older. With respiratory distress, the child's respiratory rate initially increases. A resting respiratory rate greater than 60 breaths/min is a sign of respiratory distress in a child, regardless of age. As respiratory distress progresses to failure, the child becomes more acidotic, mental status changes occur, and respiratory rate slows. Bradypnea is an ominous sign in a pediatric patient.

Work of Breathing

Children in respiratory distress exhibit increased work of breathing as evidenced by the use of accessory muscles for breathing. As work of breathing increases, intercostal, substernal, and supraclavicular retractions may be observed.

Inspiration is an active process in which muscles expand the chest. Exhalation is passive, relying on elastic recoil of the lungs and chest wall. Under normal circumstances these two processes are balanced, with expiration roughly the same length as inspiration (inspiration/expiration ratio 1:1). When air passages are narrowed by inflammation or obstruction, time required for inhalation may remain the same with an increase in effort; however, exhalation takes substantially longer than inspiration (inspiration/expiration ratio 1:2 or 1:3).

Alertness, general responsiveness to the environment, and consolability are important observations for assessing mental status with children. Inconsolability is often a sign of hypoxia; however, a restless child who becomes progressively quieter should be carefully assessed to make certain improved oxygenation rather than respiratory failure or exhaustion is causing the restlessness to abate.

Quality of Breathing

Quality of breathing includes the depth and sound of breathing. A child's chest should expand symmetrically; therefore asymmetry or inadequate expansion indicates serious problems such as pneumothorax or hemothorax, foreign body obstruction, or flail chest. To auscultate a child's chest, place the stethoscope at the anterior axillary line level with the second intercostal space on either side. This helps identify the location of any abnormal breath sounds. The small size of a child's chest and thinness of the chest wall allow sounds from one side to resonate throughout the thorax (and even into the abdomen). Therefore listening to the anterior and posterior aspects of the chest may not be as useful for pediatric assessment as it is for an adult.

Breath Sounds

Various disorders produce adventitious sounds not normally heard over the chest. Stridor is suggestive of an upper airway obstruction. Stridor is usually heard in the inspiratory phase of respiration as the child works to get air past the obstruction. Stridor will be high-pitched in croup, anaphylaxis, and foreign body aspiration. Sounds heard in the expiratory phase suggest lower airway disorders. Crackles result from passage of air through moisture or fluid. Wheezes are produced as air passes through airways narrowed by exudates, inflammation, or spasm. Bilateral wheezing suggests asthma or bronchiolitis, whereas unilateral wheezing suggests foreign body aspiration. Decreased or unequal breath sounds may be suggestive of an airway obstruction, pneumothorax, pleural effusion, or pneumonia.

Grunting is caused by early closure of the glottis during exhalation with active chest wall contraction. It is a forced expiration creating positive end-expiratory pressure (PEEP) and prevents airway collapse. Grunting is seen in diseases with diminished lung compliance such as pulmonary edema; it also occurs as a result of pain.

Monitoring

The child with a respiratory problem should be monitored carefully for changes in level of consciousness, work of breathing, and level of alertness.

Blood gas analysis gives the clearest picture of the patient's respiratory status. For pediatric patients, a venous or capillary gas sample is easier to obtain than an arterial sample and can provide helpful information on ventilatory and acid-base status. Pulse oximetry is a useful, noninvasive means of continuously measuring the oxygen saturation of hemoglobin in the capillaries and correlates well with arterial blood gas (ABG) measurement. An oxygen saturation of 90% to 93% is the lowest acceptable range in children living at sea level. At higher elevations, saturations falling into the 88% to 89% range are considered normal. Pulse oximetry's major limitation is that carbon dioxide and acid-base balance are not evaluated. Many pulse oximeters rely on analysis of hemoglobin color and may not be useful when extremity perfusion is diminished from trauma, cold ambient temperature, or vasopressors or when the number of erythrocytes is decreased, as in anemia. It can be challenging to effectively apply and monitor an infant or small child on a pulse oximeter.

Several types of probes may be used, depending on the type of oximeter available. The adhesive type of pediatric or neonatal probe is generally the most useful probe to use with the younger age-group. Common sites of application for infants include the forehead, large toe, top or bottom of the foot, or sides of the ankle.[3] In EDs across the country, it is becoming more common to see capnography used not only in the intubated patient but in the spontaneously breathing patient as well. In the spontaneously breathing patient, it can be used to determine adequacy of ventilation for patients with asthma, patients undergoing procedural sedation, or patients with altered mental status and seizures.[11]

Airway Obstruction by Foreign Body

Small children spend a good deal of time exploring their world. Small objects hold a special fascination for children and are likely to end up in their mouths. Foreign body aspiration can occur at any age but is most commonly seen in children younger than 4 years of age.[8] A child brought to the ED with sudden onset of respiratory distress should be evaluated for foreign body aspiration if no other cause is apparent. Initially, a foreign body obstruction produces choking, gagging, wheezing, or coughing. If the object becomes lodged in the larynx, the child cannot speak or breathe. If an object is aspirated into the lower airways, there may be an initial episode of choking/gagging followed by an interval of hours, days, or even weeks when the child is without symptoms. Secondary symptoms are related to the anatomic area in which the object is lodged and usually caused by a persistent respiratory infection.

Foreign body obstruction completely occluding the airway is an acute emergency. Initial treatment is immediate removal of the object using back slaps and chest thrusts for infants younger than 1 year of age. For children 1 year or older, abdominal thrusts should be used. Blind finger sweeps are not recommended to relieve upper airway obstruction; however, any visible foreign objects should be removed. Immediate cricothyrotomy or tracheostomy must be performed to open the airway if it remains obstructed. If ventilation appears adequate, allow the child to assume whatever position is most comfortable. Unless the object is observed high in the upper airway, its exact location must be determined by radiograph. Bronchoscopy may be necessary for removal. A swallowed object is allowed to pass normally through the gastrointestinal tract, unless it is long and sharp. Those objects present significant danger of intestinal perforation. Nickel-cadmium batteries must be removed because of the potential for toxic leakage. Magnets also pose a risk when more than one of them is ingested. Injury can occur when two or more magnets attract each other across the nasal septum or across loops of bowel, leading to complications such as septal necrosis, septal perforation, bowel obstruction, ulceration, volvulus, or perforation.[3,12]

Asthma

Asthma is the most common chronic illness in childhood, affecting approximately 8% of all American children.[1] This chronic lung disease is characterized by hyperreactivity of the airway, bronchospasm, widespread inflammatory changes, and mucous plugging. Wheezing, the most obvious sign of asthma, may range from mild to severe and is accompanied by tachycardia, retractions, and anxiety. Expiration may be prolonged because of narrowed airways. Obtaining a thorough history may be useful in trying to determine the cause and severity of the attack. Repeated asthma attacks are a dangerous sign because of increasing fatigue and potential complications. Recent hospitalization is likely to be an indication of a seriously ill child.

When assessing a child with asthma, evaluate respiratory rate, quality, and effort to determine the degree of respiratory distress; peak flow measurement should be obtained in older children. The child may require supplemental oxygen if saturation on room air is low and tachypnea and tachycardia are present.

Treatment of a child in the ED with moderate to severe distress involves nebulized or metered-dose inhaled β_2-agonist agents (e.g., albuterol and levalbuterol). Nebulized treatments are usually given every 20 minutes for three doses; nebulized anticholinergic agents such as ipratropium may be added to potentiate the effects of the β_2-agonists. Oral systemic corticosteroids are given to suppress and reverse airway inflammation. Adequate hydration for children with asthma is important. They are prone to fluid loss during hyperventilation because of decreased intake due to an increased work of breathing. IV fluids may be necessary for some patients.

Bronchiolitis

Bronchiolitis, a viral infection commonly found in infants younger than 24 months of age, can be a life-threatening illness in high-risk children. Those at high risk include the very young (0–3 months of age), premature infants, and children with heart or lung disease or chromosomal abnormalities. The viral infection causes an inflammatory process that produces edema in the bronchial mucosa with resultant expiratory obstruction and air trapping. The virus also causes necrosis of the epithelial cells in the upper airways, which produces thick, copious mucus. Bronchiolitis has a broad spectrum of severity. Determination of when the respiratory distress began helps predict the course of the illness because the critical period of bronchiolitis usually occurs during the first 24 to 72 hours after onset of respiratory distress. History typically includes symptoms of a cold, cough, and copious amounts of thick nasal drainage for a few days before the onset of respiratory distress. High-risk infants can present with apnea and be very ill in appearance compared with the older child. Hospitalization is necessary for high-risk infants younger than 2 months of age and those with an apneic episode.

RSV, the most common causative organism of bronchiolitis, is a highly contagious respiratory pathogen transmitted by direct contact with infected respiratory secretions or contaminated objects. The virus enters the body by contact of contaminated hands with the nose, eye, or other mucous membranes. Aerosol spread occurs but is less common. Care includes appropriate isolation precautions.

Nasal suctioning, oxygen therapy, and adequate hydration along with other appropriate supportive care measures are the mainstays of treatment. The American Pediatric Association 2015 guidelines state that the use of bronchodilators, corticosteroids, and nebulized hypertonic saline should be avoided in the ED.[13]

Croup

Croup, or laryngotracheobronchitis, is viral inflammation of the subglottic area, including the trachea and bronchi. Croup occurs most frequently in infants and children 6 months to 3 years of age but may occur in older children. It is slightly more prevalent in boys. Croup is seen most frequently in cooler months.

The inflammatory process of viral croup produces edema of the trachea and surrounding structures. Edematous airways secrete tenacious mucus, which leads to problematic removal of secretions. The child's effort to inspire air through edematous structures produces the characteristic stridor of croup.

History usually includes an upper respiratory infection for a few days followed by nocturnal onset of the characteristic "barking" cough. The child may have a hoarse voice or cry. Nursing assessment should be performed carefully to keep the child calm. The stress of crying increases the work of breathing, so both stridor and retractions markedly increase. Assessment should focus on cardiorespiratory status, hydration, anxiety, and fatigue level as well as parental anxiety.

Nursing interventions for croup focus on relieving anxiety and reducing work of breathing. The child should be kept as comfortable as possible (e.g., sitting on a parent's lap); painful interventions should be minimized. Heart rate, respiratory rate, and work of breathing should be monitored. There is no evidence to support the treatment of croup with the use of humidified air. Mist tents separate the child from their caregivers, can disperse fungus, and are not recommended.[14] Corticosteroids are administered to reduce airway inflammation and swelling, and improvement generally persists for 24 to 48 hours after a single dose of dexamethasone. Nebulized racemic epinephrine is used in moderate to severe cases to reduce mucosal edema and laryngospasm. Children should be monitored for at least 2 to 4 hours after racemic epinephrine is administered because the medication's effect may not be sustained, producing a "rebound" effect.[14] Soft-tissue radiograph of the neck may be indicated to rule out epiglottitis; croup is associated with tracheal narrowing, a "steeple sign" on neck films.

The decision for hospital admission depends on the patient's degree of respiratory distress, ability to maintain adequate hydration, ability to rest, and the degree of parental apprehension.

Epiglottitis

Epiglottitis, or supraglottic laryngitis, is the most emergent acute bacterial upper airway obstruction of childhood. This condition produces a rapid onset of inflammatory edema of the epiglottis. *Haemophilus influenzae* type B causes most pediatric cases of epiglottitis. The incidence of epiglottitis has significantly declined since the *H. influenzae* type B conjugate vaccine has become available. A child with epiglottitis typically presents in an anxious state, with respiratory distress, drooling because of difficulty swallowing, and sitting forward with the neck extended (tripod position) to maximize airway patency. The child may have audible respiratory sounds and appears flushed and toxic with a high temperature. The epiglottis becomes swollen and cherry red and can cause total airway obstruction if manipulated during examination.

The child should be allowed to assume a position maximizing his or her respiratory effort. Initially, no attempts should be made to perform invasive procedures or look down the patient's pharynx unless absolutely necessary. Most patients with severe respiratory distress from epiglottitis go directly to the operating room for intubation or tracheostomy. Hospital admission is always required for known or suspected epiglottitis. IV fluids are necessary until oral fluids can be swallowed. IV administration of antibiotics is preferred; however, IV access, fluids, and antibiotics should be deferred until the patient's airway is secured and protected.

Peritonsillar and Retropharyngeal Abscess

Other diseases with signs and symptoms similar to epiglottitis include peritonsillar abscess and retropharyngeal abscess. A peritonsillar abscess, on rare occasions, can compromise a child's airway. Retropharyngeal abscesses have a less abrupt onset than epiglottitis but also pose a substantial risk to airway patency. A child with a peritonsillar or retropharyngeal abscess requires the caregiver to frequently assess and support respiratory and circulatory function. Retropharyngeal abscesses require drainage in the operating room, whereas a peritonsillar abscess may be drained in the ED if there is danger of airway compromise. Both conditions are treated with IV antibiotics.

Pertussis

Pertussis, or whooping cough, is an acute respiratory infection caused by *Bordetella pertussis.* Whooping cough usually occurs in children younger than 4 years of age who have not been immunized. Highly contagious, whooping cough is particularly threatening to young infants, resulting in higher morbidity and mortality rates. Incidence is highest in the spring and summer.

Pertussis is usually indistinguishable from a common cold until the paroxysmal stage. During this stage, the child has a fever and whooping type of spasmodic cough that can lead to hypoxia, gagging, vomiting, and exhaustion. Petechiae above the nipple line, ear infection, atelectasis, pneumothorax, and vomiting may also be present. Hernias may appear suddenly as a result of exertion during coughing.

Excitement and crying tend to worsen the coughing paroxysms, so care should be taken to keep the child as calm as possible. Airway clearance is important in the management of pertussis and may require gentle suctioning. Humidified oxygen should be used, the child should be isolated from other patients, and antibiotic therapy should be initiated as soon as possible. Hospitalization is recommended for infants who exhibit respiratory distress and have a significant oxygen desaturation associated with coughing paroxysms. Infants may also require IV fluids for dehydration secondary to inability to feed caused by coughing.[15]

Pneumonia

Pneumonia, inflammation of the pulmonary parenchyma, is common throughout childhood but occurs more frequently in infancy and early childhood. Clinically, pneumonia may occur as a primary disease or a complication of other illnesses. Viruses cause most pneumonias in children, although bacterial pneumonia, usually caused by group B streptococci and gram-negative bacilli, is more likely to occur in the first weeks of life. Whether viral or bacterial, pathogens reach the lung and cause an inflammatory response leading to an accumulation of fluid in the lungs, tachypnea, cough, and fever. Bacterial pneumonia tends to have an abrupt onset with high fever, 101.3°F to 105.8°F (38.5°C–41°C). In viral pneumonia, fever is usually lower than 102.2°F (39°C). With bacterial pneumonia there is an increase in the number of granulocytes and bands on the white cell differential count.

Treatment varies with the child's age, suspected causative agent, severity of symptoms, and immune status of the child. Infants younger than 2 months usually require a complete septic workup and hospitalization for IV antibiotic treatment. Children with minimal distress and who are tolerating oral fluids well can usually be treated at home with oral antibiotic therapy.

Pneumothorax

A pneumothorax is a collection of air in the pleural space caused by the rupture of an alveolar bleb on the surface of the pleura and results in the partial collapse of one or both lungs. A pneumothorax may occur spontaneously or secondary to obstruction, trauma, cancer, or tuberculosis. A history of a previous spontaneous pneumothorax increases the likelihood of recurrence.

Symptoms depend on how much air escapes into the pleural space. Small amounts may be asymptomatic. A large amount of air prevents full expansion of the affected lung, causing tachypnea, dyspnea, grunting, hypoxia, and cyanosis. Most respiratory problems cause retraction of chest wall musculature; however, a pneumothorax may cause bulging of these muscles, especially intercostal muscles over the affected area. Bilateral breath sounds are usually heard in infants and small children with a pneumothorax because their thin chest wall allows breath sounds to be readily transmitted from one area to another.

Hospital admission is almost always recommended. Oxygen administration and bed rest are used in mild cases. Children with more than 40% pneumothorax usually require a chest tube with closed drainage and suction to evacuate air from the pleural space and reexpand the lung. The child must be continually assessed for development of a tension pneumothorax, which is a life-threatening problem. If a tension pneumothorax is suspected, a needle thoracentesis must immediately be done. Prepare for a chest tube insertion after the needle thoracentesis.

CARDIOVASCULAR EMERGENCIES

Causes of cardiovascular emergencies in the pediatric population differ from those in adults, but the three basic categories of cardiovascular compromise are the same: inadequate heart function (rhythm disturbances, heart failure, congenital heart disease), inadequate volume for circulation (dehydration, burns, trauma), and inadequate fluid distribution (distributive shock states such as sepsis and anaphylaxis).

Most pediatric cardiac arrests are related to respiratory arrest rather than primary cardiac arrest.[4,7] Supporting the child's respiratory efforts and intervening early can prevent potential cardiac problems.

Assessment

Blood volume in a child is 80 mL/kg, with total blood volume much less than in an adult. Loss of 1 cup (8 oz or 240 mL) of blood in a 10-kg child is equivalent to blood loss of 1 quart (32 oz or 960 mL) in an adult. With infants and children, the immature sympathetic innervation of the ventricles and the shorter and less elastic myocardial fibers keep the stroke volume at a relatively fixed rate.16 A child responds to the need for increased cardiac output with an increased heart rate. Tachycardia may initially increase cardiac output during periods of distress; however, prolonged tachycardia causes cardiac decompensation and decreases cardiac output. Close attention to heart rate, skin perfusion, and mental status is the key to early recognition of compensated shock. Capillary refill time is also recommended as a sensitive indicator of perfusion in the pediatric patient. Use of this parameter has not been studied extensively; however, normal capillary refill time is about 2 seconds. More than 3 seconds may indicate poor perfusion in a normothermic child.

Cardiovascular assessment should identify shock or conditions leading to shock requiring intervention by the emergency nurse. A history of illness or injury is important in interpreting signs and symptoms. Observing the child plays a major role. Important elements to assess include the following:

- *Skin color:* Pallor and mottling may indicate decreased perfusion caused by diminished cardiac output.
- *Capillary refill:* A delay of 3 seconds or more is abnormal.
- *Level of consciousness:* Decreased perfusion to the brain may cause restlessness, confusion, or lethargy.
- *Skin turgor:* Checking this estimates the state of hydration and, to a lesser extent, nutrition of the child. To assess, grasp the skin on the back of the hand, lower arm, or abdomen between two fingers so the child's skin is tented up. Hold the skin for a few seconds, then release it. Skin with normal turgor snaps rapidly back to its normal position. Skin with decreased turgor remains elevated and returns slowly to its normal position (tenting). This is a late sign of moderate to severe dehydration.
- *Mucous membranes:* Membranes should be moist. Dry, cracked, parched lips suggest moderate to severe dehydration.
- *Anterior fontanel:* A bulging fontanel may indicate increased intracranial pressure, whereas a sunken fontanel suggests dehydration. The anterior fontanel generally closes by 9 to 18 months of age.
- *Peripheral pulse quality:* Decreased perfusion to extremities results in weak peripheral pulses. Inappropriate distribution of fluids, as in a distributive shock state (sepsis and anaphylactic) causes bounding pulses.
- *Vital signs:* Temperature, pulse rate, respiration rate, and blood pressure. Normal vital sign parameters for the pediatric patient are listed in Table 45.2.

Vital signs should be documented as part of the baseline assessment. Children in early shock may have a normal SBP because of their strong compensatory mechanisms (tachycardia and vasoconstriction). Trending pulse pressure (systolic pressure minus diastolic pressure) provides valuable clues to perfusion status: a narrowing pulse pressure indicates further vasoconstriction; a widening pulse pressure indicates increasing vasodilation. Declining SBP is a sign of a decompensated shock state warranting immediate intervention. A child can lose a significant amount of circulating volume before hypotension ensues. SBP can be estimated using the following formula:

$$\text{Normal Systolicpressure} = 80 + (\text{age in year} \times 2)$$

$$\text{Minimal acceptable systolicpressure} = 70 + (\text{age in year} \times 2)$$

Inadequate Heart Function

Rhythm Disturbances

Children generally have young, strong hearts, so rhythm disturbances are seldom primary events. Dysrhythmias usually result from hypoxia or metabolic disturbances. Because of increased survival rates, pediatric patients with rhythm disturbances from congenital cardiac problems are seen with increasing frequency in the ED. The most common congenital problems causing rhythm disturbances are transposition of the great vessels and congenital mitral stenosis. Acquired cardiac diseases such as cardiomyopathies, rheumatic heart disease, and viral myocarditis may also cause rhythm disturbances.

Abnormal rhythms in pediatric patients are often divided into three categories: fast, slow, and absent (Table 45.3). Sinus tachycardia and supraventricular tachycardia (SVT) are two major rhythm disturbances found in children. Sinus tachycardia is caused by a variety of factors, including fever, anxiety, pain, and hypovolemia. The rate of sinus tachycardia is 140 to 220 beats/min. Treatment of sinus tachycardia is focused on the underlying cause; for example, if the child is febrile, control the fever and then reassess the heart rate. SVT is caused by a reentry mechanism and is characterized by a nonvarying heart rate higher than 220 beats/min in infants and greater than 180 beats/min in children. Infants often present with symptoms of poor feeding, rapid breathing, pale skin color, or fussiness. SVT can be initially well tolerated; however, it will ultimately lead to congestive heart failure if left untreated. Stable SVT may respond to vagal maneuvers: an example of a vagal maneuver appropriate for an infant would be putting a bag of ice water over the forehead, eyes, and bridge of the nose (not obstructing the airway).[14] An example of a vagal maneuver for an older child would be to have the child blow through an obstructed straw.[16] Adenosine should be considered if there is no response to the vagal maneuvers. Bradycardia is an ominous sign in a pediatric patient. Sinus bradycardia is frequently caused by hypoxia and should be treated aggressively with ventilation and oxygenation. A child with a heart rate of less than 60 beats/min with signs of poor perfusion requires immediate cardiac compressions.[16] Junctional and idioventricular rhythms are usually terminal rhythms. Absent, disorganized, and nonperfusing rhythms require cardiopulmonary resuscitation and advanced life support procedures.

TABLE 45.3 Rhythm Disturbances in Children.

Rhythm	Cause	Characteristics	Treatment
Fast Rhythms			
Sinus tachycardia	Fever, anxiety, pain, hypovolemia	Rapid sinus rhythm; rate 140–220 beats/min	Treat underlying cause.
Supraventricular tachycardia	Reentry mechanism	Paroxysmal sinus rhythm; P waves often undetectable; rate >220 beats/min (infant), rate >180 beats/min (child)	*Stable:* Vagal maneuvers. Consider adenosine if no response. Adenosine 0.1 mg/kg IV bolus (maximum initial dose: 6 mg). May double and repeat dose once (maximum second dose: 12 mg). If no response consider: Alternative medications (e.g., amiodarone, procainamide). Cardioversion 0.5–1 J/kg. *Unstable:* Cardioversion 0.5–1 J/kg; if not effective, increase to 2 J/kg. Sedate if possible, but do not delay cardioversion. May attempt adenosine if this does not delay cardioversion.
Ventricular tachycardia	Structural disease, hypoxia, acidosis, electrolyte imbalance, toxic ingestion (e.g., tricyclic antidepressants)	Rate ≥120 beats/min; wide QRS; no P waves	*Pulse and stable:* Amiodarone 5 mg/kg IV (max 300 mg) over 20–60 min or procainamide 15 mg/kg IV over 30–60 min or lidocaine 1 mg/kg IV bolus. Consider sedation, and cardiovert at 0.5–1 J/kg. *Pulse but unstable:* Cardioversion 0.5–1 J/kg; if not effective, increase to 2 J/kg. Sedate if possible, but do not delay cardioversion. *Pulseless:* Defibrillation at 2 J/kg, high-quality BLS for 2 minutes; if no response, repeat defibrillation using 4 J/kg followed by high-quality BLS for 2 minutes; repeat as needed.
			Epinephrine IV/IO: 0.01 mg/kg (1:10,000: 0.1 mL/kg) as soon as vascular access obtained. ET: 0.1 mg/kg (1:1000: 0.1 mL/kg). Repeat dose every 3–5 minutes. Consider antidysrhythmics: Amiodarone 5 mg/kg (max 300 mg) IV/IO. Lidocaine 1 mg/kg IV/IO. Magnesium 25–50 mg/kg IV/IO if torsades de pointes.

Continued

TABLE 45.3 Rhythm Disturbances in Children.—cont'd

Rhythm	Cause	Characteristics	Treatment
Slow Rhythms			
Sinus bradycardia	Hypoxemia, hypotension, acidosis	Sinus rhythm; slow rate (<80 beats/min in infants, <60 beats/min in children)	Ventilation, oxygenation, cardiac compressions for heart rate <60 beats/min with signs of poor perfusion. Epinephrine (1:10,000), 0.01 mg/kg IV/IO. Repeat every 3–5 minutes. If increased vagal tone or primary AV block: Atropine, 0.02 mg/kg IV; may repeat. (Minimum dose 0.1 mg; maximal total dose for child: 1 mg.) Consider cardiac pacing.
Junctional rhythm, heart blocks	Hypoxemia, hypotension, acidosis	Rare in children; slow rate; P waves may or may not be present	Ventilation, oxygenation, cardiac compressions for heart rate <60 beat/min with signs of poor perfusion. Atropine, 0.02 mg/kg IV; may repeat. (Minimum dose 0.1 mg; maximal total dose for child: 1 mg.) Epinephrine (1:10,000) 0.1 mL/kg IV. Consider cardiac pacing.
Absent/Disorganized/Nonperfusing Rhythms			
Asystole/PEA	Hypoxia, hypovolemia, acidosis, hypo/hyperkalemia, hypoglycemia, hypothermia, toxins, cardiac tamponade, tension pneumothorax, thrombosis (coronary or pulmonary), trauma	Asystole: Flat line on ECG; absent pulse; absent respirations PEA: Pulselessness, with organized electrical activity on ECG	BLS, identify/treat underlying cause. Epinephrine IV/IO 0.01 mg/kg (1:10,000): 0.1 mL/kg; ET; 0.1 mg/kg (1:1000: 0.1 mL/kg). Repeat every 3–5 minutes.
Ventricular fibrillation	Rare in infants and children; hypoxia, hypovolemia, acidosis, hypo/hyperkalemia, hypoglycemia, hypothermia, toxins, cardiac tamponade, tension pneumothorax, thrombosis (coronary or pulmonary), trauma	No identifiable P, QRS, or T waves; wavy line on ECG	Defibrillation at 2 J/kg, high-quality BLS for 2 minutes; if no response, repeat defibrillation using 4 J/kg followed by high-quality BLS for 2 minutes; repeat as needed. Epinephrine IV/IO: 0.01 mg/kg (1:10,000: 0.1 mL/kg) as soon as vascular access obtained. ET: 0.1 mg/kg (1:1000: 0.1 mL/kg). Repeat dose every 3–5 minutes. Consider antidysrhythmics: Amiodarone 5 mg/kg (max 300 mg) IV/IO. Lidocaine 1 mg/kg IV/IO. Magnesium 25–50 mg/kg IV/IO if torsades de pointes.

BLS, Basic life support (ventilations and compressions); *ET,* endotracheal tube; *IO,* intraosseous; *IV,* intravenous; *PEA,* pulseless electrical activity.

Heart Failure

Congenital heart disease accounts for the majority of children seen in the ED with heart failure (HF). Preload, afterload, and myocardial contractility are major factors in determining the amount of blood pumped through the vascular system. When the heart is not able to pump effectively because of chronic disease, rhythm disturbance, pressure on the heart, or excessive fluid volume, the fluid backs up in the system, causing signs of overload such as pulmonary edema, jugular vein distention, and enlarged liver.

Signs of HF include tachycardia, tachypnea, cough, wheezes, pulmonary crackles, cyanosis, pallor, poor appetite, and failure to thrive. Many times, infants with HF have a very rapid respiratory rate (60–100 breaths/min) but do not appear in distress. Lack of distress is evidence of the infant's ability to compensate. Observe for presence and degree of other indicators of respiratory effort such as nasal flaring, intercostal retractions, head bobbing, and expiratory grunting.

Primary treatment of HF is aimed at improving myocardial contractility and decreasing cardiac workload by using pharmacologic agents. These agents include inotropic drugs (dobutamine, milrinone, digoxin) that improve myocardial contractility, diuretics (furosemide) to reduce preload, and afterload-reducing agents (sodium nitroprusside, captopril) to reduce ventricular afterload.

Inadequate Volume

The major medical cause of hypovolemia in children is dehydration. A child who has been sick for even a short time with vomiting and diarrhea is at risk, as is a child who has been ill for several days with fever and decreased fluid intake. When output exceeds intake over time, dehydration becomes clinically significant and electrolyte imbalances occur. Electrolyte disturbances cause more nausea and vomiting, starting a downward spiral to be reversed only with medical intervention. The degree of dehydration is categorized as a percentage of lost body weight (mild—5%, moderate—10%, severe—15%). When 5% or more of the child's body mass (weight) is lost, skin and mucous membranes appear dry. It is often helpful to ask the parent about intake and output—the number of bottles the child has taken and the number of stools or wet diapers per day for small children (six to eight wet diapers per day is considered normal). Mild dehydration is commonly treated with oral rehydration. Parents may be instructed to give the child small amounts of an oral electrolyte solution at frequent intervals (a teaspoonful at a time). Changes in mental status, skin perfusion, heart rate, pulse quality, urinary output, and blood pressure occur in moderate and severe dehydration; eyes appear sunken and infants exhibit a sunken anterior fontanel. Unless fluid volume is replaced and balance between intake and output restored, the condition will progress to hypovolemic shock.

Increasing heart rate, mottled cool skin, decreasing mental status, narrowing pulse pressure, and extremely prolonged capillary refill time suggest the child's perfusion status is worsening. Resuscitation requires ensuring adequate ventilation and oxygenation, rapid bolusing with 20 mL/kg of crystalloid solution, and repeated fluid boluses until improvement is seen.[16] If vascular access cannot be rapidly obtained, intraosseous (IO) access should be attempted, and in some cases of severe decompensated shock, IO access should be the initial access. IO access can be performed safely on children of all ages.[16] IO access is a quick, safe, and dependable route for administering fluids, medications, and blood products.

Diagnostic tests may include complete blood count (CBC); determination of electrolytes, glucose, and blood urea nitrogen (BUN) values; and urinalysis. The decision to admit is based on the child's condition after evaluation and management and the ability to tolerate oral feeding.

Inadequate Fluid Distribution

Septic Shock

Sepsis, or septicemia, is a profound, life-threatening bacterial infection in the bloodstream. Septic shock occurs in patients with septicemia when inadequate tissue perfusion occurs in the wake of massive vasodilation. The massive vasodilation causes a relative hypovolemia in the intravascular space, which is why pediatric septic shock frequently responds well to early aggressive fluid resuscitation. The clinical diagnosis of septic shock is made in children with a suspected infection, manifested by hyperthermia or hypothermia, who exhibit other signs of decreased perfusion. Septic shock may be manifest as a warm shock or a cold shock state. Tachycardia and decreased mental status are seen in both shock states. Warm shock may occur, initially characterized by a flushed, ruddy appearance, bounding peripheral pulses, and flash capillary refill; cold shock is associated with mottled cool extremities, diminished peripheral pulses, and capillary refill greater than 3 seconds.[3,17]

The ABCs should be rapidly assessed and supported. The nurse must keep in mind that hypotension is a late sign of shock in infants and young children, and when present, it indicates decompensated severe shock. Skin should be inspected for petechial or purpuric lesions that would be "red flag" skin signs of septic shock caused by meningococcemia.

Management in the ED focuses on preservation of vital functions. Adequate ventilation and oxygenation are the first priority. Administer supplemental oxygen, and assist with breathing if ventilation is inadequate. Maintaining normal perfusion is a priority. Fluid infusion is best initiated with boluses of 20 to 30 mL/kg, titrated to assuring an adequate blood pressure and clinical monitors of cardiac output including HR, quality of peripheral pulses, capillary refill, level of consciousness, and urine output. Initial volume resuscitation requirements may be 10 mL/kg if rales or hepatomegaly are present but commonly are 40 to 60 mL/kg.[18] Isotonic crystalloids such as normal saline or lactated Ringer's solution are given for volume replacement.[18,19] Once the diagnosis of sepsis or septic shock is made, IV antibiotic therapy should be instituted immediately.

Ideally, all cultures (blood, urine, others) are collected before antibiotic administration. The antibiotics administered vary with the child's age and the presumed source of infection. After culture results are available, antibiotic therapy can be more specific. Sympathomimetic and inotropic drugs such as epinephrine and dopamine may be used to increase heart rate and cardiac output in patients with poor myocardial function and systemic perfusion despite adequate oxygenation and fluid resuscitation. Serum glucose level should be carefully monitored. In younger infants and children, limited glycogen stores in the liver place the child at risk for hypoglycemia. A child is considered hypoglycemic if his or her blood glucose level is less than 60 mg/dL (in a child) or less than 40 mg/dL (in a neonate). The child is admitted, usually to the intensive care unit, for continued IV fluid replacement, antibiotics, and monitoring.

Anaphylaxis

Anaphylaxis is a potentially life-threatening manifestation of immediate hypersensitivity. The severity of these reactions varies from mild urticarial to shock and death. Anaphylaxis most commonly involves the pulmonary, circulatory, cutaneous, gastrointestinal and central nervous systems.[7]

Anaphylaxis is highly likely if there is (1) sudden onset of skin or mucosal changes with acute respiratory symptoms, hypotension, or other signs of end-organ dysfunction; (2) sudden involvement of at least two body organ systems after exposure to a likely allergen or trigger for the patient; or (3) age-specific hypotension after exposure to a known allergen.[7]

Recovery from anaphylactic reactions depends on rapid recognition and institution of treatment. The goal of treatment is to provide ventilation, restore adequate circulation, and prevent further exposure by identifying and removing the cause. Establishing an airway is the first concern. The child should receive high-flow oxygen, cardiac monitoring should be initiated, and vital signs should be assessed. Epinephrine intramuscularly, 1:1000 solution: 0.01 mg/kg (0.01 mL/kg), maximum 0.3 mg (0.3 mL), should be given immediately and repeated every 5 to 15 minutes as necessary.[7,16]

Fluids are given to restore volume. The amount of fluid given should be determined by the clinical situation. Children with anaphylaxis should be hospitalized and monitored for at least 24 hours because of the risk for a biphasic reaction.

Second-line treatments, such as antihistamines and steroids, are slower acting than epinephrine and have little effect on acute blood pressure changes. They are helpful for symptomatic relief of itching, angioedema, or hives and are commonly administered in the ED setting.

Sickle Cell Disease

Sickle cell disease (SCD) is an inherited hemoglobinopathy characterized by the presence of hemoglobin S. In SCD, red blood cells that are normally round assume an irregular sickle shape when deoxygenated. These sickled cells clump together, occluding small blood vessels and causing tissue ischemia. Sickling is precipitated by multiple factors, including infection, dehydration, fatigue, cold exposure, and stress.

There are three major categories of sickle cell crisis. Vasoocclusive crises occur when small vessels in bone, soft tissue, and organs (e.g., liver, spleen, brain, lungs, penis) are occluded, causing ischemia, pain, and swelling. The first presentation of vasoocclusive crisis, usually after 2 or 3 months of age, is manifested by warmth and swelling of one or both hands or feet. Older children have pain in affected organs, visual disturbances, respiratory distress, and priapism. Management is primarily focused on correcting the precipitating cause, if identified, supporting hydration and oxygenation as needed, and providing pain management.

Aplastic crisis is characterized by impaired red blood cell production in the bone marrow. Aplastic crisis worsens the anemia of SCD and leads to high-output congestive heart failure. The diagnosis of aplastic crisis is made on the basis of CBC and reticulocyte count results. Management is focused on restoring depleted blood components.

Sequestration crisis is the most fulminant manifestation of SCD. It is less common than other crises but can be rapidly fatal. Its incidence is greater in young children who are several months to 6 years of age. Blood suddenly pools in the spleen and other visceral organs, causing severe anemia and hypovolemic shock. Emergent management is focused on the restoration of circulating blood volume.

Acute chest syndrome (ACS) is a major cause of morbidity and mortality for children with SCD. There is a higher incidence of ACS during the winter months and the peak incidence occurs in patients 2 to 4 years of age. The specific cause of ACS is not easily determined. Triggers such as a vasoocclusive crisis, infection, asthma, or postoperative complication have all been implicated. Chest pain, shortness of breath, coughing, and fever are the most common presenting complaints of those experiencing ACS.[20]

Because of the need for close monitoring, specialists care for most patients with SCD. However, a first crisis or a severe crisis may lead to treatment in the ED. Medical management is usually directed at supportive, symptomatic treatment. The main objectives are pain management, oxygenation, hydration with oral or IV solutions, electrolyte replacement, rest, blood replacement as needed, and antibiotics as required. The administration of narcotics should be anticipated for pain control because SCD is a chronic painful disease.

NEUROLOGIC EMERGENCIES

Head trauma is the most common cause of neurologic emergency in children. Seizures, shunt malfunction and, rarely, brain tumors and congenital vascular malformations can also affect mental status in the pediatric population. Infectious processes such as meningitis and sepsis are other causes of neurologic changes in children.

Assessment

When a child has an altered mental status, it is important to remember that the first priority is airway and ventilation. Neurologic assessment of pediatric patients presents special challenges, especially for the nonverbal child. When parents say their child is "not acting normal," this should be taken seriously. Early signs and symptoms of increased intracranial pressure include altered mental status, restlessness, inconsolability, headache, and vomiting. Constricted or dilated pupils and decorticate (abnormal flexion) or decerebrate (abnormal extension) posturing are late signs of increased intracranial pressure.

Numerous methods of assessing neurologic function in children have been proposed, including pediatric adaptations of the Glasgow Coma Scale (see Table 42.3). The simplest and probably the most useful in the emergency setting is the mnemonic AVPU:

- **A** Alert
- **V** responds only to Verbal stimuli
- **P** responds only to Painful stimuli
- **U** Unresponsive

Serial assessment with the AVPU mnemonic tool, together with a description of the patient's behavior, is the clearest means for documenting changes. An accurate history from parents is also helpful. When a child presents with an altered mental status, ask about trauma, previous medical problems, ingestions, headache, and signs and symptoms of infection. An altered level of consciousness in any child needs to be recognized as an emergent condition.

Treatment for children who arrive in the ED with an altered level of consciousness includes assessment of ABCs along with assessment for injury or illnesses. The child must be evaluated for signs and symptoms of increased intracranial pressure to prevent secondary central nervous system injury. Laboratory studies may be ordered to detect toxins or electrolyte abnormalities; diagnostic imaging may be ordered to rule out injury or other pathologic processes as the precipitator of the child's change in mental status.

Seizures

Seizures are involuntary movements or alteration in sensation, behavior, or consciousness caused by abnormal electrical activity in the brain. In young children, seizures associated with fever are one of the most common neurologic disorders of childhood, affecting 3% to 5% of children and accounting for 1% of all ED visits for patients younger than 18 years of age.[21] Most febrile seizures occur after 6 months of age and usually before 3 years, with increased frequency in children younger than 18 months.

The cause of febrile seizures is still uncertain. In most children, height and rapidity of temperature elevation or rapidity of the temperature drop seem to be important factors; however, seizures usually occur during temperature fluctuations rather than after prolonged elevation. Febrile seizures may accompany upper respiratory infection, gastrointestinal infection, or ear infection. Between 25% and 30% of children with simple febrile seizures have a recurrence with subsequent infections.[3]

Treatment for febrile seizures consists of ensuring the child's safety during the seizure, controlling the seizure, and reducing the temperature. Parents also need reassurance of the generally benign nature of febrile seizures.

Other seizure disorders have numerous and varied causes. Seizure disorders are idiopathic if the cause is unknown and organic or symptomatic if the cause is identifiable. Epilepsy is the diagnosis when seizures are recurrent with no apparent cause for the seizures. Patients who have seizures may exhibit a wide range of behaviors, from lip smacking and staring to violent muscular contractions or sudden loss of consciousness; urinary and bowel incontinence may also occur. Status epilepticus occurs when seizure activity is prolonged (greater than 30 minutes) or when the patient has sequential seizures without regaining consciousness between each seizure. This may be a manifestation of anoxia, infection, trauma, ingestion, or metabolic disorder. Sustained seizure activity can potentially produce cerebral anoxia and possible ischemic brain damage; therefore airway protection, oxygenation, and rapid termination of convulsive activity are priorities. Anticonvulsant medications (e.g., benzodiazepines) may be administered rectally, intranasally, or intramuscularly until seizure activity abates and vascular access can be established. Common laboratory tests include CBC, electrolytes, glucose, calcium, magnesium, BUN, anticonvulsant drug levels, urinalysis, and toxicology screen. Whether the patient is admitted to the hospital or discharged home depends on the patient's history, laboratory findings, and physical findings.

GASTROINTESTINAL AND GENITOURINARY EMERGENCIES

Gastroenteritis

Innumerable children are brought to the ED with complaints of nausea, vomiting, diarrhea, and poor feeding. Gastroenteritis is an inflammation of the gastrointestinal tract caused by bacterial, viral, or parasitic agents. Viral pathogens are the most common cause of acute gastroenteritis. Morbidity results from dehydration and electrolyte imbalances. Diagnostic tests including electrolytes, BUN, and creatinine and point-of-care glucose testing are to be performed for children with severe dehydration.[21]

Gastroenteritis associated with signs of severe dehydration/hypovolemic shock is treated with 20 mL/kg boluses of IV crystalloid solutions. Fluids boluses of 20 mL/kg should be repeated until perfusion improves. Patients whose laboratory analyses are within normal limits, those who are only mildly dehydrated, and those who are able to take fluids by mouth are generally discharged to home after rehydration. Parents are instructed to give the child small amounts of clear liquids at frequent intervals (a teaspoonful at a time). Oral rehydration fluids (such as Pedialyte, Enfalyte, or generic formulations of these solutions) are preferred; apple juice should be avoided because it is hyperosmolar and may worsen diarrhea. Studies have shown that children fed their regular diet (instead of a diet restriction like the BRAT [bananas, rice, applesauce, toast] diet) return to their preillness weight sooner than children who are diet restricted.[21] Most children seen in the ED for acute gastroenteritis should be advised to follow up with their primary care doctor.

Abdominal Pain

Other illnesses causing gastrointestinal upset or abdominal pain are infection with bacterial agents and parasites; surgical emergencies such as appendicitis, strangulated hernia, intussusception, testicular torsion, or bowel obstruction; urinary tract infection (UTI); and toxic ingestion. For the most part, ED treatment of the stable patient with abdominal pain focuses on assessing the patient, including history and vital signs, deciding whether the patient can be discharged or requires hospitalization, and determining whether the problem needs medical or surgical intervention. If the child has abdominal pain, an acute abdominal condition must be ruled out, so the child should not be allowed to drink any fluid until evaluation is complete. In general, the possibility of a surgical abdomen should be considered for any patient with abdominal pain associated with palpation or movement. Basic diagnostic tests include a CBC and urinalysis; imaging studies of the chest, abdomen, or pelvis may be needed. Adolescent female patients should be asked about pregnancy, and a menstrual history should be obtained. Assume that any female of childbearing age could be pregnant and obtain a pregnancy test to rule out gestation as the potential cause of abdominal pain.

Appendicitis

Appendicitis is inflammation of the vermiform appendix or blind sac of the cecum. It is the most common condition requiring surgical intervention during childhood. Primarily an acute condition, appendicitis can progress to perforation and peritonitis without appropriate treatment. Signs and symptoms of appendicitis vary greatly but commonly include pain beginning in the periumbilical region and migrating to the right lower quadrant, rebound tenderness, nausea, and vomiting. Appendicitis in the nonverbal child often presents very late; the appendix may be ruptured and the peritoneum contaminated by the time symptoms are recognized and the child goes to surgery.

The most important diagnostic tests are a white blood cell count with differential and urinalysis. With appendicitis, total white blood cell count is usually 15,000 to 20,000 cells/mL with bands present. Fever is usually present, varying from 99.5°F to 101.3°F (37.5°C–38.5°C). If the temperature is greater than 102.2°F (39°C), viral illness or perforation is likely. Imaging studies (e.g., abdominal computed tomography or ultrasonography) may be obtained if diagnosis is uncertain. Definitive treatment for appendicitis is surgical removal of the appendix, or appendectomy. The child should have no oral intake, and fluid and electrolyte imbalances should be corrected before the child goes to surgery. Prophylactic antibiotics may be started before surgery for patients with evidence of perforation.

Incarcerated Hernia

A hernia is a protrusion of a portion of an organ through an abdominal opening. Classic presentation is an asymptomatic bulge that becomes more prominent with crying, defecation, coughing, or laughing.[3] Danger from herniation arises when the intestine protruding through the opening is constricted until circulation is impaired. Hernias can often be manually reduced in the ED. Giving pain medication, placing the patient in Trendelenburg's position, and applying ice to the area may assist in this process. Surgical intervention is eventually required for most patients.

Intussusception

Intussusception occurs when a proximal portion of the intestine telescopes into a more distal portion of intestine. This generally occurs in infancy, most often between ages 3 months and 1 year. Telescoping prevents passage of intestinal contents, including fecal material, beyond the defect. Stools passed in this disorder contain primarily blood and mucus, resulting in the "currant jelly" stools characteristic of intussusception. The child may have intermittent spasmodic type of pain. Occasionally a sausage-shaped mass can be palpated in the abdomen.

In most cases initial treatment is nonsurgical hydrostatic reduction by barium enema concurrent with diagnostic testing. If this does not reduce the obstruction, surgical intervention is necessary.

Pyloric Stenosis

Pyloric stenosis results from hypertrophy of the circular muscle of the pylorus that causes constriction and obstruction of the gastric outlet. Although it is has been reported in infants from birth to 5 months, it most commonly occurs at 3 to 4 weeks of life; projectile, nonbilious vomiting after feeding is common. The infant is persistently hungry and easily refed. Weight loss, constipation, and dehydration result from the continuing emesis. An olive-shaped mass may be palpable in the right upper quadrant, and peristaltic waves may be visualized across the abdomen. This condition is diagnosed by history, physical examination, and abdominal ultrasonography. Management consists of correcting dehydration with IV fluid, inserting a gastric tube to decompress the stomach, and preparing the infant for a surgical pyloromyotomy.

Testicular Torsion

A prepubertal male with sudden onset of severe scrotal pain radiating to the abdomen may have testicular torsion. Twisting of spermatic vessels causes ischemia, swelling, and a high-lying testis. Patients may complain of nausea and vomiting. Scrotal edema is present, and blood pressure may be elevated because of pain and anxiety. Fever is rarely present. Diagnosis can often be made clinically, but Doppler ultrasound flow studies may also be used.

Testicular torsion is a surgical emergency. Testicular salvage is approximately 80% to 100% if detorsion is accomplished within 6 hours; salvage is less than 20% with more than 12 hours of torsion, and after 24 hours the rate of salvage approaches 0%. If the torsion has been present less than 3 or 4 hours, manual reduction by the ED physician or urologist may be possible. If surgery is indicated, make sure the patient has no oral intake and administer analgesics as ordered. Patients with suspected testicular torsion should receive a higher triage priority because of increased potential for functional recovery with early resolution of the problem.

Urinary Tract Infections

UTIs are a major concern in children. About 3% to 5% of all girls and 1% of boys will have a symptomatic UTI before puberty.[8] Neonatal UTIs usually result from a bacteremia, whereas infants and children become infected from bacteria traveling up the urethra to the bladder. The presence of a possible UTI should be considered in all febrile infants, even if there is another source of infection identified. The gold standard for obtaining a urine specimen in a child with a suspected UTI is a catheterized sample, not a bagged collection. Urinary reflux can move bacteria up into the kidneys and lead to abnormal renal function and pyelonephritis if left undetected.

ENDOCRINE EMERGENCIES

Diabetic Ketoacidosis

Diabetic ketoacidosis (DKA) is a life-threatening medical emergency characterized by hyperglycemia, dehydration, metabolic acidosis, and ketonemia or ketonuria resulting from an absolute or relative insulin deficiency. DKA is more common in young children and adolescents with type 1 diabetes mellitus than in adults and remains the most common cause of death in diabetic children. DKA is the most common presentation of diabetes in children younger than 4 years of age; overall, 20% to 40% of children newly diagnosed with type 1 diabetes present for medical care in DKA. Early symptoms of hyperglycemia, including polyuria, polydipsia, polyphagia, weight loss, and fatigue, are often subtle and are easily missed in infants or preschool children. As hyperglycemia progresses, nausea, vomiting, lethargy, altered mental status, deep rapid breathing (i.e., Kussmaul respirations), acetone odor to the breath, and abdominal pain are commonly identified, signaling the onset of DKA. In children with known type 1 diabetes, infection and noncompliance with insulin regimen are the most common precipitators of DKA. Diagnosis of this disorder is based on the result of blood gas analysis, blood glucose level, and serum and/or urine ketones.

Once the child's ABCs have been supported, management of the patient in DKA should focus on the correction of metabolic acidosis. Systematic interventions are implemented to restore fluid volume, stop ketogenesis, correct electrolyte disturbances, and avoid complications (cerebral edema, hypoglycemia, and hypokalemia). Cerebral edema is the most frequent, serious complication of pediatric DKA; children younger than 5 years of age and patients previously undiagnosed with type 1 diabetes are at high risk for developing this potentially devastating complication.

The current recommendations for the management of pediatric DKA are as follows. Initially, a bolus of 5 to 20 mL/kg of 0.9% saline is administered and repeated as necessary to restore adequate perfusion of end organs, often judged by monitoring mentation, capillary refill, and heart rate. Subsequently, the remaining fluid deficit should be replaced over a 48-hour period. Gradual correction of fluid status is advised to minimize the risk for developing cerebral edema. Insulin should be administered by continuous infusion at a rate of 0.05 to 0.1 unit/kg per hour until ketosis/acidosis is resolved. This low dose of insulin usually decreases serum glucose concentration by 50 to 75 mg/dL per hour. The insulin drip should be continued until the metabolic acidosis has resolved (pH greater than or equal to 7.3, bicarbonate greater than or equal to 18 mEq/L). Serum glucose concentrations generally decrease to the normal range before ketosis and acidosis have resolved. To prevent hypoglycemia during insulin infusion, dextrose-containing fluids should be added when the serum glucose falls below 250 to 300 mg/dL. Serum glucose levels should be checked every hour until stabilized.

Initial serum potassium levels may be low, normal, or high. Potassium levels drop as acidosis is corrected, and replacement therapy should be initiated once adequate renal function has been ensured, generally after the child's first void. Potassium is typically administered at a concentration of 30 to 40 mEq/L of fluid given adequate renal function. Potassium may be administered as potassium chloride and potassium phosphate or potassium acetate. Ongoing monitoring should include serial evaluation of vital signs, neurologic checks, intake and output, and laboratory samples (e.g., glucose, pH, electrolytes).[7]

INFECTIOUS DISEASE EMERGENCIES

Children with upper respiratory infections such as colds, sore throats, sinusitis, and ear infections are often brought to the ED. For the most part, they are rapidly discharged and followed by their private physicians. Some of the more serious infectious diseases are described in this section.

AIDS

In 2016 youth aged 13 to 24 made up 21% of the new HIV cases in the United States.[22] Infants and children with acquired immunodeficiency syndrome (AIDS) or those infected with the human immunodeficiency virus (HIV) present to the ED with numerous physical problems requiring both physiologic and psychological support. In the pediatric population, three age-groups are primarily affected. These are children exposed in utero to an infected mother, children who received blood products infected with the virus, and adolescents infected through high-risk behaviors. Most children with AIDS are younger than 2 years of age and constitute a small percentage of the total AIDS population. Most children with AIDS have recurrent bacterial and fungal infections, chronic diarrhea, chronic anemia, renal disease, cardiomyopathy, neurologic deterioration, or general failure to thrive.

Treatment is primarily supportive, aimed at prevention of infections and complications, early recognition of complications, and support of optimal general health.

Tuberculosis

Tuberculosis (TB) is caused by *Mycobacterium tuberculosis,* and the source of infection in most situations is a member of the household. It is a disease controlled in most developed countries that still remains a health hazard and leading cause of death in many parts of the world. A steady increase in new cases has occurred during the past several years, attributed in part to the influx of foreign-born people and recognition of the disease in the native-born population.

Clinical manifestations of TB are extremely variable. Fever, malaise, anorexia, weight loss, or cough may be present. Coinfection with HIV is also common. Most children with pulmonary TB have noninfectious disease; therefore they seldom require isolation. Hospitalization is seldom necessary because most children can be managed at home. Antimicrobial agents cure most cases of TB, with the limiting factor being patient compliance with drug administration. Drug therapy usually lasts 6 to 9 months. Historically, TB has been regarded with fear of infection, so it is important to clarify any misconceptions parents may have regarding this disease.

Bacteremia

The effects of bacterial invasion of the bloodstream may range from relatively mild symptoms of infection (bacteremia) to overwhelming, life-threatening infection (sepsis or septic shock). Bacteremia and septic shock represent the two extremes on a continuum of severity rather than disparate entities.

Bacteremia may occur in association with meningitis, cellulitis, or UTI. It may also occur without localized findings (occult bacteremia). Bacteremia is most common in children younger than 2 years of age and may be difficult to detect in the child younger than 2 months of age. Any child younger than 2 years of age should be suspected of bacteremia when there is fever and documented infection (white blood cell count greater than 15,000 cells/mL) without an observable focus of infection. Bacteremia may be especially difficult to detect in young infants because they do not always respond to infection with fever. Bacteremia should be suspected when a child has fever with malaise, poor feeding, irritability, or is not playful or easily consoled. The diagnostic workup commonly includes CBC, blood cultures, urinalysis, urine culture, and lumbar puncture if indicated. Broad-spectrum antibiotics are initially administered.

If the patient is discharged, careful attention should be given to the parent's ability to understand and appreciate the importance of the diagnosis and the need to continue antimicrobial therapy as prescribed. The child should be reevaluated within 24 to 48 hours. Bacteremia can progress to sepsis if the patient is not adequately treated.

Meningitis

Meningitis, acute inflammation of the meninges, is a common cause of death and disability in children. Annual incidence of meningitis is 1 case per 2000 children with a peak in children 2 months to 5 years of age.[8] Causative organisms are often bacterial, but viral meningitis also occurs. With bacterial meningitis, organisms can enter the bloodstream through focal infection or by routes such as open wounds, skull fractures, and surgical procedures. The infection spreads through the subarachnoid space, causing swelling and pain. Recognition and treatment are essential to prevent death and residual damage.

Increased intracranial pressure is a major concern in meningitis. As inflammation increases, expansion within the rigid skull causes direct pressure on the brain. Narrow passageways to the ventricles are occluded, and cerebrospinal fluid outflow is obstructed, producing altered sensorium.

Many children diagnosed with meningitis present with headache, nausea, vomiting, or poor feeding. Most children have an elevated temperature; however, infants may have normal temperature or even hypothermia. A classic sign of meningitis is nuchal rigidity, which is rarely seen in infancy. Common signs and symptoms of increased intracranial pressure may be evident, including inconsolability, restlessness, altered mental status, and seizures. A bulging fontanel is a late sign. A severely ill child may be in respiratory distress, exhibit cyanosis, and have a rash or petechiae.

In the late stages, meningitis requires aggressive intervention, including airway management, control of increased intracranial pressure, IV medication (e.g., vasopressors, mannitol, diuretics, antibiotics), and admission to the intensive care unit. Definitive diagnosis requires a lumbar puncture and laboratory analysis of cerebrospinal fluid for protein, glucose, cell count, and Gram stain.

Meningococcemia

Meningococcemia, caused by invasion of the bloodstream with *Neisseria meningitidis,* can occur with or without meningitis. The child with meningococcemia has fever, headache, and rash (usually maculopapular rash), petechiae, and purpuric lesions. Fig. 45.2 illustrates the cutaneous effects of meningococcemia. Meningococcemia can be rapidly fatal. Shock and disseminated intravascular coagulation occur very quickly; therefore rapid assessment and intervention are critical. Aggressive resuscitation, including advanced airway management, fluid bolusing, antibiotics, and vasopressors, should be anticipated. Diagnostic tests may include CBC, electrolytes, glucose, clotting studies, blood cultures, urinalysis and urine culture, and lumbar puncture. Isolation with droplet precautions should be initiated immediately upon suspicion of meningococcemia to protect caregivers from exposure to this life-threatening illness.

Lyme Disease

Lyme disease is a systemic, tick-borne illness. A skin lesion, known as erythema chronicum migrans, is present in most cases. A tick that lives primarily on white-tailed deer and white-footed field mice carries Lyme disease, caused by the spirochete *Borrelia burgdorferi.* The multisystem nature and slow evolution of the illness make diagnosis difficult. In a child with suspected Lyme disease, a history of tick bite or being in a wooded area is important. The small size of the tick may prevent the patient from realizing its presence. General malaise, aching, sore throat, or fever may cause the patient to seek treatment.

Antibiotic therapy varies, depending on clinical presentation and progression of the disease. Early Lyme disease is treated with oral doxycycline, amoxicillin, or erythromycin. More serious symptoms such as Lyme carditis, neurologic manifestations, or Lyme arthritis require IV therapy with ceftriaxone or penicillin G. Prevention of the disease involves awareness and taking precautions before and after being in areas where the ticks reside. Parents should check the child's entire body after being in a wooded area.

Skin Rashes

Children are often brought to the ED with a concern related to a rash. In fact, rashes are quite a common pediatric complaint. Most rashes, such as neonatal acne, diaper dermatitis, and viral exanthema, are not life-threatening. Other diseases have long-term consequences and should be taken seriously. Some infectious diseases that present with a skin rash are shown in Table 45.4.

OTHER CONDITIONS

Cellulitis

An injury that breaks the skin barrier, such as an insect bite, abrasion, laceration, or surgical procedure, may allow entry of organisms causing cellulitis (e.g., *Staphylococcus aureus,* group A streptococci). An inflammatory response causes

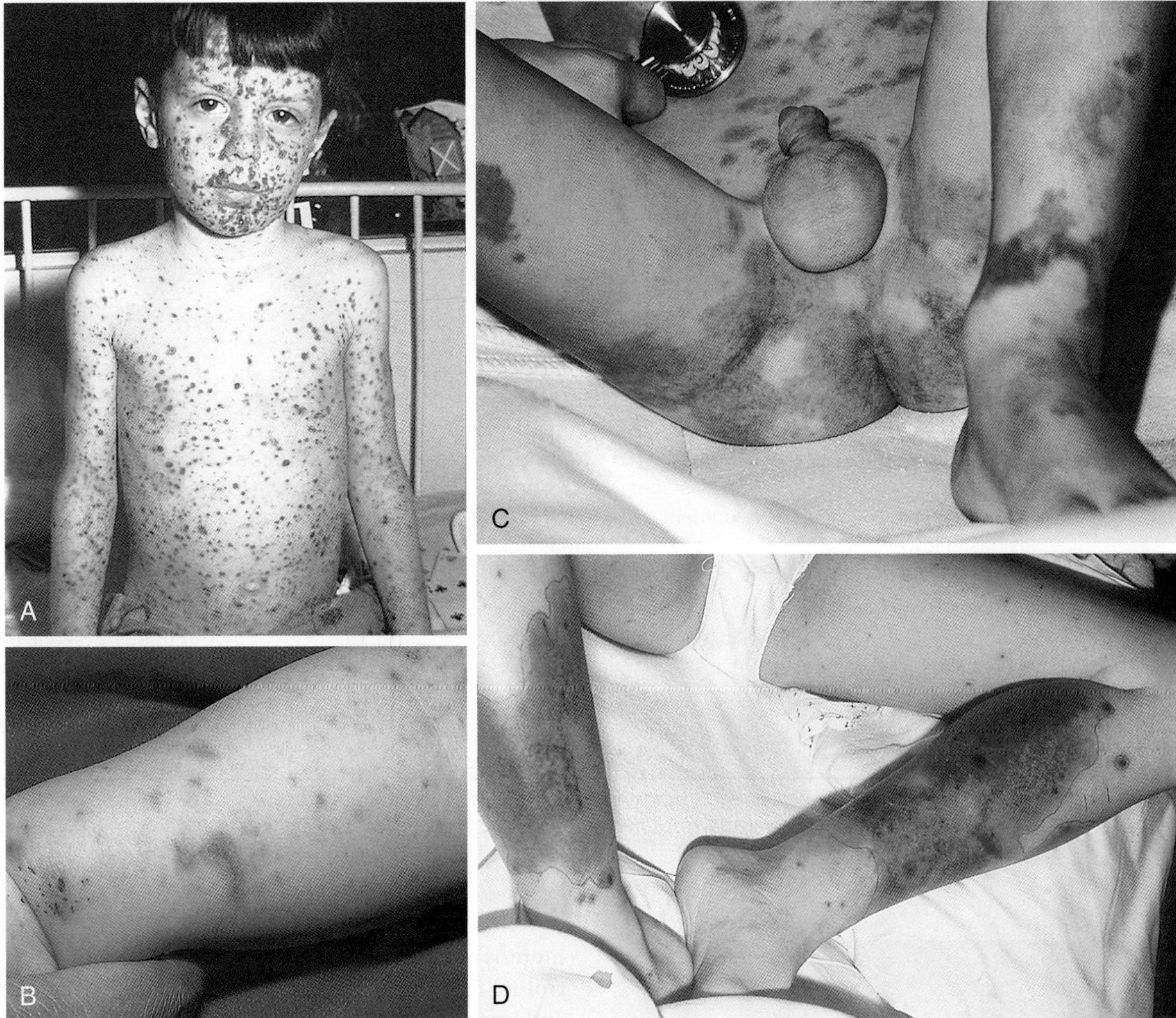

Fig. 45.2 Meningococcemia. (A) This child manifests the generalized purpuric and petechial rash characteristic of acute meningococcemia. (B) Petechiae are more apparent in this close-up of an infant. Gram stain of petechial scrapings may reveal organisms. (C and D) Purpura may progress to form areas of frank cutaneous necrosis, especially in patients with disseminated intravascular coagulation. (From Zitelli B, Davis H: *Atlas of Pediatric Physical Diagnosis.* 5th ed. St Louis, MO: Mosby; 2007.)

edema and swelling of the affected area, usually without fever. Most patients are treated on an outpatient basis. Children younger than 3 years old with facial cellulitis are more likely to have bacteremia and require IV antimicrobial therapy.

Community-acquired methicillin-resistant *Staphylococcus aureus* (CA-MRSA) infection is a common concern, especially in children with skin and soft-tissue infections. When children receive antibiotics for soft-tissue cellulitis on an outpatient basis, close follow-up to ensure clearance of the infection is vital.

Hair Tourniquets

Hair tourniquet syndrome is a relatively common finding in infants. The infant usually presents with excessive crying, or the parent or caretaker notices redness of the extremity. It is an emergency because failure to promptly remove the hair acting as a tourniquet can lead to serious infection or even amputation.

This syndrome usually affects the toes, fingers, or external genitalia, with the third toe and third finger the most commonly involved areas. Hair is more commonly associated with toes (Fig. 45.3) and external genitalia, whereas threads are more often found around fingers.

Treatment includes removal with fine scissors and forceps. If unable to remove, some physicians have used depilatory agents to dissolve the hair and material. In rare incidents, surgery may be required if the hair/thread is very deep. Usually there is no sequela after removal.

Impetigo

Impetigo is a skin infection caused by group A streptococci. It is typically found in children younger than 6 years of age. The patient has skin lesions oozing serous fluid and honey-colored crust when dry. Most cases of impetigo can be treated on an outpatient basis with topical antibiotics and good skin hygiene.

TABLE 45.4 Infections With Skin Rashes.

Characteristic	Measles (Rubeola)	Chickenpox (Varicella)	Scarlet fever	Roseola (Exanthema Subitum)	Petechial Rash (From Meningitis)
Incubation	10–11 days	10–20 days	2–4 days	10–15 days	None
Signs and symptoms	3–5 days of fever, cough, coryza, toxic appearance, conjunctivitis; Koplik's spots (mucosal lesions) appear 2 days before rash	Fever and cough, simultaneously with rash; headache; malaise	Fever for 1–2 days, sore throat, strawberry tongue, vomiting, chills, malaise	Rapid onset of high fever lasting 3–4 days in otherwise well child	May be sudden onset or preceded by fever and malaise; if sudden onset and accompanied by fever, may indicate sepsis
Exanthem (rash)	Reddish brown; begins on face, spreads downward; confluent high on body, discrete lesions in lower portions; lasts 7–10 days	Vesicles appearing in crops; trunk, scalp, face, extremities; lesions in all stages of development	Punctate, sandpaper texture; blanches on pressure; appears first in flexor areas; rash lasts 7 days	Appears discrete, rose-colored; appears after fever; begins on chest and spreads to face	Reddish purple vascular, *nonblanching* rash
Complications	Pneumonia, encephalitis, otitis media	Pneumonia, encephalitis, Reye's syndrome	Rheumatic heart disease	None	Sepsis, septic shock, long-term sequelae from increased intracranial pressure

From Centers for Disease Control and Prevention. National Hospital Ambulatory Medical Care Survey: 2015 emergency department summary tables. Centers for Disease Control and Prevention website. https://www.cdc.gov/nchs/data/nhamcs/web_tables/2015_ed_web_tables.pdf. Accessed June 11, 2019.

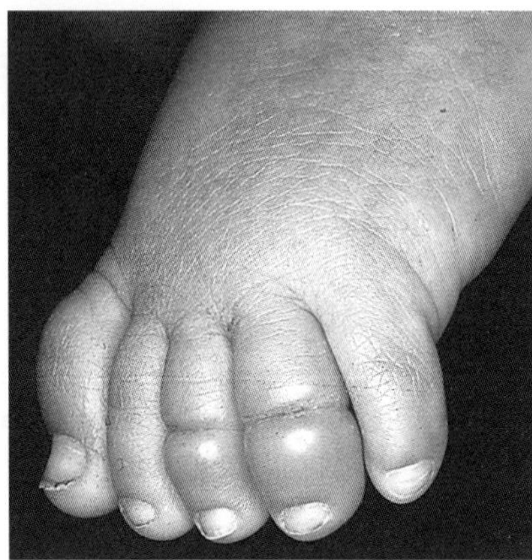

Fig. 45.3 Hair Tourniquet. The mild erythema and edema of the third and fourth toes are the result of constriction by hairs that accidentally became wrapped around them. (From Zitelli B, Davis H. *Atlas of Pediatric Physical Diagnosis.* 5th ed. St Louis, MO: Mosby; 2007.)

Scabies

Scabies is caused by the itch mite *Sarcoptes scabiei.* The major symptom of scabies is severe itching. Infestation results in eruption of wheals, papules, vesicles, and often-visible threadlike burrows. Scabies is transmitted by direct contact. Topical application of permethrin cream remains the standard treatment for children older than 2 months of age. Oral antihistamines may be required to control itching. All bedding and clothing should be removed and washed.

FAMILY PRESENCE

The Emergency Nurses Association, American Association of Critical Care Nurses, and American Heart Association are among the growing number of professional organizations supporting the option of family presence during invasive procedures and resuscitation. Family presence can be looked at as a natural extension of family-centered care, which is a fundamental part of pediatric emergency care. Well-thought-out planning is a crucial component of any family presence guideline used in the emergency care setting. Some of the key points to consider for a family presence guideline include the following[14]:

- Discuss the plan with all resuscitation team members in advance.
- One team member must be assigned to stay with the family to clarify information and answer questions.
- Have a specific space for the family member to be in during the resuscitation, and if possible, facilitate the opportunity for the family to touch their child.
- Resuscitation team members must be aware of the family presence and communicate in a sensitive way.

SUMMARY

Children seen in the ED can cause great anxiety for health care providers, especially those who are not accustomed to caring for children on a regular basis. Developing skill in pediatric triage, assessment, and care requires the emergency nurse to develop a system that is comfortable, systematic, thorough, and adaptable to the age of the child. Acquiring the habit of beginning a pediatric assessment as soon as the child enters the ED is good practice. Use information provided by the parents or caregivers because it can be very useful in painting a picture of what is normal and not normal for the child. Appreciate the differences physically, physiologically, and developmentally between adults and children, and be mindful of the differences with each child you assess. Take special care when obtaining and interpreting vital signs in pediatric patients because abnormal vital signs may be the first clues you detect telling you your patient is "sick," is not responding to interventions, or is decompensating. Showing concern and offering support for the family, including the family in the child's care whenever possible, and giving thorough, clear discharge instructions lay the groundwork for ongoing care of the child after the emergency is over.

REFERENCES

1. National Center for Health Statistics. Emergency department visits. Centers for Disease Control and Prevention website. https://www.cdc.gov/nchs/fastats/emergency-department.htm, Published 2017. Accessed June 10, 2019.
2. Harless J, Ramaiah R, Bhananker SM. Pediatric airway management. *Int J Crit Illn Inj Sci*. 2014;4(1):65–70.
3. *Emergency Nursing Pediatric Course: Provider Manual (ENPC)*. 5th ed. Des Plaines, IL: Emergency Nurses Association; 2020.
4. Shaw K, Bachur R. *Textbook of Pediatric Emergency Medicine*. 7th ed. St Louis, MO: Wolters Kluwer; 2010.
5. Burns CE, Starr NB, Dunn AM, Blosser CG, Brady MA. *Pediatric Primary Care*. St Louis, MO: Elsevier; 2017.
6. Aronson PL. Evaluation of the febrile young infant: an update. *Pediatr Emerg Med Pract*. 2013;10(2):1–17.
7. Aehlert B. *Comprehensive Pediatric Emergency Care*. Rev ed. Burlington, MA: Jones & Bartlett Learning; 2007.
8. Bernardo L, Thomas D, eds. *Core Curriculum for Pediatric Emergency Nursing*. 2nd ed. Boston, MA: Jones & Bartlett; 2009.
9. The Joint Commission. Preventing pediatric medication errors. The Joint Commission website. https://www.jointcommission.org/assets/1/18/SEA_39.PDF, Published April 11, 2008. Accessed June 10, 2019.
10. Anchor J, Settipane RA. Appropriate use of epinephrine in anaphylaxis. *Am J Emerg Med*. 2004;22(6):488–490.
11. Becker HJ, Langhan M. Capnography in the pediatric emergency department: clinical applications. *Pediatr Emerg Med Pract*. 2013;10(6):1–14.
12. Rempe B, Iskyan K, Alol M. An evidence-based review of pediatric retained foreign bodies. *Pediatr Emerg Med Pract*. 2009;6(12).
13. Ralston S, Lieberthal A, Meissner HC, et al. Clinical Practice Guideline: the diagnosis, management and prevention of bronchiolitis. *Pediatrics*. 2014;134(5):e1474–e1502.
14. Ortiz-Alvarez O. Acute management of croup in the emergency department. *Paediatr Child Health*. 2017;22(3):166–169.
15. Zibners L. Diphtheria, pertussis, and tetanus: evidence-based management of pediatric patients in the emergency department. *Pediatr Emerg Med Pract*. 2017;14(2):1–24.
16. Samson R, Schexnayder S, Hazinski M, et al. *Textbook of Pediatric Advanced Life Support*. Dallas, TX: American Academy of Pediatrics and American Heart Association; 2016.
17. Hazinski M. *Nursing Care of the Critically Ill Child*. 3rd ed. St Louis, MO: Elsevier; 2013.
18. Davis A, Carcillo J, Rajesh A, et al. American college of critical care medicine clinical practice parameters for hemodynamic support of pediatric and neonatal septic shock. *Crit Care Med*. 2017;45(6).
19. Silverman AM. Septic shock: recognizing and managing this life-threatening condition in pediatric patients. *Pediatr Emerg Med Pract*. 2015;12(4):1–25.
20. Subramaniam S, Chao J. Managing acute complications of sickle cell disease in pediatric patients. *Pediatr Emerg Med Pract*. 2016;13(11):1–28.
21. Brady K. Acute gastroenteritis: evidence-based management of pediatric patients. *Pediatr Emerg Med Pract*. 2018;15(2):1–25.
22. HIV among youth. Centers for Disease Control and Prevention website. https://www.cdc.gov/hiv/group/age/youth/index.html. Updated April 10, 2019. Accessed June 11, 2019.

46

Geriatric Emergencies

Nancy McGowan

INTRODUCTION

According to the 2010 US census, more than 40 million Americans were older than age of 65 years, with the 85-years-and-older population growing at a rate almost three times that of the general population.[1] With this increase in the geriatric population, the emergency department (ED) is uniquely positioned to provide improved care for geriatric patients. It is the role of the ED nurse to be both the patient advocate and also the patient and family educator. The ED nurse may be the person that the family of a geriatric patient trusts and is most comfortable interacting with.

Geriatric patients may present to the ED with a unique set of problems, such as issues with hearing and vision, mobility, polypharmacy, cognitive decline, depression, and social isolation. Each of these issues must be dealt with in a caring, empathetic manner. The ED can be a challenging environment for both the patient and the caregiver. Just as important, ED use will only be increasing in the future with the burgeoning Baby Boomer generation entering the geriatric population for the first time.

OVERVIEW OF THE GERIATRIC POPULATION AND PHYSIOLOGIC CHANGES OF AGING

Overall, the geriatric population accounts for 12% to 24% of all ED visits.[2] Older patients arrive with a higher level of acuity and more serious medical illnesses than other patients. They arrive more often by ambulance and have higher rates of testing and longer ED stays.[3]

When caring for the geriatric ED patient, it is important that the health care team remain aware of several important changes that older adult patients experience as they age. First, there is a change in body composition, including a decrease in bone mass, lean mass, and water content of the body. The total body fat increases, most commonly with intraabdominal fat stores. The standardized nutritional requirements of young or middle-aged adults cannot be generalized to the older adult.[4] In the older adult patient, there is a decreased response to thermal variance, with a loss of fat and thinning of skin, loss of sweat glands, decreased blood flow to the skin, and decreased muscle mass. Joints become stiffer and less flexible. There is a decrease in bone density, movement slows and becomes limited, and there is decreased coordination and muscle weakness. Endocrine changes in aging include a decrease in testosterone and estrogen.[4]

The incidence of cardiovascular disease increases progressively with age, affecting up to 80% of men and women older than 80 years.[4] The principal effects of aging on the cardiovascular system include increased arterial stiffness that produces an increase in afterload and increased blood pressure. There is a decrease in myocardial relaxation and compliance that causes a risk of diastolic heart failure and atrial fibrillation. Sinus node dysfunction increases with a decline in the conduction velocity of the atrioventricular node and infranodal conduction system, leading to an increased risk of sick sinus syndrome, atrioventricular block, left anterior fascicular block, and bundle branch block.[4] Additionally, the clinical effects of cardiovascular changes cause a decline of the body's ability to meet the increased demands associated with exercise or illness, and peak aerobic capacity declines with advancing age.[4]

Pulmonary changes in the geriatric patient include reduced airway size, reduced chest wall compliance, intercostal muscle atrophy, and a decline of forced vital capacity (FVC). Although there may be a common misperception that the geriatric population may tend to overestimate or exaggerate respiratory complications, in reality the opposite is often true. Geriatric patients may have more than one cause of their problem; for example, dyspnea, cough, and wheezing may overlap. The causes might include a combination of diseases such as asthma, emphysema, obstructive sleep apnea, heart failure, or gastroesophageal reflux disease (GERD).[4]

Urinary changes in the geriatric patient include a decrease in kidney size and weight, decrease in glomerular filtration rate (GFR), a decline in the ability to concentrate urine, and urethral mucosal atrophy.[4] Other changes in the geriatric patient's urinary tract system include bladder contractility decline, uninhibited bladder contractions, decreased bladder capacity, and prostate hypertrophy in men, which may affect urine output.[4]

When assessing geriatric patients entering an ED, it is important to recognize that their illness may be due to the following:

- instability
- incontinence
- immobility
- intellectual impairment
- iatrogenesis.[4]

Instability can be a precursor to an escalating loss of independence or an underlying disease process. **Incontinence** may be a warning sign of an underlying disease that possibly could be attributed to delirium, infection, pharmaceutical intervention, or restricted mobility.[4] **Immobility** may lead to pressure ulcers, development of pneumonia, pain, social isolation, elder abuse, and malnutrition.[4] **Intellectual impairment** may present as an abrupt change in cognitive function, as seen in delirium, or it may be a slow, chronic condition, such as dementia. An electrolyte imbalance may lead to cognitive changes and infections. Intellectual impairment may also be due to intracranial changes or myocardial dysfunction. Finally, **iatrogenic changes** may be due to a medication issue. Polypharmacy is a major concern in the care of the geriatric patient. This problem can be exacerbated by lack of provider follow-up of the medication's effectiveness, or the interaction of prescription medications with over-the-counter (OTC) supplements or medications.[4]

TRIAGE AND INITIAL ASSESS OF THE GERIATRIC PATIENT IN THE EMERGENCY DEPARTMENT

Initiating an ED triage encounter with the geriatric patient may be challenging. These patients often suffer from both acute and chronic issues and may have cognitive impairment. Obtaining a "collateral" history from caregivers or a long-term care facility can be difficult and time-consuming.[5] It is important to recognize atypical, multifactorial, and nonspecific presentations that are common for older adult patients. Obtaining a thorough assessment can be a time-consuming and intensive process.[5]

The triage period may be a valuable time for identifying problems such as dementia, frailty, or other comorbidities that may affect the care of the geriatric patient.[5]

Identification of patients with a likelihood of admission may be enhanced by the use of the ISAR score (identification of seniors at risk).[6] Box 46.1 lists reasons for undertriage of the geriatric patient.

Just as important as avoiding undertriage of the geriatric patient is the difficulty of recognition of an atypical presentation of a patient. Physiologic changes related to age can lead to a diverse response to foreign stimuli.[7] The atypical presentation of the geriatric patient can be complicated by a lack of the common classic signs and symptoms of illness, such as altered mental status, failure to eat and drink, failure to develop a fever, or lack of pain in a disease known to cause these conditions.[7] The definition of "atypical presentations" is

> *presentation of illness in a geriatric adult which includes vague, altered, or nonpresentation of the typical illness signs or symptoms.*[8]

It is important for the ED nurse who is triaging the older adult patient to recognize atypical presentations and obtain a baseline assessment if possible. Obtaining this baseline information requires patience, time, and perhaps most importantly, availability of reliable relatives or caregivers.[8]

Examples of atypical geriatric illness presentations[8] can be seen in Table 46.1.

It is vital to recognize two leading atypical presentations: lack of pain with a disease known to cause pain or the failure to develop a fever with diseases that normally present with fever.[7] The most common presenting complaint for older adults is often related to an infectious disease process, such as pneumonia/bronchitis or a urinary tract infection. The

BOX 46.1 Reasons for Under-Triage in the Geriatric Population.

- Physiologic and pharmacologic factors masking changes in vital signs with illness or injury
- Presentation with nonspecific symptoms or geriatric syndromes, such as immobility, which may be mistaken for a more trivial complaint
- Difficulties with history taking or lack of information about the patient's baseline mental and physical function
- Lack of awareness of past medical problems, which may significantly affect presentation
- Failure to appreciate symptoms and signs that may be of higher risk in the older patient, such as abdominal pain

From Grossman FF, Zumbrunn T, Frauchiger A, Delport K, Bingisser R, Nickel CH. At risk of undertriage? Testing the performance and accuracy of the emergency severity index in older emergency department patients. *Ann Emerg Med.* 2012;60(3):317–325.

TABLE 46.1 Atypical Geriatric Illness Presentations.[8]

Illness	Altered Presentation in Geriatric Patient
Infectious diseases	Absence of fever Falls Decreased appetite or fluid intake Confusion
"Silent" acute abdomen	Absence of symptoms Mild discomfort and constipation May be tachypneic or have vague respiratory symptoms
"Silent" malignancy	Back pain secondary to metastases from slow-growing breast masses Silent masses of the bowel
"Silent" myocardial infarction	Absence of chest pain Vague symptoms of fatigue, nausea, and decrease in functional status **Classic presentation: shortness of breath is a more common complaint than chest pain**
Depression	Lack of sadness Somatic complaints: appetite changes, vague gastrointestinal symptoms, constipation, and sleep disturbances

absence of fever may lead to a misdiagnosis in these patients and should always lead the triage nurse to delve further into the geriatric patient's baseline history.[7]

MAXIMIZING COMMUNICATION WITH THE GERIATRIC PATIENT

It is important to recognize that optimal communication with the patient will provide the most complete assessment and is a vital component of the triage process and definitive ongoing care. Being aware of the differing needs of the geriatric patient will improve this process and reassure the patient, family, and caregivers.

The nurse's positioning and body language are important in obtaining a history during the initial assessment. Make eye contact and take steps to appear nonthreatening. Appearing relaxed and providing appropriate physical contact, such as hand-holding, may encourage the trust of the patient.[5] Perhaps most difficult in a busy ED is the ability to remain patient. Many older adult patients may feel they are already a burden, and rushing them through an assessment will only encourage them to omit details of their history or become withdrawn, thinking they are saving time.[5]

Ensuring that any visual or hearing aids are working correctly will encourage the patient to interact with the triage nurse and provide accurate and pertinent information. Speaking slowly and distinctly will help with the assessment. When geriatric patients are cognitively impaired, maintaining eye contact as much as possible and using a friendly and positive tone of voice may help. Closed questions may be easier for the cognitively impaired patient to understand and answer.[5]

It is common for the geriatric patient to be brought to the ED from an assisted living facility, nursing home, or long-term care facility. Although the patient may arrive with documentation detailing medications, functional ability, and cognitive ability, there may be a lack of information regarding the actual reason for the patient's transfer to an acute care facility.[5] For this reason, it is vital that the triage or accepting nurse be aware of questions that should be addressed regarding the patient.

Some of these questions include the following topics:

- history of falls
- pain (what type/for how long)
- incontinence
- memory loss
- depression
- anxiety
- eyesight and hearing changes
- weight loss
- changes in eating pattern
- sleep disturbances[5]

By addressing any of these issues, the nurse is more likely to identify specific causes for a nonspecific complaint, such as urinary incontinence or frequency in a patient who presents after a fall.[5] Problems that may be attributed to "old age," such as changes in diet, may also be related to another event, such as memory loss.

POLYPHARMACY OF THE GERIATRIC PATIENT IN THE EMERGENCY DEPARTMENT

Adverse drug effects lead to 11% of ED visits in patients older than 65 years versus 1% to 4% in the general population.[9] There is no consensus definition of the term "polypharmacy," but it is generally accepted to be the presence of several daily medications, some of which may be considered inappropriate for the patient.[10] Some medications may be lifesaving; however, others may be unnecessary and in fact detrimental to an older person's health and quality of life. Polypharmacy is a risk factor for falls and places older patients at increased risk of adverse drug reactions.[5] In the United States, a large review showed that nearly 30% of older patients were taking six or more medications.[11] It is important on admission for the geriatric patient to have an accurate list of medications within the first 24 hours of admission. Patients noted to be receiving several medications should have a medication reconciliation done by either a pharmacist or a geriatric specialist.[5]

Hospital pharmacies should develop and maintain a list of high-risk medications. Although these lists should be hospital-specific, they should include these medications at a minimum[12]:

- anticoagulants and antiplatelet medications
- antihyperglycemics
- cardiac medications, including digoxin, amiodarone, β-blockers, and calcium channel blockers
- diuretics
- opiates
- antipsychotics and other psychiatric medications
- immunosuppressant medications, including chemotherapy agents

Additionally, geriatric patients being discharged from the ED who have been recognized as at risk for polypharmacy should be referred to their primary care physician for a thorough review of their medications.[12]

In assessing the geriatric patient, the ED nurse must be continually aware of the role homeostasis plays in the aging process. Homeostasis refers to the regulation of body temperature, blood pressure, blood glucose, blood pH, fluid balance, and thirst.[13] Because of decreased reserves in older adults, the ability to maintain these systems may be vulnerable. With minimal changes, the geriatric patient's body may respond to changes in homeostasis in a more exaggerated manner, moving further away from a balanced state than a younger patient. It may also take the older patient more time to return to a state of balance than a younger person would.[13]

Each individual patient responds to a specific situation differently and is also affected by the results of chronic illnesses, medications, and baseline status.[13] Homeostasis in the geriatric patient can be affected by changes in temperature, renal changes, respiratory changes, and tissue sensitivity to such hormones as insulin and antidiuretic hormones. Changes in fluid status can be affected by impairment of water conservation and sodium balance and a decrease in the thirst mechanisms and a decline in total body water.[13]

Using a "head-to-toe" assessment model, the older adult patient may exhibit several changes in status the nurse must be able to recognize as specific to this population. Cognitive status must first be examined.

In assessing neurologic status in the geriatric patient, it is important for the emergency nurse to recognize that impaired mental status occurs in approximately one-quarter of all older ED patients.[14] This impaired mental status may be due to delirium or dementia or a combination of both.[14] It may be difficult to differentiate the two pathologies. The Confusion Assessment is a quick and easy method to help determine delirium.

Confusion Assessment Tool

In the following assessment, the presence of the symptoms in questions 1 and 2 with the presence of symptoms from either question 3 or 4 indicates delirium[15]:

1. Is there evidence of an acute change in mental status from the patient's baseline?
2. Did the patient have difficulty focusing attention (for example, being easily distractible or having difficulty keeping track of what was being said)?
3. Was the patient's thinking disorganized or incoherent, such as having rambling or irrelevant conversation, unclear or illogical flow of ideas, or unpredictable switching from subject to subject?
4. Overall, how would you rate this person's level of consciousness?
   - alert (normal)
   - vigilant (hyperalert)
   - lethargic (drowsy, easily aroused)
   - stupor (difficult to arouse)
   - coma (unarousable)

In addition to the changes caused by dementia or delirium, there may be pronounced physiologic changes. The blood-brain barrier is more permeable, there are few neurons and nerve fibers, reaction times become slower, and proprioception in the lower limbs is decreased. There is also a decrease in the neurotransmission systems, the enzymes, receptors, and neurotransmitters.[13] In the older adult, the brain may be the first system showing dysfunction, with neurologic changes such as confusion, lethargy, or agitation being the sentinel signs of illness.[13]

A challenge for the ED care of the geriatric patient is the management of an agitated patient. It is vital to recognize chemical and physical restraints are critical interventions that, when used appropriately, can improve patient health and safety.[13] When used inappropriately, these techniques can actually increase the severity or length of a delirium. The treatment of a geriatric patient with agitation is very different from that of a younger patient with similar concerns.[13] It is the policy of some geriatric EDs to limit the use of chemical and physical restraints to only those situations where they are absolutely necessary. To manage the agitated geriatric patient, it is vital to use medications and alternative safety measures appropriately.[13]

When an older adult patient is diagnosed with delirium, the underlying cause must be determined. Some of these causes include the following[12]:

- infections
- urinary tract infections or pneumonia
- medications
- sedative/hypnotics, opiates, or any new medication, especially if multiple medications have recently been added
- electrolyte imbalances
- alcohol use or withdrawal

CARDIOVASCULAR ASSESSMENT OF THE GERIATRIC PATIENT

Important changes in the cardiovascular system occur with aging. The ED nurse should be aware of these changes. With age comes increased vascular stiffness and increased vascular intimal thickness, leading to atherosclerosis and hypertension.[13] Additionally, the sinoatrial node may become thicker, with a decrease in the number of pacemaker cells, leading the patient to be at risk for slow or irregular heart rates.[13] A decreased cardiovascular reserve can lead to an increased risk for heart failure and to the cardiovascular system being less able to respond to volume changes and less able to generate and maintain an altered cardiac output.[13] The use of β-blockers may aggravate this problem because of their ability to slow the heart rate and may prevent compensatory increases in heart rate and cardiac rhythm, increasing the risk of orthostatic hypertension.[13] Pain may be poorly localized. When the geriatric patient complains of pain with a cardiac event, it may be localized in the throat, shoulder, or abdomen.[13] Additionally, because the patient may be leading a sedentary lifestyle, exertional angina may be difficult to assess in the geriatric patient.[13]

Presentation of illnesses in older adult patients may be confusing to the ED nurse. Acute myocardial infarction in the older patient may be of atypical presentation, with shortness of breath, syncope, nausea, and vomiting being the presenting symptoms.[16] The ECG is nondiagnostic in 43% of patients older than 85 years.[16]

The geriatric ED patient should be assessed in the same manner as any patient presenting with cardiac symptoms. However, it must be understood that these patients may not have typical presentations that may normally indicate a cardiac event. If the patient is complaining of shortness of breath, nausea, and vomiting instead of the "typical" complaint of substernal chest pain, there should be a high index of suspicion for a cardiac event. Cardiac monitoring, oxygen, pain relief, and laboratory studies should all be provided urgently for these patients, as with any "typical" cardiac patient.

DEHYDRATION

Recognition of dehydration in the geriatric patient is an important concern for the ED nurse. It is the most common problem in the older adult and can lead to other serious issues.[8] This may be due in part to normal age-related changes, which may include decreases in total-body water, alterations in perception of thirst, and reduced renal function leading to decreased urine-concentration ability.[8] In the older adult, the signs of dehydration may be vague and difficult to recognize. Adults with feeding tubes, infection, and medication-related side effects may be more at risk for dehydration.[8] In assessing dehydration in the older adult patient, skin turgor may be an unreliable sign, and problems with incontinence may make intake/output charts unreliable.[8] A dry mouth in an older adult patient may also be an unreliable sign because many patients may be mouth breathing or have a dry mouth as a result of medications with anticholinergic properties.[8] In the older adult patient, dehydration may only be recognized as constipation or slight orthostatic hypotension. It is vital for the ED clinician to rely on a combination of signs, symptoms, and laboratory studies to recognize dehydration in these patients.[8]

THE ACUTE ABDOMEN IN THE GERIATRIC PATIENT

Acute abdominal pain in the older patient is often underrecognized, and as many as 40% of older patients are misdiagnosed.[8] In the older adult patient, some of the most common causes of acute abdominal findings include cholecystitis, bowel obstruction, diverticular disease, complications of cancer, and medication side effects.[8] In these patients, pain may be diffuse, mild, or absent. Fever and tachycardia are also frequently absent with acute abdominal diseases in the older adult.[13]

Classic signs of appendicitis, such as right lower quadrant pain, fever, nausea, and vomiting, may be absent in the older adults.[13] They may lack an elevated white blood cell count and have reduced rebound secondary to decrease abdominal wall musculature.[8] The altered sensation of pain may mean that the older patient does not present to the ED until the disease is very advanced and, in the case of appendicitis, the appendix may have ruptured.[13] By that time, geriatric patients may be very ill, leading to a higher mortality rate than in younger patients, with more than 50% of deaths associated with appendicitis happening in the older adult.[13] For these patients, this late presentation may be due to social factors, such as lack of a caregiver, lack of transportation, the fear of hospitalization, or loss of independence.[8]

INFECTION AND SEPSIS IN THE OLDER ADULT

In the older adult, the signs and symptoms of infection may be difficult to assess. Traditional signs, such as an elevated white blood cell count and fever, may not be reliable signs in the older adult.[13] It is common for an older adult to present to the ED with vague, diffuse symptoms, no sign of fever, and no localizing signs.[8] Older adults may have a lower basal body temperature due to decreased muscle mass.[8] It is vital that the nurse recognize a change in mental status or functional status, which may be the only sign of an underlying infection.

A urinary tract infection may be the best example of this phenomenon. Instead of presenting with dysuria and frequency, the older patient, whether male or female, may be exhibiting signs of confusion, incontinence, or anorexia.[8] Additionally, the patient with pneumonia may not exhibit cough or shortness of breath but instead present with confusion and a feeling of general malaise.[8] Diaphragmatic weakness, an age-related change, may predispose the older patient to pneumonia.[13] Radiologic imaging may be inconclusive for a diagnosis in the older patient. It is important for the nurse to recognize that important signs such as a productive cough, fever, and chest pain may not be present in an older patient with a developing pneumonia.[13] It is sometimes thought that if an older adult patient has developed a fever, the patient may already be septic.[17] Although leukocytosis is less common in older adults, a left shift (i.e., a greater percentage of band cells in a complete blood count [CBC] with differential) is usually observed and indicative of a bacterial infection. Attending to these subtle but important clues is important to avoid having the patient become septic, which could lead to prolonged hospitalization and even death.[8]

RENAL

In older patients, the renal system may show a decrease in the glomerular filtration rate.[13] Additionally, the ability of the kidneys to concentrate or dilute urine is diminished with aging. It is important that drug doses be adjusted to compensate for the decrease in kidney function.[13] There is also a decrease in the bladder capacity and consequently an increase in the residual bladder volume, leading to urinary frequency, urgency, or urinary tract infections.[13]

FALLS

Falls are the most common cause of ED admissions for older adult patients (15%–30%).[14] When triaging a patient after a fall, it is important to distinguish whether this fall is an isolated event or due to an underlying difficulty, such as generalized frailty, or medication problems.[14] A fall may be the first indication of another problem, such as an acute myocardial infarction, sepsis, medication toxicity, acute abdominal pain, or elder abuse.[14] Patients who are unable to remember the cause of the fall, have multiple falls, or who are unable to get up after a fall should be considered for admission to the hospital for further assessment.[14] A simple way to steer the assessment of an older adult patient after a fall is the use of the mnemonic CATASTROPHE[18]:

C: Caregiver and Housing (information about the circumstances of the fall)
A: Alcohol (including withdrawal)
T: Treatment (medications, recently added or stopped, patient adherence)
A: Affect (depression)
S: Syncope (any episodes of fainting)
T: Teetering (dizziness)
R: Recent illnesses
O: Ocular problems
P: Pain
H: Hearing
E: Environmental hazards (rugs, steps, floors)

Falls may result in fractures, with hip fractures producing a change in the older adult patient's ability to provide self-care. Falls may result in traumatic brain injuries in the older adult. Even seemingly simple falls may result in serious intracranial injuries that may be difficult to assess in the older adult patient.[14] A chronic subdural hematoma may be present for weeks or months before symptoms appear and prompt the individual to seek ED care. In 30% to 50% of the cases, the patient may be unable to recall the initial fall; it seemed so "trivial."[14] Altered mental status and headache may lead the older adult patient to seek medical care.

Brain imaging studies, such as computed tomography scans, may be used to provide a definitive diagnosis.

Several screening tools have been developed to identify older adult patients at high risk for adverse outcomes. The ISAR is one tool that can be easily used in the ED.[19] It uses a self-reporting questionnaire asking about functional dependence, recent hospitalizations, impaired memory and vision changes, polypharmacy, and functional decline.[19] Use of tools such as the ISAR will encourage the ED nurse to identify older adult patients at risk for falls, both currently and in the future.

ALCOHOL AND SUBSTANCE ABUSE

Alcohol and substance abuse disorders may account for 5% to 14% of ED visits by older patients.[20] Substance abuse in the older adult patient may be related to prescription drugs, such as benzodiazepines and opioid analgesics.[20] The ED nurse may feel uncomfortable approaching an older adult patient about possible substance abuse, but it is important for baseline information to be obtained from the patient to avoid future problems, such as withdrawal from alcohol or drugs. In the case of falls, it is vital to determine whether this fall is related to the use of alcohol or another substance.

VULNERABLE ADULTS AND ELDER ABUSE

Elder abuse is defined by the World Health Organization as "a single or repeated act, or lack of appropriate action, occurring within any relationship where there is an expectation of trust which causes harm or distress to an older person."[21]

With elder abuse, 90% of abusers are known to their victims, and the most common abusers are an adult child or a spouse.[5] (See also Chapter 49.) It is difficult to determine the prevalence of elder abuse because often the older adult person feels ashamed or embarrassed and relies on the potential abuser. Elder abuse also may be underreported by both the victims and health professionals.[5] Here are some types of abuse that may be present:

- physical: inflicting physical pain or injury
- psychological/emotional: inflicting mental pain, anguish, or distress
- financial/material: illegal theft, misuse of funds
- sexual: nonconsensual sexual contact of any kind
- neglect: refusal or failure by those responsible to provide food, shelter, health care, or protection[5]

Risk factors for elder abuse include the following:

- decreased physical health
- dementia or other cognitive impairment
- female gender
- history of violence
- increased age
- shared living arrangement
- social isolation
- having a victim or caregiver with mental health or substance abuse issues[22]

Having initial contact with a patient provides an opportunity for the ED nurse to identify and act on any suspected elder abuse.[5] Patients with cognitive impairment are at increased risk of being a victim, yet they may still be able to report abuse. Any signs of depression or anxiety should be noted, and it is critical to determine decision-making capacity. Those who lack this capacity are particularly vulnerable and may be at greatest risk.[5]

ED nurses must be aware of reporting requirements in their state and local jurisdictions. Referral should be done if there are concerns about the possibility of abuse being present.[5]

SUMMARY

The older adult ED patient is a unique individual requiring a thorough assessment. The nurse must be able to obtain a history, which is often complex. This task may take patience when the individual is cognitively or physically impaired. This skill is an important one as the population of the United States ages, and it will become more important because chronically ill patients may rely on the ED for their primary care needs.

REFERENCES

1. Pines JM, Mullins PM, Cooper JK, Feng LB, Roth KE. National trends in emergency department use, care patterns, and quality of care of older adults in the United States. *J Am Geriatr Soc.* 2013;61(1):12–17.
2. Roussel-Landrin S, Paillaud E, Alonso E, et al. The establishment of geriatric intervention group and geriatric assessment at emergency of henri-mondor hospital [in French]. *Rev Med Interne.* 2005;26(6):458–466.

3. Singal BM, Hedges JR, Rousseau EW, et al. Geriatric patient emergency visits. Part I: comparison of visits by geriatric and younger patients. *Ann Emerg Med*. 1992;21(7):802–807.
4. Moquist D. Atypical presentation of illness in the elderly. Galveston, Texas: Paper presented at: Texas Academy of Family Physicians (TAFF) Annual Session and Primary Care Summit; November 9–12, 2017.
5. Murdoch IT. Essentials of assessment and management in geriatric medicine. In: Murdoch IE, Turpin S, Johnston B, MacLullich A, Losman E, eds. *Geriatric Emergencies*. Chichester, United Kingdom: John Wiley & Sons; 2015:9–29.
6. Grossman FF, Zumbrunn T, Frauchiger A, Delport K, Bingisser R, Nickel CH. At risk of undertriage? Testing the performance and accuracy of the emergency severity index in older emergency department patients. *Ann Emerg Med*. 2012;60(3):317–325.
7. Limpawattana P, Phungoen P, Mitsungnern T, Laosuangkoon W, Tansangworn N. Atypical presentations of older adults at the emergency department and associated factors. *Arch Gerontol Geriatr*. 2016;62:97–102.
8. Pessinotto CA. Atypical presentations of illness in older adults. In: Williams BC, ed. *Current Diagnosis & Treatment: Geriatrics*. 2nd ed. New York, NY: McGraw-Hill; 2014:122–137.
9. Hohl CM, Dankoff J, Colacone A, Afilalo M. Polypharmacy, adverse drug-related events, and potential adverse drug interactions in elderly patients presenting to an emergency department. *Ann Emerg Med*. 2001;38(6):666–671.
10. Bushardt RL, Massey EB, Simpson TW, Ariail JC, Simpson KN. Polypharmacy: misleading but manageable. *Clin Interv Aging*. 2008;3(2):383–389.
11. Maher RL, Hanlon J, Hajjar ER. Clinical consequences of polypharmacy in the elderly. *Expert Opin Drug Saf*. 2014;13(1):57–65.
12. American College of Emergency Physicians, American Geriatrics Society, Emergency Nurses Association, Society for Academic Emergency Medicine. *Geriatric Emergency Department Guidelines*. Guidelines for Geriatric Emergency Department Care; 2013. https://www.acep.org/patient-care/policy-statements/geriatric-emergency-department-guidelines/. Updated January 2019. Accessed May 26, 2019.
13. Peters ML. The older adult in the emergency department: aging and atypical illness presentation. *J Emerg Nurs*. 2010;36(1):29–34.
14. Samaras NC, Chevalley T, Samaras D, Gold G. Older patients in the emergency department: a review. *Ann Emerg Med*. 2010;56(3):261–269.
15. Inouye SV, van Dyck CH, Alessi CA, Balkin S, Siegal AP, Horwitz RI. Clarifying confusion: the confusion assessment method. A new method for detection of delirium. *Ann Intern Med*. 1990;113(12):941–948.
16. Alexander KP, Newby LK, Armstrong PW, et al. Acute coronary care in the elderly, part II: ST-segment-elevation myocardial infarction: a scientific statement for healthcare professionals from the American Heart Association Council on Clinical Cardiology: in collaboration with the Society of Geriatric Cardiology. *Circulation*. 2007;115(19):2570–2589.
17. Shankar-Hari M, Phillips GS, Levy ML, et al. Developing a new definition and assessing new clinical criteria for septic shock: for the Third International Consensus Definitions for Sepsis and Septic Shock (Sepsis-3). *JAMA* 2016;315:775.
18. Sloan J. *Protocols in Primary Care Geriatrics*. 2nd ed. New York, NY: Springer; 1997.
19. McCusker JB. Detection of older people at risk screening tool: further evidence of concurrent and predictive validity. *J Am Geriatr Soc*. 1999;47:1229–1237.
20. O'Connell HC. Alcohol use disorders in elderly people–redefining an age old problem in old age. *Br Med J*. 2003;327(7416):664–667.
21. World Health Organization. Elder maltreatment. World Health Organization website. https://www.who.int/en/news-room/fact-sheets/detail/elder-abuse, Published June 8, 2018. Accessed May 26, 2019.
22. Bond MB. Elder abuse and neglect: definitions, epidemiology, and approaches to emergency department screening. *Clin Geriatr Med*. 2013;29(1):257–273.

47

Behavioral Health Emergencies

Wanda S. Pritts

Psychiatric emergencies are presenting in emergency departments (EDs) at an alarming rate. The Agency for Healthcare Research and Quality reports one in eight visits to EDs involves mental, behavioral, emotional, or substance use disorders, an increase of 15% in the last decade.[1] These emergencies take many forms in the ED. Patients may arrive with severe dysfunction of behavior, mood, thinking, or perception representing a significant threat to life, daily living, or psychological integrity. Severity is related to the patient's ability to function and adapt but also depends on the person's support systems. Working with this type of patient requires patience, understanding, and flexibility. A comprehensive discussion of psychiatric emergencies is beyond the scope of this chapter. Therefore material presented herein focuses on those conditions seen most often in the ED: agitation, anorexia, bulimia, anxiety, panic disorder (PD), depression, suicidal ideation, schizophrenia, and substance abuse with co-occurring illness.

The initial assessment for all psychiatric disorders should include vital signs, medical history, visual examination, urine toxicology screen, cognitive examination, pregnancy test for fertile women, and a cursory medical examination for medical clearance. Goals of interventions for psychiatric emergencies are to mitigate the risk to the patient and to staff. Calming the patient without sedation is most desirable.

AGITATION

Patient agitation presents a significant challenge in the ED. The potential to escalate to aggressive behavior that endangers the patient, the staff, and others requires prompt assessment and intervention.[2] The Best practices in Evaluation and Treatment of Agitation (BETA) guidelines are the comprehensive recommendations on the management of agitation, from triage, diagnosis, and interpersonal calming skills to medication choices.[2] Agitation is demonstrated by abnormal and excessive verbal, physically aggressive, or purposeless motor behaviors, heightened arousal, or other symptoms causing clinically significant disruption of a patient's ability to function.[3]

Obtaining an accurate initial history is important while assessing and establishing triggers precipitating the event. Agitation may be caused by medical and psychiatric conditions including head trauma, infection, thyroid disease, substance abuse or withdrawal, psychotic disorders, and depression. Safely identifying the etiology represents a significant challenge in the ED.[2] When possible, oxygen levels and blood glucose levels should be obtained. Treatment should include management of the agitation with verbal deescalation if possible or, if necessary, with physical or chemical restraint. Medications used to treat agitation are listed in Table 47.1. Key aspects of deescalation include

- respecting a patient's personal space
- avoiding provocation
- establishing verbal contact
- providing communication that is calm, simple, and concise
- providing orientation and reassurance
- listening to what the patient is saying
- setting clear limits while offering choices if possible
- debriefing the patient if involuntary intervention has become necessary[2]

Establishing a plan of care includes psychiatric assessment for underlying organic illness in the form of delirium or behavioral disturbance in psychiatric patients or for agitation noted in drug-related presentations, particularly those involving stimulants and hallucinogens.[3] The goal of pharmacologic intervention is to calm the patient enough to allow assessment but avoid having the patient fall sleep if possible.

Restraints

Restraints should be used in the ED to manage aggression, or any patient with a behavioral emergency, *only* when all other less-restrictive means have been exhausted. Physical restraint requires increased resources, results in longer time spent in the ED, and increases the risk of injury to both the patient and the staff.[2]

The last condition of participation published in 2007 by the Centers for Medicare and Medicaid Services (CMS) requires patient rights to explicitly include the "right to be free of restraint." The CMS definition of restraint is "any means to restrict movement of a patient."[3]

Training in restraint application and management is required in behavioral health units and for all acute hospitals. Demonstration of annual physical restraint training is required, and specifics related to restraint use and patient management must be described. Any hospital death of a patient in restraints or who has been in restraint within the past 24 hours must be reported as a sentinel event and reported directly to the regional offices of CMS. States with requirements for hospital licensing may have additional requirements related to restraint use. Use of a sitter in the ED

TABLE 47.1 Medications Used to Treat Agitation.

Generic Name	Brand Name	Indications
Olanzapine	Zyprexa	Calming but not sedating
Risperidone	Risperdal	Mood stabilizer
Haloperidol	Haldol	Second line for agitation
Ziprasidone	Geodon	Second line for agitation

may also be considered to be a "restraint" and is subject to CMS rules as well.

Reasons for restraints or seclusion must be documented and include immediate threat to life and failure of less-restrictive methods. Orders must be time specific; "restraint as needed" is not an acceptable order. Once a patient is in restraints, the patient's safety and well-being must be assessed every 15 minutes and documented.[3]

ANOREXIA NERVOSA

Anorexia nervosa is an eating disorder characterized by severe weight loss to the point of significant physiologic consequences. Diagnostic criteria include

- intense fear of obesity despite slenderness,
- overwhelming body-image perception of being fat,
- weight loss of at least 25% from baseline or failure to gain weight appropriately (resulting in weight 25% less than would be expected from the patient's previous growth curve),
- absence of other physical illnesses to explain weight loss or altered body-image perception, and
- at least 3 weeks of secondary amenorrhea or primary amenorrhea in a prepubescent adolescent.[3]

Associated physical characteristics include excessive physical activity, denial of hunger in the face of starvation, asexual behavior, and history of extreme weight loss methods (e.g., diuretics, laxatives, amphetamines, emetics). Academic success is another associated characteristic. Psychiatric characteristics include excessive dependency needs, developmental immaturity, behavior favoring isolation, obsessive-compulsive behavior, and constriction of affect. Patients with anorexia nervosa generally fall into two categories—those with extreme food restriction and those with food binge and purge behavior.[3]

Anorexia nervosa is thought to result from psychological, biologic, and environmental factors.[3] There is a high incidence of premorbid anxiety disorder in prepubescent patients who subsequently develop anorexia nervosa. The patient's altered body image results in a perception of fatness. Attempts to correct this misperception through food restriction or progressive purging lead to progressive starvation. The modern preoccupation with slenderness and beauty is thought to contribute to the mind-set of slenderness in girls and young women, although research has not proved a direct relationship.[3]

Anorexia malnutrition causes protein deficiency and disrupts multiple organ systems. Nutritional deficiencies, including hypoglycemia, severe loss of fat stores, and multiple vitamin deficiencies are common. Cardiovascular effects of anorexia include dysrhythmias, bradycardia, orthostatic hypotension, and shock. Renal aberrations lead to decreased glomerular filtration rate, elevated blood urea nitrogen, edema, metabolic acidosis, hypokalemia, and hypochloremic alkalosis resulting from vomiting. Gastrointestinal findings include constipation, delayed gastric emptying, gastric dilation and rupture, dental enamel erosion, esophagitis, and Mallory-Weiss tears. Bone marrow suppression leading to platelet, erythrocyte, and leukocyte abnormalities has been reported.[4]

The ED nurse should suspect anorexia in patients presenting with extreme weight loss and history of food refusal, amenorrhea, dehydration in an otherwise healthy individual, flat affect, or near-catatonic behavior. Patients may be depressed, so the risk for suicide should be carefully assessed. Obtain a mental health history because there is a strong association with depression and substance abuse.

Assessment

The most striking physical attribute of patients with moderate to severe anorexia is their cachectic appearance. Physical examination may reveal hypothermia, peripheral edema, and thinning hair.[4] Behaviorally, these patients have a flat affect and may display psychomotor alterations. Physical and behavioral symptoms also occur in other conditions, so it is important to rule out potentially treatable causes.

A complete blood count (CBC) may reveal normocytic, normochromic anemia resulting from bone marrow suppression from starvation. Serum chemistry determinations often indicate varying degrees of hypokalemia from laxative abuse or vomiting. In addition, dehydration can cause significant electrolyte abnormalities, including hyponatremia. Hypocalcemia from dietary deficiency of calcium and associated protein deficiency also occur. β-Human chorionic gonadotropin can determine whether pregnancy is the cause of vomiting and electrolyte abnormalities. Urinalysis is used to rule out urinary tract infections, dehydration, or renal acidosis. Positive results for fecal occult blood suggest esophagitis, gastritis, or repetitive colonic trauma from laxative abuse and a bleeding disorder or severe protein malnutrition. Serum erythrocyte sedimentation rate and thyroid function tests are unlikely to alter ED management but may be ordered to rule out inflammatory or endocrine pathologic processes.[3]

An ECG should be obtained because anorexia can precipitate several heart rhythm disturbances. Noted ECG changes include nonspecific ST- and T-wave abnormalities, atrial or ventricular tachydysrhythmias, idioventricular conduction delay, heart block, nodal rhythms, ventricular escape, premature ventricular contractions, and prolonged QTc interval. These abnormalities are attributable to starvation, ipecac toxicity, and electrolyte and neuroendocrine abnormalities. Rib fractures from repetitive vomiting in the presence of hypocalcemia do occur, so a chest x-ray examination should be obtained. Cardiomegaly from ipecac toxicity or malnutrition has been noted in many patients. Electrolyte disturbances or malnutrition can lead to development of an ileus, so abdominal x-ray films are often obtained.[4]

Treatment

Care in the ED includes rehydration, correction of electrolyte abnormalities, and appropriate referral for continuing medical and psychiatric treatment.[4] Consultations with psychiatry and adolescent medicine specialists are recommended for inpatient care and to facilitate outpatient follow-up care. No specific medications have been shown to alleviate the disordered body image characteristic of anorexia. For nutritional therapy, forced feedings with total parenteral nutrition or tube feedings may be used to replace nutrients, stabilize nutrient deficiency syndromes, and alter mood when the patient becomes nutritionally replenished.[4]

BULIMIA

Bulimia nervosa is an eating disorder characterized by eating binges followed by self-induced vomiting, laxative or diuretic abuse, prolonged fasting, or excessive exercise.[3] The patient with binge eating exhibits characteristics such as

- eating, in a discrete period of time (e.g., within any 2-hour period), an amount of food larger than most people would eat during a similar period of time under similar circumstances, or
- a perceived lack of control over eating during the episode (i.e., a feeling of being unable to stop eating or the inability to control what or how much one is eating)[3]

Some patients with anorexia nervosa also manifest bulimia; however, patients with bulimia typically have a normal weight or are overweight. Recurrent inappropriate compensatory behavior is used to prevent weight gain (e.g., self-induced vomiting; misuse of laxatives, diuretics, enemas, or other medication; fasting; excessive exercise). Determining the level of severity is based on the average frequency of binge eating and inappropriate compensatory behaviors: (1) mild severity is an average of 1 to 3 episodes per week, (2) moderate is an average of 4 to 7 episodes per week, (3) severe is an average of 8 to 13 episodes per week, and (4) extreme is an average of 14 or more episodes per week.[3] Self-evaluation is unduly influenced by body shape and weight.

Bulimia nervosa is categorized as purging type when the person regularly engages in self-induced vomiting or misuse of laxatives, diuretics, or enemas. If other inappropriate compensatory behaviors, such as fasting or excessive exercise, are used without self-induced vomiting or misuse of laxatives, diuretics, or enemas, the diagnosis is bulimia nervosa, nonpurging type. Individuals who binge eat without regular use of characteristic inappropriate compensatory behaviors of bulimia nervosa are included under the category of eating disorders not otherwise specified.[4]

Bulimia nervosa is a chronic disorder with a waxing and waning course.[4] Comorbid conditions associated with bulimia nervosa include mood disorders such as major depressive disorder and bipolar disorder, anxiety disorders, alcohol and substance abuse, and adverse events related to aggression or poor impulse control.[3]

The vast majority of patients with bulimia nervosa are women. Eating disorders also occur among men who participate in sports with a weight requirement (e.g., wrestling) or in whom low body fat is important (bodybuilders).[4] As in anorexia, a morbid fear of obesity is the overriding psychological preoccupation in bulimia nervosa. Bulimia, however, is more frequent in people with a history of obesity. The common behavior of dieting may be related to the development of bulimia. Bulimia may occur after an episode of anorexia nervosa or substance abuse. Self-loathing and disgust with the body are even more severe in bulimia than in anorexia nervosa.

Binges may occur habitually or may be triggered sporadically by unpleasant feelings of anger, anxiety, or depression. Food deprivation (i.e., dieting) also plays a role in inducing bingeing. Guilt and dysphoria are common feelings after binges; however, some patients find these binges themselves soothing. Binges are typically followed by efforts to prevent weight gain. Generally, patients attempt to prevent weight gain by self-induced vomiting; however, ingestion of ipecac syrup was occasionally used to prevent weight gain. Ipecac syrup has become difficult to purchase with manufacturers discontinuing production in 2010. Laxative or diuretic misuse is also common, although these substances almost exclusively produce fluid loss rather than calorie loss. Individuals may display extreme caloric restriction between episodes, exhibit wide fluctuations in weight, or become obese.[3]

Although the act of self-induced vomiting may occur only occasionally and may be of little consequence, a chronic pattern may develop, leading to poor overall health, decreased muscle strength, dental erosion, serious electrolyte abnormalities, cardiac arrhythmias, or death. Electrolyte abnormalities resulting from vomiting may be compounded by those from laxative-induced diarrhea or diuretic use. Chronic laxative (phenolphthalein) overdose has been reported. Menstrual irregularities may be caused by weight fluctuations, nutritional deficiency, or emotional stress.[4]

Deaths related to bulimia are thought to result from cardiac arrhythmias. Gastric or esophageal rupture, Mallory-Weiss tear, pneumomediastinum, and postbinge pancreatitis have resulted from gorging and vomiting and may be life-threatening. Diet pills can cause hypertension and cerebral hemorrhage when taken in excess. Ipecac-related deaths have been reported, probably resulting from emetine cardiotoxicity in conjunction with electrolyte imbalances.[4]

Assessment

Common complaints include muscle weakness, cramps, dizziness, carpopedal spasm, hematemesis, abdominal pain, chest pain, heartburn, sore throat, or menstrual irregularity. Patients may admit to use of diuretics for edema but often deny self-induced vomiting or laxative use. Caffeine, pseudoephedrine, phenylpropanolamine (now off the market), ginseng, thyroid replacement preparations, ma huang, and other "cleansing" or "dieter's" herbs may be used in an attempt to increase metabolic rate and calorie loss. Many "natural" or herbal remedies thought to be completely safe actually contain substances increasing blood pressure or promote electrolyte imbalance.

Vital signs may be normal. Tachycardia and hypotension, when present, suggest volume depletion, whereas hypertension should raise the suspicion of stimulant use. Physical examination may reveal signs of dehydration and erosion of tooth enamel with or without frank caries. A callus resulting from repetitive contact with the upper teeth during self-induced vomiting may be found on the dorsal surface of the index and middle finger of the patient's dominant hand. Alopecia, hypertrichosis, and nail fragility are other common skin findings.[5] Weight is frequently normal or above normal, and the remainder of the physical examination is usually normal. Specific complications, however, may be found on examination of the abdomen (e.g., epigastric tenderness, guaiac-positive stools), chest (e.g., Hamman crunch resulting from air in the mediastinal space from an esophageal tear), or extremities (e.g., edema). These symptoms can be found with other conditions, so care should be taken to rule them out.[5]

Obtain electrolyte measurements even in patients with normal weight. Hypokalemia, hypomagnesemia, and metabolic alkalosis secondary to compulsive vomiting are confirmatory for bulimia. Sodium and chloride levels may be decreased. In patients who abuse laxatives but are not vomiting, hypokalemia is associated with metabolic acidosis, whereas hypocalcemia is caused by loss of bicarbonate and calcium in diarrheal stool. Diuretic abuse can decrease serum sodium and potassium levels and increase uric acid and calcium levels. Urinary findings vary with the degree of vomiting or laxative-induced diarrhea, diuretic use, and volume status. Findings also depend on whether the condition is acute or chronic. If abdominal pain is present, serum lipase and amylase measurements are used to screen for pancreatitis. Gastric rupture should be ruled out with an upright chest x-ray film. Pneumomediastinum secondary to esophageal rupture may also be evident. If hematemesis or melena has been reported, placement of a nasogastric tube may be indicated. A pregnancy test should be obtained in all female patients of childbearing age.[5]

Treatment

Emergency nurses should anticipate and be prepared to intervene for the complications of bulimia, including volume depletion, electrolyte abnormalities, esophagitis, Mallory-Weiss tear, esophageal or gastric rupture, pancreatitis, arrhythmias, or adverse effects of medication (e.g., ipecac, appetite suppressants). Associated illnesses, including depression, anxiety disorders, and substance abuse, put patients at risk for other illness and injury. Directly question patients regarding suicidal ideation.

For patients unable to halt the dangerous sequence of dieting, bingeing, and purging, admission may be necessary to break the cycle. Psychiatric hospitalization may be necessary for patients with severe depression and suicidal ideation, weight loss greater than 30% over 3 months, failure to maintain an outpatient weight contract, or family crisis.[4] Medical admission is warranted for patients with significant metabolic disturbance or other physical complications of bingeing or purging, such as Mallory-Weiss tear, esophageal rupture, or pancreatitis. For those not requiring acute inpatient care, provide referrals to appropriate outpatient services.

Patient education topics should include body weight regulation; the effects of starvation; the effects of vomiting and laxative use; and the risks of using diet pills, amphetamines, energy pills, and diet teas claiming to be natural. The latter products often contain herbal forms of caffeine and ephedrine and have been associated with hypertension, cerebrovascular accident, and death. Phenylpropanolamine, the most common ingredient in both over-the-counter diet pills and decongestants, has been taken off the market because of the fear of severe hypertension leading to stroke and other serious pathologic processes (especially in females). Patients with serious eating disorders often mistrust health care professionals, but establishing rapport to facilitate appropriate referrals is key to assisting the patient to normalize eating behaviors.[3]

ANXIETY

Anxiety is a complex feeling of apprehension, fear, and worry often accompanied by pulmonary, cardiac, and other physical sensations.[6] Anxiety is a normal response to threatening situations. Patients experiencing severe anxiety present in the ED with PDs, phobic disorders, obsessive-compulsive disorders, acute distress, posttraumatic stress disorder, anxiety due to medication conditions, and anxiety due to substance abuse. Anxiety in its most severe form can be quite debilitating. Anxiety disorders are the most common of all psychiatric disorders and can result in functional as well as emotional impairment.[7] A heightened physiologic response and elevated catecholamine levels play an important role in the normal physiologic response of the body to stress and anxiety. Three neurotransmitters are identified with anxiety—norepinephrine, γ-aminobutyric acid (GABA), and serotonin.[6]

Assessment

Anxiety is categorized as mild, moderate, severe, or PD.[5] Organic illness, medications, drug abuse, and obvious psychotic causes of an anxious state must be ruled out and documented before treatment of anxiety.[8] Patients require ED treatment for anxiety when they are in such an acutely anxious state that they pose a danger to themselves and others. A thorough medical and psychiatric history is critical. Documentation should include any changes in behavior and somatic symptoms such as headaches, dizziness, disorientation, confusion, and syncope. Family and significant others are reliable sources of history for the patient with acute anxiety. Previous psychiatric illnesses and any current medical problems should be documented. Identify any anxiety-causing agents (e.g., caffeine, nicotine, prescribed drugs, over-the-counter medications, illicit drugs, or alcohol). Thorough physical assessment is required to identify potential life-threatening illnesses. The clinician should focus on signs and symptoms of anxiety after first eliminating organic causes.[8] Diagnostic studies are used to rule out physical causes of anxiety such as metabolic disorders. Needle marks indicate illicit drug involvement, whereas hepatomegaly, ascites, and spider angioma suggest alcohol abuse.[5]

A patient with anxiety may present as having a classic panic attack, which is characterized by a sudden onset of fear and a sense of impending doom with at least four of the following symptoms—palpitations, diaphoresis, tremulousness, shortness of breath, chest pain, dizziness, nausea, abdominal discomfort, fear of injury or going crazy, derealization (perception of altered reality), and depersonalization (perception that one's body is surreal).[5] Evaluation of mental status can be especially helpful in distinguishing functional disorders from organic disorders. Assessment should include the following:

- level of consciousness
- affect
- behavioral observation
- speech pattern and cadence
- level of attention
- language comprehension
- memory, calculation, and judgment

Anxiety states are associated with an increased prevalence of other physical illnesses. Avoid falsely attributing somatic symptoms of anxiety to other medical conditions. Laboratory tests to rule out physical illness include a CBC with differential, a serum chemistry profile, a pregnancy test, and serum or urine screens for drugs. Specific serum endocrine panels are also available to diagnose illnesses such as hyperthyroidism. An ECG can identify tachydysrhythmias and myocardial infarction as the cause of palpitations and other symptoms.[8]

While remaining vigilant for life-threatening illness, emergency nurses should reassure patients experiencing anxiety. Place the patient in a calm, quiet room for formal evaluation. Rhythmic breathing, imagery techniques, and hypnotic suggestion have been used for patients with anxiety.

Treatment

Acute anxiety has been effectively treated with the passage of time, social support, and a short course of fast-acting anxiolytics, preferably a parenteral form of benzodiazepine (Table 47.2). The efficacy of benzodiazepines in treating anxiety has implicated the GABA neurotransmitter as a primary contributor to the pathophysiology of anxiety disorders. Drugs affecting norepinephrine, such as tricyclic antidepressants and monoamine oxidase inhibitors, are efficacious in treatment of several anxiety disorders as well.[8] Chronic anxiety often requires a comprehensive approach using psychotherapy, counseling, and a wider spectrum of medications (e.g., selective serotonin reuptake inhibitors [SSRIs], serotonin-norepinephrine reuptake inhibitors, benzodiazepines, low-dose antiseizure medications, and antihistamines).[8]

TABLE 47.2 Antianxiety Medications.

Generic Name	Brand Name	Drug Class
Alprazolam	Xanax	Benzodiazepine
Chlordiazepoxide	Librium	Benzodiazepine
Clonazepam	Klonopin	Benzodiazepine
Diazepam	Valium	Benzodiazepine
Lorazepam	Ativan	Benzodiazepine
Oxazepam[a]	Serax	Benzodiazepine
Hydroxyzine hydrochloride	Atarax	Antihistamine
Hydroxyzine	Vistaril	Antihistamine

[a]May be addictive. Sudden withdrawals may cause convulsions.

Benzodiazepines should be prescribed only for motivated and cooperative individuals with reliable follow-up arrangements. β-Blockers do not reduce intrinsic anxiety but may be beneficial in treatment of associated tachycardia.

Anxiety disorders are often chronic illnesses and require follow-up psychiatric intervention for successful treatment. Any patient with anxiety who presents with suicidal ideation, homicidal ideation, or acute psychosis requires emergent psychiatric consultation.[5] Listening to the patient and allowing expression of concern makes the patient feel safe.

PANIC DISORDERS

Understanding PD is important for emergency nurses because patients with PD frequently present to the ED with various somatic complaints. It is estimated that 5% of the general population meet formal criterial for panic disorder.[9] PD most commonly has an onset in early adulthood, with the prevalence increasing during childhood and adolescence.[9] PD is defined as a minimum of three panic attacks that are of sudden onset, involve at least 4 of 12 symptoms, and occur within a 3-week period.[10] The 12 symptoms are palpitations; sweating; trembling; a sensation of shortness of breath or smothering; feelings of choking, chest pain, or discomfort; nausea or abdominal distress; feeling dizzy or faint; chills or heat sensations; paresthesias; derealization (feelings of unreality) or depersonalization (being detached from oneself); fear of losing control; or fear of dying.

Asthma cardiac dysrhythmia, or metabolic disturbances such as hypoglycemia, hypoxia, and thyroid storm can mimic panic attack. Other conditions found in the patient with PD include depression, obsessive-compulsive disorder, specific phobias, social phobia, agoraphobia (fear of being unsafe in public settings), irritable bowel syndrome, migraine, mitral valve prolapse, and alcohol and drug abuse. Panic attacks may be triggered by injury, surgery, illness, interpersonal conflict, or personal loss. Use of stimulants such as caffeine, decongestants, cocaine, and sympathomimetics (e.g., amphetamines) can precipitate panic attacks in susceptible individuals. Bouts of panic can also occur in certain settings, such as stores and public transportation, especially in patients with agoraphobia. After one has excluded somatic disease and other psychiatric disorders, confirmation of the diagnosis with a brief mental status screening examination and initiation of appropriate treatment and referral is time- and cost-effective in patients with high rates of medical resource use.[9]

Assessment

Patients in the throes of a panic attack complain of sudden onset of extreme apprehension or fear, usually with feelings of impending doom. The feelings may be so intense that normal functioning is suspended and misinterpretation of reality may occur. The attacks generally come on suddenly, are very intense, and last 10 minutes or less and then subside.[3] Assessment should include precipitating events, suicidal ideation or plan, phobias, agoraphobia, obsessive-compulsive behavior, and involvement of alcohol, illicit drugs, and medications with stimulatory effects (e.g., caffeine). Determination of a family history of panic or other psychiatric illness is indicated.

Patients with PD may manifest any one of several physical symptoms. They appear anxious and may have cool, clammy skin. Heart rate and respiratory rate are usually elevated; however, blood pressure and temperature are usually normal. Hyperventilation may be difficult to detect by observing breathing because respiratory rate and tidal volume may appear normal. Room air pulse oximetry values are normal to high normal; however, arterial blood gas analysis is indicated to rule out the presence of acid-base abnormalities. Hypoxemia with hypocapnia should raise the possibility of pulmonary embolus in the patient who appears to be having a panic attack. Laboratory studies helpful in excluding other medical disorders include serum electrolytes to exclude hypokalemia and acidosis; serum glucose to exclude hypoglycemia; cardiac markers in patients suspected of acute coronary syndromes; hemoglobin in patients with near-syncope; thyroid-stimulating hormone in patients suspected of hyperthyroidism; and urine toxicology screen for amphetamines, cocaine, and phencyclidine in patients suspected of intoxication. Chest x-ray films are useful in excluding various causes of dyspnea. An ECG should be inspected for signs of ventricular preexcitation (short PR and delta wave) and long QT interval in patients with palpitations and for ischemia, infarction, or pericarditis patterns in patients with chest pain—conditions that share symptoms with or may precipitate a panic attack.[5]

Treatment

Patients presenting to the ED who appear anxious but also complain of chest pain, dyspnea, palpitations, or near-syncope should be treated as they clinically present. Place the patient on oxygen, and monitor pulse oximetry, ECG, and frequent vital signs. Patients with PD require frequent reassurance and explanation; many may benefit from social service intervention after more serious organic causes of symptoms are ruled out. A major component of therapy involves education that the symptoms are neither from a serious medical condition nor from mental deficiency, but rather from a chemical imbalance in the fight-or-flight response.

The ED staff should listen, remain empathic, and be nonargumentative with these patients. Statements such as "It's nothing serious" and "It's related to stress" can be misinterpreted as implying lack of understanding and concern. Intravenous (IV) medication (e.g., Ativan, 0.5 mg IV every 20 minutes) may be necessary in patients with PD who, as a result of subsequent poor impulse control, pose a risk to themselves or to those around them.[8] Patients with PD are best served by referral to a qualified mental health professional, who can establish a constructive rapport with them and follow their needs on a long-term basis before beginning to give them anxiolytic medications.

Aside from IV medications required to treat acute anxiety states in the ED, the use of pharmacotherapy for patients with PD should, in most instances, be deferred to the psychiatrist who is following the patient for the long term. Benzodiazepines are optimal for ED and outpatient abortive therapy because of their immediate antipanic effects.[8] Coexisting disorders may influence medication choice (e.g., monoamine oxidase inhibitors [MAOIs], clonazepam, and SSRIs for social phobia; SSRIs or clomipramine [Anafranil] for obsessive-compulsive disorder; tricyclic antidepressants [TCAs] for depression).[8] Institution of treatment for PD in the ED is appropriate in a very limited subset of patients with PD. Those who are very motivated and cooperative and possess an understanding of the psychological nature of their disorder and whose symptoms are elicited as a response to temporary stress are good candidates. In such cases, pharmacotherapy with an oral benzodiazepine for no longer than 1 week may be appropriate.

Inpatient treatment is necessary in patients with suicidal ideation and a suicide plan or with serious alcohol or sedative withdrawal symptoms, or when potential medical disorders warrant admission (e.g., unstable angina, acute myocardial ischemia). Follow-up with a chemical dependence treatment specialist should be arranged when indicated. All discharged patients with PD should be referred to a psychiatrist, a psychologist, or another mental health professional.

DEPRESSION

Depression is a potentially life-threatening mood disorder afflicting approximately 7% of the population.[11] This holistic disorder affects the body, feelings, thoughts, and behaviors, affecting how one feels, thinks, and handles daily activities. Considerable pain and suffering significantly affect the individual's ability to function. As many as two-thirds of the people experiencing depression do not realize they have a treatable illness and therefore do not seek treatment. Mortality of depression is measurable and is the direct result of suicide, the 10th leading cause of death in the United States.[11] Almost all those who kill themselves intentionally have a diagnosable mental disorder with or without substance abuse. Ironically, substance abuse is often the result of attempted self-treatment for symptoms of depression. Most suicide attempts are expressions of extreme distress, not bids for attention.[11] These patients *must* be assessed for suicidality. Any treatment that

TABLE 47.3 Antidepressants.

Generic Name	Brand Name	Indications
Amitriptyline[a]	Elavil	Typical
Imipramine[a]	Tofranil	Typical
Doxepin[a]	Sinequan	Typical
Fluoxetine	Prozac	Atypical
Citalopram	Celexa	Atypical
Fluvoxamine	Luvox	Atypical
Sertraline	Zoloft	Atypical
Trazodone	Desyrel	Atypical
Venlafaxine	Effexor	Atypical
Bupropion	Wellbutrin	Other
Mirtazapine	Remeron	Other
Nefazodone	Serzone	Other

[a]These medications can be cardiotoxic—need baseline ECG.

initiates antidepressant medications should also require a follow-up appointment because it can take up to 2 weeks for these medications to have a noticeable effect. Antidepressant medications are listed in Table 47.3.

The development of depression is felt to be multifactorial and may be due to biologic, physiologic, genetic, or psychosocial factors. Serotonin and norepinephrine are the primary neurotransmitters involved, although dopamine has also been related to depression. A family history of depression is common. Bipolar disorder has a prominent depressive phase but is a different clinical entity from depression. Depressive syndrome frequently accompanies comorbid conditions such as schizophrenia, substance abuse, eating disorders, schizoaffective disorder, and borderline personality disorder.[3]

Assessment

Depression is often difficult to diagnose because it can manifest in many different forms. General classifications of depression include disruptive mood dysregulation disorder, introduced in 2013 as an alternative to diagnosing children and adolescents with bipolar disorder. The symptoms of disruptive mood dysregulation disorder[3,11] are constant and severe irritability and anger in individuals aged 6 to 18 years, with onset before age 10. The National Institutes of Health also recognizes the following:

- persistent depressive disorder, a depressed mood that lasts for at least 2 years;
- postpartum depression, which occurs after childbirth and has depressive symptoms ranging from mild depression and anxiety to major depression;
- psychotic depression, occurring when a person has severe depression plus some form of psychosis, such as hallucinations;
- seasonal affective disorder, characterized by the onset of depression during the winter months, when there is less natural light; and
- bipolar disorder.

Bipolar disorder is different from depression. Some individuals with bipolar disorder experience episodes of major depression, although usually they also experience extreme high-euphoric moods, or "mania," as well.[3]

The diagnosis of major depression is made when at least five of the following characteristics are present for at least 2 weeks: (1) loss of interest in usual activities, (2) depressed mood, (3) appetite increase or decrease with weight change, (4) insomnia or hypersomnia, (5) fatigue, (6) psychomotor agitation or retardation, (7) decreased ability to think, (8) recurrent thoughts of death, or (9) feelings of worthlessness. Occasionally symptoms are precipitated by life crises or other illnesses, whereas at other times depression can occur at random. Clinical depression often occurs concurrently with other medical illnesses and worsens the prognosis for these illnesses.

The emergency nurse's responsibility when caring for a patient with depression is to maintain a high index of suspicion for the diagnosis, especially in populations at risk for suicide. Primary at-risk populations include young adults and older adults; however, depression and suicide can occur in any age-group, including children.[12] Depression should be suspected as an underlying factor in drug overdose (including alcohol), self-inflicted injury, or intentionally inflicted injury when the assailant is known to the victim. In any such patient, screening for diagnostic symptoms of major depression and suicide is essential.[5]

Serotonin syndrome is a rare but potentially fatal condition caused by drugs that affect serotonin metabolism or act as serotonin receptor agonists. These drugs are commonly prescribed in the management of depression, and vigilant assessment followed by supportive treatment will make a significant effect on the duration and severity of the reaction.[13] Serotonin syndrome is thought to be caused by excess stimulation of the serotonin receptors with the following symptoms: agitation, akathisia, clonus, confusion, diaphoresis, diarrhea, significantly high fever, hyperreflexia, hypertension, increased bowel sounds, muscular rigidity, mydriasis, tachycardia, and tremor. Treatment is symptomatic and supportive; discontinue the medication and use fluid replacement and benzodiazepines to control agitation. Haloperidol should not be used for sedation because of the potential to worsen hyperthermia. External cooling measures should be applied, as well as sedation, paralysis, and intubation, as needed. Assess for the potential that the medication was an intentional overdose. Antidotal therapies may be of benefit based on the drug ingested.[13]

Treatment

Depression is a clinical diagnosis; however, symptoms associated with depression may be the result of medications, metabolic disorders, and other nutritional abnormalities. Assessment and treatment of the person with depression should rule out various treatment conditions. Laboratory tests are primarily used to rule out other diagnoses, such as renal failure, hypoglycemia, and drug toxicity. Additional diagnostic studies include computed tomography (CT) scan, magnetic resonance imaging (MRI) scan, and electroencephalogram to rule out organic brain syndrome or other central nervous system (CNS) problems. Treatment is aimed at the reduction of depressive symptoms and the restoration of function. Medication and inpatient care are recommended when there is significant concern for the patient's safety.[3]

SUICIDALITY

People at risk for suicide present with a variety of complaints: mental disorders, substance abuse, physical abuse, chronic illness, or recent losses. The Joint Commission reports inpatient suicide as the fourth most reported sentinel event and suicide as the 10th leading cause of death for people of all ages.[12] Risk factors associated with suicide include (1) biological factors; familial history of suicide or previous attempt and low serotonin levels that have been documented; (2) psychological factors; suicidal hostility seen as the wish to kill (revenge), the wish to be killed (guilt), and the wish to die (hopelessness); (3) environmental factors: the lethal combination of suicidal fantasies accompanied by loss, rage, or identification with someone who completed suicide (e.g., copycat suicide); and (4) cultural factors, religious beliefs, family values, gender issues, and attitude toward death.[3]

Assessment

Assessment is critical in determining imminent risk to the patient. Essential elements of the assessment require a complete history, including current ideation, intent, and plan; history of previous attempts; family history of suicide; history of mental illness and any current treatment; history of alcohol or substance abuse; current medical problems; recent life stressors; and any history of aggression or violence. It is also important to determine whether the patient has social supports, such as family or friends. EDs are encouraged to implement an assessment tool such as the Beck Scale, IS THE PATH WARM, or the SADD PERSONS scale to provide a consistent approach to the assessment of these patients.[14] IS THE PATH WARM consists of assessing for I-ideation, S-substance abuse, P-purposelessness, A-anxiety, T-trapped, H-hopelessness, W-withdrawal, A-anger, R-recklessness, M-mood changes.[10] These tools are not a definitive predictor of suicide but can provide some suggestions for a course of treatment based on scoring.[14]

Treatment

Despite the 2007 Joint Commission national patient safety goal requiring assessment of patients at risk for suicide, suicides continue to occur within health care settings. The Joint Commission outlines two strategies to keep patients with serious suicide ideation safe: (1) place the patient in a "safe room" that is ligature-resistant, and (2) keep the suicidal patient in the main area of the ED, initiate continuous 1:1 monitoring, and remove all objects that pose a risk for self-harm.[12] If the patient is discharged, there should be plans for immediate follow-up. "Contracting" with the patient for safety is usually part of the plan of care when the patient is in the ED. Patients with a plan for suicide should be admitted until appropriate safety measures can be implemented. Psychiatric evaluation should occur after acute medication conditions are addressed.

SCHIZOPHRENIA

Schizophrenia is a severe psychiatric disorder that has a profound effect on both the individual affected and society. Schizophrenia is characterized by diverse psychopathology with symptoms grouped as positive, negative, cognitive, and affective. Positive symptoms are the addition of things that should not be there: delusions, hallucinations, disorganized speech (associative looseness), and bizarre or disorganized behavior. The positive symptoms tend to relapse and remit, a frequent cause of ED admission. Negative symptoms are a "lack," or absence, of what would be deemed normal, seen as blunted affect, impaired motivation (avolition), reduction in spontaneous speech, poverty of thought (alogia), inability to experience pleasure or joy (anhedonia), and social withdrawal. Cognitive symptoms include exhibiting inattention, being easily distracted, or having impaired memory, poor problem-solving skills, poor decision-making skills, illogical thinking, and impaired judgment. Affective symptoms include dysphoria, suicidality, and hopelessness. The negative and cognitive symptoms frequently cause the chronic disability, with long-term effects on function, whereas the affective symptoms contribute to the high suicide rate of schizophrenia.[3,15,16]

Current diagnostic requirements are met if the syndrome continues for at least 6 months with at least 1 month in which active symptoms are present and these symptoms result in significant impairment of occupational and social functioning. Substance use disorders occur in nearly half of affected individuals.[3] Substance use is associated with higher rates of treatment nonadherence, relapse, incarceration, homelessness, violence, suicide, and a poorer prognosis. Research demonstrates that approximately 20% of people with schizophrenia have attempted suicide, with 5% to 10% dying by suicide, a rate five times that of the general population.[3] In addition to suicide, premature death may result from poor health maintenance, substance abuse, poverty, and homelessness. The onset of symptoms is insidious in about half of all patients. The prodromal phase can begin years before the full-blown syndrome. It is characterized by losses of previously achieved functioning in home, society, and occupation (e.g., poor school or work performance, deterioration of hygiene and appearance, decreasing emotional connections with others, and behaviors considered odd for this individual).

Gradual onset predicts a more severe and chronic illness course, whereas abrupt onset of hallucinations and delusional, bizarre, or disorganized thinking in previously functioning patients can lead to a better intermediate and long-term outcome. Such patients arrive in the ED in a psychotic crisis requiring acute management, often without having been previously diagnosed with a psychiatric illness. They present diagnostic dilemmas regarding organic versus psychiatric etiology and primary psychotic versus affective disorder that may be further complicated by the presence of alcohol or drug intoxication. Due to the variability of symptom expression and diagnostic requirements of chronicity, the diagnosis of schizophrenia in the ED should be provisional at best. As a diagnosis by exclusion, schizophrenia must be distinguished from the numerous psychiatric and organic disorders that also lead to psychotic behaviors.

Assessment

Schizophrenia most commonly presents with an episode of psychosis, typically occurring in adolescence or young adulthood (15–25 years of age), and in males four times more often than in females.[3] The most common causes for severe mental status changes in the ED are organic, not psychiatric. They include medications, drug intoxication, drug withdrawal syndromes, and general medical illnesses causing delirium.[3] The presence of an affective disorder (e.g., major depression, bipolar disorder, or schizoaffective disorder) must be excluded. Conditions mistaken for schizophrenia have very different prognoses and therapies. In addition, an organic cause (e.g., drug intoxication, medical illness) must be ruled out. Commonly, problems with antipsychotic medications are the chief complaint. Medical illness can cause or complicate a psychotic process. Obtain a complete medication history; many commonly prescribed medicines can cause psychotic reactions.[3]

Psychiatric and organic illness can coexist and interact at the same time in the same patient. Acute psychiatric symptoms and difficulty obtaining a reliable history can mask serious organic illness. The history obtained in the ED may relate to a complication of treatment (medication side effects) or a crisis arising from socioeconomic factors secondary to schizophrenia, such as poverty, homelessness, social isolation, and failure of support systems. Information should be elicited about the actual or potential likelihood for acts of violence. Acutely psychotic patients presenting to the ED place other patients and staff in danger. A paranoid schizophrenic patient, in response to delusions and command hallucinations, can be extremely dangerous and unpredictable. Identify threats made to others, expressions of suicidal intent, and possession of weapons at home or on the person.[15]

The patient with schizophrenia may be wildly agitated, combative, withdrawn, or severely catatonic. Conversely, he or she may appear rational, cooperative, and well controlled. Blunting of affect may be noted, or the person may be subtly odd, unkempt, or grossly bizarre in manner, dress, or affect. Physical examination with attention to vital signs, pupillary findings, hydration status, and mental status should be performed. Diagnostic evaluation is required when organic cause or drug intoxication may be related to mental status changes. Pay particular attention to fever (tachycardia can be a sign of neuroleptic malignant syndrome), heat stroke (antipsychotics inhibit sweating), and other medical illness. Look for dystonia, akathisia, tremor, and muscle rigidity. Tardive dyskinesia is a common, often irreversible sequela of long-term (and sometimes brief) antipsychotic use. The condition is characterized by uncontrollable tongue thrusting, lip smacking, and facial grimacing. Mental status is usually normal, with the sensorium clear and the person oriented to person, place, and time. Assess attention, language, memory, constructions, and executive functions.[15]

Treatment

No specific laboratory findings are diagnostic of schizophrenia; however, some studies may be necessary to rule out organic causes for psychosis or to uncover complications of schizophrenia and its treatment. Blood levels of certain psychiatric drugs, specifically lithium and mood-stabilizing antiseizure medications, can confirm compliance or indicate toxicity. Serum alcohol and toxicology tests can be useful when substance abuse is suspected, and a capillary blood glucose test can rule out a diabetic emergency. Similarly, oxygen saturation can disclose hypoxia as a potential cause of behavioral or CNS disturbances. Electrolyte levels may reveal hyponatremia secondary to water intoxication (psychogenic polydipsia), which is common in undertreated or refractory schizophrenia. A CT scan and an MRI scan can disclose abnormalities of brain structure and function in the patient with schizophrenia. Although imaging results are of interest for research, such studies have very narrow clinical relevance and may be quite a challenge to obtain.

Evolving from the efficacy of modern antipsychotic medications and budget cutting, there was a widespread closing of psychiatric beds in public psychiatric hospitals between 1955 and 1994. Approximately 90% of the people who would have been living in public psychiatric hospitals in 1955 were not there by 1994. Between 50% and 60% of those patients were diagnosed with schizophrenia.[16] Deinstitutionalization of patients with schizophrenia has had a major effect on emergency nursing. The patient with schizophrenia is now a frequent visitor to the ED, with problems ranging from disease exacerbation, medication noncompliance, or side effects to medical and socioeconomic crises arising from substance abuse, poverty, homelessness, and failed support systems.[17]

Care for the patient with schizophrenia in the ED may be limited to diagnosis and treatment of an urgent or nonurgent medical complaint. In some patients, brief medical evaluation before psychiatric, crisis intervention, or social service consultation is adequate. For others, evaluation and treatment of a psychiatric drug adverse reaction is necessary. Physical and chemical restraint are indicated when the patient represents an immediate threat to self or others and alternatives have failed. Psychiatry consultation should be obtained as soon as organic processes are ruled out to correctly diagnose or safely treat a severely disturbed patient with schizophrenia.

Antipsychotic medications (previously referred to as neuroleptics or major tranquilizers) have revolutionized the treatment of and prognosis for schizophrenia (Table 47.4). First-generation antipsychotics block dopamine receptors in the brain, whereas second-generation antipsychotics affect serotonin transmission. The second-generation drugs (e.g., risperidone, clozapine, olanzapine, quetiapine) are less likely to produce dystonia and tardive dyskinesia and more likely to improve negative symptoms.[2] However, with the possible exception of clozapine, they are no more effective than traditional agents (e.g., haloperidol, fluphenazine) in the treatment-resistant patient. Benzodiazepines also have a role in schizophrenia, especially for emergency care of the acutely psychotic patient.[2] In the case of acute withdrawal from

TABLE 47.4 Antipsychotics.

Generic Name	Brand Name	Indications
Chlorpromazine[a,b]	Thorazine	Typical
Thioridazine[a,b]	Mellaril	Typical
Haloperidol[a,b]	Haldol	Typical
Clozapine[a,b]	Clozaril	Atypical
Olanzapine[a,b]	Zyprexa	Atypical
Quetiapine[a,b]	Seroquel	Atypical
Risperidone[a,b]	Risperdal	Atypical

[a]Antiparkinsonian medications (Artane, Cogentin, amantadine, Benadryl) may be used to decrease side effects of antipsychotic medications.

[b]Neuroleptic malignant syndrome is a potentially life-threatening adverse effect that can occur with anyone taking antipsychotics. Symptoms include fever, muscle rigidity, and altered consciousness. The patient may also demonstrate decreased blood pressure, appetite, and urine output; and increased white blood cell count, sweating, and pulse rate.

alcohol, benzodiazepines are the preferred medication. This is an important consideration because it is estimated that half of all patients with schizophrenia have comorbid drug- or alcohol-abuse problems.[2] Anticholinergic medications are used to counteract dystonic and parkinsonian side effects (extrapyramidal symptoms [EPS]) of antipsychotics, particularly higher-potency agents that are less sedating but more likely to produce EPS.[15]

Schizophrenia is a complex, chronic, and disabling illness. Fewer than 20% of patients recover fully from a single psychotic episode. More than 50% of individuals who receive the diagnosis have intermittent and long-term psychiatric problems, with 20% experiencing chronic symptoms and disability. Unemployment is estimated to be 80% to 90% and life expectancy reduced by 10 to 20 years.[15] Rapid and aggressive medication therapy of acute psychotic episodes, family intervention, and cognitive behavioral therapy are correlated with a better overall prognosis.[17]

SUBSTANCE ABUSE

The World Health Organization (WHO) defines substance abuse as use of harmful or hazardous psychoactive substances, including alcohol and illicit drugs.[18] In 2013, the American Psychiatric Association replaced "substance abuse" and "substance dependence" with a single term: substance use disorder.[3] Substance use disorders are complex diseases of the brain characterized by craving, seeking, and using a substance regardless of consequences. Continuous substance use results in actual changes in the brain structure and function.[3] Substance use disorders are chronic and relapsing, and the magnitude of effect on EDs continues to rise. Population-based studies estimate that substance use disorders account for approximately 6% of all ED visits, with some research finding as many as 12.5%.[18,19] Of particular concern is that the opioid overdose epidemic continues to worsen in the United States. Drug overdose, driven by opioid addiction, is the leading cause of accidental death in the United States.[18] Opioid overdose–related deaths[20] increased 22% between 2015 and 2016 and yet again 30% from 2016 to 2017. Substance abusers are at high risk for suicide, homicide, and overdose.

Assessment

Assessment includes the following topics:

- What is the history of patient's past use, and/or what did he or she take just before coming to the ED?
- For alcohol: what was the amount consumed in the last 24 hours and the time and amount of the last drink?
- Is there any history of blackouts or seizures related to withdrawal?
- For drugs: What is the amount, timing, and route of last use?
- Has the patient been treated for substance abuse previously?
- Is there any history of withdrawal symptoms or overdoses?
- Is there any family history of drug or alcohol problems?
- Does the patient have any coexisting physical conditions?
- What is the patient's current medical status?
- Is there any history of physical or sexual abuse?
- Is there any history of violence toward self or others?
- Are there any thoughts or plans of self-harm?

Treatment

Immediate medical treatment of withdrawal or overdose symptoms should be undertaken to avert any life-threatening problems. Are there any physical complications related to drug abuse (acquired immunodeficiency syndrome [AIDS], abscesses, or hepatitis)? Once necessary medical interventions have been completed and the patient is stable, the focus of treatment should be on appropriate follow-up.

SUMMARY

Psychosocial conditions found in the ED are varied and challenging. Regardless of the presenting symptoms, it is important for the emergency nurse to treat the patient with empathy and respect while protecting the patient and others from harm. Recent decreases in federal and state funding for mental health services are a harbinger for increases in the number of patients presenting to the ED. In many situations, the patient may have no previous psychiatric history or contact with the mental health system—the ED is the "first contact." ED nurses are uniquely prepared and positioned to provide expert care and to this vulnerable population.

REFERENCES

1. Weiss AJ, Barrett ML, Heslin KC, Stocks C. *Trends in Emergency Department Visits Involving Mental and Substance use Disorders, 2006–2013. HCUP Statistical Brief #216.* Rockville, MD: Agency for Healthcare Research and Quality; 2016. https://www.hcup-us.ahrq.gov/reports/statbriefs/sb216-Mental-Substance-Use-Disorder-ED-Visit-Trends.pdf. Accessed June 4, 2019.
2. Zeller SL, Citrome L. Managing agitation associated with schizophrenia and bipolar disorder in the emergency setting. *West J Emerg Med.* 2016;17(2):165–172. https://doi.org/10.5811/westjem.2015.12.28763.
3. Halter MJ. *Varcarolis' Foundations of Psychiatric-Mental Health Nursing: A Clinical Approach.* 8th ed. St Louis, MO: Elsevier; 2018.
4. Nagl M, Jacobi C, Paul M, et al. Prevalence, incidence, and natural course of anorexia and bulimia nervosa among adolescents and young adults. *Eur Child Adolesc Psychiatry.* 2016;25:903–918. https://doi.org/10.1007/s00787-015-0808-z.
5. Pitner J. Psychiatric/psychosocial emergencies. In: *Emergency Nursing Core Curriculum.* 7th ed. St Louis, MO: Elsevier; 2018.
6. Brawman-Mintzer O, Lydiard RB. Biological basis of generalized anxiety disorder. *J Clin Psychiatr.* 1997;58(suppl 3):16–25.
7. Dark T, Flynn HA, Rust G, Kinsell H, Harman J. Epidemiology of emergency department visits for anxiety in the United States: 2009–2011. *Psychiatr Serv.* 2017;68(3):238–244. https://doi.org/10.1176/appi.ps.201600148.
8. Bystritsky A, Khalsa SS, Cameron ME, Schiffman J. Current diagnosis and treatment of anxiety disorders. *P T.* 2013;38(1):30–57.
9. Elkins RM, Pincus DB, Comer JS. A psychometric evaluation of the panic disorder severity scale for children and adolescents. *Psychol Assess.* 2014;26(2):609–618.
10. Asmundson GJ, Taylor S, Smits JA. Panic disorder and agoraphobia: an overview and commentary on DSM-5 changes. *Depress Anxiety.* 2014;31(6):480–486.
11. National Institute of Mental Health, US Department of Health and Human Services. *Depression.* National Institute of Mental Health website. www.nimh.nih.gov/health/topics/depression/index.shtml Accessed June 4, 2019.
12. The Joint Commission. *Quality and Safety. November 2017 Perspectives Preview: Special Report: Suicide Prevention in Health Care Settings.* The Joint Commission website. https://www.jointcommission.org/issues/article.aspx?Article=GtNpk0ErgGF%2B7J9WOTTkXANZSEPXa1%2BKH0/4kGHCiio%3D. Accessed June 4, 2019.
13. Bartlett D. Drug-induced serotonin syndrome. *Crit Care Nurse.* 2017;37(1):49–54. https://doi.org/10.4037/ccn2017169.
14. Patterson WM, Dohn HH, Bird J, Patterson GA, et al. Evaluation of suicidal patients: the SAD PERSONS scale. *Psychosomatics.* 1983;24(4):343–349.
15. Owen MJ, Sawa A, Mortensen PB. Schizophrenia. *Lancet.* 2016;388(10039):86–97. https://doi.org/10.1016/S0140-6736(15)01121-6.
16. Fuller-Torrey E. *Out of the Shadows: Confronting America's Mental Illness Crisis.* New York, NY: John Wiley & Sons; 1997.
17. Clinical update: psychosis and schizophrenia. *Nurs Stand.* 2014;28(30):20. https://doi.org/10.7748/ns2014.03.28.30.20.s26.
18. Emergency Nurses Association. *Position Statement: Patients With Substance Use Disorders and Addiction in the Emergency Care Setting.* https://www.ena.org/docs/default-source/resource-library/practice-resources/position-statements/patientswithsubstanceuse.pdf?sfvrsn=6c33cad2_2. Published 2016. Accessed June 4, 2019.
19. Huynh C, et al. Factors influencing the frequency of emergency department utilization by individuals with substance use disorders. *Psychiatr Q.* 2016;87(4):713–728. https://doi.org/10.1007//s11126-016-9422-6.
20. Vivolo-Kantor AM, et al. Vital signs: trends in emergency department visits for suspected opioid overdoses—United States, July 2016–September 2017. *MMWR Morb Mortal Wkly Rep.* 2018;67(9):279–285.

48

Forensic Nursing in the Emergency Department

Colleen Mary Pedrotty

FORENSIC NURSING DEFINED

Care of trauma victims in an emergency setting occurs every day and in every emergency setting. The trauma team staff are members of a unique group of health care workers specializing in providing optimal care to victims of trauma and violence. The nurse is an essential part of the team in caring for these patients and may also be asked to collect forensic evidence. The Emergency Nurses Association has worked collaboratively for many years with the International Association of Forensic Nurses, whose mission is to develop, promote, and share forensic nursing science and related information.[1]

Often the need for forensic nursing stems from trauma, which is injury to tissue caused by an extrinsic agent. A traumatic incident may be classified as intentional or unintentional.[2] Unintentional injuries remain the fifth leading cause of death across all ages in the United States. Homicide, assaults, interpersonal violence, and sexual, physical, and psychological abuse are huge public health issues. Homicide is one of the top five causes of death in people aged 1 to 44 years, the third leading cause for those 15 to 34 years of age, and the fourth leading cause in ages 1 to 10 years. Suicide is the second leading cause of death in people aged 10 to 34 years.[3] Mechanism of injury (MOI) is the result of the transfer of external energy in the environment into the body. These injuries occur as a result of motor vehicle crashes (MVCs), violence, burns, suicide, drowning, mass disasters, thermal blast, and bioterrorism.[4] Violence and crime are on the rise around the world. The World Health Organization (WHO) cites violence and crime as the fourth leading cause of death.[5]

Most victims, however, do survive the violence with minor to severe injuries.[6] Many victims will seek medical attention in the emergency department (ED). Forensic victims are victims of crime and violence who require involvement of the health care and justice systems. Victims of traumatic injuries should be treated as forensic victims until proven otherwise. ED nurses and physicians have the opportunity to identify these victims during their initial evaluation and treatment.

Forensic victims enter the ED with evidence on their clothes, body, and belongings that can assist in the investigation of a criminal incident.[7] All too often, trauma patients enter the ED arena and then the evidence is destroyed. The wounds are often exposed, irrigated, and sutured before any swabs can be obtained, which results in loss, contamination, and/or the destruction of the evidence.[7,8] This loss of evidence can compromise and violate the victim's right to justice. Victims of violence have unique needs that require sensitivity from health care workers. They often feel that what happened was their fault, or they may fear that the perpetrator will return. The nature of the ED is one of chaos—saving lives and throughput being the ultimate goal, rather than the identification and collection of evidence. If the evidence is damaged or destroyed, case progression can be compromised.[7] That is why it is so important to recognize these victims and obtain evidence without compromising lifesaving care. Health care providers need to be educated about forensic victims so they can identify and provide care that is appropriate for this population.[7,9]

HISTORY OF FORENSIC NURSING

According to Lynch, defining forensics helped establish the bases on which forensic nursing was established.[10] Forensic nursing is the application of medicolegal aspects in the scientific investigation. As early as 1974, Burgess and Holmstrom coined the phrase "rape trauma syndrome." Rape trauma syndrome included not only the acute phase but also the long-term reorganization process that occurs as a result of rape.[11] Burgess and Holmstrom also developed an intervention and treatment schema involving crisis intervention counseling. Rape was a major concern in 1976, and the National Center for the Prevention and Control of Rape was established. This organization opened up doors for reform on statutory rape, established stalking laws, improved treatment of victims, developed protocols for health care providers, and improved funding for rape crisis services. In 1976 the first Sexual Assault Examiner (SANE) program was developed in Memphis, Tennessee. In 1977 the second program started in Minneapolis, Minnesota. In 1979 Amarillo, Texas, established its program. In the 1980s, the national center was closed, which slowed down the progress[11] until 1994.

In 1992 in St Paul, Minnesota, 74 nurses, mostly sexual assault nurse examiners, came together to form the International Association of Forensic Nurses for the first-ever national convention of sexual assault nurses. The convention included nurses who were death investigators, correctional specialists, forensic psychiatric nurses, legal consultants, nurse attorneys, forensic clinical specialists, forensic gynecology nurses, and nurses in other roles. They formed the International Association of Forensic Nurses. Their goal is to improve the standard of practice, promote the development of evidence-based knowledge, and facilitate educational opportunities.[12]

EMERGENCY NURSE ROLES AND RESPONSIBILITIES

When the victim arrives at the ED, the triage acuity should indicate a high-risk situation. A level 2, using the Emergency Severity Index, is any patient who is in extreme distress (either physical or psychological).[13] Several different triage scales are available, but the urgency for patient care is the same. The staff needs to develop a trusting relationship. Listen to the patient and explain what will happen during the examination. The victim should be triaged in a private area. The only questions that should be asked are about pertinent medical history, complaint, and vital signs. The nurse should put all statements in quotation marks. Specific questions that require the patient to relive the assault are not needed. Determining the presence of physical trauma requiring immediate treatment is the initial priority. In the case of suspected sexual assault, the Sexual Assault Response Team (SART) should be notified. If it is not available, follow the policies and procedures of the facility.[14] Forensic nurses' skills include the ability to document injuries, provide photo documentation, collect and preserve forensic evidence, testify in court, and work collaboratively with other disciplines, such as advocacy and criminal justice practitioners.[15]

In the case of abuse or neglect not related to sexual assault, the triage nurse should alert other members of the multidisciplinary team. If the abuser accompanies the victim to the ED, the nurse should make every attempt to separate the victim from the abuser to conduct the interview. If the person(s) accompanying the patient attempts to block the patient's privacy, the ED nurse must intercede on the patient's behalf. The nurse should be careful not to endanger the victim or the ED staff in the process of patient care. Nurses can take action to ensure a safe environment in the ED and advocate for a safe environment upon discharge. Safe care should include ongoing education and resources to assist the ED nurse to obtain this goal.[16]

Consent

Consent must be obtained from the victim before proceeding to the kit collection in the case of sexual assault. In a medical emergency, consent is assumed and the medical team can proceed to care for the patient. When the victim is able to consent, a consent form is signed. The victim is giving permission for the nurse to collect evidence, report and surrender evidence to law enforcement, send evidence to a laboratory approved by the Federal Bureau of Investigation (FBI) for CODIS access, and take photographs of injuries. The victim has the right to refuse any part of the examination and can stop at any time during the examination. Age of consent varies from state to state. The ED nurse should know his or her state law for consent.[11] When collecting evidence from a suspected perpetrator, the law enforcement officer must present a subpoena to the ED nurse, which will give instruction on which specific specimens to obtain. Never collect an unrequested or extra forensic specimen from the perpetrator.

Forensic Interview

Once consent is obtained from the victim, the forensic interview and examination should be conducted. Ideally the forensic interview should be done first. The purpose of interviewing the victim first is to guide the examination. This approach helps the investigator decide which specimens should be obtained. The interview should be conducted in a private area so that information is not overheard by other patients or their family members. The examiner should pay close attention to details involved in the assault. Trace evidence is often difficult to find in the best of circumstances. Another purpose of a forensic examination is to assist law enforcement to obtain information about the location of the crime. The victim should be questioned about loss of consciousness, attempted strangulation, head injuries, and any experienced pain. The interview with the investigating officer and forensic nurse should be conducted together. This prevents discrepancies in the story and fatigue on the victim's part. Consistency is key in the prosecution of perpetrators.[11] All information needs to be documented clearly and legibly.

Documentation of Evidence

Documentation is a key element in the investigation and prosecution of a perpetrator. This documentation provides essential case information. A complete and accurate record of the assault is essential for investigating the crime and for presenting the case when it goes to court.[17] Wounds will have healed and the memory forgets, but the recorded words of the victim remain available if the documentation is accurate. Multiple areas of documentation are necessary for the forensic examiner to complete: patient consent, authorization to release the information, forensic interview, the examination, and chain-of-custody documentation.[18]

The first principle of a forensic examination is the principle of objectivity on the part of the examiner. It is important for the forensic examiner to maintain an unbiased approach in the care of their patient and toward documentation.[18,19] Whenever possible, the forensic examiner should avoid medical terminology and instead use terms understood by the law enforcement officer, prosecutor, defense attorney, and most important, the jurors.[18] Use the victim's words; never change their words to make it look cleaner. Use quotation marks whenever possible. For example, if the victim states that the perpetrator threatened him or her, document the entire threat in quotation marks, include the perpetrator's name in the quote. For example, say "Johnny threaten to kill me if I told anyone" as opposed to "He threaten to kill me if I told anyone." This approach helps jurors put a face and a name to the perpetrator.

Handwriting must be legible because years later the nurse will not remember many of the details of the case, and the nurse may not be able to read the handwriting. Never lead the victim during the interview; instead, direct the person. Interviewers should keep an even tone, maintain eye contact, avoid showing shock, and be aware of body expression. Documentation should include the place and time of the assault; the perpetrator's race and relationship with the victim and the number of assailants; any force or weapons involved; the type of assault (sexual and or physical); the use of objects, fingers, or the penis if sexual assault occurred; the occurrence of penetration and/or ejaculation; the use of a condom or a lubricant; quotations from the victim that may have made him or her afraid to resist; any consensual sex in the past 72 hours; activities of the victim since the assault (eating, drinking, change of clothing, shower, smoking, urination or bowel movements); and the victim's appearance and emotional response during the interview and examination. An exception to hearsay is an "excited utterance," which is a spontaneous statement made by the victim during the interview examination.[18] Never use the word "alleged" in the record. Using this word can place doubt and bias on the case. The triage nurses and physicians, who have no education in forensic documentation, need to be educated not to use this term.

Medical personnel must remain objective in their documentation, limiting bias and subjectivity. This decision is most clear when considering the patient's sexual history. A victim's past sexual activity is irrelevant to the case. The only relevant sexual activity is consensual sex in the last 72 to 96 hours. Defense attorneys in the past have attempted to use the patient's past sexual history. As a result of these tactics, all states have passed a rape shield law to prevent the patient's unrelated, past sexual history from being the focus in court. If the forensic examiner inquires about past sexual activity and then documents the sexual history, the door is opened for the defense attorney to question the examiner; even if the prosecutor objects, the victim's past sexual history is still in the juror's minds.[18]

Emergency Nurses Association Position Statement

The ED nurse has a responsibility to recognizing the effect of violence and trauma on the patient's physical and psychological responses. Emergency nurses have a duty to collaborate with all team members to develop guidelines and policies to ensure identification, collection, and preservation of evidence and to maintain the chain of custody of all evidence. ED nurses must protect victims' privacy and rights. If possible, a forensic nurse should be among the team and should be notified as soon as the victim is identified.[20]

WHAT IS FORENSIC EVIDENCE?

Forensic evidence is obtained by scientific methods, such as ballistic analysis, blood testing, DNA testing, and photography, which can be used in a court of law. This evidence can help establish the guilt or innocence of a suspect. It can also be used to link crimes that may be related to one another. DNA evidence can link one offender to several different crimes or crime scenes. This linking of crimes helps the investigators to narrow the range of possible suspects and to establish patterns.[9] Locard theory states that when a person comes in contact with another person, there is an exchange of physical material. Material left behind includes DNA, fingerprints, footprints, hair, skin cells, blood, bodily fluids, pieces of clothing, and fibers. Trace evidence, no matter how small, is factual.[21] This evidence is sometimes not visible to the human eye. Close adherence to established principles of forensic collection and examination enhances the contribution to higher crime rate detection.[19]

Gloves should be worn at all times when collecting or handling potential evidence to prevent contamination. Also, frequent changing of gloves is also necessary to prevent cross-contamination.

Collection of Evidence

Collection of evidence begins with the patient's admission that a crime was committed. Triage nurses are often the first caregivers to come in contact with victims of violence; they have the important responsibility of recognizing it and notifying the team. The first priority for these victims is medical stability. In the case of an unstable patient, the nurses often overlook crucial forensic evidence that can be lost forever. This situation, unfortunately, is a fact of the emergency needs of the victim. Every effort should be made to prevent loss of evidence from happening.

Urine/Blood Collection

If drug-facilitated sexual assault (DFSA) is suspected, the urine and blood collection should be the first to be obtained. There is variation in the speed of drug metabolism, which is why time is so important in obtaining the specimens. Some drugs can be present only for few hours; others may be present for weeks. Blood specimens are indicators of early exposure to drugs. Urine can an indicator of drugs for up to a few days. Blood and urine need to be obtained and are usually packaged separately from the sexual assault kit. Negative test results do not mean the assault did not happen but rather that collection could have been done too late to detect drugs used.[22,23]

Clothing

Clothing is usually the next item the forensic examiner needs to package. The victim stands on a paper white sheet and undresses, placing each item of clothing separately on the sheet. The paper sheet is placed in the kit as evidence. Package each piece of clothing in paper bags separately; properly label, seal, and document the evidence. Fold garments only enough so that they fit into the container. If the victim has changed clothes, make sure the investigating officer is aware of what the victim was wearing at the time of the assault. This gives the officer a description of the clothing he or she needs to retrieve, which can save time and mistakes in retrieving the wrong items. If the victim has changed clothes, it is important to submit clothing that will provide evidence, such as underwear garments. If the clothing is wet, it must be dried, but if it is soaked in blood, it may need to be dried in the police evidence room. In such cases, note the need for drying in your documentation.[14]

Gunpowder residue (GSR) on clothing can help ballistic experts determine the firearm distance. GSR may be found on an entrance wound of a victim or on clothing of the person who fired the gun. GSR on a victim's hands can determine whether the individuals are victims, perpetrators or both.[24] GSR can be removed by washing, wiping, or performing other activity before a sample can be obtained.[25,26] Shoe prints or footprints can prove the victim was at the scene. For this reason, shoes should also be saved. If the crime was committed indoors, there is no need to place shoes in an evidence bag.

Typically, the trauma team cuts all clothes off with trauma shears and throws the clothes on the floor in a pile. Avoid cutting through damaged areas of the clothing. Clothes thrown on the floor can easily become contaminated. Avoid contamination by placing a clean hospital sheet on the floor before the trauma patient's arrival. Also, each article of clothing should be kept separated to prevent cross-contamination. If the patient can undress himself or herself, have the patient do so while standing on the sheet or paper sheet. The sheets from the emergency medical services (EMS) stretcher and/or hospital stretcher should be bagged to preserve trace evidence.

Place each piece of clothing in a separate clean paper bag; do not use plastic. Paper bags are air permeable and facilitate drying of contents. Plastic bags allow moisture condensation, resulting in degradation of evidence. The investigating officer may want to examine the articles before placing the bag. The paper bags should be sealed with tape. The nurse should date and initial over the tape, designating that the nurse sealed and labeled the bags. Label the bags with a brief, detailed description of the contents. Give all bags to the officer. If any item is still wet, inform the officer. It is the officer's duty to freeze, dry, or take these items to the crime laboratory immediately.[18,24]

Stains or Other Debris

Photograph and measure the stains. If a stain is dry, moisten a cotton-tipped swab using minimal distilled water, which should be drawn up by a syringe to prevent overwetting the swab. Avoid contaminating the swab; do not touch the tip of the swab to any other surface. Do not touch the tip of the water bottle to the swab. Touch the swab firmly and rotate the swab to ensure that the stain is collected. Do not smear the stain when swabbing it. Dry the swab in a drying box. Stains on deceased individuals should not be swabbed unless permission is obtained from the local medical examiner or coroner. If a drying box is not available, an inverted Styrofoam cup will work to hold the applicator while it dries, limiting cross-contamination. Allow the specimen to dry, place it in a box, then place it in an envelope and seal it with tape. The nurse should write the appearance and location of the stain on the envelope. Then the investigator should add the date and his or her initials to the outer envelope.[1,6,19]

Loose debris, such as hair, soil, leaves, or paint, can also be collected. Take a sheet of clean white paper and place the debris on it by using swab or rubber-tipped forceps. Refold the paper and place it in a clean envelope, then seal and label the specimens.

Semen as Evidence

Unlike blood stains, semen stains are not always obvious to the naked eye. Semen stains are difficult to see even under the best circumstances. They may appear as a slightly yellow stain on light-colored fabrics or a whitish color on dark-colored fabrics. Semen stains may also appear crusty if dried; therefore, it is best to collect any item that may have semen stains, such as the victim's clothing, especially the underwear of sexual assault victims, and the suspect's clothing. Document the location of the semen stain with photography.

A blacklight, also referred to as a UV-A light or Wood's lamp, is a lamp that emits long-wave ultraviolet light. A forensic light source is an alternative light source that may cause semen stains to fluoresce when viewed through an appropriate color filter. Optimal wavelength is dependent on surface characteristics of item. Certain surfaces appear to quench the fluorescent reaction. Argon ion laser (AIL) causes a similar reaction. The nurse and the patient must wear plastic ultraviolet eye protection when using the AIL. Some clothing could fluoresce what may appear to be stains but are really a result of certain detergents or food. A 2006 study of 36 items of clothing and linens proved to have a greater yield of DNA than semen.[27,28]

In 1986 DNA analysis was first used. It was discovered by Sir Alec Jeffreys, who realized that genetic codes could be used to identify individuals. In 1985 a 15-year-old schoolgirl was raped and murdered in Carlton, Hayes Hospital. In 1986 another 15-year-old was raped and murdered in a nearby town. The DNA matched from both cases and was linked to a suspect. He was convicted of both murders. The DNA database was developed because of this case.

When a stain is discovered, the nurse should describe the stain as red or white and never assume it is blood or semen until it is tested in the laboratory.[29]

Saliva

Make sure the investigating officers are aware of the perpetrator's behavior at the crime scene, such as drinking or smoking. Cigarette butts and used beverage cans or bottles are common types of saliva-containing evidence found at crime scenes. In cases of sexual assaults, consider swabbing the breast or other bodily areas to collect any potential saliva evidence. Use a dry or moistened swab, depending on the circumstance of the stain.

Projectiles

A projectile is any object (empty or not) thrown into space by the exertion of a force. Examples of projectiles include bullets, arrows, baseballs, and other projectiles sometimes found on a victim in the ED or removed from a victim during surgery. The projectile can contain trace evidence, such as blood, hair, fibers, tissue, or paint.

A bullet has specific markings that can link the bullet to the gun used in a crime. Metal projectiles should never be handled using metal forceps without rubber tips. Metal instruments can scratch the metal surface and alter the specific marking of the gun. If rubber-tipped forceps are not available, a gloved hand can be used. Each projectile should be wrapped in soft gauze and placed in a separate rubber container or box.[24,27] The medical team should never document exit or entrance bullet wounds. The belief that entrance wounds are always smaller than exit wounds is a generality, and even forensic pathologists can struggle to differentiate entrance from exit.

Needles and Knives

Sometimes EMS will transport victims with sharp objects because of the need to scoop and run with trauma victims. The trauma team must use care when handling sharp objects so as not to injure the forensic nurse or other ED staff while preserving the integrity of the trace evidence. Needles may contain toxic substances, and a knife blade may contain fingerprints. To prevent scratching, sharp objects should not be handled using metal forceps without rubber tips. Sharp objects should be carefully packaged in appropriate cardboard boxes or test tubes. Ensure that all sharps are secured in proper preventive packaging and that investigating officers are aware of the secured sharps.[27,30,31]

Strangulation

Strangulation often occurs in intimate partner violence (IPV). Strangulation survivors may appear stable but can have insidious injuries associated with high morbidity and mortality. Strangulation attempts can result in laryngotracheal, digestive, vascular, and neurologic injuries. Signs and symptoms of strangulation are loss of memory or consciousness, petechiae of eyes or face, drooling, swelling, chest pain, hoarse voice, scratches, abrasions, voice changes, tongue swelling, finger marks, difficulty swallowing, difficulty breathing, and ringing in the ears. All marks need to be measured, photographed, and documented. If a victim has suffered from a strangulation attempt, they must be medically evaluated before the forensic examination can be done. Survivors may require admission for observation after the examination.[32]

Sexual Assault Evidence Collection Kit

ED nurses should have familiarity with the sexual assault kit (Table 48.1) used in the state in which they practice. The kits contain all the supplies needed to collect and preserve evidence and a step-by-step set of instructions. DFSA kits are separate and also contain instructions. Paper bags for clothing collection are usually separate because of their size. The nurse should follow the steps in order and document the procedure.

TABLE 48.1 Contents of a Patient Evidence[1] Recovery Kit.

Item	Number
Evidence collection procedures	
Large white envelopes	5
White paper	10
Sterile cotton-tipped applicators	10
Sterile urine specimen cups	3
Sterile gauze (4 × 4 inches)	3
Large paper bags	5
Small paper bags	5
Glass slides	3
Various sizes of cardboard boxes	3
Transparent tape	1
Rubber-tipped forceps (clean)	1
Permanent marker	1
Digital camera	
Chain of custody forms	

CHAIN OF CUSTODY

Chain of custody must be maintained throughout the forensic investigation. Every person who handles the evidence must be identified with a notation about the date of contact with the evidence. This method ensures that the integrity of the evidence has been maintained from the time of collection through the laboratory analysis and during use in the courtroom.

Without a proper chain of custody, it is possible that the evidence may be inadmissible in the court. It is imperative that the examiner maintain direct control of the evidence during collection and throughout the transfer of custody. The forensic examiner must also document when he or she places the evidence in secured storage or when transfer of evidence custody to another individual occurs. During transfer of custody, the signature of the examiner, date and time of transfer, and the full name and signature of the person accepting custody must be placed on the kit. There should also be a separate checklist signed by both parties. The same documentation has to occur with each successive transfer of the evidence. The transfer of evidence list should have separate checkboxes for photographs, clothing, sexual assault evidence kit, a tampon and/or sanitary napkin, DFSA kit, and a miscellaneous checkbox. The patient, patient advocate, family members, or support personnel should not be involved in the chain of custody.[18] If a kit does not have a transfer of evidence form, most police departments have a form available to be completed by the examiner and the investigative officer.

BODY DIAGRAMS AND PHOTOGRAPHS

Body diagrams show a clear location and size of injuries (Fig. 48.1) and should be included along with photographs and nursing documentation. Injuries should be numbered and measured. Photographs should never replace body diagrams, because they may be lost or show poor quality.

When taking photographs, be considerate of the victim's comfort and privacy. Photographs are a valuable way of collecting impression evidence. Photographs can supplement the medical forensic history, evidence documentation, and physical findings.[33] Ideally, a colposcope is the camera used during an examination. Colposcopy can magnify an area over 30 times its size.[14] It is specialized piece of equipment with a camera used in examining and collecting evidence for victims of sexual assault. It can be costly and difficult to use. A digital

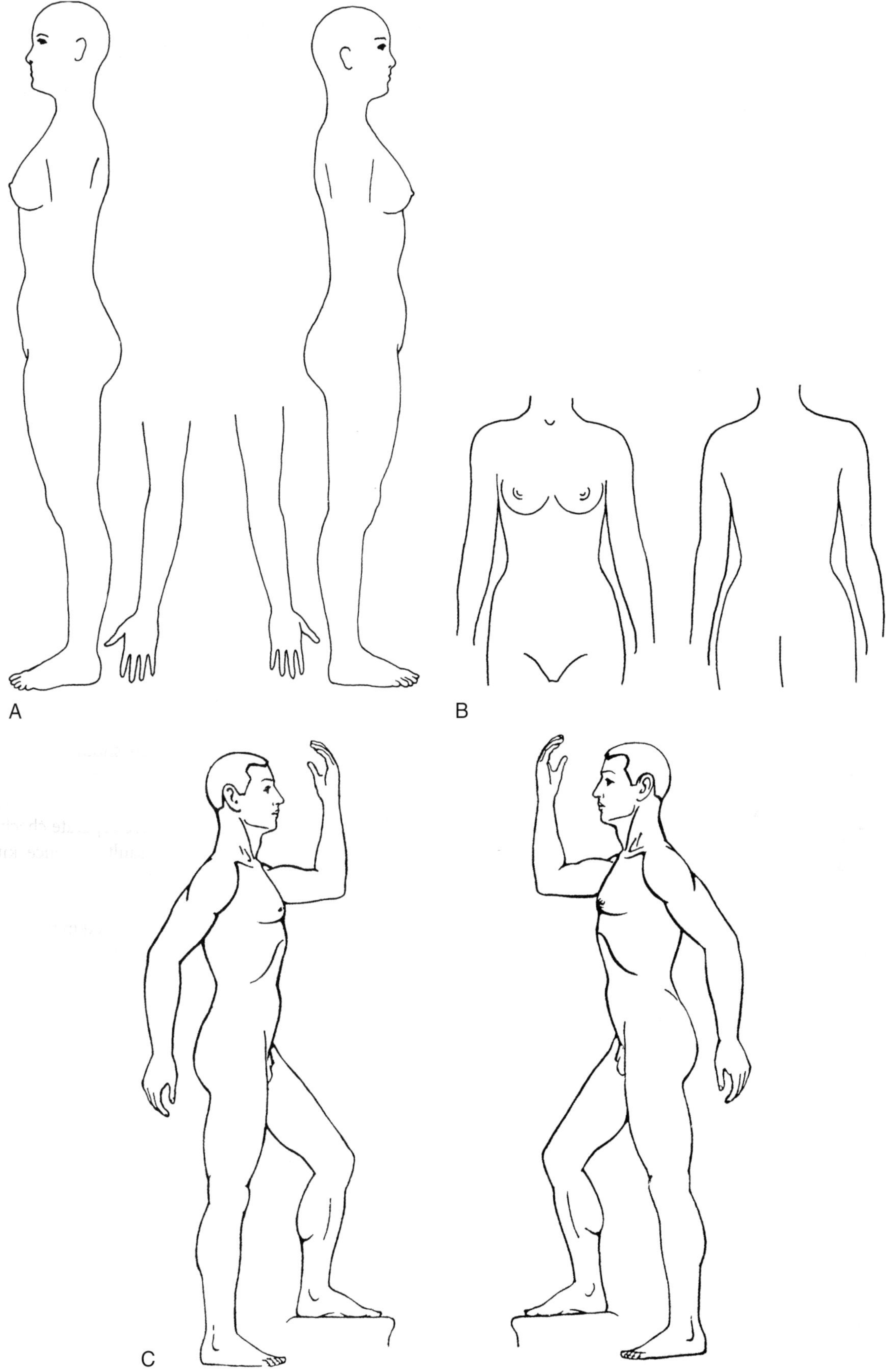

Fig. 48.1 Body Map. (A) Full body, female, lateral view. (B) Thoracic abdominal, female, anterior and posterior view. (C) Full body, male, lateral view. (D) Full body, male, anterior and posterior view. (E) Infant, ventral, dorsal, and left and right lateral view. (F) Head and face diagrams. (G) Submental view. (H) Head and skull, lateral view. (I) Head and skull, anterior and posterior view. (J) Top of head and skull. (K) Left and right hands. (L) Feet, left and right plantar surfaces. (From Lynch VA. *Forensic Nursing.* St Louis, MO: Mosby; 2006. Courtesy the Metropolitan Dade County Medical Examiner Department, Dade County, FL.)

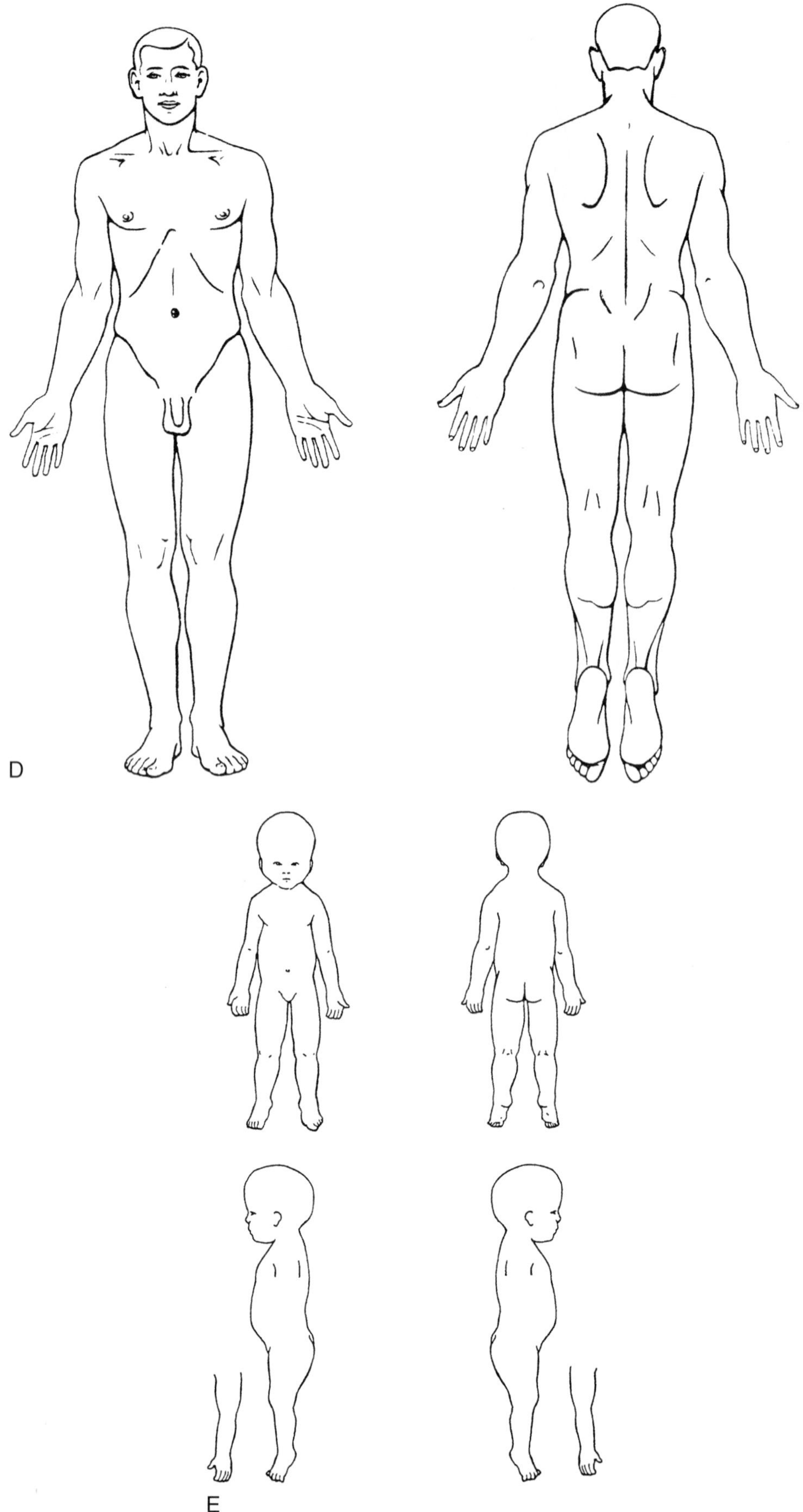

Fig. 48.1, Cont'd

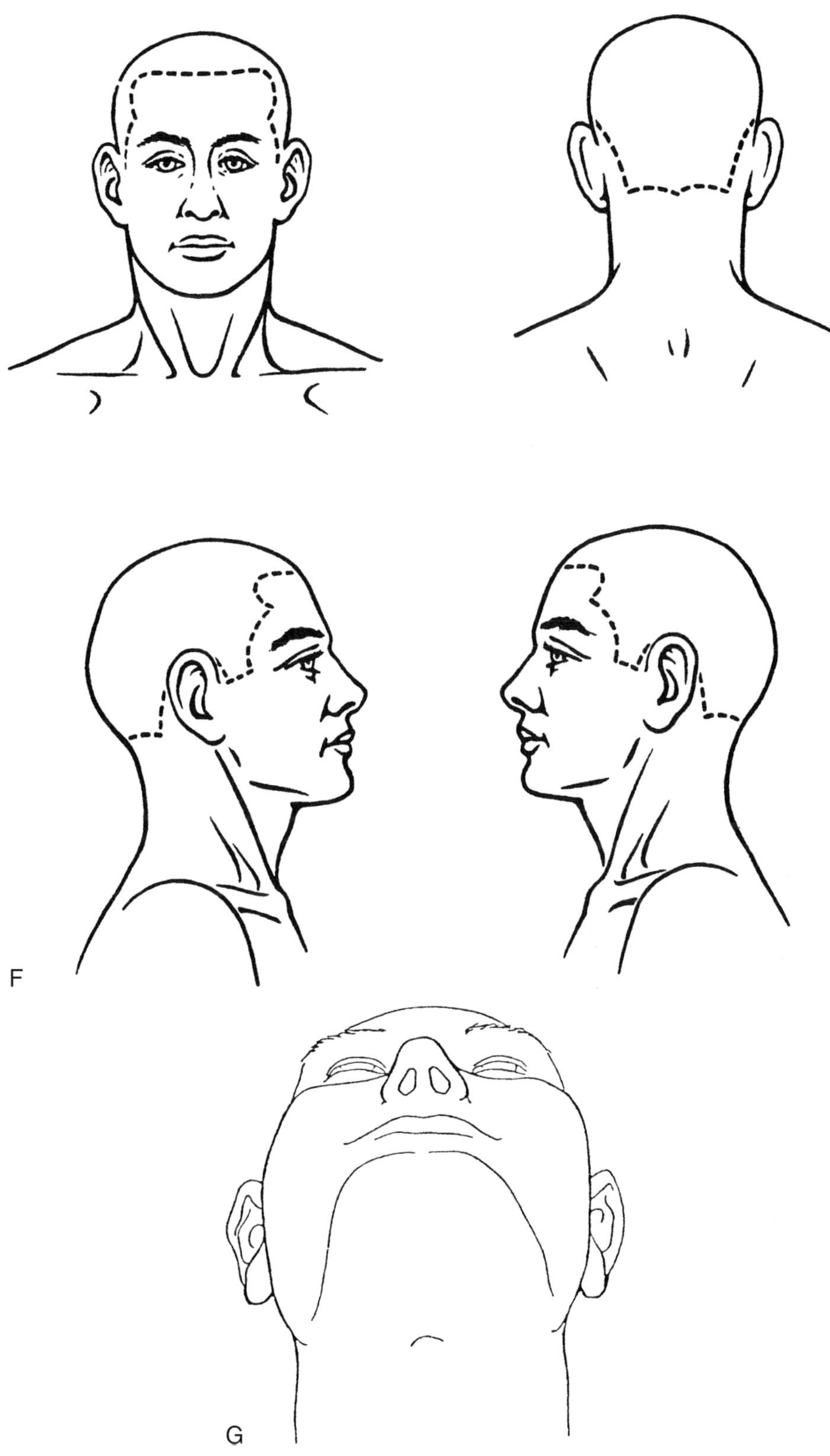

Fig. 48.1, Cont'd

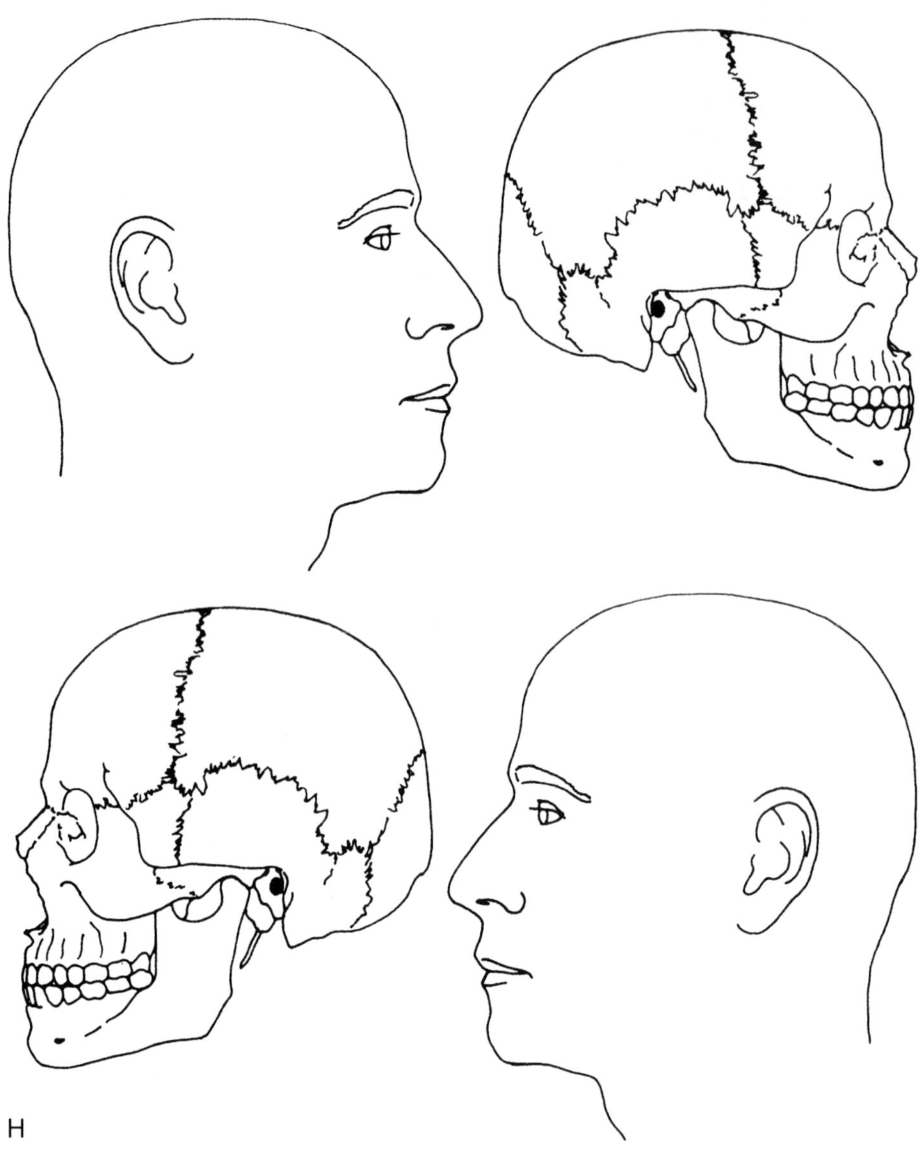

Fig. 48.1, Cont'd

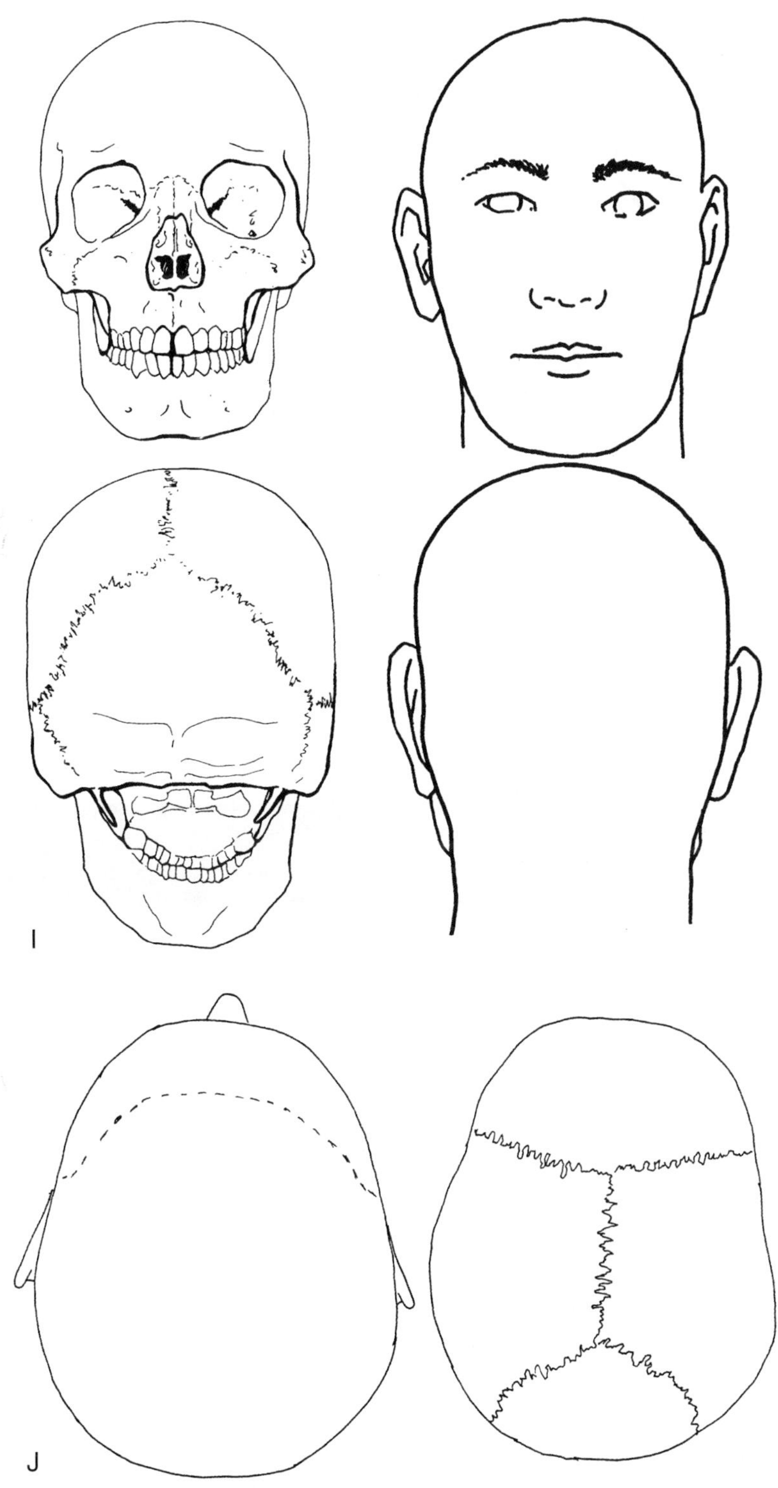

Fig. 48.1, Cont'd

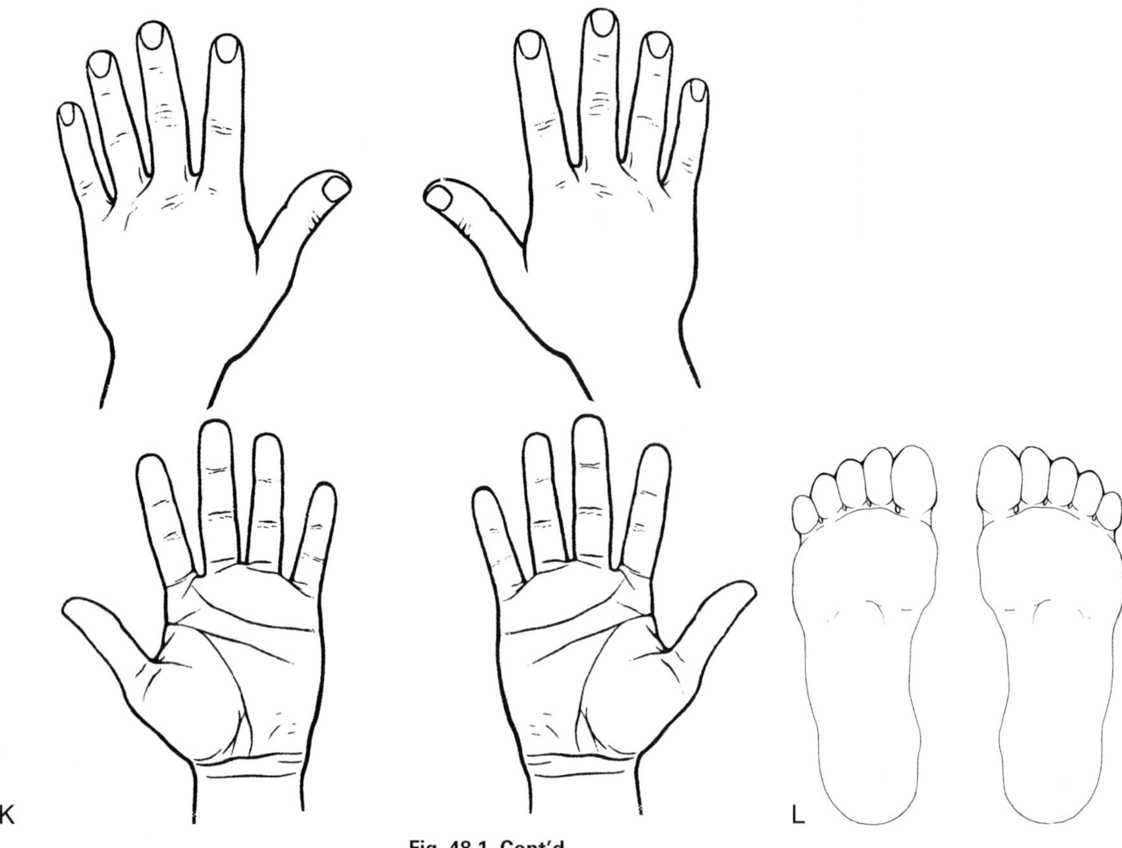

Fig. 48.1, Cont'd

camera is the most frequently used instrument for photographing. It is critical that photographic distortions are minimized. Documentation must include a photograph with and without a measurement scale. The scale should not be placed over or across the injury. A photograph of the identification bracelet should be the first photo taken during the examination and the last photo as well. The second photo should be a photograph of the victim, if permitted by the victim, from approximately 6 feet away. Close-up photographs of hands and fingernails could show trace evidence of blood, skin, or hair. Be sure to photograph any damage to nails or missing nails that occurred during the attack.[33]

Photographs should be labeled with patient's name, date, and case or medical record number. Photographic images must be stored securely on a computer, uploaded into an electronic medical record, or stored on a separate disk. The photographs should be deleted after the downloading to the medical record.

CORRECT MEDICAL TERMINOLOGY

It is imperative that all nurses use the correct terminology in their description of injuries. Abrasions can be partial- or full-thickness wounds that denude the surface of the skin. Avulsions are full-thickness wounds caused by tearing of the skin and soft tissue. A contusion (bruise) is a wound in which vessels or capillaries rupture, whereas a hematoma is bleeding under the skin causing a clot to form.[16] A senile purpura contusion is often confused with an inflicted contusion. A senile purpura contusion is one seen in the older adult population with fragile, thin skin, or it can occur with certain medications, such as steroids.[34]

Another frequent mistake is the identification of a laceration versus a cut. A laceration is an irregular and ragged wound that is caused by rupturing the skin due to compression. A cut is a cleaned-edged, well-approximated wound caused by a sharp-edged instrument such as a knife.[23,34] Blunt

BOX 48.1 Emergency Nurses Association Position Statement on Forensic Evidence Collection.

- ENA believes that it is the emergency nurse's role not only to provide physical and emotional care to patients but also to help preserve the evidence collected in the emergency department.
- ENA supports collaboration with emergency physicians, social service, and law enforcement personnel to develop guidelines for forensic evidence collection and documentation in the emergency care setting.
- ENA encourages emergency nurses to become familiar with the concepts and skills of evidence collection, photographic and written documentation, as well as testifying in legal proceedings.

ENA, Emergency Nurses Association.[21]

force trauma injuries result from impact with a dull, firm surface or object.[34] Bite injuries are ovoid patterns of bruising, abrasion, and/or lacerations. A canine tooth mark will be the most prominent or deepest part of the bite. If the distance is greater than 3 cm, it is usually an adult bite.[23] A patterned injury is one that has a pattern that reproduces characteristics of the object causing the injury. The pattern may be caused by impact of a weapon or another object on the body.[35]

The color of bruises cannot estimate the time of infliction. There is no true scientific evidence to support the determination of aging in contusion or abrasions.[34] Bruise color charts are available in some textbooks, but there is no evidence-based research supporting their use. The nurse should document what the victim states concerning the time and cause of the injury. Never get caught testifying on issues that are not evidence based.

SUMMARY

All EDs, large or small, rural, suburban, or urban, treat patients who have been victims of violence. Many victims arrive in the ED by private car and deserve the same care as patients in accredited trauma center with a SANE program. Although a growing number of formal nursing educational programs are preparing nurses to be forensic specialists, most of the forensic care of these patients will be provided by an ED nurse with basic training. The ED nurses need to know the policies and procedures for care of victims of violence and the preservation of forensic evidence. Lack of a specialized team is no excuse for further traumatizing of a victim of a violent crime.

REFERENCES

1. International Association of Forensic Nurses. *Overview*. International Association of Forensic Nurses website. https://www.forensicnurses.org/page/Overview. Accessed 4 June 2019.
2. National Association of EMTS, American College of Surgeons Committee on Trauma. Kinematics of Trauma. In: *Prehospital Trauma Life Support*. 7th ed. St Louis, MO: Mosby; 2011:44–85.
3. National Center for Health Statistics. *10 Leading Causes of Death by Age Group, United States—2016* (table). https://www.cdc.gov/injury/images/lc-charts/leading_causes_of_death_age_group_2016_1056w814h.gif. Accessed June 4, 2019.
4. New South Wales Government of Trauma and Injury Management. *Mechanism of Injury*. 2012. https://www.aci.health.nsw.gov.au/get-involved/institute-of-trauma-and-injury-management/clinical/trauma-guidelines. Accessed June 4, 2019.
5. Butchart A, Milton C. *Global Status Report on Violence Prevention*. Geneva, Switzerland: World Health Organization; 2014.
6. Cucu A, Daniel I, Paduraru D, Galan A. Forensic nursing emergency care. *Rom J Legal Med*. 2014;22(2):133–136. https://doi.org/10.4323/rjlm.2014.133.
7. Filmalter CJ. Heyns T, Ferreira R. Forensic patients in the emergency department: Who are they and how should we care for them?. *Int Emerg Nursing* 2018;40:33–36. Retrieved from https://www.researchgate.net/profile/Tanya_Heyns/publication/320436522_Forensic_patients_in_the_emergency_department_Who_are_they_and_how_should_we_care_for_them/links/5ac70c494585151e80a38ef1/Forensic-patients-in-the-emergency-department-Who-are-they-and-how-should-we-care-for-them.pdf. Accessed June 4, 2019.
8. Caleskan N, Ozden D. The knowledge levels of health personnel in Turkey regarding forensic evidence. *J Forensic Sci*. 2012;57(5):1217–1221.
9. Sekula LK. *What Is Forensic Nursing: A Practical Guide to Forensic Nursing*. Indianapolis, IN: Sigma Theta International; 2016.
10. Lynch VA. Forensic aspects of health care: new roles, new responsibilities. *J Psychol Nurs Ment Health Serv*. 1993;31(11):5–6.
11. Burgess AW, Holmstrom LL. Rape trauma syndrome. *Am J Psychiat*. 1974;136(11):1391–1506.
12. Lynch VA. Forensic nursing science. In: Hammer RM, Moynihan B, Pagliaro EM, eds. *Forensic Nursing*. Sudbury, MA: Jones and Bartlett Publishers; 2005.
13. Agency for Healthcare Research and Quality. *Emergency Severity Index (ESI): A Triage Tool for Emergency Department Care*. Version 4. 2012. https://www.ahrq.gov/sites/default/files/wysiwyg/professionals/systems/hospital/esi/esihandbk.pdf. Accessed June 4, 2019. AHRQ Publication No. 12-0014. Published November 2011.
14. Burgess AW. *Practical Aspects of Rape Investigation: A Multidisciplinary Approach*. 5th ed. New York, NY: CRC Press; 2019.
15. *History of Forensic Nursing*. The forensicnurse.com website. http//www.theforensicnurse.com/History.cfm. Accessed June 4, 2019.
16. Office of Justice Programs, Office for Victims of Crimes. Expanding forensic nursing practice. In: *SANE Program Development and Operation Guide*. https://www.ovcttac.gov/saneguide/expanding-forensic-nursing-practice/. Accessed June 4, 2019.
17. Blank-Reid C, Bokholdt ML. Special populations: the interpersonal violent trauma patient. In: *Emergency Nurses Association. Trauma Nursing Core Course*. 7th ed. Des Plaines, IL: Emergency Nurses Association; 2014:286–292.
18. Warrington D. *Crime Scene Documentation: Start to Finish*. https://www.forensicmag.com/article/2016/02/crime-scene-documentation-start-finish. Published February 2, 2016. Accessed June 4, 2019.
19. Ledray LE. *Documentation: What Should be Documented as Part of the SANE/SAFE Evidentiary Examination?* https://www.forensicmag.com/article/2016/02/crime-scene-documentation-start-finish. Accessed June 4, 2019.
20. Juszka K, Juszka K. A researcher's review of adherence to forensic examination principles in homicide cases in Poland. *Arch Med Sadowej Kryminol*. 2015;65(4):214–224.
21. Emergency Nurses Association. *Position Statement: Forensic Evidence Collection in the Emergency Care Setting*. https://www.ena.org/docs/default-source/resource-library/practice-resources/position-statements/forensic-evidence-collection-in-the-emergency-care-setting.pdf?sfvrsn=a1f89eba_4 Published 2018. Accessed June 4, 2019.
22. *Locard's Exchange Prrinciple*. https://www.forensichandbook.com/locards-evidence-principle. Published 2012. Accessed June 4, 2019.

23. LeBeau MA. *Drug Facilitated Sexual Assault and the Investigation and Prosecution of Cases.* Abington, PA: Presentation at: The Third Annual Southeastern Pennsylvania Forensic Nursing Conference; 2018.
24. Rape, Abuse & Incest National Network (RAINN). *Drug-Facilitated Sexual Assault.* RAINN website. https://www.forensichandbook.com/locards-exchange-principle/, Published Aug 12, 2012. Accessed June 4, 2019.
25. Brown K. *Practical Aspects of Rape Investigation: Multidisciplinary Approach.* 3rd ed. New York, NY: CRC Press; 2001.
26. *Examination of Gunshot Residue.* https://webpath.med.utah.edu/TUTORIAL/GUNS/GUNGSR.html(n.d.). Accessed June 4, 2019.
27. California Department of Justice: Bureau of Forensic Services. PEB 15 (Rev. 5/2014) *Physical Evidence Bulletin Gunshot Residue (GSR) Collection.* https://oag.ca.gov/sites/all/files/agweb/pdfs/cci/reference/peb_15.pdf. Accessed June 4, 2019.
28. National Forensic Science Technology Center. *Crime Scene Investigation: A Guide for Law Enforcement.* Largo, FL: National Forensic Science Technology Center; 2013. https://www.nist.gov/sites/default/files/documents/forensics/Crime-Scene-Investigation.pdf. Accessed June 4, 2019.
29. Magalhães T, Dinis-Oliveira RJ, Silva B, Corte-Real F, Nuno Vieira D. Biological evidence management for DNA analysis in cases of sexual assault. *ScientificWorld Journal.* 2015;2015:365674. https://doi.org/10.1155/2015/365674.
30. US Department of Justice Office on Violence Against Women. *A National Protocol for Sexual Assault Medical Forensic Examinations: Adults/Adolescents.* 2nd ed. US Department of Justice; 2013. https://cdn.ymaws.com/www.safeta.org/resource/resmgr/Protocol_documents/SAFE_PROTOCOL_2012-508.pdf. Accessed June 4, 2019.
31. California Department of Justice. *Firearms Evidence Collection Procedures.* www.crime-scene-investigator.net/CAfirearms.pdf. Published 1984. Accessed June 4, 2019.
32. Taliaferro E, Hawley D, McClane M, Stack G. Strangulation in intimate partner violence. In: Mitchell C, Anglin D, eds *Intimate Partner Violence: A Health-Based Perspective.* New York: Oxford University Press; 2009:217–325.
33. SAFEta.org. *Examination Process-Photography.* https://www.safeta.org/page/ExamProcessPhotogra. Accessed June 4, 2019.
34. Batalis NI. *Forensic Autopsy of Blunt Force Trauma.* Medscape website. https://emedicine.medscape.com/article/1680107-overview. Updated March 2, 2016. Accessed June 4, 2019.
35. Little D. Patterned injuries. *Pathology.* 2011;43(suppl 1):S24.

49

Abuse and Neglect

Angela Dillahunty

This chapter addresses some difficult topics that emergency nurses hope they will never have to see. However, these issues are all too prevalent in our society. As nurses, we are in an excellent position to screen, identify, treat, and provide referrals for these issues: child abuse, intimate partner violence (IPV), human trafficking, and elder abuse. But first, we must educate ourselves and others on these important health issues and have a high index of suspicion to be able to identify these victims. We must also be knowledgeable about local and state laws where we practice. And finally, we must approach these victims with empathy and in a nonjudgmental manner to be able to effectively advocate for their health and well-being.

CHILD ABUSE AND NEGLECT

Child abuse and neglect affects children of all ages, ethnicities, genders, and socioeconomic groups. Nationally, there were an estimated 4.1 million reports to child protective service agencies involving 7.4 million children in 2016. Professionals such as nurses, teachers, and law enforcement personnel submitted 64.9% of these reports. In this same year, approximately 1750 children died as a result of abuse and neglect—an increase of 7.4% over 2012 estimates. Younger children experience the highest rate of fatalities; children younger than 3 years of age account for almost three-quarters (70%) of children killed as a result of child maltreatment. Children younger than age 1 year died at a rate three times higher than children older than 1 year (20.63 per 100,000 vs. 6.5 per 100,000).[1] This figure may be conservative due to potential inaccurate determination of the manner and the cause of death.

Child abuse and neglect are a burden to society in many ways. A great deal of research has been done on the negative effect of adverse childhood experiences (ACEs; which includes various types of abuse and neglect) on individuals throughout their life span. Abused children are more likely to misuse alcohol, cigarettes, illicit drugs, and food, to become pregnant during their teenage years, have a sexually transmitted infection, experience depression, or have a suicide attempt during their lifetime. They are also more likely to be unemployed or have low incomes as adults. As they age, people who were abused during childhood have an increased risk for heart disease, asthma, stroke, and diabetes. The more ACEs a person has, the higher the likelihood of these lifelong effects.[2-6] See Fig. 49.1. One study found that women who had two or more adversities in childhood had an 80% increased risk of early death, whereas men had a 57% increased risk.[7] Tragically, abused children are also more likely to grow up to be abusive adults.[8]

There is also a significant financial burden. Each case of nonfatal child maltreatment is estimated to cost more than $200,000, whereas abuse resulting in the death of a child has an estimated impact of well over a million dollars. These costs include medical care, lost productivity, criminal justice costs, provision of special education, and the cost for investigation and services provided by child protective services. The annual cost is more than $124 billion.[9]

More often than not, abused children present to the emergency department (ED) without a declaration of abuse or neglect. This situation, along with a false presentation of the history surrounding the child's injury or illness, or a caregiver's intentional withholding of information, leads to difficulty in identifying child maltreatment. A detailed history and a thorough physical assessment are essential when identifying these small victims of maltreatment. The historical data and physical findings must be compared and evaluated to determine congruency. The interactions among the child, caregivers, and staff are also important to evaluate. Some behaviors potentially indicating a child is suffering from abuse or neglect are reviewed in Box 49.1, and Box 49.2 presents several risk factors for child maltreatment.

Neglect

The lack of visible bruises or broken bones belies the fact that ongoing child neglect is a silent, serious attack on children and results in lasting mental and physical problems. Currently, 74.8% of all abuse cases involve neglect, and 74.6% of the deaths in 2016 were attributed to neglect.[1] Neglect, defined as failure to provide for a child's basic physical, emotional, or educational needs or to protect a child from harm or potential harm,[10] may appear to the emergency nurse as a child who is unkempt, left unattended, not dressed appropriately for the weather, malnourished, or diagnosed with "failure to thrive." Identification of neglect must recognize parental attempts to provide essentials despite limited resources. Failure to provide adequate physical protection, nutrition, or health care is generally considered neglect, but neglect can also include lack of human contact and love. Recognizing neglect is often difficult because of limited, one-time contact with most ED

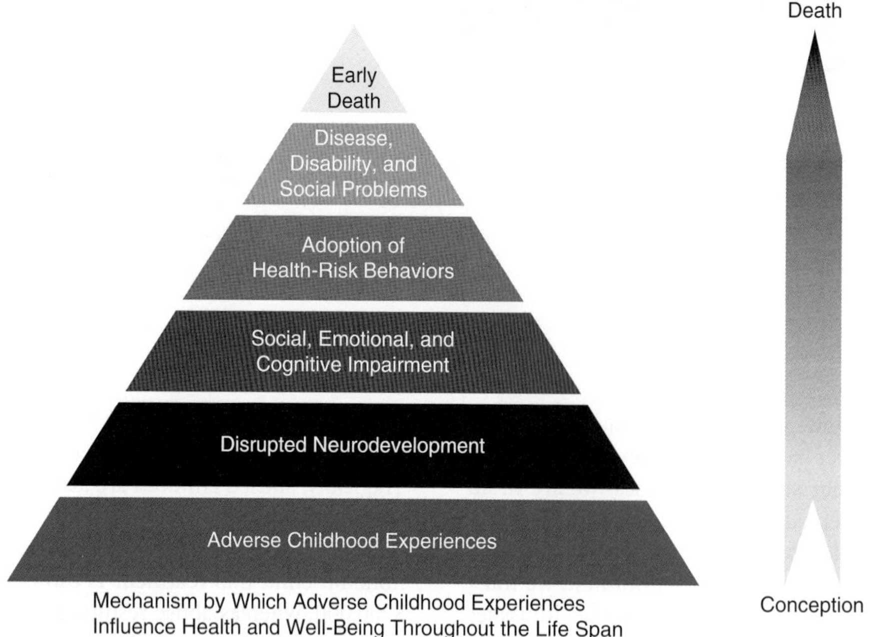

Fig. 49.1 The ACEs Pyramid represents the conceptual framework for the ACE Study. The ACE Study has uncovered how ACEs are strongly related to development of risk factors for disease and well-being throughout the life course. *ACEs*, adverse childhood experiences. (From Centers for Disease Control and Prevention. About the CDC-Kaiser ACE Study. Centers for Disease Control and Prevention website. https://www.cdc.gov/violenceprevention/acestudy/about.html. Accessed 7 June 2019.)

BOX 49.1 Indicators of Child Abuse or Neglect.

Child	Caregiver
• Extreme change in behavior (regressive, passive, or overly aggressive) • Flat affect • Does not cry during painful procedures • Appears malnourished, unkempt • Sudden drop in school performance • Sexual behavior toward adults or other children	• No explanation or a changing explanation for the child's injury • Explanation of injury does not match clinical findings • Delay in seeking health care • Uncooperative or hostile toward health care team • Inappropriate response to the seriousness of the child's condition

BOX 49.2 Risk Factors for Child Maltreatment.[9]

Child	Caregiver	Community
• Prematurity • Prenatal drug exposure • Product of unwanted pregnancy • Developmental or physical disability • Chronic illness • Difficulty with milestones (e.g., walking, toilet training)	• Childhood history of abuse • Acute or chronic stressors • Lack of parenting knowledge • Rigid or unrealistic expectations • Alcohol or substance abuse • Low self-esteem	• Social isolation • Domestic violence • Community violence • Unemployment • Homelessness • Frequent relocations

patients. However, the emergency nurse should be alert for behaviors suggestive of neglect (Box 49.3). Fig. 49.2 depicts a case of neglect.

Physical neglect accounts for the most child maltreatment in the United States. Physical neglect includes cases such as child abandonment, inadequate supervision, inadequate nutrition, and failure to adequately provide for the child's safety and physical and emotional needs. This type of neglect leads to failure to thrive, malnutrition, serious illness, physical harm from injuries due to lack of supervision, and a lifetime of low self-esteem.[11]

Medical neglect is the failure to provide appropriate health care for a child, such as providing immunizations, recommended surgery, or other interventions necessary for a serious health problem. In some cases, a parent may withhold traditional medical care because of religious beliefs. These cases generally do not fall under the definition of medical neglect; however, some states will intervene through the court system and force medical treatment for the child to save the child's life or prevent life-threatening injury. Medical neglect can lead to poor overall health and compounded medical issues.

Educational neglect occurs when a child is allowed to engage in chronic absenteeism or is of mandatory school age but not enrolled in school or receiving needed special educational training. This situation can have a negative effect on

BOX 49.3 Potential Indicators of Child Neglect.

Behavioral Findings	Physical Findings
• Begs or steals food • Falls asleep in school, is lethargic • Poor school attendance, frequent tardiness • Chronic hunger • Dull, apathetic appearance • Runs away from home • Reports no caregiver in the home • Assumes adult responsibilities	• Height and weight significantly below normal for age level • Inappropriate clothing for weather • Poor hygiene, including lice, body odor, scaly skin • Child abandoned and left with inadequate supervision • Untreated illness or injury • Lack of safe, warm, and sanitary shelter • Lack of necessary medical and dental care

From *For kids sake: a child abuse prevention and reporting kit,* rev ed, Oklahoma City, 1992, Oklahoma State Department of Health.

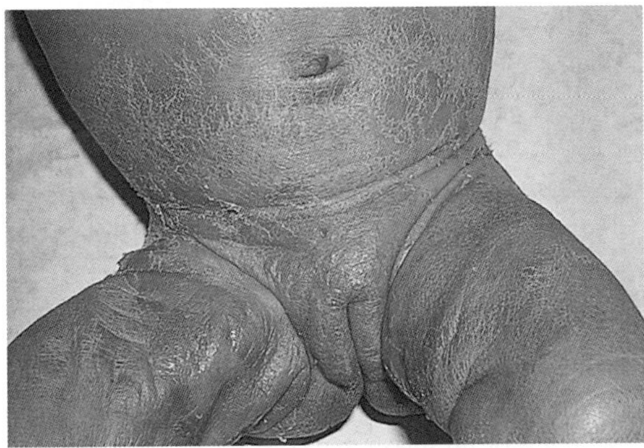

Fig. 49.2 Neglect An infant with severe failure to thrive has a badly neglected case of irritant diaper dermatitis. (From Zitelli BJ, Davis HW. *Atlas of Pediatric Physical Diagnosis.* 4th ed. St Louis, MO: Mosby; 2002.)

cognitive and intellectual development, language development, and academic achievement.[11]

Finally, emotional neglect is difficult to recognize and diagnose because of the lack of physical evidence. Emotional neglect is often typified by child behaviors such as depression, habit disorders (sucking, biting, rocking, enuresis), or conduct and learning disorders such as antisocial behaviors (e.g., cruelty). Emotional neglect includes actions such as chronic or extreme spousal abuse in the child's presence, failure to provide psychological care, and belittling and withholding of affection, all of which lead to poor self-image, alcohol or drug abuse, destructive behavior, and even suicide.[12]

Failure to Thrive

Failure to thrive is "an abnormal pattern of weight gain defined by the lack of sufficient usable nutrition and documented by inadequate weight gain over time. The decrease in the velocity of weight gain results in the child steadily falling off the expected weight curve on growth charts."[13] Although inadequate weight gain, or failure to maintain adequate weight, is the first sign of failure to thrive, continued lack of adequate nutrition results in lack of growth in head circumference and height and failure to meet developmental milestones. Failure to thrive may be organic, which is caused by a medical condition (e.g., *Giardia* organism infection, celiac disease, lead poisoning, malabsorption), or inorganic, caused by psychosocial issues.

Psychosocial causes are often linked to and reported as child neglect. Maladaptive parenting practices, chronic family illnesses, parental depression, and substance abuse among caregivers are recognized causes. Failure to thrive does not necessarily imply abuse or neglect but does require aggressive treatment and follow-up by appropriate health care professionals. If untreated, failure to thrive can lead to developmental and behavioral difficulties secondary to nutritional deprivation of the nervous system and other systems. A multidisciplinary approach in treating failure to thrive has the best opportunity for success. Family assessment, nutritional counseling, medical intervention, and family support are essential in improving patients with failure to thrive.

Assessment for Neglect

The medical evaluation for suspected neglect and failure to thrive should include a thorough history, physical examination, feeding observation, and a home visit by a health care provider. The history should review the child's family history, including genetic conditions, growth histories, endocrine disorders, caregivers' knowledge of normal growth and development, family functioning, eating patterns, types of food available in the home, and family stressors. The physical examination should include past and present growth parameters, including head circumference, using appropriate growth charts. Along with a general examination, a careful neurologic examination and observation of the child's developmental skills and interactive behaviors with parents is necessary. Diagnostic testing should be based on findings from the history and physical examination. Early intervention is vital to prevent negative cognitive and developmental outcomes.[13] Fig. 49.3 illustrates a case of failure to thrive.

Physical Abuse

Physical abuse is "the intentional use of physical force against a child that results in, or has the potential to result in, physical injury."[14] Of the four types of child maltreatment, physical abuse is second to neglect, accounting for approximately 18% of all abuse cases. In 2016, 122,067 children were confirmed victims of physical abuse in the United States.[1] Despite these statistics, physical abuse remains underreported for several reasons, including individual and community variations in what is considered abuse, inadequate knowledge among professionals in recognition of abusive injuries, and unwillingness to report suspected abuse. Perpetrators rarely admit to the abuse. Children may not be able to give a clear history of events due to young age, severe injuries, or fear of their abuser.[15] Child abuse is typically a pattern of behavior repeated over time, but it can also be a single attack.

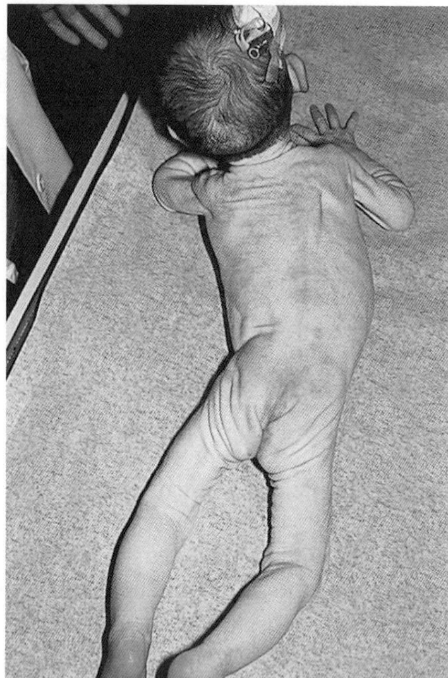

Fig. 49.3 Psychological Failure to Thrive as a Result of Neglect This 4½-month-old infant was brought to the emergency department because of congestion, where she was found to be below her birth weight and to be suffering from severe developmental delay. Note the marked loss of subcutaneous tissue manifested by the wrinkled skin folds over her buttocks, shoulders, and upper arms. (From Zitelli BJ, Davis HW. *Atlas of Pediatric Physical Diagnosis.* 4th ed. St Louis, MO: Mosby; 2002.)

The condition is characterized by injury, torture, maiming, or use of unreasonable force. Abuse may result from harsh discipline or severe punishment. Abused children may present to an ED with injuries ranging from minor to life-threatening. Box 49.4 identifies behavioral and physical indicators found in physical abuse.

Skin Injuries

In contrast to accidental injuries, inflicted injuries tend to occur on surfaces other than bony prominences. The head and the face are the most common areas where bruising is found on abused children. Any bruising on a nonmobile child is concerning for abuse, as are bruises to the ear, neck, or torso on children 4 years or younger. "TEN 4" is a mnemonic that can be helpful in remembering these concerning red flags; T = torso; E = ear; N = neck, 4 = in children ≤4 years or any bruise in an infant <4 months.[15] Location, size, and shape of bruises, lacerations, burns, or bites should be documented in the medical record and be accompanied by high-quality photographs. Measurement of skin injuries will help in determining the mechanism of injury and the object used to inflict the injury. Bite marks should be carefully measured and photographed if possible. Referral to professionals who can gather specific forensic information is ideal. Causes of burn injuries may be chemical, thermal, or electrical. The history and continuity of the burn pattern may indicate a greater probability of inflicted trauma. Unintentional scalds commonly involve hot liquids pulled or splashed onto the child's head, torso, and upper extremities. Inflicted injuries will be sharply demarcated with few or no splash marks.

BOX 49.4 Physical Abuse Findings.

Behavioral Findings	Physical Findings
• Requests or feels deserving of punishment • Afraid to go home, or requests to stay in school or daycare • Overly shy, tends to avoid physical contact with adults, especially parents • Displays behavioral extremes (withdrawal or aggressiveness) • Cries excessively or sits and stares • Reports injury by parent or caretaker • Gives unbelievable explanations for injuries • Clings to health care worker rather than parent	• Unexplained bruises or welts found most frequently, usually on face, torso, buttocks, back, or thighs; can reflect shape of object used (e.g., electrical cord, hand, belt buckle); may be in various stages of healing • Unexplained burns often on palms, soles of feet, buttocks, or back; can reflect pattern of cigarette burn, electrical appliance, or rope burn • Unexplained fractures or dislocations involving skull, ribs, and bones around joints; may include multiple fractures or spiral fractures • Other unexplained injuries such as lacerations, abrasions, human bite, or pinch marks; loss of hair or bald patches; retinal hemorrhages; abdominal injuries

Modified from *For kids sake: a child abuse prevention and reporting kit,* rev ed, Oklahoma City, 1992, Oklahoma State Department of Health.

Cranial Injuries

Head trauma is the leading cause of death for victims of child abuse and most often occurs in infants and very young children.[15] The peak incidence of abusive head trauma is found in children 1 to 2 months of age, which corresponds to the time infants spend the greatest amount of time crying as part of normal development.[16] Crying can trigger anger and frustration in some parents and caregivers, resulting in them shaking the infant or striking its head against an object, such as a wall, the floor, or furniture.[17] Abuse should be suspected in infants with a history of a minor head trauma, such as a short fall off a sofa, presenting with multiple, complex, or occipital skull fractures. Children with head injuries from inflicted trauma are more likely to have retinal hemorrhages and subdural hemorrhages than children with head injuries from accidental causes.[15]

Unfortunately, it is easy to overlook signs and symptoms of abusive head trauma. One landmark study estimated that more than one in three cases is missed.[18] Acceleration-deceleration of the head from shaking often creates a triad of injuries: subdural hemorrhage (Fig. 49.4), retinal hemorrhage (Fig. 49.5), and altered level of consciousness. There are often no external signs of trauma. Presenting symptoms can range

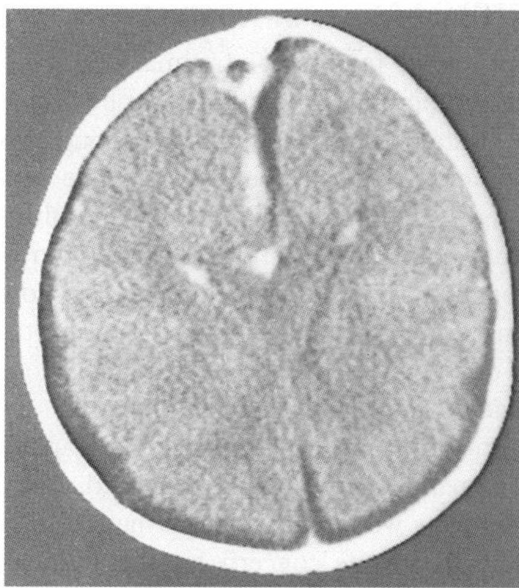

Fig. 49.4 Subdural Hematoma Secondary to Shaken Baby Syndrome (From Zitelli BJ, Davis HW. *Atlas of Pediatric Physical Diagnosis.* 4th ed. St Louis, MO: Mosby; 2002. Courtesy the Division of Neuroradiology, University Health Center of Pittsburgh.)

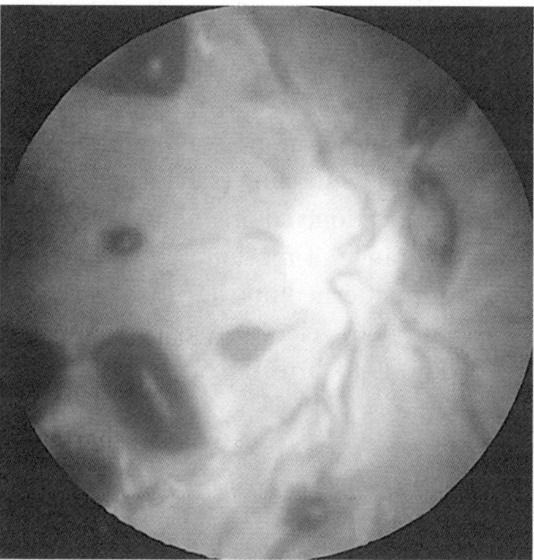

Fig. 49.5 Retinal Hemorrhages Secondary to Shaken Baby Syndrome (From Zitelli BJ, Davis HW. *Atlas of Pediatric Physical Diagnosis.* 4th ed. St Louis, MO: Mosby; 2002. Courtesy Dr. Stephen Ludwig, Children's Hospital of Philadelphia.)

from irritability, vomiting, and poor feeding to lethargy, seizures, and respiratory arrest, depending on the severity of the injury.[19] Therefore staff must have a high index of suspicion to identify patients who may have experienced this type of abuse. Even in the absence of neurologic symptoms, children younger than 2 years should have imaging studies, such as computed tomography (CT) or magnetic resonance imaging (MRI), performed when abuse is suspected.[5,20]

Skeletal Injuries

Skeletal fractures are common in childhood, leading to difficulty determining whether a fracture is unintentional or inflicted. However, accidental fractures, although common in older children, are uncommon in children <18 months of age. No single type of fracture is diagnostic for abuse, but fractures that are particularly concerning for abuse include multiple fractures in different stages of healing, old fractures that did not receive medical treatment, metaphyseal fractures, and rib fractures.[21] Rib fractures in infants can be caused by forceful squeezing of the chest. Posterior or lateral rib fractures or multiple rib fractures are especially predictive of abusive trauma.[21] Toddlers may sustain femur fractures from short falls, but these fractures are rare in nonambulatory children, as are humerus fractures. If a fracture is suspected, the skin should be carefully assessed for grab marks; however, the absence of bruising does not exclude an abusive mechanism of injury. A skeletal survey is recommended for any child younger than 2 years when abuse is suspected. Although rare, testing for medical conditions that may affect the ease and frequency of fractures should also be considered to prevent false accusations of abuse.[15]

Caregiver-Fabricated Illness

Caregiver-fabricated illness, also known as Munchausen syndrome by proxy, medical child abuse, or factitious disorder by proxy, is abuse occurring as a result of a caregiver faking or inducing injuries or illness in a child. This situation leads to unnecessary medical tests, procedures, and treatments. It is a rare form of child abuse, most often perpetrated by the child's mother. Presentation is dependent on the injuries or illness being fabricated. Apnea, anorexia, urinary tract infections, diarrhea, vomiting, or seizures are commonly reported.[22] The caregiver may invent nonexistent symptoms or may produce the symptoms via various means, such as smothering a child with a pillow to cause apnea or administering ipecac to induce vomiting. The parent often demands extensive medical evaluations and appears very concerned for the child. The child's history may also include the parents seeking health care at multiple locations and from multiple physicians. Often undetected by health care professionals, caregiver-fabricated illness can lead to emotional problems, chronic disabilities, and death.

Abuse Mimics

When abuse is suspected, physiologic or pathologic causes for physical findings should always be considered:

- Sudden infant death syndrome can appear as child abuse because of pooling of blood, mottling, and other discoloration associated with death. The definitive cause of death should be determined by a complete autopsy with appropriate ancillary studies, a review of clinical findings, and a scene investigation.
- Disorders such as erythema multiforme, Henoch-Schönlein purpura, leukemia, Wiskott-Aldrich syndrome, hemophilia, and idiopathic thrombocytopenic purpura can cause bruising or lesions resembling burns.
- Mongolian spots are benign, bluish-gray birthmarks found predominantly in African Americans, Hispanic Americans, Asians, Latinos, Native Americans, or anyone with dark pigmentation. Mongolian spots are usually located over the sacral area and buttocks but may also be located on the legs, shoulders, upper arms, and face.
- Multiple petechiae and purpuric lesions of the face can occur when vigorous crying, retching, or coughing

increases vena caval pressure. Unlike intentional choking, there are no marks around the neck.

- Bullous impetigo may appear as an infected wound or burn. This condition may reflect neglect if caregivers are apathetic about care of lesions.
- Glutaricaciduria type 1, a rare disorder of amino acid metabolism, can cause subdural hematomas and retinal hemorrhages after minimal trauma.
- Cultural or ethnic practices such as coining or cupping are used to treat pain, fever, or poor appetite. Coining—rubbing a coin over bony prominences—causes a striated "pseudoburn." Cupping (warming a cup, spoon, or shot glass in oil and then placing it on the neck, back, or ribs) can result in a petechial or purpuric rash over the affected area.
- Osteogenesis imperfecta, or "brittle bone disease," is an inherited disease characterized by abnormal collagen synthesis that can result in multiple fractures with minimal trauma and causes a tendency to bleed easily.

Obtaining a History

A detailed history should be obtained from the caregiver. If there is more than one caregiver present, it is ideal to interview them separately when possible. A history should also be obtained from a verbal child separate from family or caregivers. The history should include the sequence of events surrounding the injury, who was present, when was the last time the child was fine, onset of symptoms, and who witnessed the events. Further details such as additional symptoms, recent illness, and recent activities may also be helpful. Particular attention should be paid to determine whether the injuries are consistent with the history provided and the child's developmental abilities. Additional red flags for abuse include a delay in seeking medical care, denial of trauma in a child with obvious injury, inconsistent or changing explanations for injuries, or no history given for obvious significant injuries.[15] Make every effort to establish rapport, conveying genuine concern and understanding. A nonjudgmental approach is essential. Judgmental attitudes hinder communication and limit information. Any statements made by the patient or the caregiver regarding the injury should be documented accurately and be verbatim.

Changes in Family Dynamics

Allegations of child abuse sometimes arise during separation, divorce, and child custody proceedings. Perceptions exist that false allegations are made during divorce or custody proceedings in an attempt to place one parent in a "favored" position for child custody. Although false accusations are sometimes made, all allegations of abuse or neglect during divorce proceedings deserve serious consideration because of the increased risk for abuse during this time. A higher index of suspicion for abuse and neglect is required with divorcing families because families are experiencing increased stress as a result of the divorce process. Separation of parents increases the opportunity for sexual and physical victimization but can also provide an opportunity for a child to disclose that abuse has taken place if the abuser is out of the home.

Reporting Child Abuse or Neglect

When suspicion of intentional trauma, neglect, or sexual abuse is raised, appropriate agencies must be notified immediately. All 50 states have mandatory reporting laws for suspected abuse or neglect of a child. Each state defines child abuse and neglect differently; however, the ultimate goal, regardless of geographic location, is prevention of further injury through prompt intervention. State reporting laws grant immunity for good-faith reporting. In most states, liability exists only if the reporter knows the allegations are false or the individual acted with malicious purpose.

The health care team should inform the parents or caregivers when an inflicted injury is suspected. Avoid inflammatory statements when relaying information to caregivers; instead, relay the team's concern for the child and his or her safety. When child protective services and/or the police are contacted, simply state the team's legal responsibility to report suspicions. Health care providers must remember that investigation of child abuse allegations is the responsibility of police or the appropriate division of family services. Emergency nurses who suspect child abuse or neglect must report specific concerns and the reasons for those concerns.

Physical Examination

Identify and document all injuries, old and new, comparing historical information with clinical evidence. Measure, draw, and describe the location, color, induration, and scarring. Assess for limited range of motion, which may indicate old fractures. Look for patterned injuries such as cigarette burns, strap marks (Fig. 49.6), electrical cord marks (Fig. 49.7), imprint marks (Fig. 49.8), bruising on the buttocks (Fig. 49.9),

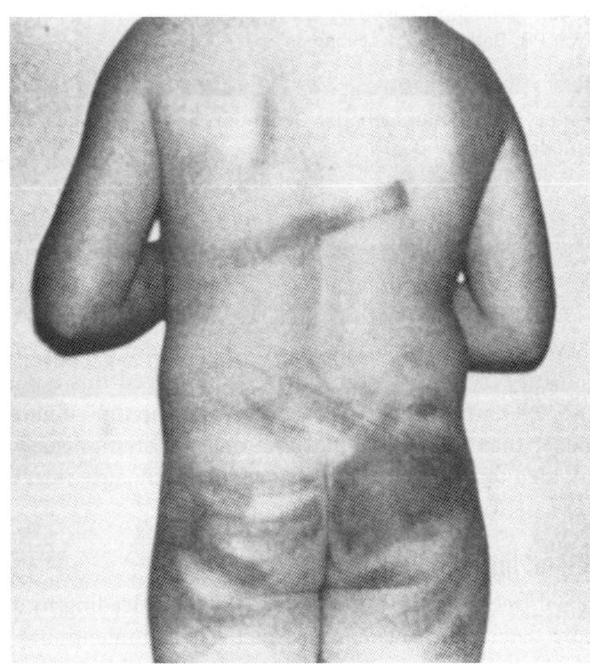

Fig. 49.6 Injuries From Strap Marks (From Rosen PR, Barkin RM, Hockberger RS, et al. *Emergency Medicine: Concepts and Clinical Practice.* 4th ed. St Louis, MO: Mosby; 1998. Courtesy J Brummitt, MD, Alberta Children's Hospital.)

or inflicted scald burns (Fig. 49.10). Measure height, weight, and head circumference and compare the measurements with those on standard growth charts. Assess the developmental level of function. An ocular and funduscopic examination is required to identify retinal hemorrhages; however, this is rarely available in an ED setting. Skeletal surveys are obtained on children younger than 2 years to rule out existing or healed fractures. Prothrombin time, partial thromboplastin time, factor XIII, fibrinogen level, platelet count, and bleeding time results are recommended to rule out an existing blood dyscrasia.

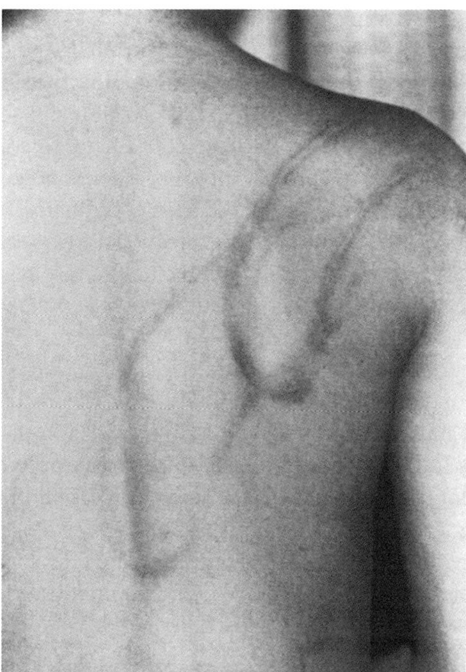

Fig. 49.7 Bruising Caused by Beating With a Looped Cord (From Rosen PR, Barkin RM, Hockberger RS, et al. *Emergency Medicine: Concepts and Clinical Practice.* 4th ed. St Louis, MO: Mosby; 1998. Courtesy J Brummitt, MD, Alberta Children's Hospital.)

Sexual Abuse

Child sexual abuse, involvement of children in sexual activities violating social taboos, is often done for gratification or profit of a significantly older person. Types of sexual abuse include, but are not limited to, fondling, digital manipulation, exhibitionism, pornography, and actual or attempted oral, vaginal, or anal intercourse. A national study found that 14% of girls and 6% of boys experienced sexual assault during childhood.[23] Unfortunately, the definition of child sexual abuse varies from state to state and there is no national reporting system, so determination of actual incidence and prevalence rates is difficult.

Many children do not disclose sexual abuse until they are adults. When children do disclose, they are often brought to an

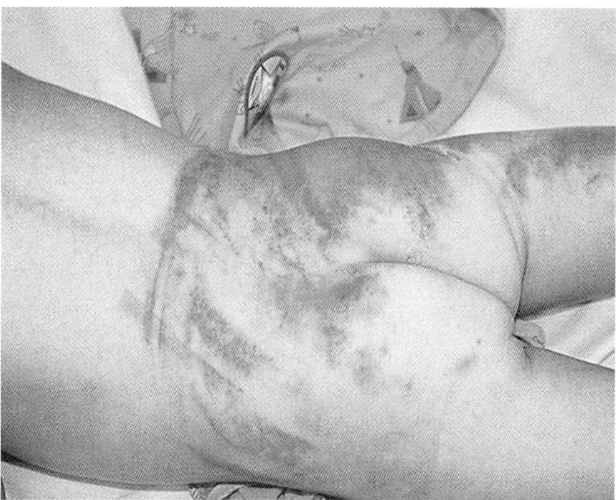

Fig. 49.9 Buttock Bruises The severe contusions of the buttocks and lower back seen in this child were inflicted by hand, hairbrush, and belt. (From Zitelli BJ, Davis HW. *Atlas of Pediatric Physical Diagnosis.* 4th ed. St Louis, MO: Mosby; 2002.)

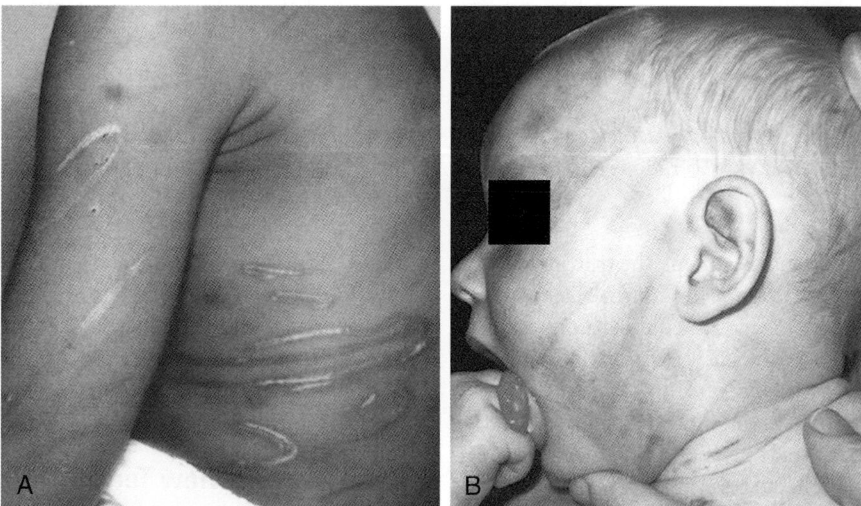

Fig. 49.8 Imprint Marks Reflecting the Weapons Used to Inflict Them (A) Hypopigmented and hyperpigmented scars that were the result of beatings with a looped electrical cord. (B) The characteristic pattern of parallel lines that results from blows with a belt. (From Zitelli BJ, Davis HW. *Atlas of Pediatric Physical Diagnosis.* 4th ed. St Louis, MO: Mosby; 2002.)

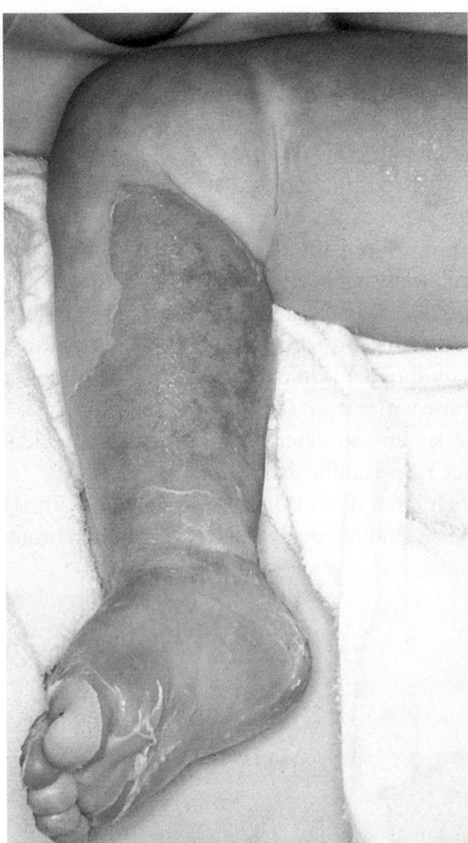

Fig. 49.10 Inflicted Scalds Close-up of severe second-degree burns of the foot and lower leg. (From Zitelli BJ, Davis HW. *Atlas of Pediatric Physical Diagnosis.* 4th ed. St Louis, MO: Mosby; 2002.)

ED for evaluation. Consequently, emergency care professionals must recognize sexual abuse, be skilled in examinations, and have medical and forensic awareness. Knowledge of normal and abnormal sexual behaviors, physical signs of sexual abuse, appropriate diagnostic tests for sexually transmitted infections, and medical conditions confused with sexual abuse is useful in the evaluation of such children. Screening and treatment protocols specifically addressing child sexual abuse are recommended for all EDs. Discussion of sexual abuse, along with recommendations for evaluation and treatment, will be discussed in depth in the chapters specifically dedicated to sexual assault (Chapter 51) and forensic considerations (Chapter 48).

Psychological Abuse

As with other forms of child maltreatment, the true incidence of psychological/emotional abuse is unknown. Definitions vary greatly from state to state, and it is difficult to precisely define what constitutes psychological abuse. That said, it may be the most prevalent type of child maltreatment.[24] Psychological abuse is defined as "intentional caregiver behavior that conveys to a child that he/she is worthless, flawed, unloved, unwanted, endangered, or valued on in meetings another's needs."[14] This type of abusive behavior may include blaming, terrorizing, isolating, confining, exploiting, ridiculing, or belittling a child. The abuse may be continual or may occur intermittently. Children who experience psychological abuse are more likely to have low self-esteem, poor academic performance, lower IQ, and difficulty maintaining friendships. They are also more likely to experience depression, attention-deficit/hyperactivity disorder, exhibit aggressive behaviors, and become suicidal.[12]

OTHER ISSUES RELATED TO CHILD ABUSE AND NEGLECT

Multidisciplinary Teams and Sexual Assault Nurse Examiners

Child abuse and neglect issues are complex and require the expertise of many professionals. Many hospitals and communities have adopted a multidisciplinary approach, using a core team with a health care provider (physician or nurse practitioner), a social worker, and a team coordinator. A consulting team may include a child psychiatrist, a developmental specialist, a psychologist, a public health coordinator, an adult psychiatrist, and an attorney. Professionals who can offer opinions on a case-by-case basis include family physicians, public health nurses, child protection workers, police officers, mental health therapists, guardians ad litem, foster parents, county attorneys, and teachers.

A cooperative approach can decrease the incidence of repeated abuse, serious injury, and child death and ensure that hospitals fulfill the legal mandate to report suspected abuse. Consistent use of trained experts increases case findings and reporting within the community while focusing treatment on the entire family. A team approach also provides expert collection of forensic evidence and court testimony and ensures continuing education across disciplines.

Testifying for Child Abuse and Neglect Cases

Health care providers are often the first professionals who become aware of child maltreatment; therefore the quality of documentation is critical to future prosecutorial decisions. The medical record and the health care professional who examined the child will almost certainly be involved if the case goes to court. Consequently, effective communication skills are essential for charting, obtaining history, handling parents, and interacting with investigators and attorneys. Testimony from medical personnel is often not considered hearsay, so they are allowed to testify as to what the child told them during a medical examination.

When health care providers receive a subpoena, the provider should contact the attorney who subpoenaed them. Find out what is expected from your testimony and discuss what you can and cannot say. If you are called as a material witness, there is an expectation to "tell what you observed." An "expert" witness is required to prepare and support expert knowledge with current scientific literature.

Child Death Review Teams

In 2016 there were 1700 child deaths due to child abuse or neglect, a rate of 2.36 per 100,000 children. Tragically, 70% of these children were younger than 3 years. Children vulnerable to serious or fatal abuse are those least visible to the community, educational programs, and protective services. Although many believe that perpetrators are those not related to the victim, approximately 78% of child fatalities occur at the hand of one or more parents. Neglect accounted for 74.6% of the deaths, with combinations of maltreatment, physical abuse, and medical neglect accounting for the rest.[1]

Child death review teams grew from an effort to determine how and why children were dying. According to the National Center for Fatality Review and Prevention,[25] the purpose of a child death review team is "to conduct a comprehensive, multidisciplinary review of child deaths, to better understand how and why children die, and to use the findings to take action that can prevent other deaths and improve the health and safety of children." In 1983 a tiny infant was beaten and eventually starved to death. A Los Angeles deputy sheriff mapped more than 52 contacts with 10 agencies. Investigations of drug abuse, domestic violence, reports of suspicious injuries, and drunken brawls were conducted; however, no agency knew the other was involved, and no one saw a need to remove the infant. After the discovery of multiagency involvement, a small group of professionals began to meet, share records, and make team decisions. Teams stood together, faced judges returning children to abusive settings, and started asking questions about siblings. Michael Durfee, a child psychiatrist, pressed for child death review teams across the country. There are now more than 1350 child death review teams across the country.[25]

The death of a child in an ED is usually unexpected and sudden. Health care providers should be sensitive to the family's needs while trying to obtain a history and conduct an examination to determine cause of death. After death has been pronounced, provide the family an opportunity to view and hold the child. Every ED should have written policies and procedures accompanied by checklists (Box 49.5) to follow in the event of a child's death. The medical examiner and the child's primary medical caregiver should be notified of the death. Autopsy requirements vary by state, but in general, autopsies should, at a minimum, be performed on suspicious, obscure, or otherwise unexplained deaths. Community resources should be offered for grief counseling. Hospital resources such as critical incident stress debriefings should be made available to all caregivers who have been emotionally stressed by a child's death.[26]

BOX 49.5 Checklist for Child Death in the Emergency Department.

- Obtain a complete history (medical, family, social)
- Describe the circumstances of death (especially when SIDS is suspected):
  - Position in which the child was put to sleep
  - Type of bed and bedding
  - Did child sleep alone or cosleep?
  - What and when child last ate
  - Position in which child was found and by whom
  - Clothing child was wearing
  - Temperature of room
- Core temperature upon arrival at ED
- Perform a complete physical examination (head to toe, including eyes, skin, and genitalia)
- Photograph any bruises or wounds if present
- Review prior medical records
- Skeletal survey
- Laboratory tests such as cultures, drug screen, and routine blood studies
- Grief support for family and ED staff
- Autopsy (documentation of circumstances and laboratory specimens should accompany body to morgue)

SIDS, Sudden infant death syndrome; *ED*, emergency department.

Prevention

Prevention of child abuse and neglect is extremely difficult. It is essential that health care providers be able to recognize children and families at risk for child maltreatment. Precursors to physical maltreatment include excessive parental physical discipline, failure to provide basic necessities such as food and a safe home, and unobtainable goals set by parents. Programs for prevention of child abuse and neglect typically focus on physical abuse, centering on the parent, parenting skills, and damaging practices. Pilot programs such as home visiting and increased public awareness have decreased physical abuse of children in some areas. Changing attitudes and modifying behaviors requires at least 6 to 12 months. To successfully reduce physical abuse and neglect within diverse populations, preventive services should begin before or shortly after birth of the first child—through support of effective child-rearing skills. Prevention efforts should tie the child's developmental level to parent enhancement education. Parents must observe and be able to model desired parental behaviors. Child safety can depend on the parent's ability to take advantage of social programs and obtain assistance as appropriate. All prevention programs must recognize and accept cultural differences.

Child abuse and neglect are complex, life-threatening situations. Medical professionals who work with children must speak out for abused children. No single agency or discipline can be solely responsible for protection of children. The community, law enforcement, child protection workers, mental health counselors, legislators, educators, health care providers, and the judicial system must work together to remove barriers to identification, treatment, and prevention of child abuse and neglect.

INTIMATE PARTNER VIOLENCE

Although recognizing, assessing, and intervening with victims of IPV in the ED can be challenging, the emergency nurse has the opportunity to affect the victim's outcome. According to the Centers for Disease Control and Prevention (CDC),[27] "intimate partner violence includes physical violence, sexual violence, stalking and psychological aggression (including coercive tactics) by a current or former intimate partner (i.e., spouse, boyfriend/girlfriend, dating partner, or ongoing sexual partner)." An intimate partner is defined as "a person with whom one has a close personal relationship that may be characterized by the partners' emotional connectedness, regular contact, ongoing physical contact and sexual behavior, identity as a couple, and familiarity and knowledge about each other's lives. The relationship may not involve all of these dimensions."[28]

Incidence

IPV occurs in adolescents and adults, in all social and cultural groups, among lesbian and gay, heterosexual, and transgendered couples, and in married and unmarried relationships. The most prevalent incidence of IPV is among women. The National Intimate Partner and Sexual Violence Survey found that 23% of women (1 in 4) and about 14% of men (1 in 7) experienced severe physical violence or had a weapon used against them in their lifetime.[29]

Although IPV affects people of all ages, it often begins in adolescence. More than half of female victims, and almost half of male victims, experienced IPV for the first time before age 25, with many being victims of IPV in adolescence or childhood.[30] Among high school students, 21% of girls and 10% of boys reported experiencing physical or sexual violence from a dating partner.[31] Although IPV may begin at an early age, it may continue to affect people throughout their life span. One study reported 1 in 10 women aged 70 or older experienced some form of abuse in the prior year.[32]

A higher incidence of lifetime risk for IPV exists for people of certain racial, ethnic, and socioeconomic groups, as well as some groups based on sexual orientation. The ethnic groups most at risk are multiracial women (58%), Native American/Alaskan Native women (48%), and black women (45%). Lifetime risk for white women is 37%, followed closely by Hispanic women at 34%. The lifetime risk of IPV for men follows a similar pattern, with multiracial men at highest risk (at 42%), followed closely by Native American/Alaskan Native men (41%) and black men (40%). White and Hispanic men have a 30% lifetime prevalence of IPV, respectively. Sexual orientation affects the lifetime prevalence for IPV, with bisexual women at highest risk (at 61%), followed by 44% of lesbian women and 35% of heterosexual women. Thirty-seven percent of bisexual men experience sexual or physical violence or stalking during their lifetime, whereas the lifetime prevalence is 26% for gay men and 29% for heterosexual men.[33] Pregnant women also note a higher incidence, with almost 1 in 6 experiencing IPV.[34] Common sites of physical abuse in pregnancy include the face, head, breasts, and abdomen. The economic impact of IPV is notable. When taking into account lost productivity across the lifetime of victims, IPV costs exceed $110 billon.[35]

Risk Factors

The group at the highest risk for IPV is young, unmarried women who experience an unplanned pregnancy.[36] In addition to the danger the mother encounters, there is significant threat of harm to the fetus. IPV during pregnancy results in an increased risk for stillbirth, preterm labor, fetal death, and poor intrauterine growth.[37]

Women who experienced abuse in childhood are more than twice as likely to experience IPV during their lifetime as those who were not abused as children. If a woman experienced both physical and sexual abuse in childhood, her risk for IPV is seven times higher.[38] Additional factors associated with an increased risk for IPV include but are not limited to

- prior history of IPV,
- young age (adolescence or young adulthood),
- low self-esteem,
- low academic achievement,
- alcohol and drug use, and
- having parents with less than a high school education.[36,39]

The following are relationship factors:

- hostile relationship or communication styles
- higher risk during a breakup of a relationship
- having friends who experience or perpetrate IPV[29]

Community and societal factors include the following:

- poverty and associated factors
- neighbors' lack of willingness to intervene when they witness IPV
- low social capital
- traditional gender norms (e.g., the belief that women should stay at home and not enter the workforce, that they should be submissive)[29]

Cycle of Violence

The central functions of IPV are intimidation and control. Control is accomplished by the perpetrator through physical, sexual, and emotional abuse, social isolation, and financial dependency. Even pets may be used to exert control over the victims. One study of women with pets who experienced IPV found more than 35% reported their pets being threatened, hurt, or killed by their abuser.[40]

The cycle of violence in an abusive relationship consists of three phases:

- *Tension-building phase:* This phase can last hours, days, or months. Tension builds. The victim typically feels as if he or she is walking on eggshells trying to please the abuser to avoid abuse. Verbal abuse and threats may occur during this phase.
- *Abusive incident:* Physical, emotional, and/or sexual violence occurs.
- *Honeymoon phase:* The abuser may express remorse or shame for his or her behavior, make promises that it will never happen again, purchase gifts for the victim, and be very affectionate. The goal is to convince the victim not to leave the relationship.[41] Eventually the honeymoon phase ends, and the cycle starts again.

Even more unfortunately, the cycle of violence can continue throughout generations. Children who witness violence in their household have an increased risk of becoming victims or perpetrators of IPV in adulthood.[29]

Effect on the Victim

In addition to causing serious injury or death, battering can have long-lasting physical, emotional, and psychological effects on the victim. As a result, the victim may exhibit depression, antisocial behavior, suicidal behavior in females, anxiety, miscarriage, low self-esteem, inability to trust men, and a fear of intimacy. Chronic stress from the abusive relationship has a negative effect on multiple body systems, including the cardiovascular and immune systems. This can result in chronic conditions such as asthma, fibromyalgia, cardiovascular disease, irritable bowel syndrome, and migraines, among others. Due to the social isolation batterers often impose, victims are isolated from social networks such as family or friends, have restricted access to services, and may experience strained relationships with health care providers and employers.

Women experiencing IPV are more likely to display negative health behaviors that present further health risks. Some noted behaviors are engaging in high-risk sexual behavior such as unprotected sex or multiple partners, using or abusing harmful substances such as alcohol or drugs, and engaging in unhealthy diet-related behaviors such as vomiting after eating or overeating.[27]

Effect on Children

Children who are exposed to violence in their environment have an increased risk for both physical and behavioral health problems. Children whose lives are touched by IPV may have resultant low self-esteem, depression, ineffective coping, higher levels of aggression, oppositional behavior, fear, anxiety, withdrawal, and poor peer and other social relationships. Also noted are lower cognitive functioning, poor school performance, lack of conflict resolution skills, and limited problem-solving skills. As they grow into adults, children who had ACEs such as being exposed to violence in their homes are at increased risk for a variety of health problems, including cardiovascular disease, stroke, and diabetes.[2-6]

Why Do Women Stay?

Understanding why a woman chooses to stay in a violent relationship is probably the most challenging aspect of providing care for the victims of IPV. It would seem obvious that the solution to the violence is to just "get out." But for the victim of IPV, this is often the solution that seems most out of reach or inconceivable. As awful as their world is, it is the world they know versus the unknown should they choose to leave. Women feel they are the "victim" and feel a loss of control over their lives. They often believe that if they just love their abuser enough and behave appropriately, things will change. Many have a negative self-concept, and they doubt they can manage on their own. These victims may be afraid they will be unable to financially support themselves or their children. They may have been prevented from working, and even if they were able to work, they may not have access to the money they earned. This may mean they have no way to pay for housing or other essentials outside the abusive relationship and, by leaving, they and their children may be left homeless.[42] There may also be cultural factors that shape what is considered acceptable and unacceptable behaviors.[43] Victims may be justifiably afraid of retaliation. The greatest risk for homicide often occurs when the victim has decided to leave or just after the victim has left. In the United States, more than half of the murders of women are related to IPV.[27] The emergency nurse repeatedly asks the questions and assists victims with knowing about available options until the victim is ready to take action.

Treatment of Batterers

Legal interventions, such as being arrested and/or prosecuted, are often the primary impetus for batterers to receive treatment. Treatment of batterers is focused on prevention and decreased recidivism. Interventions are tailored to a specific type of batterer based on psychological factors, risk assessment, or substance abuse history. The effectiveness of batterer treatment programs remains in question because of variable results.[44]

ROLE OF THE EMERGENCY NURSE

IPV is a serious problem associated with myriad health problems ranging from minor physical injury to death. Abused persons are more likely to present to an ED, may have multiple injuries, and are more likely to be hospitalized. One study found that 54% of abused women had used an ED within the previous year.[45] The ED nurse is in a unique position to screen for the abuse, assist the patient to access available community services such as shelters, counseling services, and law enforcement, and help the patient create a safety plan.

Screening

The Joint Commission (TJC) standards regarding victims of abuse recognize the importance of identifying, assessing, intervening, and initiating a referral for victims of abuse. The requirement to screen for abuse is integrated into routine care of all patients. In addition, TJC notes it is necessary to collect information and evidentiary materials for potential future actions as part of a legal process for victims of reported abuse or neglect.[46] A joint position statement from the Emergency Nurses Association (ENA) and the International Association of Forensic Nurses (IAFN) also supports routine screening for IPV.[47] The rationale for ED screening is due to use as the access point for all populations, particularly the underserved. The ED is generally a secure environment, and it affords the opportunity for greater anonymity in an environment where there is no ongoing health care relationship. The ED visit may be the only "window of opportunity" to assess and provide assistance to victims of IPV.

In addition to screening, the ENA recommends education for staff on identification of IPV and collaboration with other disciplines for improved reporting, protection, and prevention. Use of specialty staff, such as forensic nurse examiners or sexual assault nurse examiners, is also recommended.[47] For universal screening to be most effective, appropriate assessment, intervention, and referral practices must also be in place. Ideally, the patient should remain clothed at the time of screening. To introduce the topic, the health care provider may state, "Because violence is so common in many people's lives, I've begun to ask all my patients about it routinely."[46]

The Partner Violence Screen is a brief screening instrument designed for use in EDs or other urgent care settings. This screening tool includes the following questions:

1. Have you been kicked, hit, punched, or otherwise hurt by someone in the past year? If so, by whom?
2. Do you feel safe in your current relationship?
3. Is there a partner from a previous relationship who is making you feel unsafe now?[48]

The first question is nearly as sensitive and specific as the combination of the three questions. To facilitate a safe environment for disclosure, screening questions to assess for IPV should be asked in a private setting outside the presence of the family or friends accompanying the patient. Maintain a respectful and nonjudgmental tone.[48] In the busy ED setting, the first question may be asked during triage if privacy is possible. Positive answers on the initial screen itself can be explored after the patient is in the treatment area away from the partner. Escorting the patient to the bathroom for a urine sample provides an ideal opportunity to ask the patient about potential abuse.

Patient Presentation

The emergency nurse must have a high index of suspicion and be alert for physical and behavioral clues. The most common patient presentation injuries are head and neck injuries/fractures, contusions, sprains and strains, skull fractures, pregnancy complications, or open wounds of the head, neck, or trunk.[49,50] Injuries may appear inconsistent with the history provided regarding how the injury occurred, and old injuries may also be present. Patients who visit the ED as a result of IPV may also present with medical complaints such as abdominal pain, back pain, pelvic pain, urinary tract infections, headaches, anxiety, substance abuse, sexually transmitted infections, or symptoms of posttraumatic stress. Patient behaviors that may indicate possible abuse are concerns about confidentiality, comments regarding their carelessness or stupidity in getting hurt, fear of their partner leaving them in the ED, and appearing anxious to leave or to get their partner out of the room. Abusive partners present with the victims may stay very close during the assessment and interview of a patient or even respond to questions for their partner. The abuser may also be very aggressive and demanding toward staff.

Evidence Collection

Evidence helpful for prosecution may be collected, including sexual assault kits or photographs of injuries. Use of specially trained staff, such as forensic nurse examiners or sexual assault nurse examiners, if available, can increase prosecution of guilty individuals. Collaborate with law enforcement regarding evidence collection and maintaining the appropriate chain of custody. Consider testing for pregnancy or sexually transmitted infections, if appropriate.

Safety Planning and Referrals

When a patient responds positively to any of the screening questions, further assessment occurs to assess the incidence of violence and identify safety concerns. The emergency nurse assesses for the safety of the patient by asking questions such as:

- Has the physical violence increased in frequency or severity during the past 6 months?
- Has your partner ever used a weapon or threatened you with a weapon?
- Do you believe your partner is capable of killing you?
- Have you ever been beaten by your partner while you were pregnant?
- Is your partner violently and constantly jealous of you?[48]

A safety plan is a tool to help the patient prepare to leave if the situation escalates. In addition to providing information on available local resources, discussion should also include identification of a safe place to go, such as a shelter or the home of a family member or friend. It may also include establishing a code word to use to family or friends to alert them if the patient is in imminent danger, making copies of important papers, securing funds, and packing essential items to be ready for sudden departure.[51]

Initial crisis management begins immediately. Arrangements should be made to provide for advocacy services and follow-up appointments for primary care. It is ideal if a social worker or advocate can come to the ED to meet with the victim and assist in developing an initial action plan for securing the victim's safety. Information regarding available shelters and other community resources should be provided. The patient should be given resources such as websites or a phone number he or she can call 24 hours a day to get help[52] (National Domestic Violence Hotline: www.thehotline.org or 800-799-SAFE, pamphlets or cards with phone numbers), and information on local resources, such as a women's shelter. Be aware that patients may refuse cards or phone numbers because it may not be safe to bring home material mentioning IPV. If the patient will not take any material, give the number of the ED or the name of a local IPV organization to him or her to look up online.

Reassure the patient that he or she is not to blame for the battering. Many patients believe they have done something to incite the violence or are sure they can prevent further violence if they simply behave in the appropriate manner. This is a false assumption; the pattern of abuse will continue until an outside intervention stops it. Reinforce that even risk factors such as high-risk sexual activity do not make the victim responsible for the batterer's actions.

Documentation and Reporting

Documentation is a crucial step in the care of the victim of IPV. Documentation should include the responses to all screening and safety questions and incidents surrounding the injury or other physical complaints using the patient's own words in quotation marks. Include accurate descriptions of all injuries, using a body map to mark location and size, and support these with photographs. Documentation serves multiple purposes, including

- alerting other health care providers of ongoing domestic violence in a patient's life,
- serving as objective documentation that injuries not consistent with accidental origin have been observed,
- assisting those who monitor quality of care to determine the rate of screening that is occurring, and

- contributing data to hospital and clinic policy decisions so that scarce resources are allocated to the problems that patients are most typically presenting.

To summarize these key elements in caring for the victim of IPV, in 1992 the Massachusetts Medical Society developed the acronym RADAR:

- **R**outinely screen,
- **A**sk direct questions,
- **D**ocument your findings,
- **A**ssess patient safety, and
- **R**eview possible options with the victim and provide referrals.[46]

Forensic nurse examiners, already available in many EDs, are an excellent resource to assess and document injury related to IPV. Forensic nurse examiners routinely work with law enforcement, clinicians, advocacy agencies, and community services as part of a multidisciplinary team. They are well versed in principles of forensic evidence collection, photo-documentation, and legal testimony.

Emergency nurses must be familiar with the mandatory reporting laws of their state. Most states require that health care providers report when they treat patients who have been shot, stabbed, or injured. Some states have laws that specifically address IPV. The Family Violence Prevention Fund[53] provides a listing and evaluation of mandatory reporting laws for all states, which can be found online.

IPV Summary

As emergency nurses, we may feel great frustration in caring for victims of IPV, especially when victims choose to remain in a violent relationship or place themselves at risk. Although the process is often slow, many women do leave their abusive partners. Our role is not to judge, but rather to provide appropriate treatment, assess patients' current situations for safety risks, and convey to victims the awareness of options and resources to make a change should they so choose. We can be an essential part of a process supporting patient autonomy, offering hope, and empowering the patient to eventually take action to stop the cycle of violence.

HUMAN TRAFFICKING

Human trafficking generally falls into one of two broad categories: sex trafficking, which is defined as an activity "in which a commercial sex act is induced by force, fraud, or coercion, or in which the person induced to perform such act has not attained 18 years of age,"[54] and labor trafficking, defined as "the recruitment, harboring, transportation, provision, or obtaining of a person for labor or services through the use of force, fraud, or coercion for the purpose of subjection to involuntary servitude, peonage, debt bondage, or slavery."[54]

Sex trafficking includes inducing a person to participate in prostitution, marriage, or pornography through force, fraud, or coercion. Labor trafficking includes forced work in industries such as construction, food services, salon services, manufacturing, agriculture, and domestic work. A small percentage of persons are trafficked for organ procurement. Regardless of the type of human trafficking, the goal for the trafficker is economic benefit. Selling humans is highly lucrative, generating an estimated $150 billion yearly. Approximately $99 billion results from sex trafficking; $51 billion is generated by labor trafficking.[55] Having surpassed illicit arms trade in annual profit, sex trafficking is now second only to drug trafficking.

Prevalence

Trafficking, a form of slavery, is a worldwide problem. In 2016 there was estimated to be more than 40 million people on any given day who were victims. In 2011 of those persons who were identified as being trafficked globally, 40% were forced to labor, 53% were sex trafficked, 0.3% had organ removal, and 7% experienced other forms of trafficking, such as forcing children into armed combat. Women accounted for more than 70% of those affected.[56] Seventy-four percent of children involved in trafficking in the United States are trafficked for sex.[57] The vast majority of those trafficked for sexual exploitation are women, whereas a smaller percentage are men or transgender individuals. Two-thirds of those trafficked for forced labor are male.[58] During 2016 various federal law enforcement agencies in the United States investigated more than 3800 cases of human trafficking.[59] The United States, Mexico, and the Philippines have been identified as the top three countries of origin for human trafficking.[59] The United States is also a preferred destination country for traffickers, due to the high prices obtained for both labor and sex. One victim of sex trafficking can bring in as much as $750 per day for the trafficker.[58] If a person sells drugs, once they sell the drugs, they must spend some of their profit to obtain more product to sell. If a person is sold for sex, the trafficker still has the person to sell repeatedly without any additional outlay of funds.

Trafficking Versus Smuggling

Trafficking is different than smuggling. Smuggling is defined as "the importation of people in to the United States involving deliberate evasion of immigration laws. This offense includes bringing illegal aliens into the United States as well as the unlawful transportation and harboring of aliens already in the United States."[60] Smuggling involves transportation of a person and is done with the consent of the person being smuggled. The relationship between the person being smuggled with their smuggler typically ends once the destination is reached. Smuggling, however, can become trafficking if force, fraud, or coercion are used. Trafficking involves exploitation of a person and does not necessarily involve moving the person from one location to another. Domestic trafficking, which does not involve crossing country borders, is less complicated and has a lower risk of identification because there is no interaction with security checkpoints. Any transportation of the victim can be done by private vehicle on public roadways, which is easily accomplished by a single individual. Sizable operations involving large numbers of victims or transporting victims across borders is likely to involve well-organized criminal groups.[58]

Recruitment

Persons trafficked for labor may be promised high wages and a better life for work they expect to do. In some cases, they pay exorbitant fees to the person who recruited them and arranged work and/or transportation and a place to live. They are then forced to give up their wages to their trafficker to pay off their debt. At other times, they are simply not paid the wages they were promised, and instead are forced to work long hours for little or no pay. When women are trafficked for labor, they are often also sexually abused.[56]

Persons trafficked for sex may have been seeking marriage or a loving relationship, only to be forced to prostitute themselves or participate in pornography. The Internet facilitates trafficking persons for sex, particularly children and adolescents. Someone with nefarious plans may target children on the Internet, befriend them, then over time coerce and manipulate them into sharing pictures of themselves in underwear or naked. Once the first pictures are obtained, the bad actor will further coerce the child into sending more and more explicit photographs and videos by telling them the images will be shared with the child's friends and family if they do not cooperate. Traffickers may, for profit, live-stream the child performing sex acts, or they may coerce the child into meeting them, at which time the child is further victimized. The "pimp" trafficker may have one girl or may have a larger operation with multiple victims.

Traffickers may be men or women. Although most perpetrators are men, 30% of convicted traffickers globally have been women.[58] Couples may work together to recruit persons for trafficking, and families may even traffic other family members. Traffickers are good at gaining the trust of their victims and may appear as upstanding community citizens. Victims are controlled through physical violence, psychological abuse, fear, shame, and lies. Their legal papers, such as passports, may be taken from them. The victim may not speak the language of the country they are in and may be mistrustful of authorities, further isolating them. In many cases, victims are forced to use drugs as an additional measure to facilitate ease of controlling them.[61] They also may use drugs in an attempt to escape the psychological effect of the trafficking. Unfortunately, drug use by the victim makes it less likely they will be believed if they tell someone what is happening to them. Populations particularly at risk for trafficking in the United States include workers from other countries who are in the United States on temporary visas, migrant workers, undocumented persons, and persons with limited English proficiency. Children who are runaways or are homeless are also highly vulnerable. They may be forced to participate in sex for pay for food or housing just to survive. Additional at-risk populations include those with disabilities; individuals who are lesbian, gay, transgender, questioning (or queer), or intersex (LGBTQI); Alaska natives; and American Indians.[59]

Identification

ED staff are in a prime position to identify victims of human trafficking. Research has shown that more than 87% of victims came into contact with the health care system while they were being trafficked, with most of that contact being through an ED.[62] Human trafficking victims present with a wide range of symptoms. More than two-thirds of adult victims and more than half of child victims reported having a sexually transmitted infection.[62,63] More than 80% of adults and 70% of children used drugs or alcohol during the time they were trafficked.[62,63] Most experience some type of physical or sexual violence or assault. They frequently have exacerbation of untreated conditions, poor nutrition, gastrointestinal problems, and tooth loss. The psychological effect is also devastating, with more than 96% of adult victims reporting at least one mental health symptom, such as depression, anxiety, stress, bipolar disorder, guilt, shame, flashbacks, nightmares, and suicide attempts.[62] Women who are trafficked report being sold for sex an average of 13 times per day, with some reporting much larger numbers.[62] Not surprisingly, reproductive health concerns, such as pregnancy, miscarriage, and abortion, are frequently experienced by these women. Some women are forced to have abortions because their profit value may decrease while they are pregnant. Refer to Table 49.1 for additional information on potential health consequences of abuses associated with trafficking.[64]

It is important for the ED nurse to look for red flags related to the interaction of a patient with the person accompanying them to the ED. For instance, if a person insists on answering questions for the patient, refuses to leave the patient's side, or has possession of all of the documents related to the patient's identity, these behaviors should raise suspicion. A thorough history and a physical examination are also vital to identify victims of trafficking. Due to threats, fear, shame, guilt, and/or language barriers, victims rarely spontaneously report their plight.[65]

Obtaining a History

When speaking with the patient, maintain a nonjudgmental, culturally sensitive approach. Obtain a comprehensive history of events surrounding the illness or injury in a private area, maintaining confidentiality. Document the history from the patient by using direct quotes. Building trust is vital. If the patient does not speak English, use a professional interpreter. If the person accompanying the patient to the ED is the trafficker or is someone who works with the trafficker and is used as an interpreter, the patient is denied the opportunity to disclose their situation. Conflicting stories, histories that do not match the injuries, a reluctance to speak or make decisions without the consent of another person, and lack of knowledge of their location are red flags.[66]

Physical Examination

Assess for signs of abuse, such as untreated wounds or fractures. Body maps should be used to document size, color, and location of any injuries. Assess for signs of sexually transmitted infections, urinary tract infections, or injuries from sexual assault or forced abortions. Victims of labor trafficking may exhibit visual or hearing problems, respiratory complications, or skin issues from unsafe work environments. Victims may also contract diseases, such as

TABLE 49.1 **Physical, Sexual, and Psychological Abuse and Substance Misuse and Potential Health Consequences Associated With Human Trafficking.**[a]

Forms of Abuse and Risk	Potential Health Consequences[†]
Physical Abuse	
Physical deprivation (i.e., sleep, food, light, and basic necessities)	Fatigue, exhaustion
Physical restraint or confinement	Poor nutrition, malnutrition, starvation
Withholding medical or other essential care	Disability, physical and emotional
Physical assault	Injuries, acute and chronic
Murder	Death
Sexual Abuse	
Rape	Sexually transmitted infections
Forced prostitution	Urinary tract infections
Forced unprotected sex	Changes in menstrual cycle
Forced TOP, unsafe TOP	Acute or chronic pain during sex
Sexual humiliation	Vaginal injuries
Coerced misuse of oral contraceptives or other contraceptive methods	Unwanted pregnancy Complications from unsafe TOP Irritable bowel syndrome, stress syndromes
Psychological Abuse	
Intimidation	Depression, anxiety, and aggression
Lies, deception, blackmail	Suicidal thoughts, self-harm, suicide
Emotional manipulation	Memory loss, dissociation
Unsafe, unpredictable, uncontrollable events and environment	Somatic complaints
Isolation and forced dependency	Immunosuppression
	Loss of trust in others or self, problems with or changes in identity and self-esteem, guilt, shame, difficulty with intimate relationships
Substance Misuse	
Forced and coerced use of drugs and alcohol	Substance addiction and dependence
	Drug or alcohol overdose
	Direct health effects and complications of alcohol and drug use
Social Restrictions and Marginalization	
Restrictions on movement, time, and activities	Depression and anxiety
Frequent relocation	Deterioration of health and existing health problems associated with lack of treatment or delayed treatment
Denial of or control over access to health and other services	Alienation from available health services
Cultural and social exclusion	Increased physical and psychological dependence on abusers or exploitative employers
Limited access to public services, legal assistance, and health care	Adopting unhealthy coping strategies
Public discrimination and stigmatization	
Reduced income, weak negotiating power	
Economic Exploitation	
Indentured servitude	Inability to afford basic necessities and health care
Usurious charges for travel documents, housing, food, clothing, condoms, health care, other basic necessities	Potentially dangerous self-medication or forgoing of medication
Control over and confiscation of earnings	Heightened vulnerability to sexually transmitted infections, other infections, and work-related injuries

Continued

TABLE 49.1 Physical, Sexual, and Psychological Abuse and Substance Misuse and Potential Health Consequences Associated With Human Trafficking.[a]—cont'd

Forms of Abuse and Risk	Potential Health Consequences[†]
Turning victims over to authorities to prevent them from collecting wages	Physical or economic retribution for not earning enough, withholding earnings, or escape attempts
Forced or coerced acceptance of long hours, large numbers of clients, and sexual risks to meet financial demands	
Legal Insecurity	
Confiscation of travel documents, passports, tickets, and other vital documents	Exposure to dangerous conditions, dependency on traffickers and employers
Threats to expose to authorities	Poor access to medical services for acute, chronic, and preventive care
Concealment of legal status	Fear of authorities
Poor Working and Living Conditions	
Abusive work hours and practices	Injuries
Dangerous work and living conditions	Vulnerability to infection, parasites, and communicable diseases
Abusive interpersonal relationships, lack of personal safety	Exhaustion, dehydration, poor nutrition, and starvation
Nonconsensual marketing or sale, exploitation	

TOP, Termination of pregnancy.

[a]Adapted from Zimmerman C. *Trafficking in Women. The Health of Women in Post-Trafficking Services in Europe Who Were Trafficked Into Prostitution or Sexually Abused as Domestic Laborers* [PhD thesis]. University of London; 2007. https://www.annemergmed.com/article/S0196-0644(16)30054-3/fulltext

[b]Many of the forms of abuse overlap, as do their consequences. In particular, negative mental health consequences frequently result from each of the different forms of abuse. To avoid repetition, these will be highlighted primarily under "psychological abuse."

tuberculosis or hepatitis, from living in overcrowded or unsanitary conditions. Many trafficked victims abuse drugs and/or alcohol, and they may have panic attacks or exhibit hypervigilance, posttraumatic stress disorder (PTSD), or anxiety.[67] Some victims have brands or tattoos such as bar codes showing they are merchandise, the name or initials of their "owner," or various currency symbols, which may indicate their asking price.[68]

Organ Removal

Although the percentage of persons trafficked for organ removal is small, the ED nurse may encounter a patient who was the donor or recipient of an illegally harvested organ. Those who are organ donors are recruited, transported, or harbored through the use of "threat of use of force, coercion, abduction, fraud, deception, abuse of power or a position of vulnerability, or giving or receiving payments or benefits to achieve the consent of a person in control of the victim for the purpose of exploitation, including the removal of organs."[69] The World Health Organization guidelines, as well as protocols from a variety of other worldwide organizations, require that organs be donated without monetary or other rewards and prohibit their use as a commodity for monetary gain. The demand for organs for transplant far outpaces the supply, creating a lucrative market. In 2011 trade in organs was estimated to result in profits of as much as $1.2 billion annually.[69] Victims who are generally poor and uneducated may be promised large sums of money, typically for a kidney, only to receive nothing or much less than promised. They are often not informed of the full risks of the procedure and may even be told lies such as "it will grow back." They often receive little postoperative care. Organ donors are predominately from very poor countries, whereas recipients are most often from more wealthy countries, such as North America, Europe, and the Near East.[69] Persons in need of a kidney transplant may travel abroad for a transplant not knowing the details of how their organ was procured, or they may feel it is mutually beneficial to pay someone who is living in abject poverty for a kidney.

Persons who have supplied or received a trafficked organ may appear unannounced at an ED with a recently removed or transplanted organ without having received proper medical care or medication. They may lack adequate medical records regarding the procedure and may be reluctant to discuss the details. They may have infections or other complications, such as hepatitis, human immunodeficiency virus (HIV), sepsis, abscesses, or graft failure.[70] Recipients are not considered traffickers, and recipients and donors alike should receive appropriate medical care.

Reporting

All 50 states and US territories mandate reporting suspected child abuse, which includes trafficking children for labor or sex. Laws on reporting abuse of adults aged 18 years and older vary from state to state. If there is no legal obligation to report trafficking of an adult patient, discuss the risk and benefit of reporting with the patient. Support the decision regarding reporting to authorities.

Assist the patient with developing a safety plan and provide information on local and national resources available to assist and support the patient. A multidisciplinary approach is beneficial for the patient (Fig. 49.11). Involving mental health professionals, social service providers, advocates, addiction specialists, and community-based specialists for assistance with food, housing, and legal services can help patients access the tools they need to successfully leave once they make that decision.[71] National resources are important because victims may be moved from one area to another. The National Human Trafficking Resource Center[57] is a hotline and resource center available anywhere in the country 24/7 in more than 200 languages. Staff are available for live chat at www.humantraffickinghotline.org, by phone at 1-888-373-7888, or by texting HELP or INFO to 233733 (BeFree).

Human Trafficking Summary

Human trafficking is an underrecognized problem resulting in a multitude of adverse effects. ED nurses are in a unique position to identify and assist victims. Although emergency nurses routinely screen for intrapersonal violence, research has shown that few ED nurses have education on recognition of human trafficking, and screening for this patient population does not typically occur. The same study found that, although victims of violence were viewed sympathetically as "fragile," those they saw as prostitutes were viewed as "tough" and "having chosen their lifestyle" No nurses in the study expressed concern that the patient may have been forced into the lifestyle.[72] Education on human trafficking is an important step to improve recognition and rescue of victims.[73] Use of specialty staff, such as forensic nurses, can increase detection of trafficking victims.[74]

ELDER ABUSE AND NEGLECT

Elder abuse and neglect is an area sorely lacking in research. According to the National Center on Elder Abuse, research in this area is at least two decades behind that of child abuse and domestic violence.[75] Meanwhile, abuse and neglect have increased steadily as the number of older adults requiring dependent care has increased. Elder persons who experience abuse visit EDs twice as often as those who have not.[76] Sometimes the only time elders may leave their home is to obtain medical treatment for injury or illness. Because nurses spend more time with ED patients and their families than physicians do, this places ED nurses in a unique position to identify red flags for abuse and neglect.[77] The emergency nurse cultivates a sensitivity and heightened consciousness of the scope of this problem and its risk factors and approaches the suspicion of elder abuse in the same manner as suspected child abuse is addressed.

Defining Elder Abuse and Neglect

Historically, varying definitions of elder abuse and neglect, as well as varying definitions of "elderly," have contributed to the difficulty that exists with determining the prevalence of elder abuse and neglect. The CDC defines elder abuse as "an intentional act, or failure to act, by a caregiver or another person in a relationship involving an expectation of trust that causes or creates a risk of harm to an older adult (an older adult is someone age 60 or older)."[78] Elder abuse and neglect includes not only physical abuse and neglect but also may encompass sexual abuse, psychological abuse, or financial exploitation. Many elders will experience more than one type of abuse.[75]

Scope of the Problem

The US Census Bureau estimates that by 2030 there will be more than 73 million people who are age 65 or older. This equates to 20% of the population. In comparison, 2012 statistics indicate that only 14% of the population was age 65 or older.[79] The life span of the average American is increasing, whereas the US birth rate has declined. More people require care, but fewer people are available to provide care. Consequently, the literature suggests that the number of older adult abuse incidents will continue to increase.

Elder abuse occurs among men and women of all racial, ethnic, and socioeconomic groups. However, obtaining a clear, accurate picture of demographics is difficult. Significant shame and embarrassment are associated with this problem, so abused individuals may keep the problem hidden within the family. One recent study found that 1 in 10, or approximately 4.4 million persons, aged 70 or older experienced some form of physical, sexual, or psychological abuse in the previous year.[32] Other study findings confirm commonly held theories that officially reported cases of abuse are only the "tip of a much larger iceberg."

For instance, the National Elder Mistreatment Study determined that 5.2% of adults age 60 or older experienced financial abuse, but a follow-up study revealed that an alarming 87.5% of the incidents that occurred were not reported when it was perpetrated by family, friends, or acquaintances.[80] Self-neglect is the most common type of abuse reported to Adult Protective Services (APS); however, neglect may also be perpetrated by caregivers.[81] Even residents of nursing homes and residential care centers are not immune to abuse and neglect. Psychological/verbal abuse is the most commonly reported type of abuse in these facilities, followed by physical abuse.[82] Sexual abuse is also reported in both nursing homes and residential settings and is thought to be the most underreported type of abuse.[83] Perpetrators may be employees or other residents.

Most research suggests the risk of abuse decreases with age. Persons younger than age 70 are more likely to experience abuse than those older than age 70. Physical or cognitive impairment and depending on someone else for help with activities of daily living increases the risk of abuse, as does lack of social support and low income.[32] Elder persons who

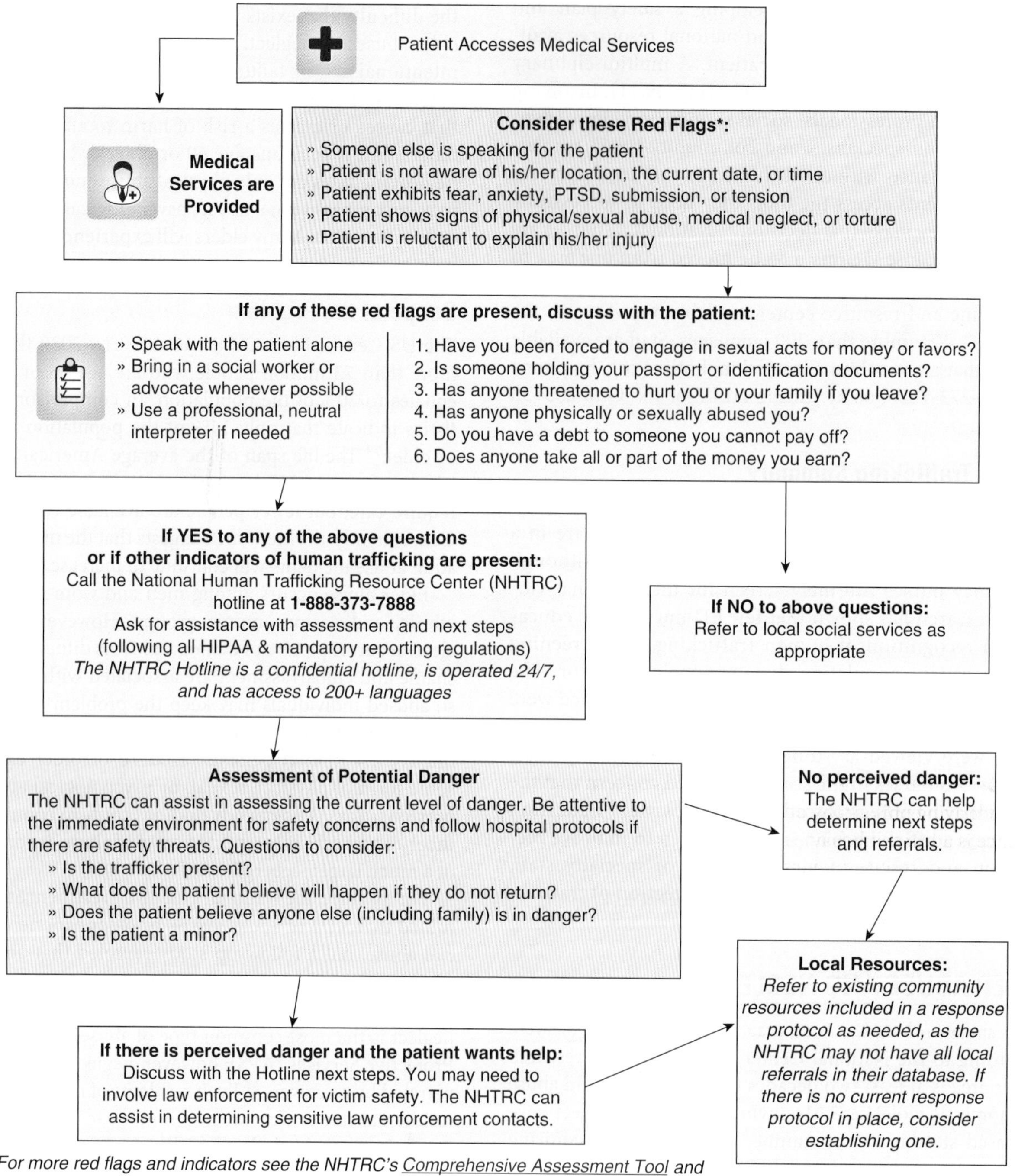

Fig. 49.11 Framework for a Human Trafficking Protocol in Health Care Settings *HIPAA,* Health Insurance Portability and Accountability Act of 1996; *PTSD,* posttraumatic stress disorder (From National Human Trafficking Resource Center. Framework for a human trafficking protocol in health care settings. Polaris, 2010. https://humantraffickinghotline.org/resources/framework-human-trafficking-protocol-healthcare-settings. Updated February 2016. Accessed June 7, 2019.)

experience abuse or neglect have a higher risk of premature death their nonabused counterparts.[84] They are also more likely to experience depression, anxiety, suicidal ideation, and generalized poor health.[85]

Abusers may be men or women of any age, but most commonly, perpetrators range in age from 30 to 59 years. Women are more likely to be perpetrators of verbal abuse and some physical violence, whereas men are more likely to subject victims to more severe physical assaults. Drug and alcohol abuse by perpetrators are common findings. Although abusers may be related in a variety of ways or be unrelated caregivers, in approximately 25% of cases, the perpetrator is the spouse of the victim. Adult sons are also often the culprit.[86]

Origin of the Problem

Four main theories may explain elder abuse: role theory, transgenerational theory, psychopathology theory, and stressed-caregiver theory.

Role Theory

As the parent ages and becomes more childlike, the child must assume a parental role. The elder who once helped the child must now take orders from that child. The psychological effect of this role reversal is significant for both generations. When role conflicts are present, the potential for abuse increases substantially. Many family caregivers find themselves "sandwiched" between providing care for their own children while providing care for their older parent(s) or spouse's parent(s), a situation creating additional stress and role conflicts.

Transgenerational Theory

The underlying philosophy of transgenerational theory is that violence is a learned behavior. If a child grows up in a family in which aggressive behavior is a part of life, the child exhibits similar behavior. If the parent abused the child, then the child, as the caregiver, abuses the parent in retribution.

Psychopathology Theory

Altered impulse control caused by psychological problems such as mental illness or drug or alcohol dependence places the elder at greater risk for abuse.

Stressed-Caregiver Theory

This is one area in which the nurse providing long-term care for older adults can abuse their charge as easily as the family caregiver can. Caregivers under stress have limited amounts of internal resources. Stress associated with the health care environment and stress in the individual's personal and family life may lead the caregiver to express stress through maltreatment of older adults.

Primary Categories of Elder Maltreatment

Physical abuse is "the intentional use of physical force that results in acute or chronic illness, bodily injury, physical pain, functional impairment, distress, or death."[78] Injuries result from slapping, shoving, hitting, beating, pushing, kicking, incorrect positioning, pinching, burning, biting, overmedicating or undermedicating, or improper use of restraints. Signs of physical abuse include bruises or grip marks around the arms or neck, lacerations, fractures, and rope marks or welts on the wrists and/or ankles.

Sexual abuse is "forced and/or unwanted sexual interaction (touching and nontouching acts) of any kind with an older adult."[78] This may include unwanted or forced contact of the genitalia with a finger, penis, or other object either under or on top of the clothing or contact between the mouth and penis. It may also include forcing an elder person to watch pornography, sexually explicit photography of an elder person, voyeurism, or sexual harassment. Signs include unexplained genital or anal bleeding or bruising, bruised breasts, or sexually transmitted infections. A sexually abused elder person may also exhibit sudden personality changes, such as depression, withdrawal, anxiety, or fear of certain people or places.

Neglect is "failure by a caregiver or other responsible person to protect an elder from harm, or the failure to meet needs for essential medical care, nutrition, hydration, hygiene, clothing, basic activities of daily living, or shelter, which results in a serious risk of compromised health and safety."[78] Signs of neglect include dehydration, malnutrition, decubitus ulcers, and poor personal hygiene.

Self-neglect encompasses behaviors of an older adult that threaten his or her own health or safety. Victims are usually depressed, confused, or extremely frail. Excluded are situations in which a mentally competent older adult makes a conscious and voluntary decision to engage in acts threatening his or her health or safety.

Psychological or emotional abuse is "verbal or nonverbal behavior that results in the infliction of anguish, mental pain, fear, or distress, that is perpetrated by a caregiver or other person who stands in a trust relationship to the elder."[78] This includes using verbal aggression, intimidation, and humiliation; making threats to deprive the elder of property or services, place the person in a nursing home, or remove financial support; making unreasonable demands; deliberately ignoring the elder; isolating the elder from family, friends, or activities; and failing to provide companionship. Findings suggestive of psychological abuse include elders who are uncommunicative and unresponsive; unreasonably fearful or suspicious; lack interest in social contacts; have chronic physical or psychiatric health problems; or exhibit emotional pain, distress, and evasiveness.

Violation of personal rights is the deprivation of inalienable rights (i.e., personal liberty, personal property, free speech, privacy, voting).

Abandonment is "the desertion or willful disregard of an older adult by anyone having care or custody of that person under circumstances in which a reasonable person would continue to provide care and custody."[78]

Financial abuse/ exploitation is "the illegal, unauthorized, or improper use of an older individual's resources by a caregiver or other person in a trusting relationship, for the benefit of someone other than the older individual."[78] This includes misuse of funds, petty theft, material exploitation, coercion of the elder to sign contracts, failure to pay bills, or declaration of the elder as incompetent to confiscate property. It may also include failure to allow the elder to access information they rightfully have access to, such as financial records or insurance information. This type of exploitation is not unique to family caregivers—it can also be perpetrated by individuals or corporations who take advantage of seniors through confusing or misleading mail or telephone offers (e.g., elders who have multiple magazine subscriptions or who get checks in the mail not realizing that their signature on the check is a contract for a service they did not solicit or a loan with an extremely high interest rate).

Risk Factors for Maltreatment

Risk factors can be divided into four broad categories: economic, caregiver related, social, and physical. An example of an economic situation might be the stress of living in cramped conditions with associated financial problems. Caregiver factors may be inexperience of the caregiver in dealing with complex needs of the frail, ill older adult; caregiver mental illness; and stress resulting from the "sandwich generation," when the addition of an older adult to the household brings sudden, unwanted, and unexpected dependency to the caregiver who has young children in the home. The greater the dependency on the caregiver, the greater the risk for abuse. Social factors may be seen in a role reversal in which the parent abused the child and now the child abuses the parent. Physical factors may include advanced age of the caregiver or the older adult and alcohol or drug abuse in the older adult or the caregiver. Research additionally shows that persons who experienced sexual or emotional abuse in childhood have a higher risk of being abused as elders.[87]

Recognizing Clues of Maltreatment

Identifying elder abuse or neglect in the ED is challenging for several reasons. The aging process, comorbid conditions, and some medications often result in a higher likelihood of fractures and bruising even in the absence of abuse, making it difficult to differentiate between accidental and inflicted injuries. Elder persons may be reluctant to make an outcry of abuse or neglect, fearing retribution from the abuser, or as a result of the desire to protect the abuser. They may also fear losing their independence or being sent to a nursing home if the abuser is someone they rely on for care. Some elder persons may not have the mental capacity to tell someone what has occurred. Emergency physicians and nursing staff typically lack formal education on identification of elder abuse. Research has shown that emergency physicians make a formal diagnosis of elder abuse in less than 0.02% of patients aged 60 or older who are evaluated in EDs, far below the estimated prevalence of 10% who experience abuse or neglect.[88]

Clues to abuse may be detected during the review of the patient's medical history, during the physical assessment, and/or by the patient's psychological status.

The history should be documented in quotation marks in the person's exact words and should be obtained from the patient privately, outside the presence of family or caregivers. Family members or caregivers are frequently the perpetrators of the abuse. The patient may be reluctant to share details of their abuse in front of their abusers or may not want to burden their family with details of what they have experienced. When talking with the suspected abuser, empathy and an understanding approach go a long way in obtaining information about the patient's care environment. Try to identify specific issues that may present problems resulting from the patient's diagnosis. For example, close monitoring for skin breakdown in a patient with dementia and frequent episodes of incontinence are challenges. In talking with this patient's caregiver, you might say, "Caring for your father in this stage of his dementia must be a real challenge at times. Do you ever feel overwhelmed with the responsibility? How do you deal with it?" It is essential to avoid confrontation in this phase of the assessment.

Physical clues may be evidenced as previously unexplained injuries, the presence of old and new bruises, injuries that do not match the history given for sustaining them, weight gain or loss, or poor personal hygiene. Alopecia secondary to repeated pulling and tugging of the person's hair or positioning of the head in one position for a long period of time is another significant finding. Blows to the eyes can cause dislocation of the lens, subconjunctival hemorrhage, or retinal detachment. Whiplash injuries may be seen after violent shaking. Patterned injuries that reflect the shape of the item that caused the injury are highly concerning for physical abuse. Consider the possibility of sexual abuse if there is difficulty walking or sitting. This may be a subtle sign, whereas bruises or lacerations of the inner thighs or genitalia are more overt findings. Pain or itching in the genital area may indicate a sexually transmitted infection. Multiple decubitus ulcers without interventions suggest neglect. Be alert to the implication "old people always get bed sores." A delay in seeking medical care for injury or illness may also be a red flag. Photographs of bruises, lacerations, and other injuries should be obtained to document type and extent of injuries.

Psychological clues of maltreatment manifest as extreme mood changes, withdrawn or agitated behavior, depression, fearfulness, insomnia or excessive sleeping, and ambivalent feelings toward family and/or caregivers. The older adult may not be given the opportunity to speak for himself or herself; the caregiver may exhibit an attitude of indifference or anger toward the older adult. The caregiver may blame the patient for his or her condition (e.g., incontinence is viewed as a deliberate act and not a result of physical dysfunction).

Health of household pets may also offer clues to the potential for abuse or neglect. The caregiver may threaten or mistreat a pet to silence its owner, or a person may want to leave a relationship but is afraid of leaving the animal behind.

Asking the Right Questions

There is no universally accepted instrument for screening for elder abuse and neglect. Recently proposed, the Senior Abuse Identification (ED Senior AID) tool, although still in need of additional validation, is helpful with this assessment. There is no score; instead it serves as a screening tool to heighten the clinician's awareness of potential elder abuse and maltreatment.

- After assessing for cognitive impairment, ask the patient, "Within the past 6 months…" have you required help with bathing, dressing, shopping, banking, or meals?
  - If the answer is yes, have you had someone who helps you with this?
  - If the answer is yes, is this person always there when you need them?
- Has anyone close to you called you names or put you down?
- Has anyone told you that you give them too much trouble?
- Has anyone close to you threatened you or made you feel bad?
- Has anyone tried to force you to sign papers or use your money against your will?
- Has anyone close to you tried to hurt you or harm you?

During the physical assessment, nurses should ask themselves if red flags or concerning findings are present.

Elements highly suggestive of abuse can be identified by asking about the following:

- bruising that occurs in unusual locations, or the presence of multiple bruises or large bruises
- burn patterns suggestive of intentional injury
- patterned injuries
- abrasions or lacerations suggestive of intentional injury
- evidence of neglect

Elements that may suggest abuse are:

- evidence of dehydration
- evidence of poor control of medical problems
- evidence of malnutrition
- swollen or tender area on palpation

Several specific circumstances should also be discussed:

- genital trauma or infection—evidence of sexual abuse
- fractures concerning for abuse
- a current problem that has been present for a long time (In this case, ask if there been an unusual delay in seeking medical attention concerning for abuse.)

Once these assessments are completed, nurses should ask themselves, "Based on all information available, including the answers the patient provided, the patient's chief complaint, and any observations you have made, do you suspect an ongoing problem of elder abuse?"[89]

Interventions for Abuse and Neglect

The Older Americans Act of 1965 and its amendments require each state to identify agencies involved in recognizing and treating abused, neglected, and exploited elders and to determine the need for appropriate services. Although all 50 states have adult protection legislation, mandatory reporting laws vary from state to state. Emergency nurses should be familiar with the reporting requirements for their specific state.

The primary goal of intervention is to protect the elder patient from immediate and future harm. A secondary and equally important goal of intervention is to break the cycle of maltreatment. The well-being of the abused individual must be considered concurrently with the coping ability of the abuser.

Interventions for family-mediated elder abuse are divided into two broad categories. First are cases in which the elder has physical or mental impairment and is dependent on the family for daily care needs. The second group comprises individuals with minimal care needs overshadowed by pathologic behavior of the caregiver. Potential intervention strategies for both categories include providing referrals to community agencies for continual monitoring of the situation, suggesting support services to decrease caregiver stress, performing close health care follow-up to prevent switching to another health care provider, and making reports to APS to facilitate removal of the individual from a harmful environment or use of 24-hour supervision through a home care agency.

Access is a major issue in assessment and intervention for alleged abuse or neglect of older adults. The competent elder has the right to make his or her own personal care decisions. The elder may choose to stay in the abusive situation despite all efforts to effect a change; this does not negate the emergency nurse's responsibility to report the suspected maltreatment. Victims of abuse often have both positive and negative feelings toward their abusers. Such ambivalence makes separation from the abuser difficult for the abuse victim.

Care needs of elders in the home increase over time; however, resources of the family in terms of psychosocial and financial reserves do not always increase at the same rate. Intervention requires a multidisciplinary team approach. Such a team is able to assess aspects of the situation such as physical injury, mental status, competency, financial irregularities, legality, treatment, assistance, protection, or prosecution. When there is a high degree of suspicion for elder abuse, consult social services or the responsible agency in your area. When appropriate, contact a home care agency to make an initial home assessment. In acute situations, the elder may require shelter or protective care.

Unfortunately, prosecuting elder abuse cases often proves challenging. Difficulties arise from diminished mental capacity of the victim; physical health of the victim; cooperation by the victim, proving undue influences; and witness intimidation.

Elder Abuse Summary

The American population is living longer. As baby boomers enter their senior years, more and more elders with mounting health problems require assistance to perform simple activities of daily living. Caregivers are frequently balancing demands of a young family, career, and aging parents.

As children, we are taught to honor our mothers and fathers and to respect and care for older adults. The notion of frail older adults facing a life of fear and pain caused by someone they love and trust may be beyond our comprehension. Similarly, understanding the frustration, fear, and sadness of the person who has gone from being a child cared for and nurtured by a parent to being the adult caring for that parent as one would a small child is also difficult to accept. For health care professionals to successfully diagnose and treat elder abuse, a nonjudgmental, open, and caring attitude toward all those involved is essential.

REFERENCES

1. US Department of Health and Human Services. *Administration for Children and Families, Administration on Children, Youth and Families*. Children's Bureau. Child maltreatment; 2016. https://www.acf.hhs.gov/sites/default/files/cb/cm2016.pdf. Accessed 10 June 2019. Published 2018.
2. Felitti VJ, Anda RF, Nordenberg D, et al. Relationship of childhood abuse and household dysfunction to many of the leading causes of death in adults: the adverse childhood experiences (ACE) study. *Am J Prev Med*. 1998;14(4):245–258.
3. Centers for Disease Control and Prevention. About adverse childhood experiences. Centers for Disease Control and Prevention website. https://www.cdc.gov/violenceprevention/acestudy/about_ace.html. Published 2016. Accessed 10 June 2019.
4. Purewal Boparai SK, Au V, Koita K, et al. Ameliorating the biological impacts of childhood adversity: a review of intervention programs. *Child Abuse Negl*. 2018;81:82–105. https://doi.org/10.1016/j.chiabu.2018.04.014.
5. Bachmann MB. The case for including adverse childhood experiences in child maltreatment education: a path analysis. *Perm J*. 2018;22:17–122. https://doi.org/10.7812/TPP/17-122.
6. Hamdullahpur HJ. Mental health among help-seeking urban women: the relationships between adverse childhood experiences, sexual abuse, and suicidality. *Violence Against Women*. 2018;24(16):1967–1981.
7. Kelly-Irving M, Lepage B, Dedieu D, et al. Adverse childhood experiences and premature all-cause mortality. *Eur J Epidemiol*. 2013;28(9):721–734. https://doi.org/10.1007/s10654-013-9832-9.
8. Levey EG. A systematic review of randomized controlled trials of interventions designed to decrease child abuse and neglect in high-risk families. *Child Abuse Neglect*. 2017;65:48–57.
9. Fang X, Brown DS, Florence CS, Mercy JA. The economic burden of child maltreatment in the United States and implications for prevention. *Child Abuse Neglect*. 2012;36(2):156–165. https://doi.org/10.1016/j.chiabu.2011.10.006.
10. Centers for Disease Control and Prevention. Violence Prevention Fast Facts: childhood Abuse & Neglect. Centers for Disease Control and Prevention website; 2018. https://www.cdc.gov-/violenceprevention/childabuseandneglect/definitions.html. Accessed 10 June 2019. Published 2018.
11. Child Welfare Information Gateway. *Acts of Omission: An Overview of Child Neglect*. Washington, DC: US Department of Health and Human Services, Children's Bureau; 2018. https://www.childwelfare.gov/pubPDFs/acts.pdf. Accessed 10 June 2019.
12. Maguire SA, Williams B, Naughton AM, et al. A systematic review of the emotional, behavioural and cognitive features exhibited by school-aged children experiencing neglect or emotional abuse. *Child Care Health Dev*. 2015;41(5):641–653. https://doi.org/10.1111/cch.12227.
13. Homan GJ. Failure to thrive: a practical guide. *Am Fam Physician*. 2016;94(4):295–299. https://www.aafp.org/afp/2016/0815/p295.html. Accessed 10 June 2019.
14. Leeb RT, Paulozzi L, Melanson C, Simon T, Arias I. *Child Maltreatment Surveillance: Uniform Definitions for Public Health and Recommended Data Elements, Version 1.0*. Atlanta, GA: Centers for Disease Control and Prevention, National Center for Injury Prevention and Control; 2008. https://www.cdc.gov-/violenceprevention/pdf/CM_Surveillance-a.pdf. Accessed 10 June 2019.
15. Christian CC. The evaluation of suspected child physical abuse. *Pediatrics*. 2015;135(5):e1337–1354. https://doi.org/10.1542/peds.2015-0356.
16. Yu YR, DeMello AS, Greeley CS, Cox CS, Naik-Mathuria BJ, Wesson DE. Injury patterns of child abuse: experience of two Level I pediatric trauma centers. *J Pediatr Surg*. 2018;53(5):1028–1032. https://doi.org/10.1016/j.jpedsurg.2018.02.043.
17. Centers for Disease Control and Prevention. Preventing Abusive Head Trauma in Children. Centers for Disease Control and Prevention website. https://www.cdc.gov/violenceprevention/childabuseandneglect/Abusive-Head-Trauma.html. Published 2018. Accessed 10 June 2019.
18. Jenny C, Hymel KP, Ritzen A, Reinert SE, Hay TC. Analysis of missed cases of abusive head trauma. *JAMA*. 1999;281(7):621–626. https://doi.org/10.1001/ama.281.7.621.
19. Narang SC, Clarke J. Abusive head trauma: past, present, and future. *J Child Neurol*. 2014;29(12):1747–1756. https://doi.org/10.1177/0883073814549995.
20. Boehnke MM, Mirsky D, Stence N, Stanley RM, Lindberg DM. Occult head injury is common in children with concern for physical abuse. *Pediatr Radiol*. 2018;48(8):1123–1129. https://doi.org/10.1007/s00247-018-4128-6.
21. Chauvin-Kimoff L, Allard-Dansereau C, Colbourne M. The medical assessment of fractures in suspected child maltreatment: infants and young children with skeletal injury. *Pediatr Child Health*. 2018;23(2):156–160. https://doi.org/10.1093/pch/pxx131.
22. Flaherty EG, MacMillan HM. Caregiver-fabricated illness in a child: a manifestation of child maltreatment. *Pediatrics*. 2013;132(3):590–597. https://doi.org/10.1542/peds.2013-2045.
23. Finkelhor D, Turner HA, Shattuck A, et al. Prevalence of childhood exposure to violence, crime, and abuse: results from the National Survey of Children's Exposure to Violence. *JAMA Pediatr*. 2015;169(8):746–754. doi:10.1001.jamapediatrics.2015.0676.
24. Kimber M, MacMillan HL. Child psychological abuse. *Pediatr Rev*. 2017;38(10):496–498.
25. National Center for Fatality Review and Prevention. National Center for Fatality Review and Prevention website. https://www.ncfrp.org/. Accessed 10 June 2019.
26. O'Malley P, Barta I, Snow S, et al. Death of a child in the emergency department. *Pediatrics*. 2014;134(1):e313–330. https://doi.org/10.1542/peds.2014-1246.
27. Centers for Disease Control and Prevention. *Intimate Partner Violence: What are the Consequences? Centers for Disease Control and Prevention website*; 2017. https://www.cdc.gov/violenceprevention/intimatepartnerviolence/consequences.html. Published 2017. Accessed 10 June 2019.
28. Breiding MJ, Basile KC, Smith SG, Black MC, Mahendra R. *Intimate Partner Violence Surveillance: Uniform Definitions and Recommended Data Elements, Version 2.0*. Atlanta, GA: National Center for Injury Prevention and Control, Centers for Disease Control and Prevention; 2015. https://www.cdc.gov/violenceprevention/pdf/ipv/intimatepartnerviolence.pdf. Accessed 10 June 2019.
29. Niolon PH, Kearns M, Dills J, et al. *Preventing Intimate Partner Violence Across the Lifespan: A Technical Package of Programs, Policies, and Practices*. Atlanta, GA: National Center for Injury Prevention and Control, Centers for Disease Control and Prevention; 2017. https://www.cdc.gov/violenceprevention/pdf/ipv-technicalpackages.pdf. Accessed 10 June 2019.

30. Brieding MJ, Smith SG, Basile KC, Walters ML, Chen J, Merrick MT. Prevalence and characteristics of sexual violence, stalking, and intimate partner violence victimization—National intimate partner and sexual violence survey, United States, 2011. *MMWR Surveill Summ.* 2014;63(8):1–18.
31. Vagi KJ, Olsen EO, Basile KC. Teen dating violence (physical and sexual) among US high school students: findings from the 2013 National Youth Risk Behavior Study. *JAMA Pediatr.* 2015;169(5):474–482.
32. Rosay AB, Mulford CS. Prevalence estimates and correlates of elder abuse in the United States: the National Intimate Partner and Sexual Violence Survey. *J Elder Abuse Negl.* 2017;29(1):1–14. https://doi.org/10.1080/08946566.2016.1249817.
33. Walters ML, Chen J, Breiding MJ. *The National Intimate Partner and Sexual Violence Survey: 2010 Findings on Victimization by Sexual Orientation.* Atlanta, GA: National Center for Injury Prevention and Control, Centers for Disease Control and Prevention; 2013. https://www.cdc.gov/violenceprevention/pdf/nisvs_sofindings.pdf. Accessed 10 June 2019.
34. Agency for Healthcare Research and Quality. Intimate Partner Violence Screening: Fact Sheet and Resources. https://www.ahrq.gov/professionals/prevention-chronic-care/healthier-pregnancy/preventive/partnerviolence.html. Accessed 10 June 2019. Published 2015.
35. Peterson C, Liu Y, Kresnow M, et al. Short-term lost productivity per victim: intimate partner violence, sexual violence, or stalking. *Am J Prev Med.* 2018;55(1):106–110. https://doi.org/10.1016/j.amepre.2018.03.007.
36. Yakubovich AR, Stockl H, Murray J, et al. Risk and protective factors for intimate partner violence against women: systematic review and meta-analyses of prospective-longitudinal studies. *Am J Public Health.* 2018;108(7):e1–e11.
37. Mogos MF, Araya WN, Masho SW, et al. The feto-maternal health cost of intimate partner violence among delivery-related discharges in the United States, 2002-2009. *J Interpers Violence.* 2016;31:444–464. https://doi.org/10.1177/0886260514555869.
38. Barrios YV, Gelaye B, Zhong Q, et al. Association of childhood physical and sexual abuse with intimate partner violence, poor general health and depressive symptoms among pregnant women. *PLoS One.* 2015;10(1):e0116609. https://doi.org/10.1371/journal.pone.0116609.
39. Devries KM, Child JC, Bacchus LJ, et al. Intimate partner violence victimization and alcohol consumption in women: a systematic review and meta-analysis. *Addiction.* 2014;109(3):379–391. https://doi.org/10.1111/add.12393.
40. Collins EA, Cody AM, McDonald SE. A template analysis of intimate partner violence survivors' experiences of animal maltreatment: implications for safety planning and intervention. *Violence Against Women.* 2018;24(4):452–476. https://doi.org/10.1177/1077801217697266.
41. National Center for Health Research. The Cycle of Domestic Violence. http://www.center4research.org/cycle-domestic-violence/. Accessed 10 June 2019.
42. Adams EN, Clark HM, Galano MM, et al. Predictors of housing instability in women who have experienced intimate partner violence. *J Interpers Violence.* 2018:886260518777001. https://doi.org/10.1177/0886260518777001.
43. Amerson R, Whittington R, Duggan L. Intimate partner violence affecting Latina women and their children. *J Emerg Nurs.* 2014;40(6):531–536. https://doi.org/10.1016/j.jen.2013.12.003.
44. Boots DP, Wareham J, Bartula A, et al. A comparison of the batterer intervention and prevention program with alternative court dispositions and 12-month recidivism. *Violence Against Women.* 2016;22(9):1134–1157. https://doi.org/10.1177/1077801215618806.
45. Anderson J, Stockman JK, Sabri B, Campbell DW, Campbell JC. Injury outcomes in African American and African Caribbean women: the role of intimate partner violence. *J Emerg Nurs.* 2015;41(1):36–42. https://doi.org/10.1016/j.jen.2014.01.015.
46. Cook County Department of Public Health. *9. The Joint Commission Requirements for IPV Assessments and Documentation.* http://cookcountypublichealth.org/violence-prevention/ipv-toolkit/9. Accessed 10 June 2019.
47. Emergency Nurses Association, International Association of Forensic Nurses. Joint Position Statement: Intimate Partner Violence. https://ena.org/docs/default-source/resource-library/practice-resources/position-statements/joint-statements/intimatepartnerviolence.pdf. Published 2018. Accessed 10 June 2019.
48. Choo EK, Houry DE. Managing intimate partner violence in the emergency department. *Ann Emerg Med.* 2015;65(4):447–451. https://doi.org/10.1016/j.annemergmed.2014.11.004.
49. Davidov DM, Larrabee H, Davis SM. United States emergency department visits coded for intimate partner violence. *J Emerg Med.* 2015;48(1):94–100. https://doi.org/10.1016/.j.jemermed.2014.07.053.
50. Sprague S, Madden K, Dosanjh S, et al. Intimate partner violence and musculoskeletal injury: bridging the knowledge gap in orthopaedic fracture clinics. *BMC Musculoskelet Disord.* 2013;14:23. https://doi.org/10.1186/1471-2474-14-23.
51. Dicola DS, Spaar E. Intimate partner violence. *Am Fam Physician.* 2016;94(8):646–651. https://www.aafp.org/afp/2016/1015/p646.html. Accessed 10 June 2019.
52. The National Domestic Violence Hotline. https://www.thehotline.org/. Accessed 10 June 2019.
53. Futures Without Violence. https://www.futureswithoutviolence.org/. Accessed 10 June 2019.
54. National Institute of Justice. Human Trafficking. https://www.nij.gov/topics/crime/human-trafficking/pages/welcome.aspx. Published 2018. Accessed 10 June 2019.
55. International Labour Organization. Profits and Poverty: The Economics of Forced Labour. http://www.ilo.org/global/topics/forced-labour/publications/profits-of-forced-labour-2014/lang—en/index.htm. Published 2014. Accessed May 23, 2018.
56. International Labour Organization. Global Estimates of Modern Slavery: Forced Labour and Forced Marriage. https://www.ilo.org/global/publications/books/WCMS_575479/lang--en/index.htm. Accessed 10 June 2019. Published 2017.
57. National Human Trafficking Resource Center. *Human Trafficking Trends in the United States, 2007-2012.* https://polarisproject.org/resources/human-trafficking-trends-2007-2012. Published 2013. Accessed 10 June 2019.
58. United Nations Office on Drugs and Crime. *Global Report on Trafficking in Persons*; 2014. https://www.unodc.org/res/cld/bibliography/global-report-on-trafficking-in-persons_html/GLOTIP_2014_full_report.pdf. Accessed 10 June 2019. Published 2016.
59. US Department of State. *Trafficking in Persons Report June*; 2017. https://www.state.gov/reports/2017-trafficking-in-persons-report/. Accessed 10 June 2019. Published 2017.
60. US Department of Homeland Security. Human trafficking and smuggling. https://www.ice.gov/factsheets/human-trafficking. Accessed 10 June 2019. Published 2013.

61. Greenbaum J, Bodrick N. Global human trafficking and child victimization. *Pediatrics*. 2017;140(6):e20173138. https://doi.org/10.1542/peds.2017-3138.
62. Lederer LW, Wetzel CA. The health consequences of sex trafficking and their implications for identifying victims in healthcare facilities. *Ann Health Law*. 2014;23(1):61–91.
63. Varma S, Gillespie S, McCracken C, Greenbaum VJ. Characteristics of child commercial sexual exploitation and sex trafficking victims presenting for medical care in the United States. *Child Abuse Negl*. 2015;44:98–105. https://doi.org/10.1016/j.chiabu.2015.04.004.
64. Shandro J, Chisolm-Straker M, Duber HC, et al. Human trafficking: a guide to identification and approach for the emergency physician. *Ann Emerg Med*. 2016;68(4):501–508. https://doi.org/10.1016.j.annemergmed.2016.03.049.
65. Hemmings S, Jakobowitz S, Abas M, et al. Responding to the health needs of survivors of human trafficking: a systematic review. *BMC Health Serv Res*. 2016;16:320. https://doi.org/10.1186/s12913-016-1538-8.
66. National Human Trafficking Resource Center. Recognizing and Responding to Human trafficking in a healthcare context. https://humantraffickinghotline.org/resources/recognizing-and-responding-human-trafficking-healthcare-context. Updated February 2016. Accessed 10 June 2019.
67. National Human Trafficking Resource Center. Framework for a Human Trafficking Protocol in Healthcare Settings; 2010. https://humantraffickinghotline.org/resources/framework-human-trafficking-protocol-healthcare-settings. Polaris. Updated February 2016. Accessed 10 June 2019.
68. Kelly A. I Carried His Name on my Body for Nine Years: The Tattooed Trafficking Survivors Reclaiming their Past. The Guardian website. https://www.theguardian.com/global-development/2014/nov/16/sp-the-tattooed-trafficking-survivors-reclaiming-their-past. Published November 15, 2014. Accessed 10 June 2019.
69. United Nations Office on Drugs and Crime. *Trafficking in Persons for the Purpose of Organ Removal*. https://www.unodc.org/documents/human-trafficking/2015/UNODC_Assessment_Toolkit_TIP_for_the_Purpose_of_Organ_Removal.pdf. Published 2015. Accessed 10 June 2019.
70. de Jong J. Indicators to identify trafficking in human beings for the purpose of organ removal. *Transp Direct*. 2016;2(2):e56. https://doi.org/10.1097/TXD. 000000000000568.
71. Tracy EE, Macias-Konstantopoulos W. Identifying and assisting sexually exploited and trafficked patients seeking women's health care services. *Obstet Gynecol*. 2017;130(2):443–453. https://doi.org/10.1097/AOG 0000000000002144.
72. Long E, Dowdell EB. Nurses' perceptions of victims of human trafficking in an urban emergency department: a qualitative study. *J Emerg Nurs*. 2018;44(4):375–383. https://doi.org/10.1016/j.jen.2017.11.004.
73. Egyud A, Stephens K, Swanson-Bierman B, DiCuccio M, Whiteman K. Implementation of human trafficking education and treatment algorithm in the emergency department. *J Emerg Nurs*. 2017;43(6):526–531. https://doi.org/10.1016/j.jen.2017.01.008.
74. Scannell MM. Human trafficking: how nurses can make a difference. *J Forensic Nurs*. 2018;14(2):117–121. https://doi.org/10.1097/JFN.0000000000000203.
75. National Center on Elder Abuse. Research: Statistics/Data. https://ncea.acl.gov/About-Us/What-We-Do/Research/Statistics-and-Data.aspx. Accessed 10 June 2019. Published 2018.
76. Dong X, Simon MA. Association between elder abuse and use of ED: findings from the Chicago Health and Aging Project. *Am J Emerg Med*. 2013;31(4):693–698. https://doi.org/10/1016/j.ajem.2012.12.028.
77. Rosen T, Hargarten S, Flomenbaum NE, Platts-Mills TF. Identifying elder abuse in the emergency department: toward a multidisciplinary team-based approach. *Ann Emerg Med*. 2017;68(3):378–382. https://doi.org/10.106/j.annemergmed.2016.01.037.
78. Hall JE, Karch DL, Crosby AE. *Elder Abuse Surveillance: Uniform Definitions and Recommended Core Data Elements for Use in Elder Abuse Surveillance, Version 1.0*. Atlanta, GA: National Center for Injury Prevention and Control, Centers for Disease Control and Prevention; 2016. https://www.cdc.gov/violenceprevention/pdf/EA_Book_Revised_2016.pdf. Accessed 10 June 2019.
79. Colby SL, Ortman JM. Projections of the Size and Composition of the U.S. Population: 2014 to 2060. https://census.gov/content/dam/Census/library/publications/2015/demo/p25-1143.pdf. Published March 2015. Accessed 10 June 2019.
80. Acierno R, Steedley M, Hernandez-Tejada MA, Frook G, Watkins J, Muzzy W. Relevance of perpetrator identity to reporting elder financial and emotional mistreatment. *J Appl Gerontol*. 2018;733464818771208. https://doi.org/10.1177/0733464818771208.
81. Dong X. Elder self-neglect: research and practice. *Clin Interv Aging*. 2017;12:949–954. https://doi.org/10.2147/CIA.S103359.
82. Castle N. An examination of resident abuse in assisted living facilities. National Criminal Reference Services, National Institute of Justice, U.S. Department of Justice. 2013. https://www.ncjrs.gov/pdffiles1/nij/grants/241611.pdf. Accessed 10 June 2019.
83. Abner EL, Teaster PB, Mendiondo MS, et al. Victim, allegation, and investigation characteristics associated with substantiated reports of sexual abuse of adults in residential care settings. *J Interpers Violence*. 2016:886260516672051. https://doi.org/10.1177/0886260516672051.
84. Yunus RM, Hairi NN, Choo WY. Consequences of elder abuse and neglect: a systematic review of observational studies. *Trauma Violence Abuse*. 2019;20(2):197–213. https://doi.org/10.1177/1524838017692798.
85. Acierno R, Hernandez-Tejada MA, Anetzberger GJ, Loew D, Muzzy W, Milis M. The National Elder Mistreatment Study: an 8-year longitudinal study of outcomes. *J Elder Abuse Negl*. 2017;29(4):254–269. https://doi.org/10.1080/08946566.2017.1365031.
86. Roberto KA. Perpetrators of late life polyvictimization. *J Elder Abuse Negl*. 2017;29(5):313–326. https://doi.org/10.1080/08946566.2017.1374223.
87. Kong J, Easton SD. Re-experiencing violence across the life course: histories of childhood maltreatment and elder abuse victimization. *J Gerontol. B Psychol Sci Soc Sci*. 2018. https://doi.org/10.1093/geronb/gby035.
88. Evans CS, Hunold KM, Rosen T, Platts-Mills TF. Diagnosis of elder abuse in U.S. emergency departments. *J Am Geriatr Soc*. 2017;65(1):91–97. https://doi.org/10.111/jgs.14480.
89. Platts-Mills TF, Dayaa JA, Reeve BB, Krajick K, Mosqueda L, Haukoos JS. Development of the Emergency Department Senior Abuse Identification (ED Senior AID) tool. *J Elder Abuse Negl*. 2018;30(4):247–270. https://doi.org/10.1080/08946566.2018.1460285.

Substance Use Disorders

Joanne Ingalls McKay

Over the past four decades, substance use disorders (SUDs) have increasingly become common as a primary and/or secondary presentation complaints for patients coming to emergency departments (EDs). This includes the abuse of and addiction to alcohol, nicotine, illicit and over-the-counter (OTC) drugs, and prescription drugs. Substance abuse results in Americans paying more than $700 billion a year in increased health care costs, crime, and lost productivity.[1] In October 2017 the opioid crisis was declared a public health emergency by the US government based on epidemic levels of illegal and prescription drug use and deaths. According to the 2017 *President's Commission on Combating Drug Addiction and the Opioid Crisis*, more than 174 Americans died every day in 2016 of substance use, and the situation was considered the "worst drug crisis in American history."[2] In 2015 there were 33,091 opioid overdose deaths in the United States, and in 2016 there were more than 42,000, a number that exceeded the number of all other drug-related deaths or traffic fatalities.[3,4] The most frequently mentioned drugs involved in these deaths were illegal and prescription opioids (heroin, oxycodone, methadone, morphine, hydrocodone, and fentanyl), benzodiazepines (alprazolam and diazepam), and stimulants (cocaine and methamphetamine).[4]

People of all ages suffer the harmful consequences of drug abuse and addiction.[5] **Babies** exposed to drugs in the womb may be born premature and underweight, which can slow the child's intellectual development and affect behavior later in life. Babies born to mothers using opioids during pregnancy can develop neonatal abstinence syndrome (NAS) and may suffer from withdrawal and require specialized detox.[6,7] **Adolescents** who abuse drugs often act out at home, fail in school, and may drop out of school and become involved in the legal system due to crime. They are at risk for unplanned pregnancies, violence, and infectious/communicable diseases. **Adults** who abuse drugs frequently have difficulty thinking clearly, remembering, and paying attention. They tend to develop poor social behaviors as a result of their drug abuse, and their work performance and personal relationships suffer. If the addict is a parent, their SUD often results in chaotic, stress-filled homes, child abuse, and/or neglect. Living with a substance-dependent person causes harm and poor development of children living in the home and can contribute to SUD for the children as they become teenagers. **Parents and siblings** of teenagers and/or young adults who abuse drugs or substances also suffer. They often have to deal with truant school behaviors, theft within the home, and involvement with the law for illegal activities perpetrated by the substance user to sustain the substance abuse. This situation affects the whole family in a very negative manner.

Emergency nurses are faced with treating and caring for patients and their families who present to the ED with substance use and abuse daily, so knowledge and understanding of the scope of the issue can help nurses manage SUD. For purposes of this chapter, specific information is presented on illicit and several OTC drugs, alcohol, and tobacco. The reader is encouraged to seek additional resources for a more comprehensive discussion of the extensive issue with the abuse of prescription drugs (narcotics, stimulants, depressants, steroids) and overdose, because those topics are not specifically covered in this chapter.

DEFINITIONS

The following definitions apply to the use of alcohol, tobacco/nicotine, prescription drugs, illegal drugs, and several OTC drugs:

- *Addiction:* a term used to indicate the most severe, chronic stage of substance use disorder, in which there is a substantial loss of self-control, as indicated by compulsive drug taking despite the desire to stop taking the drug.[8]
- *Medication-assisted treatment (MAT):* medications used to assist in the treatment of opioid, alcohol, and tobacco use disorders.[8]
- *Substance misuse:* the use of any substance in a manner, situation, amount, or frequency that can cause harm to users or to those around them. For some substances or individuals, any use would constitute misuse (e.g., underage drinking, injection drug use).[9]
- *Substance use disorder:* a diagnostic term referring to recurrent use of alcohol, tobacco, or other drugs that cause clinically and functionally significant impairment, such as health problems, disability, and failure to meet major responsibilities at work, school, or home. Depending on the level of severity, this disorder is classified as mild, moderate, or severe.[8]

Subcategories of SUD[8] include specific substances that lead to clinically significant impairment or distress affecting young and old alike:

- *Opioid use disorder (OUD):* a problematic pattern of use of opioids.
- *Tobacco use disorder (TUD):* a problematic pattern of use of tobacco products containing nicotine.
- *Alcohol use disorder (AUD):* a problematic pattern of use of alcohol.
- *Substance use disorder treatment:* a service or set of services that may include medication, counseling, and other supportive services designed to enable an individual to reduce or eliminate alcohol and/or other drug use, address associated physical or mental health problems, and restore the patient to maximum functional ability.[9]

THE SCIENCE OF ADDICTION

Scientists began studying addictive behavior as early as the 1930s and since then, people addicted to drugs were thought to be morally flawed and lacking willpower to stop abusing the substances. For decades, those views shaped society's responses to substance abuse, treating it as a moral failing rather than a health problem, which led to an emphasis on punishment rather than prevention and treatment.[5] Over the past several decades, scientific views, study of the brain, and responses to SUDs and addiction have changed dramatically.[5,10] Drug addiction is a biologically based disease that alters the pleasure center and other aspects of the brain via the neurotransmitter dopamine.[9,10] When dopamine joins with a receptor, like a key fitting into a lock, the biochemical process in the neuron is activated. This process is called chemical neurotransmission, and it allows a receptor neuron to connect with other neurons.[5] The biologic basis for addiction is the repeated process of altering chemical neurotransmission. Repeated use of these drugs affects the brain on a permanent basis. Addiction begins when the pleasure circuit is repeatedly stimulated.

A combination of factors is known to influence risk for addiction, including biology, environment, and development.[5,10,11] The more risk factors a person has, the greater is the chance that taking substances can lead to addiction. About 50% of the risk is genetic, within a range of about 40% to 60%.[5] The environment includes many different influences, including family, friends, economic status, and general quality of life. Other factors like peer pressure, physical and sexual abuse, early exposure to drugs, stress, and parental guidance can also play a part in substance use and addiction. Although taking drugs or using other substances at any age can lead to addiction, the earlier that drugs or substances are used, the more likely they will progress to addiction. Brain development continues into the mid-20s, when many important developmental and social changes occur in teens and young people. This puts teenagers at risk because the prefrontal cortex in their brain controlling decision making, judgment, and self-control is still developing, making them prone to risky behaviors, including experimentation with substances.[10,11] For decades, researchers have been mapping the electrical and chemical circuits underlying addiction, and imaging studies have shown how the brain rewires during recovery from addiction.[11] Researchers are now working on identifying strategies to heal these neural pathways.

IDENTIFICATION OF SUBSTANCE USE DISORDERS

Early identification and treatment must be initiated for people with substance use disorders. Appropriate screening tools should be used in the ED for drug, tobacco, and alcohol abuse so problems can be detected and early intervention started. Numerous validated online screening tools are available to use in assessing ED patients for substance use disorders of drugs, tobacco, and alcohol. Some are for adults or adolescents, and several are for adolescents only. A chart of evidence-based screening tools and assessments for adults and adolescents is available on the National Institute on Drug Abuse (NIDA) website.[12] EDs may wish to consider tools including the Brief Screener for Alcohol, Tobacco, and other Drugs (BSATD) tool, the Screening to Brief Intervention (S2BI) tool for adolescents, and the Tobacco, Alcohol, Prescription medication, and other Substance use (TAPS) Tool for adults.[12] The CAGE-AID Questionnaire and the AUDIT-C are both for alcohol assessment in adults only.[12] Nurse screening of ED patients is a key part of assessing for suspected or known substance use.

SPECIFIC SUBSTANCES

Emergencies related to SUD may be acute or chronic in nature. The patient may come to the ED with severe drug intoxication/overdose, acute withdrawal, an injury secondary to substance use, or seeking help for addiction. This chapter will focus on substance use and addiction rather than acute intoxication. Refer to Chapter 31 for information on other toxicologic emergencies. This chapter will include the key chemical substances emergency nurses will treat patients for as well as tobacco and alcohol use disorder. NIDA publishes an extensive list of commonly abused drugs for reference, including illicit and prescription drugs, OTC medications, alcohol, and tobacco.[13]

Chemical Substance Use

The Drug Enforcement Agency (DEA) identifies nine classes of drugs: depressants, designer drugs, drugs of concern, hallucinogens, inhalants, marijuana/cannabis, narcotics, steroids, and stimulants, most of which are discussed in the next sections.[14]

Depressants

Gamma-hydroxybutyrate (GHB)/Xyrem. GHB[13,14] is a CNS depressant approved only for use in treating narcolepsy, but it is commonly referred to as a "club drug" or "date-rape" drug because it is abused by teens and young adults at bars, parties, clubs, and "raves" (all-night dance parties) by placing it in alcoholic beverages. GHB is a substance used for sexual assault and other criminal acts because it is swallowed, often when combined with alcohol or other beverages. It comes in a colorless liquid or white powder and is odorless but may have a soapy or salty taste. GHB is produced illegally in domestic and foreign laboratories. Short-term effects include euphoria, drowsiness, decreased anxiety, confusion, and amnesia. It takes effect in 15 to 30 minutes and lasts 3 to 6 hours. Long-term effects include insomnia, anxiety, nausea, vomiting, bradycardia, lower body temperature, seizures, coma, or death.

Rohypnol (flunitrazepam). Rohypnol[13,14] is a CNS depressant belonging to the benzodiazepine class of drugs that is chemically similar to prescription sedatives such as diazepam. This drug is typically abused by teens and young adults at bars, nightclubs, concerts, and parties. It has been used to commit sexual assaults due to its ability to sedate and incapacitate unsuspecting victims. It comes in a tablet that is crushed, snorted, or dissolved in liquid. Short-term effects include drowsiness, sedation, sleep, amnesia, blackout, decreased anxiety, muscle relaxation, impaired reaction time and motor coordination, impaired mental functioning and judgment, confusion, aggression, excitability, slurred speech, headache, hypoventilation, and decreased heart rate.

Designer Drugs

Synthetic cathinones (bath salts, 3,4-methylenedioxypyrovalerone-MDPV). Synthetic cathinones[13-15] are man-made CNS stimulants chemically related to cathinone, a substance found in the khat (pronounced "cot") plant. Synthetic cathinones are chemically similar to drugs like amphetamines, cocaine, and Ecstasy/MDMA. They are unregulated, psychoactive, mind-altering substances with no legitimate medical use and are made to copy the effects of controlled substances in the brain. They are commonly bought online and in drug paraphernalia stores or gas stations and, although they are marketed as "bath salts," they should not be confused with products such as Epsom salts or Calgon products that people use during bathing. This drug looks like white or brown crystalline powder and is sold in small plastic or foil packages or bottles. It is snorted, injected, smoked with e-cigarettes or vape pens, or dropped on the tongue or into drinks. These drugs typically produce effects that include paranoia, hallucinations with sensations and images that appear real but are not, increased friendliness, increased sex drive, panic attacks, and excited delirium (extreme agitation and violent behavior). Some physiologic effects of synthetic cathinones include tachycardia, hypertension, and chest pain. The worst outcomes are associated with snorting or needle injection and have resulted in death.

Synthetic cannabinoids. Synthetic cannabinoids[13,14,16] are synthetic drugs containing man-made cannabinoid chemicals related to tetrahydrocannabinol (THC) in marijuana but are much stronger and more dangerous. They mimic THC and affect the body in a similar way as marijuana does. Synthetic cannabinoids are usually sprayed onto herbal products. These drugs frequently are marketed and sold as "herbal incense" or "potpourri," and they are popular with adolescents and young adults. Since 2009, many different types have been sold as "legal" alternatives to marijuana in head shops, gas stations, convenience stores, and on the Internet from international and national sources. Most are produced in Asia without any regulatory standards or quality control. They come as dried, shredded plant material and are usually smoked or swallowed as tea. Known side effects include agitation, anxiety, nausea, vomiting, tachycardia, increased blood pressure, tremor, seizures, hallucinations, paranoid behavior, and nonresponsiveness. They are difficult to detect or regulate because no tests are currently available to identify them in people using them.

Drugs of Concern

Over-the-counter medicines: dextromethorphan and loperamide (Imodium). Two commonly misused OTC medicines are dextromethorphan (DXM) and loperamide (Imodium).[9,13,14] DXM is a cough suppressant found in many OTC cold medicines; the most common sources of abused DXM are "extra-strength" cough syrup, dissolving strips, lozenges, chewable tablets, and gel capsules (e.g., Robitussin, Coricidin, and Nyquil). DXM is often swallowed in its original form or mixed with soda for flavor. Loperamide is meant for diarrhea and is available in tablet, capsule, powder, or liquid form. When misusing loperamide, people swallow large quantities of the medicine to cause a stimulant effect. DXM and loperamide are classified as opioids, but they both also have stimulant effects.

As with other opioids, when people overdose on DXM or loperamide, their breathing often slows or stops, and this can lead to effects on the nervous system, including coma, permanent brain damage, or death. Side effects of DXM overdose include drowsiness, dizziness, blurred vision, nausea or severe vomiting, difficulty urinating, shakiness, unsteady gait, unusual excitement, nervous behavior, or severe irritability. Side effects of loperamide include slurred speech, vision changes, sweating, hypertension, stomach pain, poor motor control, hyperexcitability, and lack of energy. These medicines are often misused in combination with other drugs, such as alcohol and marijuana. Naloxone can be given to someone who has acutely overdosed on DXM, and activated charcoal is used for DXM and loperamide if the ingestion has been within a few hours.

Kratom. Kratom[13,14] comes from a tropical tree native to Southeast Asia with leaves containing compounds with opioid-like effects. The leaves are usually crushed and then smoked, brewed with tea, chewed, or placed into gel capsules. The onset of effects typically begins within 5 to 10 minutes of use and lasts for 2 to 5 hours. Side effects include itching, nausea, vomiting, dry mouth, sweating, drowsiness, loss of appetite, and increased urination. At moderate doses and higher doses, at which opioid effects generally appear, additional adverse effects include tachycardia and the opioid side effects of dizziness, hypotension, dry mouth, sweating, and constipation. Frequent use of high doses of kratom may cause tremors, anorexia, weight loss, seizures, and psychosis. Kratom is banned in some states and jurisdictions. Kratom can be easily purchased in head shops and on the Internet. Overdoses of kratom are managed with naloxone.

Salvia. Salvia[13,14] is a hallucinogenic plant/herb in the mint family that is native to southern Mexico and Central and South America. It is sold legally in most states as *Salvia divinorum* and comes in fresh or dried leaves. Salvia is smoked, vaporized, inhaled, chewed, or brewed as tea. Short-term effects include intense hallucinations, altered visual perception/mood/body sensations, mood swings, feelings of detachment from one's body, and sweating. Salvia may also cause fear and panic, uncontrollable laughter, and a sense of overlapping realities. Addiction to salvia is unknown.

Hallucinogens

Hallucinogens are drugs causing profound distortions in a person's perception of reality and include ayahuasca, dimethyltryptamine (DMT), ketamine, lysergic acid diethylamide (LSD), mescaline (peyote), phencyclidine (PCP), psilocybin, and salvia.[13,14,17] There are no medications approved by the Food and Drug Administration (FDA) to treat addiction to any hallucinogens.

Dimethyltryptamine (DMT). DMT[13,17]is a synthetically made drug producing powerful but relatively short-lived (30–45 minutes) hallucinogenic experiences. It is available illegally as white or yellow crystalline powder and is smoked or injected. Short-term effects include intense visual hallucinations, auditory distortions, and an altered perception of time and body image. Physical effects are hypertension, tachycardia, dilated pupils, dizziness, agitation, and seizures. At high doses, coma, cardiac and respiratory arrest have occurred.

Ayahuasca. Ayahuasca[13,14,17] is a hallucinogenic tea made in the Amazon region from a DMT-containing plant and another vine brewed together. Ayahuasca plants and preparations are legal because they contain no scheduled chemicals; however, brews made using DMT-containing plants are illegal because DMT is a Schedule I drug. Short-term effects from drinking the brew include strong hallucinations with altered visual and auditory perceptions, increased heart rate and blood pressure, nausea, vomiting, a burning sensation in the stomach, tingling sensations, and increased skin sensitivity. Long-term effects have shown possible changes to the serotoninergic and immune systems, but further research is needed.

Ketamine. Ketamine[13,14] is a dissociative drug (distorts sights, sounds, and perceptions) with hallucinogenic effects that is intended to be used as an anesthetic for animals and humans. It is produced commercially for anesthesia, but most of the ketamine illegally sold in the United States is diverted or stolen from legitimate sources or smuggled from Mexico. It is a drug used most often by teens and young adults at raves and dance clubs. It is odorless and tasteless and has amnesia-inducing properties, so it has been added to drinks to facilitate sexual assault. It comes in a clear liquid and a white or off-white powder. It is snorted, swallowed, smoked (as a powder added to tobacco or marijuana), or injected. As a hallucinogen, it causes the user to feel detached from reality. Short-term effects include difficulty paying attention/learning/memory, dreamlike states, hallucinations, sedation, confusion, loss of memory, hypertension, loss of consciousness, and dangerously slowed breathing. Long-term effects can include ulcers and pain in the bladder, kidney problems, stomach pain, depression, and poor memory.

Lysergic acid diethylamide (LSD). LSD[13,14,17] is a classic and potent hallucinogen found in ergot, a fungus growing on rye and other grains and produced in illegal laboratories in the United States. It is sold on the street in tablets and capsules and in liquid form or on blotter paper with LSD added that can be sucked orally. Short-term side effects include rapid emotional swings; distortion of a person's ability to recognize reality, think rationally, or communicate with others; dilated pupils; dry mouth; enlarged pupils; hypertension; tachycardia; increased body temperature; diaphoresis; dizziness; loss of appetite; tremors; and sleeplessness. Long-term effects include frightening flashbacks, ongoing visual disturbances, acute anxiety, depression, and disorganized thinking.

Ecstasy/MDMA (3,4-methylenedioxy-methamphetamine). Ecstasy[13,14,18] is a synthetic drug made in illegal laboratories. With both hallucinogenic and stimulant effects, MDMA is often taken by adolescents and young adults. It first became popular in the 1980s with the all-night party scene (raves). It is available in different-colored tablets with imprinted logos, capsules, powder, and liquid. Users typically swallow it or crush and snort it, but it is occasionally smoked and rarely injected. It is often taken with alcohol or other drugs, takes effect within 30 to 45 minutes, and lasts 4 to 6 hours. Short-term effects include lowered inhibition, enhanced sensory perception, tachycardia, hypertension, muscle tension, nausea, faintness, chills or sweating, a loss of consciousness, or seizures. Long-term effects include long-lasting confusion; depression; problems with attention, memory, and sleep; anxiety; impulsivity; and decreased libido.

Mescaline (peyote). Mescaline[13,14,17] is an illegal substance found in the disk-shaped buttons in the crown of several cacti, including peyote. Mescaline has been used for centuries in northern Mexico and the southwestern United States as part of religious rites. It is extracted from peyote or produced synthetically. The fresh dried cactus buttons are chewed or soaked in water for the liquid. The buttons are sometimes ground into powder and put into capsules for swallowing or smoked with a leaf material such as tobacco or cannabis. Short-term effects include enhanced perception and feeling, hallucinations, euphoria followed by anxiety, increased body temperature/heart rate/blood pressure, diaphoresis, headaches, muscle weakness, and impaired coordination. Long-term effects are unknown.

Phencyclidine (PCP). PCP[13,14] is a dissociative drug originally developed as an anesthetic but discontinued due to serious adverse effects. Its common forms are white or colored powder, tablet, capsule, and a clear liquid. Common use includes injection, snorting, swallowing, and smoking (as a powder added to mint, parsley, oregano, or marijuana). Short-term effects include delusions, hallucinations, paranoia, problems in thinking, a sense of distance from one's environment, and anxiety. In low doses, the user often feels a slight increase in respiratory rate, increased blood pressure and heart rate, shallow breathing, facial flushing, diaphoresis, numbness of the hands or feet, and problems with movement. In high doses, the user experiences nausea, vomiting, drooling, loss of balance, dizziness, seizures, coma, and possibly death.

Psilocybin. Psilocybin[13,14,17] is a chemical found in certain types of fresh or dried mushrooms in tropical and subtropical regions of Mexico, South America, and the United States. The mushrooms have long, slender stems topped by caps with dark gills on the underside. They are ingested orally but can be brewed into a tea or added to other foods to mask their bitter flavor. These mushrooms produce similar effects to those of LSD, such as hallucinations, an altered perception of time, the inability to tell fantasy from reality, panic, muscle relaxation or weakness, problems with movement, enlarged pupils, nausea, vomiting, and drowsiness. Long-term effects include risk of flashbacks and memory problems. "Mushrooms" are illegal in the United States.

Inhalants

Inhalants are invisible, volatile substances found in common household products that produce chemical vapors.[9,14] More than 1000 products exist that are extremely dangerous when inhaled because they produce psychoactive or mind-altering effects. They include solvents, aerosols, gases, and nitrites found in household products.[19]

Solvents. Solvents include glue, paint thinners or removers, degreasers, dry cleaning fluid, gasoline, lighter fluid, correction fluids, and permanent markers.

Aerosols. Aerosols include spray paint, hair or deodorant sprays, aerosol computer cleaners, and vegetable oil sprays.

Gases. Gases include butane lighters, propane tanks, whipped cream aerosols, refrigerant gases, ether, chloroform, and nitrous oxide.

Nitrites. Nitrites include video head cleaner, room deodorizer, leather cleaner, and liquid aroma. They are inhaled by breathing fumes through the nose or mouth (sniffing, snorting, bagging, and huffing) most typically by middle school–aged children. Short-term effects from nitrite use include confusion, nausea, slurred speech, lack of coordination, euphoria, dizziness, drowsiness, disinhibition, lightheadedness, delusions, or headaches. Severe effects include death caused by heart failure (from sniffing butane, propane and other chemicals found in aerosols), and death from asphyxiation, suffocation, convulsions or seizures, coma, or choking. Long-term effects include liver and kidney damage; bone marrow damage; limb spasms caused by nerve damage; and brain damage from lack of oxygen that causes problems with thinking, movement, vision, and hearing. If nitrites are used during pregnancy, they can cause problems for the baby, such as low birth weight, bone problems, delayed behavioral development owing to brain problems, and altered metabolism and body composition.

Marijuana/Cannabis

Marijuana[13,14,20] is the most commonly used illegal drug in the United States[21]: 24 million people aged 12 years or older used it as of 2016. Although ED visits caused by marijuana use alone are rare, it is frequently used in combination with other drugs. Marijuana comes from the hemp plant, *Cannabis sativa,* in various forms (leaf, extracts, and oils). The main psychoactive chemical in marijuana is delta-9-tetrahydrocannabinol, commonly known as THC. The leaf variety is usually smoked as a cigarette (called a joint) or in a pipe or bong. It is also popular to mix it in foods or brew it as tea to consume orally. The extract or oil is smoked via water or oil pipe, vaporized via e-cigarette, eaten, or drunk (mixed in food or drinks). The DEA describes marijuana concentrate as a substance containing highly potent THC.[14] This concentrate is often referred to as oil or "710" ("OIL" spelled upside down and backward). THC levels in this oil can range from 40% to 80%, which is about four times stronger than what is found in a "high-grade" marijuana plant.[14,20] It is odorless, so it is difficult to detect in e-cigarettes/vape pens or food, and it is more difficult for parents, teachers, and law enforcement staff to know when it is being used.

Numerous states have legalized the sale and use of marijuana for medical or recreational purposes, but it is still illegal under federal law.[22] The short-term effects of marijuana use include sedation, bloodshot eyes, tachycardia, coughing from lung irritation, increased hunger, and decreased blood pressure. Long-term effects can include bronchitis, emphysema, bronchial asthma, or suppression of the immune system. Withdrawal symptoms include restlessness, irritability, difficulty sleeping, and decreased appetite. Withdrawal symptoms from high doses of marijuana include headache, shakiness, sweating, and abdominal pain and nausea, for which some patients seek ED care.

Narcotics

Heroin. Heroin[13,14] is an illegal opioid drug made from morphine, a natural substance extracted from the seed pod of various opium poppy plants. An estimated 948,000 people[23] were heroin users in 2016, a number that has been increasing since 2007. Many heroin users become addicted to prescription opioids first, have difficulty continuing to obtain the pills, and then switch to heroin, a less expensive and easier-to-obtain narcotic. The common form of heroin is a white or brownish powder or black sticky substance known as "black tar heroin." It is injected, smoked, or snorted. Short-term effects include euphoria, dry mouth, itching, nausea, vomiting, analgesia, and slowed breathing and heart rate. Long-term effects are collapsed veins, abscesses, pericarditis, constipation, and stomach cramps, liver or kidney disease, and pneumonia. If taken during pregnancy, it can result in miscarriage, low birth weight, or NAS. Withdrawal symptoms for heroin addicts are physically difficult and often bring them to seek treatment in the ED if they cannot get more of the drug. Symptoms include restlessness, muscle and bone pain, insomnia, diarrhea, vomiting, abdominal pain, or cold flashes with goose bumps when quitting "cold turkey". Heroin abuse has also been shown to contribute to increased transmission of infectious diseases, such as hepatitis and human immunodeficiency virus (HIV)/AIDS.

Treatment of opioid use disorder (OUD). Treatment of OUD[5,13,24] is complex. The heroin addict may present to the

ED in acute withdrawal, after an overdose, or with problems related to intravenous drug injection. Acute heroin intoxication is treated with administration of naloxone ventilatory support and intravenous fluids when appropriate. Naloxone administration can precipitate severe withdrawal in some patients, so careful monitoring is essential.[25] Post-ED treatment for heroin addiction is complex and involves the addict wanting to recover from addiction. This step often takes years and numerous failed treatment attempts before the addict achieves success. Opioid dependence and addiction to short-acting opioids such as heroin, morphine, and codeine, as well as semisynthetic opioids such as oxycodone and hydrocodone, are treated with methadone, buprenorphine, and naltrexone (short- and long-acting forms), along with ongoing behavioral therapy strategies.[5,13,26,27] People may safely take these medications for months, years, or even a lifetime. For patients presenting to the ED with OUD, research has shown that initiating medication-assisted treatment (MAT) with buprenorphine in the ED, with continuation in primary care, increased treatment retention and reduced self-reported illicit opioid use compared with brief intervention and referral.[26] The CDC noted that EDs are a critical entry point for treatment and prevention of overdose, with opportunities to improve opioid prescribing, respond to overdoses with overdose prevention education and naloxone training and distribution for friends/family, link patients to treatment and services, and start MAT in the ED.[24,26] See Table 50.1 and the "Treatment of Substance Use Disorder" section.

Stimulants

Cocaine. Cocaine[13,14] is a highly addictive illegal stimulant drug made from leaves of the coca plant from Bolivia, Peru, and Colombia. In 2016 the estimate of current users of cocaine was approximately 1.9 million people aged 12 years or older.[21] Cocaine is distributed as a white crystalline powder, and the cocaine base (crack) looks like small whitish rock crystals. The powder cocaine is snorted or injected after dissolving it in water. Cocaine base (crack) is smoked. Short-term health effects include narrowed blood vessels, enlarged pupils, increased body temperature/heart rate/blood pressure, headache, abdominal pain, nausea, euphoria, increased energy, alertness, insomnia, restlessness, anxiety, erratic and violent behavior, panic attacks, paranoia, psychosis, heart rhythm problems, heart attack, stroke, seizure, or coma. Other cocaine-related problems include agitation, paranoia, and epistaxis. Life-threatening emergencies related to cocaine include chest pain, seizures, severe hypertension, and stroke. Management of these life-threatening emergencies is no different in the patient who uses cocaine than in other patients with these problems. There is an increased risk for injury to self and others with these patients, so the ED nurse should decrease stimulation and monitor the patient carefully.

Khat. Khat[13,14] is pronounced "cot" and is made from a flowering evergreen shrub found in East Africa and southern Arabia. It contains the psychoactive chemicals cathinone and cathine that are commonly used for its stimulant effects. Khat use is illegal, but the plant is not controlled. It comes in fresh or dried leaves and is chewed or brewed as tea. Short-term effects include euphoria, increased alertness and arousal, increased blood pressure and heart rate, depression, paranoia, headaches, loss of appetite, insomnia, fine tremors, and loss of short-term memory. Long-term effects are gastrointestinal disorders, such as constipation, ulcers, and stomach inflammation, and increased risk of myocardial infarction.

Methamphetamine. Methamphetamine[13,14] is an extremely addictive CNS stimulant amphetamine drug made illegally from pseudoephedrine products. It comes in white powder or a pill; crystal meth looks like pieces of glass or shiny blue-white "rocks" of different sizes. It can be swallowed, snorted, injected, or smoked. Short-term effects include increased wakefulness and physical activity, decreased appetite, increases in respirations/heart rate/blood pressure/temperature, and arrhythmias. Chronic meth users can exhibit violent behavior, anxiety, confusion, memory loss, insomnia, and psychotic features such as paranoia, aggression, visual and auditory hallucinations, mood disturbances, and delusions, such as the sensation of insects creeping on or under their skin. They can also experience damage to the cardiovascular system, malnutrition, and severe dental problems. Babies born to pregnant women using methamphetamine can experience premature delivery, separation of the placenta from the uterus, low birth weight, lethargy, and heart and brain problems. Methamphetamine abuse has also been shown to contribute to increased transmission of infectious diseases, such as hepatitis and HIV/AIDS.

TOBACCO USE

Cigarette/Cigar/Pipe Tobacco

Nicotine[13] is an addictive stimulant in cigarettes and other forms of tobacco that increases dopamine release in the brain.[28] As of 2017, nearly 40 million US adults smoke cigarettes, and approximately 4.7 million middle school and high school students use at least one tobacco product, including e-cigarettes.[29] More than 16 million Americans live with a smoking-related disease.[29] Tobacco use is the leading cause of preventable disease, disability, and death in the United States. Cigarette smoking is the most common form of tobacco use in the United States and is on the decline. Cigarette smoking accounts for more than 480,000 deaths every year.[30] Secondhand smoke is also a significant health risk for children and adults. Nonsmokers exposed to secondhand smoke are 25% to 30% more likely to develop coronary heart disease, and many have died of heart disease or cancer.[31]

Hookah Tobacco

Another increasingly popular form of tobacco use among youth and college students over the past 20 years is the use of water pipes, commonly called hookahs. Hookah tobacco[13,32,33] is usually smoked in groups at homes or in hookah lounges/cafes using the same mouthpiece passed from person to person. Hookahs are used to smoke specially made tobacco in different flavors, such as apple, mint, cherry, chocolate, coconut,

TABLE 50.1 **Pharmacotherapies Used to Treat Opioid, Alcohol, and Tobacco Use Disorders.**

Medication	Used For	Dosage Information	Application
Buprenorphine-Naloxone (Suboxone)	OUD	Sublingual/buccal film 2 mg/0.5 mg, 4 mg/1 mg, 8 mg/2 mg, and 12 mg/3 mg Sublingual tablet: 1.4 mg/0.36 mg, 2 mg/0.5 mg, 2.9/0.71 mg, 5.7 mg/1.4 mg, 8 mg/2 mg, 8.6 mg/2.1 mg, 11.4 mg/2.9 mg Buccal film: 2.1 mg/0.3 mg, 4.2 mg/0.7 mg, 6.3 mg/1 mg	Used for detoxification or maintenance of abstinence for individuals aged 16 or older. Physicians who wish to prescribe buprenorphine must obtain a waiver from SAMHSA and be authorized to prescribe by the State.
Buprenorphine Hydrochloride (Subutex, Probuphine, Sublocade)	OUD	Sublingual tablet: 2 mg, 4 mg, 8 mg, and 12 mg Probuphine implants: 80 mg × four implants for a total of 320 mg	This formulation is indicated for treatment of opioid dependence and is preferred for induction. However, it is considered the preferred formulation for pregnant patients, patients with hepatic impairment, and patients with sensitivity to naloxone. It is also used for initiating treatment in patients transferring from methadone, in preference to products containing naloxone, because of the risk of precipitating withdrawal in these patients. For those already stable on low- to moderate-dose buprenorphine. The administration of the implant dosage form requires specific training and must be surgically inserted and removed.
Methadone (Dolophine, Methadose)	OUD	Tablet: 5 mg, 10 mg Tablet for suspension: 40 mg Oral concentrate: 10 mg/mL Oral solution: 5 mg/5 mL, 10 mg/5 mL Injection: 10 mg/mL	Methadone used for the treatment of opioid addiction in detoxification or maintenance programs is dispensed only by Opioid Treatment Programs (OTPs) certified by SAMHSA and approved by the designated state authority. Under federal regulations it can be used in persons under age 18 at the discretion of an OTP physician.
Naltrexone (Revia/ Vivitrol)	OUD and AUD	Revia: Tablet daily: 25 mg, 50 mg, and 100 mg Vivitrol: Extended-release injectable suspension monthly: 380 mg/vial	Provided by prescription. Naltrexone blocks opioid receptors, reduces cravings, and diminishes the rewarding effects of alcohol and opioids. Extended-release injectable naltrexone is recommended to prevent relapse to opioids or alcohol. The prescriber need not be a physician, but must be licensed and authorized to prescribe by the state. Has not been shown to affect the use of cocaine or other nonopioid drugs of abuse.
Acamprosate (Campral)	AUD	Delayed-release tablet three times a day: 333 mg	Acamprosate is used in the maintenance of alcohol abstinence. The prescriber need not be a physician, but must be licensed and authorized to prescribe by the state.
Disulfiram (Antabuse)	AUD	Tablet daily: 250 mg, 500 mg	When taken in combination with alcohol, disulfiram causes severe physical reactions, including nausea, flushing, and heart palpitations. The knowledge that such a reaction is likely if alcohol is consumed acts as a deterrent to drinking.

Continued

TABLE 50.1 Pharmacotherapies Used to Treat Opioid, Alcohol, and Tobacco Use Disorders.—cont'd

Medication	Used For	Dosage Information	Application
Bupropion Hydrochloride (Zyban)	TUD	Initial dose: 150 mg daily for 6 days, increased to 150 mg twice daily on day 7 through 7–12 weeks total.	It is recommended that treatment is started while the patient is still smoking and a "target stop date" set in the second week.
Varenicline (Chantix)	TUD	Days 1–3: 0.5 mg once daily Days 4–7: 0.5 mg twice daily Days 8–end of treatment: 1 mg daily for 12 weeks	This option provides three different quit approaches that vary from quitting on day 8, by day 35, and by day 84.
Nicotine replacement (patch, gum, lozenge)	TUD	21-mg patch/day weeks 1–6, then 14-mg patch/day weeks 7–8, then 7-mg patch/day weeks 9–10 Gum: Chew gum slowly until tingly feeling, then park gum in cheek until tingly feeling leaves. Then chew gum slowly until tingly feeling returns and park gum in cheek. Remove gum in 30 min. Do not repeat gum until 60 min passes. Lozenge: Dissolve slowly over 20–30 min without chewing; use at least 9 lozenges daily for 6 weeks but no more than 20/day	If 10 or fewer cigarettes/day, start patch with 14 mg for 6 weeks, then 7 mg for 2 weeks, then stop.

AUD, Alcohol use disorder; *OUD*, opioid use disorder; *SAMHSA*, Substance Abuse and Mental Health Services Administration; *TUD*, tobacco use disorder.

From US Department of Health and Human Services. Facing Addiction in America: The Surgeon General's Report on Alcohol, Drugs, and Health. Washington, DC: US Department of Health and Human Services; 2016. https://addiction.surgeongeneral.gov/sites/default/files/surgeon-generals-report.pdf. Accessed June 11, 2019.

National Institute on Drug Abuse. Treatment approaches for drug addiction. https://www.drugabuse.gov/publications/drugfacts/treatment-approaches-drug-addiction, Revised January 2019. Accessed June 11, 2019.

licorice, cappuccino, and watermelon. Many users think hookah smoking is less harmful than cigarette smoking, but it has many of the same health risks, if not more. Because of the way the hookah is used when the tobacco is exposed to high heat from burning charcoal, the users tend to absorb more of the toxic chemicals that are also found in cigarette smoke than cigarette smokers do. Use of these pipes is linked to lung/oral/bladder cancer and respiratory and heart diseases.

Electronic Cigarettes

The use of e-cigarettes[13,34] by adolescents and adults has escalated in the United States. E-cigarettes are known by different names, such as e-cigs, e-hookahs, vape pens, vapes, mods, tank systems, and electronic nicotine delivery systems (ENDS). Most e-cigarettes contain nicotine, which is addictive and also toxic to developing fetuses. E-cigarette aerosol can contain chemicals harmful to the lungs. E-cigarettes have also caused unintended injuries when defective e-cigarette batteries have ignited or exploded.[35] Children and adults have been poisoned by swallowing, breathing, or absorbing e-cigarette liquid through their skin or eyes.

Smokeless Tobacco

Smokeless tobacco[13,36,37] is defined as any finely cut, ground, powdered, or leaf tobacco intended to be placed in the oral cavity. There are numerous types of smokeless tobacco such as chewing tobacco (loose leaf, plug, and twist/roll), dissolvables (lozenges, sticks, strips, orbs), and snuff (moist, dry and packets called snus). Using smokeless tobacco can lead to nicotine addiction; cancer of the mouth (tongue, cheek, gums), esophagus, and pancreas; diseases of the mouth, such as gum disease and tooth loss; increased risks for early delivery and stillbirth when used during pregnancy; nicotine poisoning in children; and increased risk for death from heart disease and stroke.

Medications for Tobacco Use Disorder

Together with the use of behavioral therapies for tobacco use disorder (TUD), there are three medications approved to treat tobacco use disorders (See Table 50.1).

Nicotine Replacement Therapy

Nicotine replacement therapy (NRT) includes medications available OTC or by prescription and is used to treat nicotine withdrawal symptoms when a person is quitting nicotine substances.[9,13,38] These medications assist with reducing nicotine withdrawal symptoms such as irritability, anger, depression, anxiety, and decreased concentration. Such OTC medications tend to have little effect on craving for cigarettes because nicotine delivered through chewing gum containing nicotine, via transdermal patch, or in lozenges has a slower onset of action than does the systemic delivery of nicotine through smoked tobacco. The nicotine inhaler and nasal spray deliver nicotine more rapidly to the brain and work faster, so they are available only by prescription.

Bupropion Hydrochloride (Zyban)

Bupropion hydrochloride (Zyban)[13,38] was originally developed and approved as an antidepressant and was also found to help people quit smoking. This medication can be used at the same dose for nicotine withdrawal and depression treatment.

Varenicline Tartrate (Chantix)

Varenicline tartrate (Chantix)[13,38] is a nicotine partial agonist that reduces craving for cigarettes and has been helpful in smoking cessation. The smoker continues to smoke during the first week of taking the medication, and it is advised that he or she stops using nicotine on the established quit date. This medication is taken for a 12-week treatment period. Some users complain that they experience intense dreams/nightmares and they quit using the medication. Bupropion and varenicline are available only as prescription medications. Counseling and medication together are effective for treating tobacco dependence and more effective than using either one alone.

ALCOHOL USE

The excessive use of alcohol[9,38,39] is a significant public health issue in the United States. Ethyl alcohol (ethanol) is an intoxicating ingredient in beer, wine, and liquor that is produced by fermenting yeast, sugar, and starches.[13] About 17 million adults aged 18 and older currently have an alcohol use disorder (AUD) affecting 1 in 10 children who live in a home with a parent who has a drinking problem.[13] Alcohol is a widely used and abused depressant drug, and its effects vary from person to person, depending on a variety of factors, including amount consumed, frequency of drinking, age, one's health status, and family history. There are three levels of drinking identified: moderate alcohol consumption, binge drinking, and heavy use.[39] Moderate consumption is defined as up to one drink per day for women and up to two drinks per day for men. Binge drinking is a pattern of drinking that brings blood alcohol concentration (BAC) levels to 0.08g/dL. This happens after four drinks for women and five drinks for men in about 2 hours. Heavy use is binge drinking on 5 or more days in the past month.

Alcohol's effects on the body are numerous and have been written about for decades. Short-term effects may include injuries and risky behavior, including drunk driving, inappropriate sexual behavior, impaired judgment, coordination and reflexes, slurred speech, memory problems, and death. Long-term effects of overusing alcohol affect the whole body and include arrhythmias; stroke; hypertension; cirrhosis and fibrosis of the liver; and mouth, throat, liver and/or breast cancer.[40] Women who drink alcohol excessively can also have pregnancy-related effects such as fetal alcohol syndrome (FAS).[39]

Treatment for AUD

As a result of significant advances in the field of alcohol research over the past 60 years, there are a variety of methods available for treating AUD.[9,13,27,38] Providers usually collaborate with the person to determine the best combination of treatment (medications, mutual support groups, and/or behavioral therapies). The following three medications are approved by the FDA to treat alcohol use disorder:

- Acamprosate (Campral) reduces symptoms of protracted withdrawal (cravings) and has been shown to help those who have achieved abstinence go on to maintain abstinence for several weeks to months.
- Naltrexone (Revia) blocks the effects of opioids and is also used to reduce cravings.
- Disulfiram (Antabuse) changes the way the body metabolizes alcohol, resulting in an unpleasant reaction that includes flushing, nausea, and/or vomiting if a person takes the medication and then consumes alcohol. See Table 50.1 for further information on these medications.

TREATMENT OF SUBSTANCE USE DISORDER

The ED nurse's primary responsibility is to treat the acute illness or injury and also to address the need for detoxification and/or rehabilitation therapy. The ED nurse must be acutely aware of his or her role in assessment and identification of SUD so that medical treatment and/or referral can be initiated to aid in recovery. The diagnosis of a SUD is made by a trained professional based on 11 symptoms defined in the fifth edition of the *Diagnostic and Statistical Manual of Mental Disorders* (DSM-5).[8] Multiple components are commonly used when individualizing a treatment program based on the type of SUD, including MAT,[13,38] inpatient and residential treatment, individual and group counseling, intensive outpatient treatment, partial hospital programs, case or care management, recovery support services, 12-step programs (i.e., AA, NA), peer support groups, and drug courts, which are becoming increasingly effective.[39] Medications approved by the FDA to treat opioid, tobacco, and alcohol use disorders are in Table 50.1. Other therapies noted earlier are used in developing the individually identified treatment plan.

NURSING CONSIDERATIONS

Emergency nurses should continue to educate themselves and others about substance abuse disorders. Drug abuse knows no social boundaries and is rampant in the United States. The Emergency Nurses Association has a position statement, *Patients With Substance Use Disorders and Addiction in the Emergency Care Setting.*[41] It is important for ED nurses to provide care and services:

> *Emergency nurses participate in the development of emergency department management plans and prescriptive guidelines designed to address the immediate needs of patients with substance use disorders, abuse, and addiction and provide them with appropriate treatment.*

> *As part of the emergency discharge planning phase, nurses educate individuals and their families affected by substance use disorders, abuse, and addiction regarding prevention, treatment options, and rehabilitation services currently available in the community....*[41]

If you suspect the patient is abusing drugs, report your findings to the physician managing the patient's care so that appropriate management can be initiated. Screen all patients for substance use. Request a urine or blood specimen to screen for drugs of abuse for patients who present with unusual or erratic behavior. Ensure a safe environment for the patient, visitors, and staff working in the ED. The potential for violence increases in individuals under the influence of drugs. Patients often present for treatment of injuries associated with high-risk behaviors, such as assaults, penetrating trauma, blunt trauma, and sexually transmitted infections rather than drug abuse. Treat potentially life-threatening injuries and then evaluate the patient for drug-related problems. Patients with acute signs and symptoms of drug abuse need medical intervention for the effects of the drug taken. Consultation or referral to a drug treatment center is indicated for substance use treatment after the patient is medically cleared.

SUDs remain a significant challenge for emergency nurses. The emergency nurse must be knowledgeable of licit and illicit drug abuse warning signs. Caring for this patient population is challenging and consumes many emergency care resources. Emergency nurses should be prepared to advocate for, as well as treat and educate, patients who experience substance use disorders and injuries by having resources available for patients and families.

REFERENCES

1. National Institute on Drug Abuse. Trends & statistics. https://www.drugabuse.gov/related-topics/trends-statistics, Updated April 2017. Accessed June 12, 2019.
2. President's Commission on Combating Drug Addiction and the Opioid Crisis. *Final Report Draft, The President's Commission on Combating Drug Addiction and the Opioid Crisis.* https://www.whitehouse.gov/sites/whitehouse.gov/files/images/Final_Report_Draft_11-1-2017.pdf, Published November 1, 2017. Accessed June 12, 2019.
3. Centers for Disease Control and Prevention, National Center for Health Statistics. Provisional Counts of Drug Overdose Deaths, as of 8/6/2017. https://www.cdc.gov/nchs/data/health_policy/monthly-drug-overdose-death-estimates.pdf, Published 2017. Accessed June 12, 2019.
4. Hedegaard H, Warner M, Miniño AM. *Drug Overdose Deaths in the United States, 1999–2016.* Hyattsville, MD: National Center for Health Statistics; 2017. NCHS Data Brief No. 294. https://www.cdc.gov/nchs/products/databriefs/db294.htm. Accessed June 12, 2019.
5. National Institute on Drug Abuse. Drugs, brains, and behavior: the science of addiction. https://www.drugabuse.gov/publications/drugs-brains-behavior-science-addiction, Published July 1, 2014. Updated July 2018. Accessed June 12, 2019.
6. McQueen K, Murphy-Oikonen J. Neonatal abstinence syndrome. *N Engl J Med.* 2016;375:2468–2479. https://doi.org/10.1056/NEJMra1600879.
7. National Institute on Drug Abuse. Dramatic increases in maternal opioid use and neonatal abstinence syndrome. https://www.drugabuse.gov/related-topics/trends-statistics/infographics/dramatic-increases-in-maternal-opioid-use-neonatal-abstinence-syndrome, Published September 2015. Updated January 2019. Accessed June 12, 2019.
8. American Psychiatric Association. *Diagnostic and Statistical Manual of Mental Disorders (DSM-5).* 5th ed. Washington, DC: American Psychiatric Publishing; 2013.
9. US Department of Health and Human Services. *Facing Addiction in America: The Surgeon General's Report on Alcohol, Drugs, and Health.* Washington, DC: US Department of Health and Human Services; 2016. https://addiction.surgeongeneral.gov/sites/default/files/surgeon-generals-report.pdf, Accessed June 12, 2019.
10. Volkow ND, Koob G, McLellan AT. Neurobiologic advances from the brain disease model of addiction. *N Engl J Med.* 2016;374(4):363–371. https://doi.org/10.1056/NEJMra1511480.
11. Bourzac K. Neuroscience: rewiring the brain. *Nature.* 2015;522:S50–S52. https://www.nature.com/articles/522S50a.pdf. Accessed June 12, 2019.
12. National Institute on Drug Abuse. Chart of Evidence-Based Screening Tools for Adults and Adolescents. https://www.drugabuse.gov/nidamed-medical-health-professionals/screening-tools-resources/chart-screening-tools. Updated June 2018. Accessed June 12, 2019.
13. National Institute on Drug Abuse. Commonly abused drugs charts. https://www.drugabuse.gov/drugs-abuse/commonly-abused-drugs-charts, Published January 2018. Updated July 2018. Accessed June 12, 2019.
14. Drug Enforcement Administration and US Department of Justice. *Drugs of Abuse: A DEA Resource Guide*; 2017. https://www.dea.gov/sites/default/files/2018-06/drug_of_abuse.pdf. Accessed June 12, 2019.
15. National Institute on Drug Abuse. Synthetic Cathinones ("Bath Salts"). https://www.drugabuse.gov/publications/drugfacts/synthetic-cathinones-bath-salts, Updated February 2018. Accessed June 12, 2019.
16. National Institute on Drug Abuse. Synthetic Cannabinoids (K2/Spice). https://www.drugabuse.gov/publications/drugfacts/synthetic-cannabinoids-k2spice, Updated February 2018. Accessed June 12, 2019.
17. National Institute on Drug Abuse. How do Hallucinogens (LSD, Psilocybin, Peyote, DMT, and Ayahuasca) Affect the Brain and Body? https://www.drugabuse.gov/publications/hallucinogens-dissociative-drugs/how-do-hallucinogens-lsd-psilocybin-peyote-dmt-ayahuasca-affect-brain-body, Published February 2015. Accessed June 12, 2019.
18. Passie T, Benzenhofer U. The history of MDMA as an underground drug in the United States, 1960–1979. *J Psychoactive Drugs.* 2016;48(2):67–75. https://www.semanticscholar.org/paper/The-History-of-MDMA-as-an-Underground-Drug-in-the-Passie-Benzenhöfer/5d2b3c8c2b030ca828cff15c2ef64bce6cd294d4. Accessed June 12, 2019.
19. National Institute on Drug Abuse. Inhalants. https://www.drugabuse.gov/publications/drugfacts/inhalants, Updated February 2017. Accessed June 12, 2019.
20. Substance Abuse and Mental Health Services Administration. Know the risks of Marijuana. https://www.samhsa.gov/marijuana, Updated November 21, 2016. Accessed June 13, 2019.

21. Substance Abuse and Mental Health Services Administration. *Key Substance use and Mental Health Indicators in the United States: Results from the 2016 National Survey on Drug Use and Health*. Rockville, MD: Center for Behavioral Health Statistics and Quality; 2017. https://www.samhsa.gov/data/report/key-substance-use-and-mental-health-indicators-united-states-results-2016-national-survey. HHS Publication SMA 17-5044, NSDUH Series H-52. Accessed June 13, 2019.
22. Governing. State Marijuana laws in 2019 map; 2019. http://www.governing.com/gov-data/state-marijuana-laws-map-medical-recreational.html. Accessed June 13, 2019.
23. Adams, K.T., et al. Substance Abuse Center for Behavioral Health Statistics and Quality. Results from the 2016 National Survey on Drug Use and Health: Detailed Tables. SAMHSA. https://www.samhsa.gov/data/sites/default/files/NSDUH-DetTabs-2016/NSDUH-DetTabs-2016.htm, Published September 7, 2017. Accessed June 13, 2019.
24. Centers for Disease Control and Prevention. Opioid Overdoses Treated in Emergency departments. www.cdc.gov/vitalsigns/opioid-overdoses/. Published March 2018. Accessed June 13, 2019.
25. National Institute on Drug Abuse. Opioid Overdose Reversal with Naloxone (Narcan, Evzio). https://www.drugabuse.gov/related-topics/opioid-overdose-reversal-naloxone-narcan-evzio, Updated April 2018. Accessed June 13, 2019.
26. D'Onofrio GD, Chawarski MC, O'Connor PG, et al. Emergency department–initiated buprenorphine with opioid dependence with continuation in primary care: outcomes during and after intervention. *J Gen Intern Med*. 2017;32(6):660–666.
27. Substance Abuse and Mental Health Services Administration. Medication-Assisted Treatment (MAT). https://www.samhsa.gov/medication-assisted-treatment, Updated April 26, 2019. Accessed June 13, 2019.
28. National Institute on Drug Abuse. Tobacco, Nicotine, and E-Cigarettes. https://www.drugabuse.gov/publications/research-reports/tobacco-nicotine-e-cigarettes/nicotine-addictive, Updated January 2018. Accessed June 13, 2019.
29. Centers for Disease Control and Prevention. Smoking & tobacco use. Data and statistics. https://www.cdc.gov/tobacco/data_statistics/index.htm, Updated February 28, 2019. Accessed.
30. Centers for Disease Control and Prevention. Current Cigarette Smoking and Tobacco use Among Adults in the United States. https://www.cdc.gov/tobacco/data_statistics/fact_sheets/adult_data/cig_smoking/index.htm, Updated February 4, 2019. Accessed June 13, 2019.
31. US Department of Health and Human Services. *The Health Consequences of Involuntary Exposure to Tobacco Smoke: A Report of the Surgeon General*. Atlanta, GA: Centers for Disease Control and Prevention, National Center for Chronic Disease Prevention and Health Promotion, Office on Smoking and Health; 2006. https://www.ncbi.nlm.nih.gov/books/NBK44324/. Accessed June 13, 2019.
32. American Lung Association. *An Emerging Deadly Trend: Waterpipe Tobacco Use*. http://www.lungusa2.org/embargo/slati/Trendalert_Waterpipes.pdf, Published 2007. Accessed June 13, 2019.
33. Centers for Disease Control and Prevention. Smoking & Tobacco use: Hookahs. https://www.cdc.gov/tobacco/data_statistics/fact_sheets/tobacco_industry/hookahs/, Published 2018. Accessed June 13, 2019.
34. Centers for Disease Control and Prevention. Smoking and Tobacco use: Electronic Cigarettes. https://www.cdc.gov/tobacco/basic_information/e-cigarettes/index.htm, Published 2018. Accessed June 13, 2019.
35. US Department of Health and Human Services. *E-Cigarette Use Among Youth and Young Adults: A Report of the Surgeon General*. Rockville, MD: US Department of Health and Human Services; 2016. https://www.cdc.gov/tobacco/data_statistics/sgr/e-cigarettes/pdfs/2016_sgr_entire_report_508.pdf. Accessed June 13, 2019.
36. World Health Organization. *IARC Monographs on the Evaluation of Carcinogenic Risks to Humans. Vol 89: Smokeless Tobacco and Some Tobacco-Specific N-Nitrosamines*. Lyon, France: International Agency for Research on Cancer; 2007.
37. Piano MR, Benowitz NL, Fitzgerald GA, et al. Impact of smokeless tobacco products on cardiovascular disease: implications for policy, prevention, and treatment: a policy statement from the American Heart Association. *Circulation*. 2010;122(15):1520–1544.
38. National Institute on Drug Abuse. Treatment Approaches for Drug Addiction. https://www.drugabuse.gov/publications/drugfacts/treatment-approaches-drug-addiction, Updated January 2019. Accessed June 13, 2019.
39. Substance Abuse and Mental Health Services Administration. Behavioral health treatments and services. https://www.samhsa.gov/treatment, Published 2015. Updated January 30, 2019. Accessed June 13, 2019.
40. National Institute on Alcohol Abuse and Alcoholism. Alcohol's Effects on the Body. https://www.niaaa.nih.gov/alcohol-health/alcohols-effects-body, Published 2018. Accessed June 13, 2019.
41. Emergency Nurses Association. *ENA Position Statement: Patients with Substance use Disorders and Addiction in the Emergency Care Setting*. Des Plaines, IL: Emergency Nurses Association; 2016. https://www.ena.org/docs/default-source/resource-library/practice-resources/position-statements/patientswithsubstanceuse.pdf?sfvrsn=6c33cad2_6. Accessed June 13, 2019.

51

Sexual Assault

Colleen Mary Pedrotty

Every 98 seconds, an American is sexually assaulted. The definition of sexual assault varies depending on the state.[1] In 2011, the Federal Bureau of Investigation (FBI) defined sexual assault to include both genders and oral and anal assault.[2] The Uniform Crime Reporting (UCR) definition of sexual assault is "Penetration, no matter how slight, of the vagina or anus with any body part or object or oral penetration by sex organ of another person, without consent of the person."[2] This definition, even though more comprehensive than before, does not address force. Force can also refer to the perpetrator's use of emotion, psychological factors, or manipulation to coerce the victim.[3] Often, victims will consent to the act for fear of threats to family.[3] This often happens in spousal sexual assault cases.

The second and even less defined term in sexual assault is the consent. The Rape, Abuse & Incest National Network (RAINN) has consent listed by individual states, each with its own definition.[1] Some states have a one-paragraph definition; other states have several pages. This disconnect often makes for difficulty in prosecution of perpetrators, especially in case of intimate partner rapes. Rape is not a crime of passion, but about power and control.[3] Conventional wisdom holds that women who dress provocatively draw attention to themselves and put themselves in harm's way.[3] Victimology studies the harms caused to victims in commission of crimes and the relative scope for compensation to the victim.[4]

The term "victimization" refers to a process whereby an external force comes in contact with a person, rendering that person to feel pain, sometimes causing injury, either of which can be short-lived or which might cause extended suffering and sometimes death.[4] According to the Bureau of Justice Statistics, in 2015 the annual number of victimizations in the United States is about 5 million.[5] Four theories are presently being looked at as possible causes of victimization: victim precipitation theory, lifestyle theory, deviant place theory, and routine activities theory.[3]

Victim precipitation theory suggests that the victim may actually initiate, either passively or actively, the criminal act ultimately leading to injury or death.[3,4,6] Lifestyle theory suggests individuals are targeted based on their lifestyle choices, which expose them to criminal offenders and situations in which crimes may be committed.[3,4,6] The deviant place theory purports that greater exposure to dangerous places makes one more likely to become the victim of a crime.[3,4] Routine activities theory suggests that the rate of victimization is through a set of situations reflecting the routines of typical individuals, availability of suitable targets, absence of capable guardians, and the presence of motivated offenders. According to routine activities theory, the presence of one or more high-risk situations creates a higher risk of victimization.[3,4,6]

A more accepted theory, which does not include victim blaming, finds its roots in the writings of criminologists such as Marvin Wolfgang[6] and suggests that the interactions of the victim make him or her vulnerable to a crime. Recent work by the World Society of Victimology (WSV) focused on victimization. The purpose of this society is to ensure victims' basic rights with fairness, respect, dignity, notification of court proceedings, a chance to be present for important judicial proceedings, prompt return of stolen property, protection from intimidation and harassment, and restitution and/or compensation for the crime.[7] This shift has changed the way society looks at the victim of sexual assault, shifting some of the focus off of blaming the victim and placing blame on the perpetrator.[7] Again, sexual assault is not a crime of passion, but about power and control. Rape and sexual assault are motivated by interpersonal aggression and by conflict and psychological issues.[1]

There are different types of rapists, such as the power-assertive rapist, the anger/anger excitement rapist, the sadistic rapist, and opportunist, to name just a few.[3,8,9] The power-assertive rapist is the most common type. The objective is to control but not harm. This rapist will be repetitive and attack frequently. The most dangerous types are anger excitement and/or sadistic rapists. These rapists want to harm the victim. Murder is the ultimate gratification. Most rapists have no race or gender classification.[3,8,9] However, the classification of the crime by the FBI does have a purpose, which is to standardize terminology, facilitate communication, educate, and develop a database.[2]

Anyone can be a victim of sexual assault. Findings from research indicate that 17% to 18% of women and 3% of men experience a rape or attempted rape in their life.[2] In rural settings, incidence of rape can be as high as 30%.[1] The response to these numbers has dramatically changed the approach to sexual assault by the medical and legal system. Before the 1970s, patients who were sexually assaulted were treated by untrained medical personal.[10] Victims often sat in emergency department (ED) waiting rooms for hours. Treatment varied from one ED to another, and there was little communication between law enforcement, the medical team, and prosecutors.[10] The US Department of Justice believes that only 15.8% to 35% of sexual assaults are reported to the police.[2] According to RAINN, some of the reasons victims did not report were as follows: 20% feared retaliation, 13% believed the police would not do anything to help, and 2% believed the police could not help them.[1] Rape against males was not placed in the FBI definition until 2012. Although rapes of men are less frequent than of women, they are just as devastating.[2] About 3% of American men have experienced an attempted or completed rape.[3] A 2011 survey reported that lesbian and bisexual women are three times more likely than heterosexual women to be sexually assaulted, and gay men may be 15 times as likely as heterosexual men.[11] Lesbian, gay, bisexual, transgender, and queer (LGBTQ) persons and heterosexual men are sexually assaulted for the same reasons as heterosexual women. All survivors need the same level of compassion and recognition.[11]

MYTHS AND MISCONCEPTIONS

Many of the misconceptions surrounding rape are that the victims did something to make them responsible for the end result.[3] Another myth is that if victims drink too much or uses drugs, they deserve to be raped. The law is clear that the person must have the capacity to give consent. Alcohol and drugs take away the ability to give informed consent. Another misconception is that rape occurs only if the perpetrator uses physical force and also that there should be injuries. Very few sexual assaults cause physical injury. Sometimes the perpetrator will use threats of harm or harm to others. Some victims are unable to fight due to shock or believe that fighting will make it worse. Another myth about rape is that if two people had consensual sex with each other before, it is always okay. Consent must be given every time people engage in sex. One of the worst myths about sexual assault and rape is that people who were sexually abused as children are likely to become the abuser. The majority of those who are abused will never sexually assault another person. Women are most likely to be raped after dark by a stranger, so some believe women should not go out after dark. Rape is about control and power.[3]

RAPE-TRAUMA SYNDROME

Rape-trauma syndrome is a cluster of reactions that are emotional, physical, and behavioral and are seen in victims of attempted or completed rape. The syndrome, first described in 1974, has three stages. The acute stage is intense, and the victim expresses disbelief and shock. Victim responses vary in a range of emotional reactions such as restlessness, tenseness, crying, or sobbing. Another victim can appear calm, composed, or with a subdued affect. This stage occurs in the days or weeks after the rape. The second stage is the outward adjustment stage in which the victim seems to resume normal life but suffers with internal turmoil. Signs can be numbness, disorganization, dulled senses, vomiting, obsession, hysteria, sleep disorders, and anxiety. This stage can last months and even years after a rape. The third stage is renormalization, at which point the survivors recognize rape is no longer the focus of their life.[12]

The Sexual Assault Survivor in the Emergency Department

When the survivor arrives at the ED, the victim needs to be triaged as a high-priority, high-risk level 2 patient due to extreme physical or psychological distress.[13] The staff needs to develop a trusting relationship, listen to the patient, and explain what will happen during the examination. Victims should be triaged in a private area. The only questions to ask are about the pertinent medical history and the overall complaint. The nurse should put all statements in quotes. Specific questions requiring the patient to relive the assault are not needed. Determining the presence of physical trauma requiring immediate treatment is the initial priority. If a sexual assault response team (SART) is available, it should be notified. If not, follow the facility policies and procedures.[3] Placing victims immediately into a private treatment space helps them feel safe.

The extent of emotional injury cannot be estimated. Each person's response to a sexual assault is different. Individuals may laugh, cry, tell a joke, or become catatonic. Patients may blame themselves for fighting back or for not fighting back. Inform the patients that their actions helped get them through the ordeal, regardless of what action was taken. Patients may believe they caused the rape by trusting the perpetrator. Remind the survivor that they did not cause the assault. All of these reactions are signs of the trauma. Remind survivors of their bravery in coming forward and in stopping the cycle of the perpetrator. The more power given back to the victim, the less the feeling of helplessness. There should be clear guidelines in taking care of the victim that remain the same for all victims.[3,7]

Most states have a kit with a step-by-step instruction sheet and standard documentation forms.[14] Copies must be given to law enforcement, the criminalistics laboratory, and the hospital. This standardized paperwork and kit help ensure evidence is collected in the same way.[14]

Sexual Assault Response Team

The SART is a specialized team developed to address the lack of support for victims of sexual assault. Before the movement to use SARTs, nontrained physicians and nurses would care for the victims of sexual assault.[2,3] The victim would spend countless hours sitting in the waiting room. The nurses and physicians had no guidelines or understanding of the crime these victims endured. The lack of care led to the formation of a specialized, trained team. The team is identified as SART, which consists of a sexual assault examiner (SANE), a rape crisis advocate, law enforcement officers, and legal counsel personnel. Some programs have started with a nurse shadowing a physician but did not include formal training. In 1992 the International Forensic Nurses Association (IFNA) was established to provide specialized guidelines for SANEs.[15]

The SANE receives specialized training in using interviewing techniques, conducting an examination, collecting material for a forensic kit, providing sexually transmitted infection (STI) prophylaxis, offering pregnancy prevention medication, and giving discharge instructions. The SANE works with specialized advocates and law enforcement to make the experience more victim centered. Law enforcement and SANEs conduct interviews together if possible to prevent inconsistency and decrease victim fatigue.[3,5] SANE personnel become the medical and legal experts in the field of sexual assault. Often, SANEs are on call and respond when a sexual assault victim presents to the ED or free-standing clinics. This in no way means that EDs without SARTs cannot take care of the victims.

Individual hospitals can educate and train selected nurses to care for sexual assault survivors. Identified personnel may conduct the complete evidentiary examination independently or in conjunction with a physician. Department policies are developed to reflect this practice.

The Examination Begins

After the victim is triaged and placed in a safe, secure room, a medical screening examination must be done to rule out an emergency medical condition. One nurse should be assigned to care for this victim. The victim should be given the option to contact a support person, and an advocate from the rape crisis team should be called, if agreed upon by the victim. Law enforcement personnel may be asked to leave during the physical examination. Privacy is of the utmost importance.[13]

Consent

Consent in an emergency situation is assumed. In the case of sexual assault, consent for care and treatment related to the assault should be obtained as soon as possible.[1,3] The nurse can allow the victim to read the consent form, or the nurse can read the consent form to the victim. The consent form can be overwhelming to the victim. The victim is consenting to more than just care but also to photographs of injury. The victim has the right to refuse any part of the examination or photographs.

Some victims are too young to consent. Each state has its own standards for care of a minor. Medical personnel should be aware of the age of consent in the state where they practice. The victim can also agree to examination but can remain a Jane Doe for the purposes of the medical record.

Never force the victim into the consent. Victims should not be forced to sign any part of the consent. This is a form of victimization. Victims must be informed if the hospital is required to notify law enforcement. Obtaining consent can be delayed if the victim is intoxicated or drugged. Care is still administered, but the forensic examination and interview may be delayed.[1,3]

History

Medical history should be obtained before the examination is started.[3] This history helps the nurse determine the type of evidence collection required. Examinations performed within 72 hours of the sexual assault are optimal, but evidence has been obtained up to 5 to 6 days afterward. Questions should be asked in a way the victim understands. Never change the victim's words to make the statement more professional. Write only what the patient tells you and use quotes whenever possible. The reason for the forensic interview is to guide the examination, as per the victim's account. It allows the examiner to focus on the forensic collection of the evidence and where to look for additional evidence. If the victim was drugged or intoxicated, the examiner must complete a comprehensive, thorough examination.[3]

If drug-facilitated sexual assault (DFSA) is suspected, a special collection container is used, which is usually not part of the kit. The DFSA specimen collection requires blood and urine samples because most drugs have a short half-life. Signs and symptoms commonly found in patients who have experienced a drug-facilitated sexual assault include the following:

- recalls having a drink but cannot recall what happened afterward,
- suspects someone had sex with them but cannot remember the entire incident or cannot remember with whom,
- feels more intoxicated then usual after drinking the same amount of alcohol as in the past,
- wakes up without underwear or an article of clothing,
- wakes up with loss of memory or account for a time period.[16]

The number one substance used in DFSA is ethanol. So, when questioning a victim with the signs and symptoms in the preceding list, ask how many drinks the victim had over what period of time. Ask what the victim was drinking. Was there anything different about the drink? Was the drink ever left unobserved? This approach can help corraborate the victim's history. Obtain a urine specimen for drug and pregnancy testing as soon as possible after the victim arrives. Remember that the half-life is short for many DFSA drugs.[17]

Physical Examination and Evidence Collection

Before asking the victim to undress, note the person's appearance and the condition of their clothing. The victim is asked to stand on a white paper sheet and undress. Place each article of clothing in paper bags. Label each bag with a description of the clothing article and victim demographics. Unless they are a part of the evidence, shoes and coats are not submitted to the crime laboratory. All articles must be dry before inserting them in the bag. If clothing is saturated with blood or other secretions, drying may occur in the police evidence room.[3] All bags must be sealed with evidence tape. The paper drape that the victim undressed on is also placed in a paper evidence bag. All evidence is turned over to law enforcement, and nurses must make sure to document the number of evidence bags given to the officer.[3,14]

The victim is then dressed in a gown and a head-to-toe assessment is done, looking for signs of injury. The use of a Wood's lamp or ultraviolet light, if available, can be used to uncover trace evidence. Semen may appear as orange or blue-green on the skin. The area should be swabbed with a moistened cotton-tipped applicator. Injuries may appear as a red mark but over time will change color. Follow-up photographs may be necessary at a later date and are usually done by the police department. Next, an oral (buccal) swab will be obtained for the victim's deoxyribonucleic acid (DNA) or, in some areas, blood is obtained. Then an oral swab is collected if oral penetration occurred. Fingernail scrapings are also collected for perpetrator DNA.[3,14]

Documentation of all injuries should include the color and size of injuries such as bruising, scratches, laceration, abrasions, bite marks, and swelling. Bruising is not staged or dated because such a practice is very inaccurate. Use body figures, usually available in the sexual assault kit, to document the location, size, and description of injuries. Caution should be taken when reporting Wood's lamp findings because other materials such as lint also fluoresce. Oral swabs are taken for evidence of semen and as a reference sample. Reference samples include saliva, blood, semen, pubic hair, and body hair. The criminalistics laboratory results of these reference samples are compared with specimens from potential suspects.[3,14]

For the female patient, the pelvic examination begins with a visual examination of the external structures. The external genitalia are examined for signs of injury or foreign materials and swabbed for semen or saliva. If the patient is male, the scrotum and penis need to be swabbed. For females, the hymen is examined and, if not visualized, a urinary catheter can be inserted with the balloon inflated just past the hymenal tissue. A speculum is inserted so the vaginal wall and cervix can be inspected. Swabs are then taken of the vaginal wall and cervix.[3,14] All swabs and slides must be labeled to identify the patient and the source along with the time, date, location of collection, and the name of the person collecting the evidence.

Photographs are then used to detect and document genital trauma.[3] The colposcope provides magnification and visualization but is not always available. Documentation should indicate if the injury is apparent without use of the colposcope.

Pubic hair can be collected. Pubic hair is no longer pulled or cut, in most states. During the pelvic examination, swabs and slides are taken.[3]

Rectal examination and inspection are done.[3] Swabs are obtained. Anoscopy is performed if sodomy has occurred or is suspected. The swabs and/or slides should be placed in a drying device, if available. The specimens are then bagged and labeled and placed in the kit. The nurse should limit handling of evidence and take care not to leave any of his or her own DNA on the evidence. A good way to do that is frequent changing of gloves.[3] All equipment contacting evidence must be cleaned.

Chain of Custody

Chain of custody must be maintained during and after the examination. The nurse must be able to prove the evidence was never left alone and that there was no tampering.[3] Documentation in the record must reflect chain of custody information. The evidence needs to be transferred from nurse to law enforcement officer. The kit must be signed for by the officers and the nurse. All transfers of evidence must be included in the paperwork. Evidence must be properly stored in the police evidence room at the correct temperature.

BOX 51.1 Medication Prophylaxis in Sexual Assault.

Ceftriaxone (Rocephin), a third-generation cephalosporin, 250 mg intramuscularly in a single dose for treatment of possible exposure to gonorrhea

OR

Cefixime (Suprax) 400 mg orally in a single dose and metronidazole (Flagyl) 2 g orally in a single dose for treatment of possible bacterial vaginosis and trichomoniasis postassault (send home with patient if alcohol ingestion in previous 24 hours)

AND azithromycin (Zithromax; macrolide) 1 g orally in a single dose for treatment of possible exposure to chlamydia

AND emergency contraception (consider: Plan B, Plan B One-Step, ella)

Pregnancy prophylactic treatment can be a one-time dose or two separate doses, depending on the hospital protocol

Antiemetic of choice

After Examination

After the examination, the victim is likely exhausted. The ideal situation is that the victim is able to be escorted to a private area to shower and change clothes. An appropriate change of clothes should be offered that is size appropriate. The hospital may provide new clothes. Victims do not want to wear used clothes or scrubs. Used clothes or scrubs are a reminder of the assault. Victims are often afraid neighbors will see them and know what happened.

Medication management for postassault care is important to consider. The Centers for Disease Control and Prevention (CDC) currently recommends prophylactic treatment for trichomoniasis, bacterial vaginosis, gonorrhea, and chlamydial infections.[18] See Box 51.1. Prophylaxis for human immunodeficiency virus (HIV) and hepatitis B should be considered for victims at high risk for exposure. HIV is a serious concern for these high-risk victims. The prompt initiation of the non-occupational post exposure prophylaxis (n-PEP) is crucial in these high-risk victims, and any delay increases the exposure.[19] Additionally, consent for pregnancy prevention should be obtained after a negative pregnancy test result and after the patient is informed of associated risks.

Follow-up Care

Follow-up should be done in 10 days to 2 weeks.[3] Referral to a gynecologist or nearby clinic is essential. Cultures can be obtained at this time. At the follow-up appointment, timelines for HIV testing can be discussed. Many established specialized teams include follow-up care as part of their overall program. An advocate in a SART program may be available at the time of the follow-up examination and can assess the patient's need for counseling. They can also accompany a victim to court.[3]

LEGAL ASPECTS

Legal aspects of the case can take weeks, months, or even years before the case is in the legal arena.[3] The nurse may be called to be a fact witness to the examination and may receive a subpoena from the district attorney's office or a defense attorney representing the accused. The nurse most often gives only facts about the case and must refrain from expressing bias through opinions or emotions. Before the court hearing, the nurse should review the record and communicate with the legal representative. The nurse with a master's degree should have a professional curriculum vitae (CV) brought to the courtroom. The nurse should be prepared to describe his or her education, experience, and sexual assault training. Attire in the courtroom should be professional and businesslike. When on the witness stand, the nurse should be professional, answer only what is asked, never add anything, always face the jury with confident eye contact, never become defensive or out of control, and never interrupt the judge. When answering questions, be confident and calm.[3] In some cases, the nurse will be qualified by the judge as an expert witness. An expert witness is allowed to give opinion testimony and offer conclusions regarding his or her findings.

SUMMARY

The emergency nurse has an opportunity to give sensitive and specialized care for victims of one of the most heinous crimes committed against other human beings. Although not all hospitals have a SART program, it is the duty of the nursing profession, in conjunction with other members of the medical community and law enforcement, to care for these victims.

REFERENCES

1. Rape, Abuse & Incest National Network. Sex crimes: definitions and penalties, Pennsylvania. RAINN website. https://apps.rainn.org/policy/policy-crime-definitions.cfm?state=Pennsylvania&group=3. Published December 2017. Accessed May 26, 2019.
2. US Department of Justice. Federal Bureau of Investigation website. Attorney General Eric Holder announces revisions to the Uniform Crime Report's definition of rape. https://archives.fbi.gov/archives/news/pressrel/press-releases/attorney-general-eric-holder-announces-revisions-to-the-uniform-crime-reports-definition-of-rape. Published January 6, 2012. Accessed May 26, 2019.
3. Burgess AW. *Practical Aspects of Rape Investigation: A Multidisciplinary Approach*. 5th ed. New York, NY: CRC Press; 2017.
4. Seigel L. *Criminology*. 11th ed. Belmont, CA: Wadsworth; 2012.
5. Truman JL, Morgan RE. Criminal victimization, 2015. Bureau of Justice Statistics. https://www.bjs.gov/content/pub/pdf/cv15.pdf. Updated March 22, 2018. Accessed May 26, 2019.
6. Dempsey JP, Fireman GD, Wang E. Transitioning out of peer victimization in school children: gender and behavioral characteristics. *J Psychopathol Behav Assess*. 2006;28(4):271–280. https://doi.org/10.1007/s10862-005-9014-5.
7. World Society of Victimology. About us. World Society of Victimology website. http://www.worldsocietyofvictimology.org/about-us/. Published 2018. Accessed May 26, 2019.
8. *Psychology Today* staff. A round-up of rapists. *Psychology Today* website. https://www.psychologytoday.com/us/articles/199211/round-rapists. Published November 1, 1992. Reviewed June 6, 2016. Accessed May 26, 2019.
9. Hope for Healing. Types of rapists. Hope for Healing website. http://hopeforhealing.org/types.html. n.d. Accessed May 26, 2019.
10. Antognoli-Toland P. Comprehensive program for examination of sexual assault victims by nurses: a hospital-based project in Texas. *J Emerg Nurs*. 1985;11(3):132.
11. Pennsylvania Coalition Against Rape. *About Sexual Violence*. Pennsylvania Coalition Against Rape website. 2018. https://www.pcar.org/about-sexual-violence/lgbtq. Published 2018. Accessed May 26, 2019.
12. Burgess AW, Holmstrom LL. Rape trauma syndrome. *Am J Psychiatry*. 1974;136(11):1391–1506.
13. Agency for Healthcare Research and Quality. Emergency Severity Index (ESI): a triage tool for emergency department care. Version 4. https://www.ahrq.gov/sites/default/files/wysiwyg/professionals/systems/hospital/esi/esihandbk.pdf. Published 2012. Accessed May 26, 2019.
14. US Department of Justice. *A National Protocol for Sexual Assault Medical Forensic Examinations: Adults/Adolescents*. 2nd ed. https://www.ncjrs.gov/pdffiles1/ovw/241903.pdf. Published April 2013. Accessed May 26, 2019.
15. International Forensic Nurses Association. International Forensic Nurses Association website. https://www.forensicnurses.org. Published 2018. Accessed May 26, 2019.
16. LeBeau MA. Drug-facilitated sexual assault: the investigation and prosecution of cases. Paper presented at: The Third Annual Southeastern Pennsylvania Forensic Nursing Conference. Abington, PA. June 1, 2018.
17. Rape Abuse, Incest National Network. RAINN website. Drug-facilitated sexual assault. https://www.rainn.org/articles/drug-facilitated-sexual-assault. Published 2018. Accessed May 26, 2019.
18. Centers for Disease Control and Prevention. *2015 Sexually Transmitted Diseases Treatment Guidelines*. Centers for Disease Control and Prevention website. https://www.cdc.gov/std/tg2015/default.htm. Published 2015. Accessed May 26, 2019.
19. Scannell M, MacDonald AE, Berger A, et al. The priority of administering HIV postexposure prophylaxis in cases of sexual assault in an emergency department. *J Emerg Nurs*. 2018;44(2):117–122.

INDEX

Note: Page numbers followed by "f" indicate figures "t" indicate tables and "b" indicate boxes.

I

T

W

X

Y

Z